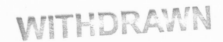

PHYSIOLOGY

PHYSIOLOGY

Editors

ROBERT M. BERNE, MD, DSc (Hon)

Professor Emeritus
Department of Molecular Physiology and Biological Physics
University of Virginia Health Sciences Center
Charlottesville, Virginia

MATTHEW N. LEVY, MD

Professor Emeritus of Physiology and Biomedical Engineering
Case Western Reserve University
Cleveland, Ohio

Associate Editors

BRUCE M. KOEPPEN, MD, PhD
Professor of Medicine and Physiology
Dean, Academic Affairs and Education
University of Connecticut Health Center
Farmington, Connecticut

BRUCE A. STANTON, PhD
Professor
Department of Physiology
Dartmouth Medical School
Hanover, New Hampshire

FOURTH EDITION
with 1096 illustrations

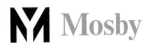 Mosby

A *Harcourt Health Sciences Company*
St. Louis   Philadelphia   London   Sydney   Toronto

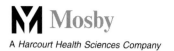

A Harcourt Health Sciences Company

Editor: Emma D. Underdown
Developmental Editors: Christy Wells, Kathleen Scogna, Linda Caldwell
Project Manager: Linda Clarke
Associate Production Editor: Deborah Ann Cicirello
Senior Composition Specialist: Joan Herron
Designer: Carolyn O'Brien
Manufacturing Manager: William A. Winneberger, Jr.
Cover Art: Hyperdesign, Inc.

FOURTH EDITION

Printed in the United States of America

Mosby, Inc.
11830 Westline Industrial Drive
St. Louis, Missouri 63146

Library of Congress Cataloging-in-Publication Data

Physiology / edited by Robert M. Berne . . . [et al.]. -- 4th ed.
       p. cm.
     Includes bibliographical references and index.
     ISBN 0-8151-0952-0
     1. Human physiology.   I. Berne, Robert M.
     [DNLM: 1. Physiology.   QT 4 P5783 1998]
   Q34.5.P496 1998
   612--dc21
   DNLM/DLC   97-38215

00 01 02 / 9 8 7 6 5 4 3 2

Contributors

ROBERT M. BERNE, MD, DSc (Hon)

Professor Emeritus
Department of Molecular Physiology and Biological Physics
University of Virginia Health Sciences Center
Charlottesville, Virginia
Section IV, The Cardiovascular System

SAUL M. GENUTH, MD

Professor of Medicine
Case Western Reserve University School of Medicine
Chief, Division of Endocrinology
PHS–Mount Sinai Medical Center
Cleveland, Ohio
Section VIII, The Endocrine System

BRUCE M. KOEPPEN, MD, PhD

Professor of Medicine and Physiology
Dean, Academic Affairs and Education
University of Connecticut Health Center
Farmington, Connecticut
Section VII, The Kidney

HOWARD C. KUTCHAI, PhD

Professor, Department of Molecular Physiology and Biological
    Physics
University of Virginia School of Medicine
Charlottesville, Virginia
Section I, Cellular Physiology
Section VI, The Gastrointestinal System

MATTHEW N. LEVY, MD

Professor Emeritus of Physiology and Biomedical Engineering
Case Western Reserve University
Cleveland, Ohio
Section IV, The Cardiovascular System

RICHARD A. MURPHY, PhD

Professor
Department of Molecular Physiology and Biological Physics
University of Virginia Health Sciences Center
Charlottesville, Virginia
Section III, Muscle

BRUCE A. STANTON, PhD

Professor
Department of Physiology
Dartmouth Medical School
Hanover, New Hampshire
Section VII, The Kidney

NORMAN C. STAUB, Sr., MD

Professor Emeritus
Department of Physiology
University of California at San Francisco School of Medicine
San Francisco, California
Section V, The Respiratory System

WILLIAM D. WILLIS, Jr., MD, PhD

Professor and Chairman
Department of Anatomy and Neurosciences
Cecil H. and Ida M. Green Chair and Director
Marine Biomedical Institute
The University of Texas Medical Branch
Galveston, Texas
Section II, The Nervous System

Reviewers

MARIA L. CAMARDA-VOIGHT, MD

Resident, Internal Medicine
Stritch School of Medicine
Loyola University
Chicago, Illinois

JOANN S. KAPLAN

Medical Student
College of Human Medicine
Michigan State University
East Lansing, Michigan

JOHN LIM, MD

Resident, Internal Medicine
School of Medicine
Washington University
St. Louis, Missouri

NOEL NUSSBAUM, PhD

Professor
Department of Physiology and Biophysics
Wright State University
Dayton, Ohio

EDWARD K. STAUFFER, PhD

Associate Professor
Department of Medical and Molecular Physiology
School of Medicine
University of Minnesota
Duluth, Minnesota

JOHN L. WALKER, PhD

Professor
Department of Physiology
School of Medicine
University of Utah
Salt Lake City, Utah

Dedicated to

Alex, Ari, Chris, Daniel, Kyle, Madelyn, Maggie,
Molly, Nicolas, Sarah, Todd, and Tracy

Preface

The fourth edition of this text, like the previous editions, emphasizes broad concepts and minimizes the compilation of isolated facts. Each of the chapters in this edition has been altered significantly to make the text as lucid, accurate, and current as possible. We have revised many of the illustrations and we have substituted many new ones in an effort to assist the readers in comprehending some of the more difficult physiological concepts and to introduce them to some of the modern techniques that are being used to acquire physiological knowledge. Finally, in keeping with our emphasis on broad principles, we have highlighted the important mechanistic homologies and critical interactions among the various organ systems wherever possible. We have tried to maintain similar goals and formats among the various sections of the book, without altering materially the writing styles of the section authors. We hope that this will actually enhance the overall readability of the book.

Physiology is distinguished from the other basic biomedical sciences by its concern with the function of the intact organism and its emphasis on the processes that regulate the important properties of living systems. In the healthy human, many variables are maintained within narrow limits. The list of controlled variables includes body temperature, blood pressure, ionic composition of the body's various fluid compartments, blood glucose levels, and oxygen and carbon dioxide contents of the blood. This ability to maintain the relative constancy of such critical variables, even in the face of substantial environmental changes, is known as homeostasis. A central goal of physiological research is the elucidation of the mechanisms responsible for homeostasis.

In Section I, Cellular Physiology, and at the beginnings of several other sections, certain important physiochemical principles of physiology are analyzed in detail. Among these principles we have included considerable information about major advances in cellular and molecular biology. To emphasize the clinical relevance of selected advances, we have directed the readers' attention to specific diseases in which the applicable physiological mechanism plays an important role. Interspersed throughout each chapter, these clinical examples have been highlighted by enclosing them in colored boxes.

When important principles could be represented profitably by equations, the bases of the equations and the major underlying assumptions have been stated. This approach provides students with a more quantitative understanding of these principles. However, because some of the readers might not favor a rigorous analytical approach to certain topics or might not have the requisite mathematical background, these more extensive mathematical analyses have been presented in gray boxes.

Section II, The Nervous System, provides a functional neuroanatomic framework for its presentation of contemporary cellular neurophysiology. Substantial attention has been directed toward the sensory and motor systems because of their relevance to clinical problems. The theoretical foundation common to all sensory systems has been constructed so as to facilitate the learning of the various components.

Throughout Section III, Muscle, we have refrained from describing the three types of muscle in sequence, but instead we have emphasized and integrated their common characteristics. We have stressed that the basic mechanisms of contraction are similar in skeletal, cardiac, and smooth muscles, and that the differences lie mainly in the relative importance of certain critical components of those basic processes.

To clarify cardiovascular physiology, in Section IV, The Cardiovascular System, we have dissected the entire system initially into its major components. One such component, namely blood composition and function, has been condensed and simplified, and it has been included in this section, whereas previously it had been treated as a separate section. In the subsections related to the heart and vasculature, we have first examined the functions of these individual components in isolation. Toward the end of the cardiovascular section, we have analyzed the system as a whole and have described how the various parts of this closed loop system interact under certain important physiological and pathophysiological conditions.

Section V, The Respiratory System, emphasizes the physical principles that underly the mechanics of breathing and the processes of gas exchange between the blood and the alveoli and between the blood and the peripheral tissues. Also the various neural and chemical processes that regulate respiration have been described in detail.

Section VI, The Gastrointestinal System, considers first the details about the motility and secretions of the gastrointestinal tract, and then analyzes how these functions are integrated by neural, endocrine, and paracrine mechanisms. Dysfunction of certain critical mechanisms has been shown to be involved in the pathogenesis of various important gastrointestinal disturbances.

In Section VII, The Kidney, homologies influence the presentation of factual material. The mechanisms whereby the kidneys handle a few important solutes have been described in detail. The specific information about the transport of the myriad substances that pass through the kidneys has been condensed.

In Section VIII, The Endocrine System, homologies in the functioning of the various endocrine glands are emphasized. Discussions of the male and female gonads have been included in a common chapter to highlight the similarities between the Sertoli cell functions in spermatogenesis and the granulosa cell functions in oogenesis.

Again, the framework of this textbook comprises firmly established facts and principles. Isolated phenomena generally are ignored unless they are considered to be highly significant, and experimental methods are described sparsely unless they are essential for comprehension. Although controversies exist in virtually all areas of physiology, such controversies are not considered unless they provide a deeper understanding of the subject. The authors of each section have presented what they believe to be the most likely mechanism responsible for the phenomenon under consideration. We have adopted this compromise to achieve brevity, clarity, and simplicity. We have not documented the specific sources for the assertions that appear throughout the book, but we have provided references at the end of each chapter. These references have been selected because they provide a current and comprehensive review of the topic, a clear and detailed description of important mechanisms, or a complete and current bibliography of the subject.

At the end of each chapter, we have included summary statements of the important facts and concepts. We have also included Self-Study Problems, which are essay-type questions. At the end of the book, we have provided the answers to these essay questions (Apppendix A), and have added a substantial set of multiple choice questions and answers that relate to the contents of the entire book (Appendix B, Mini-Exam).

We wish to express our appreciation to all of our colleagues and students who have provided constructive criticism during the revision of this book.

Robert M. Berne
Matthew N. Levy

Contents

PHYSIOLOGY

CELLULAR PHYSIOLOGY

Howard C. Kutchai

Cellular Membranes and Transmembrane Transport of Solutes and Water

■ *Cellular Membranes*

Membranes are a prominent part of all cells. Every cell is surrounded by a plasma membrane that separates it from the extracellular environment. The plasma membrane serves as a permeability barrier that allows the cell to maintain an interior composition far different from the composition of the extracellular fluid. The plasma membrane also contains enzymes, receptors, and antigens that play important roles in the cell's interaction with other cells and with hormones and other regulatory agents in the extracellular fluid.

Membranes also enclose the various organelles of eukaryotic cells. These membranes divide the cell into discrete compartments within which particular biochemical processes take place. Many vital cellular processes actually take place in or on the membranes of the organelles. Examples of these membrane-localized processes include electron transport and oxidative phosphorylation, which occur on, within, and across the mitochondrial inner membrane.

Most biological membranes have certain features in common. However, in keeping with the diversity of membrane functions, the composition and structure of the membranes differ from one cell to another and among the membranes of a single cell.

■ *Membrane Structure*

The most abundant constituents of cellular membranes are proteins and phospholipids. A **phospholipid** molecule consists of a polar head group and two nonpolar, hydrophobic fatty acyl chains (Fig. 1-1, *A*). In an aqueous environment, phospholipids tend to orient with their hydrophobic fatty acyl chains away from contact with water. This orientation can be seen in the **lipid bilayer** (Fig. 1-1, *B*). Many phospholipids, when dispersed in water, spontaneously form lipid bilayers. Most of the phospholipid molecules in biological membranes have a lipid bilayer structure.

The **fluid mosaic model** of membrane structure shown in Fig. 1-2 is consistent with many of the properties of biological membranes. Note the bilayer structure of most of the membrane phospholipids. Note also that proteins are abundant in the membrane. These membrane proteins are of two major classes: (1) **integral** or **intrinsic membrane proteins** that are embedded in the phospholipid bilayer and (2) **peripheral** or **extrinsic membrane proteins** that are associated with the surface of the membrane. In general, the peripheral membrane proteins associate with the membrane by means of charge interactions with integral membrane proteins. When the ionic composition of the medium is altered, peripheral proteins are often removed from the membrane. Integral membrane proteins are embedded in the membrane by means of hydrophobic interactions with the interior of the membrane. The only substances that can disrupt these hydrophobic interactions are detergents, which make the integral proteins soluble by interacting hydrophobically with nonpolar amino acid side chains.

As the term *fluid mosaic model* suggests, cellular membranes are fluid structures. Many of the constituent molecules of cellular membranes are free to diffuse in the plane of the membrane. Most lipids and proteins move freely in the bilayer plane, but they "flip-flop" from one phospholipid monolayer to the other at much slower rates. A large, hydrophilic membrane component is unlikely to flip-flop if it must be dragged through the nonpolar interior of the lipid bilayer.

Sometimes, membrane components are not free to diffuse in the plane of the membrane. For example, acetyl-

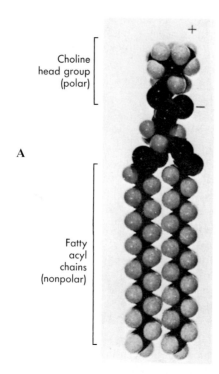

Choline head group (polar)

Fatty acyl chains (nonpolar)

A

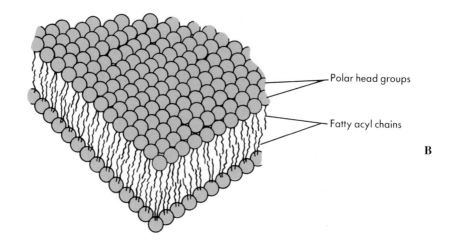

Polar head groups

Fatty acyl chains

B

■ **Fig. 1-1 A,** Structure of a membrane phospholipid molecule, in this case a phosphatidylcholine. **B,** Structure of a phospholipid bilayer. The circles represent the polar head groups of the phospholipid molecules. The wavy lines represent the fatty acyl chains of the phospholipids.

■ **Fig. 1-2** Schematic representation of the fluid mosaic model of membrane structure. The integral proteins are embedded in the lipid bilayer matrix of the membrane, and the peripheral proteins are associated with the external surfaces of integral membrane proteins.

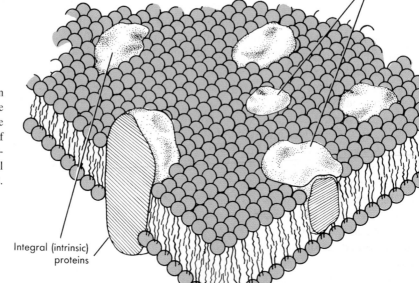

Peripheral (extrinsic) proteins

Integral (intrinsic) proteins

choline receptors (integral membrane proteins) are sequestered at the motor endplate of skeletal muscle. Different membrane proteins are confined to the apical and basolateral plasma membranes of epithelial cells. In some cells, cytoskeleton appears to tether certain membrane proteins. For example, the **anion exchanger,** a major protein of the human erythrocyte membrane, is bound to the spectrin network that undergirds the membrane via a protein called **ankyrin.**

If the motor nerve that innervates a skeletal muscle is accidentally severed, the acetylcholine receptors are no longer sequestered at the motor endplate. Instead, they spread out over the entire plasma membrane of the muscle cells. The entire surface of the cell then becomes excitable by acetylcholine, a phenomenon known as **denervation supersensitivity.**

Membrane Composition

Lipid Composition

Major phospholipids. In animal cell membranes, the *phospholipid bilayer is primarily responsible for the passive permeability properties of the membrane.* The most abundant phospholipids in these membranes are often the choline-containing phospholipids: the **lecithins** (phosphatidylcholines) and the **sphingomyelins.** Next in abundance are frequently the **amino phospholipids:** phosphatidylserine and phosphatidylethanolamine. Other important phospholipids that are present in smaller amounts are **phosphatidylglycerol, phosphatidylinositol,** and **cardiolipin.**

Certain phospholipids that are present in *tiny* amounts in the plasma membrane play vital roles in cellular signal transduction processes. **Phosphatidylinositol bisphosphate,** when cleaved by a receptor-activated phospholipase C, releases **inositol trisphosphate (IP$_3$)** and **diacylglycerol.** IP$_3$ is released into the cytosol, where it acts on receptors in the endoplasmic reticulum to cause release of stored Ca^{++}, which affects a wide variety of cellular processes. Diacylglycerol remains in the plasma membrane, where it participates, along with Ca^{++}, in activating **protein kinase C,** an important signal transduction protein.

Cholesterol. Cholesterol is a major component of plasma membranes. Its steroid nucleus lies parallel to the fatty acyl chains of membrane phospholipids. Cholesterol functions as a "fluidity buffer" in the plasma membrane. It tends to keep the fluidity of the acyl chain region of the phospholipid bilayer in an intermediate range in the presence of agents, such as alcohols and general anesthetics, that would otherwise make the biological membranes more fluid.

Glycolipids. Although **glycolipids** are not abundant in plasma membranes, they have important functions. Glycolipids are found mostly in plasma membranes, where their carbohydrate moieties protrude from the external surface of the membrane. The carbohydrate parts of glycolipids frequently function as receptors or antigens.

The receptor for **cholera toxin** (Chapter 39) is the carbohydrate moiety of a particular glycolipid, ganglioside (G$_{M1}$). The A and B blood group antigens (Chapter 20) are the carbohydrate moieties of other gangliosides on the human erythrocyte membrane.

Asymmetry of lipid distribution. In many membranes, the lipid components are not distributed uniformly across the bilayer. For example, the glycolipids of the plasma membrane are located almost exclusively in the outer monolayer. Phospholipids are also distributed asymmetrically between the inner and outer monolayers of membranes. In the red blood cell membrane, for example, the outer monolayer contains most of the choline-containing phospholipids, whereas the inner monolayer contains most of the amino phospholipids.

Membrane Proteins

The protein composition of membranes may be simple or complex. The functionally specialized membranes of the sarcoplasmic reticulum of skeletal muscle and the disks of the rod outer segment of the retina contain only a few different proteins. In contrast, plasma membranes, which perform many functions, may have more than 100 different protein constituents. Membrane proteins include enzymes, transport proteins, and receptors for hormones and neurotransmitters.

Glycoproteins. Some membrane proteins are glycoproteins with covalently bound carbohydrate side chains. As with glycolipids, the carbohydrate chains of glycoproteins are located on the external surfaces of plasma membranes. The carbohydrate moieties of membrane glycoproteins and glycolipids have important functions. The negative surface charge of cells is caused by the negatively charged sialic acid of glycolipids and glycoproteins.

Fibronectin is a large fibrous glycoprotein that helps cells attach, via cell surface glycoproteins called **integrins,** to proteins of the extracellular matrix. This linkage allows communication to take place between the extracellular matrix and the cell's cytoskeleton during embryonic development.

The major membrane proteins of enveloped **viruses** are glycoproteins. Their carbohydrate moieties appear as "spikes" that stud the outer surface of the virus. These "spikes" are necessary for the binding of the virus to a host cell.

Asymmetry of membrane proteins. The Na$^+$, K$^+$-ATPase (also called the Na$^+$, K$^+$-pump) of the plasma membrane and the Ca^{++}-ATPase (also called the Ca^{++} pump) of the sarcoplasmic reticulum membrane are examples of the asymmetric distribution of membrane proteins. In both of these pumps, the cleavage of ATP occurs on the cytoplasmic face of the membrane, and some of the energy liberated is used to pump ions in specific directions across the membrane. The Na$^+$, K$^+$-ATPase pumps K$^+$ into the cell and Na$^+$ out of the cell, whereas the Ca^{++}-ATPase actively pumps Ca^{++} into the sarcoplasmic reticulum.

Membranes as Permeability Barriers

Biological membranes serve as *permeability barriers.* Most of the molecules present in living systems are highly soluble in water and poorly soluble in nonpolar solvents. Not surprisingly, molecules are also poorly soluble in the nonpolar environment that exists within the interior of the lipid bilayer of biological membranes. As a consequence, biological membranes pose a formidable barrier to most water-soluble molecules. This barrier allows the maintenance of large concentration differences of many substances between the cytoplasm and the extracellular fluid. However, the plasma membrane is also permeable to some substances. Thus, although it keeps out many substances, it also allows the selective passage of other substances.

The localization of various cellular processes in certain organelles depends on the barrier properties of cellular membranes. For example, the inner mitochondrial membrane is impermeable to the enzymes and substrates of the tricarboxylic acid cycle, and thus it allows the localization of the tricarboxylic cycle in the mitochondrial matrix. Much as the walls of a house separate rooms with different functions, barriers imposed by cellular membranes organize the chemical and physical processes within the cell.

The permeability function of membranes, which allows the passage of important molecules across membranes at controlled rates, is central to the life of the cell. Examples include the uptake of nutrient molecules, the discharge of waste products, and the release of secreted molecules. As discussed in the next section, molecules may move from one side of a membrane to another without actually moving through the membrane itself. In other cases, molecules cross a particular membrane by passing through or between the molecules that make up the membrane.

■ Transport across, but not through, Membranes

■ Endocytosis

Endocytosis is the process that allows material to enter the cell without passing through the plasma membrane (Fig. 1-3); it includes phagocytosis and pinocytosis. The uptake of particulate material is termed **phagocytosis** ("cell eating") (Fig. 1-3, *A*). The uptake of soluble molecules is called **pinocytosis** ("cell drinking") (Fig. 1-3, *B*).

Sometimes, special regions of the plasma membrane are involved in endocytosis. In these regions, the cytoplasmic surface of the plasma membrane is covered with bristles made primarily of a protein called **clathrin.** These clathrin-covered regions are called **coated pits,** and their endocytosis gives rise to **coated vesicles** Fig. 1-3, *C*). The coated pits are involved in **receptor-mediated endocytosis.** In this process, specific membrane receptor proteins in the coated pits recognize and bind to the protein to be taken up. This binding often leads to aggregation of receptor-ligand complexes, and the aggregation triggers endocytosis. *Endocytosis is an active process that requires metabolic energy.* Endocytosis can also occur in regions of the plasma membrane that do not contain coated pits.

Most cells cannot synthesize cholesterol, which is needed for synthesis of new membranes (see Chapter 51). Cholesterol is carried in the blood predominantly in low-density lipoproteins (LDLs). Many cells have LDL receptors in their plasma membranes. When LDL binds to these receptors, the receptor-LDL complexes migrate to coated pits, where they aggregate and are taken into the cell by receptor-mediated endocytosis. Individuals who lack LDL receptors or have defective LDL receptors have high levels of cholesterol-laden LDL in their blood. Consequently, such individuals tend to develop arterial disease (**atherosclerosis**) at an early age, which increases the risk of early heart attacks.

■ Exocytosis

Molecules can be ejected from cells by **exocytosis,** a process that resembles endocytosis in reverse. The release of neurotransmitters from the presynaptic nerve endings (discussed in more detail in Chapter 4) takes place by exocytosis. Exocytosis is responsible for the

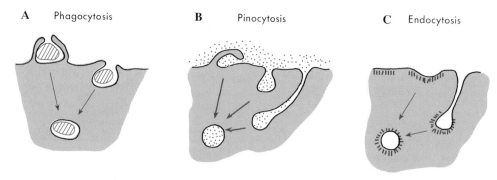

■ **Fig. 1-3** Schematic depiction of endocytotic processes. **A,** Phagocytosis of a solid particle. **B,** Pinocytosis of extracellular fluid. **C,** Receptor-mediated endocytosis by coated pits. (Redrawn from Silverstein SC et al: *Annu Rev Biochem* 46:669, 1977. With permission by Annual Reviews.)

release of secretory proteins by many cells. A well-studied example is the release of pancreatic enzymes from the acinar cells of the pancreas. These proteins are stored in secretory vesicles in the cytoplasm of pancreatic cells. *A stimulus to secrete causes the secretory vesicles to fuse with the plasma membrane and to release the vesicle contents by exocytosis.*

■ *Fusion of Membrane Vesicles*

The contents of one type of organelle can be transferred to another organelle by fusion of the membranes of the organelles. In some cells, secretory products are transferred from the endoplasmic reticulum to the Golgi apparatus by fusion of vesicles. In this process, endoplasmic reticulum vesicles fuse with membranous sacs of the Golgi apparatus. Fusion of phagocytic vesicles with lysosomes allows the phagocytosed material to be digested by proteolytic enzymes in the lysosomes. The turnover of many normal cellular constituents involves their destruction in lysosomes, followed by their resynthesis.

Influenza viruses have membrane proteins that undergo a dramatic conformational change that allows the insertion of a "fusion peptide" into the host cell. The fusion peptide promotes the fusion of the viral membrane with the plasma membrane of the host cell, allowing entry of the viral genome into the host cell.

■ *Transport of Molecules through Membranes*

The traffic of molecules through biological membranes is vital for most cellular processes. Some molecules move through biological membranes simply by diffusing among the molecules that make up the membrane. Other molecules move through membranes via specific transport proteins in the membrane.

Oxygen, for example, is a small molecule that is fairly soluble in nonpolar solvents. It crosses biological membranes by diffusing among membrane lipid molecules. Glucose, on the other hand, is a much larger molecule that is not very soluble in the membrane lipids. Glucose enters cells via specific glucose transport proteins in the plasma membrane.

■ *Diffusion*

Diffusion occurs because of the random thermal motion of atoms or molecules, also called **Brownian motion.** Diffusion eventually results in the uniform distribution of the atoms or molecules. Imagine a container divided into two compartments by a removable partition (Fig. 1-4). A much larger number of molecules of a compound is placed on side A than on side B, and then the partition is removed. Every molecule is in random thermal motion. The probability that a molecule that is located initially on side A will move to side B in a given time is equal to the probability that a molecule initially located on side B will end up on side A. Because many more molecules are present on side A, the total number of molecules moving from side A to side B will be greater than the number moving from side B to side A. Eventually, the number of molecules on side A will decrease, whereas the number of molecules on side B will increase. This process of net diffusion of molecules will continue until the concentration of molecules on side A equals that on side B. Thereafter the rate of diffusion of molecules from A to B will equal that from B to A, and no further net movement will occur; a dynamic equilibrium exists.

Range of diffusion. Diffusion is rapid when the distance over which it takes place is small. A rule of thumb is that a typical molecule takes 1 msec to diffuse 1 μm. However, the time required for diffusion increases with the square of the distance over which diffusion occurs. *Thus, a tenfold increase in the diffusion distance means that it will take 100 times longer for diffusion to reach a given degree of completion.*

Table 1-1 shows the results of calculations for a typical, small, water-soluble solute. Diffusion is extremely rapid on a microscopic scale of distance. For macroscopic distances, however, diffusion is rather slow. A cell that is 100 μm away from the nearest capillary can receive nutrients from the blood by diffusion about 5 seconds or so, which is sufficiently fast to satisfy the metabolic demands of many cells. However, a skeletal muscle cell that is 1 cm long cannot rely on diffusion for the intracellular transport of vital metabolites. It would take 14 hours for the diffusion of these metabolites to be completed, and this time requirement is not feasible for efficient cellular metabolism. Some nerve fibers are longer than 1 m. To overcome this difficulty, intracellular axonal transport systems are involved in transporting important molecules along nerve fibers. Because of the slowness of diffusion over macroscopic distances, even small multicellular organisms have evolved circulatory systems to bring the individual cells of the organisms within a reasonable diffusion range of nutrients.

Diffusion coefficient. The **diffusion coefficient** (D) is proportional to the speed with which the diffusing molecule can move in the surrounding medium. The larger the molecule and the more viscous the medium, the smaller is D. For small molecules, D is inversely proportional to $MW^{1/2}$. (*MW* refers to molecular weight). For macromolecules, D is inversely proportional to $MW^{1/2}$. *Thus, a protein that has one eighth the mass of another molecule will have a diffusion coefficient only two times larger than the larger molecule.*

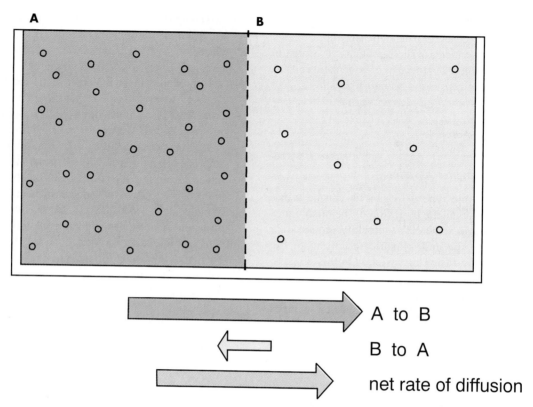

■ **Fig. 1-4** Chambers A and B are separated by a partition with holes in it. The concentration of molecules in chamber A is much greater than that in chamber B. For this reason the rate of diffusion of molecules from A to B is much greater than that from B to A. There is thus a net flux of molecules from A to B.

■ **Table 1-1** The time required for diffusion to occur over various diffusion distances*

Diffusion distance (μm)		Time required for diffusion	
1		0.5	msec
10		50	msec
100		5	sec
1000	(1 mm)	8.3	min
10,000	(1 cm)	14	hr

*The time required for the "average" molecule (with diffusion coefficient taken to be 1×10^{-5} cm^2/sec) to diffuse the required distance was computed from the Einstein relation.

For large spherical molecules the diffusion coefficient is approximated by the Stokes-Einstein equation

$$D = kT/6\pi r\eta$$

where

k	=	Boltzmann's constant
T	=	absolute temperature
r	=	radius of the macromolecule
η	=	viscosity of the medium

The numerator, kT, is directly proportional to the kinetic energy of the average diffusing molecule. The denominator is proportional to the viscous drag encountered by the molecule as it diffuses. The inverse proportionality of D to the radius of the molecule implies that D is inversely proportional to the cube root of the molecular weight.

Diffusion across a membrane. Diffusion leads to a state in which the concentration of the diffusing species is constant in space and time. Diffusion across cellular membranes tends to equalize the concentrations on the two sides of the membrane (Fig. 1-4). The diffusion rate across a membrane is proportional to the area of the membrane and to the difference in concentration of the diffusing substance on the two sides of the membrane. **Fick's first law of diffusion** states that

$$J = -DA\frac{\Delta C}{\Delta x} \qquad (1-1)$$

where

J = net rate of diffusion in moles or grams per unit time
D = diffusion coefficient of the diffusing solute in the membrane

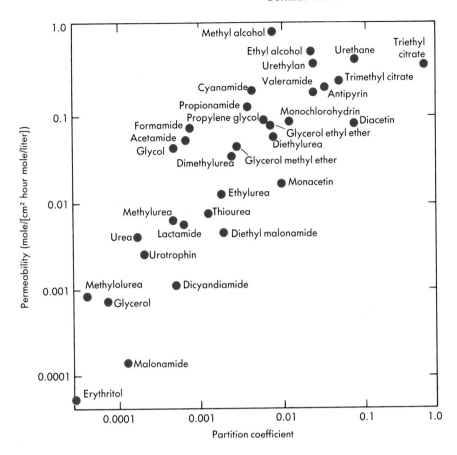

■ **Fig. 1-5** Illustration of the permeability of the plasma membrane of the alga *Chara ceratophylla* to various nonelectrolytes as a function of the lipid solubility of the solutes. Lipid solubility is represented on the abscissa by the olive oil/water partition coefficient. (Redrawn from Christensen HN: *Biological transport*, ed 2, Menlo Park, Calif, 1975, WA Benjamin. Data from Collander R: *Trans Faraday Soc* 33:985, 1937.)

A = area of the membrane
Δc = concentration difference across the membrane
Δx = thickness of the membrane

Diffusive permeability of cellular membranes

Permeability to lipid-soluble molecules. The plasma membrane serves as a diffusion barrier that enables the cell to maintain cytoplasmic concentrations of many substances that differ greatly from their extracellular concentrations. As early as the turn of the twentieth century, the relative impermeability of the plasma membrane to most water-soluble substances was attributed to its "lipoid nature."

The lipoid character of the plasma membrane can be demonstrated by experiments showing that compounds that are soluble in nonpolar solvents (e.g., benzene or olive oil) enter cells more readily than do water-soluble substances of similar molecular weight. Fig. 1-5 shows the relationship between membrane permeability and solubility in a nonpolar solvent for a number of different solutes. The ratio of the solubility of the solute in olive oil to its solubility in water is used as a measure of solubility in nonpolar solvents. This ratio is called the *olive oil/water partition coefficient. The permeability of the plasma membrane to a particular substance increases with the "lipid solubility" of the substance.* For compounds with the same olive oil/water partition coefficient, permeability decreases with increasing molecular weight.

As described previously, the fluid mosaic model of membrane structure envisions the plasma membrane as a lipid bilayer with proteins embedded in it (Fig. 1-2). The data shown in Fig. 1-5 support the idea that the lipid bilayer is the principal barrier to substances that permeate the membrane by simple diffusion.

Fat-soluble vitamins are absorbed by the epithelial cells of the small intestine by simply diffusing across their luminal plasma membranes. Water-soluble vitamins, by contrast, do not readily diffuse across biological membranes, and thus special membrane transport proteins are required for absorption of water-soluble vitamins (see Chapter 39).

Permeability to water-soluble molecules. Very small, uncharged, water-soluble molecules pass through cell membranes much more rapidly than is predicted by their lipid solubility. For example, water permeates cell membranes about 100 times more rapidly than is predicted from its molecular radius and its olive oil/water partition coefficient. There are two reasons for the unusually high permeability to water. First, certain very small water-soluble molecules can pass between adjacent phospholipid molecules without actually dissolving in the region occupied by the fatty acid side chains. Second, the plasma membranes of most cells contain membrane proteins that form channels permitting a high rate of water flow.

The permeability of membranes to uncharged, water-soluble molecules decreases as the size of the molecules increases. Most plasma membranes are essentially impermeable to water-soluble molecules whose molecular weights are greater than about 200.

Because of their charge, ions are relatively insoluble in lipid solvents, and thus membranes are not very permeable to most ions. Ionic diffusion across membranes occurs mainly through protein **ion channels** that span the membrane. Some ion channels allow only specific ions to pass, whereas others allow all ions below a certain size to pass. *Some ion channels are controlled by the voltage difference across the membrane; others are controlled by neurotransmitters or other regulatory molecules* (see Chapters 3 and 4).

Although some water-soluble molecules such as sugars and amino acids are essential for cellular survival, they do not cross plasma membranes appreciably by simple diffusion. Plasma membranes have specific proteins that allow the transfer of vital metabolites into or out of the cell. The characteristics of membrane **protein-mediated transport** across membranes are discussed later.

■ *Osmosis*

Osmosis is defined as the flow of water across a **semipermeable membrane** from a compartment in which the solute concentration is lower to one in which the solute concentration is greater. A semipermeable membrane is defined as a membrane permeable to water but impermeable to solutes. *Osmosis takes place because the presence of solute decreases the chemical potential of water.* Water tends to flow from where its chemical potential is higher to where its chemical potential is lower.

Decreasing the chemical potential of water (because of the presence of solute) also reduces vapor pressure, lowers the freezing point, and increases the boiling point of the solution as compared with pure water. Because these properties, as well as osmotic pressure, depend primarily on the concentration of the solute present rather than on its chemical nature, they are called **colligative properties.**

Osmotic pressure. In Fig. 1-6 a semipermeable membrane separates a solution from pure water. Water flows from side B to side A by osmosis because the presence of solute on side A reduces the chemical potential of water in the solution. Pushing on the piston will increase the chemical potential of the water in the solution on side A and slow the net rate of osmotic water flow. If the force on the piston is increased gradually, a pressure is eventually reached at which net water flow stops. Application of still more pressure will cause water to flow in the opposite direction. *The pressure on side A that is just sufficient to keep pure water from entering is called the osmotic pressure of the solution on side A.*

The osmotic pressure of a solution depends on the number of particles in solution. Thus, the degree of ionization of the solute must be taken into account when osmotic pressure is calculated. A 1-M solution of glucose, a 0.5-M solution of NaCl, and a 0.333-M solution of $CaCl_2$ have approximately the same osmotic pressure. (Actually, their osmotic pressures will differ somewhat because of the deviations of real solutions from ideal behavior.) One form of **van't Hoff's law** for calculation of osmotic pressure is

$$\pi = RT(\Phi ic) \qquad (1\text{-}2)$$

where

π	=	osmotic pressure
R	=	ideal gas constant
T	=	absolute temperature
Φ	=	osmotic coefficient
i	=	number of ions formed by dissociation of a solute molecule
c	=	molar concentration of solute (moles of solute per liter of solution)

The osmotic coefficient (Φ) accounts for the deviation of the solution from the ideal. Φ depends on the particu-

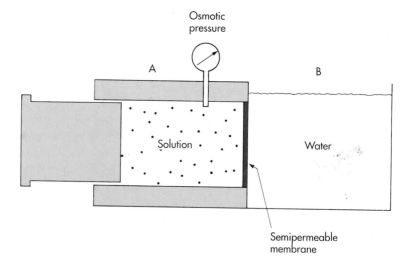

■ **Fig. 1-6** Schematic representation of the definition of osmotic pressure. When the hydrostatic pressure applied to the solution in chamber A is equal to the osmotic pressure of that solution, there will be no net water flow across the membrane.

lar compound, its concentration, and the temperature. Values of Φ may be greater or less than 1. It is less than 1 for electrolytes of physiological importance, and for all solutes Φ approaches 1 as the solution becomes more and more dilute. *The term Φic can be regarded as the osmotically effective concentration, and Φic is called the osmolarity of the solution,* with units in osmoles per liter. Sometimes a less precise estimate of osmotic pressure is computed assuming that Φ is equal to 1.

Values of Φ can be obtained from handbooks that list values of Φ for different substances as functions of concentration. Solutions of proteins deviate greatly from ideal behavior, and different proteins may deviate to different extents. Values of the osmotic coefficient depend on the concentration of the solute and on its chemical properties. Table 1-2 lists osmotic coefficients for several solutes. These values apply, to a first approximation, to concentrations of these solutes in the extracellular fluids of mammals.

Sample calculations

1. What is the osmotic pressure at 0° C of a 154-mM NaCl solution?

$$\pi = RT(\Phi ic)$$

Using $\Phi = 0.93$ for NaCl from Table 1-2, we obtain

$$\pi = 22.4 \text{ L-atm/mole} \times 0.93 \times 2 \times 0.154 \text{ mole/L}$$
$$= 6.42 \text{ atm}$$

2. What is the osmolarity of this solution?

osmolarity $= \Phi ic$
$= 0.93 \times 2 \times 0.154$ mole/L $= 0.286$ osmolar
$= 286$ milliosmolar

■ **Table 1-2**   Osmotic coefficients (Φ) of certain solutes of physiological interest

Substance	i	Molecular weight	Φ
NaCl	2	58.5	0.93
KCl	2	74.6	0.92
HCl	2	36.6	0.95
NH_4Cl	2	53.5	0.92
$NaHCO_3$	2	84.0	0.96
$NaNO_3$	2	85.0	0.90
KSCN	2	97.2	0.91
KH_2PO_4	2	136.0	0.87
$CaCl_2$	3	111.0	0.86
$MgCl_2$	3	95.2	0.89
Na_2SO_4	3	142.0	0.74
K_2SO_4	3	174.0	0.74
$MgSO_4$	2	120.0	0.58
Glucose	1	180.0	1.01
Sucrose	1	342.0	1.02
Maltose	1	342.0	1.01
Lactose	1	342.0	1.01

Reproduced with permission from Lifson N, Visscher MB: *Osmosis in living systems.* In Glasser O, editor: *Medical physics,* vol 1, Chicago, 1944, Mosby–Year Book.

Measurement of osmotic pressure. The osmotic pressure of a solution can be obtained by determining the pressure required to prevent water from entering the solution across a semipermeable membrane (Fig. 1-6). It is easier, however, to estimate the osmotic pressure from another colligative property, such as depression of the freezing point. The equation that describes the osmolarity (Φic) of a solution in terms of the depression of the freezing point of water by the solute is

$$\Phi ic = \Delta T_f / 1.86 \qquad (1\text{-}3)$$

where ΔT_f is the freezing point depression in degrees centigrade. When the freezing point depression of a multicomponent solution is determined, the effective osmolarity (in osmoles per liter) of the solution as a whole can be obtained.

If the total osmotic pressures of two solutions (as measured by freezing point depression or by the osmotic pressure developed across a semipermeable membrane) are equal, the solutions are said to be **isoosmotic** (or **isosmotic**). If solution A has greater osmotic pressure than solution B, A is said to be **hyperosmotic** with respect to B. If solution A has less total osmotic pressure than solution B, A is said to be **hypoosmotic** to B.

Osmotic swelling and shrinking of cells. The plasma membranes of most of the cells of the body are relatively impermeable to many of the solutes of the extracellular fluid but are highly permeable to water. Therefore, when the osmotic pressure of the extracellular fluid is increased, water leaves the cells by osmosis and the cells shrink. When water leaves the cell, the cellular solutes become more concentrated until the effective osmotic pressure of the cytoplasm is again equal to that of the extracellular fluid. Conversely, if the osmotic pressure of the extracellular fluid is decreased, water enters the cells. The cells will continue to swell until the intracellular and extracellular osmotic pressures are equal.

Red blood cells are often used to illustrate the osmotic properties of cells, because they are readily obtained and are easily studied. Within a certain range of external solute concentrations, the red cell behaves as an osmometer, because its volume is inversely related to the solute concentration in the extracellular medium. In Fig. 1-7 the red cell volume (the fraction of its normal volume in plasma) is plotted against the concentration of NaCl solution in which the red cells are suspended. At an NaCl concentration of 154 mM (308 mM osmotically active particles), the volume of the cells is the same as their volume in plasma; this concentration of NaCl is said to be **isotonic** to the red cell.

Isotonic NaCl solution (also known as isotonic saline) is used for intravenous rehydration or for administration of drugs to patients. Almost every patient undergoing surgery will be given an intravenous drip of isotonic saline.

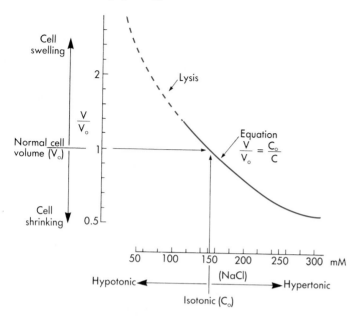

■ **Fig. 1-7** The osmotic behavior of human red blood cells in NaCl solutions. At 154 mM NaCl (isotonic), the red cell has its normal volume. It shrinks in more concentrated (hypertonic) solutions and swells in more dilute (hypotonic) solutions. V_o and C_o are the red cell volume and intracellular solute concentration, respectively, for the red cell in the blood or in an isotonic solution. V and C are, respectively, the cell volume and intracellular solute concentration in a solution that is not isotonic.

A concentration of NaCl greater than 154 mM is called **hypertonic** (greater strength, causes cells to shrink); and a solution less concentrated than 154 mM is called **hypotonic** (cells swell). When red cells have swollen to about 1.4 times their original volume, some cells lyse (burst). At this volume, the properties of the red cell membrane abruptly change; hemoglobin leaks from the cell, and the membrane becomes transiently permeable to most other molecules as well.

The intracellular substances of the red blood cell that produce an osmotic pressure that just balances the osmotic pressure of the extracellular fluid include hemoglobin, K^+, organic phosphates (e.g., ATP and 2,3-diphosphoglycerate), and glycolytic intermediates. The chemical nature of the cell's contents is not important. The red cell behaves as if it were filled with a solution of impermeant molecules with an osmotically effective concentration of 286 milliosmolar, which is the same as the osmolarity of isotonic saline:

$$\Phi_{NaCl}\, i_{NaCl}\, C_{NaCl} = 0.93 \times 2 \times 0.154 \text{ M} =$$
$$0.286 \text{ osmolar} = 286 \text{ milliosmolar} \qquad (1\text{-}4)$$

Osmotic effects of permeant solutes. In contrast to impermeant solutes, permeant solutes are those that are able to pass through the plasma membrane. Because of this ability, permeating solutes eventually equilibrate across the plasma membrane. For this reason, permeating solutes exert only a transient effect on cell volume.

Consider a red blood cell placed in a large volume of 0.154 M NaCl that contains 0.050 M glycerol. Initially, because the extracellular fluid contains NaCl and glycerol, the osmotic pressure of the extracellular fluid will exceed that of the cell interior, and the cell will shrink. With time, however, glycerol will equilibrate across the plasma membrane of the red cell, and the cell will swell back toward its original volume. However, *the steady-state volume of the cell is determined only by the impermeant solutes in the extracellular fluid.* In this case, the concentration of impermeant solute of the extracellular fluid (NaCl) is 154 M, which is isotonic to the red blood cells. Therefore, the final volume of the cell will be equal to the normal red cell volume. *Because the red cell ultimately returns to its normal volume, the solution (0.050 M glycerol in 0.154 M NaCl) is isotonic. Because the red cell initially shrinks when put in this solution, the solution is hyperosmotic with respect to the normal red cell.* The transient changes in cell volume depend on equilibration of glycerol across the membrane. Had we used urea (a more rapidly permeating substance), the cell would have reached steady-state volume sooner.

The following rules help predict the volume changes a cell will undergo when suspended in solutions of permeant and impermeant solutes:

1. *The steady-state volume of the cell is determined only by the concentration of impermeant solutes* in the extracellular fluid.
2. *Permeant solutes cause only transient changes* in cell volume.
3. The greater the permeability of the membrane to the permeant solute, the more rapid is the time course of the transient changes.

Magnitudes of osmotic flows caused by permeating solutes. In the preceding example, we saw that permeant solutes, such as glycerol, exert only a transient osmotic effect on cells. It is sometimes necessary to determine the rate of the osmotic flow caused by a particular permeant solute.

When a difference of *hydrostatic pressure* (ΔP) causes water to flow across a membrane, the rate of water flow (V_w) is

$$V_w = L\Delta P \qquad (1\text{-}5)$$

where L is a constant of proportionality, called the **hydraulic conductivity.**

Osmotic flow of water across a membrane is directly proportional to the osmotic pressure difference ($\Delta\pi$) of the solutions on the two sides of the membrane; thus,

$$V_w = L\Delta\pi \qquad (1\text{-}6)$$

Equation 1-6 is true only for osmosis caused by *impermeant* solutes. *Permeant solutes cause less osmotic flow. The greater the permeability of a solute, the less is the osmotic flow it causes.* Table 1-3 shows the osmotic water flows induced across a porous membrane by

■ **Table 1-3** Osmotic water flow across a porous dialysis membrane caused by various solutes*

Gradient producing the water flow	Net volume flow ($\mu l/min$)*	Solute radius (Å)	Reflection coefficient (σ)
D_2O	0.06	1.9	0.0024
Urea	0.6	2.7	0.024
Glucose	5.1	4.4	0.205
Sucrose	9.2	5.3	0.368
Raffinose	11	6.1	0.440
Inulin	19	12	0.760
Bovine serum albumin	25.5	37	1.02
Hydrostatic pressure	25		

Data from Durbin RP: *J Gen Physiol* 44:315, 1960. Reproduced from *The Journal of General Physiology* by copyright permission of The Rockefeller University Press.

*Flow is expressed as microliters per minute caused by a 1-M concentration difference of solute across the membrane. The flows are compared with the flow caused by a theoretically equivalent hydrostatic pressure.

solutes of different molecular size. The solutions have identical freezing points, so the total osmotic pressures are the same. Table 1-3 demonstrates that the larger the solute molecule, the more impermeable the membrane is to the solute, and the greater the osmotic water flow it causes.

Reflection coefficients. Equation 1-6 can be rewritten to take solute permeability into account by including σ, the **reflection coefficient.**

$$V_w = \sigma L \Delta \pi \qquad (1\text{-}7)$$

σ is a dimensionless number that ranges from 1 for completely impermeant solutes to 0 for extremely permeant solutes. σ is a property of a particular solute and a particular membrane and represents the osmotic flow induced by the solute as a fraction of the theoretical maximal osmotic flow (Table 1-3).

The mechanism by which the kidney produces urine that is more concentrated than the extracellular fluid (see Chapter 41) requires that various parts of the nephron have different reflection coefficients for important solutes, such as NaCl and urea. The osmotic water flows induced by NaCl and urea in a particular segment of the nephron depend on the values of σ of the epithelium in that segment to these solutes.

■ *Protein-Mediated Membrane Transport*

Some substances enter or leave cells via intrinsic proteins of the plasma membrane called *carriers* or *channels.* Transport via such protein carriers or channels is called **protein-mediated transport** or simply **mediated trans-**

port. Specific ions or molecules may cross the membranes of mitochondria, endoplasmic reticulum, and other organelles by mediated transport. There are two types of mediated transport: **active transport** and **facilitated transport.** Although these processes have several properties in common, the principal distinction between them is that *active transport is capable of "pumping" a substance against a gradient of concentration (or electrochemical potential), whereas facilitated transport tends to equilibrate the substance across the membrane.*

■ *Properties of Mediated Transport*

1. A substance that is transported by mediated transport is transported *much more rapidly* than other molecules that are of similar molecular weight and lipid solubility that cross the membrane by simple diffusion.

2. The transport rate shows **saturation kinetics.** As the concentration of the transported compound is increased, the rate of transport at first increases, but eventually a concentration is reached after which the transport rate increases no further (Fig. 1-8). At this point, the transport system is said to be saturated with the transported compound. Saturation behavior of the rate (J) of mediated transport is represented by a Michaelis-Menten type of equation:

$$J = \frac{J_{max}[S]}{K_m + [S]} \qquad (1\text{-}8)$$

where J_{max} is the maximal rate of transport, [S] is the concentration of the transported substance in the compartment from which it is being removed, and K_m is the apparent Michaelis constant for the transporter. When $[S] = K_m$, $J = J_{max}/2$, so K_m can be defined as the concentration of the transported compound required for half-maximal transport.

3. The mediating protein has **chemical specificity:** only molecules with the requisite chemical structure are transported. The specificity of most transport systems is not absolute, and in general it is broader than the specificity of most enzymes. However, the *lock-and-key* relationship between an enzyme and its substrate can be applied to transport proteins as well.

4. Structurally related molecules may compete for transport. Typically, the presence of one transport substrate will decrease the transport rate of a second substrate by competing for the transport protein. This competition is analogous to **competitive inhibition** of an enzyme.

5. Transport may be inhibited by compounds that are not structurally related to transport substrates. An inhibitor may bind to the transport protein in a way that decreases the affinity of the protein for the normal transport substrate. For example, the compound **phloretin** does not resemble a sugar molecule, yet it strongly inhibits red cell sugar transport. Active transport systems, which

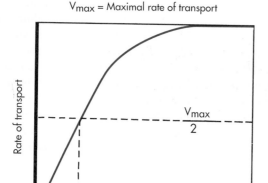

V_max = Maximal rate of transport

■ **Fig. 1-8** Transport via a transport protein shows saturation kinetics. As the concentration of the transported substance increases, the rate of its transport approaches a maximal value, the V_{max} for the transporter. The concentration of the transported substance required for the transport rate to be half-maximal is termed the K_m of the transporter.

require some link to metabolism, may be inhibited by metabolic inhibitors. The rate of Na^+ transport out of cells by the Na^+, K^+-ATPase is decreased by substances that interfere with ATP generation.

■ *Facilitated Transport*

Sometimes called *facilitated diffusion,* facilitated transport occurs via a transport protein that does not require an input of *energy.* Facilitated transport has all the properties discussed previously except one: it is not generally depressed by metabolic inhibitors. Because facilitated transport processes are not linked to energy metabolism, they cannot move substances against concentration gradients. Instead, *facilitated transport systems act to equalize concentrations of the transported substances* on the two sides of the membrane.

Monosaccharides enter muscle cells by facilitated transport. Glucose, galactose, arabinose, and 3-O-methyl-glucose compete for the same carrier. The rate of transport of all these substances shows saturation kinetics. The nonphysiological stereoisomer L-glucose enters the cells very slowly, and nontransported sugars, such as mannitol or sorbose, enter muscle cells very slowly, if at all. Phloretin inhibits sugar uptake, and insulin stimulates it.

Current evidence suggests that most transport proteins span the membrane and are multimeric. Fig. 1-9 depicts a hypothetical model that has been proposed for the monosaccharide transport protein that spans the membrane of the human red blood cell. Conformational changes of the protein, induced by monosaccharide binding, may allow a sugar molecule to enter and leave the central cavity of the transport protein.

■ *Active Transport*

Active transport processes have most of the properties of facilitated transport. In addition, *active transport systems allow the concentration of their substrates against concentration or electrochemical potential gradients. Because this process requires energy, active transport processes must be linked to energy metabolism in some way.* Active transport systems may use ATP directly, or they may be linked indirectly to metabolism. Because they depend on an input of energy, active transport processes may be inhibited by any substance that interferes with energy metabolism.

Primary active transport. An active transport process that is linked directly to cellular metabolism, for example, by using ATP to power the transport, is called **primary active transport.**

An example of a primary active transporter is the **Na^+, K^+-ATPase.** The **Na^+, K^+-ATPase** *uses ATP directly* to power the transport of Na^+ into and K^+ out of cells. In the cytoplasm of most animal cells, the concentration of Na^+ is much less and the concentration of K^+ is much greater than their extracellular concentrations. These concentration gradients are maintained by the action of the Na^+, K^+-ATPase in the plasma membrane. The Na^+, K^+-ATPase transports three sodium ions out of the cell and transports two potassium ions into the cell for each molecule of ATP hydrolyzed.

Transport of Na^+ and K^+ by the Na^+, K^+ pump takes place by a process that has been described as *molecular peristalsis.* The cyclic phosphorylation and dephosphorylation of the protein cause it to alternate between two conformations, E1 and E2. In the E1 conformation, the ion-binding sites of the protein have a high affinity for Na^+ and a low affinity for K^+, and the binding sites face the cytoplasm. In the E2 conformation, the ion-binding sites face the extracellular fluid, and their affinities favor the binding of K^+ and the dissociation of Na^+. The Na^+, K^+-ATPase alternates between the E1 and the E2 conformations, and transports K^+ into the cell and Na^+ out of the cell.

The Na^+, K^+-ATPase's use of the energy in the terminal phosphate bond of ATP to power the transport cycle classifies it as a primary active transport system. A transport process powered by some other high-energy metabolic intermediate or linked directly to a primary metabolic reaction would also be classified as primary active transport.

Secondary active transport. The previous section emphasized that energy is required to create a concentration gradient of a transported substance. Once created, *a concentration gradient represents a store of chemical potential energy that can be harnessed to do work* (see Chapter 2). In many cell types, the concentration gradient of Na^+ created by the Na^+, K^+-ATPase is used to actively transport other solutes into the cell. Many cells import neutral, hydrophilic amino acids by membrane transport proteins that link the inward transport of Na^+ down its

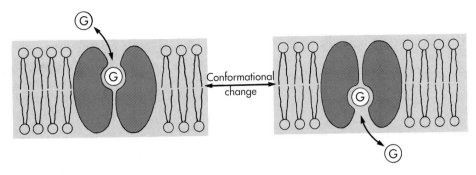

■ **Fig. 1-9** Hypothetical model of a transport protein. This is a model of the mechanism of monosaccharide transport by the sugar transport protein of the human red blood cell. The protein is postulated to be a dimer. Binding of sugars is proposed to cause conformational changes that allow sugar molecules to enter and leave the central cavity of the transport protein.

electrochemical potential gradient to the inward transport of amino acids against their concentration gradients (Fig. 1-10). The energy for the transport of the amino acid is not provided directly by ATP or some other high-energy metabolite *but is provided indirectly from the gradient of Na⁺* that is itself actively transported. Hence, the amino acid is said to be transported by **secondary active transport.** In the secondary active transport of amino acids, both the rate of amino acid transport and the extent to which the amino acid accumulates in the cell depend on the electrochemical potential gradient of Na^+.

In the small intestine, glucose and galactose are absorbed by Na^+-powered secondary active transport. The presence of Na^+ in the lumen enhances the absorption of glucose, and vice versa. In severe diarrheal illnesses, oral rehydration therapy is frequently employed. Patients drink a solution containing both NaCl and glucose, along with K^+ and HCO_3^-. The absorption of Na^+ and glucose in the small intestine helps to drive the osmotic absorption of water and thus facilitates the rehydration of the patient.

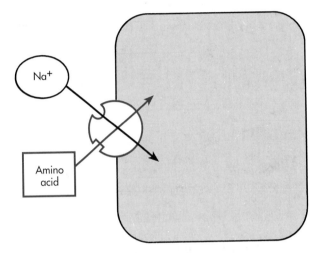

■ **Fig. 1-10** Many cells take up neutral amino acids by secondary active transport. The transport protein binds both Na^+ and the amino acid. Na^+ is transported down its electrochemical gradient, and the transport protein uses the energy released by Na^+ flux to transport the amino acid against a concentration gradient.

■ *Other Membrane Transport Processes*

Ion-transporting ATPases. Ion-transporting ATPases are central to the lives of all cells, from Archaebacteria to *Homo sapiens.* There are three major classes of ion-transporting ATPases: **P-type, V-type,** and **F-type ATPases.**

P-type ATPases. These ATPases are so named because their transport cycle involves a phosphorylated intermediate. The Na^+, K^+-ATPase, discussed above, is a P-type ATPase. So are the Ca^{++}-ATPases of the sarcoplasmic reticulum, endoplasmic reticulum, and plasma membrane, and the H^+, K^+-ATPases of the gastric parietal cell, the intercalated cell of the kidney, and the epithelial cells in the colon. P-type ATPases are also known as E1-E2 ATPases because their transport cycle involves two distinct classes of conformational states. As noted, the inter-

conversion between the E1 and E2 states is driven by the phosphorylation (ATP is the phosphoryl donor) and dephosphorylation of the transporter.

V-type ATPases. The membranes of various intracellular organelles, such as lysosomes, endosomes, secretory vesicles, and storage granules, contain V-type ATPases. The V-type ATPases actively accumulate H^+ in the vesicle lumen. Acidification of the vesicle lumen is essential for the function of lysosomes and for the storage of neurotransmitters in synaptic vesicles.

F-type ATPases. The inner mitochondrial membrane contains an F-type ATPase, known as **ATP synthase.** Whereas P- and V-type ATPases hydrolyze ATP and use some of the energy released to actively transport ions, the ATP synthase generally uses the energy of the H^+ gradient that is established across the mitochondrial inner membrane by electron transport to synthesize ATP. (Because all chemical reactions are reversible, under appropriate conditions P- and V-type ATPase can use the energy of ion gradients to produce ATP, and F-type ATPases can use ATP to actively transport H$^+$.) In the normal economy of animal cells, the mitochondrial ATP synthase is the major source of ATP, and the P- and V-type ATPases are major consumers of ATP (Fig. 1-11).

Calcium transport. Under most circumstances, the concentration of Ca^{++} in the cytosol of cells is maintained at low levels, 10^{-7} M or less, whereas the concentration of Ca^{++} in extracellular fluids is approximately 10^{-3} M. Because Ca^{++} is an important second messenger, the cytosolic level of Ca^{++} is subject to complex regulation. Many hormones and agonists elevate the intracellular level of Ca^{++} by opening Ca^{++} channels in the plasma membrane and/or in the membranes of intracellular Ca^{++}-storage vesicles. Among the membrane transport proteins that participate in regulating the level of cytosolic Ca^{++} are Ca^{++}-ATPases located in plasma membranes and in the membranes of endoplasmic and sarcoplasmic reticulum, and Na$^+$-Ca^{++} exchange proteins of plasma membranes.

Ca^{++}-ATPases. Plasma membranes contain a Ca^{++}-ATPase that helps maintain the large gradient of Ca^{++} between the cytosol and the extracellular fluid. The plasma membrane Ca^{++}-ATPase is a relative of the Ca^{++}-ATPase that is responsible for sequestering Ca^{++} in the sarcoplasmic reticulum of muscle (see Chapter 17). The plasma membrane Ca^{++}-ATPase shares several important structural and mechanistic properties with the Ca^{++}-ATPase of the sarcoplasmic reticulum and with the Na$^+$, K$^+$-ATPase of plasma membranes. The plasma membrane Ca^{++}-ATPase is regulated by **calmodulin.** In the presence of micromolar Ca^{++}, the complex of Ca^{++} with calmodulin binds to a specific site on the plasma membrane Ca^{++}-ATPase. This binding causes an autoinhibitory peptide domain to dissociate from the ATP-binding site, and thus activates the Ca^{++}-ATPase.

In addition, *most cells store Ca^{++} in endoplasmic reticulum or other intracellular storage vesicles,* such as the sarcoplasmic reticulum of muscle cells. Ca^{++} is concentrated in these vesicles by Ca^{++}-ATPases that are members of a closely related family of Ca^{++}-ATPases called SERCA (sarcoplasmic and endoplasmic reticulum Ca^{++}-ATPases). The best characterized SERCA Ca^{++}-ATPase is the Ca^{++}-ATPase of fast skeletal muscle.

Na$^+$-Ca^{++} exchange. Certain electrically excitable cells, such as those of the heart, have an additional mechanism for controlling the level of intracellular Ca^{++}. A sodium/calcium exchange protein in their plasma membranes uses the energy in the Na$^+$ gradient to extrude Ca^{++} from the cell. In heart cells, the decrease in intracellular Ca^{++} that occurs in each diastole is caused by both the sodium/calcium exchange protein and the Ca^{++}-ATPase of the sarcoplasmic reticulum. The Na$^+$-Ca^{++} exchanger is stimulated at micromolar levels of Ca^{++} by binding of the Ca^{++}-calmodulin complex to a specific site of the exchanger protein.

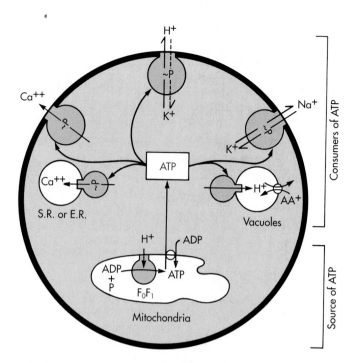

■ **Fig. 1-11** Ion-transporting ATPases are the major sources and among the major consumers of ATP in cells. The F-type ATPase of mitochondria, ATP synthase, is the major source of ATP. P-type and V-type ATPases consume a significant fraction of the ATP utilized by cells. *S.R.,* Sarcoplasmic reticulum; *E.R.,* endoplasmic reticulum. (Modified from Pedersen PL, Carafoli E: *Trends Biochem Sci* 12:146, 1987.)

In most cells, the rate at which Ca^{++} leaks into the cell down its electrochemical potential gradient is slow: therefore, the energy cost of maintaining a low intracellular level of Ca^{++} is also low. This low-energy expenditure contrasts with the cost of pumping Na$^+$ and K$^+$; *running the Na$^+$, K$^+$ pump is a major item in the energy budget of many cells.* Kidneys have an extremely high metabolic rate; the largest fraction of the energy expended by the kidney is consumed by the Na$^+$, K$^+$-ATPase.

Na$^+$-H$^+$ exchange. Most cells contain a protein that mediates the one-for-one exchange of Na$^+$ for H$^+$ across the plasma membrane. This protein, the Na$^+$-H$^+$ exchanger, functions to prevent acidification of the cytosol. When the pH of the cytosol is nearly neutral, the Na$^+$-H$^+$ exchanger has a low affinity for H$^+$ and is almost inactive. Acidification of the cytosol increases the affinity of the protein for H$^+$. Na$^+$ flows into the cell down its electrochemical potential gradient in exchange for the outward transport of H$^+$, and as a result the pH of the cytosol rises toward neutrality.

Treatment of cells with certain growth factors, tumor promoters, and mitogens results in phosphorylation of the Na$^+$-H$^+$ exchanger and increases its affinity for H$^+$. Increased affinity for H$^+$ causes the exchanger to be active at neutral pH and results in persistent alkalinization of the cytosol. The activation of the Na^+-H^+ exchanger is apparently required for the stimulation of cell division by mitogens, but the mechanism by which alkalinization contributes to an increased rate of cell division is not yet understood.

Anion exchange. Essentially all cells contain **anion exchange proteins** in their plasma membranes. Three members of the family of anion exchange proteins have been found in animal cells; the best characterized is the band 3 protein of human erythrocytes. These proteins mediate the exchange of an intracellular anion for an extracellular anion. A number of different univalent anions are transported. Physiologically, the anions present at highest concentrations are Cl^- and HCO_3^-. Hence, the anion exchange protein, especially in red blood cells, is often called the **chloride-bicarbonate exchanger.**

The chloride-bicarbonate exchanger plays an important role in the transport of CO_2 from the tissues to the lungs and the unloading of CO_2 from the blood in the lungs (see Chapter 35).

The anion exchanger is also involved in regulation of cell pH. Alkalization of the cytosol shifts the equilibrium of carbonic acid toward elevated bicarbonate. Consequently, elevated cell pH activates the efflux of bicarbonate in exchange for chloride and thereby shifts the cytosolic pH back toward neutrality. *Cytosolic pH is thus maintained at near-neutral levels by the combined actions of the anion exchanger (which responds to alkalinization of the cytosol) and the Na^+-H^+ exchanger (which is activated by acidification of cytosol).*

Na^+, K^+, Cl^- cotransport. Many cells, both epithelial and nonepithelial, contain a plasma membrane protein that mediates the simultaneous transport ("cotransport") of Na^+, K^+, and Cl^- from the extracellular fluid to the cytosol. The stoichiometry is 1 Na^+ : 1 K^+ : 2 Cl^-, and thus the transport is electroneutral. The entry of Na^+ into the cell down its electrochemical potential gradient provides the energy for the active uptake of K^+ and Cl^-. In many cell types, Na^+, K^+, Cl^- cotransport plays a role in volume regulation. The cotransporter is activated by cell shrinking, which leads to an influx of Na^+, K^+, and $Cl-$ and thereby generates an osmotic force to restore cell volume.

The Na^+, K^+, Cl^- cotransporter is specifically inhibited by drugs, such as **furosemide** and **bumetanide,** known as **loop diuretics.** Loop diuretics inhibit the Na^+, K^+, Cl^- cotransporter in the thick ascending limb of the loop of Henle, and thereby interfere with the reabsorption of Na^+ and Cl^- from the thick ascending limb (see Chapter 41). Because the reabsorption of

Na^+ and Cl^- plays a primary role in the ability of the kidney to produce a urine of low volume and high concentration, loop diuretics are among the most powerful diuretics.

Facilitated transport of glucose. Glucose is the primary fuel for most of the cells of the body, but glucose diffuses across plasma membranes very slowly. The plasma membranes of many cell types contain transport proteins that mediate the facilitated transport of glucose and related monosaccharides. Red blood cells, hepatocytes, adipocytes, and muscle cells (skeletal, cardiac, smooth) all possess glucose transporters. Glucose uptake by these cell types does not depend on the electrochemical potential difference of Na^+ across the plasma membrane or in any direct way on cellular metabolism. Cells of adult humans contain three distinct, but highly homologous, isoforms of glucose transporters.

Stimulation of glucose transport by insulin. In adipocytes and muscle cells, the rate of transport of glucose across the plasma membrane is increased by insulin. *Insulin increases the rate of glucose transport by prompting the insertion of more glucose transport proteins into the plasma membrane.* The source of the newly inserted protein is a preformed pool of transporters in the membranes of the endoplasmic reticulum within the cell (Fig 1-12).

In **type I diabetes mellitus,** also known as **insulin-dependent diabetes,** pancreatic β cells secrete very little insulin in response to elevations of blood glucose. In the absence of insulin, muscle and adipose cells must rely on the slow diffusion of glucose. Because transport of glucose into these cells is the rate-limiting step in glucose metabolism, muscle and fat cells are impaired in their ability to metabolize glucose. Consequently, in type I diabetes, these cells must turn to other fuels, such as fats, to satisfy their energy demands.

Metabolic regulation of glucose transport. The glucose uptake capacity of several different cell types is modulated in accordance with metabolic requirements. In red cells and certain neurons, glucose transport is stimulated by decreased levels of ATP and increased levels of adenosine diphosphate (ADP) and adenosine monophosphate (AMP). Anoxia in cardiac muscle and exercise in skeletal muscle stimulate glucose transport. These responses may involve the insertion of additional glucose transporters into the plasma membrane, but most of the response is attributable to stimulation of preexisting transporters in the membrane.

The stimulation of glucose uptake in skeletal muscle by exercise does not depend on insulin. Insulin-dependent diabetics can diminish the amount of insulin required to regulate their blood glucose levels by engaging in regular exercise.

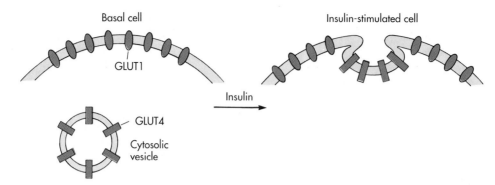

■ **Fig. 1-12** Schematic depiction of the stimulation of glucose transport in muscle or fat cells by insulin. In the basal state glucose transporters are present in the plasma membrane (the GLUT1 isoform of the glucose transporter) and in a pool of intracellular vesicles (the GLUT4 isoform). Upon stimulation by insulin, many of the intracellular vesicles fuse with the plasma membrane, thereby increasing the total number of glucose transporters in the plasma membrane.

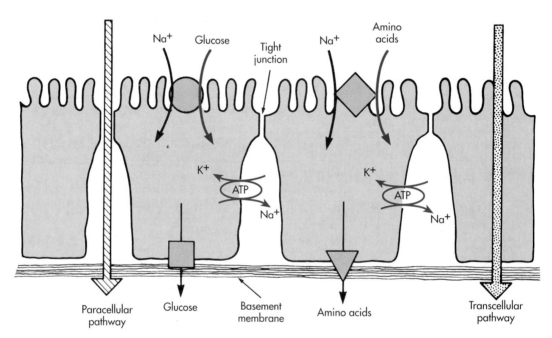

■ **Fig. 1-13** Epithelial transport processes that occur in the small intestine and renal tubules. Epithelia are polarized so that the transport processes on one side of the cell differ from those on the other side. Glucose and neutral amino acids enter the epithelial cell at the brush border via Na^+-powered secondary active transport, but they leave the cell across the basolateral membrane by facilitated transport.

Amino acid transport. Most of the cells in the body synthesize proteins and therefore require amino acids. The synthesis of proteins is required for the turnover of cells and tissues and in processes such as wound healing. Several different amino acid transport proteins are present in plasma membranes. The amino acid transport systems include *three distinct classes of transporters:* for neutral, for basic, and for acidic amino acids (see Chapter 39). Amino acid transport proteins overlap significantly in specificities, and the distribution of the different transport proteins varies from one cell type to another. Some of these transport proteins are secondary active transporters powered by the concentration gradient of Na^+;

others are facilitated transport proteins. Certain amino acid transporters in the brush border membranes of the jejunum and the renal proximal tubule are found only in epithelial cell types. Other amino acid transporters are present in almost all cell types.

■ *Transport across Epithelia*

Epithelial cells are polarized with respect to their transport properties. The transport properties of the plasma membrane facing one side of the epithelial cell layer are different from those of the membrane facing the other side.

The epithelial cells of the small intestine (see Chapter 39) and the proximal tubule of the kidney (see Chapter 41) provide good examples of this polarity. The composition of membrane transport proteins in the brush border membrane that faces the lumen of the small bowel or the renal tubule differs from the transport protein composition of the basolateral plasma membrane of the cell. The **tight junctions** that join the epithelial cells side to side prevent mixing of the transport proteins of the luminal and basolateral plasma membranes. The brush border plasma membranes of these epithelia contain very few Na$^+$, K$^+$-ATPase molecules, which reside mainly in the basolateral plasma membrane. Glucose (and galactose) and neutral amino acids enter these epithelial cells at the brush border by secondary active transporters driven by the Na$^+$ gradient. However, these substances leave the cells at the basolateral membrane primarily by facilitated transporters (Fig. 1-13).

The tight junctions that join the cells are leaky to water and small water-soluble molecules and ions. There are thus two types of pathways for transport across the epithelia: (1) **transcellular** pathways, through the cells, and (2) **paracellular** pathways, between the cells (Fig. 1-13).

■ *Summary*

1. Biological membranes are phospholipid bilayers. Integral membrane proteins are embedded in the bilayer, and peripheral membrane proteins adhere to the surfaces of the membrane. Membranes serve as permeability barriers that separate the cell from the extracellular environment and divide the cell into biochemically specialized compartments.

2. Endocytosis and exocytosis permit material to enter or leave the cell without passing through the membrane.

3. Diffusion is an effective biological transport process over *microscopic* distances. Only very small water-soluble molecules and lipid-soluble molecules can diffuse across biological membranes at appreciable rates.

4. Gradients of solutes across membranes power the flow of water by osmosis. The steady-state volume of cells is determined by impermeant solutes, while permeant solutes have only transient effects. The osmotic water flow caused by a particular solute depends on the permeability of the membrane to that solute: the greater the permeability of the membrane to the solute, the less is the osmotic water flow.

5. Biological membranes contain proteins (transporters) that transport various classes of molecules. Facilitated transporters allow the transported substance to equilibrate across the membrane. Active transporters can pump the transported substances against a concentration or energy gradient. Active transport is an energy-requiring process and must be linked to metabolism.

6. Primary active transport proteins are directly linked to metabolism, frequently by consuming ATP. The Na$^+$, K$^+$-ATPase of the plasma membrane hydrolyzes ATP and uses some of the energy released to actively import K$^+$ and extrude Na$^+$.

7. Secondary active transport proteins use the gradient of another substance, frequently Na$^+$, to power the transport of substances such as sugars and amino acids.

8. Ion-transporting ATPases are central to the economy of the cell. The F-type ATPases of mitochondria are the primary producers of ATP. The P- and V-type ATPases of plasma and organellar membranes are major consumers of ATP.

9. Calcium ions are key second messengers. The resting cellular level of Ca^{++} is maintained at submicromolar levels. Calcium ATPases in the plasma membrane, endoplasmic reticulum, and sarcoplasmic reticulum and sodium-calcium exchange proteins in plasma membranes play key roles in regulating the basal level of cytosolic Ca^{++}.

10. Several types of transport proteins mediate the exchange of ions across membranes. Na$^+$-H$^+$ exchangers and anion exchangers in the plasma membranes of cells help maintain cytosolic pH near neutral. Plasma membrane Na$^+$, K$^+$, Cl$^-$ cotransporters maintain cellular volume.

11. Facilitated transport of glucose into muscle and fat cells is rate-limiting for glucose metabolism. Insulin stimulates glucose transport into these cells by promoting the insertion of additional glucose transporters into the plasma membrane.

12. Epithelial cells contain different transporters in the plasma membranes that face the opposite sides of the tissue. In most epithelia, significant transport of water and solutes occurs via the tight junctions (which are somewhat leaky) between the cells.

■ *Self-Study Problems*

1. (a) Write the form of Fick's first law of diffusion that describes diffusion of a substance across a membrane. (b) What is the meaning of the symbols in the equation? (c) State in words what the equation says.

2. (a) How does the lipid solubility of solute molecules affect their ability to permeate biological membranes? (b) For molecules of similar lipid solubility, how does molecular weight influence permeability? (c) What is the approximate molecular weight above which permeation of water-soluble substances by diffusion occurs at negligible rates? (d) How do water-soluble molecules that are much larger than this cut-off enter and leave cells?

3. Define: osmosis, osmotic pressure, semipermeable membrane.

4. (a) Write van't Hoff's law. (b) Assuming that the osmotic coefficient (Φ) is equal to 1.0, what is the approximate osmotic pressure (0° C) of a 0.01-M $CaCl_2$ solution? (c) Under what conditions does the assumption that the osmotic coefficient equals 1.0 apply most precisely? (d) What is the osmotic coefficient used for? (e) If the osmotic coefficient (Φ) for $CaCl_2$ is 0.86, what is a better estimate of the osmotic pressure of a 0.01-M $CaCl_2$ solution?

5. List the three rules that help to describe the osmotic behavior of cells in response to solutes, both impermeant and permeant.

6. (a) List the properties of protein-mediated transport across membranes that distinguish mediated transport from simple diffusion. (b) Differentiate active transport from facilitated transport. (c) Distinguish primary active transport from secondary active transport.

■ *Bibliography*

Journal articles

Carruthers A: Facilitated diffusion of glucose, *Physiol Rev* 70:1135, 1990.

Christensen HN: Role of amino acid transport and countertransport in nutrition and metabolism, *Physiol Rev* 70:43, 1990.

Fambrough DM: The sodium pump becomes a family, *Trends Neurosci* 11:325, 1988.

Finkelstein A: Water movement through membrane channels, *Curr Top Membr Transp* 21:295, 1984.

Griffith JK: Membrane transport proteins: implications of sequence comparisons, *Curr Opin Cell Biol* 4:684, 1992.

Handler JS: Overview of epithelial polarity, *Annu Rev Physiol* 51:729, 1989.

Henderson PJF: The 12-transmembrane helix transporters, *Curr Opin Cell Biol* 5:708, 1993.

Lodish HF: Anion-exchange and glucose transport proteins: structure, function, and distribution, *Harvey Lect* 82:19, 1988.

Mercer RW: Structure of the Na, K-ATPase, *Int Rev Cytol* 137C:139, 1993.

Pedersen PL, Carafoli E: Ion motive ATPases. I. Ubiquity, properties, and significance to cell function, *Trends Biochem Sci* 12:146, 1987.

Sachs G, Munson K: Mammalian phosphorylating ion-motive ATPases, *Curr Opin Cell Biol* 3:685, 1991.

Walter A, Gutknecht J: Permeability of small nonelectrolytes through lipid bilayer membranes, *J Membr Biol* 90:207, 1986.

Wright EM, Hager KM, Turk E: Sodium co-transport proteins, *Curr Opin Cell Biol* 4:696, 1992.

Books and monographs

Andreoli TE et al, editors: *Physiology of membrane disorders,* ed 2, New York, 1986, Plenum Press.

Finean JB, Michell RH, editors: *Membrane structure,* New York, 1981, Elsevier/North-Holland Biomedical Press.

Finkelstein A: *Water movement through lipid bilayers, pores, and plasma membranes: theory and reality,* New York, 1987, John Wiley.

Kaplan JH, De Weer P, editors: *The sodium pump: structure, mechanism, and regulation, 44th Symposium of the Society of General Physiologists,* New York, 1990, Rockefeller Press.

Kotyk A, Janacek K, Koryta J: *Biophysical chemistry of membrane functions,* New York, 1988, Wiley Interscience.

Läuger P: *Electrogenic ion pumps,* Sunderland, Mass, 1991, Sinauer Associates.

Martonosi AN, editor: *The enzymes of biological membranes,* ed 2, New York, 1985, Plenum Press.

Stein WH: *Channels, carriers, and pumps: an introduction to membrane transport,* San Diego, 1990, Academic Press.

Ionic Equilibria and Resting Membrane Potentials

Most animal cells maintain an electrical potential difference (voltage) across their plasma membranes. *The cytoplasm is usually electrically negative* relative to the extracellular fluid. This electrical potential difference across the plasma membrane in a resting cell is called the **resting membrane potential.** The resting membrane potential plays a central role in the excitability of nerve and muscle cells and in certain other cellular responses. The major goal of this chapter is to explain how the resting membrane potential is generated. First, however, it is necessary to describe the principles of ionic equilibria.

■ *Ionic Equilibria*

■ *Electrochemical Potentials of Ions*

In Fig. 2-1, a membrane separates aqueous solutions in two chambers (A and B). The ion X^+ is at a higher concentration on side A than on side B. If no electrical potential difference exists between side A and side B, X^+ tends to diffuse from side A to side B, just as if it were an uncharged molecule. If, however, side A is electrically negative with respect to side B, the situation is more complex. Although X^+ still tends to diffuse from side A to side B because of the concentration difference, now X^+ also tends to move in the opposite direction (from B to A) because of the electrical potential difference across the membrane. *The direction of net X^+ movement depends on whether the effect of the concentration difference or the effect of the electrical potential difference is larger. By comparing the two tendencies— concentration and electrical—one can predict the direction of net X^+ movement.*

The quantity that allows us to compare the relative contributions of ionic concentration and electrical potential to the movement of an ion is called the **electrochemical potential (μ)** of an ion. The electrochemical potential difference of X^+ across the membrane is defined as

$$\Delta\mu\,(X^+) = \mu_A\,(X^+) - \mu_B\,(X^+) = RT\ln\frac{[X^+]_A}{[X^+]_B}$$
$$+ zF\,(E_A - E_B)\quad(2\text{-}1)$$

where

$\Delta\mu$	=	electrochemical potential difference of the ion between sides A and B of the membrane
R	=	ideal gas constant
T	=	absolute temperature
$\ln\dfrac{[X^+]_A}{[X^+]_B}$	=	natural logarithm of concentration ratio of X^+ on the two sides of the membrane
z	=	charge number of the ion (+ 2 for Ca^{++}, 1 for Cl, etc.)
F	=	Faraday's number
$E_A - E_B$	=	electrical potential difference across the membrane

The first term on the right side of equation 2-1, $RT\ln[X^+]_A/X^+]_B$, is the tendency of X^+ ions to move from A to B *because of the concentration difference,* and the second term, $zF(E_A - E_B)$, is the tendency of the ions to move from A to B *because of the electrical potential difference.* The first term represents the potential energy difference between a mole of X^+ ions on side A and a mole of X^+ ions on side B as a result of the concentration difference. The second term represents the potential energy difference between a mole of X^+ ions on side A and a mole of X^+ ions on side B caused by the electrical potential difference between A and B. Thus, $\Delta\mu\,(X^+)$ *describes the difference in potential energy that exists between a mole of X^+ ions on side A and a mole of X^+ ions on side B that results from both concentration and electrical potential differences;* hence the name **electrochemical potential difference.** The unit of electrochemical potential, and of both terms on the right hand side of equation 2-1, is *energy/mole.*

The X⁺ ions tend to move spontaneously from a higher to a lower electrochemical potential. We defined $\Delta\mu$ as the electrochemical potential of the ion on side A minus that on side B. If $\Delta\mu$ is positive, the ions tend to move from A to B; if $\Delta\mu$ is zero, there is no net tendency for the ions to move at all; if $\Delta\mu$ is negative, the ions tend to move from side B to side A.

If μ_A is *greater* than μ_B, ions tend to flow spontaneously *from side A to side B. To cause ions to flow from B to A, work must be done.* This work is expressed in equation 2-1: $\mu_A(X^+) - \mu_B(X^+)$. $\mu_A - \mu_B$ is the minimal amount of work that must be done to cause 1 mole of ions to flow from B to A. Conversely, when ions flow from A to B, energy is dissipated. *This energy can be harnessed to perform work.* The maximal amount of work that can be done by 1 mole of ions flowing from A to B is $\mu_A - \mu_B$. *An electrochemical potential difference of an ion across a membrane thus represents potential energy that can be harnessed to perform work.*

What sort of work can be done by the electrochemical potential energy stored in an ion gradient? In Chapter 1, we saw that the electrochemical potential of the Na⁺ gradient across the plasma membrane powers the secondary active transport of sugars and amino acids. In mitochondria, the action of the electron transport enzymes creates an electrochemical potential gradient of H⁺ across the mitochondrial inner membrane. The H⁺ ions flow back into the mitochondrial matrix via the ATP synthase enzyme complex in the mitochondrial inner membrane. The ATP synthase uses the energy released by the H⁺ ions to drive the synthesis of ATP. Drugs, such as the poison **dinitrophenol,** that increase the permeability of the mitochondrial inner membrane to H⁺ collapse the H⁺ gradient and prevent the synthesis of ATP.

■ *Electrochemical Equilibrium and the Nernst Equation*

In equation 2-1, $\Delta\mu$ may be thought of as the net force on the ion, whereas $RT\ln [X^+]_A/[X^+]_B$ is the force caused by the concentration difference, and $zF(E_A - E_B)$ is the force caused by the electrical potential difference. *When the latter two forces are equal and opposite, $\Delta\mu = 0$, and there is no net force on the ion.* When there is no net force on the ion, no net movement of the ion occurs, and the ion is said to be in **electrochemical equilibrium** across the membrane. *At equilibrium, $\Delta\mu = 0$.* From equation 2-1, therefore, at equilibrium:

$$RT\ln \frac{[X^+]_A}{[X^+]_B} + zF (E_A - E_B) = 0 \qquad (2\text{-}2)$$

Solving for $E_A - E_B$, we obtain

$$E_A - E_B = - \frac{RT}{zF} \ln \frac{[X^+]_A}{[X^+]_B} = \frac{RT}{zF} \ln \frac{[X^+]_B}{[X^+]_A} \qquad (2\text{-}3)$$

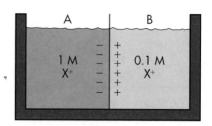

■ **Fig. 2-1**   X⁺ is present at 1 M in chamber A and at 0.1 M in chamber B. A concentration force for X⁺ tends to cause X⁺ to flow from A to B. However, chamber A is electrically negative with respect to chamber B, so an electrical force tends to cause X⁺ to flow from B to A.

Equation 2-3 is called the **Nernst equation.** Because the condition of equilibrium was assumed in its derivation, *the Nernst equation is satisfied only for ions at equilibrium.* The equation is used to compute the electrical potential difference, $E_A - E_B$, *required to produce an electrical force, $zF(E_A - E_B)$, that is equal and opposite to the concentration force,* $RT/zF \ln [X^+]_A/[X^+]_B$.

Use of Nernst equation. In using the Nernst equation, it is often convenient to convert the equation to a form that involves logarithm to the base 10 (log) rather than natural logarithms (ln). The formula for this conversion is $\ln y = 2.303 \log y$. Because biological electrical potentials are usually expressed in millivolts (mV), the units of R may be selected so that RT/F comes out in millivolts. At 29.2° C, the quantity 2.303 RT/F is equal to 60 mV. Because this quantity is proportional to the absolute temperature, it changes by approximately 1/273 (0.36%) for each centigrade degree. Thus, the value of 60 mV for 2.303 RT/F holds approximately for most experimental conditions in biology, and a useful form of the Nernst equation is

$$E_A - E_B = \frac{-60 \text{ mV}}{z} \log \frac{[X^+]_A}{[X^+]_B}$$

$$= \frac{60 \text{ mV}}{z} \log \frac{[X^+]_B}{[X^+]_A} \qquad (2\text{-}4)$$

Examples of uses of the Nernst equation

Example 1. In Fig. 2-2, K⁺ is 10 times more concentrated in chamber A than in chamber B. The following is a calculation of the electrical potential difference *that must exist between the chambers for K⁺ to be in equilibrium across the membrane.* Because we have specified that K⁺ should be in equilibrium, the Nernst equation will hold:

$$E_A - E_B = \frac{-60 \text{ mV}}{+1} \log \frac{[K^+]_A}{[K^+]_B} = - (60 \text{ mV}) \log \frac{0.1}{0.01}$$

$$= -60 \text{ mV} \log (10) = -60 \text{ mV} \qquad (2\text{-}5)$$

The Nernst equation tells us that *at equilibrium,* side A *must* be 60 mV negative relative to side B. We can see that this polarity is correct because the electrical force tends to drive K⁺ from B to A, which counteracts the ten-

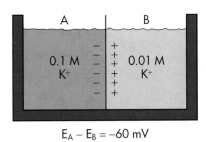

$$E_A - E_B = -60 \text{ mV}$$

■ **Fig. 2-2** A membrane separates chambers containing different K^+ concentrations. At an electrical potential difference $(E_A - E_B)$ of -60 mV, K^+ is in electrochemical equilibrium across the membrane.

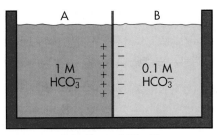

$$E_A - E_B = +100 \text{ mV}$$

■ **Fig. 2-3** A membrane separates chambers that contain different HCO_3^- concentrations. $E_A - E_B = +100$ mV. HCO_3^- is not in electrochemical equilibrium. If $E_A - E_B$ were $+60$ mV, HCO_3^- would be in equilibrium. $E_A - E_B$ (*+100 mV*) is stronger than it needs to be ($+60$ mV) to just balance the tendency for HCO_3^- to move from A to B because of its concentration difference. Thus, net movement of HCO_3^- from B to A will occur.

dency for K^+ to move from A to B because of the concentration difference.

This example shows that *an electrical potential difference of about 60 mV is required to balance a tenfold concentration difference of a univalent ion.* This example thus provides a useful rule of thumb.

Example 2. When ions are not in equilibrium, the Nernst equation can be used to predict the direction in which ions will flow. For example, in Fig. 2-3 the Nernst equation can help decide whether HCO_3^- is in equilibrium. If HCO_3^- is not in equilibrium, the Nernst equation can predict the direction of net flow of HCO_3^-.

First, we must see if HCO_3^- is in equilibrium. The Nernst equation tells us the electrical potential difference, $E_A - E_B$, that will just balance the concentration difference of HCO_3^- across the membrane:

$$
\begin{aligned}
E_A - E_B &= \frac{-60 \text{ mV}}{-1} \log \frac{[HCO_3^-]_A}{[HCO_3^-]_B} \\
&= +(60 \text{ mV}) \log \frac{1}{0.1} \quad (2\text{-}6) \\
&= -60 \text{ mV} \log (10) = -60 \text{ mV}
\end{aligned}
$$

Thus, a potential difference of $+60$ mV between A and B would just balance the tendency of HCO_3^- to move from A to B because of its concentration difference. However, in our example, $E_A - E_B$ is *actually* $+100$ mV. HCO_3^- is not in equilibrium. Now we can predict the direction in which HCO_3^- will flow. Although the electrical force is oriented in the right direction to balance the concentration force, it is 40 mV *larger* than it needs to be to just balance the concentration force. Because the electrical force on HCO_3^- is larger than the concentration force, the electrical force will determine the direction of net HCO_3^- movement. Net HCO_3^- flow will occur from B to A.

In brief, the Nernst equation can be used to predict the direction that ions tend to flow:

1. If the potential difference measured across a membrane is *equal* to the potential difference calculated from the Nernst equation for a particular ion, that ion is *in electrochemical equilibrium* across the membrane, and no net flow of that ion will occur across the membrane.

2. If the measured electrical potential is of the same sign (positive or negative) as that calculated from the Nernst equation for a particular ion but is *larger* in magnitude than the calculated value, the electrical force is larger than the concentration force, and net movement of that particular ion tends to occur in the direction *determined by the electrical force.* Fig. 2-3 meets this condition.

3. When the electrical potential difference is of the same sign but is *numerically less* than that calculated from the Nernst equation for a particular ion, the concentration force is larger than the electrical force, and net movement of that ion tends to occur in the direction *determined by the concentration difference.*

4. If the electrical potential difference measured across the membrane is of the *opposite sign* to that predicted by the Nernst equation for a particular ion, the electrical and concentration forces are in the same direction. Thus, that ion *cannot be in equilibrium,* and it will tend to flow in the direction determined by both electrical and concentration forces.

■ *Gibbs-Donnan Equilibrium*

The cytoplasm of a cell typically contains proteins, organic polyphosphates, nucleic acids, and other ionized substances that cannot permeate the plasma membrane. Most of these impermeant intracellular ions are *negatively charged* at physiological pH. The steady-state properties of this mixture of permeant and impermeant ions are described by the **Gibbs-Donnan equilibrium.**

Fig. 2-4 *(top)* represents a model of a cell with impermeant anions. A membrane separates a solution of KCl from a solution of KY. Y^- is an anion to which the membrane is completely impermeable. The membrane is permeable to water, K^+, and Cl^-. Suppose that initially chamber A contains a 0.1-M solution of KY and that chamber B contains an equal volume of 0.1 M KCl. Because $[Cl^-]_B$ exceeds $[Cl^-]_A$, Cl^- flows from chamber B to chamber A. Negatively charged Cl^- ions flowing from side B to side A will create an electrical potential difference (side A negative) that will then cause K^+ also to flow from side B to side A. Given enough time, K^+ and Cl^- will come into equilibrium. At equilibrium, both $\Delta\mu_{K^+}$ and $\Delta\mu_{Cl^-}$ must equal zero. When *both* K^+ and Cl^- are at equilibrium,

$$[K^+]_A[Cl^-]_A = [K^+]_B[Cl^-]_B \qquad (2\text{-}7)$$

Equation 2-7 is called the **Donnan relation** or the **Gibbs-Donnan equation** and it holds for any univalent cation and anion pair in equilibrium between the two chambers. If other univalent ions that could attain an equilibrium distribution were present, the same reasoning and an equation similar to equation 2-7 would apply to cation-anion pairs of these ions also.

The derivation of the Gibbs-Donnan equation follows from the definition of electrochemical potential. When both K^+ and Cl^- have reached equilibrium, the electrochemical potential difference of each ion across the membrane will be zero. Recalling that $z = 1$ for K^+ and $z = -1$ for Cl^-,

$$\Delta\mu_{K^+} = RT \ln \frac{[K^+]_A}{[K^+]_B} + F(E_A - E_B) = 0$$

$$\Delta\mu_{Cl^-} = RT \ln \frac{[Cl^-]_A}{[Cl^-]_B} - F(E_A - E_B) = 0$$

Adding these two equations and doing some algebra yields

$$\ln \frac{[K^+]_A}{[K^+]_B} = -\ln \frac{[Cl^-]_A}{[Cl^-]_B} = \ln \frac{[Cl^-]_B}{[Cl^-]_A}$$

Which gives

$$\frac{[K^+]_A}{[K^+]_B} = \frac{[Cl^-]_A}{[Cl^-]_B}, \text{ so that } [K^+]_A[Cl^-]_A = [K^+]_B[Cl^-]_B$$

For the model situation we are considering, application of the Gibbs-Donnan equation will result in the final concentrations shown in Fig. 2-4 *(bottom)*.

In this Gibbs Donnan equilibrium, both K^+ and Cl^- (but not Y^-) are in electrochemical equilibrium. Because they are in electrochemical equilibrium, both K^+ and Cl^- satisfy the Nernst equation. Therefore, we can use the Nernst equation to calculate the equilibrium transmembrane potential difference for either K^+ or Cl^-. Applying the Nernst equation to either K^+ or Cl^- results in

$$E_A - E_B = -60 \text{ mV } \log(2) = -18 \text{ mV} \qquad (2\text{-}8)$$

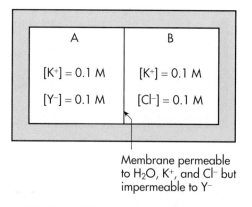

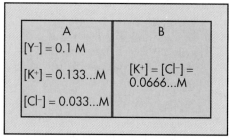

■ **Fig. 2-4** *Top,* Before a Gibbs-Donnan equilibrium is established, a membrane separates two aqueous compartments. The membrane is permeable to water, K^+, and Cl^- but impermeable to Y^-. *Bottom,* Ion concentrations after Gibbs-Donnan equilibrium has been attained.

The presence of the impermeant Y^- anions results in a negative electrical potential in the chamber that contains them. In a typical cell *the impermeant anions in the cytoplasm contribute on the order of -10 mV to the resting membrane potential of the cytoplasm relative to the extracellular fluid.*

Note that only the permeant ions (K^+ and Cl^- in this example) attain equilibrium. The impermeant anion, Y^-, cannot reach an equilibrium distribution. It may not be evident that water also will not achieve equilibrium, unless provision is made for that to occur. The sum of the concentrations of K^+ and Cl^- ions on side A in the preceding example exceeds that on side B. *This is a general property of Gibbs-Donnan equilibria.* When the impermeant Y^- is taken into account as well, the total concentration of osmotically active ions is considerably greater on side A than on side B. Water will tend to flow by osmosis from side B to side A until the total osmotic pressure of the two solutions is equal. Then, however, ions will flow to set up a new Gibbs-Donnan equilibrium, and this requires that there be more osmotically active ions on the side with Y. All the water from side B will end up on side A unless water is restrained from moving.

Water can be restrained from moving by enclosing the solution on side A in a rigid container (Fig. 2-5). Then, as fluid flows from side B to side A, pressure will build up in chamber A. This pressure will oppose further osmotic

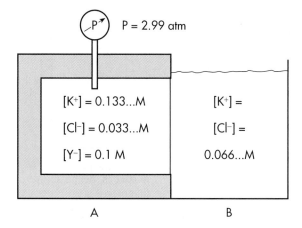

P = 2.99 atm

[K⁺] = 0.133...M   [K⁺] =

[Cl⁻] = 0.033...M   [Cl⁻] =

[Y⁻] = 0.1 M   0.066...M

A   B

■ **Fig. 2-5** A hydrostatic pressure of 2.99 atmospheres is required to prevent water from flowing from chamber B to chamber A in the Gibbs-Donnan equilibrium in Fig. 2-4. This 2.99-atmosphere is equal to the osmotic pressure in chamber A minus that in chamber B.

water flow. The pressure in chamber A at equilibrium will be equal to the difference between the total osmotic pressures of the solutions in chambers A and B.

An example of a structure that restrains the movement of water is the rigid cell wall of plant cells. The cell wall allows turgor pressure to build up in the cell and partly compensates for the osmotic effects of the Gibbs-Donnan equilibrium. If a cell wall were not present, the Gibbs-Donnan equilibrium would cause osmotic pressure in the cytoplasm to build up in excess of the osmotic pressure in the extracellular fluid. This build-up of pressure would threaten the maintenance of the normal cellular volume. Animal cells, which do not have cell walls, have evolved other ways that involve ion transport processes to deal with the osmotic consequences of the Gibbs-Donnan equilibrium, which are discussed in the next section.

■ *Regulation of Cell Volume*

Both K⁺ and Cl⁻ are nearly in equilibrium across many plasma membranes, and their distribution is influenced by the predominantly negatively charged impermeant ions, such as proteins and nucleotides, in the cytoplasm. This being the case, why does the osmotic imbalance discussed previously not cause animal cells to swell and finally burst? One reason is that *these cells actively pump Na⁺ out of the cytoplasm into the extracellular fluid. The extrusion of Na⁺ decreases the osmotic pressure of the cytoplasm and increases that of the extracellular fluid.* Much of the pumping of Na⁺ is accomplished by the Na⁺, K⁺-ATPase in the plasma membrane. The Na⁺, K⁺-ATPase splits a molecule of ATP and uses some of the energy released to extrude 3 Na⁺ from the cytoplasm and to pump 2 K⁺ into the cell. Whereas K⁺ is only slightly removed from an equilibrium distribution,

Na⁺ is pumped out against a large electrochemical potential difference.

When the ATP production of a cell is compromised (such as in the presence of metabolic inhibitors or low O₂ levels), or when the Na⁺, K⁺-ATPase is specifically inhibited, Na⁺ enters the cell more rapidly than it can be pumped out. As a result, the cell swells.

The plasma membranes of red blood cells of patients with **hereditary spherocytosis** (HS) are about three times more permeable to Na⁺ than red cells of normal individuals. The level of Na⁺, K⁺-ATPase in the erythrocyte membranes of HS patients is also substantially elevated. When HS red blood cells have sufficient glucose to maintain normal ATP levels, they extrude Na⁺ as rapidly as it diffuses into the cell cytosol, and the red blood cell volume is maintained. However, when HS erythrocytes are delayed in the venous sinuses of the spleen, where glucose and ATP are present at low levels, the intracellular ATP concentration falls, and Na⁺ cannot be pumped out by the Na⁺, K⁺-ATPase as rapidly as it enters. The red blood cells swell owing to the osmotic effect of elevated intracellular Na⁺ concentration. The spleen targets these swollen erythrocytes, and as a consequence, HS patients become anemic.

■ *Resting Membrane Potentials*

Communication between nerve cells depends on an electrical disturbance, called an **action potential,** that is propagated in the plasma membrane of the nerve cell. In striated muscle, an action potential propagates rapidly over the entire cell surface and allows the cell to contract synchronously. The action potential in nerve and muscle cells and the ionic mechanisms that account for its properties are discussed in Chapter 3. All cells that can produce action potentials have sizable resting membrane potentials (cytoplasm negative) across their plasma membranes. Inexcitable cells also have negative resting membrane potentials, but these potentials are smaller in magnitude than those of excitable cells.

The resting membrane potential of a skeletal muscle cell is about −90 mV. By convention, we express membrane potential difference as the voltage in the cytoplasm minus that in the extracellular fluid. A negative value denotes that the cytoplasm is electrically negative relative to the extracellular fluid. The resting membrane potential is necessary for the cell to fire an action potential.

Ions that are actively transported are not in electrochemical equilibrium across the plasma membrane. As shown later in the chapter, the flow of ions across the plasma membrane, down their electrochemical potential gradients, is directly responsible for generating much of the resting membrane potential. To understand how the electrochemical potential gradient of an ion gives rise to a transmembrane difference in electrical potential, let us first consider a model system known as a **concentration cell.**

Concentration Cells

In Fig. 2-6, the membrane that separates chambers A and B is permeable to cations but not to anions. Initially, no electrical potential difference exists across the membrane. K^+ flows from A to B because of the concentration force acting on it. Cl^- has the same force on it, but it cannot flow because the membrane is impermeable to anions. The flow of K^+ from A to B will transfer net positive charge to side B and leave a very slight excess of negative charges behind on side A. *Side A will thus become electrically negative to side B* (Fig. 2-6). This electrical force is in direct opposition to the concentration force on K^+. The more K^+ that flows, the larger will be the opposing electrical force. *Net K^+ flow will stop when the electrical force just balances the concentration force, i.e., when the electrical potential difference is equal to the equilibrium (Nernst) potential for K^+.* That is, when

$$E_A - E_B = \frac{-60 \text{ mV}}{+1} \log \frac{[K^+]_A}{[K^+]_B}$$

$$= -(60 \text{ mV}) \log \frac{0.1}{0.01} = -60 \text{ mV} \quad (2\text{-}9)$$

Only a very small amount of K^+ flows from A to B before equilibrium is reached. This amount of K^+ is small because the separation of positive and negative charges across the membrane requires a large amount of work. The potential difference that builds up to oppose further K^+ movement is a manifestation of that work.

The K^+ concentration difference in this example acts like a battery. The natural tendency for any ion that can flow is to seek equilibrium; thus, K^+ tends to flow until its equilibrium potential difference is established. As explained later, when more than one type of ion can permeate a membrane, *each ion "strives" to make the transmembrane potential difference equal to its equilibrium potential. The more permeant the ion, the greater is its ability to force the electrical potential difference toward its equilibrium potential.*

Distribution of Ions across Plasma Membranes

In most tissues, a number of ions are not in equilibrium between the extracellular fluid and the cytoplasm. Table 2-1 lists the concentrations of Na^+, K^+, and Cl^- in the extracellular fluid and in the cytoplasmic water of frog skeletal muscle. Intracellular ion concentrations for mammalian muscle are similar to those for frog muscle.

Cl^- is nearly in equilibrium across the plasma membrane of a skeletal muscle cell. We know this because the

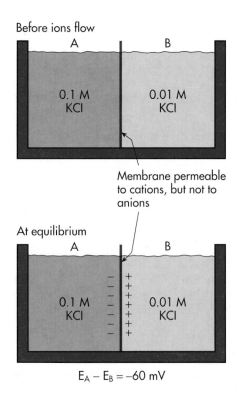

■ **Fig. 2-6**   *Top,* A concentration cell. A membrane, which is permeable to cations but not to anions, separates KCl solutions of different concentrations. *Bottom,* The concentration cell after electrochemical equilibrium has been established. The flow of an infinitesimal amount of K^+ generated an electrical potential difference across the membrane that is equal to the equilibrium potential for K^+.

equilibrium potential of chloride, as calculated from the Nernst equation, is about equal to the measured transmembrane potential difference. K^+ has a concentration force that tends to make it flow out of the cell. The electrical force on K^+ opposes the concentration force. If the $E_{in} - E_{out}$ transmembrane potential in frog muscle were -105 mV (equal to the equilibrium potential for K^+), electrical and concentration forces on K^+ would exactly balance. However, because the actual transmembrane potential is only -90 mV, the concentration force on K^+ is greater than the electrical force. Therefore, K^+ has a *net tendency* to flow out of the cell. Na^+ is the ion farthest from an equilibrium distribution. Both the concentration and the electrical forces on Na^+ tend to cause it to flow into the cell. The larger the difference between the measured membrane potential and the equilibrium potential for an ion, the larger is the net force that tends to make that ion flow. We return to this concept later in this chapter, when we discuss how these ions maintain the resting membrane potential.

Active Ion Pumping and Resting Potential

The Na^+, K^+-ATPase located in the plasma membrane uses the energy within the terminal phosphate ester bond

■ **Table 2-1**   Distribution of Na^+, K^+, and Cl^- across the plasma membranes of frog muscle and squid axon

	Extracellular fluid (mM)	*Cytoplasm (mM)*	*Approximate equilibrium potential (mV)*	*Actual resting potential (mV)*
Frog muscle				
$[Na^+]$	120	9.2	+67	
$[K^+]$	2.5	140	−105	
$[Cl^-]$	120	3 to 4	−89 to −96	−90
Squid axon				
$[Na^+]$	460	50	+58	
$[K^+]$	10	400	−96	
$[Cl^-]$	540	About 40	About −68	−70

Data from Katz B: *Nerve, muscle, and synapse,* New York, 1966, McGraw-Hill Book Co. With permission of McGraw-Hill Book Co.

of ATP to extrude Na^+ actively from the cell and to take K^+ actively into the cell. The Na^+, K^+-ATPase is responsible for the high intracellular K^+ concentration and the low intracellular Na^+ concentration. Because the pump moves a greater number of Na^+ ions out than K^+ ions in (3 Na^+ to 2 K^+), *it causes a net transfer of positive charge out of the cell and thus contributes to the resting membrane potential. Because it brings about net movement of charge across the membrane, the pump is termed **electrogenic**.*

The size of the pump's electrogenic contribution to the resting potential can be estimated by completely inhibiting the pump with a cardiac glycoside, such as **ouabain.** Such studies show that in some cells, the electrogenic Na^+, K^+-ATPase is responsible for a large fraction of the resting potential. In most vertebrate nerve and skeletal muscle cells, however, the direct contribution of the pump to the resting potential is usually small—less than 5 mV. The resting membrane potential in nerve and skeletal muscle results mainly from the diffusion of ions down their electrochemical potential gradients. The ionic gradients are maintained by active ion pumping. In other types of excitable cells, electrogenic pumping of ions may contribute more to the resting membrane potential. In certain smooth muscle cells, for example, the electrogenic effect of the Na^+, K^+-ATPase is responsible for 20 mV or more of the resting membrane potential.

Cardiac glycosides, such as **digitalis** and related drugs, are able to increase the strength of contraction of the heart (see Chapter 23). These compounds inhibit the Na^+, K^+-ATPase. As a result of this inhibition, the intracellular level of Na^+ in cardiac cells is elevated. Each contraction of the heart is initiated by an increase in the cytosolic concentration of Ca^{++} (see Chapter 24). For cardiac muscle to relax, Ca^{++} must be removed from the cytosol. The removal of Ca^{++} from the cytosol of the cardiac cells is accomplished by its being pumped into the sarcoplasmic reticulum (SR) by a Ca^{++}-ATPase in the SR membrane and out across the plasma membrane by a plasma membrane Ca^{++}-ATPase and by Na^+-Ca^{++} exchangers in the plasma membrane. The Ca^{++}-ATPase pumps Ca^{++} into the SR; the Na^+-Ca^{++} exchangers pump the Ca^{++} from the SR out across the plasma membrane. (These ion transporters were described in Chapter 1.) Because cardiac glycosides increase the elevated cytosolic Na^+ concentration, the Na^+-Ca^{++} exchanger is not as effective in extruding Ca^{++} from the cell. Consequently, the Ca^{++}-ATPase can accumulate more Ca^{++} in the SR, so that more Ca^{++} is released from the SR to power the next cardiac contraction, which is stronger than normal because of the greater peak level of Ca^{++} in the cytosol.

■ *Generation of Resting Membrane Potential by Ion Gradients*

The earlier discussion of concentration cells shows how an ion gradient can act as a battery. When a number of ions are distributed across a membrane, and all are removed from electrochemical equilibrium, *each ion will tend to force the transmembrane potential toward its own equilibrium potential, as calculated from the Nernst equation. The more permeable the membrane to a particular ion, the greater strength that ion will have in forcing the membrane potential toward its equilibrium potential.* In frog muscle (Table 2-1), the Na^+ concentration difference can be regarded as a battery that tries to make the transmembrane potential equal to + 67 mV. The K^+ concentration difference resembles a battery that attempts to make the transmembrane potential equal to −105 mV. The Cl^- concentration difference resembles a battery trying to make the transmembrane potential equal to −90 mV.

■ *Chord Conductance Equation*

How the interplay of ion gradients creates the resting membrane potential (E_m) is illustrated by a simple mathematical model. If we consider the distribution of K^+, Na^+, and Cl^- across the plasma membrane of a cell, the following equation predicts the transmembrane potential difference across the membrane:

$$E_m = \frac{g_K}{\Sigma g} E_K + \frac{g_{Na}}{\Sigma g} E_{Na} + \frac{g_{Cl}}{\Sigma g} E_{Cl} \qquad (2\text{-}10)$$

where

$$\Sigma g = (g_K + g_{Na} + g_{Cl})$$

The g's represent the conductances of the membrane to the ions indicated by the subscripts and the E's represent the *equilibrium potentials* of the ions denoted by their subscripts. *Conductance is the reciprocal of resistance (g = 1/R).* The more permeable the membrane to a particular ion, the greater is the conductance of the membrane to that ion.

Equation 2-10 is called the **chord conductance equation.** *It states that the membrane potential is a weighted average of the equilibrium potentials of all the ions to which the membrane is permeable,* in this case K⁺, Na⁺, and Cl⁻. The weighting factor for each ion is the individual conductance of the ion in question divided by the total ionic conductance of the membrane, Σg, or the sum of all the individual ion conductances. *Note that the sum of the weighting factors for the ions must equal 1, so that if one weighting factor becomes larger, the others must become smaller. The chord conductance equation shows that the greater the conductance of the membrane to a particular ion, the greater is the ability of that ion to bring the membrane potential toward the equilibrium potential of that ion.*

The chord conductance equation can be derived fairly simply. As we have seen, if the transmembrane voltage is equal to the equilibrium potential for a particular ion, there will be no net flow of that ion across the membrane. However, if the membrane potential is *not* equal to the equilibrium potential for a given ion, the difference between the membrane potential and the ion's equilibrium potential can be regarded as the driving force for that ion. Because ions bear charge, ionic flow is equivalent to electrical current. Applying Ohm's law, the net current of an ion across a membrane is equal to the conductance (g) of the membrane to the ion times driving force on the ion ($E_m - E_{eq}$).

For K⁺, Na⁺, and Cl⁻

$$\begin{aligned} I_K &= g_K (E_m - E_K) \\ I_{Na} &= g_{Na} (E_m - E_{Na}) \\ I_{Cl} &= g_{Cl} (E_m - E_{Cl}) \end{aligned} \qquad (2\text{-}11)$$

where E_m is the membrane potential and I's are currents, g's are conductances, and E's are the equilibrium potentials of the ions denoted by the subscripts.

In the steady state, when E_m is constant, there is no net ionic current across the membrane. If there were net current, E_m would change. If we assume that K⁺, Na⁺, and Cl⁻ are the only important ions, the requirement that net ionic current be zero leads to

$$I_K + I_{Na} + I_{Cl} = 0 \qquad (2\text{-}12)$$

Substituting from equation 2-11 gives

$$g_K(E_m - E_K) + g_{Na}(E_m - E_{Na}) + g_{Cl}(E_m - E_{Cl}) = 0 \ (2\text{-}13)$$

Solving this equation for E_m gives

$$E_m = \frac{g_K}{\Sigma g} E_K + \frac{g_{Na}}{\Sigma g} E_{Na} + \frac{g_{Cl}}{\Sigma g} E_{Cl} \qquad (2\text{-}14)$$

where $\Sigma g = g_K + g_{Na} + g_{Cl}$.

For the frog muscle fiber discussed earlier, the transmembrane potential = −90 mV. The membrane potential is much closer to the equilibrium potential of K⁺ to [(E_K) (−105 mV)] than to E_{Na} (+67 mV), because in the resting cell g_K is larger than g_{Na}. The chord conductance equation predicts that, in resting muscle, g_K is about 10 times larger than g_{Na}. This prediction has been confirmed by ion flux measurements with radioactive tracers. In other types of excitable cells, the relationship between g_K and g_{Na} may be somewhat different. Other ions also may play a role in generating the resting membrane potential. Resting membrane potentials vary from about −10 mV or so in human erythrocytes to around −40 mV in some types of smooth muscle and up to −90 mV or more in vertebrate skeletal muscle and cardiac ventricular cells.

We have seen that K⁺ has the largest resting conductance and thus has the largest influence on the resting membrane potential. For this reason, changes that occur in the concentration of K⁺ in a patient's extracellular fluid will affect the resting membrane potentials of all cells. An increase in extracellular K⁺ will partially depolarize cells (decrease the magnitude of the resting membrane potential), whereas a decrease in the level of extracellular K⁺ will hyperpolarize cells (increase the magnitude) of the resting membrane potential. Either a depolarization or a hyperpolarization of cardiac cells (see Chapter 23) may lead to **cardiac arrhythmias,** some of which are life-threatening. **Hypokalemia** (low serum K⁺) may be a result of long-term use of diuretics. **Hyperkalemia** (elevated serum K⁺) occurs in acute renal failure and in a disorder called **hyperkalemic periodic paralysis,** which is characterized by episodes of muscle weakness and flaccid paralysis.

■ Roles of Na⁺,K⁺-ATPase in Establishing Resting Membrane Potential: Direct vs. Indirect

The Na⁺, K⁺-ATPase establishes gradients of Na⁺ and K⁺ across the plasma membranes of cells. Because the amount of Na⁺ pumped out is larger than the amount of K⁺ pumped in, the pump transfers net charge across the membrane and in this way *contributes directly* to the resting membrane potential. However, in vertebrate skeletal and cardiac muscle and in nerve, this *electrogenic activity of the pump is directly responsible* for only a small fraction of the resting membrane potential. The major portion of the resting membrane potential in these tissues is a result of the diffusion of Na^+ and K^+ down their electrochemical potential gradients, with each ion tending to bring the transmembrane potential toward its own equilibrium potential. This contribution to the resting membrane potential is *indirectly* caused by the Na^+, K^+-ATPase. Therefore, the relative magnitudes of the direct and indirect contributions of the Na^+, K^+-ATPase to the resting membrane potential vary from one cell type to another.

■ *Summary*

1. An ion tends to flow across a membrane if there is a concentration difference of that ion or an electrical potential difference across the membrane. The electrochemical potential difference ($\Delta\mu$) of an ion across a membrane includes the contributions of both the concentration difference and the electrical potential difference to the tendency of the ion to flow across the membrane.

2. An electrochemical potential difference of an ion across a membrane represents a difference of chemical potential energy. This potential energy difference can be harnessed to do work.

3. An ion that is distributed in equilibrium across a membrane will satisfy the Nernst equation. We can use the Nernst equation to tell whether an ion is in equilibrium or to compute what the electrical potential difference across the membrane would have to be for a particular ion to be in equilibrium.

4. Cytoplasm contains an excess of negative ions that are impermeant to the plasma membrane. A permeant univalent ion pair X^+, Z^- that can attain equilibrium across the membrane will satisfy the Gibbs-Donnan equilibrium, which is represented by the relationship: $[X]_{in}[Z]_{in} = [X]_{out}[Z]_{out}$, where "in" and "out" refer to cytoplasm and extracellular fluid, respectively.

5. All cells have a negative resting membrane potential, that is, the cytoplasm is electrically negative relative to the extracellular fluid. The diffusion of ions across the plasma membrane down their electrochemical potential gradients contributes to the resting membrane potential.

6. The flow of each ion across the plasma membrane tends to bring the resting membrane potential toward the equilibrium potential for that ion. The more conductive the membrane to a particular ion, the greater will be the ability of that ion to bring the membrane potential toward its equilibrium potential. This is described by the chord conductance equation.

7. Three processes contribute to generating the resting membrane potential: (a) ionic diffusion as just described (major), (b) the electrogenic effect of the Na^+, K^+-ATPase (variable in importance), and (c) the Gibbs-Donnan equilibrium (minor in excitable cells).

■ *Self-Study Problems*

1. Write the equation that defines the electrochemical potential difference of an ion X^+ across a membrane. Which is the "concentration term"? Which is the "electrical term"?

2. Write the Nernst equation and define the symbols in it. What does it imply when we say that "an ion satisfies the Nernst equation"?

3. Chambers A and B are separated by a membrane. Chamber A contains 1 M KNO_3 and chamber B contains 0.1 M KNO_3. If K^+ is in equilibrium across the membrane, what is the electrical potential difference, $E_A - E_B$? Which side is electrically positive?

4. Write down the Donnan relation for the ions X^+ and Y^-. If the transmembrane distribution of a cation-anion pair (both univalent) satisfies the Donnan relation, what does this imply?

5. Define an electrogenic membrane transport process. Is the Na^+, K^+-ATPase an electrogenic ion pump? Why?

6. The following data apply to the sartorius muscle of the South American spotted tree frog:

Ion	Intracellular concentration	Extracellular concentration	Relative resting membrane conductance
Na^+	12	120	0.05
K^+	120	4	0.5
Cl^-	4	120	0.45

What is the resting membrane potential (sign and magnitude) of this cell? Is the inside negative or positive relative to the outside?

■ *Bibliography*

Books and monographs

Aidley DJ: *The physiology of excitable cells,* ed 3, Cambridge, 1990, Cambridge University Press.

Hille B: *Ion channels of excitable membranes,* ed 2, Sunderland, Mass, 1992, Sinauer Associates.

Junge D: *Nerve and muscle excitation,* ed 2, Sunderland, Mass, 1981, Sinauer Associates.

Kandel ER, Schwartz JH: *Principles of neural science,* ed 3, New York, 1991, Elsevier Science.

Katz B: *Nerve, muscle, and synapse,* New York, 1966, McGraw-Hill.

Keynes RD, Aidley DJ: *Nerve and muscle,* ed 2, New York, 1991, Cambridge University Press.

Läuger P: *Electrogenic ion pump,* Sunderland, Mass, 1991, Sinauer Associates.

Nicholls JG, Martin AR, Wallace BG: *From neuron to brain,* ed 3, Sunderland, Mass, 1992, Sinauer Associates.

Shepherd GM: *Neurobiology,* ed 2, New York, 1988, Oxford University Press.

Generation and Conduction of Action Potentials

An **action potential** is a rapid change in the membrane potential followed by a return to the resting membrane potential (Fig. 3-1). Although the size and shape of action potentials differ considerably from one excitable tissue to another, the following generalizations can be drawn about action potentials:

- An action potential is propagated with the same shape and size along the whole length of a nerve or muscle cell.
- The action potential is the basis of the signal-carrying ability of nerve cells.
- In muscle cells, an action potential allows the entire length of these long cells to contract almost simultaneously.
- Voltage-dependent ion channel proteins in the plasma membrane are responsible for action potentials. Different action potentials in the cell types shown in

Fig. 3-1 occur because these cells have different populations of voltage-dependent ion channels.

This chapter describes how action potentials are generated and conducted in cells. Within this general discussion, the different action potentials of different excitable cells are also discussed and explained.

■ Membrane Potentials

■ Observations of Membrane Potentials

Our current knowledge about the ionic mechanisms of action potentials comes from experiments on the squid giant axon. The large diameter (up to 0.5 mm) of the squid giant axon makes it a convenient model for electrophysiological research with intracellular electrodes. The frog sartorius muscle is another useful preparation.

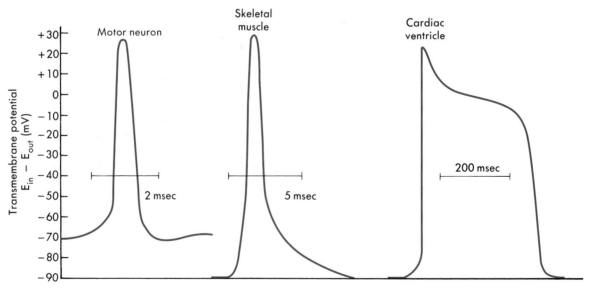

■ Fig. 3-1 Action potentials from three vertebrate cell types. Note the different time scales. (Redrawn from Flickinger CJ et al: *Medical cell biology,* Philadelphia, 1979, WB Saunders.)

When a microelectrode (tip diameter <0.5 μm) is inserted through the plasma membrane of a single muscle cell of a frog sartorius muscle, a potential difference is observed between the tip of the microelectrode inside the cell and an electrode placed outside the cell. The internal electrode is approximately 90 mV negative with respect to the external electrode. This 90-mV potential difference is the **resting membrane potential** of the muscle fiber. By convention, membrane potentials are expressed as the intracellular potential minus the extracellular potential; therefore the membrane potential of the frog sartorius muscle cell is −90 mV. In the absence of perturbing influences, the resting membrane potential remains at −90 mV.

■ *Subthreshold Responses: The Local Response*

Fig. 3-2 illustrates the results of an experiment in which the membrane potential of an axon of a shore crab is perturbed by passing rectangular pulses of current across the plasma membrane. Current pulses are depolarizing or hyperpolarizing, depending on the direction of current flow. The terms **depolarizing** and **hyperpolarizing** may be confusing. A change of the membrane potential from −90 mV to −70 mV is a depolarization because it *decreases* the potential difference, or polarization, across the cell membrane. Conversely, a change in the membrane potential from −90 mV to −100 mV *increases* the polarization of the membrane; this change in potential is a hyperpolarization.

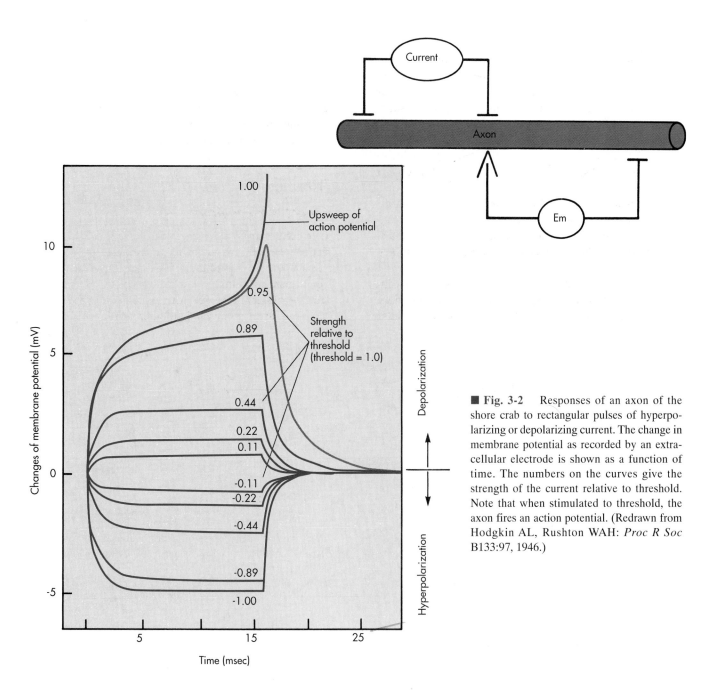

■ **Fig. 3-2** Responses of an axon of the shore crab to rectangular pulses of hyperpolarizing or depolarizing current. The change in membrane potential as recorded by an extracellular electrode is shown as a function of time. The numbers on the curves give the strength of the current relative to threshold. Note that when stimulated to threshold, the axon fires an action potential. (Redrawn from Hodgkin AL, Rushton WAH: *Proc R Soc B*133:97, 1946.)

The larger the current that passes across the plasma membrane, the larger is the change in the membrane potential. Fig. 3-2 shows that when the depolarizing current pulses reach above a certain **threshold** strength, the cell fires an action potential.

When subthreshold current pulses are passed across the plasma membrane, the size of the potential change observed *depends on the distance of the recording electrode from the point of current passage* (Fig. 3-3, *A*). *The closer the recording electrode to the site of current passage, the larger is the potential change observed.* The size of the potential change is found to *decrease exponentially with distance* from the site of current passage (Fig. 3-3, *B*). In other words, the potential change is said to be **conducted with decrement.** The distance over which the potential change decreases to 1/e (37%) of its maximal value is called the **length constant** or space constant. (*e* is the base of natural logarithms and is equal to 2.7182.) *A length constant of 1 to 3 mm is typical for mammalian nerve or muscle cells.* Because these potential changes are observed primarily near the site of current passage and the changes are not propagated along the length of the cell (as are action potentials), they are called **local responses.**

■ *Action Potentials*

If progressively larger depolarizing current pulses are applied to the plasma membrane, a **threshold membrane potential** can be reached at which a different sort of response, the action potential, occurs (Figs. 3-2 and 3-4). For example, the threshold value for the squid giant axon is near −55 mV. When the membrane potential reaches this value, an action potential is triggered. The action potential differs from the local response in two important ways: (1) it is a *much larger response*, in which the polarity of the membrane potential actually reverses (the cell interior becomes positive with respect to the exterior); and (2) *the action potential is propagated without decrement* down the entire length of the nerve or muscle fiber. *The size and shape of an action potential remain the same* as it travels along the fiber. Unlike a local response, it does not decrease in size with distance. In addition, when a stimulus larger than the threshold stimulus is applied, the size and shape of the action potential still do not change; the size of the action potential does not increase with increased stimulus strength. A stimulus either fails to elicit an action potential (a subthreshold stimulus that leads to a local response) or it

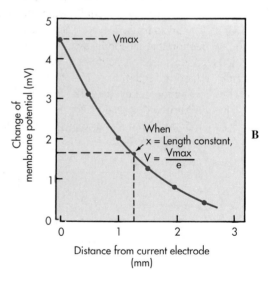

■ **Fig. 3-3**   **A,** Responses of an axon of a shore crab to a subthreshold rectangular pulse of current recorded extracellularly by an electrode located different distances from the current-passing electrode. As the recording electrode is moved farther from the point of stimulation, the response of the membrane potential is slower and smaller. **B,** The maximal change in membrane potential from **A** is plotted versus the distance from the point of current passage. The distance over which the response falls to 1/e (37%) of the maximal response is called the **length constant.** (**A** redrawn from Hodgkin AL, Rushton WAH: *Proc R Soc* B133:97, 1946.)

produces a full-sized action potential. For this reason, the action potential is described as an **all-or-none response.**

■ *Ionic Mechanisms of Action Potentials*

■ *Action Potentials in Squid Giant Axon*

The form of an action potential of a squid giant axon is shown in Fig. 3-4. When the membrane is depolarized to the threshold, *depolarization becomes explosive.* This depolarization completely depolarizes the membrane and even **overshoots,** so that the membrane potential reverses from negative to positive. The peak of the action potential reaches about +50 mV. The membrane potential then returns toward the resting membrane potential almost as rapidly as it was depolarized. After repolarization, a transient hyperpolarization occurs that is known as the **hyperpolarizing afterpotential.** It persists for about 4 msec. The following section discusses the ionic currents that cause the phases of the action potential.

■ *Ionic Mechanism of Action Potential in the Squid Giant Axon*

In Chapter 2, we saw that the resting membrane potential was the weighted sum of the equilibrium potentials for Na^+, K^+, Cl^-, and so forth. The weighting factor for each ion is the fraction that its conductance contributes to the total ionic conductance of the membrane (the chord conductance equation, equation 2-10). In the squid giant axon, the resting membrane potential (E_m) is about -70 mV. The equilibrium potential of K^+ (E_K) is about -100 mV in the squid axon. An increase in g_K would therefore hyperpolarize the membrane, while a decrease in g_K

would tend to depolarize the membrane. E_{Cl} is about -70 mV, so an increase in g_{Cl} would stabilize E_m at -70 mV. An increase in g_{Na} of sufficient magnitude would cause depolarization and reversal of the membrane polarity, because E_{Na} is about $+65$ mV in the squid giant axon.

In a giant squid model, the action potential of the axon is caused by successive increases in plasma membrane conductance to sodium and potassium ions. The conductance to Na^+, g_{Na}, increases very rapidly during the early part of the action potential (Fig. 3-5). Sodium conductance peaks at about the same time as the action potential peaks, and then decreases rapidly. The potassium conductance, g_K, increases more slowly, peaks at about the middle of the repolarization phase, and then returns more slowly to resting levels.

As described in Chapter 2, the chord conductance equation shows that the membrane potential is a result of the opposing tendencies of the K^+ gradient to bring the resting membrane potential toward the equilibrium potential for K^+, and of the Na^+ gradient to bring the resting membrane potential toward the equilibrium potential for Na^+. *Increasing the conductance of either ion will increase its ability to pull the resting membrane potential toward its equilibrium potential.* The rapid increase in g_{Na} during the early phase of the action potential causes the membrane potential to move toward the equilibrium potential for Na^+ ($+65$ mV). The peak of the action potential reaches only about $+50$ mV because g_{Na} quickly decreases toward resting levels and because the increase in g_K, which occurs later, provides an opposing tendency to the depolarization.

The rapid return of the membrane potential toward the resting potential is caused by the rapid decrease of g_{Na} and the continued increase in g_K. These conductance changes decrease the size of the Na^+ term in the chord conductance equation and increase the size of the K^+ term. During the hyperpolarizing afterpotential, when the

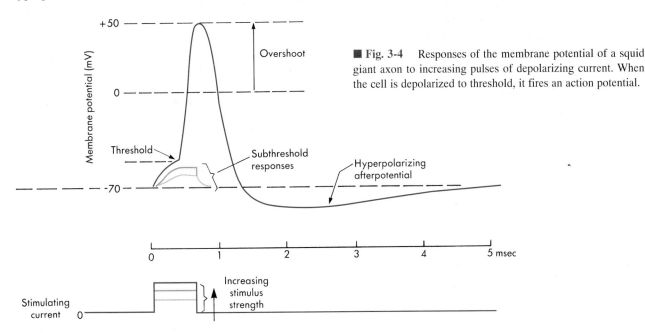

■ **Fig. 3-4** Responses of the membrane potential of a squid giant axon to increasing pulses of depolarizing current. When the cell is depolarized to threshold, it fires an action potential.

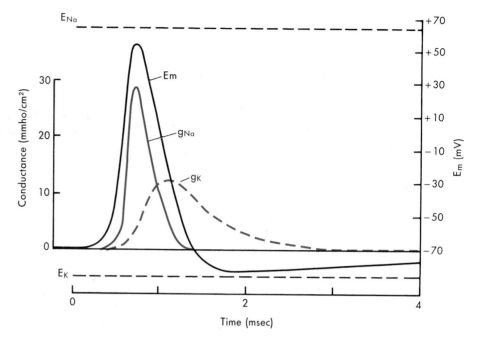

■ **Fig. 3-5** The action potential (E_m) of a squid giant axon is shown on the same time scale with the associated changes in the conductance of the axon membrane to sodium and potassium ions. (Redrawn from Hodgkin AL, Huxley AF: *J Physiol* 117:500, 1952.)

membrane potential is actually more negative than the resting potential (more polarized), g_{Na} has returned to baseline levels, but g_K remains elevated above resting levels. Thus, the resting membrane potential is pulled closer to the K$^+$ equilibrium potential (-100 mV) as long as g_K remains elevated.

■ *Ion Channels and Gates*

Hodgkin and Huxley proposed that the ion currents pass through separate Na$^+$ and K$^+$ channels, each with distinct characteristics, in the plasma membrane. Subsequent research supports this interpretation and has determined some of the properties of proteins that form the channels. Also the amino acid sequences of several K$^+$ and Na$^+$ channels have been determined. Research is ongoing and our knowledge of the structure of ion channels is rapidly expanding (Fig. 3-6). Although the three-dimensional structure of the Na$^+$ channel remains unknown, its intramembrane domain is known to consist of several α helices that span the membrane and probably surround the ion channel. The Na$^+$ channel has both an **activation gate** and an **inactivation gate,** which accounts for the changes in g_{Na} during an action potential (Fig. 3-6). Groups of charged amino acid residues that form the activation and inactivation gates have been tentatively identified.

It is believed that to enter a channel's narrowest part, known as the **selectivity filter,** an ion must shed most of the water it acquires through hydration. To strip a K$^+$ or Na$^+$ ion of its associated water molecules, negative amino acid residues that line the pore of the channel must have a particular geometry; this precise geometry is different for K$^+$ and Na$^+$. In fact, this geometry is believed to confer specificity on an ion channel.

Tetrodotoxin (TTX), one of the most potent poisons known, specifically blocks the Na$^+$ channel. TTX binds to the extracellular side of the sodium channel. Tetraethylammonium (TEA$^+$), another poison, blocks the K$^+$ channel. TEA$^+$ enters the K$^+$ channel from the cytoplasmic side and blocks the channel because TEA is unable to pass through it.

The ovaries of certain species of puffer fish, also known as blowfish, contain TTX. Raw puffer fish is a highly prized delicacy in Japan. Connoisseurs of puffer fish enjoy the tingling numbness of the lips caused by minuscule quantities of TTX present in the flesh. Sushi chefs who are trained to remove the ovaries safely are licensed by the government to prepare puffer fish. Despite these precautions, each year several people die from eating improperly prepared puffer fish.

Saxitoxin is another blocker of Na$^+$ channels that is produced by reddish-colored dinoflagellates that are responsible for so-called **red tides.** Shellfish eat the dinoflagellates and concentrate saxitoxin in their tissues. A person who eats these shellfish may experience life-threatening paralysis within 30 minutes after the meal.

■ *Behavior of Individual Ion Channels*

One way to study the behavior of individual ion channels is to incorporate either purified ion channel proteins or bits of membrane into planar lipid bilayers that separate two aqueous compartments. Electrodes placed in the aqueous compartments can then be used to monitor or impose currents and voltages across the membrane. Under some conditions only one, or only a few, ion chan-

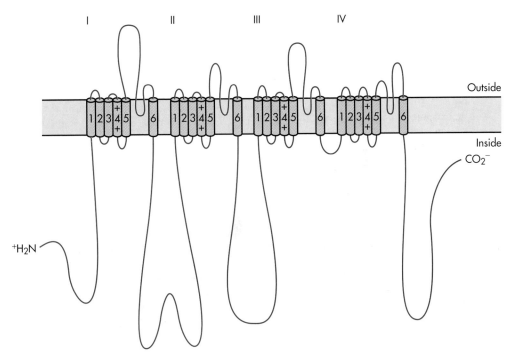

■ Fig. 3-6 A two-dimensional model of the voltage-dependent Na^+ channel protein. The cylinders represent transmembrane α helices. There are 4 repeats of 6-cylinder domains of homologous α helices. The S4 helices, marked with plus signs, function as voltage sensors, and movements of these helices are responsible for activation (opening) of the channel. The intracellular loop connecting domains III and IV functions as the inactivation gate: after depolarization, with a slight delay, this loop apparently swings up into the mouth of the channel to block ion conduction. Note that part of the extracellular loop connecting helices 5 and 6 in each domain is inserted into the membrane. These segments participate in forming the extracellular mouth of the ion channel and in determining ion selectivity.

nel(s) of a particular type may be present in the planar membrane. The ion channels spontaneously oscillate between two conductance states, an open state and a closed state (Fig. 3-7).

Another way to study individual ion channels involves the use of so-called **patch electrodes.** A fire-polished microelectrode is placed against the surface of a cell, and suction is applied to the electrode. A high-resistance seal is formed around the tip of the electrode. The sealed patch electrode can then be used to monitor the activity of whatever channels happen to be trapped inside the seal. Sometimes, the patch trapped inside the electrode contains more than one functional ion channel of a particular type (Fig. 3-8).

Both these techniques have contributed greatly to our knowledge about the behavior of ion channels. During an action potential in a skeletal muscle cell, a rapid influx of Na^+ ions occurs that lasts for only about 1 msec. The duration of this inward Na^+ current resembles the duration of the change in the Na^+ conductance shown in Fig. 3-5. The overall Na^+ current that flows into the muscle cell is caused by the opening of thousands of Na^+ channels in response to the depolarization. However, the behavior of each individual Na^+ channel is actually random, like the

behavior of the channels shown in Figs. 3-7 and 3-8. *The probability of each channel being in the open state is increased when the membrane is depolarized to threshold.* In response to a step depolarization of a muscle cell plasma membrane (Fig. 3-9), some of the Na^+ channels open, some do not open at all, and some open more than once. However, when the currents of a large number of channels are averaged (Fig. 3-9, *B*), it appears as if all the Na^+ channels open in response to the depolarization and then promptly close. In other words, the "average channel" opens (activates) quickly in response to depolarization: after a short time delay, the channel then closes (inactivates), even though the applied depolarization is maintained.

■ *Action Potentials in Cardiac and Smooth Muscle*

Cardiac muscle. An action potential in a cardiac ventricular cell is shown schematically in Fig. 3-1 (see also Chapter 22). The initial rapid depolarization and overshoot is caused by the rapid entry of Na^+ into the cell through channels that are very similar to the Na^+ chan-

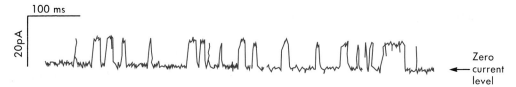

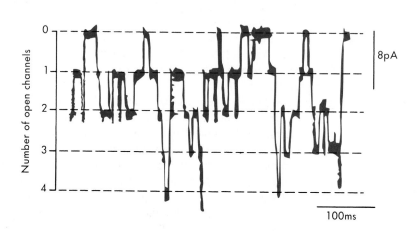

■ **Fig. 3-7**   Ionic current through a single ion channel from rat muscle incorporated into a planar lipid bilayer membrane. The channel opens and closes spontaneously. The fraction of time this channel spends in the open state is a function of calcium ion concentration and membrane potential. (Reproduced from Moczydlowski E, Latorre R: *J Gen Physiol* 82:511-542, 1983, by copyright permission of the Rockefeller University Press.)

■ **Fig. 3-8**   A current recording from a patch electrode on a muscle cell plasma membrane. The five different current levels show that this particular patch of membrane contains four different ion channels, each opening and closing independently of the others. (Redrawn from Hammill OP et al: *Pflugers Arch* 391:85, 1981.)

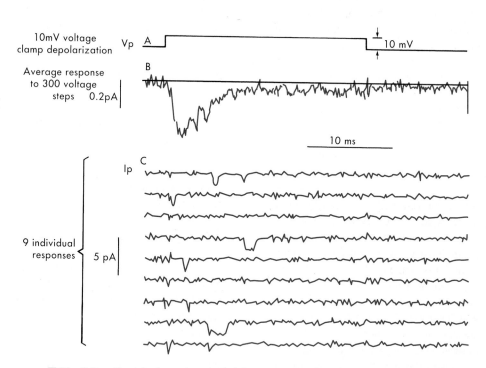

■ **Fig. 3-9**   A patch electrode recorded the currents that flowed in small patches of rat muscle membrane in response to a 10-mV depolarization (trace *A*). Tetraethylammonium was used to block potassium channels that might have been present in the patch. The traces in curve *C* show responses to nine individual 10-mV depolarizations. The tracing in *B* is the average of 300 individual responses. Note that this average response resembles the summed response of thousands of sodium channels, as seen in measurements of whole cell Na^+ currents during an action potential. (Redrawn by permission from Sigworth FJ, Neher E: *Nature* 287:447-449. Copyright 1980 Macmillan Journals.)

nels of nerve and skeletal muscle. The Na^+ channels are called **fast channels.** After the initial depolarization and overshoot, the cardiac ventricular action potential enters a plateau phase. The plateau is caused by another set of channels that are distinct from the fast Na^+ channels. Because these channels open and close much more slowly than the fast Na^+ channels, they are sometimes called **slow channels.** The slow channels belong to a particular class of Ca^{++} channels called **L-type Ca^{++} channels.** The Ca^{++} that enters the ventricular cell through the L-type Ca^{++} channels during the plateau phase helps to initiate cell contraction by stimulating the release of more Ca^{++} from the sarcoplasmic reticulum of the cell. The repolarization of the ventricular cell is brought about by the closing of the L-type Ca^{++} channels and by a much-delayed opening of K^+ channels. The ionic mechanisms of cardiac action potentials are discussed in more detail in Chapter 22.

Smooth muscle. Action potentials vary considerably among different types of smooth muscle (see Chapter 19). Characteristically, action potentials in smooth muscle have slower rates of depolarization and repolarization and less overshoot than skeletal muscle action potentials. Most smooth muscle cells lack Na^+ channels. The depolarizing phase of smooth muscle action potentials is caused primarily by Ca^{++} channels, like those that contribute to the plateau phase in cardiac cells. Like the cardiac Ca^{++} channels, these channels open and close slowly. The Ca^{++} that enters via these channels is often vital for excitation-contraction coupling in smooth muscle, because some smooth muscle cells have little sarcoplasmic reticulum. Repolarization is caused by the closing of the slow Ca^{++} channels and a simultaneous delayed opening of K^+ channels.

■ *Properties of Action Potentials*
■ *Voltage Inactivation*

If a neuron or skeletal muscle cell is partially depolarized, for example, by increasing the concentration of K^+ in the extracellular fluid, its action potential has a slower rate of rise and a smaller overshoot than does the action potential of the normally polarized cell. This is a result of two factors: (1) a smaller electrical force driving Na^+ into the depolarized cell, and (2) voltage inactivation of some of the Na^+ channels. In response to depolarization of the membrane, g_{Na} first increases and then, a short time later, decreases. The decrease in g_{Na} is caused by **voltage inactivation.** In other words, the inactivation gates of Na^+ channels close soon after the activation gates open. Once the Na^+ channels are inactivated, the membrane must be repolarized toward the normal resting membrane potential before the channels can be reopened. As the membrane potential is restored toward normal resting levels, more and more of the Na^+ channels again become capable of being activated.

The explosive depolarizing phase of the action potential may be compared with a chemical explosion. Just as a chemical explosion requires a critical mass of material, *the spike of the action potential can be generated only if a critical number of Na^+ channels are recruited.* When a cell is only partly depolarized, the pool of activatable Na^+ channels is reduced; consequently, a stimulus may not be able to recruit a sufficient number of Na^+ channels to generate an action potential. In effect, this **voltage inactivation** of the action potential results from voltage inactivation of the Na^+ channels. *Voltage inactivation of Na^+ channels partially accounts for the important properties of excitable cells, such as refractory periods and accommodation.*

■ *Refractory Periods*

During much of the action potential, the membrane is completely refractory to further stimulation. *When a membrane is refractory, it is unable to fire a second action potential, no matter how strongly the cell is stimulated.* This unresponsive state is called the **absolute refractory period** (Fig. 3-10). The cell is refractory because a large fraction of its Na^+ channels is voltage inactivated and cannot be reopened until the membrane is repolarized.

During the latter part of the action potential, the cell is able to fire a second action potential, *but a stronger than normal stimulus is required.* This period is called the **relative refractory period.** Early in the relative refractory period, before the membrane potential has returned to the resting potential level, some Na^+ channels are still voltage inactivated. Therefore, a stronger than normal stimulus is required to open the critical number of Na^+ channels needed to trigger an action potential. Throughout the relative refractory period, the conductance to K^+ is elevated, which opposes depolarization of the membrane. This increase in K^+ conductance also contributes to the refractoriness.

■ *Accommodation*

When a nerve or muscle cell is depolarized slowly, the normal threshold may be passed without an action potential being fired; this property is called **accommodation.** Na^+ and K^+ channels are both involved in accommodation. During slow depolarization, some of the Na^+ channels that are opened by depolarization have enough time to become voltage inactivated before the threshold potential is attained. *If depolarization is slow enough, the critical number of open Na^+ channels required to trigger the action potential may never be attained.* In addition, K^+ channels open in response to the depolarization. The increased g_K tends to repolarize the membrane, making it still more refractory to depolarization.

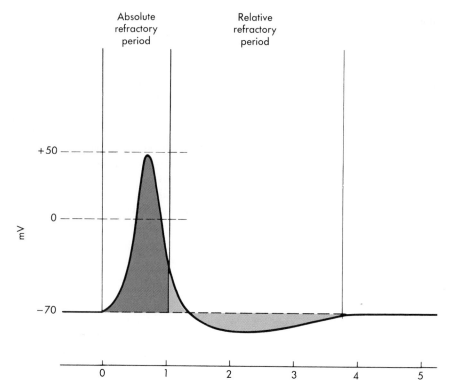

■ **Fig. 3-10**   The action potential of nerve and the associated absolute and relative refractory periods.

In an inherited disorder called **primary hyperkalemic paralysis,** patients have episodes of painful spontaneous muscle contractions, followed by periods of paralysis of the affected muscles. These symptoms are accompanied by elevated levels of K+ in the plasma and extracellular fluid.

The elevation of extracellular K+ causes depolarization of skeletal muscle cells. Initially, the depolarization brings muscle cells closer to threshold, so that spontaneous action potentials and contractions are more likely. As depolarization of the cells becomes more marked, the cells accommodate because of the voltage-inactivated Na+ channels. Consequently, the cells become unable to fire action potentials and are unable to contract in response to action potentials in their motor axons.

■ *Conduction of Action Potentials*

A principal function of neurons is to transmit nerve impulses in the form of action potentials. The axons of the motor neurons of the ventral horn of the spinal cord conduct action potentials from the cell body of the neuron to a number of skeletal muscle fibers. The distance from the motor neuron to one of the muscle fibers it innervates may be longer than 1 m.

Action potentials are conducted along a nerve or muscle fiber by local current flow, just as occurs in electrotonic conduction of subthreshold potential changes. Thus, the same factors that govern the velocity of electrotonic conduction also determine the speed of action potential propagation.

■ *The Local Response: Conduction with Decrement*

Fig. 3-11, *A* shows the membrane of an axon or muscle fiber that has been depolarized in a small region. In this region, the external surface of the membrane is negative relative to the adjacent membrane, and the internal face of the depolarized membrane is positively charged relative to neighboring internal areas. These potential differences cause **local currents** to flow (Fig. 3-11, *B*), which depolarize the membrane adjacent to the initial site of depolarization. These newly depolarized areas then cause current flows that depolarize other segments of the membrane still farther removed from the initial site of depolarization. This spread of depolarization is called the **local response,** and this mechanism of conduction is known as **electrotonic conduction.**

A subthreshold depolarization will be conducted electrotonically but will diminish in strength as it moves

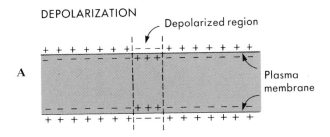

DEPOLARIZATION

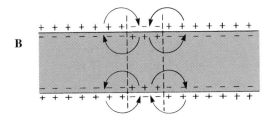

SPREAD OF DEPOLARIZATION

■ **Fig. 3-11**   Mechanism of electrotonic spread of depolarization. **A,** The reversal of membrane polarity that occurs with local depolarization. **B,** The local currents that flow to depolarize adjacent areas of the membrane and allow conduction of the depolarization.

along the cell. Thus, it is **conducted with decrement. As** shown in Fig. 3-3, *B,* an electrotonically conducted signal dies away to 37% of its maximal strength over a distance of one **length constant** (about 1 to 2 mm) and decreases to almost nothing over about 5 mm.

How is this length constant determined? A nerve or muscle fiber has some of the properties of an electrical cable. In a perfect cable, the insulation surrounding the core conductor prevents all loss of current to the surrounding medium, so that a signal is transmitted along the cable with undiminished strength (Fig. 3-12). If we compare an unmyelinated nerve or muscle fiber with an electrical cable, the plasma membrane will be the insulation, while the cytoplasm will be the core conductor. The membrane has a resistance (r_m) much higher than the resistance of the cytoplasm (r_{in}), but (partly because of its thinness) the plasma membrane is not a perfect insulator. *The higher the ratio of r_m to r_{in}, the less current is lost across the plasma membrane, the better the cell can function as a cable, and the longer the distance that a signal can be transmitted electrotonically without significant decrement. r_m/r_{in} determines the length constant of a cell: the length constant is equal to $\sqrt{r_m/r_{in}}$.*

■ *Action Potential as Self-Reinforcing Signal*

Many nerve and muscle fibers are much longer than their length constants (1 to 2 mm). Skeletal muscle cells can be as long as 1 to 2 cm; nerve axons can be 1 m in length. Conduction with decrement will not work for these long

cells. For the action potential to conduct an electrical impulse with undiminished strength along the full length of these cells, the action potential reinforces itself as it is conducted along the fiber. The action potential may be said to be **propagated,** as well as conducted.

Propagation involves the generation of "new" action potentials as they spread along the length of the cell. As we saw in Fig. 3-11, the conduction of the action potential occurs via local circuit currents by the electrotonic mechanism. When the areas on either side of the depolarized region reach threshold, these areas also fire action potentials, which locally reverses the polarity of the membrane potential. The areas of the fiber adjacent to these areas are next brought to threshold by the local current flow, and these areas in turn fire action potentials. In short, propagation involves a cycle of depolarization. This cycle occurs by local current flow followed by generation of an action potential in a region of the cell membrane; this action potential is then conducted along the length of the fiber, with "new" action potentials being generated as they spread. *In this way, the action potentials are regenerated as they spread, and the action potential propagates over long distances, keeping the same size and shape.*

Because the shape and size of the action potential usually do not change, *only variations in the frequency of the action potentials can be used as the "code" for information transmission along axons.* The maximal frequency is limited by the duration of the absolute refractory period (about 1 msec) to about 1000 impulses per second in large mammalian nerves.

■ *Conduction Velocity*

The speed of electrotonic conduction in a nerve or muscle fiber is determined by the electrical properties of the cytoplasm and of the plasma membrane that surrounds the fiber. The same electrical properties determine the velocity of propagation of an action potential. Therefore, although the following discussion focuses on the mechanism of electrotonic conduction, it applies equally well to the mechanism of propagation of the action potential.

Effect of fiber diameter on conduction. Fibers that are larger in diameter have a greater conduction velocity. This effect is principally caused by a decrease in resistance to conduction. As the radius (and hence the cross-sectional area) of a fiber increases, the cytoplasm along the length of the fiber becomes less resistant to conduction. Thus, action potential will be conducted faster along fibers with large diameters.

Effect of myelination on conduction. In vertebrates, certain nerve fibers are coated with **myelin;** such fibers are said to be **myelinated.** Myelin consists of the plasma membranes of **Schwann cells,** which wrap around and insulate the nerve fiber (Fig. 3-13). The myelin sheath consists of several to more than 100 layers of Schwann

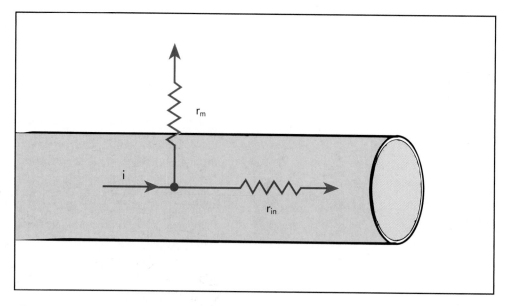

■ **Fig. 3-12**   An axon or a muscle fiber resembles an electrical cable. Currents that flow across the membrane resistance (r_m) are lost from the cable. Currents that flow through the longitudinal resistance (r_{in}) carry the electrical signal along the cable. The larger the ratio r_m/r_{in}, the more efficient is signal transmission along the fiber and the larger is the length constant of the cell.

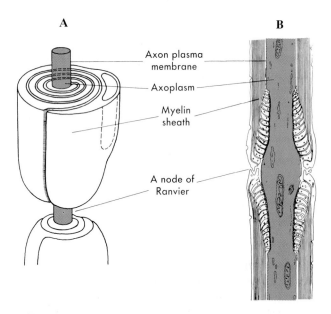

A

Axon plasma membrane

Axoplasm

Myelin sheath

A node of Ranvier

B

■ **Fig. 3-13**   The myelin sheath. **A,** Schematic drawing of Schwann cells wrapping around an axon to form a myelin sheath. **B,** Drawing of a cross-section through a myelinated axon near a node of Ranvier.

cell plasma membranes. Gaps occur in the myelin sheath every 1 to 2 mm. These gaps are known as **nodes of Ranvier,** which are about 1 μm wide. *By altering the electrical properties of the nerve fiber, myelin functions to increase the conduction velocity of the fiber.*

An unmyelinated squid giant axon with a 500-μm diameter has a conduction velocity of 25 m/sec. If conduction velocity were directly proportional to fiber radius, a human nerve fiber with a 10-μm diameter would conduct at a velocity of 0.5 m/sec. With this conduction velocity, a reflex withdrawal of the foot from a hot coal would take about 4 seconds. Although our nerve fibers are much smaller in diameter than squid giant axons, our reflexes are much faster than 4 seconds. The myelin sheath that surrounds certain vertebrate nerve fibers is responsible for the greatly increased conduction velocity over that of unmyelinated fibers of similar diameters. A 10-μm myelinated fiber has a conduction velocity of about 50 m/sec, which is twice that of the 500-μm squid giant axon. The high conduction velocity permits reflexes that are fast enough to allow us to avoid dangerous stimuli.

How much does myelin contribute to increased conduction velocity? *A myelinated axon has a greater conduction velocity than an unmyelinated fiber that is 100 times larger in diameter* (Fig. 3-14). The myelin sheath increases the velocity of action potential conduction by (1) increasing the length constant of the axon, (2) decreasing the capacitance of the axon, and (3) restricting the generation of action potentials to the nodes of Ranvier. In short, myelination greatly alters the electrical properties of the axon.

The many wrappings of membrane around the axon increase the effective membrane resistance, so that r_m/r_{in}, and thus the length constant is much greater. Less of the conducted signal is lost through the electrical insulation of the myelin sheath, so that the amplitude of a conducted signal declines less with distance along the axon. The myelin-wrapped membrane has a much smaller electrical capacitance than the naked axonal

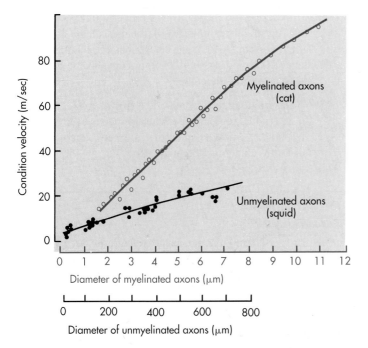

■ **Fig. 3-14** Conduction velocities of myelinated and unmyelinated axons as functions of axon diameter. Myelinated axons are from cat saphenous nerve at 38° C. Unmyelinated axons are from squid and are at 20° to 22° C. Note that myelinated axons have greater conduction velocities than unmyelinated axons 100 times greater in diameter. (Based on data from Gasser HS, Grundfest H: *Am J Physiol* 127:393, 1939 [myelinated axons] and Pumphrey RJ, Young JZ: *J Exp Biol* 15:453, 1938 [unmyelinated axons].)

membrane, so that the local currents can more rapidly depolarize the membrane as a signal is conducted. *For this reason, the conduction velocity is greatly increased by myelination.* Because of the increase in length constant and in conduction velocity, *an action potential is conducted with little decrement and at great speed from one node of Ranvier to the next.*

The resistance to the flow of ions across the many layers of Schwann cell membrane that make up the myelin sheath is so high that the ionic currents are effectively localized to the short stretches of naked plasma membrane that occur at the nodes of Ranvier. In fact, *the action potential is regenerated only at the nodes of Ranvier* (1 to 2 mm apart), rather than being regenerated at each area along the fiber, as is the case in an unmyelinated fiber. The action potential is rapidly conducted from one node to the next (in about 20 μsec) and "pauses" to be regenerated at each node. Because the action potential appears to "jump" from one node of Ranvier to the next, the process is called **saltatory** (from the Latin word *saltare,* to leap) **conduction.**

Myelinated axons are also more metabolically efficient than unmyelinated axons. The sodium-potassium pump extrudes the sodium that enters and reaccumulates the potassium that leaves the cell during action potentials. In myelinated axons, ionic currents are restricted to the small fraction of the membrane surface at the nodes of Ranvier. For this reason, far fewer Na+ and K+ ions traverse a unit area of fiber membrane, and much less ion pumping—and energy expenditure—is required to maintain Na+ and K+ gradients.

In some diseases, known as **demyelinating disorders,** the myelin sheath deteriorates. In **multiple sclerosis,** scattered progressive demyelination of axons in the central nervous system results in loss of motor control. The neuropathy common in severe cases of **diabetes mellitus** is caused by demyelination of peripheral axons. When myelin is lost, the length constant, which is dramatically increased by myelination, becomes much shorter. Hence, the action potential loses amplitude as it is electrotonically conducted from one node of Ranvier to the next. If demyelination is sufficiently severe, the action potential may arrive at the next node of Ranvier with insufficient strength to fire an action potential. The axon will then fail to propagate action potentials.

■ *Summary*

1. Different cell types have differently shaped action potentials because their populations of voltage-dependent ion channels differ.

2. The action potential in a squid giant axon is generated by the rapid opening and subsequent voltage inactivation of voltage-dependent Na+ channels and the delayed opening and closing of voltage-dependent K+ channels.

3. Ion channels are integral membrane proteins that have ion-selective pores. Charged polypeptide regions of an ion channel protein act as gates that activate and inactivate the channel.

4. An ion channel typically has two states: high conductance (open) and low conductance (closed). The channel oscillates randomly between the open and closed states. For a voltage-dependent channel, the fraction of time the channel spends in the open state is a function of the transmembrane potential difference.

5. Cardiac and smooth muscle cells have L-type Ca++ channels that open and close slowly and are responsible for the long duration of the action potential in these cell types.

6. The voltage inactivation of Na+ channels is an important factor in the absolute and relative refractory periods and in the accommodation of an excitable cell to a slowly rising stimulus.

7. Local circuit currents produce electrotonic conduction. Both subthreshold signals and action potentials are conducted along the length of a cell by local circuit currents.

8. A subthreshold signal is conducted with decrement. It dies away to 37% of its maximal strength over a distance of 1 length constant. The length constant is equal to $\sqrt{r_m/r_{in}}$. A typical value for the length constant is 1 to 2 mm.

9. The action potential is propagated, rather than merely conducted; it is regenerated as it moves along the cell. In this way, an action potential remains the same size and shape as it is conducted.

10. The velocity of conduction is determined by the electrical properties of the cell. A large-diameter cell has a faster conduction velocity.

11. Myelination dramatically increases the conduction velocity of a nerve axon. Because of myelination, an action potential is conducted very rapidly and with little decrement from one node of Ranvier to the next. Action potentials are regenerated only at the nodes of Ranvier; the internodal membrane cannot fire an action potential. Because it takes much longer to generate an action potential at each node than it does for the action potential to be conducted between nodes, the action potential appears to jump from node to node; this form of conduction is called saltatory conduction.

■ Self-Study Problems

1. (a) Draw a typical action potential from a squid giant axon (membrane potential in mV vs. time in msec). Label: resting potential, threshold, spike, overshoot, and the hyperpolarizing afterpotential. (b) On your drawing of the action potential, superimpose the time courses of the conductance changes of Na$^+$ and K$^+$ that occur during the action potential. (c) What are the approximate values of the membrane potential at: the resting potential, threshold, peak of the overshoot? (d) What is the approximate duration of the action potential?

2. (a) Why does the overshoot fall short of E_{Na}? (b) What causes the absolute refractory period? (c) What causes the relative refractory period? (d) Why does the action potential have a threshold?

3. What is the role of the Na$^+$, K$^+$-ATPase in generating a single action potential?

4. (a) Describe the mechanisms of electrotonic conduction (the local response). (b) What is meant by the length constant? (c) What determines the length constant? (d) How large is the length constant for a typical nerve of muscle cell?

5. (a) Describe saltatory conduction. (b) What happens in the internodal regions? (c) What happens at the nodes of Ranvier? (d) Why does the internodal membrane fail to fire an action potential?

■ Bibliography

Journal articles

Barchi RL: Probing the molecular structure of the voltage-dependent sodium channel, *Annu Rev Neurosci* 11:455, 1988.

Bean BP: Classes of calcium channels in vertebrate cells, *Annu Rev Physiol* 51:367, 1989.

Catterall WA: Structure and function of voltage-sensitive ion channels, *Science* 242:50, 1988.

Catterall WA: Cellular and molecular biology of voltage-gated sodium channels, *Physiol Rev* 72:S15, 1992.

Jan LY, Jan YN: Structural elements involved in specific K$^+$ channel functions, *Annu Rev Physiol* 54:537, 1992.

Neher E, Sakmann B: The patch clamp technique, *Sci Am* 266(3):28, 1992.

Perney TM, Kaczmarek LK: The molecular biology of K$^+$ channels, *Curr Opin Cell Biol* 3:663, 1991.

Stuhmer W: Structure-function studies of voltage-gated ion channels, *Annu Rev Biophys Biophys Chem* 20:65, 1991.

Books and monographs

Aidley DJ: *The physiology of excitable cells,* ed 3, Cambridge, 1990, Cambridge University Press.

Hille B: *Ionic channels of excitable membranes,* ed 2, Sunderland, Mass, 1992, Sinauer Associates.

Hodgkin AL: *The conduction of the nervous impulse,* Springfield, Ill, 1964, Charles C Thomas.

Kandel ER, Schwartz JH: *Principles of neural science,* ed 3, New York, 1991, Elsevier.

Katz B: *Nerve, muscle, and synapse,* New York, 1966, McGraw-Hill.

Levitan IB, Kaczmarek LK: *The neuron: cell and molecular biology,* New York, 1991, Oxford University Press.

Nicholls JG, Martin AR, Wallace BG: *From neuron to brain,* ed 3, Sunderland, Mass, 1992, Sinauer Associates.

Stevens CF: *Neurophysiology: a primer,* New York, 1966, John Wiley.

CHAPTER
4

Synaptic Transmission

Excitable cells are those that are able to generate action potentials, which are rapid changes in the electrical potential of the cell membrane. Excitable cells such as muscle cells and nerve cells communicate by transmitting electrical signals. A **synapse** is the site at which electrical signals are transmitted from one cell to another. There are two types: electrical and chemical synapses. At an **electrical synapse,** two excitable cells communicate by the direct passage of an electrical current between them. This form of communication is called **electrotonic** transmission. **Gap junctions** link electrotonically coupled cells and provide low-resistance pathways for current flow directly between the cells.

Electrical signals are also transferred between excitable cells by means of **chemical synapses.** At a chemical synapse, an action potential causes the release of **transmitter substance** from the presynaptic neuron. The transmitter diffuses across the extracellular **synaptic cleft** and binds to receptors on the membrane. The time it takes for these events to occur in chemical synapses is called the **synaptic delay.**

■ *Neuromuscular Junction*

The synapses between the axons of motor neurons and skeletal muscle fibers are called **neuromuscular junctions, myoneural junctions,** or **motor endplates.** The neuromuscular junction was the first vertebrate synapse to be well characterized. In the following discussion, the neuromuscular junction serves as a model chemical synapse. An understanding of the structure and function of this junction provides the basis for understanding other, more complex synaptic interactions among neurons in the central nervous system.

■ *Structure of the Neuromuscular Junction*

As the motor nerve approaches the neuromuscular junction, it loses its myelin sheath and divides into fine terminal branches (Fig. 4-1). The terminal branches of the motor axon lie in **synaptic troughs** on the surfaces of the muscle cell. The plasma membrane of the muscle cell lining the trough is arranged into numerous **junctional folds.** The axon terminal branches contain many smooth-surfaced **synaptic vesicles** that contain **acetylcholine,** the neurotransmitter employed at this synapse. The axon terminal and the muscle cell are separated by the **junctional cleft,** which contains a carbohydrate-rich amorphous material.

Acetylcholine receptor molecules are concentrated near the mouths of the junctional folds. The synaptic vesicles in the nerve terminals and specialized release sites (called **active zones**) on the prejunctional membrane are situated directly opposite the mouths of the junctional folds. **Acetylcholinesterase,** the enzyme that cleaves acetylcholine into acetate and choline, is distributed on the external surface of the postjunctional membrane.

■ *Overview of Neuromuscular Transmission*

Neuromuscular transmission begins when an action potential is conducted down the motor axon to the presynaptic axon terminal. Depolarization of the plasma membrane of the axon terminal transiently opens voltage-gated calcium channels. Ca^{++} from the interstitial fluid flows down its electrochemical potential gradient into the axon terminal. The increased concentration of Ca^{++} in the axon terminal causes synaptic vesicles to fuse with the plasma membrane and to empty their acetylcholine into the synaptic cleft by exocytosis. Acetylcholine then diffuses across the synaptic cleft and binds to a specific acetylcholine receptor protein on the external surface of the muscle plasma membrane of the motor endplate. *The binding of acetylcholine with the receptor protein transiently increases the conductance of the postjunctional membrane to Na^+ and K^+. Ionic currents (Na^+ and K^+) result in a transient depolarization of the endplate region.* This transient depolarization is called the **endplate potential** **(EPP)** (Fig. 4-2). The EPP is transient because acetylcholine is quickly hydrolyzed

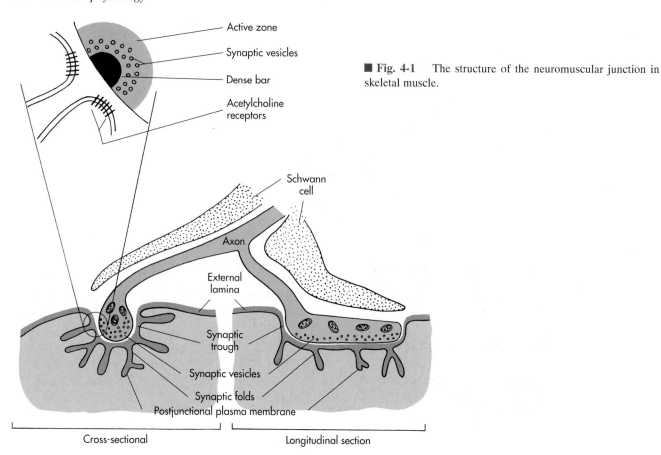

■ **Fig. 4-1** The structure of the neuromuscular junction in skeletal muscle.

into choline and acetate. The hydrolysis of acetylcholine is catalyzed by the enzyme **acetylcholinesterase,** which is present in high concentration on the postjunctional membrane. The steps involved in neuromuscular transmission are listed in Box 4-1.

> The importance of the influx of Ca^{++} into the axon terminal to initiate the release of transmitter is illustrated by the disease **Lambert-Eaton syndrome.** Patients with this syndrome have circulating antibodies against the type of voltage-gated Ca^{++} channels present in nerve terminals, and thus experience muscular weakness and diminished stretch reflexes.

Although it is depolarized during the course of neuromuscular transmission, *the postjunctional plasma membrane of the neuromuscular junction is not electrically excitable and does not itself fire action potentials.* After the postjunctional plasma membrane is depolarized, *regions of the muscle cell membrane immediately adjacent to the neuromuscular junction are depolarized by electrotonic conduction (Fig. 4-2, B). When these regions reach threshold, action potentials are generated.* Action potentials are propagated along the muscle fiber at high velocity and initiate the chain of events that leads to muscle contraction (see Chapter 18).

■ *Synthesis of Acetylcholine*

Acetylcholine is produced by condensation of acetyl coenzyme A (acetyl CoA) and choline. The enzyme choline *O*-acetyltransferase, found in the motor neuron, catalyzes this reaction. In fact, motor neurons and their axons are among the few cells able to synthesize acetylcholine; most other cells are unable to make this neurotransmitter.

Although acetyl CoA is produced by the neuron, as it is by most cells, *choline is not synthesized by the motor neuron. Instead, choline is obtained by active uptake from the extracellular fluid.* The plasma membrane of the motor neuron has an Na^+-coupled secondary active transport system that can accumulate choline against a large electrochemical potential gradient.

■ *Quantal Release of Transmitter*

Acetylcholine is not released continuously by the prejunctional nerve ending; rather, it is released in packets, *with each packet corresponding to the release of one synaptic vesicle.* The amount of acetylcholine contained in one vesicle is called a **quantum** of acetylcholine.

The quantal release of acetylcholine can be demonstrated by the small, spontaneous depolarization known

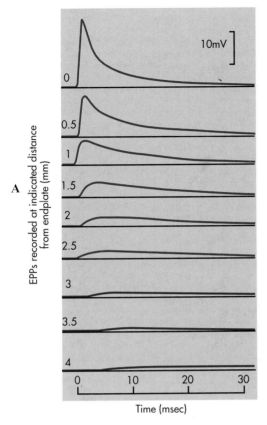

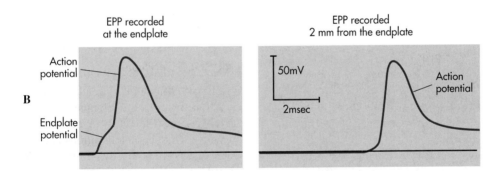

■ **Fig. 4-2** **A,** Endplate potentials *(EPPs)* in a frog sartorius muscle. The preparation was treated with curare to bring the EPP just below threshold for eliciting an action potential. The EPP, recorded at increasing distances from the neuromuscular junction, decreases in amplitude and rate of rise. **B,** Intracellular recordings made at the motor endplate *(left panel)* and 2 mm away *(right panel)* in a muscle fiber of frog extensor digitorum longus. When the motor nerve was stimulated, an EPP occurred, which triggered an action potential. Both the EPP and the resultant action potential can be recorded at the endplate, but 2 mm away from the endplate only the action potential can be seen because the EPP is conducted with decrement and has substantially decayed before reaching this point on the muscle fiber. (**A** redrawn from Fatt P, Katz B: *J Physiol* 115:320, 1951; **B** redrawn from Fatt P, Katz B: *J Physiol* 117:109, 1952.)

Box 4-1 Summary of events that occur during neuromuscular transmission

Action potential in presynaptic motor axon terminals
↓
Increase in Ca++ permeability and influx of Ca++ into axon terminal
↓
Release of acetylcholine from synaptic vesicles into synaptic cleft
↓
Diffusion of acetylcholine to postjunctional membrane
↓
Combination of acetylcholine with specific receptors on postjunctional membrane
↓
Increase in permeability of postjunctional membrane to Na+ and K+ causes EPP
↓
Depolarization of areas of muscle membrane adjacent to endplate and initiation of an action potential

---

EPP, Endplate potential.

as **miniature endplate potentials (MEPPs.)** MEPPs occur *even if the motor neuron is not stimulated* (Fig. 4-3). *An MEPP is caused by the spontaneous release of one quantum of acetylcholine into the junctional cleft.* The frequency at which MEPPs occur is random; average frequency is about 1 per second. The frequency of MEPPs may vary, but their amplitudes are within a relatively narrow range (Fig. 4-3).

Unlike EPPs, each MEPP depolarizes the postjunctional membrane by only about 0.4 mV on average, not nearly enough to trigger an action potential in the adjacent muscle plasma membrane. Despite this major difference, MEPPs and EPPs share several similarities. The MEPP has the same time course as an EPP that is evoked by an action potential in the nerve terminal. The MEPP is also similar to the EPP in its responses to most drugs. For example, the EPP and MEPP are both prolonged by drugs that inhibit acetylcholinesterase, and both are similarly depressed by compounds that compete with acetylcholine for binding to the receptor protein.

The quantal release of acetylcholine can be demonstrated in another way as well. If the extracellular concentration of Ca^{++} is reduced to low levels, much less Ca^{++} enters the nerve terminal in response to an action potential, and consequently very few synaptic vesicles release their acetylcholine. Under these conditions, the size of the EPP varies in small steps, and each step is the size of an MEPP.

Miniature endplate potentials

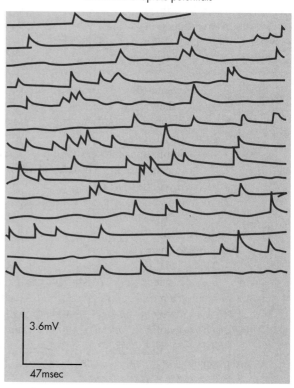

3.6mV

47msec

■ **Fig. 4-3** Spontaneous miniature endplate potentials (MEPPs) recorded at a neuromuscular junction in a fiber of frog extensor digitorum longus. (Redrawn from Fatt P, Katz B: *Nature* 166:597, 1950.)

■ *Action of Cholinesterase and Reuptake of Choline*

Acetylcholinesterase is concentrated on the external surface of the postjunctional membrane and in the external lamina. Drugs that inhibit this enzyme are called **anticholinesterases.** *In the presence of an anticholinesterase, the EPP is larger and dramatically prolonged.*

As we have seen, the motor neuron cannot synthesize choline. Therefore, its reuptake from the synaptic cleft provides the choline necessary for the resynthesis of acetylcholine. **Hemicholiniums** are drugs that block the choline transport system and inhibit choline uptake. Prolonged treatment with hemicholiniums depletes the store of transmitter and ultimately decreases the acetylcholine content of the quanta.

■ *Ionic Mechanism of the Endplate Potential*

The cation channels that acetylcholine opens in the postjunctional membrane differ from the voltage-gated cation channels of nerve and muscle in that they operate independently of the membrane potential. *The postjunctional channels are gated by the action of acetylcholine rather than by the transmembrane potential.* Acetyl-

choline receptors thus belong to the superfamily of **ligand-gated ion channels.**

Acetylcholine is the "go-between" that transmits the incoming electrical signal across the synapse. It performs this function by increasing the permeability of the postsynaptic membrane to both Na^+ and K^+. At the cell's resting potential, the driving force for Na^+ to enter the cell is much larger than the net force that causes K^+ to leave the cell. Thus, a net inward ionic current will flow through the open acetylcholine receptor protein channels, which then depolarizes the postjunctional membrane.

■ *Acetylcholine Receptor Protein*

The acetylcholine receptor protein has been extensively studied. The development of methods for isolating and purifying hydrophobic membrane proteins and the availability of snake venom neurotoxins that tightly bind to the acetylcholine receptor have been essential in these studies.

So-called **α toxins** in cobra venoms are responsible for paralyzing snakes' prey. These toxins bind to the acetylcholine binding site on the acetylcholine receptor protein and they prevent acetylcholine from binding and thereby inhibit its action. Poison arrows whose tips are dipped in **curare,** an α toxin extracted from certain plants, are used by some South American Indians to paralyze their prey.

Each motor endplate contains 10^7 to 10^8 acetylcholine receptor proteins; they are highly concentrated near the mouths of the postjunctional folds. The acetylcholine receptor protein is an integral membrane protein that spans the hydrophobic lipid matrix of the postjunctional membrane. Cholinesterase, on the other hand, is only loosely associated with the surface of the postjunctional membrane by hydrophilic interactions. The acetylcholine receptor consists of five subunits (Fig. 4-4), two of which are identical. Therefore, each receptor contains four different polypeptide chains.

Patients with a disorder called **myasthenia gravis** are unable to maintain prolonged contraction of skeletal muscle. These individuals have circulating antibodies against the acetylcholine receptor protein. Treatment with anticholinesterases markedly improves the ability of these patients to maintain muscle contractions.

Acetylcholine receptor proteins are highly concentrated in the postjunctional membrane; very few acetylcholine receptors are located elsewhere on the muscle plasma membrane. The mechanisms responsible for localizing the acetylcholine receptors in the postjunctional membrane are not completely understood, but it is clear that the motor neuron plays a role.

If a motor axon is severed, the acetylcholine receptors in all the muscle cells it formerly innervated tend to spread out over the entire plasma membrane. The muscle cell then becomes sensitive to acetylcholine applied anywhere on its surface; this phenomenon is known as **denervation supersensitivity.**

■ *Synapses between Neurons*

Chemical transmission between neurons has many of the same properties that characterize the neuromuscular junction. Electrical synapses are also present in the central nervous systems of animals, from invertebrates to mammals.

■ *Electrical Synapses*

At an electrical synapse, a change in the membrane potential of one cell is transmitted to the other cell by the direct flow of current. Because current flows directly between two cells that make an electrical synapse, trans-

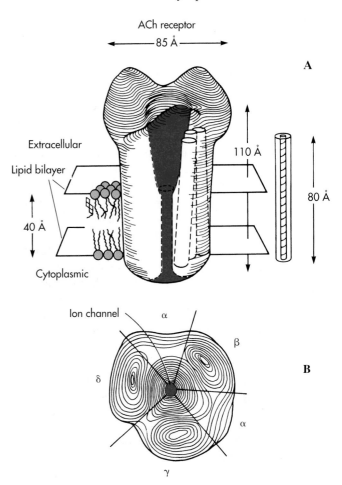

■ **Fig. 4-4** A model of the structure of the nicotinic acetylcholine receptor protein. **A,** Viewed from the side and **B,** viewed looking down on the acetylcholine receptor from the extracellular surface. The closed curves are electron density profiles. Five subunits surround a central ion channel. Shown are two α subunits and one each of β, γ, and δ subunits. A binding site for acetylcholine is located on each α subunit. (Redrawn from Kistler J et al: *Biophys J* 37:371, 1982.)

mission takes place with essentially *no synaptic delay.* Usually, electrical synapses allow conduction in both directions. In this respect they differ from chemical synapses, which must be unidirectional. Certain electrical synapses conduct more readily in one direction than in another; this property is called **rectification.**

Cells that form electrical synapses typically are joined by **gap junctions.** Gap junctions are plaquelike structures that form when the plasma membranes of coupled cells are very close together (less than 3 nm). Freeze-fracture electron micrographs of gap junctions display regular arrays of intramembrane protein particles. *These intramembrane particles consist of six subunits surrounding a central channel that is accessible to water.* The hexagonal array is called a **connexon.** Each of the six subunits is a single protein (one polypeptide chain) called a **connexin** (MW about 25,000). At the gap junction, the connexons of the coupled cells are aligned to form **connexon channels** (Fig. 4-5, *A*). The channels allow the passage of water-soluble molecules up to molecular weights of 1200 to 1500 from one cell to the other. In electrical synapses, these channels are the pathways for electrical current flow between the cells.

Cells that are electrically coupled may become uncoupled by the closing of the connexon channels. The channels may close in response to increased intracellular concentration of Ca^{++} or H^+ in one of the cells or in response to depolarization of one or both of the cells. A model for the mechanism that closes the channels is shown in Fig. 4-5, *B*.

Electrical synapses are widespread in the peripheral and central nervous systems of invertebrates and vertebrates. Electrical synapses are particularly useful in reflex pathways in which rapid transmission between cells (little synaptic delay) is necessary or when the synchronous response of a number of neurons is required. *Among the many non-neuronal cells that are coupled by gap junctions are hepatocytes, myocardial cells, intestinal smooth muscle cells, and the epithelial cells of the lens.*

■ *Chemical Synapses*

When one neuron makes a chemical synapse with another, the presynaptic nerve terminal characteristically broadens to form a **terminal bouton.** At the synapse itself, the presynaptic and postsynaptic membranes are closely apposed and lie parallel to one another. *Substantial structures stabilize the synapse.* In fact, when nervous tissue is disrupted, the relationship of the presynaptic and postsynaptic membranes at the synapse is often preserved.

Because of the structure and organization of chemical synapses, conduction is necessarily one way. The one-way conduction of chemical synapses contributes to the organization of the central nervous systems of vertebrates. The synaptic delay at chemical synapses, which is about 0.5 msec, is mainly caused by the time required for the release of transmitter. In polysynaptic pathways, synaptic delay accounts for a significant fraction of the total conduction time.

The mode of transmission at chemical synapses is similar to that at the neuromuscular junction in that transmission involves the release of a transmitter substance from the presynaptic cell. *At chemical synapses, the transmitter released by the presynaptic neurons alters the conductance of the postsynaptic plasma membrane to one or more ions.* A change in the conductance of the postsynaptic membrane to an ion not in equilibrium across the membrane alters the current carried by that ion, and the change in ionic current alters the membrane potential of the postsynaptic cell. *In most cases, transmitters produce their effects by increasing the conduc-*

tance of the postsynaptic membrane to one or more ions. However, some transmitters may decrease the postsynaptic conductance to specific ions.

The postsynaptic plasma membrane is specialized for chemical sensitivity rather than electrical sensitivity. Action potentials are not produced at the synapse. The change in postsynaptic membrane potential caused by the alteration in ion currents—whether a depolarization or hyperpolarization—is conducted electrotonically over the membrane of the postsynaptic neuron. Eventually, the depolarization or hyperpolarization is conducted to the **axon hillock,** the part of the neuron where its axon originates, and thence to the **initial segment,** the part of the

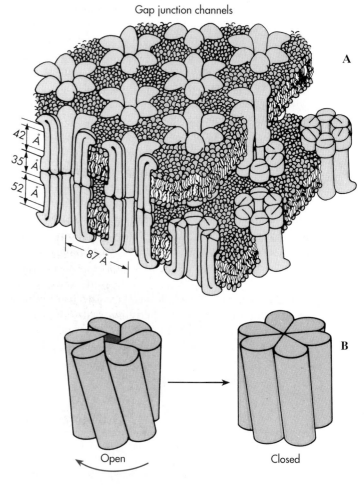

Gap junction channels

Open → Closed

■ **Fig. 4-5** **A,** A model for the structure of the gap junction channels. Each plasma membrane contains connexons, each of which consists of a hexagonal array of six connexin polypeptides. The connexons of the two membranes are aligned at the gap junction to form channels between the cytosolic compartments of the two cells. **B,** A model of the opening and closing of the gap junction channel. The individual connexin subunits of the connexon are proposed to twist relative to one another to open and close the central channel. (**A** redrawn from Makowski L et al: *J Cell Biol* 74:629, 1977, by copyright permission of The Rockefeller University Press. **B** redrawn from Unwin PNT, Zampighi G: *Nature* 283:45, 1980, by permission from Macmillan Journals.)

axon very near to the neuronal cell body. *In many neurons, the* **axon hillock–initial segment** *region of the cell has a lower threshold than the rest of the plasma membrane of the postsynaptic cell* (Fig. 4-6). An action potential will be generated at that site if the sum of all the inputs to the cell exceeds threshold. Once the action potential has been generated, it is conducted over the surface of the postsynaptic cell body and is propagated along its axon.

Input-Output Relations

The neuromuscular junction represents a simple type of synapse in which one action potential in the presynaptic cell (the input) elicits a single action potential in the postsynaptic cell (the output). In other types of synapses, the output may differ from the input. *Synapses can be classified as one-to-one, one-to-many, or many-to-one, on the basis of the relationship between input and output.*

In a **one-to-one** synapse, such as the neuromuscular junction, the input and the output are the same. A single action potential in the presynaptic cell evokes a single action potential in the postsynaptic cell. Because the output matches the input, no integration occurs at this type of synapse.

In a **one-to-many** synapse, a single action potential in the presynaptic cell elicits many action potentials in the postsynaptic cell. In these types of synapses, axon collaterals of motor neurons make one-to-many synapses on **Renshaw cells** in the spinal cord. One action potential in the motor neuron is thus able to induce the Renshaw cell to fire a burst of action potentials. The burst of action potentials in the Renshaw cell inhibits the motor neuron and prevents it from being fired too frequently.

In a **many-to-one** synaptic arrangement, one action potential in a presynaptic cell is not sufficient to make the postsynaptic cell fire an action potential. *The nearly simultaneous arrival of presynaptic action potentials from several input neurons that synapse on the same postsynaptic cell is necessary to depolarize the postsynaptic cell to threshold.* The spinal motor neuron has this type of synaptic organization. One hundred or more presynaptic axons synapse on each spinal motor neuron (Fig. 4-7). *Some of these axons carry excitatory inputs that depolarize the postsynaptic cell and bring it closer to its threshold. Other axons carry inhibitory inputs that hyperpolarize the motor neuron and take it farther away from threshold.*

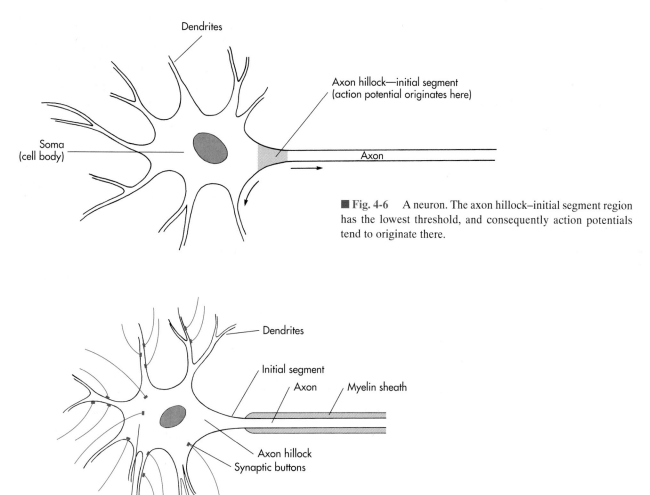

■ **Fig. 4-6** A neuron. The axon hillock–initial segment region has the lowest threshold, and consequently action potentials tend to originate there.

■ **Fig. 4-7** A spinal motor neuron with multiple synapses on both soma and dendrites.

■ *Excitatory and Inhibitory Postsynaptic Potentials*

The changes in postsynaptic potential caused by an action potential in a single presynaptic input to a spinal motor neuron amount to about 1 to 2 mV. *Thus, no one excitatory input can bring the motor neuron to threshold.* A transient depolarization of the postsynaptic neuron evoked by an action potential in a presynaptic axon is called an **excitatory postsynaptic potential (EPSP)** (Fig. 4-8). The transient *hyperpolarization* elicited by an action potential in an inhibitory input is called an **inhibitory postsynaptic potential (IPSP)** (Fig. 4-8). At any instant, the postsynaptic cell *integrates* the various inputs. If the momentary sum of the inputs depolarizes the postsynaptic cell to its threshold, it will fire an action potential. The process of integration at the level of a single postsynaptic neuron of the various inputs is called **summation.**

■ *Summation of Synaptic Inputs*

Summation of inputs can occur by either spatial summation or temporal summation (Fig. 4-9, *A*). **Spatial summation** occurs when *two separate inputs* arrive almost simultaneously. The two postsynaptic potentials are then added. If the two inputs are EPSPs, they will depolarize the postsynaptic cell about twice as much as either input alone. However, *if one input is an EPSP and the other is an IPSP, they tend to cancel one another.* Even postsynaptic potentials from synapses at opposite ends of the postsynaptic cell body act in this way.

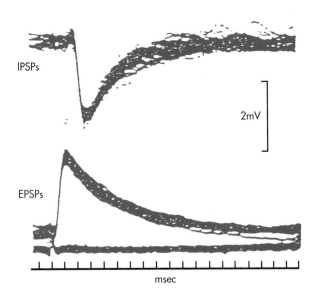

■ **Fig. 4-8** Inhibitory postsynaptic potentials *(IPSPs)* and excitatory postsynaptic potentials *(EPSPs)* recorded with a microelectrode in a cat spinal motor neuron in response to stimulation of appropriate peripheral afferent fibers. Forty traces are superimposed. (Redrawn from Curtis DR, Eccles JC: *J Physiol* 145:529, 1959.)

Both postsynaptic potentials (EPSPs and IPSPs) are conducted rapidly over the entire cell membrane of the postsynaptic cell body with almost no decrement (i.e., the potentials do not decrease in magnitude). EPSPs and IPSPs are able to maintain their magnitude because the dimensions of the cell over which they travel (less than 100 μm) are much smaller than the length constant (about 1 to 2 mm) for electrotonic conduction (see Chapter 3). In contrast, synaptic potentials that originate in fine dendritic branches decrease in magnitude as they are conducted to the cell body; the finer the dendrite, the greater is the decrement.

Temporal summation occurs when two or more action potentials in a *single presynaptic neuron* occur in rapid succession, so that the resultant postsynaptic potentials overlap in time (Fig. 4-9, *B*). A train of impulses in a single presynaptic neuron can change the potential of the postsynaptic cell in a stepwise manner. In this situation, each stepwise change in the postsynaptic potential is caused by one of the presynaptic impulses.

Integration at the spinal motor neuron takes place because many positive and negative inputs impinge on a single motor neuron. Integration permits fine control of the firing pattern of the spinal motor neuron.

■ *Modulation of Synaptic Activity*

The responses of a postsynaptic neuron to single stimulations of a particular presynaptic neuron are relatively constant in magnitude and time course. However, *when a presynaptic axon is stimulated repeatedly, the postsynaptic response may increase with each stimulation.* This phenomenon is called **facilitation** (Fig. 4-10, *A*). As shown in Fig. 4-10, *B*, the extent of facilitation depends on the frequency of presynaptic impulses. Facilitation dies away rapidly, within tens to hundreds of milliseconds after stimulation stops.

When a presynaptic neuron is stimulated **tetanically** (many stimuli at high frequency) for several seconds, **posttetanic potentiation** occurs. Posttetanic potentiation, like facilitation, is an enhancement of postsynaptic response, but it lasts longer (Fig. 4-10, *C*): tens of seconds to several minutes after cessation of tetanic stimulation.

Facilitation and posttetanic potentiation are the result of the effects of repeated stimulation on the presynaptic neuron. These phenomena do not involve a change in the sensitivity of the postsynaptic cell to transmitter. Rather, with repeated stimulation, an increased number of quanta of transmitter is released. Increased levels of intracellular calcium ions enhance transmitter release during repetitive stimulation.

Repetitive stimulation of certain synapses in the brain increases the efficacy of transmission at those synapses. This phenomenon, called **long-term potentiation,** can persist for days to weeks. Long-term potentiation is believed to be involved in the storage of memories. The increased synaptic efficacy that occurs in long-term potentiation probably involves both presynaptic (greater transmitter release) and postsynaptic (greater sensitivity to transmitter) changes.

When a synapse is repetitively stimulated for a long time, a point is reached at which each successive presynaptic stimulation elicits smaller postsynaptic responses. This phenomenon is called **synaptic fatigue** (neuromuscular depression at the motor endplate). The postsynaptic cell at a fatigued synapse responds normally to transmitter applied from a micropipette; thus, the defect is presynaptic. In some cases, a decrease in quantal content (the amount of transmitter per synaptic vesicle) contributes to synaptic fatigue. A fatigued synapse typically recovers within a few seconds.

■ Ionic Mechanisms of Postsynaptic Potentials in Spinal Motor Neurons

Much of our knowledge of synaptic mechanisms in the mammalian central nervous system is derived from studies of cat spinal motor neurons.

Excitatory postsynaptic potentials (EPSPs). The EPSP (Fig. 4-8) of the cat spinal motor neuron is caused by a *transient increase of the conductance of the postsynaptic membrane to both Na+ and K+* in response to the neurotransmitter. At the cell's resting potential, the driving force for Na+ to enter the cell is much greater than

the force for K+ to leave. Hence, in response to the neurotransmitter, a net inward flow of ions occurs; inward Na+ current depolarizes the postsynaptic cell.

Inhibitory postsynaptic potentials. The IPSP (Fig. 4-8) of cat spinal motor neurons is caused by an *increased Cl− conductance* of the postjunctional membrane. At rest, the net tendency is for Cl− to enter the cell. The increase in Cl− conductance that results from the release of transmitters at the inhibitory synapse allows Cl− to enter the postsynaptic cell and hyperpolarize it.

Presynaptic inhibition. Inhibitory interactions are vital in stabilizing the central nervous system. In addition to the postsynaptic inhibition, another type of inhibition called **presynaptic inhibition** operates at synapses. If an inhibitory input to a spinal motor neuron is stimulated tetanically and then an excitatory input to the same neuron is stimulated once, the EPSP elicited by the excitatory input may be reduced in magnitude after the inhibitory volley. This type of inhibition is believed to occur by a mechanism in which axon collaterals of the inhibitory axons synapse on the excitatory nerve terminals (Fig. 4-11). Action potentials in the inhibitory nerve depolarize the excitatory nerve terminal for a long time. Although this depolarization brings the excitatory nerve terminal closer to threshold, the partial depolarization causes less Ca++ to enter the cell, which in turn decreases the amount of transmitter released in response to an action potential. The smaller the amount of neurotransmitter released, the less is the magnitude of the excitatory postsynaptic potential.

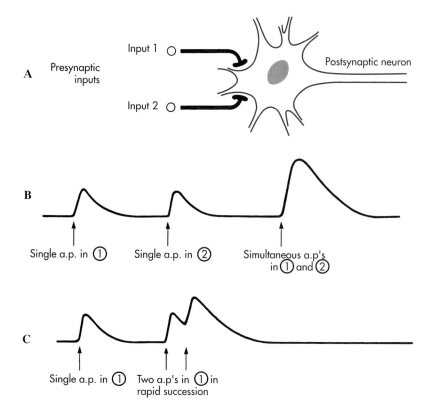

A
Presynaptic inputs

Input 1

Input 2

Postsynaptic neuron

B

Single a.p. in ①   Single a.p. in ②   Simultaneous a.p.'s in ① and ②

C

Single a.p. in ①   Two a.p.'s in ① in rapid succession

■ **Fig. 4-9** **A,** Spatial and temporal summation at a postsynaptic neuron with two synaptic inputs (*1* and *2*). **B,** Spatial summation. The postsynaptic potentials in response to single action potentials (a.p.'s) in inputs *1* and *2* occurring separately and simultaneously. **C,** Temporal summation. The postsynaptic response to two impulses in rapid succession in the same input.

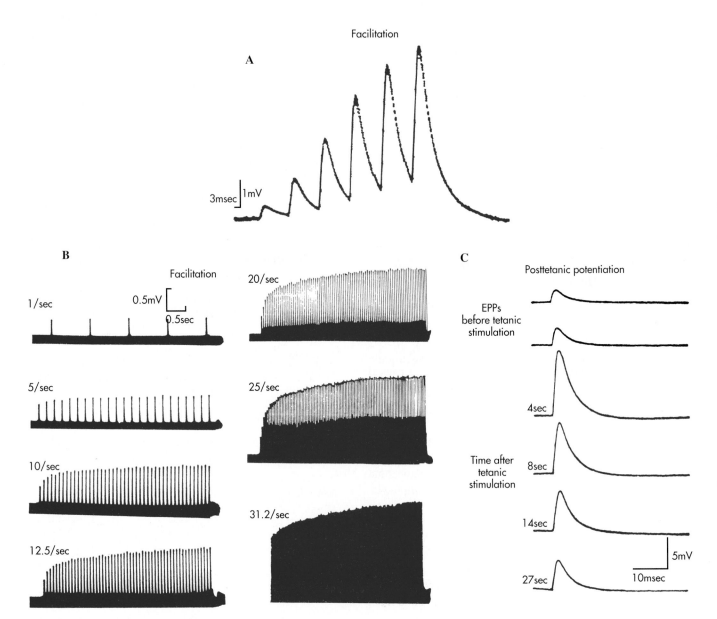

■ **Fig. 4-10** **A,** Facilitation at a neuromuscular junction. EPPs at a neuromuscular junction in toad sartorius muscle were elicited by successive action potentials in the motor axon. Neuromuscular transmission was depressed by 5 mM Mg++ and 2.1 μM curare, so that action potentials did not occur. **B,** EPPs at a frog neuromuscular junction elicited by repetitively stimulating the motor axon at different frequencies. Note that facilitation failed to occur at the lowest frequency of stimulation (1/sec) and that the degree of facilitation increased with increasing frequency of stimulation in the range of frequency employed. Neuromuscular transmission was inhibited by bathing the preparation in 12 to 20 mM Mg++. **C,** Posttetanic potentiation at a frog neuromuscular junction. The top two traces indicate control EPPs in response to single action potentials in the motor axon. Subsequent traces indicate EPPs in response to single action potentials after tetanic stimulation (50 impulses/sec for 20 seconds) of the motor neuron. The time interval between the end of tetanic stimulation and the single action potential is shown on each trace. The muscle was treated with tetrodotoxin to prevent generation of action potentials. (**A** redrawn from Belnave RJ, Gage PW: *J Physiol* 266:435, 1977; **B** redrawn from Magelby KL: *J Physiol* 234:327, 1973; **C** redrawn from Weinrich D: *J Physiol* 212:431, 1971.)

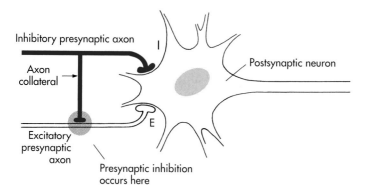

■ **Fig. 4-11** Presynaptic inhibition. Axon collaterals of the inhibitory axon *(I)* synapse on the excitatory axon terminal *(E)*. An action potential in the inhibitory axon depolarizes the excitatory axon terminal. The depolarized excitatory axon terminal will release less transmitter in response to an action potential in the excitatory neuron *(E)*.

■ *Neurotransmitters and Neuromodulators*

■ *Identification of Transmitter Substances*

Researchers working on identifying neurotransmitters call compounds that may function as neurotransmitters **candidate** or **putative neurotransmitters.** These putative neurotransmitters are usually concentrated in specific neurons or in specific neuronal pathways. Much of the research performed on putative neurotransmitters involves noting the specific responses to the microapplication of putative transmitters to particular areas of the central nervous system. Their application indicates the location of the putative transmitter and the neurons that respond to it, as well as the neuron's specific responses, which can provide clues about the functions of a putative neurotransmitter.

It is often difficult to *prove* that a substance is the transmitter at a particular synapse. *A putative transmitter (X) must satisfy the following criteria before it is accepted as a proven transmitter at a particular synapse:*

1. The presynaptic neurons must contain X and must be able to synthesize it.
2. X must be released by the presynaptic neurons in response to appropriate stimulation.
3. Microapplication of X to the postsynaptic membrane must mimic the effects of stimulation of the presynaptic neuron.
4. The effects of presynaptic stimulation and of microapplication of X should be altered in the same way by drugs.

Some transmitters have rapid and transient effects on the postsynaptic cell. Other transmitters have effects that are much slower in onset and that last for minutes or even hours. Most known neurotransmitters fall into three major chemical classes: amines, amino acids, and oligopeptides.

■ *Neurotransmitters*

Acetylcholine. As discussed previously, acetylcholine is the transmitter used by all motor axons that arise from the spinal cord. Acetylcholine also plays a central role in the autonomic nervous system; it is the transmitter for all autonomic preganglionic neurons as well as for postganglionic parasympathetic fibers. The Betz cells of the motor cortex use acetylcholine as their transmitter. The basal ganglia, which are involved in the control of movement, contain high levels of acetylcholine, and thus it is likely that acetylcholine is an important neurotransmitter in the basal ganglia. In addition, acetylcholine may be the transmitter in many other central neural pathways.

Deficits in pathways involving acetylcholine (**cholinergic pathways**) in the brain have been implicated in some forms of **senile dementia** (e.g., **Alzheimer's disease**). Treatment with long-lasting anticholinergic drugs that penetrate the blood-brain barrier may improve cognitive function in some individuals suffering from dementia.

Biogenic amine transmitters. Among the amines that may serve as neurotransmitters are **norepinephrine, epinephrine, dopamine, serotonin,** and **histamine.**

Dopamine, norepinephrine, and epinephrine are **catecholamines,** and they share a common biosynthetic pathway that starts with the amino acid tyrosine. Tyrosine is converted to L-dopa by the enzyme tyrosine hydroxylase. L-Dopa is converted to dopamine by a specific decarboxylase. In dopaminergic neurons, the pathway stops here. In noradrenergic neurons, another enzyme, dopamine β-hydroxylase, converts dopamine to norepinephrine. Norepinephrine is the primary transmitter for postganglionic sympathetic neurons. Chromaffin cells in the adrenal medulla add a methyl group to norepinephrine to produce the hormone epinephrine.

Neurons that contain high levels of dopamine are prominent in the midbrain regions known as the **substantia nigra** and the **ventral tegmentum.** Some of the axons of these neurons terminate in the **corpus striatum,** where they participate in controlling complex movements. The degeneration of dopaminergic synapses in the corpus striatum occurs in **Parkinson's disease** and may be a major cause of the muscular tremors and rigidity that characterize this disease. Treatment of some Parkinson's patients with L-dopa, a precursor of dopamine, improves motor control.

In contrast, the hyperactivity of dopaminergic synapses may be involved in some forms of **psychosis. Chlorpromazine** and related antipsychotic drugs inhibit the dopamine receptors on postsynaptic membranes and thus diminish the effects of dopamine released from presynaptic nerve terminals.

Serotonin (5-hydroxytryptamine)-containing neurons are present in high concentration in certain nuclei located in the brainstem. Serotonergic neurons may be involved in temperature regulation, sensory perception, onset of sleep, and control of mood. Serotonergic neurons have been implicated in the aggressive behavior of certain animal species.

Histamine is present in certain neurons in the hypothalamus. The functions of these presumably histaminergic neurons are not yet known.

Amino acid transmitters. Glycine, the simplest amino acid, is an inhibitory neurotransmitter released by certain spinal interneurons.

γ-Aminobutyric acid (GABA) is not incorporated into proteins, nor is it present in all cells (as are the other naturally occurring amino acids). *GABA is produced from glutamate by a specific decarboxylase present only in certain neurons in the central nervous system.* Among the cells that contain GABA are some neurons in the basal ganglia, cerebellar Purkinje cells, and certain spinal interneurons. *In all known cases, GABA functions as an inhibitory transmitter. It is the most common transmitter in the brain.* GABA may be the neurotransmitter at as many as one third of the synapses in the brain.

The postsynaptic receptors for glycine and GABA are both ligand-gated Cl^- channels that allow the influx of Cl^- to hyperpolarize the postsynaptic neuron.

General **anesthetics** prolong the open time of GABA receptor chloride channels and thus prolong the inhibition of the postsynaptic neurons at GABA-ergic synapses. GABA receptors may be a principal target of general anesthetics.

Glutamate and **aspartate,** dicarboxylic amino acids, strongly excite many neurons in the brain. Glutamate is the most common excitatory neurotransmitter in the brain. Five classes of **excitatory amino acid (EAA) receptors** have been identified.

Nitric oxide (NO). NO is a transmitter at synapses between inhibitory motor neurons of the enteric nervous system and gastrointestinal smooth muscle cells (see Chapter 37). NO also functions as a neurotransmitter in the central nervous system. It is an unusual neurotransmitter because it is neither packaged into synaptic vesicles nor released by exocytosis. It is highly permeant and simply diffuses from its site of production to neighboring cells. The enzyme **NO synthase** catalyzes the production of NO as a product of the oxidation of arginine to citrulline. This enzyme is stimulated by an increase in cytosolic Ca^{++}.

In addition to serving as a neurotransmitter, NO functions as a cellular signal transduction molecule in both neurons and non-neuronal cells (such as vascular smooth muscle, see Chapter 27). One way NO functions as a signal transduction molecule is by regulating guanylyl cyclase, the enzyme that produces cyclic guanosine monophosphate (GMP) from guanosine triphosphate (GTP). NO binds to a heme group in soluble guanylyl cyclase and potently stimulates the enzyme. The stimulation of this enzyme leads to an elevation of cyclic GMP in the target cell. The cyclic GMP can then influence multiple cellular processes.

■ *Neuroactive Peptides*

Certain cells release peptides that act at very low concentrations to excite or inhibit neurons. To date, more than 25 of these so-called **neuroactive peptides** or **neuropeptides,** ranging from 2 to about 40 amino acids long, have been identified. Some of these neuropeptides are listed in Box 4-2. Neuropeptides typically affect their target neurons at lower concentrations than the "classical" neurotransmitters discussed previously, and the actions of neuropeptides usually last longer than those of neurotransmitters.

Neuropeptides may act as hormones, as neurotransmitters, or as neuromodulators. In fact, a number of neuropeptides are more familiar as hormones, which are substances that are released into the blood and that reach their target cells via the circulation. A number of neuropeptides act as true transmitters at particular synapses and as neuromodulators at other synapses. Both neurotransmitters and neuromodulators are typically released near the surface of a target cell and diffuse to the target cell. A neurotransmitter, as discussed earlier, acts to change the conductance of the target cell to one or more ions, thereby changing the membrane potential of the target cell. A neuromodulator, on the other hand, modulates synaptic transmission. A neuromodulator may act presynaptically to change the amount of transmitter released in response to an action potential, or it may act on the postsynaptic cell to modify its response to the neurotransmitter. Box 4-3 lists differences between nonpeptide neurotransmitters and peptide neurotransmitters.

In many instances, neuropeptides coexist in the same nerve terminals with classical transmitters (Table 4-1). In some of these cases, the neuropeptide is released along with the transmitter in response to nerve stimulation.

Synthesis of neuropeptides. Nonpeptide neurotransmitters are synthesized in nerve terminals by pathways that involve soluble enzymes and simple precursors. Neuropeptides are synthesized in the neuronal cell body. They are encoded in the cell's DNA and transcribed into messenger RNA (mRNA); synthesis of the neuropeptide takes place on polyribosomes bound to the endoplasmic reticulum where the mRNA is translated. Secretory vesicles containing the neuropeptide are released from the mature face of the Golgi complex. The secretory vesicles are moved by **fast axonal transport** (Fig. 4-12) to the axon terminal, where they function as synaptic vesicles.

Some neuropeptides are synthesized as preprohormones (see also Chapter 45). Cleavage of a signal sequence converts a preprohormone to a prohormone. Proteolytic cleavage of the prohormone may then release one or more active peptides. In some cases, one prohormone may contain several active peptide sequences. For example, the prohormone of the opioid peptide, β-endorphin, is a 31,000-dalton polypeptide that contains several active sequences. One cleavage of the prohormone releases adrenocorticotropic hormone (ACTH) and β-lipotropin. Cleavage of ACTH releases yet another hormone, melanocyte-stimulating hormone (α-MSH), and cleavage of β-lipotropin releases α-MSH and a number of active β-endorphins.

Opioid peptides. Opiates are drugs derived from the juice of the opium poppy.

Opiates are useful therapeutically as powerful **analgesics** (pain relievers). They exert their analgesic effect by binding to specific opiate receptors. The binding of opiates to their receptors is stereospecifically inhibited by a morphine derivative called **naloxone.**

Compounds that are not derived from the opium poppy, but that exert direct effects by binding to opiate receptors, are called **opioids.** *Operationally, opioids are defined as direct-acting compounds whose effects are stereospecifically antagonized by naloxone.*

Box 4-2 Some neuroactive peptides

Gut-brain peptides

Vasoactive intestinal polypeptide (VIP)
Cholecystokinin octapeptide (CCK-8)
Substance P
Neurotensin
Methionine enkephalin
Leucine enkephalin
Motilin
Insulin
Glucagon

Hypothalamic-releasing hormones

Thyrotropin-releasing hormone (TRH)
Luteinizing hormone–releasing hormone (LHRH)
Somatostatin (growth hormone releasing-inhibiting factor, or SRIF)

Pituitary peptides

Adrenocorticotropin (ACTH)
β-Endorphin
α-Melanocyte-stimulating hormone (α-MSH)

Others

Dynorphin
Angiotensin II
Bradykinin
Vasopressin
Oxytocin
Carnosine
Bombesin

Modified from Snyder SH: *Science* 209:976, 1980. Copyright 1980 by American Association for the Advancement of Science.

Box 4-3 Distinctions between classical nonpeptide neurotransmitters and peptide neurotransmitters

Nonpeptide transmitters	**Peptide transmitters**
Synthesized and packaged in nerve terminal	Synthesized and packaged in cell body; transported to nerve terminal by fast axonal transport
Synthesized in active form	Active peptide formed when it is cleaved from a much larger polypeptide that contains several neuropeptides
Present in small, clear vesicles	Present in large, electron-dense vesicles
Released into a synaptic cleft	May be released some distance from the postsynaptic cell
	There may be no well-defined synaptic structure
Action terminated because of uptake by presynaptic terminal by Na$^+$-powered active transport	Action terminated by proteolysis or by the peptide diffusing away
Typically, action has short latency and short duration (msec)	Action may have long latency and may persist for many seconds

The three major classes of endogenous opioid peptides in mammals are **enkephalins, endorphins,** and **dynorphins.** Enkephalins are the simplest opioids; they are pentapeptides. Dynorphin and the endorphins are somewhat longer peptides that contain one or the other of the enkephalin sequences at their N-terminal ends.

Opioid peptides are widely distributed in neurons of the central nervous system and intrinsic neurons of the gastrointestinal tract. Within these neurons, opioid peptides are found in vesicles that resemble synaptic vesicles. The endorphins are discretely localized in particular structures of the central nervous system, whereas the enkephalins and dynorphins are more widely distributed. Opioids inhibit neurons in the brain involved in the perception of pain. Opioid peptides are among the most potent analgesic (pain-relieving) compounds known.

Nonopioid neuropeptides. Most of the known neuropeptides are not opioids. **Substance P,** a peptide of 11 amino acids, is present in specific neurons in the brain, in primary sensory neurons, and in plexus neurons in the wall of the gastrointestinal tract. Substance P was the first so-called **gut-brain peptide** to be discovered. The wall of the gastrointestinal tract is richly innervated with neurons that form networks or plexuses (see also Chapter 37). The intrinsic plexuses of the gastrointestinal tract exert primary control over its motor and secretory activities. These enteric neurons contain many of the neuropeptides, including substance P, that are found in the brain and spinal column. Substance P is involved in pain transmission and has a powerful effect on smooth muscle.

Substance P is probably the transmitter employed at synapses made by primary sensory neurons (their cell bodies are in the dorsal root ganglia) with spinal interneurons in the dorsal horn of the spinal column. Enkephalins act to decrease the release of substance P at these synapses and thereby inhibit the pathway for pain sensation at the first synapse in the pathway.

■ **Table 4-1**   Examples of the coexistence within the same nerve terminal of a classical transmitter and a neuropeptide*

Transmitter	Peptide
Acetylcholine	Vasoactive intestinal peptide (VIP)
Norepinephrine	Somatostatin
	Enkephalin
	Neurotensin
Dopamine	Cholecystokinin (CCK)
	Enkephalin
Epinephrine	Enkephalin
Serotonin	Substance P
	Thyrotropin-releasing hormone (TRH)

Reprinted by permission of the publisher from Schwartz JH: *Chemical messengers: small molecules and peptides.* In Kandel ER, Schwartz JH, editors: *Principles of neural science,* New York, 1981, Elsevier. Copyright 1981 by Elsevier Science Publishing.

*Evidence for the coexistence of a classical transmitter substance with a neuroactive peptide has been reported for these combinations. With the information thus far available, it is not yet possible to determine the specificity of the pairs and their physiological significance.

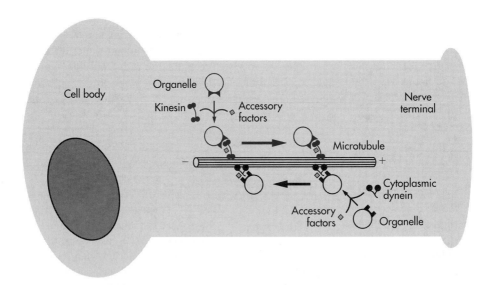

■ **Fig. 4-12**   Fast axonal transport of membrane vesicles. The network of microtubules that runs the length of the axon serves as the pathway for fast axonal transport of vesicles from the cell body to the nerve terminal and in the reverse direction. Most of the microtubules are oriented with their plus (rapidly growing) ends toward the nerve terminal. Kinesin and dynein are microtubule-associated motor proteins that function to transport the vesicles toward the nerve terminal and the cell body, respectively. Other proteins, called accessory factors, are required for transport of vesicles. (Modified from Sheetz MP, Steuer ER, Schroer TA: *Trends Neurosci* 12:474, 1990.)

Vasoactive intestinal polypeptide (VIP) is a member of a family of neuropeptides related to the hormone **secretin.** VIP was first discovered as a gastrointestinal hormone, but it is now known to be a neuropeptide also.

VIP is widely distributed in the central nervous system and in the intrinsic neurons of the gastrointestinal tract. In neurons in the brain, VIP has been localized in synaptic vesicles. VIP may function as an inhibitory transmitter of vascular and nonvascular smooth muscle and as an excitatory transmitter to glandular epithelial cells.

Secretin, glucagon, and **gastric inhibitory polypeptide (GIP),** whose functions as gastrointestinal hormones have been well characterized, have sequence homology with VIP. Although these peptides have also been found in particular neurons in the central nervous system, their functions in these neurons remain undetermined.

Cholecystokinin (CCK) is a member of a group of neuropeptides that includes **gastrin** and **cerulein,** which have similar C-terminal sequences. CCK is a well-known gastrointestinal hormone that elicits contraction of the gallbladder (see Chapter 38). One form of CCK is present in particular neurons of the central nervous system.

Neurotensin is present in enteric neurons and in the brain. When neurotensin is injected into cerebrospinal fluid at low concentrations, it lowers body temperature. Thus, neurotensin may function in temperature regulation.

■ Other Neuromodulators

Some important neuromodulators are not peptides. Purines and purine nucleotides (adenosine triphosphate [ATP]) and nucleosides (adenosine) function as neuromodulators in the central, autonomic, and peripheral nervous systems. Substances that serve as neurotransmitters may also act as neuromodulators. In some cases, a transmitter binds to receptors on the presynaptic neuron that released it, thereby regulating its own release.

■ Neurotransmitter Receptors

■ Inhibitory Receptors: GABA and Glycine Receptors

The most common inhibitory synapses in the central nervous system use either glycine or GABA as their transmitter. Glycine-mediated inhibitory synapses predominate in the spinal cord, while GABA-ergic synapses are the most numerous synapses in the brain.

GABA and glycine receptors, and most other neurotransmitter receptors, belong to a superfamily of **ligand-gated ion channels.** The probability of these channels opening and the average time a channel stays open are controlled by the concentration of the neurotransmitter for which the receptor is specific. The nicotinic acetylcholine receptor (Fig. 4-4) is the best studied member of the ligand-gated ion channel superfamily.

Despite their different ion specificities, important similarities exist between GABA and glycine receptors and the nicotinic acetylcholine receptor. All these channels are composed of five subunits that surround a central ion channel. The protein subunits share similarities in amino acid sequence and in tertiary structure. Although these channels contain five distinct subunits, only one or two subunit isoforms are typically required to form a functional ion channel. Different cell types in the central nervous system may have different receptor subtypes that consist of different combinations of subunit isoforms. Evolution appears to have created a variety of subunit isoforms from which a particular cell type can pick and choose in constructing its own multimeric ligand-gated receptor subtype.

GABA and glycine receptors are ligand-gated Cl^- channels that mediate Cl^- influx into neurons. The Cl^- current hyperpolarizes and thus inhibits the neurons. Two major types of GABA receptors have been identified—$GABA_A$ and $GABA_B$ receptors. The $GABA_A$ receptor is a GABA-mediated Cl^- channel. The $GABA_B$ receptor is not an ion channel itself but modulates the ion channel function of another protein. Five distinct protein subunits can form $GABA_A$ receptors, and different $GABA_A$ receptor subtypes are composed of different combinations of the subunits.

$GABA_A$ receptors are the targets of two major classes of drugs: **benzodiazepines** and **barbiturates.** Benzodiazepines (e.g., diazepam) are widely used antianxiety and relaxant drugs. Barbiturates are used as sedatives and anticonvulsants. Both classes of drugs bind to distinct sites on $GABA_A$ receptors and enhance the opening of the receptors' Cl^- channels in response to GABA.

■ Excitatory Amino Acid Receptors

Glutamate is the major neurotransmitter that mediates synaptic excitation in the central nervous system. Glutamate receptors are also known as **excitatory amino acid (EAA) receptors.** At present, five subtypes of EAA receptors have been recognized (Table 4-2) and classified principally by the synthetic amino acid analogs to which they bind tightly and specifically. Four of the subtypes are ligand-gated ion channels; the fifth subtype is a receptor (called the **metabotropic EAA receptor**) that is indirectly linked to an ion channel.

Two EAA receptors, the **AMPA** and **NMDA** receptors, are widely distributed in the central nervous system. Stimulation of AMPA receptors by glutamate or another agonist elicits an EPSP caused by flow of Na^+ and K^+. Stimulated NMDA receptors permit flow of Ca^{++} as well as Na^+ and K^+. NMDA receptors are blocked by extracellular Mg^{++} at physiological levels. The Mg^{++} block is relieved when the cell is depolarized. Thus, physiologi-

■ **Table 4-2**   Different classes of excitatory amino acid receptors

Receptor class	Properties
AMPA	Widely distributed in CNS; channel-selective Na^+ and K^+; formerly known as quisqualate receptor
NMDA	Widely distributed in CNS; channel-selective Ca^{++}, Na^+, and K^+; blocked by Mg^{++}; block relieved by depolarization
Kainate	Present in specific areas of CNS
L-AP4	Not widely distributed; may function as a presynaptic glutamate receptor that inhibits glutamate release
Metabotropic	Not an ion channel; mobilizes IP_3 and increases intracellular Ca^{++}

CNS, Central nervous systems.

cally, the first response to glutamate is depolarization of the postsynaptic cell by glutamate acting on AMPA receptors. This depolarization relieves the Mg^{++} block of NMDA receptors, which then respond by permitting Ca^{++} influx and further depolarization of the postsynaptic cell. NMDA receptors are also regulated by glycine, which binds to the receptor to enhance current flow in response to glutamate.

■ *Summary*

1. The neuromuscular junction is the best-characterized chemical synapse in vertebrates. Acetylcholine released by the prejunctional nerve terminal binds to acetylcholine receptors in the postjunctional membrane to open ion channels conductive to Na^+ and K^+. The resultant ion flow across the postjunctional membrane causes a depolarization, called an endplate potential.

2. The endplate potential is terminated by the hydrolysis of acetylcholine by the enzyme acetylcholinesterase. When acetylcholine is hydrolyzed, the choline liberated in the synaptic cleft is actively transported back into the nerve terminal.

3. The release of acetylcholine is quantal. A quantum corresponds to the amount of acetylcholine in a single presynaptic vesicle.

4. Direct electrical transmission between neighboring cells is mediated by gap junctions.

5. An action potential in an excitatory input to a spinal motor neuron causes an excitatory postsynaptic potential that depolarizes the motor neuron and brings it closer to threshold. An action potential in an inhibitory input causes an inhibitory postsynaptic potential that hyperpolarizes the motor neuron.

6. The efficacy of synaptic transmission depends on the timing and frequency of action potentials in the presynaptic neuron. Facilitation, posttetanic potentiation, and long-term potentiation are examples of increased efficacy of synaptic transmission in response to previous multiple stimulations of a synapse.

7. Acetylcholine, biogenic amines, glutamate, glycine, and-aminobutyric acid (GABA) are important neurotransmitters in the central nervous system.

8. Glycine and γ-aminobutyric acid are the major transmitters at inhibitory synapses in the central nervous system.

9. Glutamate is the major excitatory neurotransmitter in the central nervous system. There are five classes of excitatory amino acid (EAA) receptors.

10. Many neuroactive peptides function as neuromodulators or neurotransmitters in the central nervous system.

■ *Self-Study Problems*

1. List the general sequence of events that occur in neuromuscular transmission at the neuromuscular junction.

2. What is meant by the term quantal transmission? What is a miniature endplate potential (MEPP)? What are MEPPs due to?

3. Define facilitation. Define posttetanic potentiation.

4. What terminates the endplate potential? What effect will an inhibitor of acetylcholinesterase have on the endplate potential?

5. What is meant by "integration" at a spinal motor neuron?

■ *Bibliography*

Journal articles

Amara SG, Kuhar, MJ: Neurotransmitter transporters: recent progress, *Annu Rev Neurosci* 16:73, 1993.

Barnard EA: Receptor classes and the transmitter-gated ion channels, *Trends Biochem Sci* 17:368, 1992.

Baxter DA, Byrne JH: Ionic conductance mechanisms contributing to electrophysiological properties of neurons, *Curr Opin Neurobiol* 1:105, 1991.

Bennett MK, Scheller RH: A molecular description of synaptic vesicle membrane trafficking, *Annu Rev Biochem* 63:63, 1994.

Bredt DS, Snyder SH: Nitric oxide: a physiologic messenger molecule, *Annu Rev Biochem* 63:175, 1994.

Changeux JP: The nicotinic acetylcholine receptor: an allosteric protein prototype of ligand-gated ion channels, *Trends Pharmacol Sci* 11:485, 1990.

Froehner SC: Regulation of ion channel distribution at synapses. *Annu Rev Neurosci* 16:347, 1993.

Gingrich JA, Caron MG: Recent advances in the molecular biology of dopamine receptors, *Annu Rev Neurosci* 16:299, 1993.

Hökfelt T: Neuropeptides in perspective: the last ten years, *Neuron* 7:867, 1991.

Hollman M, Heinemann S: Cloned glutamate receptors, *Annu Rev Neurosci* 17:31,1994.

Jahn R, Sudhof TC: Synaptic vesicles and exocytosis, *Annu Rev Neurosci* 17:219, 1994.

Jessel TM, Kandel ER: Synaptic transmission: a bi-directional and self-modifiable form of cell-cell communication, *Cell* 72(Suppl 1):1, 1993.

Kennedy MB: The biochemistry of synaptic regulation in the central nervous system, *Annu Rev Biochem* 63:571, 1994.

Kupferman I: Functional studies of cotransmission, *Physiol Rev* 71:683, 1991.

Lester HA: The permeation pathway of neurotransmitter-gated ion channels, *Annu Rev Biophys Biomol Struct* 21:267, 1992.

Nakanishi S, Masu M: Molecular diversity and functions of glutamate receptors, *Annu Rev Biophys Biomol Struct* 23:319, 1994.

Nicoll RA, Malenka RC, Kauer JA: Functional comparison of neuroreceptor subtypes in mammalian central nervous system, *Physiol Rev* 70:513, 1990.

Sakmann B: Elementary steps in synaptic transmission revealed by currents through single ion channels, *Science* 256:28, 1992.

Schuman EM, Madison DV: Nitric oxide and synaptic function, *Annu Rev Neurosci* 17:153, 1994.

Stevens CF: Quantal release of neurotransmitter and long-term potentiation, *Cell* 72(Suppl):55, 1993.

Unwin N: Neurotransmitter action: opening of ligand-gated ion channels, *Cell* 72(Suppl):31, 1993.

Young AB, Fagg GE: Excitatory amino acid receptors in the brain: membrane binding and receptor autoradiographic approaches, *Trends Pharmacol Sci* 11:126, 1990.

Books and monographs

Aidley DJ: *The physiology of excitable cells,* ed 3, Cambridge, 1990, Cambridge University Press.

Eccles JC: *The physiology of synapses,* Berlin, 1964, Springer-Verlag.

Hall Z: *An introduction to molecular neurobiology,* Sunderland, Mass, 1991, Sinauer Associates.

Kandel ER, Schwartz JH: *Principles of neural science,* ed 3, New York, 1991, McGraw-Hill.

Katz B: *Nerve, muscle, and synapse,* New York, 1966, McGraw-Hill.

Levitan IB, Kaczmarek LK: *The neuron: cell and molecular biology,* New York, 1991, Oxford University Press.

Morell P, editor: *Myelin,* ed 2, New York, 1984, Plenum Press.

Nicholls JG, Martin AR, Wallace BG: *From neuron to brain,* ed 3, Sunderland, Mass, 1992, Sinauer Associates.

Membrane Receptors, Second Messengers, and Signal Transduction Pathways

Basic cellular processes are regulated by a host of substances. Some regulatory substances, such as steroid hormones, enter the cell and influence the transcription of certain genes. Other regulatory substances exert their influences from outside the cell. This chapter discusses these extracellular regulatory substances and the ways in which they influence cellular processes.

■ *Overview*

The first step in the action of extracellular regulatory substances is to bind to specific protein **receptors** on the extracellular surface of the plasma membrane of the target cells. For example, the neurotransmitters discussed in Chapter 4 bind to a receptor in order to bring about a response. The receptor is a ligand-gated ion channel, and the response of the cell is a ligand-induced ionic current. In this example, the ligand-gated ion channel is both the receptor and the **effector** for the action of the neurotransmitter.

■ *Signal Transduction Pathways*

For most regulatory molecules, however, a more complex series of events takes place between the binding of a regulatory substance to its specific membrane receptor and its final effects on cellular function. Extracellular regulatory molecules exert their effects on cells via **signal transduction pathways.** In these pathways, the binding of a regulatory substance to its plasma membrane receptor alters the activities of particular cellular proteins and ultimately causes a cellular response. Although many regulatory substances exist, there are relatively few signal transduction pathways. Our knowledge of these pathways is increasing at such a rapid rate that a comprehensive discussion of this subject is beyond the scope of this book. Therefore, only the most common and the best understood signal transduction pathways are emphasized, especially those that are relevant to topics discussed in subsequent chapters.

■ *Extracellular Regulatory Substances*

The extracellular regulatory compounds we consider in this chapter are often classified as endocrine, neurocrine, or paracrine substances. **Endocrine** regulatory substances **(hormones)** are released by endocrine cells. Hormones reach their target cells, which may be far from the endocrine cells, via the bloodstream. **Neurocrine** regulators are released by neurons in the immediate vicinity of the target cells. Neurotransmitters are neurocrine substances, as are most of the neuromodulators discussed in Chapter 4. **Paracrine** substances are released by cells that are not immediately adjacent to the target cells, but they are sufficiently close for the paracrine substance to reach the target cells by diffusion. For example, histamine is a paracrine agonist of gastric HCl secretion (see Chapter 38). Histamine is released by enterochromaffin-like (ECL) cells in the gastric mucosa, and it reaches the acid-secreting parietal cells by diffusion.

Paracrine regulators are secreted by one cell type, and they act upon cells of a different type. However, some cells release regulators that act on that cell itself or on its neighbors of the same cell type. This type of regulation is called **autocrine** regulation. For example, certain nerve terminals release autocrine substances that act on receptors on the nerve terminal to influence the subsequent release of neurotransmitter.

■ *Types of Signal Transduction Pathways*

This section provides a brief overview of some of the major signal transduction pathways that have been characterized. After this section, the discussion turns to a more detailed description of each of these pathways.

■ *Protein Kinases and Phosphatases in Signal Transduction Pathways*

Frequently, the final step in a signal transduction pathway is the phosphorylation of particular proteins that play central roles in eliciting cellular responses. When these effector proteins are phosphorylated, their activities may be enhanced or suppressed. **Protein kinases** in the cell are responsible for phosphorylating particular proteins, whereas **protein phosphatases** catalyze the removal of phosphates from proteins. The state of phosphorylation of an effector protein depends on the balance of the activities of the kinase that phosphorylates it and the phos-

phatase that dephosphorylates it. Protein phosphatases are discussed later in this chapter.

Often, a signal transduction pathway alters its activity of a protein kinase in response to the binding of the regulatory molecule, often called an **agonist,** to its membrane receptor. The major classes of agonist-activated protein kinases are shown in Fig. 5-1.

Among the receptor-mediated signals that regulate the activities of protein kinases are the following **second messengers: cyclic AMP, cyclic GMP, Ca⁺⁺, inositol-1, 4, 5-trisphosphate (IP₃),** and **diacylglycerols.** Cells contain protein kinases that are modulated by each of these second messengers. In second messenger signaling mechanisms, binding of an agonist to its membrane receptor often changes the intracellular level of a second messenger, which then modulates the activity of a protein kinase. In the following paragraphs, we discuss some of these second messengers and the protein kinases they modulate.

Cells contain protein kinases whose activities are enhanced by the second messengers, cyclic AMP and cyclic GMP. These kinases are called **cyclic AMP–dependent protein kinases** and **cyclic GMP–dependent protein kinases,** respectively.

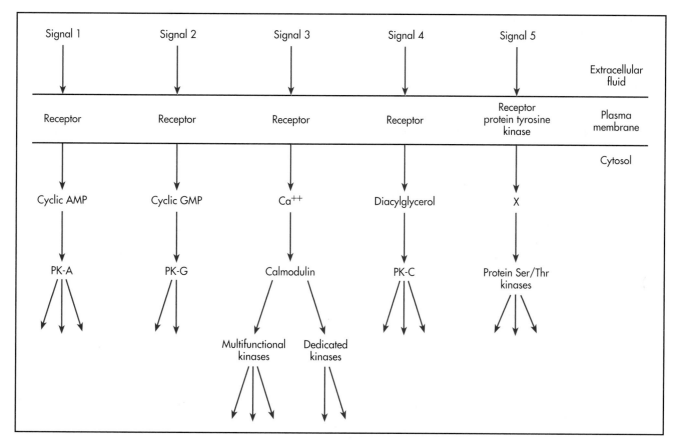

■ **Fig. 5-1** Frequently the final step in a signal transduction pathway is the phosphorylation of an effector protein by a protein kinase. Five major signal transduction pathways of mammalian cells that involve protein kinases are depicted in this diagram. *PK-A,* Cyclic AMP–dependent protein kinase; *PK-G,* cyclic GMP–dependent protein kinase; *PK-C,* protein kinase C; *X,* signaling pathways described later. (Adapted from Cohen P: *Trends Biochem Sci* 17:408, 1992.)

The activities of **calmodulin-dependent protein kinases** are enhanced when they bind to a complex consisting of Ca++ and a protein called **calmodulin.** Calmodulin is a protein (MW 16,700) that is present in all cells; in some cells calmodulin accounts for 1% of the total cellular protein. Calmodulin binds four Ca++ ions; the Ca++-calmodulin complex then regulates a host of other intracellular proteins, many of which are not kinases.

Protein kinases of the **protein kinase C** family are activated by Ca++, diglycerides, certain membrane phospholipids, and certain breakdown products of membrane phospholipids.

Insulin and some **growth factors** bind to membrane receptors that are themselves protein kinases. We discuss these receptors, called protein tyrosine kinase receptors, on p 63.

■ *G Protein–Mediated Signal Transduction Pathways*

Many hormones, neuromodulators, and other regulatory molecules that alter cellular processes do so by signal transduction pathways that involve **heterotrimeric GTP-binding proteins,** also called **G proteins.** (Another class of GTP-binding proteins, monomeric GTP-binding proteins, are discussed later.) A G protein is a molecular switch (Fig. 5-2) that can exist in two states. In its activated ("on") state, a G protein has a higher affinity for GTP. In the inactivated ("off") state, G protein preferentially binds GDP. When agonist molecules bind to them, some membrane receptors interact with a G protein to promote conversion of the G protein to its activated state by binding GTP. The activated G protein can then interact with many **effector proteins,** most notably enzymes or ion channels, to alter their activities. The activated G protein has GTPase activity, so that the bound GTP is eventually hydrolyzed to GDP, and the G protein reverts to its inactive state (Fig. 5-2).

Among the most important targets of activated G proteins are molecules that change the cellular concentrations of the second messengers cyclic AMP, cyclic GMP, Ca++, IP3, and diacylglycerol (Fig. 5-3). G protein–mediated mechanisms are powerful modulators of **adenylyl cyclase** and **cyclic GMP phosphodiesterase,** the enzymes responsible for the synthesis of cyclic AMP and the breakdown of cyclic GMP, respectively. Ca++ channels may be modulated directly by G proteins or indirectly by second messenger–dependent protein kinases. Other effectors that are modulated by G proteins include certain K+ channels and phospholipases C, A₂, and D.

In brief, the G protein–protein kinase–mediated signal transduction pathway involves the following events (Fig. 5-3):

1. A hormone or other regulatory molecule binds to its plasma membrane receptor.
2. The ligand-bearing receptor interacts with a G protein and activates it, and the activated G protein binds GTP.
3. The activated G protein interacts with one or more of the following: adenylyl cyclase; cyclic GMP phosphodiesterase; Ca++ or K+ channels; or phospholipases C, A2, or D to activate or inhibit them.
4. The cellular level of one or more of the following second messengers increases or decreases: cyclic AMP, cyclic GMP, Ca++, IP_3, or diacylglycerol.
5. The increase or decrease of the concentration of a second messenger changes the activity of one or more second messenger–dependent protein kinases such as cyclic AMP–dependent protein kinase, cyclic GMP–dependent protein kinase, calmodulin-dependent protein kinase, or protein kinase C; or the change in second messenger concentration activates an ion channel.
6. The level of phosphorylation of an enzyme or an ion channel is altered, or an ion channel activity changes and brings about the final cellular response.

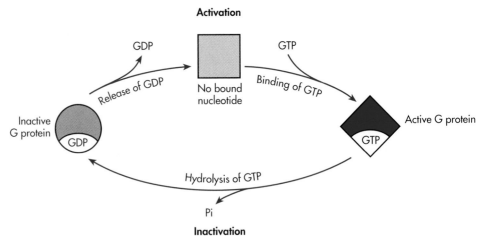

■ **Fig. 5-2** The activity cycle of a GTP-binding protein (G protein). The inactive form of the G protein *(circle)* binds GDP. Interaction of the G protein with a ligand-bearing membrane receptor promotes a conformational change leading to the release of GDP and the binding of GTP. The GTP bound form of the G protein *(diamond)* is the active form that interacts with proteins such as adenylyl cyclase and ion channels to alter their activities. The G protein has an intrinsic GTPase activity; hydrolysis of GTP converts the G protein back to its inactive state.

Membrane Phospholipids and Signal Transduction Pathways

Another class of extracellular agonists binds to receptors that activate, via a G protein called G_q, the β isoform of **phospholipase C.** This isoform cleaves phosphatidyl-inositol-4,5-bisphosphate (a phospholipid present in minute quantities in the plasma membrane) into **inositol-1,4,5-trisphosphate (IP_3)** and **diacylglycerol** (Fig. 5-4). Both IP_3 and diacylglycerol are second messengers. IP_3 binds to specific ligand-gated Ca^{++} channels in the endoplasmic reticulum and releases Ca^{++}, thus increasing its cytosolic concentration. The Ca^{++} channel of the endoplasmic reticulum has a structure similar to that of the Ca^{++} channel of the sarcoplasmic reticulum, which is involved in excitation-contraction coupling in skeletal and cardiac muscle (see Chapters 18 and 23). Diacylglycerol, together with Ca^{++}, activates another important class of protein kinases called **protein kinase C.** Among the substrates of protein kinase C are proteins involved in the control of cellular division.

The enzymes **phospholipase A_2 (PLA_2)** and **phospholipase D** are also activated by some agonists via G protein–dependent pathways. These enzymes act on membrane phospholipids, and products of these reactions also activate protein kinase C (discussed later). PLA_2 cleaves the no. 2 fatty acid from membrane phospholipids. Because some of the phospholipids contain arachidonic acid, PLA_2-mediated cleavage of these phospholipids releases significant amounts of **arachidonic acid.**

Arachidonic acid is an effector molecule in its own right, as well as the precursor for the cellular synthesis of **prostaglandins, prostacyclins, thromboxanes,** and **leukotrienes,** which are important classes of potent regulatory molecules. Arachidonic acid can also be produced from the breakdown of diacylglycerols.

Prostaglandins, prostacyclins, and thromboxanes are synthesized from arachidonic acid via the **cyclooxygenase-dependent pathway.** Leukotrienes are derived from arachidonic acid via the **lipoxygenase-dependent pathway.** One of the anti-inflammatory actions of corticosteroids (see Chapter 51) is to inhibit the phospholipase A_2 that releases arachidonic acid from phospholipids. Aspirin and other nonsteroidal anti-inflammatory agents inhibit the oxidation of arachidonic acid by cyclooxygenase.

Protein Tyrosine Kinases

Proteins with intrinsic **protein tyrosine kinase** activity represent another family of membrane receptors that are not linked to G proteins. When an agonist (such as a growth factor) binds to these receptors, their tyrosine kinase activity is stimulated and they phosphorylate specific effector proteins on particular tyrosine residues. The other protein kinases that have previously been discussed only phosphorylate proteins on serine and threonine residues. The receptor for the hormone insulin and receptors for many growth factors are tyrosine kinases. Most

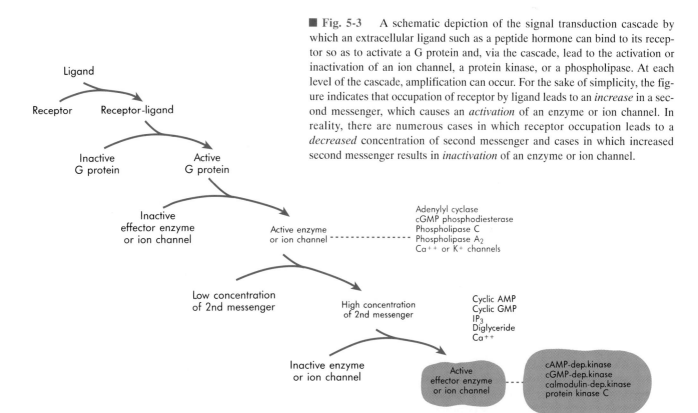

■ **Fig. 5-3** A schematic depiction of the signal transduction cascade by which an extracellular ligand such as a peptide hormone can bind to its receptor so as to activate a G protein and, via the cascade, lead to the activation or inactivation of an ion channel, a protein kinase, or a phospholipase. At each level of the cascade, amplification can occur. For the sake of simplicity, the figure indicates that occupation of receptor by ligand leads to an *increase* in a second messenger, which causes an *activation* of an enzyme or ion channel. In reality, there are numerous cases in which receptor occupation leads to a *decreased* concentration of second messenger and cases in which increased second messenger results in *inactivation* of an enzyme or ion channel.

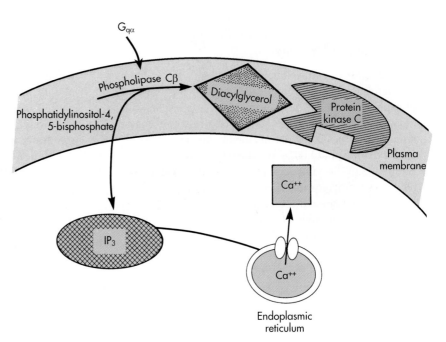

■ **Fig. 5-4** The signal transduction pathway activated by the hydrolysis of inositol phospholipids of the plasma membrane. Some agonists bind to receptors that activate the G_q class of heterotrimeric G proteins. Activated G_q stimulates the activity of phospholipase $C\beta$ to hydrolyze the minor membrane phospholipid phosphatidylinositol-4,5-bisphosphate. This cleavage releases IP_3 and diacylglycerol, both of which are second messengers. IP_3 binds to a specific Ca^{++} channel in the endoplasmic reticulum membrane, causing Ca^{++} to be released. Diacylglycerol, together with Ca^{++}, activates protein kinase C to phosphorylate important cellular effector proteins.

growth factor receptors dimerize when a growth factor binds to them. Dimerization activates the tyrosine kinase activity. Often, the activated receptors phosphorylate themselves, a process called autophosphorylation.

■ *G Protein–Linked Membrane Receptors*

Membrane receptors that mediate agonist-dependent activation of G proteins make up a protein family with more than 500 members. This family includes α- and β-adrenergic receptors, muscarinic acetylcholine receptors, serotonin receptors, adenosine receptors, olfactory receptors, rhodopsin, and receptors for most peptide hormones. The members of the G protein–coupled receptor family (Fig. 5-5) have seven transmembrane α helices, each consisting of 22 to 28 predominantly hydrophobic amino acids.

Many subtypes of G protein–linked receptors exist for certain ligands, such as acetylcholine, epinephrine, norepinephrine, and serotonin. The subtypes can often be distinguished by differing affinities for competing agonists and antagonists.

The remainder of this chapter focuses in more detail on the mechanisms of these signal transduction pathways.

■ *GTP-Binding Proteins (G Proteins)*

As we have seen, GTP-binding proteins, also known as G proteins, bind and hydrolyze GTP. They serve as molecular switches that regulate a host of intracellular processes. The active form of a G protein has a high

affinity for GTP (Fig. 5-2). The intrinsic GTPase activity of the G protein hydrolyzes GTP, which causes the G protein to revert to its inactive GDP-bound form. Active G proteins modulate many vital cellular activities by binding to and modifying the activity of certain important enzymes and ion channels. Two classes of G proteins are known: **heterotrimeric G proteins** and **monomeric GTP-binding proteins** (also called **low-molecular-weight** or **small G proteins**).

■ *Heterotrimeric G Proteins*

A heterotrimeric G protein has three subunits: an α subunit (40,000 to 45,000 daltons), a β subunit (about 37,000 daltons), and a γ subunit (8,000 to 10,000 daltons). Currently, we know of about 20 different genes that encode subunits, at least four genes that encode β subunits, and about seven genes that encode γ subunits in mammals. The function and specificity of a G protein are usually, but not always, determined by its subunit. In most G proteins, the β and γ subunits are tightly associated with one another. Some heterotrimeric G proteins and the signal transduction pathways they mediate are listed in Table 5-1.

Heterotrimeric G proteins function as intermediaries between the plasma membrane receptors for over 100 different extracellular regulatory substances (e.g., hormones, neuromodulators) and the intracellular processes they control. Simply put, binding of the regulatory substance to its receptor activates the G protein; the activated G protein then either stimulates or inhibits an enzyme or an ion channel.

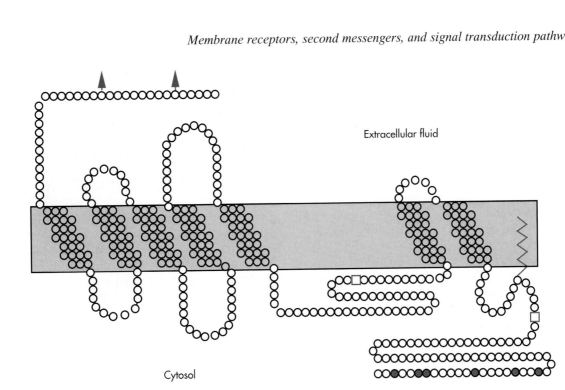

■ **Fig. 5-5** Proposed structure of the human β_2-adrenergic receptor. Sites for *N*-linked glycosylation of the extracellular domain are indicated by arrows. Phosphorylation of the receptor promotes its desensitization (bound agonist elicits diminished response). Colored circles indicate serine and threonine residues near the C terminus that are phosphorylated by β-adrenergic receptor kinase. Colored squares indicate amino acids that are phosphorylated by cyclic AMP–dependent protein kinase. The colored zigzag line represents covalently bound palmitic acid. (Modified from Dohlman HG et al: *Annu Rev Biochem* 60:653, 1991.)

■ **Table 5-1** Selected mammalian heterotrimeric GTP-binding proteins classified on the basis of their α subunits*

G protein	Activated by receptors for	Effectors	Signalling pathways
G_s	Epinephrine, norepinephrine, histamine, glucagon, ACTH, luteinizing hormone, follicle-stimulating hormone, thyroid-stimulating hormone, and others	Adenylyl cyclase Ca^{++} channels	↑ cAMP ↑ Ca^{++} influx
G_{olf}	Odorants	Adenylyl cyclase	↑ cAMP (olfaction)
G_{t1} (rods)	Photons	cGMP phosphodiesterase	↓ cGMP (vision)
G_{t2} (cones)	Photons	cGMP phosphodiesterase	↓ cGMP (color vision)
G_{i1}, G_{i2}, G_{i3}	Norepinephrine, prostaglandins, opiates, angiotensin, many peptides	Adenylyl cyclase Phospholipase C Phospholipase A$_2$ K$^+$ channels	↓ cAMP ↑ Inositol trisphosphate, diacylglycerol, Ca^{++} Arachidonate release Membrane polarization
G_q	Acetylcholine, epinephrine	Phospholipase Cβ	↑ Inositol trisphosphate, diacylglycerol, Ca^{++}

Adapted from Bourne HR, Sanders DA, McCormick F: *Nature* 348:125, 1990.

ACTH, Adrenocorticotropic hormone.

*There is more than one isoform of each class of α subunit; more than 20 distinct α subunits have been identified.

In most G proteins the subunit is the "business end" of the heterotrimeric G protein (Fig. 5-6). The activation of most G proteins involves a conformation change in the subunit. Inactive G proteins exist primarily as $\alpha\beta\gamma$ heterotrimers, with GDP in their nucleotide-binding sites.

The interaction of the heterotrimeric G protein with a ligand-bearing receptor causes an α subunit to change to the active form, which has a higher affinity for GTP and a lower affinity for the $\beta\gamma$ pair. Therefore, the activated α subunit releases GDP, binds GTP, and then dissociates from $\beta\gamma$. In most G proteins, the dissociated α subunit then interacts with the next protein in the signal transduction pathway. *In some G proteins, however, the $\beta\gamma$ dimer appears to be responsible for all or some of the receptor-mediated response.*

Regulation of adenylyl cyclase. Cyclic AMP was the first of the second messengers to be discovered, and the regulation of adenylyl cyclase, the enzyme that produces cyclic AMP, is the prototype for G protein–mediated signal transduction pathways.

Adenylyl cyclase is subject to both positive and negative control by G protein–mediated pathways (Fig. 5-6). In positive control, the binding of a stimulatory ligand, such as epinephrine acting through β-adrenergic receptors, results in activation of heterotrimeric G proteins with α subunits of the type called α_s (s for stimulatory). Activation of the G_s-type G protein by the ligand-bearing receptor causes its α_s subunit to bind GTP and then to dissociate from $\beta\gamma$. α_s then interacts with adenylyl cyclase to activate it.

Other regulatory substances, such as epinephrine acting at α_2 receptors and adenosine acting on α_1 receptors, participate in negative or inhibiting control of adenylyl cyclase. These regulatory substances activate G_i-type G proteins that have α subunits of a type called $\boldsymbol{\alpha_i}$ (*i* for inhibitory). Binding of the inhibitory ligand to its receptor activates the G_i-type G protein and causes its α_i subunit to dissociate from the $\beta\gamma$ dimers. The activated α_i binds to and inhibits adenylyl cyclase. In addition, the $\beta\gamma$ dimers may bind to free α_s subunits. In this way, the binding of $\beta\gamma$ dimers to free α_s subunits further diminishes the stimulation of adenylyl cyclase by blocking the action of stimulatory ligands.

Cholera causes a watery diarrhea that can rapidly lead to dehydration and death if not promptly treated. The diarrhea is caused by a toxin produced by the bacterium **Vibrio cholerae.** A component of the cholera toxin enters the cells and catalyzes the covalent addition of ADP-ribose to the $G_s\alpha$ subunit. This reaction permanently activates G_s, which results in persistent activation of adenylyl cyclase. As a consequence, cyclic AMP is permanently elevated. The brush border membrane that faces the lumen of the small intestine contains an electrogenic chloride channel that opens when cyclic AMP levels are elevated (see Chapter 39). The persistent activation of this Cl^- channel causes Cl^-, Na^+, and water to pour into the lumen of the small intestine. The result of this secretion is the persistent watery diarrhea of as much as 20 L per day that characterizes cholera.

Direct modulation of ion channels by G proteins. In Chapter 4, several ligand-gated ion channels that are modulated directly by an extracellular agonist, such as acetylcholine or γ-aminobutyric acid, were discussed. Other ion channels are regulated by second messenger–mediated mechanisms that involve G proteins. The regulation of these ion channels takes place after G proteins are activated in the second step of the signal transduction cascade.

Some ion channels, however, are *directly modulated by G proteins and do not involve a second messenger.* The binding of acetylcholine to M_2 muscarinic receptors in the heart and in certain neurons, for instance, leads to the activation of a specific class of K^+ channels. In this example, acetylcholine binding to the muscarinic recep-

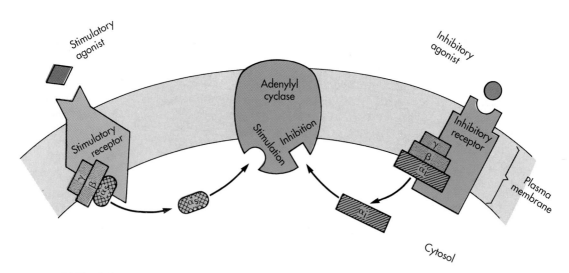

■ **Fig. 5-6**   Adenylyl cyclase may be stimulated or inhibited via signal transduction pathways. Receptors for agonists that stimulate adenylyl cyclase activate G_s, whose α_s subunit dissociates from $\beta\gamma$ and then interacts with adenylyl cyclase to stimulate it. Receptors for agonists that inhibit adenylyl cyclase activate G_i, whose α_i subunit inhibits adenylyl cyclase.

tor leads to activation of a G protein of the G_i subclass. The activated α_i subunit then dissociates from the $\beta\gamma$ dimer. *The $\beta\gamma$ dimer directly interacts with a particular class of K^+ channels* to increase their probability of opening. The action of acetylcholine on muscarinic receptors to increase K^+ conductance of the pacemaker cells in the sinoatrial node of the heart is one of the major mechanisms whereby parasympathetic nerves cause slowing of the heartbeat (see Chapter 24).

■ *Monomeric GTP-Binding Proteins*

Cells contain another family of GTP-binding proteins called **monomeric GTP-binding proteins;** they are also known as **low-molecular-weight G proteins** or **small G proteins** (MW 20,000 to 35,000 daltons). Table 5-2 lists the major subfamilies of monomeric GTP-binding proteins and some of their properties. The Ras-like and Rho-like monomeric GTP-binding proteins are involved in the signal transduction pathways that link growth factor receptor tyrosine kinases to their intracellular effects. Among the processes that are regulated by pathways that involve monomeric GTP-binding proteins are polypeptide chain elongation in protein synthesis, proliferation and differentiation of cells, neoplastic transformation of cells, control of the actin cytoskeleton and linkages between the cytoskeleton and the extracellular matrix, transport of vesicles among different organelles, and exocytotic secretion.

Monomeric GTP-binding proteins, like their heterotrimeric cousins, are molecular switches that alternate between an "on" (activated) state and an "off" (inactivated) state (Fig. 5-2). However, the activation and inactivation of the monomolecular GTP-binding proteins involve additional regulatory proteins that are not known to operate on the heterotrimeric G proteins (Fig. 5-7). Monomeric GTP-binding proteins are activated by **guanine nucleotide–releasing proteins (GNRPs)** and inactivated by **GTPase–activating proteins (GAPs).** Therefore, activation and inactivation of monomeric GTP-binding proteins are probably controlled by signals that influence the activity of GNRPs or GAPs, rather than by direct effects on the monomeric G protein.

■ *Second Messenger–Dependent Ion Channels*

Most cellular responses mediated by G protein–coupled pathways involve second messenger–dependent protein kinases. However, in some responses, the second messenger acts directly on an ion channel to produce a response. Some cells have a class of K^+ channels that are directly activated by the level of Ca^{++} inside the cell. These channels open in response to the binding of a second messenger. When intracellular Ca^{++} rises, **Ca^{++}-activated K^+ channels** are activated, which leads to repolarization or hyperpolarization of the cell. Both vision and olfaction involve ion channels that are gated by second messengers.

Visual transduction (see Chapter 9) depends on cyclic GMP–gated ion channels. When a person is in a dark room, the level of cyclic GMP in rod photoreceptors is high. Consequently, the **cyclic GMP–activated Na^+ channels** in the rod plasma membrane are open, and the entry of Na^+ into the rod cell maintains its depolarized state. **Rhodopsin** is a member of the family of G protein–coupled receptors and it is activated by light. When activated, it interacts with and activates a heterotrimeric G protein called **transducin (G_t).** Activated transducin interacts with cyclic GMP phosphodiesterase to greatly increase its activity and this effect rapidly decreases the intracellular cyclic GMP concentration. Hence, the cyclic GMP-activated Na^+ channels close and the rod cell is hyperpolarized. Hyperpolarization of rod cells is necessary for visual signals to be conducted to the brain.

Olfaction (see Chapter 11) involves cyclic AMP–gated ion channels. Humans and other vertebrates are able to distinguish a large number of different **odorants.** Many of these odorants interact with G protein–coupled receptors in the plasma membrane of olfactory receptor cells. The odorant-bearing receptor activates G_{olf}, a heterotrimeric G protein. Activated G_{olf}, in turn, stimulates adenylyl cyclase to produce cyclic AMP. Elevated cyclic AMP levels activate **cyclic AMP–gated Na^+ channels** in the plasma membrane of the olfactory receptor cell. Na^+ inflow leads to depolarization of the receptor, which may trigger an action potential in the axon of the olfactory receptor.

■ **Table 5-2**   Subfamilies of monomeric GTP-binding proteins and some of the intracellular processes they regulate

Subfamily	*Cellular effects*
Ras-like proteins	Control growth and differentiation
Rho-like proteins (including Rac)	Control polymerization of actin filaments and their assembly into particular structures such as focal adhesions
Rab-like proteins	Control vesicle trafficking by helping target vesicles to particular membranes
ARF-like proteins	Regulate the assembly and disassembly of vesicle coat proteins and thereby control vesicle traffic

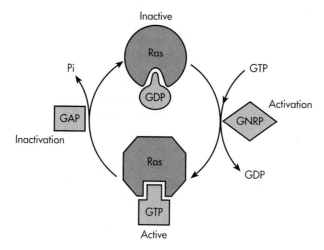

■ **Fig. 5-7**   The activity cycle of Ras, a monomeric GTP-binding protein. Other monomeric GTP-binding proteins have a similar activity cycle. The activation of Ras is stimulated by a **GNRP** (guanine nucleotide–releasing protein), which promotes the binding of GTP and the release of GDP, thereby activating the small G protein. The inactivation of Ras is promoted by a **GAP** (GTPase-activating protein), which stimulates the hydrolysis of the bound GTP, thus inactivating Ras.

■ *Second Messenger–Dependent Protein Kinases*

Cyclic AMP was first identified as a second messenger during investigations of the mechanisms involved in the hormonal control of glycogen synthesis and breakdown (see Chapters 46 and 47). Researchers found that the hormonal regulation of glycogen metabolism involves the phosphorylation of rate-determining enzymes that participate in these metabolic pathways by cyclic AMP–dependent protein kinases.

■ *Cyclic AMP–Dependent Protein Kinase*

In the absence of cyclic AMP, cyclic AMP–dependent protein kinase is composed of four subunits: two regulatory subunits and two catalytic subunits. Most cell types contain the same catalytic subunit, but their regulatory subunits differ significantly. The presence of the regulatory subunits greatly inhibits the enzymatic activity of the complex. Therefore, activation of the enzymatic activity of cyclic AMP–dependent protein kinase must involve the dissociation of the regulating subunits from the complex.

Activation takes place when micromolar levels of cyclic AMP are present. Each regulatory subunit binds two molecules of cyclic AMP. The binding of cyclic AMP induces a conformational change in the regulatory subunits and diminishes their affinity for binding the cat-

alytic subunits. Hence, the regulatory subunits dissociate from the catalytic subunits, and the catalytic subunits become activated (Fig. 5-8). The active catalytic subunit phosphorylates target proteins on particular serine and threonine residues.

Comparison of the amino acid sequence of cyclic AMP–dependent protein kinase with representatives of the other classes of protein kinases shows that, despite vast differences in their regulatory properties, the different classes of protein kinases share a common core with high amino acid homology (Fig. 5-9). The core structure includes the ATP-binding domain and the enzyme's active center, where the transfer of phosphate from ATP to the acceptor protein occurs. Regions of the kinases outside the catalytic core are involved in regulation of the kinase activities.

The crystal structure of the catalytic subunit of cyclic AMP–dependent protein kinase has also been determined. The catalytic core that is conserved among all known protein kinases consists of two lobes. The smaller of the two lobes contains an unusual ATP-binding site, whereas the larger lobe contains the peptide-binding site. Many protein kinases also contain a regulatory region known as a **pseudosubstrate domain.** The amino acid sequence of this site resembles the phosphorylation sites of substrate proteins. The pseudosubstrate region binds to the active site of the protein kinase and inhibits the phosphorylation of true substrates of the protein kinase. Activation of the kinase may involve phosphorylation or a noncovalent allo-

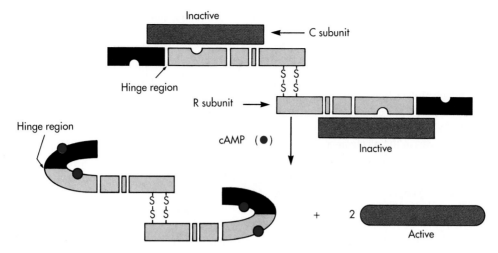

■ **Fig. 5-8**   Activation of cyclic AMP–dependent protein kinase. The two regulatory subunits (R subunit) of the R_2C_2 complex are held together by two disulfide bonds. Binding of two molecules of cyclic AMP to each R subunit causes flexion in a hinge region of each R subunit and the release of the two active catalytic subunits (C subunits). (Adapted from Taylor S: *J Biol Chem* 264:8443, 1989.)

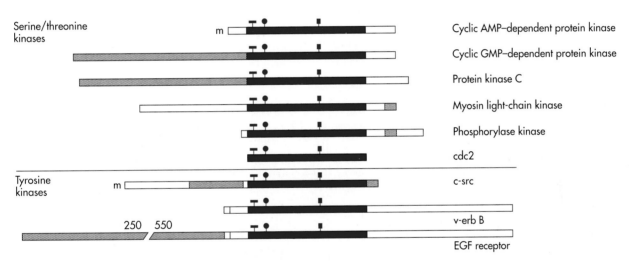

■ **Fig. 5-9**   The protein kinase family. All known protein kinases share a common catalytic core *(solid color)* that contains ATP- and peptide-binding domains and the active site where phosphoryl transfer occurs. Conserved residues are aligned with lysine 72 *(colored circle)*, aspartate 184 *(colored square)*, and the glycine-rich loop *(small colored rectangle)* of the catalytic subunit of cyclic AMP–dependent protein kinase. Regions important for regulation are cross-hatched. Sites of covalent attachment of myristic acid are indicated by *m*. This fatty acid helps to anchor the protein kinase to the plasma membrane. (Adapted from Taylor S et al: *Annu Rev Cell Biol* 8:429, 1992.)

steric modification of the protein kinase to remove the inhibition of the pseudosubstrate domain.

■ *Calmodulin-Dependent Protein Kinases*

A host of vital cellular processes, including release of neurotransmitters, secretion of hormones, and muscle contraction, are regulated by the cytosolic level of Ca^{++}. One way that Ca^{++} exerts control over these processes is by binding to the protein calmodulin. The Ca^{++}-calmodulin complex can then influence the activity of many different proteins, among them a group of protein kinases known as **calmodulin-dependent protein kinases** (Fig. 5-10). Some calmodulin-dependent protein kinases, such as myosin light chain kinase and phosphorylase kinase, have only one cellular substrate. Others are multifunctional and phosphorylate more than one substrate protein.

Myosin light chain kinase plays a central role in the regulation of contraction of smooth muscle (see Chapter

19). Elevation of the cytosolic Ca^{++} concentration in a smooth muscle cell stimulates the activity of myosin light chain kinase; the resultant phosphorylation of the regulatory light chains of myosin allows contraction of smooth muscle cells to proceed.

Calmodulin-dependent protein kinase II is among the most abundant proteins in the nervous system; it accounts for as much as 2% of total protein in certain regions of the brain. This kinase participates in the mechanism by which an increase in Ca^{++} concentration in a nerve terminal causes exocytotic release of neurotransmitter. Its preferred substrate is a protein called **synapsin I**, which is present in nerve terminals and binds to the external surface of synaptic vesicles. When synapsin I is bound to vesicles, it apparently prevents exocytosis; phosphorylation of synapsin I causes it to dissociate from the vesicles and allows the vesicle to release neurotransmitter by exocytosis.

■ *Protein Kinase C*

Protein kinase C plays a vital role in the control of certain cellular processes. For example, the primary action of certain lipophilic tumor-promoting substances, most notably the **phorbol esters,** is to activate protein kinase

C directly. This activating of protein kinase C powerfully stimulates cell division in many cell types. It also converts normal cells with controlled growth properties into transformed cells that grow uncontrollably. These transformed cells thus resemble tumor cells.

The best-known pathway of activation of protein kinase C is as follows. In an unstimulated cell, much of the protein kinase C is present in the cytosol and is inactive. When cytosolic levels of Ca^{++} rise, Ca^{++} binds to protein kinase C. This binding of Ca^{++} causes protein kinase C to bind to the inner surface of the plasma membrane, where it can be activated by the diacylglycerol that is produced by the hydrolysis of phosphatidylinositol bisphosphate. Membrane phosphatidylserine is also a potent activator of protein kinase C, once the enzyme has bound to the membrane.

About 10 different isoforms of protein kinase C have been discovered (Table 5-3). Although particular subtypes are present in many or most mammalian cells, the γ and ϵ subtypes are found predominantly in certain cells of the central nervous system. In addition to being differentially distributed among the cells and tissues of the body, the subtypes of protein kinase C also appear to be differentially regulated (Table 5-3). Some of the subtypes may be bound to the plasma membrane in unstimulated

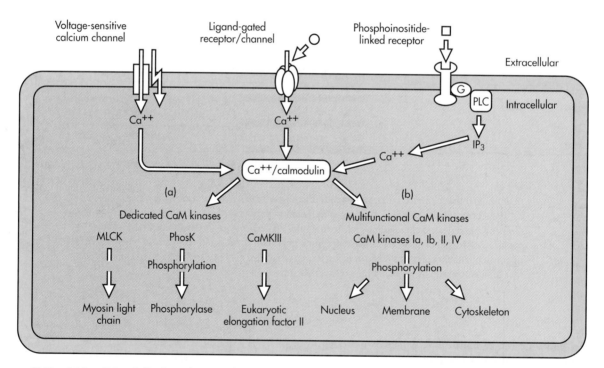

■ **Fig. 5-10**   Calmodulin-dependent protein kinases are the final steps in many signal transduction pathways that are elicited by an increase in cytosolic Ca^{++} levels. Cytosolic Ca^{++} may rise because of Ca^{++} influx via a voltage- or ligand-gated ion channel or by the release of Ca^{++} from internal stores by IP3. The complex of Ca^{++} with calmodulin activates calmodulin-dependent protein kinases. Dedicated calmodulin (CaM)-dependent protein kinases phosphorylate specific effector proteins such as the regulatory light chain of myosin, phosphorylase, and elongation factor II. Multifunctional calmodulin-dependent protein kinases phosphorylate multiple proteins of the nucleus or cytoskeleton or membrane proteins. *PLC,* Phospholipase C; *MLCK,* myosin light chain kinase; *PhosK,* phosphorylase kinase; *CaMKIII,* calmodulin-dependent kinase III. (Adapted from Schulman H: *Curr Opin Cell Biol* 5:247, 1993.)

cells and thus do not require elevated Ca++ for activation. Some of the isoforms of protein kinase C are activated by arachidonic acid, by other unsaturated fatty acids, or by lysophospholipids.

An initial, short-lived activation of protein kinase C may be caused by diacylglycerol, released when phospholipase Cβ is activated, and by Ca++, released from internal stores by IP$_3$ (Fig. 5-11). A longer-lasting activation of protein kinase C may be caused by receptor-activated phospholipases A$_2$ and D. These enzymes act primarily on phosphatidylcholine, the major membrane phospholipid. Phospholipase A$_2$ cleaves the number 2 fatty acid from phosphatidylcholine to liberate a fatty acid (mostly unsaturated fatty acids) and a lysophosphatidylcholine. Both of these products activate certain protein kinase C isoforms (Table 5-3). Receptor-activated phospholipase D cleaves phosphatidylcholine to produce phosphatidic acid and choline. The phosphatidic acid is further broken down to diacylglycerol, which participates in long-term stimulation of protein kinase C.

■ **Table 5-3**   Properties of mammalian isozymes of protein kinase C

Group	Subspecies	Apparent molecular mass (Da)	Activators	Tissue expression
cPKC	α	76,799	Ca++, DAG, PS, FFA, LysoPC	Universal
	βI	76,790	Ca++, DAG, PS, FFA, LysoPC	Some tissues
	βII	76,933	Ca++, DAG, PS, FFA, LysoPC	Many tissues
	γ	78,366	Ca++, DAG, PS, FFA, LysoPC	Brain only
nPKC	δ	77,517	DAG, PS	Universal
	ϵ	83,474	DAG, PS, FFA	Brain and others
	η (L)	77,972	?	Lung, skin, heart
	θ	81,571	?	Skeletal muscle (mainly)
aPKC	ζ	67,740	PS, FFA	Universal
	λ	67,200	?	Ovary, testis, and others

Adapted from Asaoka Y et al: *Trends Biochem Sci* 17:414, 1992.
DAG, Diacylglycerol; *PS,* phosphatidylserine; *FFA, cis*-unsaturated fatty acids; *LysoPC,* lysophosphatidylcholine.

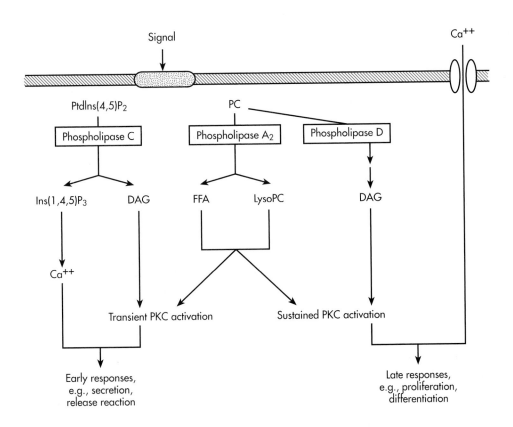

■ **Fig. 5-11** Activation of protein kinase C (PKC) by degradation of membrane phospholipids. Rapid and transient activation of PKC is effected by IP$_3$ *[Ins (1,4,5) P$_3$]* and diacylglycerol *(DAG)* formed by the degradation of phosphatidylinositol bisphosphate *[PtdIns(4,5)P$_2$]* by a specific receptor-activated phospholipase C. Slower and more sustained activation of PKC is caused by degradation of phosphatidylcholine *(PC)* by receptor-activated phospholipases A$_2$ and D. Free fatty acids (FFA), lysolecithin *(lysoPC)*, and diacylglycerol *(DAG)* released by these enzymes acting on PC stimulate PKC. (Adapted from Asaoka Y et al: *Trends Biochem Sci* 17:414, 1992.)

■ *Tyrosine Kinases*

■ *Receptor Tyrosine Kinases*

The receptors for certain peptide hormones and growth factors are proteins with a glycosylated extracellular domain, a single transmembrane sequence, and an intracellular domain with protein tyrosine kinase activity. Members of this superfamily (Fig. 5-12) of peptide receptors include the receptors for insulin and related growth factors, epidermal growth factor (EGF), nerve growth factor (NGF), platelet-derived growth factor (PDGF), colony-stimulating factor (CSF), fibroblast growth factor (FGF), and hepatocyte growth factor (HGF). The binding of hormone or growth factor to its receptor triggers multiple cellular responses, including Ca^{++} influx, increased Na^+-H^+ exchange, stimulation of the uptake of sugars and amino acids, and stimulation of phospholipase $C\beta$ and hydrolysis of phosphatidylinositol bisphosphate.

The known protein–tyrosine kinase receptors fall into eight subfamilies, four of which are shown in Fig. 5-12. In general, the mechanism by which these receptors trigger cellular responses begins with the binding of ligand (the hormone or growth factor) to the receptor, which results in dimerization of the receptor-ligand complexes. The dimerization enhances binding affinity and activates the protein–tyrosine kinase activity of the receptor. Each monomer in a dimer phosphorylates the other monomer on multiple tyrosine residues. The tyrosines that are phosphorylated reside in the kinase insert regions of subfamilies III and IV or in the carboxyl terminal tail of the receptor. (In contrast to receptor tyrosine kinases, phosphorylation of the receptor protein on serines or threonines by other kinases, such as protein kinase C, may diminish the tyrosine kinase activity of the receptor.) In subclass II receptors, the insulin receptor family, the unliganded receptor exists as a disulfide-linked dimer, and binding of insulin results in a conformational change of both "monomers." This conformational change enhances insulin binding and activates the receptor's tyrosine kinase activity, which leads to enhanced autophosphorylation of the receptor.

Protein tyrosine kinases that are "out of control" play a central role in cell transformation and cancer. In some cell types, growth factor receptor mutation causes the receptor to actively phosphorylate tyrosines, regardless of the presence or absence of the growth factor. Other tumor cells secrete a growth factor and overexpress its receptor. This situation leads to abnormally high rates of protein–tyrosine kinase activity.

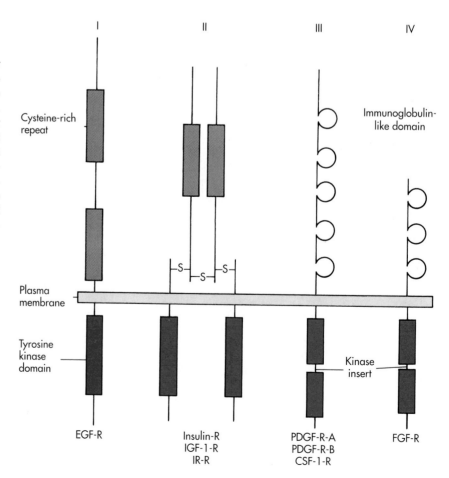

■ **Fig. 5-12** The structures of four subfamilies of receptor protein–tyrosine kinases are depicted; eight subfamilies have been identified. Subfamilies I and II have extracellular domains with cysteine-rich repeat sequence domains *(light color)*, while the extracellular domains of subclasses III and IV have immunoglobulin-like regions *(loops)*. The protein–tyrosine kinase domains *(solid color)* are the most conserved sequences. A short intracellular region, the kinase insert region (quite variable in length), and the carboxyl terminal tail are sites of regulation of protein kinase activity. *EGF,* Epidermal growth factor; *IGF-1,* insulin-like growth factor-1; *IR,* insulin-related protein; *PDGF,* platelet-derived growth factor; *CSF-1,* colony-stimulating factor-1; *FGF,* fibroblast growth factor. (Adapted from Ullrich A, Schlessinger J: *Cell* 61:203, 1990.)

Monomeric GTP-binding proteins of the Ras family (Table 5-2) are involved in coupling the binding of mitogenic ligands and their tyrosine–protein kinase receptors to the intracellular effects on cell proliferation that result. When Ras is inactive, cells cannot respond to the growth factors that operate via receptor tyrosine kinases.

Mutations in Ras may produce overactive forms of Ras that constitutively activate the effectors that ultimately lead to cell division. These effectors are normally active only in the presence of growth factors. As a result of the continued activation of these effectors, cell growth may be uncontrolled. Approximately 30% of human cancers involve mutated Ras proteins.

Activation of Ras by an activated receptor tyrosine kinase in turn activates a signal transduction pathway that ultimately turns on the transcription of certain key genes that promote cell growth. The **MAP (mitogen–activated protein) kinase cascade** (Fig. 5-13) is involved in the responses to activated Ras. Protein kinase C also activates the MAP kinase cascade. Thus, the MAP kinase cascade is an important point of convergence for multiple

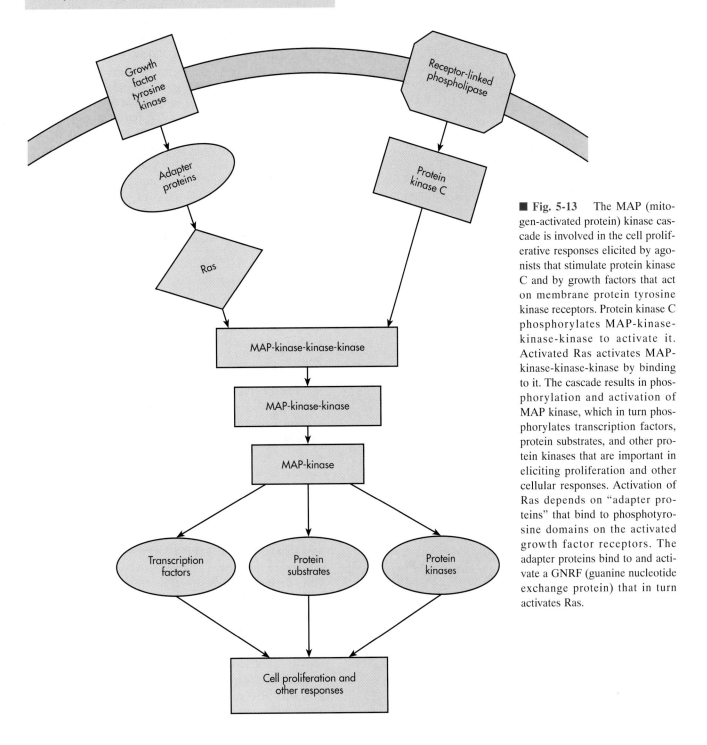

■ **Fig. 5-13** The MAP (mitogen-activated protein) kinase cascade is involved in the cell proliferative responses elicited by agonists that stimulate protein kinase C and by growth factors that act on membrane protein tyrosine kinase receptors. Protein kinase C phosphorylates MAP-kinase-kinase-kinase to activate it. Activated Ras activates MAP-kinase-kinase-kinase by binding to it. The cascade results in phosphorylation and activation of MAP kinase, which in turn phosphorylates transcription factors, protein substrates, and other protein kinases that are important in eliciting proliferation and other cellular responses. Activation of Ras depends on "adapter proteins" that bind to phosphotyrosine domains on the activated growth factor receptors. The adapter proteins bind to and activate a GNRF (guanine nucleotide exchange protein) that in turn activates Ras.

effectors that promote cellular proliferation. Moreover, there is significant cross-talk between the protein kinase C and the tyrosine kinase pathways near their starting points. For example, the γ isoform of phospholipase C is activated by binding to activated Ras; this activation turns on protein kinase C via activation of phospholipid hydrolysis.

■ *Receptor-Associated Tyrosine Kinases*

The receptors for **growth hormone, prolactin,** and **erythropoetin** (as well as receptors for interferon and many cytokines) are not themselves protein kinases. However, upon activation, these receptors form signaling complexes with intracellular tyrosine kinases that bring about their intracellular effects (Fig. 5-14). Because they are not true receptor tyrosine kinases but merely bind to

them, these receptors are called **receptor-associated tyrosine kinases.** The mechanism by which these receptors induce intracellular effects begins when a hormone binds to the receptor, which induces dimerization of the hormone receptor. The receptor dimer binds one or more members of the **Janus family of tyrosine kinases (JAK).** The JAKs then cross-phosphorylate one another and also phosphorylate the receptor. Members of the **signal transducers and activators of transcription (STAT) family** bind to phosphotyrosine domains on the complex of receptor and JAK proteins. The STAT proteins are phosphorylated by the JAKs and then dissociate from the signaling complex. Finally, the phosphorylated STAT proteins form dimers that move to the nucleus to activate the transcription of certain genes.

Specificity of the receptor for each hormone derives partly from the particular members of the JAK and STAT family that are recruited to the signaling complex. In some instances, the signaling complex also activates the MAP kinase cascade via the same adapter proteins used by the receptor tyrosine kinases. Some of the responses to receptor tyrosine kinase ligands also involve the JAK-STAT pathway.

■ *Protein Phosphatases and Their Modulation*

Phosphorylation of proteins is one of the most important means by which protein activities are regulated. The extent of phosphorylation of a regulated protein results from the activities of the protein kinase that phosphorylates that protein and the protein phosphatase that dephosphorylates it. In addition to the different types of protein kinases that we have discussed, all cells also contain **protein phosphatases** that reverse the effects of protein phosphorylation. In keeping with the classification of protein kinases, protein phosphatases are classified as **serine-threonine protein phosphatases** or **tyrosine protein phosphatases.**

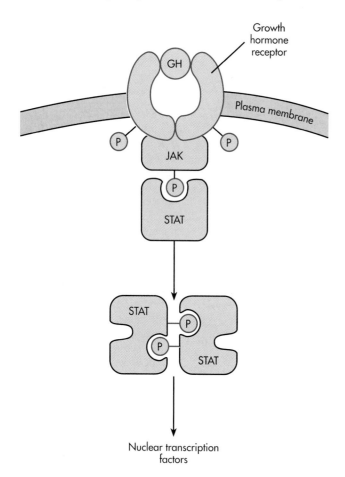

■ **Fig. 5-14** Receptors for growth hormone *(GH)*, prolactin, and certain other ligands have no intrinsic tyrosine kinase activity. The growth hormone receptor dimerizes in response to GH binding. The dimeric receptor binds one or more JAK tyrosine kinases, which phosphorylate themselves and the receptor. STAT tyrosine kinases bind to the complex and are phosphorylated. The phosphorylated STATs dissociate as dimers that are translocated to the nucleus, where they phosphorylate key transcription factors. *JAK,* Janus family of tyrosine kinases; *STAT,* signal transducers and activators of transcription.

■ *Serine-Threonine Protein Phosphatases*

The serine-threonine protein phosphatases are a large family of structurally related molecules. Currently, they are classified as type 1 **(PP-1)** or type 2 **(PP-2).** The type is based on the subunit of phosphorylase kinase they prefer to dephosphorylate. PP-1s prefer the β subunit, while PP-2s prefer the α subunit of phosphorylase kinase (Table 5-4). The PP-2s are subclassifed into PP-2A, PP-2B, and PP-2C, based on their regulation by divalent cations. PP-2A does not require divalent cations for activity. PP-2B has an absolute requirement for the Ca^{++}-calmodulin complex. PP-2C absolutely requires Mg^{++}. PP-2B is also called **calcineurin,** and it is especially abundant in certain regions of the brain. PP-1 and the PP-

2s can also be distinguished by their inhibition by **okadaic acid** (Table 5-4), a complex fatty acid produced by marine dinoflagellates. Okadaic acid is as potent a tumor promoter as the phorbol esters, presumably because both okadaic acid and phorbol esters enhance the phosphorylation of certain substrates of protein kinase C.

PP-1s and PP-2s contain a catalytic core with a significantly homologous amino acid sequence. The PP-2s appear to be mainly cytosolic enzymes. In contrast, PP-1 in the liver is bound to glycogen particles; in muscle, PP-1 is bound to glycogen, to the sarcoplasmic reticulum, and to the myofibrils (the contractile proteins). Cytosolic PP-1 is relatively inactive. Protein subunits of PP-1 are responsible for the binding of PP-1 to specific cellular structures, and this binding appears to direct the activity of PP-1 toward particular physiological substrates.

The activity of PP-1 is also regulated by two classes of **endogenous inhibitor proteins: I-1** and **I-2.** I-1 is an effective inhibitor only when it is phosphorylated by protein kinase A. Phosphorylated I-1 has a high affinity for PP-1. By binding PP-1 and removing it from the subunit that attaches it to glycogen or other cellular structure, it inactivates PP-1. The complex regulation of PP-1 suggests that it plays a key role in cellular regulation.

■ *Protein Tyrosine Phosphatases*

Protein tyrosine phosphatases (PTPases) are not structurally homologous to serine-threonine protein phosphatases. In contrast, we have noted that all the protein kinases apparently derive from a common ancestor protein kinase. Fig. 5-15 schematically depicts four of the 65 PTPases currently known. Note that, while two of the PTPases are small cytosolic proteins, two other PTPases are larger transmembrane proteins. On the basis of their structures, the transmembrane PTPases are probably receptors whose PTPase activity is modulated by extracellular ligands.

Both of the transmembrane PTPases shown in Fig. 5-15 are important molecules. **CD45** is the leukocyte common antigen that is crucial in cell-mediated immune responses. **LAR** (leukocyte common antigen-related protein) has extracellular sequences that are highly homologous to the neural cell adhesion molecule (N-CAM), which is important in the development of the nervous system.

■ *Atrial Natriuretic Peptide Receptor–Guanylyl Cyclases*

Atrial natriuretic peptide (ANP) is released by cells of the atrium of the heart in response to an elevation of atrial pressure (see Chapters 24 and 42). This hormone then acts to increase the excretion of NaCl and water by the kidney (see Chapter 42) and to diminish the constriction of certain blood vessels. The membrane receptor to which ANP binds bears discussion because it does not

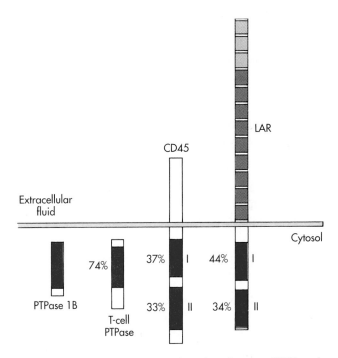

■ **Fig. 5-15** Protein tyrosine phosphatases (PTPases) schematically depicted. About 65 different PTPases have been identified. Shown are two small cytosolic PTPases: PTPase 1B from human placenta and T-cell PTPase from human T lymphocytes. Also shown are two transmembrane PTPases: CD45 (the leukocyte common antigen) and LAR (leukocyte common antigen-related protein). The solid-colored cytosolic segments of each protein are the PTPase catalytic domains. The extracellular domains of LAR are homologous to N-CAM (neural cell adhesion molecule). The lighter-colored domains are homologous to the IgG-like domains; the intermediate-colored domains are homologous to the non–IgG-like domains of N-CAM. (Adapted from Tonks NK, Charbonneau H: *Trends Biochem Sci* 14:497, 1989.)

■ **Table 5-4**   Properties of subtypes of serine-threonine protein phosphatases

Subtype	PP-1	PP-2A	PP-2B	PP-2C
Preference for the α or β subunit of phosphorylase kinase	β subunit	α subunit	α subunit	α subunit
Inhibition by I-1 and I-2	Yes	No	No	No
Absolute requirement for divalent cations	No	No	Yes (Ca^{++})	Yes (Mg^{++})
Stimulation by calmodulin	No	No	Yes	No
Inhibition by okadaic acid (K_i)	Yes (20 nM)	Yes (0.2 nM)	Yes (5 μM)	No
Phosphorylase phosphatase activity	High	High	Very low	Very low

Adapted from Cohen P: *Annu Rev Biochem* 58:453, 1989.

depend on a signal transducing protein to bring about its intracellular effects. Earlier in this chapter, we described the actions of certain extracellular agonists that bind to membrane receptors and either stimulate adenylyl cyclase via G_s heterotrimeric G proteins or inhibit adenylyl cyclase via G_i. Membrane receptors for ANP are notable because *the receptors themselves* possess guanylyl cyclase activity. This activity is stimulated when ANP is bound to the receptor.

ANP receptors have an extracellular ANP-binding domain, a single transmembrane helix, and an intracellular guanylyl cyclase domain. The binding of ANP to the receptor stimulates the guanylyl cyclase activity and elevates intracellular levels of the second messenger cyclic GMP without the intermediation of a G protein or any other signal transducing protein.

The elevated cyclic GMP concentration that occurs when ANP binds to its receptor stimulates cyclic GMP–dependent protein kinase. In contrast to the cyclic AMP–dependent protein kinase, which has regulatory and catalytic subunits, the regulatory and catalytic domains of cyclic GMP–dependent protein kinase reside on a single polypeptide chain. Cyclic GMP–dependent kinase then phosphorylates intracellular proteins to cause various cellular responses.

■ Nitric Oxide

Nitric oxide (NO) is a paracrine mediator that is released by endothelial cells and by certain neurons. Because NO is rapidly oxidized, its biological lifetime is only several seconds. For this reason, NO affects only cells in the immediate vicinity of the cell that produces it. NO stimulates a soluble guanylyl cyclase in the target cell and thereby elevates the intracellular concentration of cyclic GMP in the target cell, thus stimulating cyclic GMP–dependent protein kinase.

The production of NO is catalyzed by **NO synthase,** a Ca^{++}-calmodulin-dependent enzyme that accelerates the conversion of arginine to citrulline plus NO. An increase in cytosolic Ca^{++} levels is often the stimulus for enhanced formation and release of NO. NO is released by nerve terminals of cerebellar granule cells and acts on postsynaptic cerebellar Purkinje cells. NO is also released by endothelial cells in response to agonists such as acetylcholine, which acts on muscarinic receptors to increase intracellular Ca^{++}. NO released by these endothelial cells causes vasodilation in nearby vascular smooth muscle cells (see Chapter 27). In addition, NO is one of the neurotransmitters released by neurons of the enteric nervous system. Acting on gastrointestinal smooth muscle cells, NO inhibits their contractile activity (see Chapter 37).

■ Summary

1. Many regulatory substances exert their effects on cellular processes via signal transduction pathways.

2. Heterotrimeric GTP-binding proteins serve as intermediaries between a receptor that has been activated by binding an agonist and enzymes and ion channels whose activity is modulated in response to agonist binding.

3. A GTP-binding protein is activated by interacting with an agonist-bearing receptor. It then changes the activity of an enzyme or an ion channel, and thereby alters the intracellular concentration of a second messenger, such as cyclic AMP, cyclic GMP, Ca^{++}, IP_3, or diacylglycerol.

4. An increased level of one or more second messengers may increase the activity of a second messenger–dependent protein kinase: cyclic AMP–dependent protein kinase, cyclic GMP–dependent protein kinase, calmodulin-dependent protein kinase, or protein kinase C.

5. Many cellular processes are regulated via the phosphorylation of enzymes and ion channels.

6. Certain membrane receptors for hormones and growth factors are protein tyrosine kinases or are associated with tyrosine kinases that are activated by binding of the agonist.

7. Monomeric GTP-binding proteins are intermediaries between the binding of growth factors to their protein–tyrosine kinase receptors and the downstream effects on cellular proliferation. The small G proteins also regulate the function of the actin cytoskeleton and intracellular vesicular trafficking.

8. Protein phosphatases, which are themselves subject to complex regulation by agonists and second messengers, reverse the effects of protein phosphorylation.

■ Self-Study Problems

1. Describe the cycle of activation and inactivation of a heterotrimeric G protein.

2. Describe the stimulation and inhibition of adenylyl cyclase by heterotrimeric G proteins.

3. Describe the best-known pathway for activation of protein kinase C.

4. Concisely describe the pathway by which binding of an extracellular peptide growth factor to its receptor tyrosine kinase leads to enhanced cellular proliferation.

■ *Bibliography*

Journal articles

Berridge MJ: Inositol trisphosphates and calcium signalling, *Nature* 361:315, 1993.

Birnbaumer L: Receptor-to-effector signaling: roles for beta gamma dimers as well as alpha subunits, *Cell* 71:1069, 1992.

Bourne HR, Sanders DA, McCormick F: The GTPase superfamily: conserved structure and molecular mechanism, *Nature* 349:117, 1991.

Brown AM, Birnbaumer L: Ionic channels and their regulation by G protein subunits, *Annu Rev Physiol* 52:197, 1990.

Charbonneau H, Tonks NK: 1002 protein phosphatases?, *Annu Rev Cell Biol* 8:463, 1992.

Cohen P: Signal integration at the level of protein kinases, protein phosphatases and their substrates, *Trends Biochem Sci* 17:408, 1992.

Fantl WJ, Johnson DE, Williams LT: Signalling by receptor tyrosine kinases, *Annu Rev Biochem* 62:453, 1993.

Ferris CD, Snyder SH: Inositol 1,4,5-trisphosphate–activated calcium channels, *Annu Rev Physiol* 54:469, 1992.

Hall A: The cellular functions of small GTP-binding proteins, *Science* 249:635, 1990.

Hall A: Ras-related proteins, *Curr Opin Cell Biol* 5:265, 1993.

Harden TK: G-protein regulated phospholipase C: identification of component proteins, *Adv Sec Messenger Phosphoprot Res* 26:11, 1992.

Hepler JR, Gilman AG: G proteins, *Trends Biochem Sci* 17:383, 1992.

Hille B: G-protein–coupled mechanisms and nervous signaling, *Neuron* 9:187, 1992.

Iniguez-Lluhi J, Kleuss C, Gilman AG: The importance of G protein beta-gamma subunits, *Trends Cell Biol* 3:230, 1993.

Lamb TD, Pugh EN Jr: G protein cascades: gain and kinetics, *Trends Neurosci* 15:291, 1992.

Lefkowitz RJ: G-protein receptor kinases, *Cell* 74:409, 1993.

Linder ME, Gilman AG: G proteins, *Sci Am* 267:36, 1992.

Lowy DR, Willumsen BM: Function and regulation of Ras, *Annu Rev Biochem* 62:851, 1993.

Meldolesi J: Multifarious IP$_3$ receptors, *Curr Biol* 2:393, 1992.

Michell RH: Inositol lipids in cellular signalling mechanisms, *Trends Biochem Sci* 17:274, 1992.

Nishida E, Gotoh Y: The MAP kinase cascade is essential for diverse signal transduction pathways, *Trends Biochem Sci* 18:128, 1993.

Nishizuka Y: Signal transduction: crosstalk, *Trends Biochem Sci* 17:367, 1992.

Nishizuka Y: Intracellular signaling by hydrolysis of phospholipids and activation of protein kinase C, *Science* 258:607, 1992.

Posada J, Cooper JA: Molecular signal integration. Interplay between serine, threonine, and tyrosine phosphorylation, *Mol Biol Cell* 3:583, 1992.

Ruderman JV: MAP kinase and the activation of quiescent cells, *Curr Opin Cell Biol* 5:207, 1993.

Schlessinger J, Ullrich A: Growth factor signaling by receptor tyrosine kinases, *Neuron* 9:383, 1992.

Schulman H: The multifunctional Ca^{2+}/calmodulin-dependent protein kinases, *Curr Opin Cell Biol* 5:247, 1993.

Sternweis PC, Smrcka AV: Regulation of phospholipase C by G proteins, *Trends Biochem Sci* 17:502, 1992.

Szabo G, Otero AS: G-protein-mediated regulation of K$^+$ channels in heart, *Annu Rev Physiol* 52:293, 1990.

Tang W-J, Gilman AG: Adenylyl cyclases, *Cell* 70:869, 1992.

Taylor CW, Marshall ICB: Calcium and inositol 1,4,5-trisphosphate receptors: a complex relationship, *Trends Biochem Sci* 17:403, 1992.

Taylor SS et al: Structural framework for the protein kinase family, *Annu Rev Cell Biol* 8:429, 1992.

Walton KM, Dixon JE: Protein tyrosine phosphatases, *Annu Rev Biochem* 62:101, 1993.

Books and monographs

Alberts B et al: *Molecular biology of the cell,* ed 3, New York, 1994, Garland.

Barritt GJ: *Communication within animal cells,* Oxford, 1992, Oxford Science Publications.

Cohen P, Klee C, editors.: *Calmodulin (Molecular aspects of cellular regulation,* vol 5), New York, 1988, Elsevier.

Hardie DG: *Biochemical messengers: hormones, neurotransmitters and growth factors,* London, 1990, Chapman & Hall.

Houslay MD, Milligan G, editors: *G-proteins as mediators of cellular signalling processes,* 1990, New York, John Wiley.

Lodish H et al: *Molecular cell biology,* ed 3, New York, 1995, Scientific American Books.

Michell RH, Drummond AH, Downes CP, editors: *Inositol lipids in cell signaling,* New York, 1989, Academic Press.

Peroutka SJ, editor: *G-protein–coupled receptors,* Boca Raton, Fla, 1994, CRC Press.

THE NERVOUS SYSTEM

William D. Willis, Jr.

CHAPTER

6

The Nervous System and Its Components

The nervous system is a communications network that allows an organism to interact with its environment. In a broad sense, the term *environment* includes both the external environment (the world outside the body) and the internal environment (the contents of the body). The nervous system includes sensory components that detect environmental events, integrative components that process and store sensory and other data, and motor components that generate movements and glandular secretions.

■ *Organization of the Nervous System*

At the microscopic level of organization, the nervous system consists of a highly complex aggregation of cells. Some cells, called **neurons,** form the communications network of the nervous system. Neurons are specialized for receiving incoming signals and transmitting signals to other neurons or to effector cells.

Other cells in the nervous system perform supportive functions. These supportive cells are the **neuroglia** (meaning "nerve glue"). Several types of neuroglia exist in the nervous system. One type helps maintain an appropriate local environment for neurons; another type ensheathes axons to increase the speed of propagation of action potentials.

Before discussing the microscopic components of the nervous system, we must gain a broad overview of the structures in which these cells are found. The nervous system can be divided into peripheral and central parts, each with further subdivisions.

■ *The Peripheral Nervous System*

The **peripheral nervous system (PNS)** is the interface between the central nervous system and either the environment or the excitable cells. The PNS includes both **sensory** components formed by sensory receptors and primary afferent neurons and **motor** components formed by somatic and autonomic motor neurons.

Sensory receptors are those structures that sense the interactions of various forms of environmental energy with the body. Sensory receptors are located at the peripheral ending of **primary afferent neurons.** Information obtained by the sensory receptors is transmitted to the central nervous system (CNS) by these **afferent neurons** via **dorsal roots** or **cranial nerves.** The cell bodies of dorsal roots and cranial nerves are located in **dorsal root ganglia** or **cranial nerve ganglia.** *A ganglion in the peripheral nervous system is an aggregation of neuronal cell bodies with a similar function.*

The motor component of the PNS consists of **somatic motor neurons** and autonomic neurons. The cell bodies of somatic motor neurons are located in the spinal cord or brainstem. These neurons innervate skeletal muscle fibers. They typically have long dendrites (see p 86) and receive many synaptic connections. The motor neurons that supply a given muscle are located in a particular motor nucleus. *A nucleus is a collection of neurons in the CNS with a similar function* (as distinguished from the nucleus found in an individual cell). For instance, the **facial motor nucleus** contains neurons that innervate the facial muscles. The axons of somatic motor neurons leave the CNS through either a ventral root in the spinal cord or a cranial nerve.

Autonomic motor neurons innervate smooth muscle fibers and glands and include both **preganglionic** and **postganglionic neurons** of the **sympathetic** and **parasympathetic** nervous systems (see Chapter 15). Preganglionic neurons are located in CNS either within the spinal cord or in the brainstem. In contrast to somatic motor neurons, these preganglionic neurons do not directly synapse with their effectors (the smooth muscles and glands). Instead, preganglionic neurons synapse with postganglionic neurons, and the postganglionic neurons then synapse with the effectors.

The neural components of the PNS are described in more detail in Chapter 7.

■ *The Central Nervous System*

The **central nervous system (CNS)** performs many functions. It gathers and processes information about the environment from the PNS, organizes reflex and other behavioral responses, and plans and executes voluntary movements.

The CNS is also the site of so-called "higher" cognitive functions. Memories are processed and stored in the CNS, and it is also the site of learning and thinking. The CNS is composed of the **spinal cord** and the **brain** (Figs. 6-1 and 6-2). The spinal cord is subdivided into a series of regions, each region consisting of a number of segments. The regions of the spinal cord are cervical, thoracic, lumbar, sacral, and coccygeal.

The brain is subdivided into five regions based on embryologic development: the **myelencephalon,** the **metencephalon,** the **mesencephalon,** the **diencephalon,** and the **telencephalon** (Table 6-1). In the adult brain, the myelencephalon includes the **medulla oblongata** (or medulla); the metencephalon includes the **pons** and **cerebellum;** the mesencephalon is the **midbrain;** the diencephalon includes the **thalamus** and **hypothalamus;** and the telencephalon includes the **basal ganglia** and the **cerebral cortex** (Figs. 6-2 and 6-3). The cerebral cortex is further divided into lobes (named after the overlying bones of the skull): **frontal, parietal, temporal,** and **occipital.** The **cerebral hemispheres** on the two sides of the cerebral cortex are connected across the midline by a massive bundle of axons called the **corpus callosum** ("hard body").

The external surface of the CNS is covered by several layers of connective tissue that form the **pia mater,** the **arachnoid,** and the **dura mater.** These layers protect the CNS. The space between the pia mater and arachnoid, the **subarachnoid space,** contains **cerebrospinal fluid (CSF).**

Some of the functions of different parts of the CNS are given in Table 6-1.

■ *Environment of the Neuron*

The local environment of most neurons is carefully controlled to protect them from extreme variations in the composition of the extracellular fluid that bathes them. This control is provided by regulation of the CNS circulation (see Chapter 30), the blood-brain barrier, the buffering function of neuroglia, and the exchange of substances between the CSF and the extracellular fluid of the CNS.

The cranial cavity contains the brain, blood, and CSF (Fig. 6-4). The human brain weighs about 1350 g; approximately 15%, or 200 ml, is extracellular fluid. The intracranial blood volume is about 100 ml, as is the cranial volume of CSF. Thus, the extracellular fluid space in the cranial cavity totals approximately 400 ml.

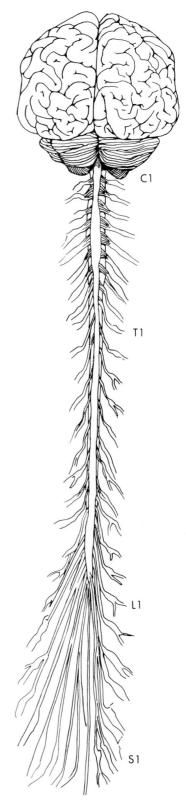

■ **Fig. 6-1**   Brain and spinal cord with attached spinal nerves. Note the relative size of various components. *C1, T1, L1,* and *S1,* First cervical, thoracic, lumbar, and sacral segments, respectively. (Redrawn from Williams PL, Warwick R: *Functional neuroanatomy of man,* Edinburgh, 1975, Churchill Livingstone.)

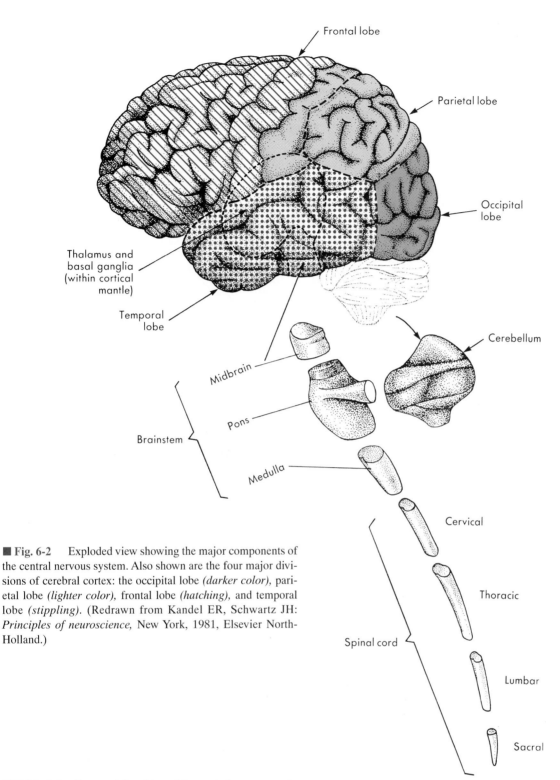

Frontal lobe

Parietal lobe

Occipital lobe

Thalamus and basal ganglia (within cortical mantle)

Temporal lobe

Cerebellum

Midbrain

Pons

Brainstem

Medulla

Cervical

Thoracic

Spinal cord

Lumbar

Sacral

■ **Fig. 6-2** Exploded view showing the major components of the central nervous system. Also shown are the four major divisions of cerebral cortex: the occipital lobe *(darker color),* parietal lobe *(lighter color),* frontal lobe *(hatching),* and temporal lobe *(stippling).* (Redrawn from Kandel ER, Schwartz JH: *Principles of neuroscience,* New York, 1981, Elsevier North-Holland.)

■ **Table 6-1** Parts and functions of the central nervous system

Region	Subdivision	Function
Spinal cord		Sensory input; reflex organization; somatic and autonomic motor output
Myelencephalon	Medulla	Cardiovascular control; respiratory control; brainstem reflexes
Metencephalon	Pons	Respiratory and urinary bladder control; vestibular control of eye movements
	Cerebellum	Motor control; motor learning
Mesencephalon	Midbrain	Acoustic relay; control of eye movements; motor control
Diencephalon	Thalamus	Sensory and motor relay to cerebral cortex
	Hypothalamus	Autonomic and endocrine control
Telencephalon	Basal ganglia	Motor control
	Cerebral cortex	Sensory perception; cognition; learning and memory; motor planning and voluntary movement

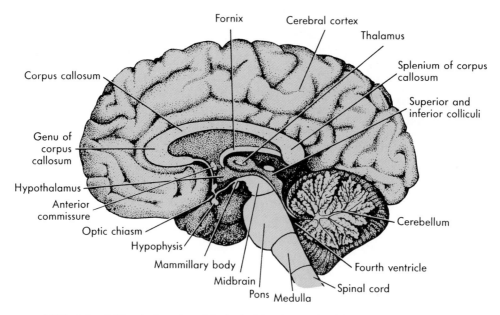

■ **Fig. 6-3**   Midsagittal section of the brain. Note the relationships among the cerebral cortex, cerebellum, thalamus, and brainstem plus the location of various commissures. (Redrawn from Kandel ER, Schwartz JH: *Principles of neuroscience,* New York, 1981, Elsevier North-Holland.)

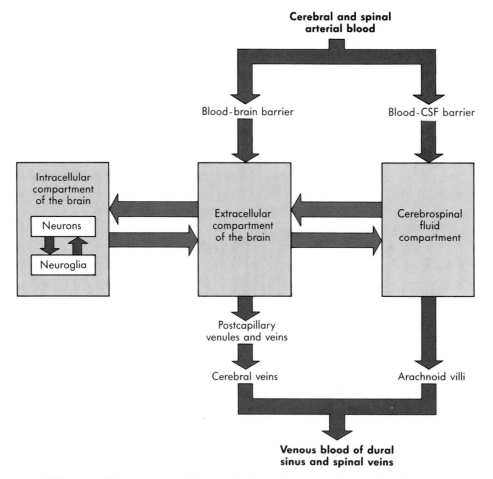

■ **Fig. 6-4**   The structural and functional relationships involved in the blood-brain and blood-CSF (cerebrospinal fluid) barriers. Substances entering the neurons and glial cells (i.e., intracellular compartment) must pass through the cell membrane. Arrows indicate direction of fluid flow under normal conditions.

The Blood-Brain Barrier

The movement of large molecules and highly charged ions from the blood into the brain and spinal cord is severely restricted (Fig. 6-4). The restriction is at least partly caused by the barrier action of tight junctions between the capillary endothelial cells of the CNS. Neuroglia called **astrocytes** (see p 88) may also help limit the movement of certain substances. For example, astrocytes take up potassium ions and thus regulate the K^+ concentration in the extracellular space. Certain transport mechanisms remove particular substances, such as penicillin, from the CNS.

> The blood-brain barrier can be disrupted by pathology of the brain. For example, **brain tumors** may allow substances that are otherwise excluded to enter the brain from the circulation. This fact can be exploited radiologically by introducing into the circulation an opaque substance that normally cannot penetrate the blood-brain barrier. Leakage of the substance into the volume of brain occupied by the brain tumor can be used to outline the tumor.

Cerebrospinal Fluid

The tissue of both the brain and spinal cord contain a series of spaces called **ventricles** that are filled with CSF (Fig. 6-5). CSF cushions the brain and regulates the extracellular environment of neurons. The CSF is formed largely by the **choroid plexuses,** which are covered by specialized ependymal cells. The choroid plexuses are located in the lateral, third, and fourth ventricles. The **lateral ventricles** are within the two cerebral hemispheres. These connect with the **third ventricle** through the **interventricular foramina** (of Monro). The third ventricle lies in the midline between the diencephalon on the two sides. The **cerebral aqueduct** (of Sylvius) traverses the midbrain and connects the third ventricle with the **fourth ventricle.** The fourth ventricle is interposed between the pons and medulla below and the cerebellum above. The **central canal** of the spinal cord continues caudally from the fourth ventricle, but in adult humans it is generally not patent.

The CSF escapes from the ventricular system into the **subarachnoid space** through three apertures in the roof of the fourth ventricle: the **medial aperture** (of Magendie) and the two **lateral apertures** (of Luschka). After leaving the ventricular system, the CSF circulates through the **subarachnoid space** that surrounds the brain and spinal cord. Regions where these spaces are distended are called **subarachnoid cisterns.** An example is the **lumbar cistern,** which surrounds the lumbar and sacral spinal roots below the end of the spinal cord. *The lumbar cistern is the target for lumbar puncture,* a proce-

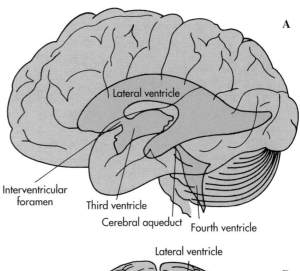

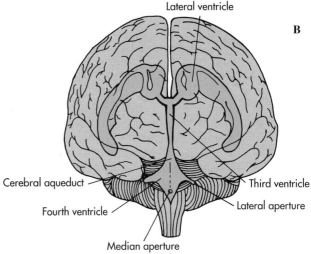

■ **Fig. 6-5** The ventricular system in situ as seen from the side (**A**) and from the front (**B**).

dure used clinically to sample the CSF. A large part of the CSF is removed by bulk flow through the valvular **arachnoid villi** into the dural venous sinuses in the cranium.

The total volume of the CSF contained within the cerebral ventricles is approximately 35 ml, while that contained in the subarachnoid spaces is about 100 ml. About 0.35 ml of CSF is produced each minute. At this rate, the CSF turns over approximately four times daily.

When a person is recumbent, the pressure in the CSF column is about 120 to 180 mm H_2O. The rate at which CSF is formed is relatively independent of the pressure in the ventricles and subarachnoid space, as well as of the systemic blood pressure. However, the absorption rate of CSF is a direct function of CSF pressure.

The extracellular fluid within the CNS communicates directly with the CSF. Thus, the composition of the CSF affects the composition of the extracellular environment of neurons in the brain and spinal cord. The main constituents of CSF in the lumbar cistern are listed in Table 6-2. For comparison, the concentrations of the same constituents in the blood are also given. As this table shows, the CSF has a lower concentration of K^+, glucose, and

■ **Table 6-2**   Constituents of CSF and blood

Constituent	Lumbar CSF	Blood
Na$^+$ (mEq/L)	148	136-145
K$^+$ (mEq/L)	2.9	3.5-5
Cl$^-$ (mEq/L)	120-130	100-106
Glucose (mg/dl)	50-75	70-100
Protein (mg/dl)	15-45	6-8 $\times$ 10^3
pH	7.3	7.4

Modified from Willis WD, Grossman RG: *Medical neurobiology,* ed 3, St Louis, 1981, Mosby–Year Book.

protein but a greater concentration of Na$^+$ and Cl$^-$ than does blood. Furthermore, CSF contains practically no blood cells. The increased concentration of Na$^+$ and Cl$^-$ enables the CSF to be isotonic to blood despite the much lower concentration of protein in the CSF.

Obstruction of the circulation of CSF leads to increased CSF pressure and **hydrocephalus,** an abnormal accumulation of fluid in the cranium. In hydrocephalus, the ventricles become distended, and if the pressure increase is sustained, brain substance is lost. When the obstruction is located within the ventricular system or in the roof of the fourth ventricle, the condition is called **noncommunicating hydrocephalus.** If the obstruction is in the subarachnoid space or arachnoid villi, it is known as **communicating hydrocephalus.**

■ General Functions of the Nervous System

The functions of the nervous system include **sensory detection, information processing,** and **behavior.** *Learning and memory are special forms of information processing that permit behavior to change appropriately in response to environmental challenges based on past experience.* Although other systems, such as the endocrine and immune systems, share these functions, the nervous system is specialized to perform these functions.

Proper functioning of the nervous system depends on the **excitability** of its neurons. An excitable cell (such as a neuron) receives and transmits information in the form of electrical signals. Excitability is manifested by such electrical events as **action potentials, receptor potentials,** and **synaptic potentials** (see Section I). Chemical events often accompany these electrical phenomena.

Sensory detection is the process whereby neurons **transduce** environmental energy into neural signals. Sensory detection is accomplished by special neurons called **sensory receptors.** Various forms of energy can be sensed, including mechanical forces, light, sound, chemicals, temperature, and (in some animals) electrical fields.

Information processing includes, among other events, the following:
1. Transmission of information in neural networks
2. Transformation of signals by combining them with other signals (**neural integration**)
3. Storage of information in and retrieval of information from memory
4. Use of sensory information for **perception**
5. Thought processes
6. Learning
7. Planning and implementation of motor commands
8. Emotions

Information processing, including learning and memory, depends on **intercellular communication** in neural circuits. These communication mechanisms involve both electrical and chemical events.

Behavior consists of the totality of the organism's responses to its environment. Behavior may be an entirely internal act, such as **cognition,** but it is often readily observable as a motor act, such as a **movement** or an **autonomic response.** In humans, a particularly important set of behaviors are those involved in **language.**

How are these highly complex functions carried out? Whether simple or complex, each response is communicated by neurons organized into neural pathways. The remainder of this chapter is devoted to the cellular mechanisms that allow neurons to interact (see Section I).

■ Cellular Components of the Nervous System

The functional unit of the nervous system is the **neuron** (Fig. 6-6). The typical neuron has a receptive surface consisting of a **cell body,** or **soma,** and several branchlike **dendrites** that receive **synapses,** or neuron-to-neuron connections. Its **axon** makes synaptic connections with other neurons or with effector cells. The communications network of the nervous system consists of **neural circuits** made up of synaptically interconnected neurons.

Neurons communicate with each other by means of **action potentials** propagated along the axons in the neural circuits (see Chapter 3). Action potentials are passed from one neuron to the next by **synaptic transmission.** In synaptic transmission, an action potential that reaches the **presynaptic ending** usually causes the release of a **neurotransmitter** substance, which either **excites** the **postsynaptic cell** to discharge one or more action potentials or **inhibits** the activity of the postsynaptic cell. Axons not only transmit information in neural circuits but also convey chemical substances toward the synaptic terminals by **axonal transport** (see p 92).

The other cellular elements of the nervous system are the **neuroglia** (Fig. 6-7), or supportive cells. Neuroglial cells in the human CNS outnumber neurons by an order of magnitude: there are about 10^{13} neuroglia and 10^{12}

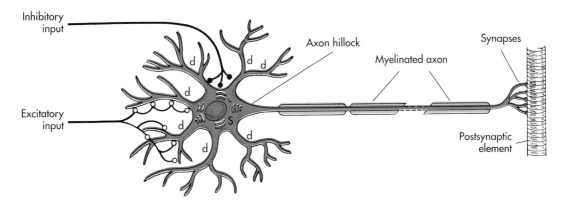

■ **Fig. 6-6** Schematic diagram of an idealized neuron and its major components. Most afferent input from axons of other cells terminates in synapses on the dendrites *(d)*, although some may terminate on the soma *(S)*. Excitatory terminals tend to terminate more distally on dendrites than do inhibitory ones, which often terminate on the soma. (Redrawn from Williams PL, Warwick R: *Functional neuroanatomy of man,* Edinburgh, 1975, Churchill Livingstone.)

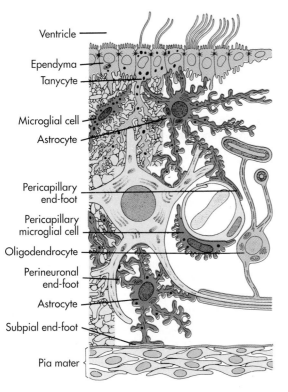

■ **Fig. 6-7** Schematic representation of non-neural elements in the central nervous system. Two astrocytes *(darker color)* are shown ending on a neuron's soma and dendrites. They also contact the pial surface and/or capillaries. An oligodendrocyte *(lighter color)* provides the myelin sheaths for axons. Also shown are microglia *(darker color)* and ependymal cells *(lighter color).* (Redrawn from Williams PL, Warwick R: *Functional neuroanatomy of man,* Edinburgh, 1975, Churchill Livingstone.)

neurons in the CNS. Neuroglia do not participate directly in the short-term communication of information through the nervous system, but they do assist neurons in this function. For example, some types of neuroglial cells provide certain axons with **myelin sheaths** that signifi-

cantly speed up the conduction of action potentials along axons (see p 90). This increase in conduction velocity allows these axons to communicate rapidly with other cells over relatively long distances.

■ *Neuron Structure*

The soma. The soma contains the **nucleus** and **nucleolus** of the neuron (Fig. 6-8). It also possesses a well-developed biosynthetic apparatus for manufacturing membrane constituents, synthetic enzymes, and other chemical substances necessary for the specialized functions of nerve cells. The neuronal biosynthetic apparatus includes **Nissl bodies,** which are stacks of rough endoplasmic reticulum, and a prominent **Golgi apparatus.** The soma also contains numerous **mitochondria** and cytoskeletal elements, including **neurofilaments** and **microtubules. Lipofuscin** is a pigment formed from incompletely degraded membrane components; it accumulates with aging in some neurons. A few groups of neurons in the brainstem (e.g., in the **substantia nigra** and the **locus caeruleus**) contain **melanin** pigment.

Dendrites. Dendrites are extensions of the cell body. In some neurons, the dendrites are more than 1 mm long, and they account for more than 90% of the surface area. The proximal dendrites (near the cell body) contain Nissl bodies and parts of the Golgi apparatus. However, the main cytoplasmic organelles in dendrites are microtubules and neurofilaments. Traditionally, dendrites have not been regarded as electrically excitable. However, we now know that the dendrites of many neurons have voltage-dependent conductances. These conductances often depend on calcium channels that, when activated, produce calcium spikes.

The axon. The axon arises from the soma (or sometimes from a dendrite) in a specialized region called the **axon hillock.** The axon hillock and axon differ from the

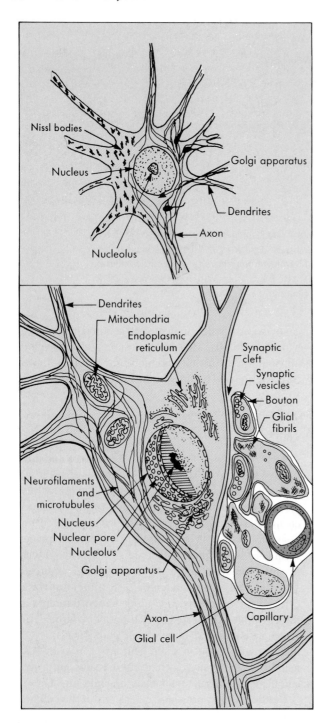

■ **Fig. 6-8** Organelles of the neuron. The smaller drawing on top shows the organelles typical of a neuron, as seen with the light microscope. The portion of the illustration to the left of the soma represents structures seen with a Nissl stain. These include the nucleus and nucleolus, Nissl bodies in the cytoplasm of the cell body and proximal dendrites, and as a negative image, the Golgi apparatus. The absence of Nissl bodies in the axon hillock and axon is also shown. To the right of the soma are structures seen with a heavy-metal stain: these include neurofibrils. The appropriate heavy-metal stain may demonstrate the Golgi apparatus (not shown). On the surface of the neuron several synaptic endings are indicated, as stained by the heavy metal. The large drawing shows structures visible at the electron microscopic level. The nucleus, nucleolus, chromatin, and nuclear pores are represented. Mitochondria, rough endoplasmic reticulum, Golgi apparatus, neurofilaments, and microtubules are in the cytoplasm. Along the surface membrane are such associated structures as synaptic endings and astrocytic processes.

■ *Types of Neurons and Neuroglia*

Types of neurons. Many different kinds of neurons exist. These different neurons perform specific communication functions; often their morphology reflects their function (Fig. 6-9). For example, **dorsal root ganglion cells** receive information from sensory endings in receptor organs rather than by synaptic transmission. Hence, their cell bodies lack dendrites (Fig. 6-9, *E*) and receive no synaptic endings. The axon branches near the cell body, and one branch (the **peripheral process**) traverses a peripheral nerve to supply a sensory receptor; the other branch (the **central process**) reaches the spinal cord through a **dorsal root** or the brainstem through a **cranial nerve.**

Other neurons, such as the **pyramidal cells** of the cerebral cortex and the **Purkinje cells** of the cerebellar cortex, function in information processing (Fig. 6-9, *A* and *B*). These neurons have greatly expanded dendritic surfaces covered with dendritic spines, and they receive enormous numbers of synaptic endings.

Types of neuroglia. Neuroglial cells support the activity of neurons (Fig. 6-10). Neuroglia include **astrocytes** and **oligodendroglia** in the CNS and **Schwann cells** and **satellite cells** in the PNS. **Microglia** and **ependymal cells** are also considered central neuroglial cells.

Astrocytes (their name reflects their star shape) regulate the microenvironment of neurons in the CNS, although they contact only part of the surfaces of central neurons (Fig. 6-7). However, their processes surround groups of synaptic endings, isolating them from adjacent synapses. The **foot processes** of astrocytes contact capillaries and the connective tissue at the surface of the CNS, the **pia mater** (Fig. 6-7). These foot processes may help limit the free diffusion of substances into the CNS.

soma and proximal dendrites in that they lack rough endoplasmic reticulum, free ribosomes, and Golgi apparatus. The axon contains smooth endoplasmic reticulum and a prominent cytoskeleton.

Neurons can be classified according to the length of their axons. In **Golgi type 1 neurons,** axons are short and, as with dendrites, terminate near the soma. In **Golgi type 2 neurons,** axons are long and may extend for more than a meter.

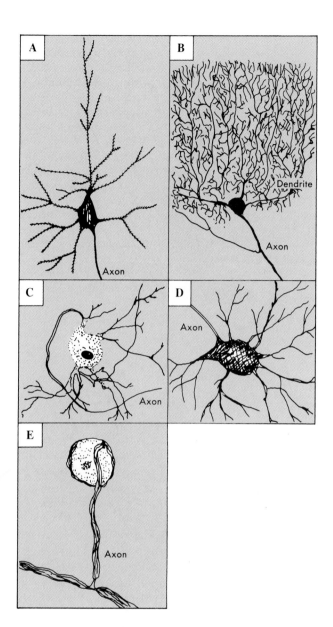

■ **Fig. 6-9** Various forms of neurons. **A,** Neuron characterized by a cell body that has a roughly pyramidal shape. This type of neuron, called a pyramidal cell, is typical of the cerebral cortex. Note the many spinous processes lining the surface of the dendrites. **B,** Cell type first described by the Czechoslovakian neuroanatomist Purkinje and since known as the Purkinje cell. Purkinje cells are characteristic of the cerebellar cortex. The cell body is pear shaped, with a rich dendritic plexus originating from one end and the axon from the other. The fine branches of the dendrites are covered with spines (not shown). **C,** A sympathetic postganglionic motor neuron. **D,** An α motor neuron of the spinal cord. Both **C** and **D** are multipolar neurons with radially arranged dendrites. **E,** A sensory dorsal root ganglion cell; no dendrites are present. The axon branches into a central and a peripheral process. Because the axon results from fusion of two processes during embryonic development, these cells are described as pseudounipolar neurons rather than unipolar.

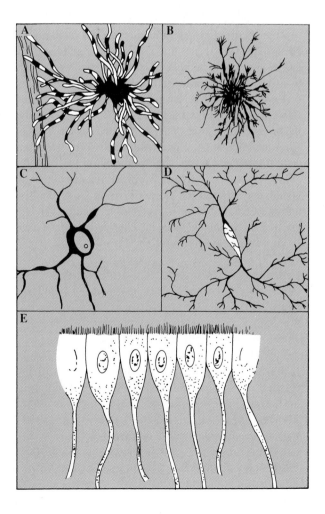

■ **Fig. 6-10** Different types of neuroglial cells of the central nervous system. **A,** Fibrous astrocyte. **B,** Protoplasmic astrocyte. Note the glial foot processes in association with a capillary in **A.** **C,** An oligodendrocyte. Each of the processes is responsible for the production of one or more myelin sheath internodes about central axons. **D,** Microglial cell. **E,** Ependymal cells.

Astrocytes can actively take up K⁺ ions and neurotransmitter substances, which they then metabolize. Thus, they serve to buffer the extracellular environment of neurons from ions and neurotransmitters. The cytoplasm of astrocytes contains glial filaments, which help provide mechanical support for CNS tissue. After injury, astrocytic processes containing these glial filaments become hypertrophic and form a glial "scar."

Other neuroglia serve to insulate the axons of neurons. Although some axons are not insulated, others are coated with an insulated sheath called the **myelin sheath.** The myelin sheath is a spiral, multilayered wrapping of the cell membrane. In the CNS, the cells whose membranes make up the myelin sheaths of myelinated axons are called **oligodendroglia** (Fig. 6-11, *A*). In the PNS, membranes of Schwann cells make up the myelin sheath (Fig. 6-11, *B*).

Some **unmyelinated** cells may be surrounded by neuroglial cells. In the PNS, for instance, unmyelinated axons are embedded within **Schwann** cells, although they are not ensheathed by myelin (Fig. 6-12). In the CNS, unmyelinated axons are bare.

Myelin increases the speed of conduction of the action potential, in part because they limit the flow of ionic current during action potentials to the **nodes of Ranvier** (the junction between adjacent sheath cells). The action potential "jumps" from node to node, a process called **saltatory conduction** (see Chapter 3).

Other neuroglial cells include **satellite cells,** which encapsulate dorsal root and cranial nerve ganglion cells and regulate their microenvironment in a manner similar to astrocytes, and **microglia,** which are latent phagocytes. When the CNS is damaged, microglia help remove the cellular products of the damage. They are assisted by neuroglia and by other phagocytes that invade the CNS from the circulation. **Ependymal cells** form the epithelium that separates the CNS from CSF in the ventricles (Fig. 6-7). Many substances diffuse readily across the ependyma between the extracellular space of the brain and the CSF. The CSF is secreted in large part by specialized ependymal cells of the choroid plexuses located in the ventricular system (see p 85).

Cells that give rise to glial cells are called glial precursor cells. These precursors are present in the adult brain and can still divide and differentiate. Sometimes, however, these glial precursor cells give rise to intrinsic **brain tumors.** Brain tumors can be derived from astrocytes (the slowly growing **astrocytoma** and the rapidly fatal **glioblastoma multiforme),** from oligodendroglia (**oligodendroglioma**), and from ependymal cells (**ependymoma**). Meningeal cells can give rise to slowly growing tumors (**meningiomas**) that compress brain tissue, as can Schwann cells (**acoustic neurinomas**). In the infant brain, neurons that are still dividing can sometimes give rise to **neuroblastomas.**

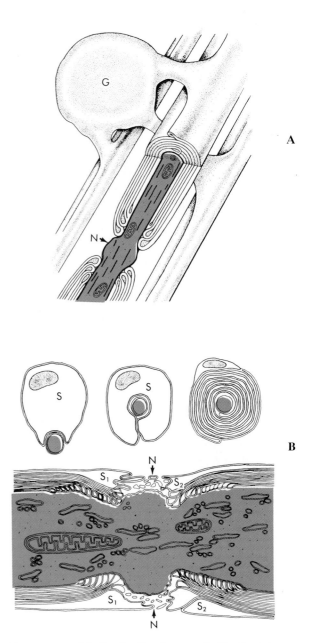

■ **Fig. 6-11**   Myelin sheaths of axons. **A,** Myelinated axons in the central nervous system. A single oligodendrocyte *(G)* emits several processes, each of which winds in a spiral fashion around an axon to form the myelin sheath. The axon *(color)* is shown in cutaway. The myelin from a single oligodendrocyte ends before the next wrapping from another oligodendrocyte. The bare axon between sheaths is the node of Ranvier *(N)*. Conduction of action potentials is saltatory down the axon, skipping from node to node. **B,** Myelinated axon in the peripheral nervous system. A Schwann cell forms a myelinated sheath for peripheral axons in much the same fashion as oligodendrocytes do for central ones, except that each Schwann cell myelinates a single axon. The top shows a cross-sectional view of progressive stages in myelin sheath formation by a Schwann cell *(S)* around an axon *(color)*. The bottom shows a longitudinal view of a myelinated axon *(color)*. The node of Ranvier *(N)* is shown between adjacent sheaths formed by two Schwann cells *(S₁* and *S₂)*. (Redrawn from Patton HD et al: *Introduction to basic neurology,* Philadelphia, 1976, WB Saunders.)

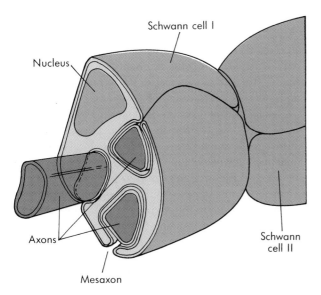

Schwann cell I

Nucleus

Axons

Mesaxon

Schwann cell II

■ **Fig. 6-12** Three-dimensional impression of the appearance of a Remak's bundle. The cut face of the bundle is seen to the left. One of the three unmyelinated axons is represented as protruding from the bundle. A mesaxon is indicated, as is the nucleus of the Schwann cell. To the right, the junction of adjacent Schwann cells is depicted.

Nutrients are delivered to these cerebral cells and wastes are removed by the vascular system. Although capillaries and other blood vessels are abundant in nervous tissue, diffusion of many substances between the blood and the CNS is limited by the blood-brain barrier (see p 85).

■ *Neuronal Transmission of Information*

A major role of axons is to transmit information from the cell body and dendrites of a neuron to synapses on other neurons or effector cells. The information is generally transmitted as a series of nerve impulses.

The conduction velocity of an axon is the speed at which an action potential is propagated (see Chapter 3). *The conduction velocity depends on the diameter of the axon and whether the axon is myelinated or unmyelinated.* Unmyelinated axons are generally less than 1 μm in diameter and conduct at less than 2.5 m/sec. It would take about 1 second for a signal from a sensory receptor in a person's foot to reach the spinal cord via an unmyelinated axon with a conduction velocity of 1 m/sec. Myelinated axons have diameters of 1 to 20 μm and conduct at 3 to 120 m/sec. A spinal motor neuron with an axon that conducts at 100 m/sec would trigger the contraction of a toe muscle in about 10 msec.

Not all neurons have axons. In the CNS, for example, certain neurons that lack axons (**amacrine cells**) send information to the synaptic terminals by intracellular electrical current flow rather than by generating action potentials. This current flow produces a **local potential,**

which decays over a short distance (millimeters to hundreds of micrometers, depending on the **length constant;** see Chapter 3) of the neuron involved. Local potentials differ from action potentials in that they are nonpropagating and therefore cannot spread over long distances. In contrast, action potentials can propagate over long distances along axons.

Signaling via local potentials is also characteristic of sensory receptors, which produce **receptor potentials,** and of communications between nerve cells by **synaptic potentials.**

Coding. Information conveyed by axons may be encoded in several ways. A **labeled line** is a set of neurons dedicated to a general function, such as a particular sensory modality. For example, the visual pathway includes neurons in the retina, the lateral geniculate nucleus of the thalamus, and the visual areas of the cerebral cortex. Fiber tracts carrying visual signals include the optic nerve and optic tract and the optic radiation. The normal stimulus that activates the visual system is light striking the retina. Neurons of the retina process the information and then transmit signals along the visual pathway. However, mechanical or electrical stimulation of neurons in the visual pathway will also produce a visual sensation, although this sensation is usually distorted. Thus, neurons of the visual system are a labeled line and when activated cause a visual sensation.

Motor pathways also provide examples of labeled lines. For example, certain neurons of the cerebral cortex, when activated, cause motor neurons to the muscles of the hand to discharge and the hand muscles to contract, whereas other cortical neurons cause movements of the foot.

A second way in which information is encoded by the nervous system is through neural maps. A **somatotopic map** is formed by arrays of neurons in the sensory or motor systems that (1) receive information from corresponding locations on the body surface or (2) issue motor commands to move particular parts of the body. In the visual system, points on the retina are represented by neuronal arrays that form **retinotopic maps.** In the auditory system, the frequency of sounds is represented in **tonotopic maps.**

A third method for encoding information is by means of patterns of nerve impulses, which are sequences of nerve impulses that result in synaptic transmission of information to a new set of neurons. In this encoding mechanism, the code is the temporal structure of the sequence of nerve impulses. Several different types of nerve impulse codes have been proposed. A commonly used code depends on the **mean discharge frequency.** For example, in many sensory systems, increases in the intensity of a stimulus cause a greater frequency of discharge of the sensory neurons. Other candidate codes depend on the **time of firing,** the **temporal pattern,** and the **duration of bursts.** Other codes have also been proposed.

Synaptic transmission. Neurons communicate with each other at specialized junctions called **synapses** (see Chapter 4). Typically, synapses are formed between the terminals of the axon of one neuron and the dendrites of another; these are called **axodendritic.** However, other types of synapses occur, including **axosomatic, axoaxonal,** and **dendrodendritic** synapses. The synapse between a motor neuron and a skeletal muscle fiber is called an **endplate** or **neuromuscular junction.**

Axonal transport. Membrane and cytoplasmic components that are made in the biosynthetic apparatus of the soma and proximal dendrites must be distributed along the axon (especially to the presynaptic elements of synapses) to replenish secreted or inactivated materials. However, many axons are too long to allow efficient movement of substances from the soma to the synaptic endings simply by diffusion. A special transport mechanism, called **axonal transport,** accomplishes this distribution.

Several types of axonal transport exist. Membrane-bound organelles and mitochondria are transported relatively rapidly by **fast axonal transport.** Substances (e.g., proteins) that are dissolved in cytoplasm are moved by **slow axonal transport.** In mammals, fast axonal transport proceeds as rapidly as 400 mm/day, whereas slow axonal transport occurs at about 1 mm/day. Synaptic vesicles, which travel by fast axonal transport, can travel from the soma of a motor neuron in the spinal cord to a neuromuscular junction in a person's foot in about 2 1/2 days. In comparison, the movement of many soluble proteins over the same distance takes nearly 3 years.

Axonal transport requires metabolic energy and involves the presence of calcium ions in the axon. The cytoskeleton, particularly the microtubules, provides a system of guidewires along which membrane-bound organelles move (Fig. 6-13). The way these organelles are attached to microtubules is similar to the linkage between thick and thin filaments of skeletal muscle fibers; the calcium ions trigger the movement of the organelles along the microtubules.

Axonal transport occurs in both directions. Transport from the soma toward the axonal terminals, called **anterograde axonal transport** (Fig. 6-14, *A*), allows the replenishment of synaptic vesicles and enzymes responsible for neurotransmitter synthesis in synaptic terminals. Transport in the opposite direction is called **retrograde axonal transport** (Fig. 6-14, *B*); this process returns synaptic vesicle membrane to the soma for lysosomal degradation.

Certain viruses and toxins can be conveyed by axonal transport along peripheral nerves. For example, **varicella-zoster virus,** the virus that causes chickenpox, invades dorsal root ganglion cells. The virus may lie dormant within these neurons for many years until some change in immune status occurs. The virus may then be transported along sensory axons to the skin, where a new outbreak of skin lesions occurs, resulting in **shingles** (or *Herpes zoster*), a painful rash in the dermatomal distribution of one or more spinal nerves. **Tetanus toxin** also travels by axonal transport. *Clostridium tetani* bacteria may grow in a dirty wound, and if the person is not vaccinated against tetanus toxin, the toxin may travel by retrograde axonal transport within motor neurons. If the toxin escapes into the extracellular space of the spinal cord ventral horn, it can block the synaptic receptors for inhibitory amino acid neurotransmitters, and thereby cause tetanic convulsions.

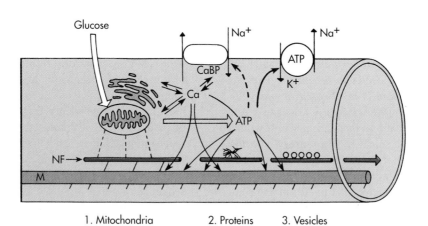

1. Mitochondria   2. Proteins   3. Vesicles

■ **Fig. 6-13**   It has been proposed that axonal transport depends on the movement of transport filaments. Energy is required and is supplied by glucose. Mitochondria control the level of cations in the axoplasm by supplying adenosine triphosphate *(ATP)* to the ion pumps. An important cation for axonal transport is calcium. Transport filaments *(red bars at bottom of drawing)* move along the cytoskeleton (microtubules, *M,* or neurofilament, *NF*) by means of cross-bridges. Transported components attach to the transport filaments.

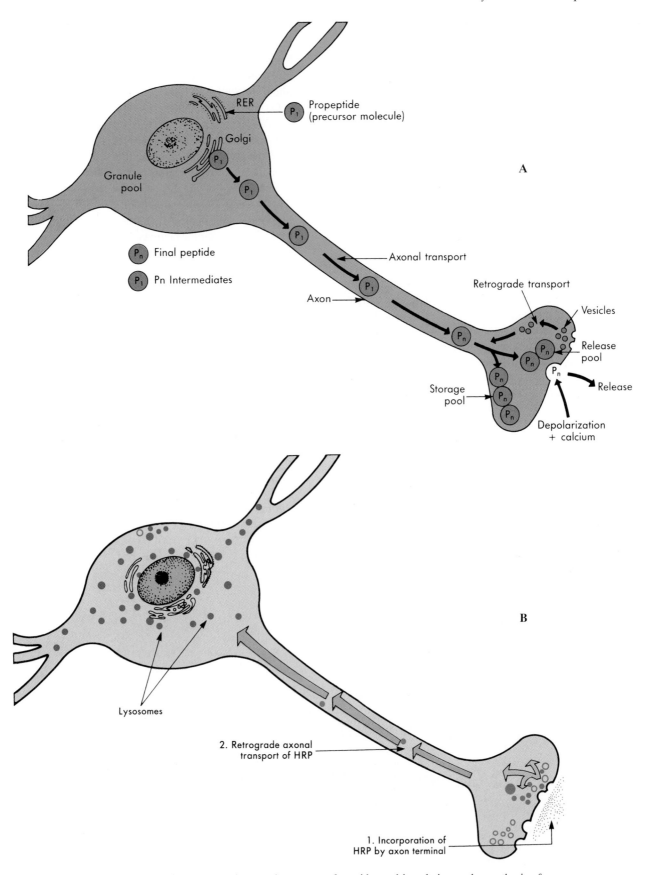

■ Fig. 6-14 **A,** Anterograde axonal transport of peptides and its relation to the synthesis of peptides in the cell body and their release from terminals. *RER,* Rough endoplasmic reticulum. **B,** Schematic summary of incorporation, retrograde axonal transport, and lysosomal accumulation of horseradish peroxidase *(HRP)* in neurons.

■ *Nervous Tissue Reactions to Injury*

Injury to nervous tissue elicits responses by neurons and neuroglia. Severe injury causes cell death. Because neurons are postmitotic cells, they cannot be replaced.

■ *Degeneration*

If an axon is transected, the soma of the neuron attempts to repair the axon by making new structural proteins. This is called the **axonal reaction.** In uninjured neurons, Nissl bodies in the soma stain well with basic aniline dyes that attach to the ribonucleic acid of the ribosomes. During the axonal reaction (Fig. 6-15, *B*), the cisterns of the rough endoplasmic reticulum become distended with the products of protein synthesis. The ribosomes appear disorganized, and the Nissl bodies are stained weakly by basic aniline dyes. This process, called **chromatolysis,** produces an alteration in staining (Fig. 6-15, *C*). The soma may swell and become rounded, and the nucleus may assume an eccentric position. These morphologic changes reflect the cytologic processes that accompany increased protein synthesis.

The axon distal to the transection dies (Fig. 6-15, *C*). Within a few days the axon and all the synaptic endings formed by the axon disintegrate. If the axon has been myelinated, the myelin sheath fragments are eventually phagocytosed and removed. However, the neuroglial cells that had formed the myelin sheath remain viable. This sequence of events was originally described by Waller and is called **wallerian degeneration.**

If the axons that provide the sole or predominant synaptic input to a neuron or an effector cell are interrupted, the postsynaptic cell may degenerate and even die. The best-known example of this process is the atrophy of skeletal muscle fibers after interruption of their innervation by motor neurons.

■ *Regeneration*

After an axon is lost through injury, many neurons can regenerate a new axon. The proximal stump of the damaged axon develops **sprouts** (Fig. 6-15, *C*). In the PNS, these sprouts elongate and grow along the path of the original nerve if this route is available (Fig. 6-15, *D*). The Schwann cells in the distal stump of the nerve not only

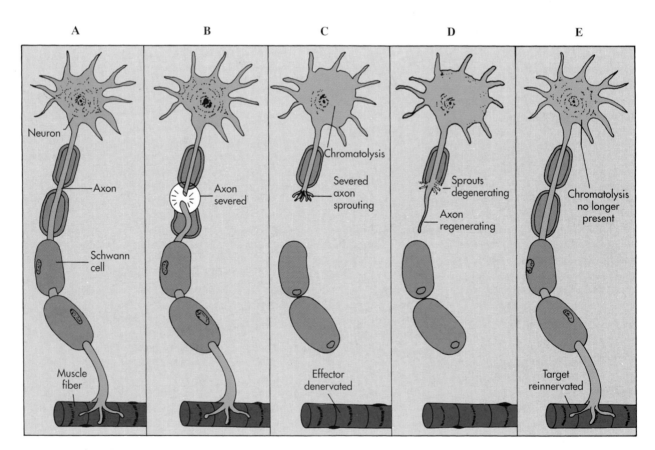

■ **Fig. 6-15**   **A,** Normal motor neuron innervating a skeletal muscle fiber. **B,** The motor axon has been severed and the motor neuron is undergoing chromatolysis. **C,** This is associated in time with sprouting and **(D)** with regeneration of the axon. The excess sprouts degenerate. **E,** When the target cell is reinnervated, chromatolysis is no longer present.

survive the wallerian degeneration but also proliferate and form rows along the course previously taken by the axons. **Growth cones** of the sprouting axons find their way along the rows of Schwann cells and may eventually reinnervate the original peripheral target structures (Fig. 6-15, *E*). The Schwann cells then remyelinate the axons. The rate of regeneration is limited by the rate of slow axonal transport to about 1 mm/day.

In the CNS, transected axons also sprout. However, the oligodendroglia are unable to form a path along which the sprouts can grow because a single oligodendroglial cell myelinates many central axons (in contrast to the Schwann cells in the PNS, each of which provides myelin for only a single axon). Alternatively, different chemical signals may affect peripheral and central attempts at regeneration differently. Another obstacle in axonal regeneration in the CNS is the formation of glial scars by astrocytes.

Trophic factors. A number of proteins affect the growth of axons and the maintenance of synaptic connections. The best studied of these substances is **nerve growth factor (NGF).** NGF was initially thought to enhance the growth of and maintain many neurons of neural crest origin, including small dorsal root ganglion cells and autonomic postganglionic neurons. However, it is now believed that NGF also influences some neurons in the CNS. Other growth factors have also been described, including **brain-derived growth factor, neurotrophin 3, neurotrophin 4, neurotrophin 5,** and **ciliary neurotrophic factor.** Some of these growth factors affect the growth of large dorsal root ganglion cells or motor neurons. It seems likely that a large assortment of growth factors will be discovered to play important roles in the growth and maintenance of neurons in both the peripheral and central nervous systems. Knowledge of these factors may be useful in understanding a number of neurodegenerative diseases and may also help researchers design therapies for these diseases.

NGF is secreted by target cells and binds to special receptors located on the neurons that synapse with the target cells. The bound NGF and receptor are internalized within the neurons, and the NGF is transported retrogradely to the soma. There, NGF may directly act on the nucleus and affect the production of enzymes responsible for neurotransmitter synthesis and axonal growth. NGF receptors include both a low-affinity form and the higher-affinity tyrosine kinase receptor known as TRK$_A$. Other neurotrophic factors bind to the same low-affinity receptor or different high-affinity tyrosine kinase receptors known as TRK$_B$ or TRK$_C$.

■ *Summary*

1. Sensory, integrative, and motor components of the nervous system allow the body to communicate with the environment.

2. The neuron is the functional unit of the nervous system. Information is conveyed through neural circuits by action potentials in neurons and by synaptic transmission between neurons.

3. Neuroglial cells regulate the microenvironment of neurons and provide myelin sheaths that speed conduction velocities.

4. The peripheral nervous system (PNS) includes sensory receptors, primary afferent neurons, somatic motor neurons, and autonomic preganglionic and postganglionic neurons.

5. The central nervous system (CNS) includes the spinal cord and the brain. The brain includes the medulla, pons, cerebellum, midbrain, thalamus, hypothalamus, basal ganglia, and cerebral cortex.

6. CNS extracellular fluid composition is regulated by the cerebrospinal fluid (CSF), the blood-brain barrier, and the astrocytes.

7. Choroid plexuses form CSF. CSF leaves the ventricles through the roof of the fourth ventricle, traverses the subarachnoid space, and returns to the circulation through arachnoid villi.

8. The composition of CSF differs from that of blood. CSF has a lower concentration of K^+, glucose, and protein and a higher concentration of Na^+ and Cl^-; CSF normally lacks blood cells. Its production is relatively independent of ventricular and blood pressure, but its absorption is a function of CSF pressure.

9. General functions of the nervous system include excitability, sensory detection, information processing, and behavior. Different types of neurons are specialized for different functions.

10. Neuroglial cells include astrocytes (which regulate CNS microenvironment), oligodendroglia (which form CNS myelin), Schwann cells (which form PNS myelin), ependymal cells (which line the ventricles), and microglia (which are CNS macrophages).

11. Neurons contain a nucleus and nucleolus, Nissl bodies (rough endoplasmic reticulum), Golgi apparatus, mitochondria, neurofilaments, and microtubules. Most neurons have dendrites and an axon: dendrites receive synaptic contacts from other neurons, and the axon makes synaptic contacts with other neurons.

12. Neurons encode information by labeled lines, neural maps, and patterns of nerve impulses.

13. Chemical substances are distributed along axons by fast or slow axonal transport; the direction of axonal transport may be anterograde or retrograde.

14. Damage to the axon of a neuron causes an axonal reaction in the cell body (chromatolysis) and wallerian degeneration of the axon distal to the injury.

Regeneration of PNS axons is more likely than that of CNS axons.

15. The growth and maintenance of axons are affected by trophic factors, such as nerve growth factor.

■ *Self-Study Problems*

1. What are the main subdivisions of the central nervous system, based on the embryologic origins of these? What adult structures belong in each?

2. What would happen to cerebrospinal fluid pressure if the outflow of CSF to the venous system by way of the arachnoidal granulations were blocked? If CSF accumulated, what would this do to the volume of brain tissue and blood contained within the skull?

3. What are the types of cells found in central nervous tissue? What are the main functions of each?

4. What are some of the ways in which information is coded in messages conducted through neural circuits?

5. Distinguish between the different types of axonal transport.

■ *Bibliography*

Journal articles

Bray GM, Rasminsky M, Aguayo AJ: Interactions between axons and their sheath cells, *Annu Rev Neurosci* 4:127, 1981.

Butt AM, Ransom BR: Visualization of oligodendrocytes and astrocytes in the intact rat optic nerve by intracellular injection of lucifer yellow and horseradish peroxidase, *Glia* 2:470, 1989.

Fawcett JW, Keynes RJ: Peripheral nerve regeneration, *Annu Rev Neurosci* 13:43, 1990.

Gehrmann J, Matsumoto Y, Kreutzberg GW: Microglia: intrinsic immuneffector cell of the brain, *Brain Res Rev* 20:269, 1995.

Ip NY, Yancopoulos GD: The neurotrophins and CNTF: two families of collaborative neurotrophic factors, *Annu Rev Neurosci* 19:491, 1996.

Landis DMD: The early reactions of non-neuronal cells to brain injury, *Annu Rev Neurosci* 17:133, 1994.

Lewin GR, Barde YA: Physiology of the neurotrophins, *Annu Rev Neurosci* 19:289, 1996.

Matthews G: Neurotransmitter release, *Annu Rev Neurosci* 19:219, 1996.

Partridge WM: Brain metabolism: a perspective from the blood-brain barrier, *Physiol Rev* 63:1481, 1983.

Udin SB, Fawcett JW: Formation of topographic maps, *Annu Rev Neurosci* 11:289, 1988.

Vallee RB, Bloom GS: Mechanisms of fast and slow axonal transport, *Annu Rev Neurosci* 14:59, 1991.

Books and monographs

Cajal SR: *Degeneration and regeneration of the nervous system,* New York, 1959, Hafner.

Cajal SR: *Histology of the nervous system of man and vertebrates,* New York, 1995, Oxford University Press.

Kandel ER, Schwartz JH, Jessell TM: *Principles of neural science,* ed 3, New York, 1991, Elsevier.

Kettenmann H, Ransom BR, editors: *Neuroglia,* New York, 1995, Oxford University Press.

Millen JW, Woollam DHM: *The anatomy of the cerebrospinal fluid,* New York, 1962, Oxford University Press.

Nicholls JG, Martin AR, Wallace BG: *From neuron to brain,* ed 3, Sunderland, Mass, 1992, Sinaer Associates.

Paxinos G, editor: *The human nervous system,* San Diego, 1990, Academic Press.

Peters A, Palay SL, Webster H deF: *The fine structure of the nervous system,* ed 3, New York, 1991, Oxford University Press.

Shephard GM, editor: *The synaptic organization of the brain,* ed 3, New York, 1990, Oxford University Press.

Whitfield IC: *Neurocommunications: an introduction,* New York, 1984, John Wiley & Sons.

Willis WD, Grossman RG: *Medical neurobiology,* ed 3, St Louis, 1981, Mosby–Year Book.

CHAPTER

7

The Peripheral Nervous System

The central nervous system (CNS) analyzes sensory information transmitted from sensory receptors that are located at the ends of primary afferent neurons. On the basis of this information, the CNS produces motor commands that are transmitted (1) by motor axons from somatic motor neurons to skeletal muscle fibers or (2) by autonomic preganglionic and postganglionic neurons to cardiac muscle, smooth muscle, or glands. The CNS thus senses and analyzes the environment in order to generate behavior appropriate to the environment.

The axons of primary afferent neurons, somatic motor neurons, and autonomic motor neurons all pass through the peripheral nervous system (PNS) (Fig. 7-1). The PNS serves as a bridge between the environment and the CNS. This chapter discusses the sensory and somatic motor components of the PNS. Details about the composition and destination of particular peripheral nerves can be found in a standard textbook of gross anatomy. The peripheral and central components of the autonomic nervous system are discussed in Chapter 15.

■ Sensory Components of the Peripheral Nervous System

■ Sensory Receptors

Sensory receptors are specialized neurons that serve as transducers of environmental energy. Some sensory receptors (e.g., the photoreceptor cells in the eye) provide information to the organism about its external environment. Other sensory receptors (e.g., baroreceptors that sense blood pressure in the arteries) provide information about the internal environment. In general, this information is then transmitted to the CNS by trains of nerve impulses along primary afferent neurons. As mentioned in Chapter 6, the cell bodies of primary afferent neurons are located in dorsal root and cranial nerve ganglia. Each primary afferent neuron has both a peripheral process that extends distally through a peripheral nerve to reach the appropriate sensory receptor(s) and a central

process that enters the CNS through a dorsal root or a cranial nerve (Fig. 7-1, *A*).

Types of sensory receptors. Sensory receptors can be classified in several different ways. One such way relates to whether they provide information about the external environment (**exteroceptors**), the internal environment (**interoceptors**), or the position of the body in space (**proprioceptors**). Another, more detailed classification is shown in Table 7-1.

Transduction. Sensory systems are designed to respond to the environment. The environmental event that excites sensory receptors is called a **stimulus.** Excited sensory receptors then relay information about the stimulus to the CNS. The **response** to the stimulus is the effect the stimulus has on the organism.

Responses can be recognized at several functional levels of the nervous system, including receptor potentials in sensory receptors, the transmission of action potentials along axons in sensory pathways, synaptic events in sensory neural networks, motor activity triggered by sensory stimulation, and ultimately behavioral events. The process that enables a sensory receptor to respond usefully to a stimulus is called **sensory transduction.**

The environmental events that trigger sensory transduction are always some form of energy, such as mechanical, thermal, or chemical energy. Sensory receptors are specialized for the transduction of one form of energy. In addition, some organisms are able to transduce forms of energy that other organisms cannot. For instance, although humans cannot sense electrical or magnetic fields, many fish have electroreceptors, and both fish and birds may use the earth's magnetic field for orientation during migration.

In all sensory receptors, transduction occurs when the properties of the sensory receptor neuron membrane are altered in some way by a stimulus. Fig. 7-2 shows how different types of stimuli can alter the membrane properties of sensory receptor neurons specialized to transduce such stimuli. For example, in Fig. 7-2, *A,* a **chemoreceptor** responds when a molecule of a *chemical stimulant* reacts with **receptor molecules** on the plasma membrane

■ **Fig. 7-1** **A,** A diagram of the spinal cord, spinal roots, and spinal nerve. A primary afferent neuron is shown with its cell body in the dorsal root ganglion and its central and peripheral processes distributing, respectively, to the spinal cord gray matter and to a sensory receptor in the skin. A motor neuron is shown to have its cell body in the spinal cord gray matter and to project its axon out of the ventral root to innervate a skeletal muscle fiber. **B,** A sympathetic preganglionic neuron is shown to have its cell body in the spinal cord gray matter. The axon courses out of the ventral root and enters a sympathetic ganglion through a white communicating ramus. The preganglionic axon synapses on a ganglion cell, and the ganglion cell sends its process, the postganglionic axon, through a gray communicating ramus into the spinal nerve. The postganglionic axon is shown to terminate on an arteriole in the body wall.

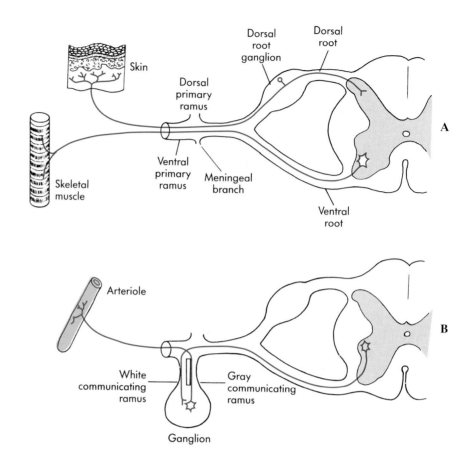

■ **Table 7-1** Classification of sensory receptors

Special	Vision, audition, taste, olfaction, balance
Superficial	Touch, pressure, flutter, vibration, tickle, warmth, cold, pain, itch
Deep	Position, kinesthesia, deep pressure, deep pain
Visceral	Hunger, nausea, distention, visceral pain

From Willis WD, Grossman RG: *Medical neurobiology,* ed 3, St Louis, 1981, Mosby–Year Book.

of the sensory receptor. (Note the distinction between a sensory receptor, which consists of one or more cells, and a receptor molecule, which is a protein inserted into the membrane of a cell.) The reaction between the chemical stimulant and the receptor molecules opens ion channels, enabling the influx of an ionic current that depolarizes the sensory receptor. In Fig. 7-2, *B,* the ion channel of a **mechanoreceptor** opens in response to the application of a *mechanical force* along the membrane. An influx of current flows through the ion channels and depolarizes the sensory receptor. Fig. 7-2, *C* shows the ion channel of a **photoreceptor** cell or a cell that responds to *light.* The ion channel is open in the dark. When a photon of light is absorbed by a special pigment on the disc membrane, the ion channel closes. Thus, an influx of current occurs in the dark and is appropriately called the **dark current;** the current ceases when light is applied. When the current stops, the photoreceptor hyperpolarizes.

As illustrated in Fig. 7-3, sensory transduction generally produces a receptor potential in the peripheral end of the sensory afferent neuron. This receptor potential is usually a depolarizing event that results from inward ionic current flow, and it brings the membrane potential of the sensory receptor toward or past the threshold needed to trigger an action potential. For example, in Fig. 7-3, a mechanical stimulus distorts the peripheral terminal mechanoreceptor and causes an inward current flow at the end of the axon and longitudinal and outward ionic current flow along the axon. The outward current produces a depolarization (the receptor potential), which may or may not exceed the threshold needed to trigger an action potential. In this example, the action potential is generated in a trigger zone at the first node of Ranvier of the afferent fiber.

In some sensory receptors, the receptor potential produced by sensory transduction is not a depolarization but a hyperpolarization. For example, in photoreceptors (as mentioned above) the receptor potential is hyperpolarizing. Details about how information is transmitted in the visual system are discussed in Chapter 9.

In some sensory receptors, the primary afferent fiber terminates on a separate, peripherally located sensory cell rather than comprising the sensory receptor itself. For example, primary afferent fibers of the cochlea of the inner ear end on **hair cells.** Sensory transduction in such sense organs is made more complex by this arrangement.

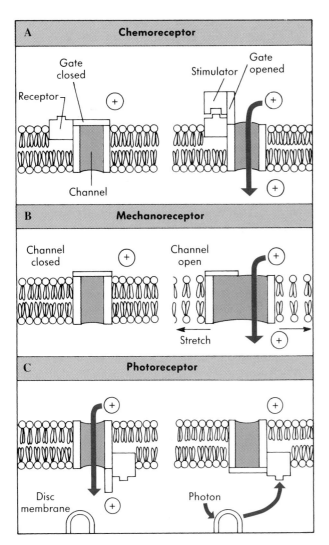

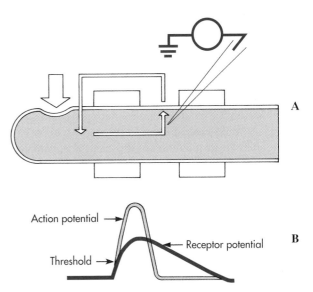

■ **Fig. 7-3 A,** The current flow produced by stimulation of a mechanoreceptor at the site indicated by the arrow and an intracellular recording from a node of Ranvier. **B,** The receptor potential produced by the current and an action potential that may be superimposed on the receptor potential if the latter exceeds threshold.

■ **Fig. 7-2 A to C,** Conceptual models of transducer mechanisms in three types of receptors. (See text.)

In the cochlea, a receptor potential arises in the hair cells in response to sound (see Chapter 10). This receptor potential is oscillatory. During each oscillation, the membrane of the hair cell is depolarized. This depolarization triggers the release of an excitatory neurotransmitter from the hair cell onto the primary afferent terminal. The result of this complex process is a **generator potential,** which in turn depolarizes the primary afferent fiber. The generator potential brings the membrane potential of the primary afferent fiber toward or beyond the threshold needed to trigger a nerve impulse.

Adaptation. **Adaptation** is a characteristic property of sensory receptors. It is far more efficient for sensory receptors to specialize in signaling one particular kind of sensory information. In **slowly adapting receptors,** a long-lasting stimulus produces a prolonged, repetitive discharge in the primary afferent neurons that supply the sensory receptors. However, the same stimulus produces only a short-lived response (one or a few discharges) in **rapidly adapting receptors.** These different rates of adaptation occur because a prolonged stimulus may produce either a sustained or a transient receptor potential depending on the type of sensory receptor. In other words, different sensory receptors analyze different features of a stimulus. These differences in analysis are reflected in different adaptation rates. For example, if the skin is indented, a slowly adapting receptor may respond repetitively at a rate proportional to the amount of indentation (Fig. 7-4). On the other hand, rapidly adapting cutaneous receptors that respond best to transient mechanical stimuli may respond to the velocity or acceleration, rather than to the amount of skin indentation.

Receptive fields. The relationship between the location of a stimulus and the activation of particular sensory neurons is a major theme in sensory physiology. The **receptive field** of a sensory neuron is the region that, when stimulated, causes the neuron to fire an action potential. For example, a sensory receptor might be activated by indentation of only a small area of skin. That area is the **excitatory receptive field** of the sensory receptor.

Neurons in the CNS are often excited by stimulation of a receptive field several times as large as that of a sensory receptor. The reason CNS sensory neurons often have larger receptive fields than do sensory receptors is that CNS sensory neurons may receive information from many sensory receptors, each with a slightly different receptive field. The receptive field of the CNS neuron is thus the sum of the receptive fields of the sensory receptors that influence the CNS neuron. The location of the receptive field is determined by the location of the sensory transduction apparatus that actually signals information about the stimulus to the sensory neuron.

Generally, the receptive fields of sensory receptors are excitatory. However, a central sensory neuron can have either an excitatory or an **inhibitory receptive field.** For example, the somatosensory neuron illustrated in Fig. 7-5 has both excitatory and inhibitory receptive fields. This neuron is located in the SI (primary) somatosensory cerebral cortex. Inhibition of this neuron is mediated by inhibitory interneurons.

Sensory coding. Sensory neurons encode stimuli. In the process of sensory transduction, one or more aspects of the stimulus must be encoded in a way that can be

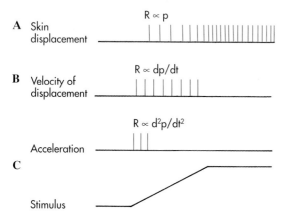

A Skin displacement
$$R \propto p$$

B Velocity of displacement
$$R \propto dp/dt$$

Acceleration
$$R \propto d^2p/dt^2$$

C

Stimulus

■ **Fig. 7-4** Responses of slowly and rapidly adapting mechanoreceptors to displacement of the skin. The discharges of the primary afferent fibers supplying the receptors in response to the ramp and hold stimulus *(bottom)* are termed the response *(R)*. **A,** *R* is proportional to skin position *(p)*. The receptor is slowly adapting and signals skin displacement. **B,** *R* is a function of the velocity of displacement *(dp/dt)*. **C,** *R* is a function of the acceleration *(d²p/dt²)*. These receptors are rapidly adapting but signal different, dynamic features of the stimulus.

interpreted by the CNS. The nature of the code is based on (1) the sensory receptors that are activated, (2) the responses of the sensory receptors to the stimulus, and (3) information processing in the sensory pathway. Some aspects of stimuli that may be encoded include the **sensory modality, spatial location, threshold, intensity, frequency,** and **duration.** Other aspects of stimuli that are encoded are presented in the discussion of particular sensory systems in later chapters.

A **sensory modality** is a readily identified type of sensation. For example, a sustained mechanical stimulus applied to the skin results in sensations of **touch** or **pressure,** and transient mechanical stimuli may evoke sensations of **flutter** or **vibration.** Other cutaneous modalities include cold, warmth, and pain. Vision, audition, position, sense, taste, and smell are examples of noncutaneous sensory modalities. Coding for modality is signaled by labeled-line sensory channels in most sensory systems (see Chapter 6). A **labeled-line** sensory channel consists of a set of neurons devoted to a particular sensory modality.

The **spatial location** of a stimulus is another way in which sensory information is coded. Often, the location of a stimulus is signaled by the activation of the sensory neurons whose receptive fields are affected by the stimulus (Fig. 7-6, *A*). In some cases, an inhibitory receptive field or a contrasting border between an excitatory and an inhibitory receptive field can localize the stimulus. Resolution of two different adjacent stimuli may depend on excitation of partially separate populations of neurons and on inhibitory interactions (Fig. 7-6, *B*).

A **threshold stimulus** is the weakest stimulus that a sensory receptor can reliably detect. For detection, a stimulus must produce receptor potentials large enough to activate one or more primary afferent fibers. Weaker intensities of stimulation can produce subthreshold receptor potentials; however, such stimuli would not

■ **Fig. 7-5** Excitatory and inhibitory receptive fields of a central somatosensory neuron located in the SI (primary) somatosensory cerebral cortex. The excitatory receptive field is on the forearm and is surrounded by an inhibitory receptive field. The graph shows the response to an excitatory stimulus and the inhibition of that response by a stimulus applied in the inhibitory field.

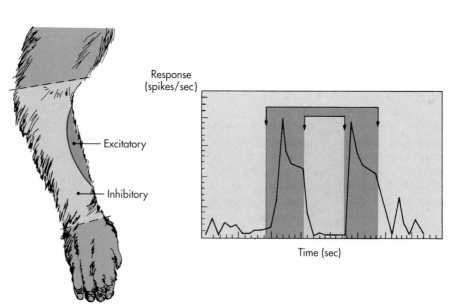

Excitatory

Inhibitory

Response (spikes/sec)

Time (sec)

excite central sensory neurons and so could not be perceived. Furthermore, the number of primary afferent neurons that must be excited for sensory detection depends on the requirements for **spatial** and **temporal summation** in the sensory pathway (see Chapter 4). In some sensory systems, a stimulus at threshold for detection must be much greater than the threshold for activation of the most responsive primary afferent neurons. Thus, a stimulus that excites some primary afferent neurons may not be perceived. On the other hand, if a stimulus is perceived, at least one primary afferent neuron must be excited beyond threshold.

An example of a difference in the thresholds for sensory receptors and for perception is in the peripheral encoding of pain. Painful stimuli generally activate sensory receptors called **nociceptors.** Recordings have been made from nociceptors in human nerves by a technique called microneurography. In this technique, a microelectrode is inserted into a peripheral nerve in a conscious subject. When recordings are taken from an individual nerve fiber, it is sometimes possible to demonstrate that the receptive field is that of a nociceptor. However, activation of the nociceptor under observation may not cause pain. Two alternative explanations may account for this absence of pain. Nociceptive processing may require spatial summation, and thus more than one nociceptive afferent axon must be activated in order to produce pain. Alternatively, nociceptive processing may rely on temporal summation, in which case a single nociceptor must be activated more than once. In fact, it appears that a single cutaneous nociceptor must fire at a rate of 3 Hz or more before pain is perceived, and pain is greater when more than one nociceptor is activated.

Another aspect of stimuli that can be encoded is the stimulus **intensity.** Stimulus intensity may be encoded by the mean frequency of the firing of sensory neurons. The relationship between stimulus intensity and response can be plotted as a stimulus-response function. For many sensory neurons, the stimulus-response function approximates an exponential curve (Fig. 7-7). The general equation for such a curve is

$$\text{Response} = \text{constant} \times (\text{stimulus} - \text{threshold stimulus})^n$$

The exponent, n, can be less than, equal to, or greater than 1. Stimulus-response functions with fractional exponents are found for many mechanoreceptors (Fig. 7-7). **Thermoreceptors,** which detect changes in *temperature,* have linear stimulus-response curves (exponent of 1).

One-point stimulus

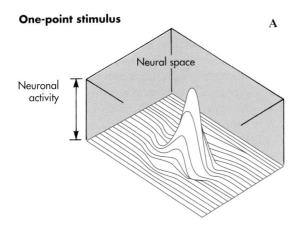

Two-point stimulus

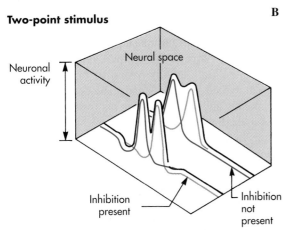

■ **Fig. 7-6 A,** Representation of the activity of a large population of neurons distributed three-dimensionally in neural space. The activity is in response to stimulation of a point on the skin. Note that an excitatory peak is surrounded by an inhibitory trough; these are determined by the excitatory and inhibitory fields of sensory neurons in the central pathways. **B,** The activity in response to stimulation of two adjacent points on the skin. Note that the sum of the activity *(black line)* is separated better into two peaks when inhibition is present than when it is not.

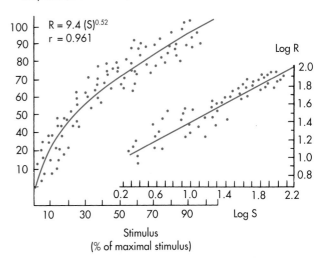

■ **Fig. 7-7** Stimulus-response function for slowly adapting cutaneous mechanoreceptors. The rate of discharge is plotted against stimulus strength (normalized to maximal). The plots are on linear and on log-log scales. The stimulus-response function is R = 9.4(S).$^{0.52}$

Nociceptors, which detect *painful* stimuli, may have linear or positively accelerating stimulus-response functions; that is, the exponent for these curves is 1 or more.

> The positively accelerating stimulus-response functions of nociceptors help explain the urgency experienced as pain increases. The processing of pain in CNS nociceptive pathways is also characterized by positively accelerating curves.

Another way in which stimulus intensity is encoded is by the number of sensory receptors activated. A stimulus at the threshold for perception may activate just one or a few primary afferent neurons of an appropriate class, whereas a strong stimulus of the same type may excite many similar receptors. Central sensory neurons that receive input from this particular class of sensory receptor would be more powerfully activated as more primary afferent neurons discharge. Greater activity in central sensory neurons is perceived as a stronger stimulus.

Stimuli of different intensities may also activate different sets of sensory receptors. For example, a weak mechanical stimulus applied to the skin might activate only mechanoreceptors, whereas a strong mechanical stimulus might activate both mechanoreceptors and nociceptors. In this case, the sensation evoked by the stronger stimulus would be more intense, and the quality would be different.

Stimulus **frequency** can be encoded by the intervals between the discharges of sensory neurons. Sometimes the intervals between discharges correspond exactly to the intervals between stimuli (Fig. 7-8). In other cases, a given neuron may discharge at intervals that are multiples of the interstimulus interval.

Stimulus **duration** may be encoded in slowly adapting sensory neurons by the duration of enhanced firing. The beginning and end of a stimulus may be signaled by transient discharges of rapidly adapting sensory receptors.

■ *Primary Afferent Neurons*

The peripheral processes of primary afferent neurons that supply different types of sensory receptors have characteristic ranges of conduction velocity. For example, some sensory receptors in muscle are supplied by the largest myelinated axons in the PNS, the **group I** afferent fibers. Other sensory receptors in muscle are innervated by medium-sized **(group II)** or small **(group III)** myelinated axons or by unmyelinated **(group IV)** axons. The largest myelinated axons that supply cutaneous sensory receptors are comparable in size with the medium-sized muscle afferent fibers. Sometimes these fibers are called group II fibers, but more commonly they are referred to as **Aβ** afferent fibers. Small myelinated and unmyelinated cutaneous afferent fibers are classed as **Aδ** fibers and **C** fibers, respectively.

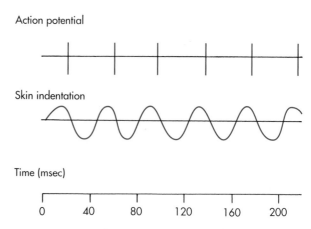

■ Fig. 7-8   Coding for the frequency of stimulation. Discharge of a rapidly adapting cutaneous mechanoreceptor in phase with a sinusoidal stimulus. The action potentials are shown at the top and the stimulus in the middle trace.

Table 7-2 lists some of the types of sensory receptors associated with differently sized peripheral processes of primary afferent neurons that supply muscle or skin. The terminology used for differently sized axons that supply joints is the same as for muscle, and that for viscera is the same as for skin.

■ *Somatic Motor Components of the Peripheral Nervous System*

Contractions of skeletal muscle fibers allow the body to move. Skeletal muscle fibers are innervated by large neurons in the ventral horn of the spinal cord or in cranial nerve nuclei called **α motor neurons.** These large, multipolar neurons range in size up to 70 microns in diameter (Fig. 7-9). They usually have 7 to 11 dendrites that may each exceed 1 mm in length. The dendrites are oriented radially and extend as far in the rostrocaudal direction as in the transverse plane.

Axons of the neurons leave the spinal cord through the ventral roots. As the axon passes ventrally, it may give off one or more recurrent collateral fibers that synapse on **Renshaw cells** (see Chapter 12), which are inhibitory interneurons in the ventral horn named after their discoverer. The motor axons are distributed to the appropriate skeletal muscles through peripheral nerves, and terminate at synapses on skeletal muscle fibers at **neuromuscular junctions** or **endplates.**

A given skeletal muscle is supplied by a group of α motor neurons located in a **motor nucleus** (Fig. 7-10, *A*). In the ventral horn, a motor nucleus is typically a sausage-shaped array of motor neurons that extend over several spinal cord segments (Fig. 7-10, *B*). Motor nuclei that supply different muscles are arranged somatotopically in the ventral horn (Fig. 7-11). Motor nuclei that

■ Table 7-2   Types of sensory receptors

Type	Group	Subgroup	Diameter (μm)	Conduction velocity (m/sec)	Tissue supplied	Function
Afferent						
A	I	Ia	12-20	72-120	Muscle	Afferents from muscle spindle primary endings
		Ib			Muscle	Afferents from Golgi tendon organs
	II		6-12	36-72	Muscle	Afferents from muscle spindle secondary endings
	Beta				Skin	Afferents from pacinian corpuscles, touch receptors
	III		1-6	6-36	Muscle	Afferents from pressure-pain endings
	Delta				Skin	Afferents from touch, temperature, and pain receptors
C	IV		<1	0.5-2	Muscle	Afferents from pain receptors
	Dorsal root				Skin	Afferents from touch, pain, and temperature receptors

From Willis WD, Grossman RG: *Medical neurobiology,* ed 3, St Louis, 1981, Mosby–Year Book.

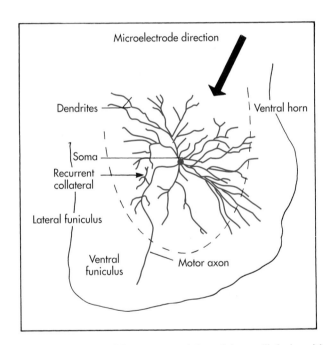

■ **Fig. 7-9**   α Motor neuron injected intracellularly with horseradish peroxidase. The small arrow indicates a recurrent collateral of the motor axon. The large arrow shows the direction followed by the microelectrode.

supply the axial muscles of the body are located in the medial part of the ventral horn in the cervical and lumbosacral enlargements and in the most ventral part of the ventral horn in the upper cervical, thoracic, and upper lumbar segments of the spinal cord. Motor nuclei that innervate the limb muscles are located in the lateral part of the ventral horn in the cervical and lumbosacral enlargements. The most distal muscles are supplied by motor nuclei located in the dorsolateral part of the ventral horn, whereas more proximal muscles are innervated by motor nuclei in the ventrolateral ventral horn. The set of α motor neurons that innervates a muscle is called the **motor neuron pool** of the muscle.

Each skeletal muscle fiber in mammals is supplied by just one α motor neuron. However, a given α motor neuron may innervate a variable number of skeletal muscle fibers, depending on the fineness of control the muscle requires. For highly regulated muscles, such as the eye muscles, an α motor neuron may supply only a few skeletal muscle fibers. However, for a proximal limb muscle, such as the quadriceps femoris, a single α motor neuron may innervate thousands of skeletal muscle fibers.

*A **motor unit** is an α motor neuron, its motor axon, and all the skeletal muscle fibers that it supplies.* The motor unit can therefore be thought of as the basic unit of movement. Under normal conditions, when an α motor neuron discharges, all the muscle fibers of the motor unit contract. A given α motor neuron may participate in a variety of reflexes and in voluntary movements. Because decisions about whether or not the synaptic input from a variety of sources will cause particular muscle fibers to contract are made at the level of the α motor neuron (in mammals), the motor neuron has been termed the **final common pathway.**

Another type of motor neuron is called the γ **motor neuron.** γ Motor neurons are smaller than α motor neurons and have a soma diameter of about 35 microns. Their dendrites are simpler and oriented mostly in the transverse plane. The γ motor neurons that project to a particular muscle are located in the same motor nucleus as the α motor neurons that supply that muscle. γ Motor neurons do not supply ordinary skeletal muscle fibers.

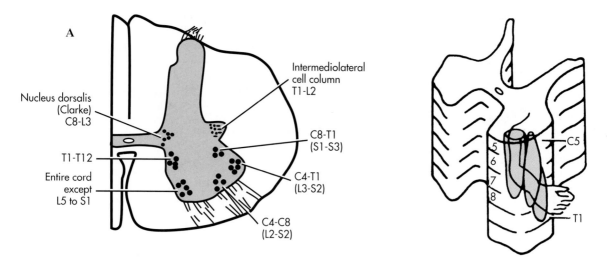

■ **Fig. 7-10**   Diagrammatic illustration of the topographic organization of the motor neurons and the muscles they innervate. **A,** A transverse section of the spinal cord with the positions of various cellular columns and their longitudinal extents. **B,** Three longitudinal columns of motor neurons *(color)* at cervical levels in relation to the parts of the arm they innervate. It should be appreciated that the more proximal muscles of the arm are innervated by more ventromedially situated motor neurons and the more distal muscles by more dorsolaterally situated motor neurons. (Redrawn from Brodal A: *Neurological anatomy,* ed 3, New York, 1981, Oxford University Press.)

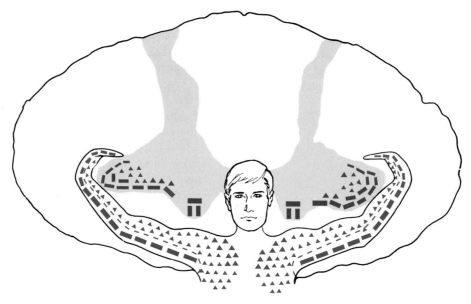

■ **Fig. 7-11**   Somatotopic organization of spinal cord motor neurons. Motor neurons to axial muscles are in the medial ventral horn. In the lateral part of the motor nucleus, motor neurons to more proximal muscles are indicated by the larger symbols. Extensor muscles are supplied by motor neurons indicated by solid rectangles, and flexor muscles by motor neurons indicated by triangles.

Instead, they synapse on the specialized striated muscle fibers, the **intrafusal muscle fibers,** that are found within muscle spindles (see Chapter 12).

Table 7-3 shows the sizes of the axons of somatic motor neurons and their conduction velocities.

The skeletal muscle fibers that belong to a given motor unit are called a **muscle unit.** All the muscle fibers in a muscle unit are of the same histochemical type; that is, they are either all type I, all type IIB, or all type IIA. The contractile properties of these muscle fiber types are summarized in Table 7-4. Motor units that twitch slowly and resist fatigue are classified as **S** (slow) and have type I fibers. S motor units depend on oxidative metabolism for their energy supply and have weak contractions (Fig.

Motor unit type	FF	FR	S
Histochemical profile	FG	FOG	SO

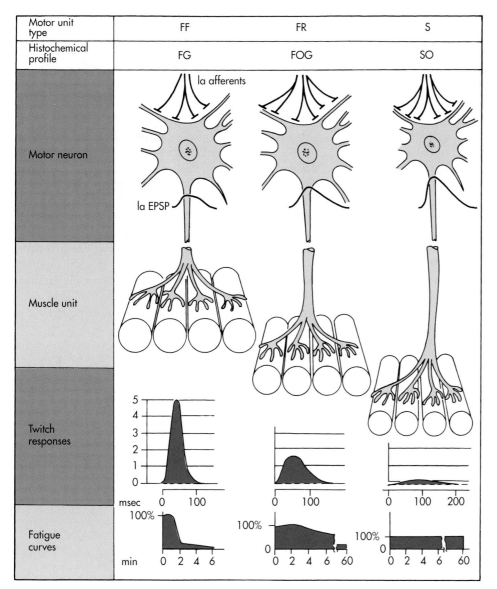

Motor neuron			
Muscle unit			
Twitch responses			
Fatigue curves			

■ **Fig. 7-12** Summary of features of motor units in a mixed muscle (medial gastrocnemius of cat). Relative sizes are shown for motor neurons, muscle fibers, monosynaptic excitatory postsynaptic potentials evoked by volleys in group Ia afferent fibers, and twitch responses. *EPSP,* Excitatory postsynaptic potential; *FG,* fast glycolytic; *FOG,* fast oxidative-glycolytic; *SO,* slow oxidative; *FF,* fast fatigable; *FR,* fast fatigue resistant; *S,* slow.

■ **Table 7-3** Characteristics of axons of somatic motor neurons

Type	Group	Subgroup	Diameter (μm)	Conduction velocity (m/sec)	Tissue supplied	Function
A	α		12-20	72-120	Muscle	Motor supply of extrafusal skeletal muscle fibers
	γ		2-8	12-48	Muscle	Motor supply of intrafusal muscle fibers

From Willis WD, Grossman RG: *Medical neurobiology,* ed 3, St Louis, 1981, Mosby–Year Book.

7-12). Muscle units with fast twitches are **FF** (fast, fatigable) or **FR** (fast, fatigue resistant). FF muscle units have type IIB fibers, use glycolytic metabolism, and contract strongly; however, these fibers fatigue easily. FR muscle units have type IIA fibers, rely on oxidative metabolism, and resist fatigue; their contractions are of intermediate force.

■ **Table 7-4** Muscle fiber contractile properties

Type	Speed	Strength	Fatigability	Motor unit
I	Slow	Weak	Fatigue resistant	S
IIB	Fast	Strong	Fatigable	FF
IIA	Fast	Intermediate	Fatigue resistant	FR

From Berne RM, Levy MN, editors: *Principles of physiology,* ed 2, St Louis, 1996, Mosby–Year Book.

A clinically useful way to monitor the activity of motor units is by means of **electromyography.** An electrode is placed within a skeletal muscle to record the summed action potentials of the skeletal muscle fibers of a muscle unit (Fig. 7-13). If no spontaneous activity is noted, the patient is asked to contract the muscle voluntarily to increase the activity of motor units in the muscle. As the force of voluntary contraction increases, more motor units are **recruited,** and contractile strength is affected by the rate of discharge of active α motor neurons.

Electromyography is used for a variety of purposes. For example, the conduction velocity of motor axons can be estimated by measuring the difference in latency of motor unit potentials when a peripheral nerve is stimulated at two sites separated by a known distance. Another use is to observe **fibrillation potentials** that occur when muscle fibers are denervated. Fibrillation potentials are spontaneously occurring action potentials in single muscle fibers.

These potentials can be contrasted with **motor unit potentials,** which are larger and have a longer duration. Motor unit potentials represent the action potentials in a set of muscle fibers belonging to a motor unit.

The first motor units to be activated, either by voluntary effort or during reflex action (see Chapter 12), are those with the smallest motor axons (Fig. 7-14); these motor units generate the smallest contractile forces and allow the initial contraction to be finely graded. As more motor units are recruited, the α motor neurons with progressively larger axons become involved and generate progressively larger amounts of tension. This orderly recruitment of motor units is called the **size principle,** because the motor units are recruited in order of motor axon size. The size principle depends on the fact that small α motor neurons are activated by excitatory postsynaptic potentials that are greater than those in large α motor neurons (Fig. 7-12).

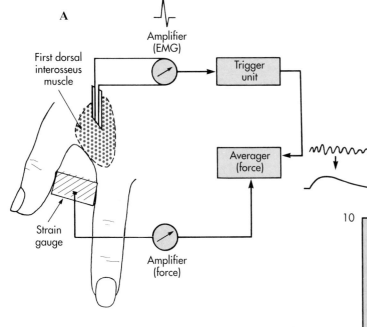

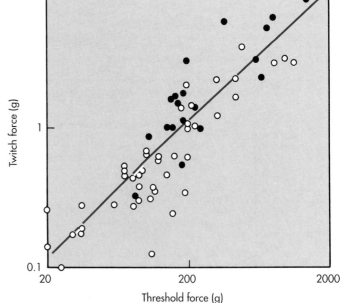

■ **Fig. 7-13**   Relationship between the threshold for recruitment and the force developed by a motor unit as studied during voluntary contraction of the first dorsal interosseus muscle of the human. **A,** Experimental arrangement for detecting the force developed by a single motor unit during voluntary contraction. The action potential of the motor unit is used to trigger an averager, which then samples the muscle force. **B,** Weaker motor units are recruited before stronger ones. (From Milner-Brown HS, Stein RB, Yemm R: *J Physiol (Lond)* 230:359, 1973.)

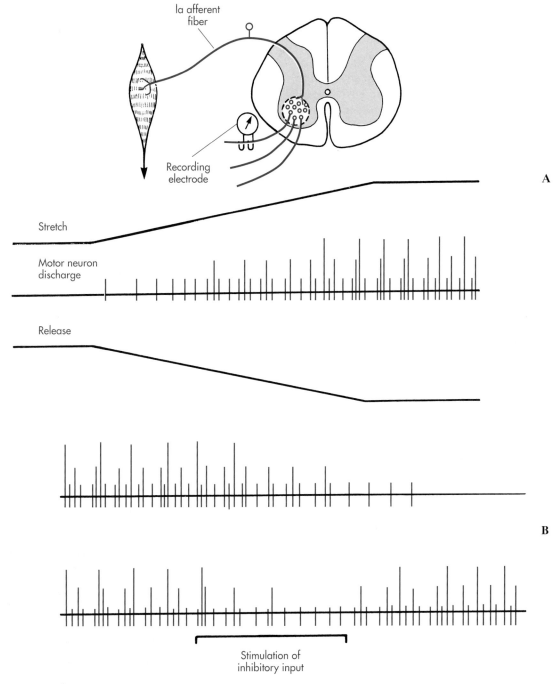

■ **Fig. 7-14** The size principle in the recruitment of motor neurons. The schematic at the top shows Ia afferent fiber from a muscle spindle and recording electrodes on a dissected ventral root filament arising from a homonymous motor neuron. **A,** Excitation. As a muscle is stretched, the increased activity of the Ia afferent fibers first recruits the smaller motor neurons. As the stretch increases, successively larger motor neurons are recruited. On release from stretch, the larger motor neurons stop discharging first and the smaller motor neurons last. **B,** Inhibition. Activating an inhibitory input to the motor neuron pool silences first the larger motor neurons and then successively smaller motor neurons. (From Eyzaguirre C, Fidone SJ: *Physiology of the nervous system: an introductory text,* ed 2, Chicago, 1975, Mosby–Year Book.)

■ *Summary*

1. The peripheral nervous system (PNS) contains the axons of primary afferent neurons, somatic motor neurons, and autonomic preganglionic and postganglionic neurons.

2. The cell bodies of primary afferent neurons are in dorsal root or cranial nerve ganglia.

3. Sensory receptors include exteroceptors, interoceptors, and proprioceptors. Stimuli are environmental events that excite sensory receptors; responses are the effects of stimuli; sensory transduction is the process by which stimuli are detected.

4. Sensory transduction is accomplished in different ways by different sensory receptors. In general, it involves the production of a receptor potential.

5. Sensory receptors may be slowly or rapidly adapting.

6. A receptive field is the region that, when stimulated, causes a response in sensory neurons.

7. Sensory receptors encode modality, spatial location, threshold, intensity, frequency, and duration of stimuli.

8. Primary afferent fibers can be subdivided according to the different receptor types that they supply and by their size.

9. α Motor neurons innervate skeletal muscle fibers; a motor unit includes an α motor neuron, its axon, and a set of skeletal muscle fibers.

10. γ Motor neurons are smaller than α motor neurons and supply intrafusal muscle fibers in muscle spindles.

11. Muscle fibers in a motor unit form a muscle unit; all the muscle fibers of a muscle unit are of the same histochemical type (slow; fast, fatigable; or fast, fatigue resistant).

12. The activity of motor units can be monitored by electromyography.

13. Motor units are recruited in an orderly fashion during voluntary or reflex activity; the first units to be recruited are those with the smallest motor axons and contractile force (size principle).

■ *Self-Study Problems*

1. What is a receptive field?

2. Describe some of the ways in which sensory receptors encode different aspects of a stimulus.

3. What is a motor unit and what are some characteristics of motor units?

4. What is the size principle and what is its functional meaning?

■ *Bibliography*

Journal articles

Westbury DR: A comparison of the structures of alpha- and gamma-spinal motoneurones of the cat, *J Physiol (Lond)* 325:79, 1982.

Books and monographs

Akoev GN, Andrianov GN: *Synaptic transmission in the mechano- and electroreceptors of the acousticolateral system.* In Ottoson D, editor: *Progress in sensory physiology 9,* Berlin, 1989, Springer-Verlag.

Belmonte C, Cervero F: *Neurobiology of nociceptors,* New York, 1996, Oxford University Press.

Binder MD, Mendell LM, editors: *The segmental motor system,* New York, 1990, Oxford University Press.

Boivie J, Hansson P, Lindblom U, editors: *Touch, temperature, and pain in health and disease: mechanisms and assessments,* Seattle, 1994, IASP Press.

Burke RE: *Motor units: anatomy, physiology and functional organization.* In Brookhart JM, Mountcastle VB, editors: *Handbook of physiology: the nervous system,* vol II, part 1, Bethesda, Md, 1981, American Physiological Society, p 345.

Henneman E, Mendell LM: *Functional organization of motoneuron pool and its inputs.* In Brookhart JM, Mountcastle VB, editors: *Handbook of physiology: the nervous system,* vol II, part 1, Bethesda, Md, 1981, American Physiological Society, p 423.

Lindauer M, Martin H: *The biological significance of the earth's magnetic field.* In Ottoson D, editor: *Progress in sensory physiology 5,* Berlin, 1985, Springer-Verlag.

Mountcastle VB: *Central nervous system mechanisms in mechanoreceptive sensibility.* In Brookhart JM, Mountcastle VB, editors: *Handbook of physiology: the nervous system,* vol III, part 2, Bethesda, Md, 1984, American Physiological Society, p 789.

Shepherd GM: *Neurobiology,* ed 3, New York, 1994, Oxford University Press.

Willis WD, Coggeshall RE: *Sensory mechanisms of the spinal cord,* ed 2, New York, 1991, Plenum Press.

Willis WD, Grossman RG: *Medical neurobiology,* ed 3, St Louis, 1981, Mosby–Year Book.

The Somatosensory System

In primitive brains, subcortical and extrathalamic sensory structures were crucial to sensory processing. Comparable structures continue to be important in the advanced brains of modern mammals, even though the role of the cerebral cortex and thalamus in sensory processing has expanded enormously. For example, the reticular formation in the brainstem is one of the major sensory-motor integration systems in nonmammalian vertebrates. In mammals, it continues to play a role in sensory processing and it contributes to the arousal mechanism, selective attention, and motor control. Another example is the optic tectum, which is the most important structure in the visual system of nonmammalian vertebrates. The tectum still has important visual functions in mammals, although the highly evolved visual cortex has been added.

In this and the following chapters, the sensory systems of mammals are considered. Emphasis is placed on the more recently evolved components of most of these sensory systems that depend on thalamocortical interactions. However, the more primitive components are also discussed where appropriate.

receives information from first-order neurons (usually several or many) and transmits information to the thalamus. The information is transmitted along second-order neurons by local neural processing circuits and by the biophysical properties of the second-order neurons. The axon of a second-order neuron typically crosses the midline to ascend to the thalamus. Thus sensory information that originates on one side of the body reaches the opposite (contralateral) side of the thalamus.

The **third-order neuron** of a sensory pathway resides in one of the sensory nuclei of the thalamus. Again, local circuits in the thalamus and intrinsic membrane properties of the third-order neurons may transform information received from the second-order neurons before the signals are transmitted to the cerebral cortex.

Fourth-order neurons in the appropriate sensory receiving areas of the cerebral cortex and **higher-order neurons** in the same and other cerebral cortical areas process the information further. At some undetermined site in the cerebral cortex, the sensory information results in **perception,** which is a conscious awareness of the stimulus.

■ *Sensory Pathways*

A sensory pathway is simply a set of sensory neurons arranged in series (Fig. 8-1). First-, second-, third-, and higher-order neurons are the sequential elements in a given sensory pathway. In addition, several parallel sensory pathways are often involved in transmitting similar sensory information.

The **first-order neuron** in a sensory pathway is a primary afferent neuron. The peripheral endings of this neuron form a sensory receptor (or receive input from an accessory sensory cell, such as a hair cell). Thus, the first-order neuron responds to a stimulus, transduces it, and then transmits encoded information to the central nervous system (CNS). The soma of a primary afferent neuron is often located in a dorsal root or cranial nerve ganglion.

The **second-order neuron** of a sensory pathway is generally located in the spinal cord or brainstem. It

■ *The Somatovisceral Sensory System*

The somatosensory system, or more appropriately the somatovisceral sensory system, transmits information from sensory receptor organs in the skin, muscles, joints, and viscera to the CNS. Information arising from these sensory receptors reaches the CNS via first-order neurons, which, as we have noted, are primary afferent neurons. The cell bodies of the primary afferent neurons are located in dorsal root or cranial nerve ganglia. Each ganglion cell gives off an axon that branches into a peripheral process and a central process. The **peripheral process** terminates peripherally as a sensory receptor (or on an accessory cell). The **central process** enters either the spinal cord through a dorsal root or the brainstem through a cranial nerve. The central process typically gives rise to numerous collateral branches that end synaptically on several second-order neurons.

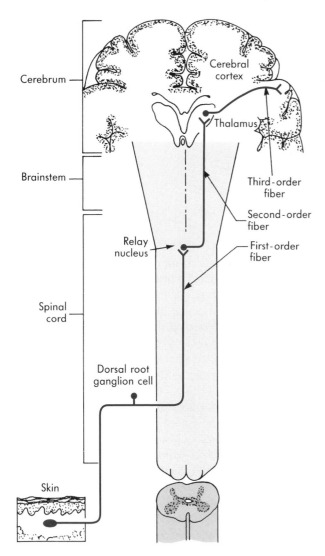

■ **Fig. 8-1** General arrangement of sensory pathways. First-, second-, and third-order neurons are shown. Note that the axon of the second-order neuron crosses the midline, so that sensory information from one side of the body is transmitted to the opposite side of the brain.

The processing of somatovisceral sensory information involves a number of CNS structures, including the spinal cord, brainstem, thalamus, and cerebral cortex. The ascending pathways are composed of second-order neurons located in the spinal cord and brainstem that project to the contralateral thalamus. The most important ascending somatosensory pathways that carry somatovisceral information from the body are the dorsal column–medial lemniscus pathway and the spinothalamic tract. The main somatosensory projection that represents the face is the trigeminothalamic tract. Ancillary somatosensory pathways include the spinocervicothalamic pathway, the postsynaptic dorsal column pathway, the dorsal spinocerebellar tract, the spinoreticular tract, and the spinomesencephalic tract. All these pathways are discussed later in this chapter.

The sensory modalities mediated by the somatovisceral sensory system include touch-pressure, flutter-vibration, proprioception (position sense and joint movement), thermal sense (warmth and cold), pain, and visceral distention.

■ *Sensory Receptors*

■ *Cutaneous Receptors*

Cutaneous receptors can be subdivided according to the type of stimulus to which they respond. The major types of cutaneous receptors include mechanoreceptors, thermoreceptors, and nociceptors.

Mechanoreceptors. Mechanoreceptors respond to mechanical stimuli such as stroking or indenting the skin, and they can be rapidly adapting or slowly adapting. Rapidly adapting cutaneous mechanoreceptors include **hair follicle receptors** in hairy skin, **Meissner's corpuscles** in glabrous (nonhairy) skin, and **pacinian corpuscles** in subcutaneous tissue (Fig. 8-2, *A*). Hair follicle receptors and Meissner's corpuscles respond best to stimuli repeated at rates of about 30 to 40 Hz, whereas pacinian corpuscles respond best to stimuli repeated at about 250 Hz. Slowly adapting cutaneous mechanoreceptors include **Merkel cell endings** and **Ruffini endings** (Fig. 8-2, *B*). Merkel cell receptors have punctate receptive fields, whereas Ruffini endings can be activated by stretching the skin, even at some distance away from the receptor terminals. The axons of all of these receptor types are myelinated. Most of the axons are Aβ fibers, although one class of hair follicle receptor, the down hair receptor, is supplied by Aδ fibers.

Some mechanoreceptors, C mechanoreceptors, are innervated by unmyelinated axons. These mechanoreceptors respond best to slowly moving stimuli, such as stroking. The C mechanoreceptors have only recently been found in humans, although they are common in other mammals, such as cats.

Thermoreceptors. Thermoreceptors are sensitive to the temperature of the skin. The two types of thermoreceptors in the skin are **cold** and **warm receptors.** Both types are slowly adapting, although they also discharge phasically when skin temperature changes rapidly (Fig. 8-3, *A*). Thermoreceptors are among the few receptor types that discharge spontaneously under normal circumstances. The receptors are active over a broad range of temperatures (Fig. 8-3, *B*). At a moderate skin temperature, such as 35° C, both cold and warm receptors may be active. However, as the skin is warmed, the cold receptors become inactive; conversely, as the skin is cooled, the warm receptors become inactive. Warm receptors also stop discharging as the temperature reaches the **noxious** (damaging) range (above 45° C). Therefore, these receptors cannot signal heat pain.

The stimulus-response curve for cold receptors in Fig. 8-3, *B* shows that the mean discharge frequencies of these

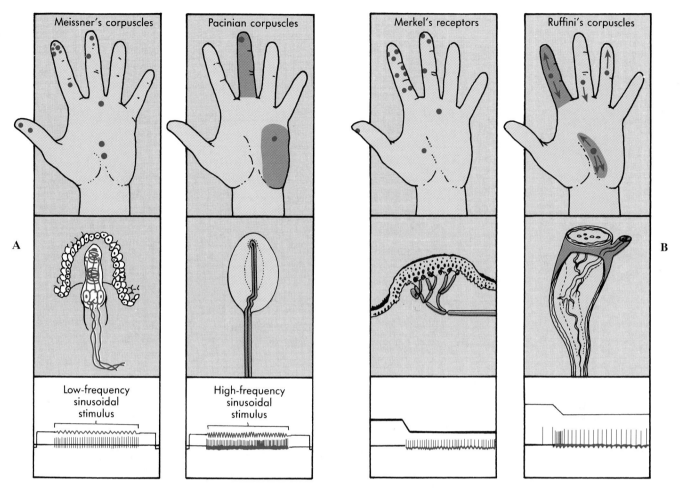

■ **Fig. 8-2** The receptive fields of several types of cutaneous mechanoreceptors are shown in the top row of drawings. **A,** Rapidly adapting mechanoreceptors: Meissner's corpuscles and pacinian corpuscles. **B,** Slowly adapting mechanoreceptors: Merkel's receptors and Ruffini's corpuscles. The second row of drawings shows the morphology of the receptors; the third row, the responses to sinusoidal stimuli (**A**) or to step indentations of the skin (**B**).

fibers do not allow the CNS to discriminate between temperatures at points above and below the peak of the curve. However, over a certain range of temperatures, cold receptors discharge in bursts (Fig. 8-3, *A*). These bursts may provide information that allows the CNS to distinguish between the activity of cold receptors exposed to higher and lower temperatures. In addition, another class of high-threshold cold receptors is activated when the temperature of the skin is lowered to a certain point. Most cold fibers are supplied by Aδ fibers and most warm receptors by C fibers.

Nociceptors. Nociceptors respond to stimuli that threaten or produce damage to the organism. The two major classes of cutaneous nociceptors are the **Aδ mechanical nociceptors** and the **C-polymodal nociceptors,** although several other types also exist. As their names suggest, the Aδ mechanical nociceptors are supplied by finely myelinated afferent fibers and the C-polymodal nociceptors by unmyelinated fibers. The Aδ mechanical nociceptors respond to strong mechanical

stimuli, such as pricking the skin with a needle or crushing the skin with forceps. They typically do not respond to noxious thermal or chemical stimuli unless they have previously been sensitized (see below). C-polymodal nociceptors, on the other hand, respond to several types of noxious stimuli, including mechanical, thermal (Fig. 8-4), and chemical stimuli.

Sensitization of nociceptors is the process by which afferent fibers that supply the receptors become more responsive. Nociceptors become sensitized after they respond to a given noxious stimulus. Sensitized nociceptors respond more vigorously to repeated stimulation by the noxious stimulus because their threshold for activation is lower (Fig. 8-4). This more vigorous response can lead to **hyperalgesia,** an increase in the pain produced by stimulation at a given intensity and a decrease in the pain threshold. The nociceptors may also develop a background discharge; this type of discharge produces spontaneous pain.

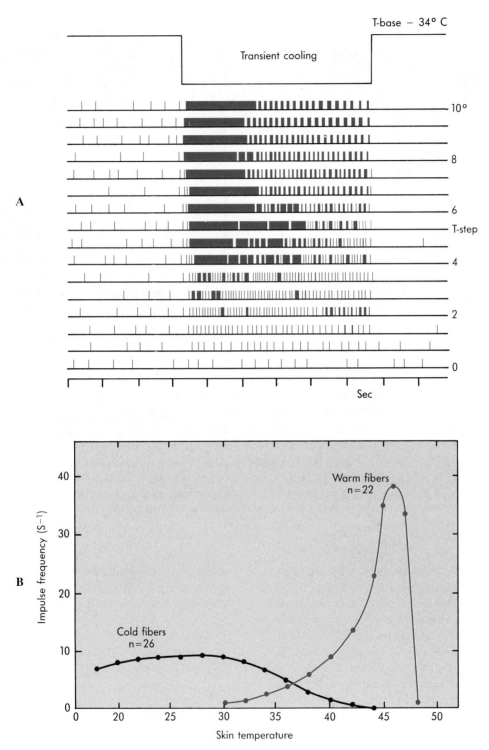

■ **Fig. 8-3** **A,** Responses recorded from the afferent supplying a cold receptor after graded cooling pulses. **B,** Average static discharge rates for populations of cold and warm receptors. (**A** from Darian-Smith I, Johnson KD, Dykes R: "Cold" fiber population innervating palmar and digital skin of the monkey: response to cooling pulses, *J Neurophysiol* 36:325, 1973; **B** from Hensel H, Kenshalo DR: *J Physiol* 204:99, 1969.)

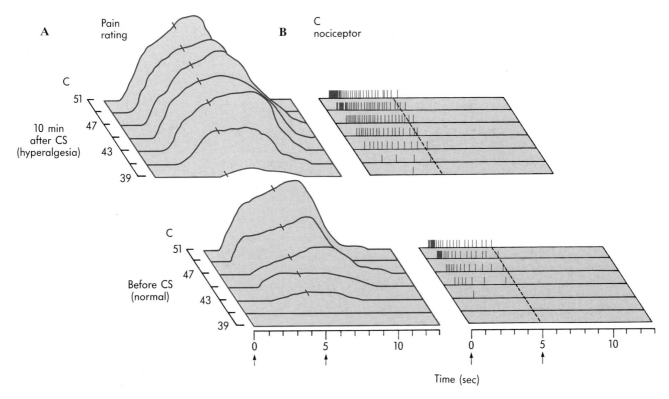

■ Fig. 8-4 **A,** Curves show magnitude ratings of pain in a human in response to heat pulses applied to the hairy skin before and after a mild burn. Arrows indicate the beginning and end of the stimuli. *CS,* Conditioning stimulus. **B,** Responses of a C-polymodal nociceptor innervating the hairy skin in a monkey in response to the same heat pulses before and after the mild burn. (From LaMotte RH, Thalhammer JG, Robinson CJ: *J Neurophysiol* 50:1, 1983.)

Sensitization occurs when chemical products, such as K⁺, bradykinin, serotonin, histamine, and eicosanoids (prostaglandins and leukotrienes) are released near nociceptor terminals after tissue damage or during inflammation. For example, a noxious stimulus applied to the skin may destroy cells near a nociceptor (Fig. 8-5, *A*). The dying cells release K^+, which depolarizes the nociceptor. Dying cells also release proteolytic enzymes that react with circulating globulins to form bradykinin. Bradykinin then binds to a receptor on the membrane of the nociceptor and activates a second messenger system, which in turn sensitizes the ending. Other chemical agents, such as serotonin released from platelets, histamine from mast cells, and eicosanoids from various cellular elements, also contribute to sensitization, either by opening ion channels or by activating second messenger systems. Many of these substances also act on blood vessels, immune cells, platelets, and other effectors that participate in inflammation.

Activation of a nociceptor terminal can also release chemicals, such as the peptide **substance P** (SP) and calcitonin gene-related peptide (CGRP), from other terminals of the same nociceptor through an **axon reflex** (Fig. 8-5, *A*). A nerve impulse estab-

lished in one branch of a nociceptor conducts centrally through the parent axon. However, it also spreads antidromically into other branches of the axon in the skin. As the nerve impulse invades these peripheral branches of the nociceptor, SP and CGRP are released into the skin (Fig. 8-5, *B*). SP and CGRP cause several effects, including vasodilation and increased capillary permeability. The effects of SP and CGRP augment the effects of other agents released from damaged cells and from platelets, mast cells, and invading leukocytes. The resultant inflammation leads to a typical series of changes in the skin, such as reddening and warming caused by the increased blood flow, swelling caused by **neurogenic edema,** and pain and tenderness due to the sensitization of nociceptors. These responses constitute the classic signs and symptoms of inflammation: **rubor** (redness), **calor** (heat), **tumor** (swelling), and **dolor** (pain).

■ *Muscle, Joint, and Visceral Receptors*

Skeletal muscle also contains several types of sensory receptors. Skeletal muscle sensory receptors are chiefly

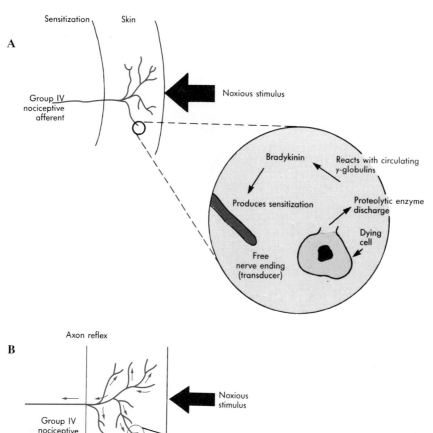

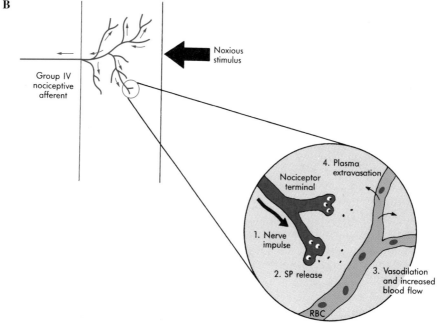

■ **Fig. 8-5** **A,** Sensitization of the terminals of a nociceptor. A noxious stimulus causing damage to cells results in the local release of proteolytic enzymes that react with circulating proteins to produce bradykinin. Bradykinin then binds to a receptor on the membrane of the nociceptive afferent fiber and sensitizes it (after activation of a second messenger system). The nociceptor is now more responsive to further stimulation. Other agents that would have similar effects include prostaglandins, serotonin, histamine, leukotrienes, and K+ ions, although these have different actions at the membrane level (e.g., serotonin would act on a receptor that opens an ion channel). **B,** Release of substance P *(SP)* and calcitonin gene-related peptide (CGRP) from a nociceptor after an axon reflex causes changes in the local environment. One action is vasodilation, resulting in reddening of the skin and warming. Another is increased capillary permeability, resulting in plasma extravasation. *RBC,* Red blood cell.

mechanoreceptors and nociceptors, although some muscle receptors may possess thermosensitivity or chemosensitivity. The best studied muscle receptors are the **stretch receptors,** which include muscle spindles and Golgi tendon organs. Although these receptors are important in sensing movement and position, called **proprioception,** they may be even more important in motor control. Their structure and function are discussed in Chapter 12. Nociceptors in muscle respond to pressure applied to the muscle and to release of metabolites, especially during ischemia (decreased blood flow). Muscle nociceptors are supplied by medium-sized and small myelinated (group II and III) axons or by unmyelinated (group IV) afferent fibers. Other muscle receptors with fine afferent fibers are regarded as **ergoreceptors,** which sense the work of muscles.

Joints are associated with several types of sensory receptors, such as rapidly and slowly adapting mechanoreceptors and nociceptors. The rapidly adapting mechanoreceptors are pacinian corpuscles, which respond to transient mechanical stimuli, including vibration. The slowly adapting receptors are Ruffini endings, which respond best to extreme movements of a joint. These endings signal pressure or torque applied to the joint. Joint mechanoreceptors are innervated by medium-sized (group II) afferent fibers. Joint nociceptors are activated by hyperextension or hyperflexion, although many articular nociceptors fail to respond to joint movements under normal conditions. If sensitized by inflammation, however, they respond to movements or to weak pressure stimuli, which normally do not activate these receptors. Joint nociceptors are innervated by finely myelinated (group III) or unmyelinated (group IV) primary afferent fibers.

The viscera are sparsely supplied with sensory receptors. The few visceral receptors are usually involved in reflexes and have little to do with sensory experience. However, some visceral mechanoreceptors are responsible for the sensation of distention, and visceral nociceptors signal visceral pain. Pacinian corpuscles are present in the mesentery and in the capsules of visceral organs such as the pancreas. These receptors presumably signal transient mechanical stimuli. Whether some forms of visceral pain result from overactivity of mechanoreceptor afferent fibers is still controversial. Some viscera, however, clearly have specific nociceptors. It is likely that some visceral nociceptors are inactive under normal circumstances but become active after sensitization by damage or inflammation.

■ *Microneurography*

The sensory functions of various cutaneous sensory receptors have been studied in human subjects by a technique known as microneurography. In this technique, a fine metal microelectrode is inserted into a nerve trunk in the arm or leg. When a recording can be made from a single sensory axon, the receptive field of the fiber is mapped. Many of the sensory receptors that have been studied in experimental animals have also been found in humans.

In some humans, it has been possible to do just the opposite, that is, stimulate the sensory axon through the microelectrode. In these experiments, the subject is asked to locate the perceived receptive field of the sensory axon, which turns out to be identical to the mapped receptive field. Repetitive stimulation is usually required to evoke a sensation, but subjects perceive the sensations produced by individual nerve fibers as pure sensations that match the properties of the receptors. The quality of

the sensations remains the same no matter what the frequency of stimulation. For example, stimulation of the afferent fiber of a Meissner's corpuscle causes a sensation of flutter, of a pacinian corpuscle a sensation of vibration, and of a Merkel's receptor a sensation of maintained touch. If the frequency of stimulation is increased to Meissner's or pacinian corpuscles, the perceived frequency of flutter or of vibration increases. However, an increase in the frequency of stimulation of Merkel endings augments the intensity of the touch or pressure sensation. Normally, the quality of the sensation does not change, for example, to pain.

The axons of most Ruffini endings so far tested do not produce a sensation when stimulated, but a few have recently been shown to cause sensations of either touch or position of a finger joint. Central summation is probably required for most Ruffini endings to produce a sensation, and the sensation can be either touch-pressure or proprioception.

Activation of individual Aδ nociceptors causes pricking pain. Stimulation of C-polymodal nociceptors produces either burning pain or, in some cases, itch. The sensory effects of C fibers probably result from activation of more than one afferent fiber.

■ *Dermatomes, Myotomes, and Sclerotomes*

Primary afferent fibers in the adult are distributed systematically both peripherally and centrally. The pattern of innervation is determined during embryologic development. During development, the mammalian embryo becomes segmented, and each body segment is called a **somite.** A somite is innervated by an adjacent segment of the spinal cord or, in the case of a somite of the head, by a cranial nerve. The portion of a somite destined to form skin is called a **dermatome.** Similarly, the part of a somite that will form muscle is a **myotome,** and the part that will form bone, a **sclerotome.** Viscera are also supplied by particular segments of the spinal cord or particular cranial nerves.

Many dermatomes become distorted during development, chiefly because of the rotation of the upper and lower extremities as they are formed and also because humans maintain an upright posture. However, the sequence of dermatomes can readily be understood if depicted on the body in a quadrupedal position (Fig. 8-6).

Although a dermatome receives its densest innervation from its corresponding spinal cord segment, the dermatome is also supplied by several adjacent spinal segments. Thus, transection of a single dorsal root causes little sensory loss in the corresponding dermatome. Anesthesia of any given dermatome requires interruption of several successive dorsal roots.

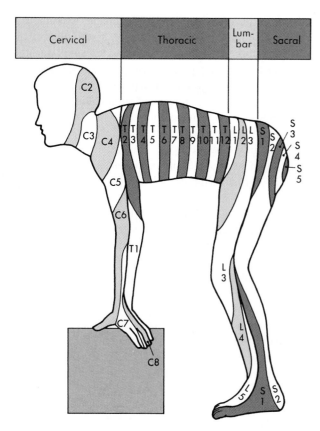

■ Fig. 8-6 Dermatomes represented on a drawing of a person assuming a quadrupedal position.

■ *Spinal Roots*

As shown in Fig. 8-7, axons of the peripheral nervous system (PNS) enter or leave the CNS through the spinal roots (or through cranial nerves). The **dorsal root** on one side of a given spinal segment is composed entirely of the central processes of dorsal root ganglion cells. The **ventral root** consists chiefly of motor axons, including α motor axons, γ motor axons, and at certain segmental levels, autonomic preganglionic axons. Ventral roots also contain many primary afferent fibers; the role of these fibers is still unclear.

Just before they penetrate the spinal cord, the large myelinated primary afferent fibers assume a medial position in the dorsal root, whereas the fine myelinated and unmyelinated fibers shift to a lateral position (Fig. 8-7). The large, medially placed afferent fibers enter the dorsal column, where they bifurcate to send one branch rostrally and another branch caudally. These branches travel through several segments, and some ascend to the medulla as part of the dorsal column–medial lemniscus pathway (see p 117). The axons in the dorsal funiculus give off collaterals that pass ventrally into the gray matter of the spinal cord. These collaterals transmit sensory information to neurons in the dorsal horn and also provide the afferent limb of reflex pathways.

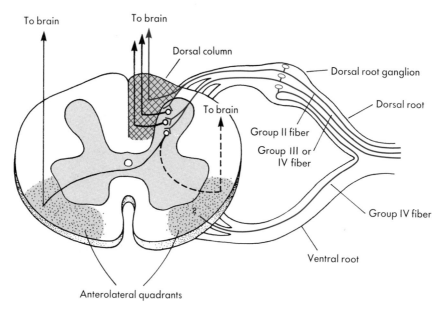

■ Fig. 8-7 Entry of large and small primary afferent fibers into the spinal cord. Primary afferent fibers have their cell bodies in the dorsal root ganglion. The central processes of the large fibers enter the spinal cord through the medial part of the dorsal root and join the dorsal funiculus. Collaterals synapse in the spinal cord gray matter. The central processes of small afferent fibers enter the cord through the lateral part of the dorsal root (or in some cases through the ventral root). Collaterals from primary afferent axons in the dorsolateral fasciculus synapse in the dorsal horn. Some of the second-order neurons project to the brain, either through the contralateral ventrolateral funiculus or through ipsilateral pathways in the dorsal or lateral funiculus.

■ *The Trigeminal Nerve*

The arrangement of primary afferent fibers that supply the face is comparable with that of fibers that supply the body. Peripheral processes of neurons in the trigeminal ganglion pass through the ophthalmic, maxillary, and mandibular divisions of the trigeminal nerve to innervate dermatome-like regions of the face. The trigeminal nerve also innervates the oral and nasal cavities and the cranial dura mater.

The large myelinated fibers that supply mechanoreceptors of the face and structures of the oral and nasal cavities synapse in the main sensory nucleus of the trigeminal nerve. Small myelinated and unmyelinated primary afferent fibers of the trigeminal nerve descend through the brainstem in the spinal tract of the trigeminal nerve and terminate in the spinal nucleus. The cell bodies of primary afferent fibers from stretch receptors in muscles of the head are located in the mesencephalic nucleus of the trigeminal nerve. This arrangement is exceptional because all other primary afferent cell bodies in the somatovisceral sensory system are located in peripheral ganglia. The central processes synapse in the motor nucleus of the trigeminal nerve.

Elderly people are sometimes susceptible to a chronic pain condition known as **trigeminal neuralgia.** People with this condition experience spontaneous episodes of severe, often lancinating pain in the distribution of one or more branches of the trigeminal nerve. Often, the pain is triggered by weak mechanical stimulation in the same region. A major contributing factor to this pain state appears to be mechanical damage to the trigeminal ganglion by an artery that impinges on the ganglion. Surgical displacement of the artery can resolve the condition.

■ *Somatosensory Pathways of the Dorsal Spinal Cord*

■ *The Dorsal Column–Medial Lemniscus Pathway*

The ascending branches of many large myelinated primary afferent nerve fibers travel rostrally in the dorsal funiculus all the way to the medulla. Axons that innervate sensory receptors of the lower extremity and the lower trunk ascend in the gracile fasciculus, whereas fibers from receptors of the upper extremity and upper trunk ascend in the cuneate fasciculus. These axons are the first-order neurons of the dorsal column–medial lemniscus pathway (Fig. 8-8).

Second-order neurons that receive synaptic input from the ascending branches of primary afferent fibers in the dorsal funiculus are located in the dorsal column nuclei,

which include the gracile and cuneate nuclei. Neurons in the dorsal column nuclei respond similarly to the primary afferent fibers that synapse on them. Some of these neurons behave like rapidly adapting receptors that respond to the same kinds of stimuli that activate hair follicle afferents and Meissner's corpuscles, such as hair move-

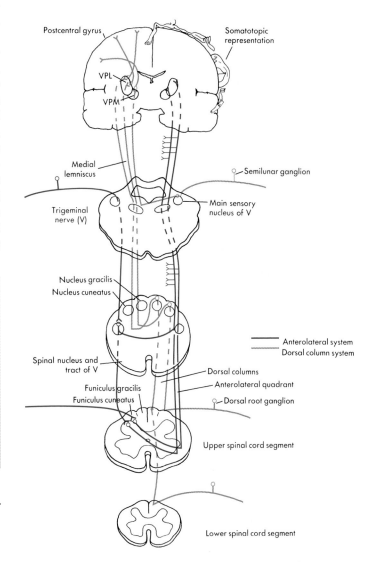

■ **Fig. 8-8** Schematic representation of some central connections in the dorsal column and anterolateral systems. For simplicity, only the primary fibers are shown in the dorsal columns. Both trigeminal and spinal components are shown. The dorsal column system is shown in lighter color and the anterolateral system in darker color. Note the somatotopic arrangement throughout the neuraxis for the dorsal column system. Fibers that enter dorsal roots at higher spinal segments ascend in the dorsal columns more laterally, and this relationship is preserved throughout; furthermore, the trigeminal component merges with the spinal component in the medial lemniscus next to fibers that represent the highest cervical spinal segments. Consequently, an accurate map of the body surface exists throughout, including the cortical areas of the postcentral gyrus. *VPL,* Ventral posterolateral nucleus; *VPM,* ventral posteromedial nucleus.

ment or transient mechanical stimuli applied to glabrous skin. Others discharge at high frequencies when vibratory stimuli are applied to their receptive fields, and thus resemble pacinian corpuscles. Still other neurons in the dorsal column nuclei have slowly adapting responses to cutaneous stimuli and behave like Merkel's cell or Ruffini endings. Many neurons in the cuneate nucleus are activated by stretching muscles.

The three main differences between the responses of dorsal column neurons and of primary afferent neurons are as follows: (1) dorsal column neurons have larger receptive fields because multiple primary afferent fibers synapse on a given dorsal column neuron, (2) dorsal column neurons sometimes respond to more than one type of sensory receptor owing to the convergence of several different types of primary afferent fibers on the second-order neurons, and (3) dorsal column neurons often have inhibitory receptive fields mediated through interneuronal circuits in the dorsal column nuclei.

Neurons in the dorsal column nuclei project their axons through the medial lemniscus to the contralateral thalamus (Fig. 8-8). The third-order neurons are located in the ventral posterolateral (VPL) nucleus. Third-order neurons in the thalamus then project to the somatosensory areas of the cerebral cortex.

The pathway in the trigeminal system that is equivalent to the dorsal column–medial lemniscus pathway involves a relay from primary afferent fibers that supply the face in the main sensory nucleus of the trigeminal nerve (Fig. 8-8). Second-order neurons in this nucleus send their axons through the trigeminothalamic tract to the ventral posteromedial (VPM) nucleus of the contralateral thalamus, and third-order neurons of the VPM nucleus project to the somatosensory cerebral cortex.

■ *Other Somatosensory Pathways of the Dorsal Spinal Cord*

Three other pathways that carry somatosensory information ascend in the dorsal part of the spinal cord on the same side as the afferent input: (1) the spinocervical tract, (2) the postsynaptic dorsal column pathway, and (3) the dorsal spinocerebellar tract.

The neurons that give rise to the **spinocervical tract** are located in the dorsal horn of the spinal cord. These cells receive input largely from hair follicle afferent fibers, although many of these cells are activated by nociceptors also. These cells project to the lateral cervical nucleus, a relay nucleus in the upper cervical spinal cord. Cells in the lateral cervical nucleus project to the contralateral VPL nucleus in the thalamus, and information is relayed from there to the somatosensory cerebral cortex.

Neurons that give rise to the **postsynaptic dorsal column pathway** are also located in the dorsal horn. These cells may receive input from mechanoreceptors of vari-

ous kinds, including pacinian corpuscles and slowly adapting cutaneous mechanoreceptors, and from nociceptors. The axons ascend in the dorsal funiculus to the dorsal column nuclei. From here, the sensory pathway proceeds through the medial lemniscus to the contralateral VPL nucleus and then to the somatosensory cerebral cortex.

The **dorsal spinocerebellar tract** (DSCT) responds to input from muscle and joint receptors of the lower extremity. The neurons that give rise to the DSCT are located in Clarke's column, a nucleus found in lamina VII at segmental levels T1 to L3. Other DSCT cells are found in the dorsal horn in the lumbosacral spinal cord. The main destination of the DSCT is the cerebellum. However, it also provides proprioceptive information from the leg to the VPL nucleus of the thalamus via a relay in a medullary nucleus known as nucleus z, which is located just rostral to the gracile nucleus. Proprioceptive information from the upper extremity is signaled by the dorsal column pathway.

■ *Sensory Functions of the Dorsal Spinal Cord Pathways*

The sensory qualities mediated by dorsal spinal cord pathways include flutter-vibration, touch-pressure, and proprioception. Each of these qualities of sensation depends on the activity in a set of sensory neurons that collectively form a labeled-line sensory channel. A sensory channel may involve several parallel ascending pathways, and it includes certain primary afferent neurons and sensory processing mechanisms at spinal cord, brainstem, thalamic, and cerebral cortical levels.

Flutter-vibration is a complex sensation. "Flutter" refers to the sensation evoked by mechanical stimuli that have low-frequency components. In clinical testing, flutter often involves sensory responses to transient applications of a wisp of cotton or a brief tap on the skin. The sensory receptors that detect flutter include hair follicles and Meissner's corpuscles. Several parallel ascending sensory tracts convey information used for flutter sensation. These tracts include the dorsal column–medial lemniscus pathway, the spinocervical tract, and the postsynaptic dorsal column pathway. In addition, the spinothalamic tract in the ventral part of the cord is partly responsible for flutter sensation, as discussed later in the chapter.

Vibratory sense involves recognition of stimuli with high-frequency components. A common clinical test of vibratory sense is to ask a subject to tell whether a tuning fork placed against a bony prominence is vibrating. High-frequency vibration is detected primarily by pacinian corpuscles. The information is transmitted through the dorsal column–medial lemniscus pathway.

Touch-pressure involves the recognition of maintained skin indentation. The receptors for touch-pressure include Merkel's cell and Ruffini endings. The ascending pathways that convey information from these receptors include the dorsal column–medial lemniscus and the postsynaptic dorsal column pathways.

Proprioception involves the sensing of both **joint movement** and **joint position.** The sensory information arises from receptors in muscle, joints, and skin. For proximal joints, such as the knee, the most important sensory information is derived from the activity of muscle spindles in the muscles that move the joint. In distal joints, such as joints of the fingers, Ruffini endings in skin and joint receptors also contribute. All the information required for proprioception in the upper extremity ascends in the dorsal column–medial lemniscus pathway. However, a major part of the information needed for proprioception in the lower extremity depends on the DSCT and its relay in the nucleus z.

Visceral distention is the sense of filling of such viscera as the urinary bladder. Information about visceral distention arises from stretch receptors in the wall of the viscus and is transmitted via the dorsal column–medial lemniscus pathway.

A lesion that interrupts pathways that ascend in the dorsal part of the spinal cord results in deficits in tactile discrimination, vibratory sense, and position sense. Particularly affected is the ability to recognize figures drawn on the skin (graphesthesia) and tactile recognition of objects placed in the hand (stereognosis). Some tactile function remains that allows localization of a tactile stimulus and flutter sensation. Cutaneous pain and temperature sensations are unaffected.

■ *Somatosensory Pathways of the Ventral Spinal Cord*

■ *Spinothalamic Tract*

The spinothalamic tract is the most important sensory pathway for pain and thermal sensations. It also contributes to tactile sensation. The first-order neurons of the spinothalamic tract are primary afferent fibers from nociceptors, thermoreceptors, and mechanoreceptors. The second-order neurons are located in the spinal cord (rather than in the medulla, as in the dorsal column–medial lemniscus pathway). The axons of the spinothalamic tract neurons cross to the opposite side within the spinal cord and ascend to the brain in the ventral part of the lateral funiculus (Fig. 8-8). They terminate on third-order neurons in the thalamus.

The neurons that give rise to the spinothalamic tract are located chiefly in spinal cord laminae I and V. Most spinothalamic tract neurons receive an excitatory input from nociceptors in the skin, but many can also be ex-

cited by noxious stimulation of muscle or viscera. Effective stimuli include noxious, mechanical, thermal, and chemical stimuli. Some spinothalamic tract neurons are excited by activity in cold or warm thermoreceptors or in sensitive mechanoreceptors. Thus, different spinothalamic tract neurons respond in a manner appropriate for signaling noxious, thermal, or mechanical events.

Wide-dynamic-range cells and high-threshold cells. Some nociceptive spinothalamic tract cells receive a convergent excitatory input from several different types of sensory receptors. For example, a given spinothalamic neuron may be activated weakly by tactile stimuli but more powerfully by noxious stimuli (Fig. 8-9). Such neurons are called **wide-dynamic-range cells** because they are activated by stimuli with a wide range of intensities. Wide-dynamic-range neurons mainly signal noxious events, the weak responses to tactile stimuli perhaps

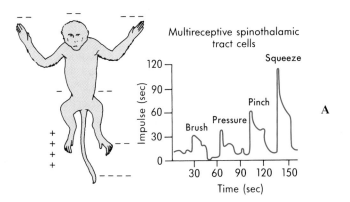

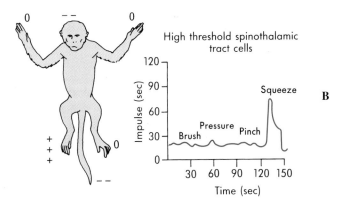

■ **Fig. 8-9** **A,** Responses of a wide-dynamic-range or multireceptive spinothalamic tract cell. **B,** Responses of a high-threshold spinothalamic tract cell. The figures indicate the excitatory (*plus signs*) and inhibitory (*minus signs*) receptive fields. The graphs show the responses to graded intensities of mechanical stimulation. *Brush* is with a camel's hairbrush repeatedly stroked across the receptive field. *Pressure* is applied by attachment of an arterial clip to the skin. This is a marginally painful stimulus to a human. *Pinch* is by attachment of a stiff arterial clip to the skin and is distinctly painful. *Squeeze* is by compressing a fold of skin with forceps and is damaging to the skin.

being ignored by higher centers. However, in pathological conditions, these neurons may be activated sufficiently to evoke a sensation of pain. This "selective" activation would explain some pain states in which the activation of mechanoreceptors causes pain (**mechanical allodynia**). Other spinothalamic tract cells are activated only by noxious stimuli. Such neurons are often called **nociceptive-specific** or **high-threshold cells** (Fig. 8-9).

Neurotransmitters that activate spinothalamic tract cells. The neurotransmitters released by nociceptors that activate spinothalamic tract cells include the excitatory amino acid glutamate and several peptides, such as substance P (SP), calcitonin gene-related peptide (CGRP), vasoactive intestinal polypeptide (VIP), and others. Glutamate appears to act as a fast transmitter by its action on non-*N*-methyl-D-aspartic acid excitatory amino acid (non-NMDA) receptors. However, with repetitive stimulation, glutamate can also cause a build-up of activity or wind-up through an action mediated by NMDA receptors. SP appears to act as a neuromodulator. Through a combined action with an excitatory amino acid, such as glutamate, SP can produce a long-lasting increase in the responses of spinothalamic tract cells. CGRP seems to increase SP release and to prolong its action by inhibiting its enzymatic degradation.

Pain inhibition. Spinothalamic tract cells often have inhibitory receptive fields. Inhibition may result from weak mechanical stimuli, but usually the most effective inhibitory stimuli are noxious ones. The nociceptive inhibitory receptive fields may be very large and may include most of the body and face (Fig. 8-9). Such receptive fields may account for the ability of various physical manipulations, including transcutaneous electrical nerve stimulation and acupuncture, to suppress pain. Neurotransmitters that can inhibit spinothalamic tract cells include the inhibitory amino acids, gamma-aminobutyric acid (GABA) and glycine, as well as monoamines and the endogenous opioid peptides (see p 126).

The **gate control theory of pain** explains how innocuous stimuli may inhibit the responses of dorsal horn neurons that transmit information about painful stimuli to the brain. In this theory, pain transmission is prevented by innocuous inputs mediated by large myelinated afferent fibers, whereas pain transmission is enhanced by inputs carried over fine afferent fibers. The inhibitory interneurons of lamina II serve as the gating mechanism. The circuit diagram originally proposed has been criticized, but the basic notion of a gating mechanism is still viable.

Noxious stimuli applied to large areas of the body can also inhibit the discharges of nociceptive dorsal horn neurons. In this kind of inhibition, the stimuli activate inhibitory pathways that ascend to the brain, which in turn activates pathways that descend from the brainstem (see later description of the endogenous analgesia system). This type of inhibitory system is referred to as *diffuse noxious inhibitory control.*

■ *Other Somatosensory Pathways of the Ventral Spinal Cord*

Two other pathways that transmit somatosensory information ascend in the ventrolateral part of the spinal cord: the spinoreticular tract and the spinomesencephalic tract.

The neurons that give rise to the **spinoreticular tract** are often difficult to activate. However, when receptive fields are found, they are generally large and sometimes bilateral. The stimuli that are effective in activating the fields include noxious stimuli. The reticular formation is involved in attentional mechanisms and arousal (see Chapter 16). The reticular formation projects to the intralaminar complex of the thalamus and thence to wide areas of the cerebral cortex. Reticulospinal projections also contribute to the descending systems that control pain transmission.

Many cells of the **spinomesencephalic** tract respond to noxious stimuli, and their receptive fields may be small or large. The terminations of this tract are located in several midbrain nuclei, including the **periaqueductal gray,** which is an important component of the endogenous analgesia system (see p 126). Motivational-affective responses may also result from activation of the periaqueductal gray and reticular formation. For example, stimulation in the periaqueductal gray can cause vocalization and aversive behavior. Information from the midbrain is relayed not only to the thalamus but also to the amygdala, a part of the limbic system. This pathway is one of several pathways by which noxious stimuli can trigger emotional responses.

■ *Sensory Functions of the Ventral Spinal Cord Pathways*

The main sensory modalities mediated by ventral spinal cord pathways are pain and thermal sensations. These pathways also contribute to flutter. Although the most essential pathway for flutter-vibration is the dorsal column–medial lemniscus pathway, the spinothalamic tract can provide sufficient information for flutter, but not for vibratory, sensation. However, the spinothalamic tract alone is insufficient for recognition of the direction of a tactile stimulus, and discrimination is much less accurate than when the dorsal column–medial lemniscus pathway is intact. The contributions of these two tracts to the recognition of tactile stimulus can be tested clinically by drawing numbers on the fingertip (graphesthesia). Graphesthesia is lost when the dorsal column–medial lemniscus pathway is interrupted but not when the spinothalamic tract is interrupted.

Thermal sense includes the two submodalities of cold and warm. Thermal sense appears to depend on input from cold and warm receptors to spinothalamic tract cells in lamina I of the dorsal horn. Sectioning the spinothalamic tract causes a loss of thermal sense on the contralateral side of the body.

Pain that results from stimulation of nociceptors is mediated partly by spinothalamic tract cells and partly by the spinoreticular and spinomesencephalic tracts. Pain is a complex phenomenon that includes both sensory-discriminative and motivational-affective components. That is, pain is a sensory experience that is accompanied by emotional responses and by somatic and autonomic motor adjustments. Presumably, the sensory-discriminative component of pain depends on the spinothalamic tract projection to the VPL nucleus and further transmission of nociceptive information to the SI and SII regions of the cerebral cortex (see p 124). Sensory processing at these and higher levels of the cortex results in perception of the quality of pain (e.g., pricking, burning, or aching), the location of the painful stimulus, the intensity of the pain, and its duration.

The motivational-affective responses to painful stimuli include attention and arousal, somatic and autonomic reflexes, endocrine responses, and emotional changes. These responses collectively account for the unpleasant nature of painful stimuli. The motivational-affective responses depend on activity transmitted in several ascending pathways, including the component of the spinothalamic tract that projects to the medial thalamus, the spinoreticular tract, and the spinomesencephalic tract. In addition, several recently discovered pathways that connect the spinal cord directly with the hypothalamus (spinohypothalamic tract) and the basal forebrain (spinotelencephalic tract) may play a role in motivational-affective responses to painful stimuli.

Both the sensory-discriminative and the motivational-affective components of pain are lost on the contralateral side of the body when the spinothalamic tract is interrupted. It was this observation that motivated the development of the surgical procedure known as **anterolateral cordotomy.** This procedure was formerly used to treat pain in many individuals, especially those suffering from cancer pain. This operation is now used infrequently because of improvements in drug therapy and because pain often returns months to years after an initially successful cordotomy. The return of pain may reflect either an extension of the disease or the development of a central pain state (see later discussion). In addition to the loss of pain sensation, anterolateral cordotomy produces a loss of cold and warmth sensations on the contralateral side of the body. Careful testing may reveal a minimal tactile deficit as well, but the intact sensory pathways of the dorsal part of the spinal cord provide sufficient tactile information so that any loss caused by interruption of the spinothalamic tract is insignificant.

Pain

Transmission of pain and the response to it have been discussed in previous sections of this chapter. Here, we discuss various aspects of pain in more detail, including referred pain, central pain, and pain that originates in the trigeminal nerve distribution.

As previously mentioned, primary afferent nociceptors may become sensitized after the skin is injured. A painful stimulus may therefore become even more painful because the nociceptive afferents are more readily activated and discharge more frequently in response to a given stimulus. This state is known as **primary hyperalgesia.** In addition, a surrounding area of skin may also become tender owing to the sensitization of nociceptive neurons in the spinal cord, including spinothalamic tract cells. If a noxious stimulus evokes more pain than in normal skin, the condition is called **secondary hyperalgesia.** If a normally innocuous tactile or thermal stimulus evokes pain, the condition is called **allodynia.** Central sensitization of nociceptive neurons is believed to be caused in part by the activation of second messenger systems in dorsal horn neurons.

Referred Pain

Referred pain is defined as pain that is perceived as coming from an area remote from its actual origin. For example, in angina pectoris, the pain is caused by ischemia of the heart. However, the ischemic heart pain may be referred to the inner aspect of the left arm. Referred pain originates from deep structures, including muscle and viscera, and is poorly localized. In contrast, pain that originates from the skin is generally well localized, presumably because spinothalamic tract cells have relatively discrete cutaneous receptive fields. Also, the ascending system through which they signal is somatotopically organized. In angina pectoris, the area of pain referral is in the T1 dermatome, which corresponds to the spinal cord level that provides the main sensory innervation of the heart.

One explanation of referred pain is that many spinothalamic neurons receive excitatory input not only from the skin but also from muscle and viscera. The spinal cord segments that innervate the dermatomes containing the cutaneous receptive field of these neurons correspond to the segments that innervate the muscle or viscus. The activity in a population of spinothalamic tract cells may be interpreted by a person as originating in somatic structures, based on his or her learning this association during childhood. Subsequently, activation of these neurons by pathological input from visceral nociceptors is misinterpreted as resulting from stimulation of superficial parts of the body.

Central Pain

Pain sometimes occurs in the absence of nociceptor stimulation. This type of pain is most likely to occur after damage to peripheral nerves or to parts of the CNS involved in transmitting nociceptive information. Examples of pain secondary to neural damage are phantom limb pain and "thalamic pain" (see later). **Phantom limb pain** follows amputation in some individuals and is clearly not caused by activation of nociceptors, because these receptors are no longer present in the area in which pain is felt. Similarly, lesions of the thalamus or at other levels of the spinothalamocortical pathway may cause severe spontaneous pain, yet interruption of the nociceptive pathway by the same lesion may prevent or reduce pain evoked by peripheral stimulation. The mechanism of such pain caused by neural damage is poorly understood, but the pain appears to depend on changes in the activity and response properties of neurons further in the nociceptive system.

Trigeminal Nociceptive System

Sensory processing of nociceptive and thermoreceptive information that originates from the face, oral cavity, and dura mater is organized in a fashion similar to that for the trunk and limbs. Pain in the trigeminal distribution is of particular importance because it includes both tooth pain and headache.

The primary afferent fibers that supply nociceptors and thermoreceptors in the head enter the brainstem through the trigeminal nerve (some also enter through the facial, glossopharyngeal, and vagus nerves) and descend through the brainstem to the upper cervical spinal cord through the spinal tract of the trigeminal nerve (Fig. 8-8). Some mechanoreceptive afferent fibers also join the spinal tract. Axons in the spinal tract synapse on second-order neurons in the spinal nucleus. These neurons transmit information concerning pain and temperature sensations that originate from the face, oral cavity, and dura mater to the contralateral VPM nucleus through the trigeminothalamic tract. The VPM nucleus in turn projects to the somatosensory cerebral cortex. The spinal nucleus also projects to the central lateral nucleus of the intralaminar complex.

Higher Processing of Somatosensory Information

Thalamus

The medial lemniscus and the spinothalamic tract synapse in the VPL nucleus of the thalamus. Several other parallel sensory tracts, such as the spinocervical tract and the pathway through nucleus z, also terminate in the VPL nucleus. The trigeminothalamic tracts from the main sensory and spinal nuclei of the trigeminal nerve synapse in the VPM nucleus of the thalamus.

The responses of many neurons in the VPL and VPM nuclei resemble those of first- and second-order neurons in the ascending tracts. The responses may be dominated by a particular type of sensory receptor, and the receptive field may be small, although generally larger than that of a primary afferent fiber. The receptive fields are contralateral to the thalamic neuron, and the location of the thalamic neuron is systematically related to that of the receptive field. In other words, the VPL and VPM nuclei are somatotopically organized. The lower extremity is represented by neurons in the lateral part of the VPL nucleus, the upper extremity by neurons in the medial part of the VPL nucleus, and the face by neurons in the VPM nucleus (Fig. 8-10).

Thalamic neurons often have inhibitory, as well as excitatory, receptive fields. The inhibition may actually take place in the dorsal column nuclei or in the dorsal horn of the spinal cord, but inhibitory circuits are also located within the thalamus. The VPL and VPM nuclei contain inhibitory interneurons (in primates, but not in rodents), and some of the inhibitory interneurons in the reticular nucleus of the thalamus project into the VPL and VPM nuclei. The inhibitory neurons intrinsic to the VPL and VPM nuclei and in the reticular nucleus use GABA as their inhibitory neurotransmitter.

An interesting difference between neurons in the VPL and VPM nuclei and sensory neurons at lower levels of the somatosensory system is that thalamic neuron excitability depends on the stage of the sleep-wake cycle and on the presence or absence of anesthesia. During a state of drowsiness or during barbiturate anesthesia, thalamic neurons tend to undergo an alternating sequence of excitatory and inhibitory postsynaptic potentials. The alternating bursts of discharges in turn intermittently excite neurons in the cerebral cortex. Such excitation results in an alpha rhythm or in spindling in the electroencephalogram (see Chapter 16). This alternation of excitatory and inhibitory postsynaptic potentials during these two states may reflect the level of excitation of thalamic neurons by excitatory amino acids acting at non-NMDA and NMDA receptors. It may also reflect the inhibition of the thalamic neurons by recurrent pathways through the reticular nucleus.

The spinothalamic tract and the part of the trigeminothalamic tract that originates in the spinal nucleus of the trigeminal nerve project to the central lateral nucleus of the intralaminar complex of the thalamus. The intralaminar nuclei are not somatotopically organized, and they project diffusely to the cerebral cortex, as well as to the basal ganglia. The projection of the central lateral nucleus to the SI cortex (see below) may be involved in arousal of this part of the cortex and in selective attention.

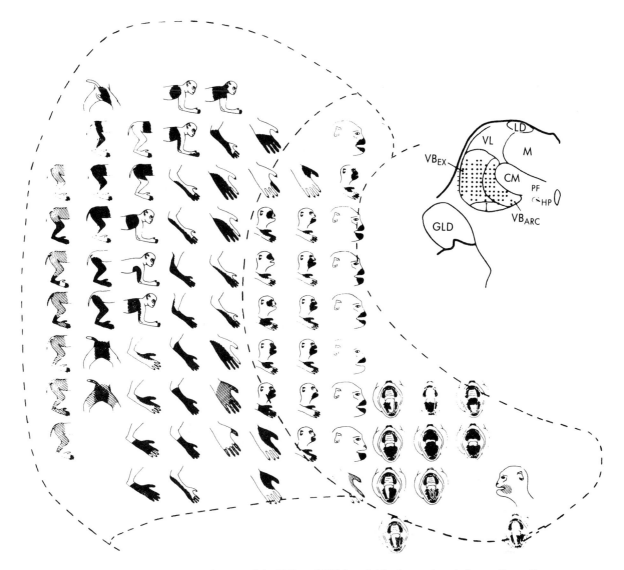

■ **Fig. 8-10** Somatotopic map of the VPL and VPM nuclei in the monkey thalamus. Recordings were made from small groups of neurons and the receptive fields were mapped using weak mechanical stimuli. The figurines show the receptive fields for multiunit activity in the VPL and VPM nuclei (demarcated by the dashed lines). The locations of the recording sites are shown by the dots on the drawing of a section through the thalamus on one side. VB_{EX}, VPL; VB_{ARC}, VPM; *VL*, ventral lateral; *LD*, lateral dorsal; *M*, medial dorsal; *CM*, center median; *PF*, parafascicular; *GLD*, dorsal lateral geniculate; *HP*, habenulopeduncular tract. (From Mountcastle VB, Henneman E: *J Comp Neurol* 97:409, 1952.)

Destruction of the VPL or VPM nuclei diminishes sensation on the contralateral side of the body or face. The sensory qualities that are lost are those mainly transmitted by the dorsal column–medial lemniscus pathway and its trigeminal equivalent. The sensory-discriminative component of pain sensation is also lost, but the motivational-affective component of pain is still present if the medial thalamus is intact, presumably because of the medial spinothalamic and spinoreticulothalamic projection. In some individuals, a lesion of the somatosensory thalamus results in a central pain state known as "thalamic pain." However, pain indistinguishable from thalamic pain can also be produced by brainstem or cortical lesions.

■ *Somatosensory Cortex*

Third-order sensory neurons in the VPL and VPM nuclei of the thalamus project to the somatosensory cortex. The main somatosensory receiving areas of the cortex are called the SI and SII areas. The SI cortex occupies much of the postcentral gyrus; the SII cortex is in the superior bank of the lateral fissure.

The **SI cortex,** like the somatosensory thalamus, has a somatotopic organization (Fig. 8-11). The **SII cortex** also contains a somatosensory map, as do several other less understood areas of cortex. The face is represented in the lateral part of the postcentral gyrus, above the lateral fissure. The hand and the rest of the upper extremity are represented in the dorsolateral part of the postcentral gyrus and the lower extremity on the medial surface of the hemisphere. The map of the surface of the body and face of a human on the postcentral gyrus is called a **sensory homunculus.** The map is distorted, because the greatest volume of neural tissue is devoted to the densely innervated regions, such as the perioral area and the thumb and other digits.

The sensory homunculus is essentially an expression of place coding of somatosensory information. A locus in the SI cortex encodes the location of a somatosensory stimulus on the surface of the body or face. For example, the brain knows that a certain part of the body has been stimulated because certain neurons in the dorsolateral part of the postcentral gyrus are activated.

The SI cortex has several morphologic and functional subdivisions, each of which has a somatotopic map like that shown in Fig. 8-11. These subdivisions were originally described by Brodmann, being based on the arrangements of neurons in the various layers of the cortex as seen in Nissl-stained preparations. The subdivisions are therefore known as Brodmann's areas 3a, 3b, 1, and 2. Cutaneous input dominates in areas 3b and 1, whereas muscle and joint input dominates in areas 3a and 2. Thus, separate cortical zones are specialized for the processing of tactile and proprioceptive information. The inputs to these cortical areas come from distinct parts of the VPL and VPM nuclei (Fig. 8-12). For example, the cutaneous input from the extremities comes from the core of the VPL nucleus, whereas the muscle and joint input comes from a "shell" region.

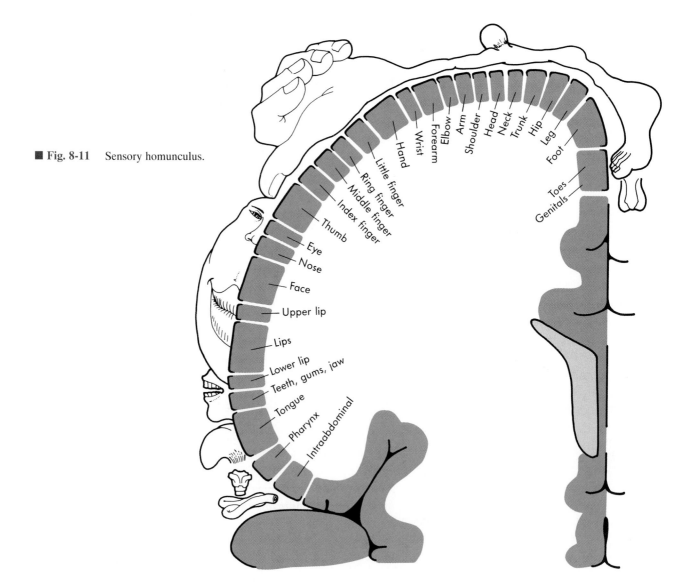

■ **Fig. 8-11**   Sensory homunculus.

Within any particular area of the SI cortex, all the neurons along a line perpendicular to the cortical surface have similar response properties and receptive fields. The SI cortex is thus said to have a **columnar organization.** A comparable columnar organization has also been demonstrated for other primary sensory receiving areas, including the primary visual and auditory cortices (see Chapters 9 and 10). Nearby cortical columns in the SI cortex may process information for different sensory modalities. For example, the cutaneous information that reaches one cortical column in area 3b may come from rapidly adapting mechanoreceptors, whereas the information that reaches a neighboring column may come from slowly adapting mechanoreceptors.

Besides being responsible for the initial processing of somatosensory information, the SI cortex also plays a preliminary role in higher-order processing, such as feature extraction. For example, certain neurons in area 1 respond preferentially to a stimulus that moves in one direction across the receptive field but not to one that moves in the opposite direction (Fig. 8-13). Such neurons presumably contribute to the perceptual ability to recognize the direction of an applied stimulus.

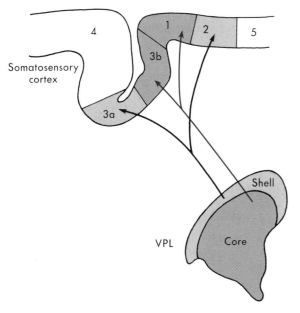

■ **Fig. 8-12**   Schematic relationships in thalamocortical projection from the VPL nucleus to areas of somatosensory cortex. A core region *(color)* of the VPL nucleus projects primarily to cortical areas 1 and 3b, and a "shell" region projects primarily to areas 2 and 3a. (Redrawn from Jones EG, Friedman DP: *J Neurophysiol* 48:521, 1982.)

■ *Association Cortex*

The SI cortex is connected with many other cortical areas, such as the SII cortex, the motor cortex, supplementary sensory and motor cortices, and the parietal association cortex. The parietal association cortex also receives input from other sensory systems, notably from the visual system. A major function of the parietal association cortex is the relationship of the body to extrapersonal space. For example, this part of the cortex on one side helps to coordinate hand and eye movements on the contralateral side. In humans, the posterior parietal cortex of the nondominant hemisphere is particularly involved in spatial relations, whereas that in the dominant hemisphere is concerned with language (see Chapter 16).

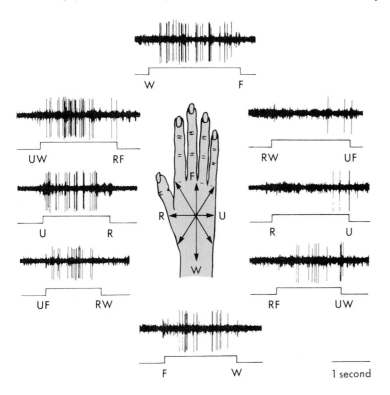

■ **Fig. 8-13**   Feature extraction by cortical neurons. The responses were recorded from a neuron in the somatosensory cortex of a monkey. The direction of a stimulus was varied, as shown by the arrows in the drawing. Note that the responses were greatest when the stimulus moved in the direction from *UW* to *RF* and least from *RW* to *UF. R,* Radial side; *U,* ulnar side; *F,* fingers; *W,* wrist. (From Costanzo RM, Gardner EP: *J Neurophysiol* 43:1319, 1980.)

A lesion of the SI cortex in humans causes sensory changes similar to those produced by a lesion of the somatosensory thalamus. However, usually only a part of the cortex is involved, and therefore *the sensory loss may be confined, for example, to the face or to the leg, depending on the location of the lesion with respect to the sensory homunculus.* The sensory modalities most affected are discriminative touch and position sense. Graphesthesia and stereognosis are particularly disturbed. Pain and thermal sensation may be relatively unaffected, although a loss of pain may follow cortical lesions. Conversely, cortical lesions can result in a central pain state that resembles thalamic pain.

A lesion of the parietal association cortex on the nondominant side causes deficits in the ability to relate to extrapersonal space. When an affected person is asked to copy geometric figures, the figures are distorted. For example, the numbers of a clock face may all be drawn on the side of the clock that corresponds to the normal side of the person with the lesion (**constructional apraxia**). The person may deny the contralateral side of the body (**neglect syndrome**) and have difficulty in dressing on that side. The individual with a lesion may also have difficulty reading maps, driving, or performing other activities that require spatial orientation.

■ *Centrifugal Control of Somatovisceral Sensation*

Sensory experience is not just the passive detection of environmental events. Instead, it more often depends on exploration of the environment. Tactile cues are sought by moving the hand over a surface. Visual cues result from scanning visual targets with the eyes. Thus, sensory information is often received as the result of activity in the motor system. Furthermore, transmission in pathways to the sensory centers of the brain is regulated by descending control systems. These systems allow the brain to control its input by filtering incoming sensory messages. Important information can be attended to and unimportant information ignored.

The tactile and proprioceptive somatosensory pathways are regulated by descending pathways that originate in the SI and motor regions of the cerebral cortex. For example, corticobulbar projections to the dorsal column nuclei help control sensory input that is transmitted by the dorsal column–medial lemniscus pathway.

Of particular interest is the descending control system that regulates the transmission of nociceptive information. This system presumably suppresses excessive pain under certain circumstances. For example, it is well known that soldiers on the battlefield, accident victims, and athletes in competition often feel little or no pain at the time a wound occurs or a bone is broken. At a later time, pain may develop and become severe. Although the descending regulatory system that controls pain is part of a more general centrifugal control system that modulates all forms of sensation, the pain control system is so important medically that it is distinguished as a special system called the **endogenous analgesia system.**

Several centers in the brainstem and the descending pathways from these centers contribute to the endogenous analgesia system. For example, stimulation in the periaqueductal gray, the locus coeruleus, or the medullary raphe nuclei inhibits nociceptive neurons at spinal cord and brainstem levels, including spinothalamic tract and trigeminothalamic tract cells (Fig. 8-14, *A*). Other inhibitory pathways originate in the sensorimotor cortex, the hypothalamus, and the reticular formation.

The endogenous analgesia system can be subdivided into two components: those that use one of the endogenous **opioid peptides** as neurotransmitters or modulators, and those that do not. The endogenous opioids are neuropeptides that activate one of several types of opiate receptors. Some of the endogenous opioids include enkephalin, dynorphin, and β-endorphin. Opiate analgesia can generally be prevented or reversed by the narcotic antagonist naloxone. Naloxone is often used to test whether or not analgesia is mediated by an opioid mechanism.

The opioid-mediated endogenous analgesia system can be activated by exogenous administration of morphine or other opiate drugs. Thus, one of the oldest medical treatments for pain depends on the triggering of a sensory control system. Opiates typically inhibit neural activity in nociceptive pathways. Two sites of action have been proposed for opiate inhibition, presynaptic and postsynaptic (Fig. 8-14, *B*). The presynaptic action of opiates on nociceptive afferent terminals is thought to prevent the release of excitatory transmitters, such as SP. The postsynaptic action produces an inhibitory postsynaptic potential. How can an inhibitory neurotransmitter activate descending pathways? One hypothesis is that the descending analgesia system is under tonic inhibitory control by inhibitory interneurons in both the midbrain and the medulla. The action of opiates would inhibit the inhibitory interneurons and thereby disinhibit the descending analgesia pathways.

Some endogenous analgesia pathways operate by neurotransmitters other than opioids and thus are unaffected by naloxone. One way of engaging a nonopioid analgesia pathway is through certain forms of stress. The analgesia so produced is a form of **stress-induced analgesia.**

Many neurons in the raphe nuclei use serotonin as a neurotransmitter. Serotonin can inhibit nociceptive neurons and presumably plays an important role in the endogenous analgesia system. Other brainstem neurons release catecholamines, such as norepinephrine and epinephrine, in the spinal cord. These catecholamines also inhibit nociceptive neurons; therefore, catecholaminer-

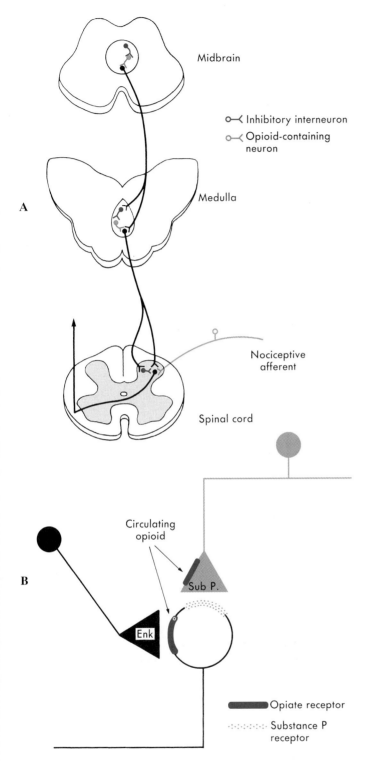

gic neurons may contribute to the endogenous analgesia system. Furthermore, these monoamine neurotransmitters interact with endogenous opioids. Undoubtedly, many other substances are involved in the analgesia system. In addition, there is evidence for the existence of endogenous opiate antagonists that can prevent opiate analgesia.

■ *Summary*

1. Sensory pathways are composed of serially connected neurons. The cell bodies of first-order neurons are located in sensory nerve ganglia; these neurons connect peripherally to a sensory receptor and centrally to second-order neurons. Higher-order neurons are located in the thalamus and cortex.

2. Skin contains mechanoreceptors, thermoreceptors, and nociceptors. Mechanoreceptors may be rapidly or slowly adapting. Thermoreceptors include cold and warm receptors. Aδ and C-polymodal nociceptors may be sensitized by release of chemical substances from damaged cells. Muscle, joints, and viscera have mechanoreceptors and nociceptors.

3. The spinocervical tract, the postsynaptic dorsal column pathway, and the part of the dorsal spinocerebellar tract that relays in nucleus z act in parallel with the dorsal column–medial lemniscus pathway. These dorsal spinal cord pathways signal the sensations of flutter-vibration, touch-pressure, and proprioception.

4. The spinothalamic tract includes nociceptive, thermoreceptive, and tactile neurons; the cell bodies of these neurons are located mostly in the dorsal horn. The axons cross, ascend in the ventrolateral funiculus, and synapse in the VPL and intralaminar nuclei of the thalamus. The equivalent trigeminal pathway relays in the spinal nucleus and projects to the contralateral VPM and intralaminar nuclei.

5. The spinothalamic relay in the VPL nucleus helps account for the sensory-discriminative aspects of pain. Parallel nociceptive pathways in the ventrolateral funiculus are the spinoreticular and spinomesencephalic tracts; these and the spinothalamic projection to the medial thalamus contribute to the motivational-affective aspects of pain.

6. Referred pain is explained by convergent input to spinothalamic tract cells from the body wall and from viscera. Damage to a peripheral nerve or to the central nociceptive pathway may result in neurogenic pain, such as phantom limb pain or thalamic pain.

7. The VPL and VPM nuclei are somatotopically organized and contain inhibitory circuits. The somatosensory cortex includes the SI and SII regions; these regions are also somatotopically organized. The SI cortex is further

■ **Fig. 8-14** **A,** Some of the neurons thought to play a role in the endogenous analgesia system. Neurons in the midbrain periaqueductal gray activate the raphe-spinal tract, which in turn inhibits nociceptive spinal neurons, such as those of the spinothalamic tract. Interneurons containing opioid substances are involved in the system at each level. **B,** Possible presynaptic and postsynaptic sites of action of enkephalin *(Enk)*. The presynaptic action might prevent the release of substance P (Sub P) from nociceptors. (Redrawn from Henry JL. In Porter R, O'Connor M, editors: *Ciba Foundation Symposium 91*, London, 1982, Pitman.)

subdivided into regions that process different kinds of information. The SI cortex contains columns of neurons with similar receptive fields and response properties. Some SI neurons are involved in feature extraction. The association cortex of the parietal lobe is concerned with extrapersonal space.

8. Transmission in somatosensory pathways is regulated by descending control systems. The endogenous analgesia system regulates nociceptive transmission, using such transmitters as the endogenous opioid peptides, norepinephrine, and serotonin.

■ *Self-Study Problems*

1. What types of cutaneous mechanoreceptors are responsible for signaling flutter and vibration?

2. What is unusual about the discharges of cold receptors?

3. What laminae of the spinal cord gray matter make up the dorsal horn? In which laminae do nociceptive primary afferent fibers terminate?

4. What is the gate control theory of pain? What are some of the limitations of this theory?

5. What is the significance of the sensory homunculi found in the VPL and VPM nuclei and in the somatosensory cortex?

■ *Bibliography*

Journal articles

Besson JM, Chaouch A: Peripheral and spinal mechanisms of nociception, *Physiol Rev* 67:67, 1987.

Boivie J, Leijon G, Johansson I: Central post-stroke pain—a study of the mechanisms through analysis of the sensory abnormalities, *Pain* 37:173, 1989.

Constanzo RM, Gardner EP: A quantitative analysis of responses of direction-sensitive neurons in somatosensory cortex of awake monkeys, *J Neurophysiol* 43:1319, 1980.

Fields HL, Heinricher MM, Mason P: Neurotransmitters in nociceptive modulatory circuits, *Annu Rev Neurosci* 14:219, 1991.

Johnson KPO, Hsiao SS: Neural mechanisms of tactual form and texture perception, *Annu Rev Neurosci* 15:227, 1992.

LaMotte RH, Thalhammer JG, Robinson CJ: Peripheral neural correlates of magnitude of cutaneous pain and hyperalgesia: a comparison of neural events in monkey with sensory judgements in human, *J Neurophysiol* 50:1, 1983.

Northcutt RG: Evolution of the telencephalon in nonmammals, *Annu Rev Neurosci* 4:301, 1981.

Schaible HG, Schmidt RF: Effects of an experimental arthritis on the sensory properties of fine articular afferent units, *J Neurophysiol* 54:1109, 1985.

Torebjork HE, Vallbo AB, Ochoa J: Intraneural microstimulation in man: its relation to specificity of tactile sensations, *Brain* 110:1509, 1987.

Books and monographs

Akil H, Lewis JW: *Neurotransmitters and pain control,* Basel, 1987, Karger.

Belmonte C, Cervero F, editors: *Neurobiology of nociceptors,* Oxford, 1996, Oxford University Press.

Boivie J, Hansson P, Lindblom U, editors: *Touch, temperature, and pain in health and disease: mechanisms and assessments,* Seattle, 1994, IASP Press.

Bonica JJ: *The management of pain,* Philadelphia, 1990, Lea & Febiger.

Creutzfeldt OD: *Cortex cerebri,* Oxford, 1995, Oxford University Press.

Foreman RD: *Organization of the spinothalamic tract as a relay for cardiopulmonary sympathetic afferent fiber activity.* In Ottoson D, editor: *Progress in sensory physiology 9,* Berlin, 1989, Springer-Verlag.

Gebhart G, editor: *Visceral pain,* Seattle, 1995, IASP Press.

Jones EG: *The thalamus,* New York, 1985, Plenum Press.

Light AR: *The initial processing of pain and its descending control: spinal and trigeminal systems,* Basel, 1992, Karger.

Mountcastle VB: Central nervous system mechanisms in mechanoreceptive sensibility. In Brookhart JM, Mountcastle VB, editors: *Handbook of physiology,* section 1: *The nervous system,* vol 3, *Sensory processes,* part 2, Bethesda, Md, 1984, American Physiological Society.

Penfield W, Jasper H: *Epilepsy and the functional anatomy of the human brain,* Boston, 1954, Little, Brown.

Wall PD, Melzack R: *Textbook of pain,* ed 3, Edinburgh, 1994, Churchill Livingstone.

Willis WD: *Control of nociceptive transmission in the spinal cord,* Berlin, 1982, Springer-Verlag.

Willis WD: *The pain system,* Basel, 1985, Karger.

Willis WD, editor: *Hyperalgesia and allodynia,* New York, 1992, Raven Press.

Willis WD, Coggeshall RE: *Sensory mechanisms of the spinal cord,* ed 2, New York, 1991, Plenum Press.

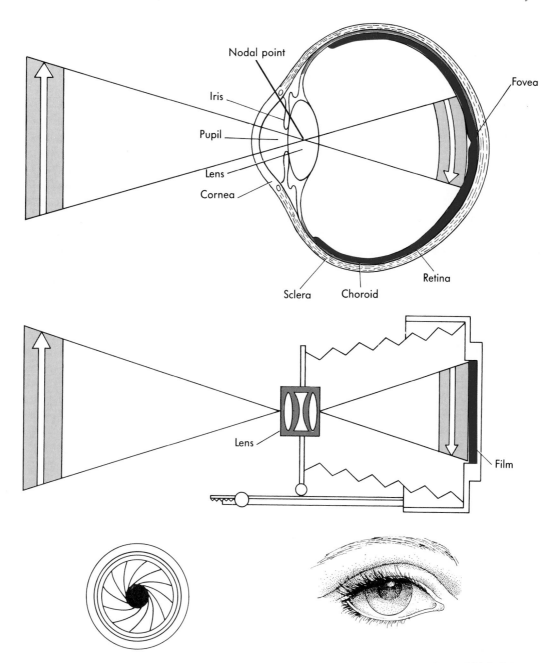

■ **Fig. 9-5**   Similarity between the optics of the eye and of a camera. (Redrawn from Wald G: *Sci Am* 183:32, 1950.)

However, the retina is far more complex than film. It processes a continuous sequence of images and also provides the brain with clues about the movement of visual targets, threats, the light-dark cycle, and other features of the visual environment.

Although the optic axis of the human eye passes through the nodal point of the lens and reaches the retina at a point between the fovea and the optic disc (Fig. 9-2), the eye is directed by the oculomotor system at a point on the visual target called the **fixation point.** Light from the fixation point passes through the nodal point and is focused on the fovea; this light courses along the visual axis. Light from the remainder of the visual target is focused on the retina surrounding the fovea (Fig. 9-5).

Proper focus of light on the retina depends not only on the lens but also on the iris. As mentioned earlier, *the iris acts like the diaphragm in a camera not only in regulating the amount of light entering the eye, but more importantly in controlling the depth of field of the image and the amount of spherical aberration produced by the lens.* When the pupil is constricted, the depth of field is increased, and the light is directed through the central part of the lens where spherical aberration is minimal. Pupillary constriction occurs automatically (i.e., it is a reflex) when the eye accommodates for near vision. Thus, when a person reads or does other fine visual work, the quality of the image is improved by the optical system of the eye. Another factor that affects the quality of the image is light scatter. Light scatter is minimized in the eye by restriction of the light path and absorption of stray light by pigment in the choroid and the retinal pigment layer. Again, the eye is similar in these respects to a camera. In a camera, light scatter is also prevented by limiting the light path and by covering the interior of the camera with black paint.

Defects in focusing are caused by a discrepancy between the size of the eye and the refractive power of the dioptric media. For example, in **myopia** (near-sightedness), the images of distant objects are focused in front of the retina (Fig. 9-6). This problem is corrected by concave lenses. Conversely, in **hypermetropia** (far-sightedness), the images of distant objects are focused behind the retina, a problem that can be corrected with convex lenses (Fig. 9-6). Although temporary focusing is also possible by accommodation, it may fatigue the ciliary muscles and cause eye strain. In **astigmatism,** an asymmetry exists in the radii of curvature of different meridians of the cornea or lens (or sometimes of the retina). Astigmatism can often be corrected by lenses with appropriately matched radii of curvature.

As an individual ages, the elasticity of the lens gradually declines. As a result, accommodation of the lens for near vision becomes progressively less effective, a condition called **presbyopia.** A young person can change the power of the lens by as much as 14 D. However, by the time a person reaches 40 years of age, the amount of accommodation halves, and after 50 years it decreases to 2 D or less. Presbyopia can be corrected by convex lenses.

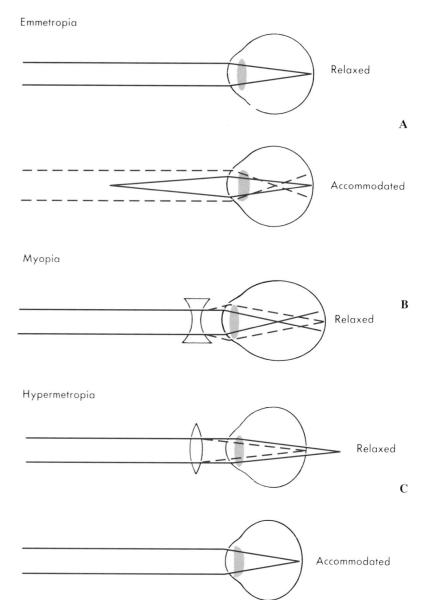

Emmetropia

Relaxed

A

Accommodated

Myopia

B

Relaxed

Hypermetropia

Relaxed

C

Accommodated

■ **Fig. 9-6** Accommodation and disorders of accommodation. **A,** The eye is emmetropic (has normal accommodation). Light rays from a distant visual target are focused on the retina *(above),* and rays from a nearby target can be focused when the eye is accommodated *(below).* **B,** The image of a distal visual target is focused in front of the retina unless a concave lens is used. **C,** The image is focused behind the retina unless a convex lens is employed *(above)* or the eye is accommodated *(below).*

■ *The Retina*

■ *Layers of the Retina*

The retina is a layered structure, the ten layers of which are shown in Fig. 9-7. The retina begins just inside the choroid with the **pigment epithelium** (layer 1). As mentioned, the pigment epithelium absorbs stray light, reducing light scatter. The pigment cells have tentacle-like processes that extend into the photoreceptor layer and surround the outer segments of the rods and cones. These processes prevent transverse scatter of light between photoreceptors. In addition, they probably serve a mechanical function in maintaining contact between layers 1 and 2. Other important functions of pigment cells include phagocytosis of the ends of the outer segments of the rods, which are continuously shed, and reconversion of metabolized photopigment into a form that can be reused after transport back to the photoreceptors (see p 137).

The **outer** and **inner segments** of the photoreceptors form layer 2 of the retina (Fig. 9-7). The structure of photoreceptors is described on p 136.

The junction between layers 1 and 2 of the retina in adults represents the surface of fusion between the anterior and posterior walls of the embryonic optic cup. Because this junction is structurally weak, it can separate, resulting in **retinal detachment.** Retinal detachment causes loss of vision due to the displacement of the retina from the focal plane of the eye. It can also lead to death of the photoreceptor cells, which are maintained by the blood supply of the choroid (the photoreceptor layer itself is avascular).

The photoreceptors form an organized surface that light strikes. Light rays that originate from different parts of the visual target correspond point to point to particular photoreceptors. Therefore, the geometry of the retina, and in particular that of the photoreceptors, must be maintained for normal vision. Retinal glial cells known as **Müller cells** play an important role in maintaining the geometry of the retina. Müller cells are oriented radially, parallel to the light path through the retina. The outer ends of the Müller cells form tight junctions with the inner segments of the photoreceptors. The numerous connections made between Müller cells and the inner segments give the appearance of a continuous layer in the light microscope (Fig. 9-7). This layer is called the **external limiting membrane** (layer 3 of the retina).

Inside the external limiting membrane is a layer of nuclei (Fig. 9-7) called the **outer nuclear layer** (layer 4 of the retina). This layer contains the nuclei of the rods and cones.

The next layer of the retina (layer 5) is called the **outer plexiform layer** (Fig. 9-7). This layer is a synaptic zone that contains presynaptic and postsynaptic elements of synapses between the photoreceptors and retinal interneurons, including bipolar cells and horizontal cells.

The next layer of the retina is the **inner nuclear layer** (layer 6 of the retina). This layer contains the cell bodies and nuclei of a number of cell types, including

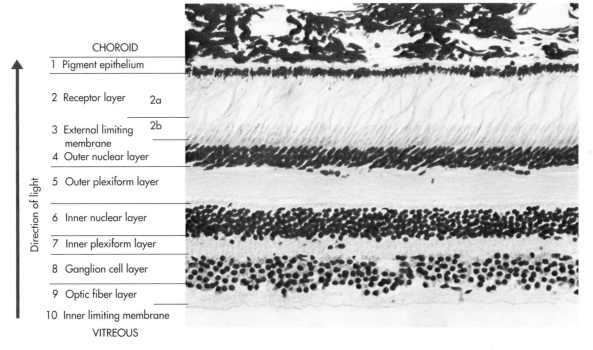

CHOROID
1 Pigment epithelium
2 Receptor layer　2a
3 External limiting membrane　2b
4 Outer nuclear layer
5 Outer plexiform layer
6 Inner nuclear layer
7 Inner plexiform layer
8 Ganglion cell layer
9 Optic fiber layer
10 Inner limiting membrane
VITREOUS

Direction of light

■ **Fig. 9-7**　Layers of the retina (from a macaque). The arrow at the left shows the direction of light impinging on the retina. (Nissl stain; courtesy of R.E. Weller.)

the retinal interneurons (bipolar cells, horizontal cells, amacrine cells, and interplexiform cells) and the Müller cells.

The next layer is the **inner plexiform layer** (layer 7 of the retina). This layer is another synaptic zone that contains the presynaptic and postsynaptic elements of synapses between some of the retinal interneurons, including the bipolar and amacrine cells, and the ganglion cells.

Layer 8 of the retina is the **ganglion cell layer.** As mentioned, the ganglion cells are the output cells of the retina. They transmit visual information to the brain.

The axons of the retinal ganglion cells form the **optic fiber layer** (layer 9 of the retina). The axons pass across the vitreous surface of the retina, avoiding the macula, and then enter the optic disc. They leave the eye in the optic nerve. The portions of the ganglion cell axons that are in the optic fiber layer are unmyelinated, but the axons become myelinated after they reach the optic disc and nerve. The lack of myelination of the axons where they cross the retina is a specialization that helps permit light to pass through the inner retina with minimal distortion.

The innermost layer of the retina is the **inner limiting membrane** (layer 10 of the retina). This layer is formed by projections of the Müller cells.

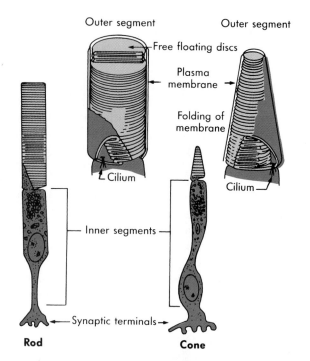

■ **Fig. 9-8**   Rods and cones. The drawings at the bottom show the general features of a rod and a cone. The insets show the outer segments in more detail.

■ *Structure of Photoreceptors: Rods and Cones*

The photoreceptors include the rods and the cones. Each photoreceptor cell is composed of a cell body, an inner and an outer segment that extends into layer 2, and a synaptic terminal (Fig. 9-8). The outer segments of rods are longer than those of cones, and they contain stacks of freely floating membrane discs rich in rhodopsin molecules (10^8 per rod outer segment). The outer segments of cones also contain membranous discs associated with photopigment. However, the outer segments of cones are not as long as those of rods, and the disc membranes consist of infoldings of the surface membrane. *Rods contain much more photopigment than do cones. The greater photopigment content of rods accounts in part for their greater sensitivity to light.* A single photon of light can elicit a rod response, whereas several hundred photons are required for a cone response.

The inner segments of the photoreceptors are connected to the outer segments by a modified cilium that contains nine pairs of microtubules but lacks the two central pairs of microtubules characteristic of most cilia. The inner segments contain a number of organelles, including numerous mitochondria.

The photopigment is synthesized in the inner segment and incorporated into the membranes of the outer segment. In rods, the pigment is inserted into new membranous discs (three new discs are formed per hour) that are then displaced distally until they are eventually shed at the apex of the outer segment. There, they are phago-

cytized by the pigment cell epithelium. This process determines the rodlike shape of the outer segments of rods. In cones, the photopigment is inserted randomly into the membranous folds of the outer segment, and shedding comparable with that seen in rods does not take place.

■ *Regional Variations in the Retina*

Fovea. *The depression in the macula lutea, known as the fovea, is the region of the retina that has the highest visual resolution.* Correspondingly, the image from the fixation point is focused on the fovea. The retinal layers in the foveal region are unusual, as several of them appear to be pushed aside (Fig. 9-9). This arrangement allows light to reach the photoreceptors without having to pass through the inner layers of the retina, and thereby reduces the distortion of the image. An additional specialization of the fovea is the unusually long and thin cone outer segments. This cone shape permits a high packing density. In fact, cone density is maximal in the fovea (Fig. 9-10). The cones provide high visual resolution, which matches the high quality of the image provided to the fovea.

Optic disc

As mentioned, the axons of the retinal ganglion cells cross the retina in the optic fiber layer (layer 9) and

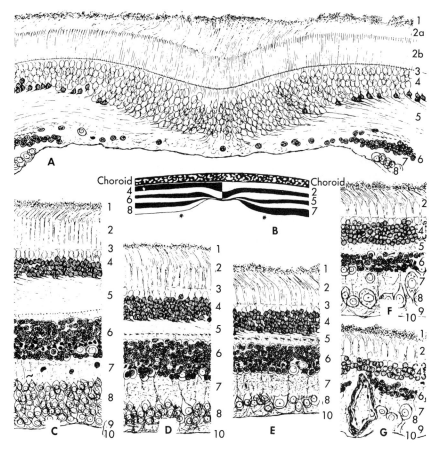

■ Fig. 9-9   Section through the fovea of a retina from a macaque monkey. The layers of the retina are numbered. (From Polyak S: *The vertebrate visual system,* Chicago, 1957, University of Chicago Press.)

enter the optic nerve at the optic disc. The axons in the optic fiber layer pass around the macula and avoid the fovea, as do the blood vessels that supply the inner layers of the retina (Fig. 9-4). The optic disc can be visualized on physical examination by use of an **ophthalmoscope.** The normal optic disc has a slight depression in its center. Changes in the appearance of the optic disc are important clinically. For example, the depression may be exaggerated by loss of ganglion cell axons **(optic atrophy),** or the optic disc may protrude into the vitreous space because of edema **(papilledema)** caused by increased intracranial pressure.

The optic disc lacks photoreceptors and therefore photosensitivity. Thus, the optic disc is a "blind spot" in the visual surface of the retina. The blind spot is normally ignored by the subject, both because the corresponding part of the visual field can be seen by the contralateral eye and because of the psychological process in which incomplete visual images tend to be completed perceptually. However, the blind spot can be mapped, as demonstrated in Fig. 9-11.

■ Visual Pigments

Light must be absorbed for it to be detected by the retina. Light absorption is accomplished by the visual pigments, which are located in the outer segments of rods and cones. The pigment found in the outer segments of rods is **rhodopsin,** or visual purple (because it has a purple appearance after green and blue light have been absorbed). Three variants of visual pigment are found in different cone types. Rhodopsin absorbs light best at a wavelength of 500 nm, whereas the cone pigments (Fig. 9-12) absorb best at 420 nm (blue), 531 nm (green), or 558 nm (red). However, the absorption spectra of these visual pigments overlap considerably.

Rhodopsin contains a chromophore called **retinal,** which is the aldehyde of **retinol,** or vitamin A. Retinol is derived from carotenoids, such as β-carotene, the orange pigment found in carrots. Like other vitamins, retinol cannot be synthesized by humans; instead, it is derived from food sources. Individuals with severe vitamin A deficiency suffer from **"night blindness,"** a condition in which vision in poor illumination is defective.

Rhodopsin is formed when an isomer of retinal known as 11-*cis* retinal combines with a glycoprotein known as opsin. When rhodopsin absorbs light, it is "boosted" to a higher energy level. This boost causes a series of chemical changes that lead to isomerization of 11-*cis* retinal to all-*trans* retinal, release of the bond with opsin, and conversion of the retinal to retinol. The separation of all-*trans* retinal from opsin causes bleaching of the visual pigment; i.e., it loses its purple color.

Visual adaptation. Light adaptation is associated with *a reduction in the amount of rhodopsin, which in turn reduces visual sensitivity.* Light adaptation occurs rapidly, within seconds. Light adaptation favors cone vision because the rhodopsin in rods bleaches more readily than do the cone pigments. (Cones have a special mechanism by which a reduction in Ca++ concentration occurs during light adaptation and permits cAMP synthesis and the reopening of Na+ channels; see p 140).

Bleached rhodopsin must be regenerated. As all-*trans* retinal is formed during light adaptation, it is transported to the retinal pigment cell layer, where it is reduced, isomerized, and esterified. As all-*cis* retinal is reconverted back to 11-*cis* retinal, it is transported back to the photoreceptor layer, taken up by outer segments of rods, and recombined with opsin to regenerate the bleached rhodopsin. *The regeneration of photopigment is one mechanism involved in* **dark adaptation,** *a process that results in an increase in visual sensitivity.* Cones adapt more rapidly to darkness than do rods, but their adapted threshold is relatively high. Thus, cones do not function when the ambient light level is low. By contrast, rods adapt to darkness slowly, but their sensitivity is high. Within 10 minutes in a dark room, rod vision is more sensitive than cone vision.

Dark adaptation is familiar to moviegoers, who must wait several minutes after entering a darkened theater before they can see an empty seat. While the theater is dark and rod vision is in use, visual acuity is low and colors are not distinguished (scotopic vision). When the movie is projected, light adaptation allows cone function to resume (photopic vision), and visual acuity and color vision are restored.

Color vision. The three visual pigments in cone outer segments have opsins that differ from the opsin found in rhodopsin. As a result of these differences, the three types of cone pigments absorb light best in the

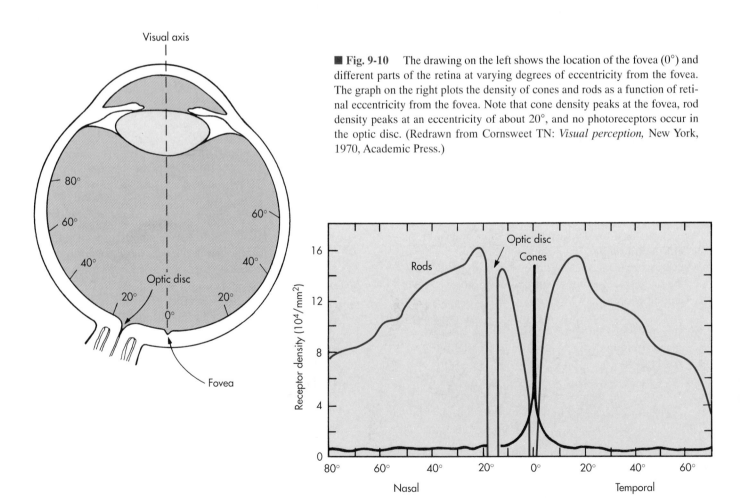

■ **Fig. 9-10**　The drawing on the left shows the location of the fovea (0°) and different parts of the retina at varying degrees of eccentricity from the fovea. The graph on the right plots the density of cones and rods as a function of retinal eccentricity from the fovea. Note that cone density peaks at the fovea, rod density peaks at an eccentricity of about 20°, and no photoreceptors occur in the optic disc. (Redrawn from Cornsweet TN: *Visual perception,* New York, 1970, Academic Press.)

blue, green, or red parts of the visible light spectrum (Fig. 9-12). According to the **trichromasy theory,** the differences in absorption are presumed to account for color vision. The basis of the trichromasy theory is that any color can be produced by a suitable mixture of three other colors. Because three types of cone pigments exist, it has been proposed that these pigments in some way provide for a neural analysis of color mixing. However, a neural system must also exist for the analysis of color brightness, because absorption of light by a visual pigment depends in part on the wavelength and in part on the intensity of the light. A given wavelength of light at a particular intensity may be absorbed by two or three of the visual pigments found in cones. However, absorption by one of the pigments will be greater than that by the others. If the intensity of the light is changed, but not the wavelength, the ratio of absorption will remain constant. By comparing the effectiveness of absorption of light of different wavelengths by the different types of cones, the visual system can distinguish different colors. At least two different kinds of cones are required for color vision. The presence of three kinds decreases the ambiguity in distinguishing colors when all three absorb light, and it ensures that at least two types of cones will absorb most wavelengths of visible light.

Observations on color blindness are consistent with the trichromasy theory. In **color blindness,** a genetic defect (sex-linked recessive), one or more cone mechanisms are lost. Normal people are **trichromats,** because they have three cone mechanisms. Individuals who have lost one of the cone mechanisms are called **dichromats.** When the long wavelength cone mechanism is lost, the resultant condition is called **protanopia;** loss of the medium wavelength system causes **deuteranopia;** loss of the short wavelength system, **tritanopia. Monochromats** have lost all three cone mechanisms (or in some cases, two cone mechanisms).

Other theories of color vision have also been proposed. The **opponent-process theory** is based on the observation that certain pairs of colors are perceived as if these colored lights activate opposing neural processes. Green and red are opposed, as are yellow and blue and black and white. For example, if a gray area is surrounded by a green ring, the gray area appears to acquire a reddish color. Furthermore, a greenish-red or a bluish-yellow color does not exist. These observations have led to the proposal that neurons activated by green are inhibited by red. Similarly, neurons excited by blue are inhibited by yellow. Neurons with these characteristics are in fact found both in the retina and at higher levels of the visual pathway.

A recent theory, the **retinex** theory, attributes color vision to the combined action of neural activity at several levels of the visual system, including the retina and cerebral cortex. All of these theories of color vision may be applicable.

■ **Fig. 9-11** If one eye is closed and the page is held about 30 cm from the open eye, when one of the symbols is fixated, the other will disappear as the page is moved back and forth. For the right eye, the fixation point should be the circle and for the left eye the cross.

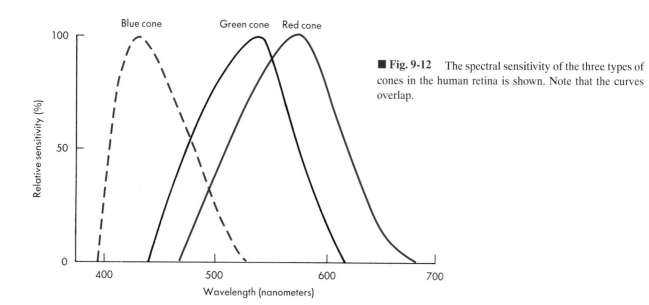

■ **Fig. 9-12** The spectral sensitivity of the three types of cones in the human retina is shown. Note that the curves overlap.

■ *Visual Transduction*

The transduction of visual signals involves the hyperpolarization of the rods and cones. Transmission of visual signals thus differs from the usual manner in which signals are transducted, in which a depolarization occurs in the sensory receptors.

When light is absorbed by rhodopsin, the signal is amplified by a special transduction mechanism in the rods. This amplification mechanism, along with the large amount of photopigment in rod outer segments, accounts for the extraordinary sensitivity of rods, which can detect a single photon after full dark adaptation. In the dark, rods have open sodium channels (Fig. 9-13). A net influx of Na+ results in a continuous current, called the **dark current.** The dark current causes the rods to be maintained in a constant state of depolarization (the "resting potential" is about −40 mV). As a consequence of this constant depolarization, neurotransmitter (considered to be glutamate) is tonically released at the rod synapses on bipolar and horizontal cells. The intracellular Na+ concentration is kept at a steady-state level by the pumping action of Na+, K+-ATPase.

Absorption of light activates a G protein, called **transducin,** which in turn activates **cyclic guanosine monophosphate (cGMP) phosphodiesterase.** This enzyme, which is associated with the rhodopsin-containing discs, hydrolyzes cGMP to 5′-GMP and lowers the cGMP concentration in the rod cytoplasm. cGMP normally keeps the sodium channels open. A reduction in cGMP concentration therefore causes the channels to close and the membrane to hyperpolarize. Amplification is the result of the ability of a single rhodopsin molecule to activate hundreds of transducin molecules; in addition, each phosphodiesterase molecule hydrolyzes thousands of cGMP molecules per second.

Similar events occur in cones, but the membrane hyperpolarization occurs more quickly than in rods, perhaps because the intracellular distances are shorter in cones.

■ *Retinal Circuitry*

A diagram of the basic circuitry of the retina is shown in Fig. 9-14. Photoreceptors *(R)* synapse on the dendrites of bipolar cells *(B)* and horizontal cells *(H)* in the outer plexiform layer. The horizontal cells make transverse connections with bipolar cells, and they receive input from interplexiform cells *(I).* Bipolar cells synapse on the dendrites of ganglion cells *(G)* and the processes of amacrine cells *(A)* in the inner plexiform layer. Amacrine cells connect with ganglion cells, other amacrine cells, and interplexiform cells.

Several features of this circuitry are noteworthy. The input to the retina is provided by light striking the photoreceptors. The output is carried by the axons of retinal

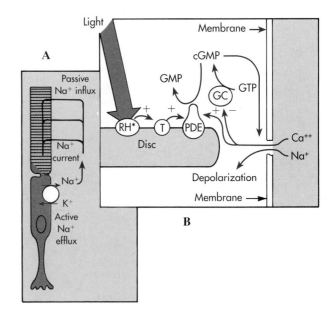

■ **Fig. 9-13** **A,** Drawing of a rod. The flow of dark current is indicated, as well as the Na pump. **B,** The sequence of second messenger events that follow absorption of light. *Rh,* Rhodopsin; *T,* transducin; *PDE,* phosphodiesterase; *GC,* guanylate cyclase; *cGMP,* cyclic guanosine monophosphate; *GTP,* guanosine triphosphate.

ganglion cells to the brain. Information is processed within the retina by the interneurons. The most direct pathway through the retina is from the photoreceptors to the bipolar cells and then to the ganglion cells. A more indirect pathway involves the photoreceptors, bipolar cells, amacrine cells, and ganglion cells. Horizontal cells provide lateral interactions between adjacent pathways. Interplexiform cells allow interactions to occur from the inner to the outer retina.

■ *Contrasts in Rod and Cone Pathway Functions*

Rod and cone pathways have several important functional differences, based partly on the differences in their phototransduction mechanisms and partly on retinal circuitry.

As we have previously observed, rods have more photopigment and a better signal amplification system than do cones, and there are many more rods than cones. Thus, rods function better in dim light (scotopic vision). However, they contain a single photopigment and so cannot signal color differences. Furthermore, many rods converge on single bipolar cells. Therefore, rods cannot provide high-resolution vision, because the effective receptive field for the rod pathway is large. In bright light, rhodopsin is bleached. Hence, rods no longer function under photopic conditions because of light adaptation. *Loss of rod function results in night blindness.*

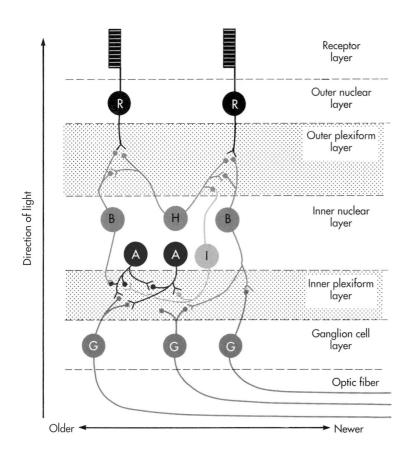

Direction of light

Older ◄───────────► Newer

Receptor
layer

Outer nuclear
layer

Outer plexiform
layer

Inner nuclear
layer

Inner plexiform
layer

Ganglion cell
layer

Optic fiber

■ **Fig. 9-14** Basic retinal circuitry. The arrow at the left indicates the direction of light through the retina. *R*, Photoreceptors; *B*, bipolar cells; *H*, horizontal cells; *A*, amacrine cells; *I*, interplexiform cells; *G*, ganglion cells.

Cones have a higher threshold to light and so are not activated in dim light after dark adaptation. However, they operate very well in daylight. They provide high-resolution vision because only a few cones converge on bipolar cells in the cone pathways, and no convergence occurs in the fovea (the cones make one-to-one connections to bipolar cells). As a result of the reduced convergence, cone pathways have very small receptive fields. Therefore, the cone pathways can resolve stimuli that originate from sources very close to each other. Cones also respond to sequential stimuli with good temporal resolution. Finally, cones have three different cone photopigments. Thus, they can discriminate among wavelengths and can participate in color vision. Loss of cone function results in functional blindness (rod vision is not sufficient for normal activities).

■ *Synaptic Interactions*

The distances within the retina are short. Hence, most of the activity in retinal circuits involves just receptor and synaptic potentials and not action potentials. Only the ganglion cells and some amacrine cells generate action potentials. It is unclear why amacrine cells generate action potentials, but ganglion cells must generate them in order to transmit information to the brain.

The receptor potential in photoreceptors is hyperpolarizing, and synaptic potentials in the retina can be either hyperpolarizing or depolarizing. Hyperpolarizing events reduce neurotransmitter release from the synaptic terminals of a retinal interneuron, whereas depolarizing events increase neurotransmitter release.

■ *Receptive Field Organization*

The activation of the receptive fields of retinal ganglion cells constitutes an important step in visual information processing, because these fields reflect the characteristics of visual signals that are conveyed to the brain. Fig. 9-15 shows how the receptive fields of photoreceptors and retinal interneurons determine the receptive fields of the retinal ganglion cells.

In Fig. 9-15, *A*, the receptive field of a photoreceptor is indicated by a circle with a minus sign. The small circle indicates that the receptive field is small and circular, and the minus sign indicates that light in the receptive field will hyperpolarize the photoreceptor cell.

The receptive field of a horizontal cell is shown in Fig. 9-15, *B* as a larger circle with minus signs. Light reaching any of the photoreceptors that converge on this horizontal cell will hyperpolarize it. The sequence of events is as follows: light hyperpolarizes one or more photoreceptors, these photoreceptors release less excitatory neurotransmitter, and the horizontal cell is hyperpolarized because of the reduction in tonic excitatory drive (i.e., it is disfacilitated).

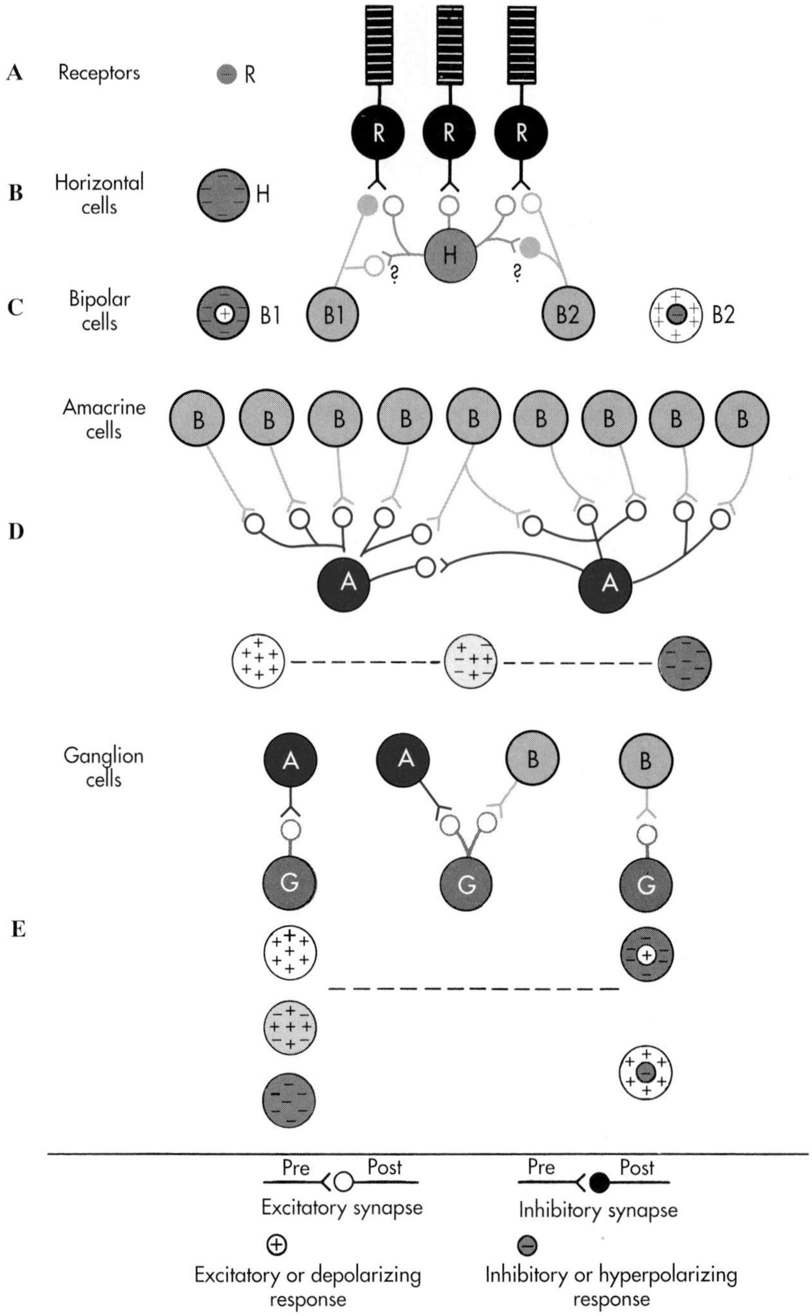

■ **Fig. 9-15** **A** to **E** show the receptive fields and neural circuitry determining them for photoreceptors *(R),* horizontal cells *(H),* bipolar cells *(B),* amacrine cells *(A),* and ganglion cells *(G).* Hyperpolarizing events are shown by minus signs and depolarizing events by plus signs.

The receptive fields of two different types of bipolar cells are shown in Fig. 9-15, *C.* The bipolar cell on the left *(B1)* has a centrally located excitatory receptive field *(shown by the white circle containing a plus sign),* surrounded by an inhibitory receptive field *(gray annulus containing minus signs).* This type of receptive field is described as having a **center-surround organization,** and this particular arrangement is called an **on-center, off-surround** receptive field (abbreviated "on-center"). The bipolar cell at the right in Fig. 9-15, *C* labeled *B2* has an "off-center," on-surround (or simply off-center) receptive field. In other words, its excitatory receptive field *(designated by plus signs)* surrounds a central inhibitory region *(designated by minus signs).*

The responses of bipolar cells depend on input from one or more photoreceptors and from horizontal cells. The response to stimulation of the center of the receptive field reflects direct connections from one or a few photoreceptors. If the neurotransmitter tonically released by the photoreceptor hyperpolarizes the bipolar cell, light striking the photoreceptor and hyperpolarizing it will reduce the release of the neurotransmitter, and the bipolar cell will be depolarized (disinhibited). On the other hand, if the neurotransmitter tonically released by the photoreceptor is depolarizing, the bipolar cell will be hyperpolarized (disfacilitated, just like the horizontal cell in Fig. 9-15, *B).* The surround response results when light impinges on adjacent photoreceptors and changes the activity of horizontal cells. The pathway through the horizontal cells results in a response that is opposite in sign to that produced directly by the photoreceptors that mediate the center response.

The neurotransmitter used in the retinal pathway from photoreceptor cells to bipolar cells and to horizontal cells is an excitatory amino acid, probably glutamate. Excitatory amino acids depolarize off-center bipolar cells, as well as horizontal cells, through activation of ionotropic glutamate receptors. They hyperpolarize on-center bipolar cells through an action on metabotropic glutamate receptors.

If light strikes photoreceptors that cause the surround response, in addition to those responsible for the center response, the bipolar cell may not respond at all because of the opposing actions from the center and surround. On the other hand, light moving across the receptive field will sequentially cause dramatic changes in the activity of the bipolar cell as it crosses the receptive field from surround to center and then again to surround.

The receptive fields of amacrine cells are shown in Fig. 9-15, *D.* The amacrine cells receive input from different combinations of on-center and off-center bipolar cells. Thus their receptive fields are mixtures of on-center and off-center regions. There are many different types of amacrine cells, and at least eight neurotransmitters are known to be released by the amacrine cells.

Fig. 9-15, *E* shows the receptive fields of ganglion cells. Ganglion cells may receive a dominant input from amacrine cells *(left),* a mixed input from amacrine and bipolar cells *(middle),* or a dominant input from bipolar cells *(right).* When the amacrine cell input dominates, the receptive fields of ganglion cells tend to be diffuse and either excitatory or inhibitory. On the other hand, when the input is dominated by bipolar cells, the ganglion cells have a center-surround organization similar to that of bipolar cells.

■ *P, M, and W Cells*

Experimental studies have shown that, on the basis of a number of features, retinal ganglion cells in cats can be subdivided into three general types, called X cells, Y cells, and W cells. X and Y cells are fairly homogeneous groups, whereas W cells are heterogeneous. In primates, cells equivalent to X cells are called P cells, because they project to the *parvocellular* layers of the lateral geniculate nucleus (LGN); cells equivalent to Y cells are known as M cells, because they project to the *magnocellular* layers of the LGN. Because human retinas more closely resemble those of subhuman primates, the terms P and M cells are used here. P and M cells have center-surround receptive fields; hence, they are presumably controlled predominantly by bipolar cells. Some W cells also have center-surround receptive fields, but many have diffuse receptive fields. Thus,

they are probably influenced chiefly through amacrine cell pathways.

The different types of ganglion cells have strikingly different shapes (Fig. 9-16). P (or X) cells have medium-sized cell bodies and axons and restricted dendritic trees. On the other hand, M (or Y) cells have larger cell bodies and axons and much more extensive dendritic trees than those of P cells. W cells have small cell bodies and axons but extensive dendritic trees.

Several physiological differences among these cell types correspond to the morphologic differences (Table 9-1). For example, P (or X) cells have smaller receptive fields (corresponding to the smaller dendritic trees) and more slowly conducting axons than M (or Y) cells. In addition, P cells tonically respond to visual stimuli, show more linear summation of responses than do M cells, and respond better to small stimuli than to large stimuli. M cells have phasic, nonlinear responses to complex stimuli; such responses cannot be predicted from the responses to simple stimuli. P cells respond differently to different wavelengths of light, whereas M cells are not sensitive to differences in wavelength. On the other hand, M cells are more sensitive to brightness than P cells. W cells have large, diffuse receptive fields and slowly conducting axons; they respond poorly to visual stimuli.

■ *The Visual Pathway*

The retinal ganglion cells transmit information to the brain via the optic nerve, optic chiasm, and optic tract (Fig. 9-1). Fig. 9-17 shows the relationships between a visual target *(arrow),* the retinal images of the target in the two eyes, and the projections of retinal ganglion cells to the two hemispheres of the brain. The eyes and the optic nerves, chiasm, and tract are viewed from above.

The visual target, an arrow, is in the **visual fields** of both eyes (Fig. 9-17). The visual target in this case is so long that it extends into the monocular segments of each retina (i.e., one end of the target can be seen only by one eye and the other end only by the other eye). The fixation point is shown by the shaded circle at the center of the target. The image of the target is reversed on the retinas by the lens system. The left half of the visual target is imaged on the nasal retina of the left eye and the temporal retina of the right eye. Thus, the left visual field is seen by the left nasal retina and the right temporal retina. Similarly, the right half of the visual target is imaged on and seen by the left temporal retina and the right nasal retina.

The projections of retinal ganglion cells may be uncrossed or crossed, depending on the location of the ganglion cell. For example, a given axon from the left retina may pass through the left optic nerve, the left side of the optic chiasm, and the left optic tract to terminate in the brain on the left side. Alternatively, an axon in the left retina may pass through the left optic nerve, cross to the

■ **Table 9-1**   Properties of retinal ganglion cells

Properties	X cells (P cells)	Y cells (M cells)	W cells
Cell body and axon	Medium-sized	Large	Small
Dendritic tree	Restricted	Extensive	Extensive
Receptive field			
Size	Small	Medium	Large
Organization	Center-surround	Center-surround	Diffuse
Adaptation	Tonic	Phasic	Poorly responsive
Linearity	Linear	Nonlinear	
Wavelength	Sensitive	Insensitive	Insensitive
Luminance	Insensitive	Sensitive	Sensitive

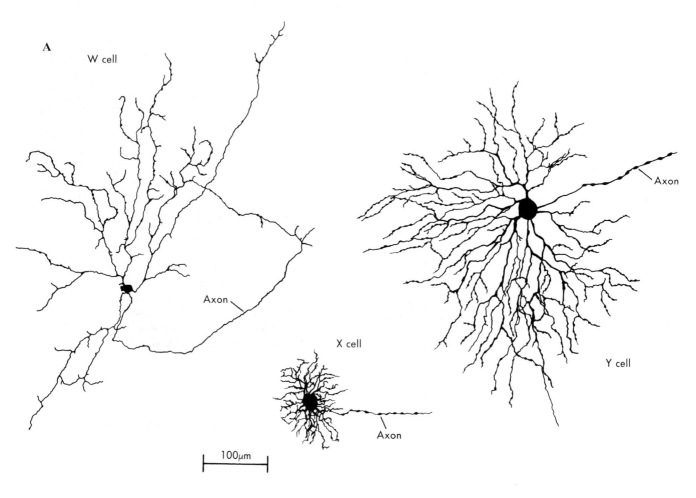

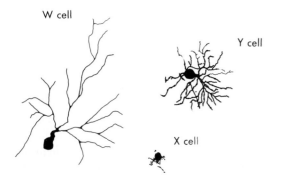

■ **Fig. 9-16**   X, Y, and W cells. **A,** Cells in cat retina. **B,** Cells in monkey retina. (**A** from Stanford LR, Sherman SM: *Brain Res* 297:381, 1984; **B** redrawn from Perry VH et al: *Neuroscience* 12:1101, 1984 and Perry VH, Cowey A: *Neuroscience* 12:1125, 1984.)

opposite side in the optic chiasm, and then pass through the right optic tract to end in the right side of the brain. *Axons that remain uncrossed arise from ganglion cells in the temporal retina, whereas axons that do cross arise from ganglion cells in the nasal retina.*

This arrangement results in the representation of the left field of vision in the right side of the brain and of the right field of vision in the left side of the brain (Fig. 9-17).

The axons of retinal ganglion cells can synapse in any of several nuclei of the brain. The main pathway for vision relays in the **lateral geniculate nucleus (LGN),** one of the sensory nuclei of the thalamus. The LGN in turn projects to the **primary visual cortex** or **striate cortex** by way of the **optic radiations** or **geniculostriate tract** (Fig. 9-18). As the optic radiation passes caudally, it fans out, and some of the fibers loop forward in the temporal lobe as **Meyer's loop**. The axons in Meyer's loop carry information derived from the lower half of the appropriate hemiretinas. Thus, the axons in Meyer's loop represent the contralateral upper visual field. Axons that pass directly caudally through the parietal lobe in the optic radiation represent the contralateral lower visual field.

The optic radiation ends in the striate cortex, which is located dorsal and ventral to the calcarine fissure in the occipital lobe. The gyrus dorsal to the calcarine fissure is the **cuneus,** and that ventral is the **lingual gyrus.** The cuneus receives information from the upper part of the appropriate hemiretinas, and the lingual gyrus receives information from the lower hemiretinas. Thus, the cuneus represents the contralateral lower visual field and the lingual gyrus the upper visual field.

■ *Visual Field Defects*

Interruption of the visual pathway at any level will cause a defect in the appropriate part of the visual field (Fig. 9-19). For example, a lesion of the retina in one eye produces localized blindness, a **scotoma,** in that eye. Complete interruption of the optic nerve results in complete blindness; partial interruption of the optic nerve causes a scotoma. Damage to the optic nerve fibers as they cross in the optic chiasm results in loss of vision in both temporal fields of vision, a condition known as **bitemporal hemianopsia.** This condition occurs because the crossing fibers originate from ganglion cells in the nasal halves of each retina. A lesion of the entire optic tract, LGN, optic radiation, or visual cortex on one side causes loss of vision in the entire contralateral visual field, or **homonymous hemianopsia.** Partial lesions produce partial visual field defects. For example, a lesion of Meyer's loop causes a loss of vision in the contralateral upper visual field, an upper **homonymous quadrantanopsia** ("pie in the sky" visual defect). A lesion of the striate cortex may not destroy all of the neurons that represent the macula, and the result is sometimes a homonymous hemianopsia with **macular sparing.**

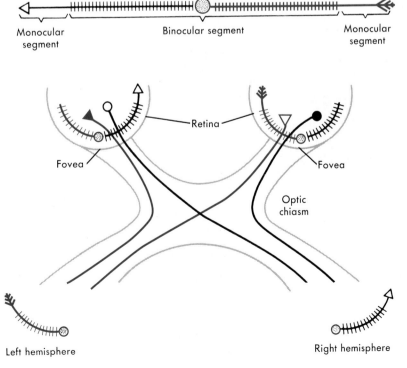

■ Fig. 9-17 Relationships between a visual target, images on the retinas of the two eyes, and the projections of the ganglion cells carrying visual information about these images. The image is so large that it extends into the monocular segments of the eyes where the image is seen in only one eye.

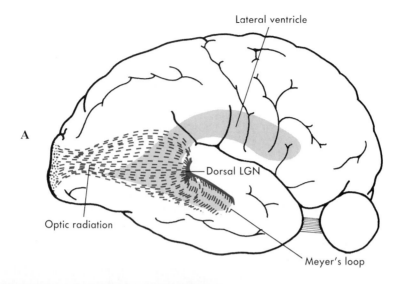

A

Lateral ventricle

Dorsal LGN

Optic radiation

Meyer's loop

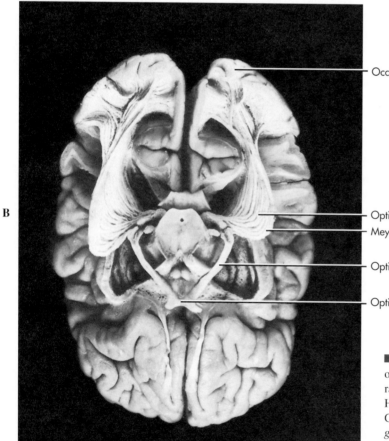

B

Occipital lobe

Optic radiations

Meyer's loop

Optic tract

Optic chiasm

■ **Fig. 9-18**   Geniculostriate tract. **A,** The course of the optic radiation in a lateral view. **B,** Dissection of the optic radiation, including Meyer's loop. (**A** redrawn from Sandford HS, Blair JHL: *Arch Neurol Psychiat* 42:21, 1939; **B** from Gluhbegovic N, Williams TH: *The human brain: a photographic guide,* New York, 1980, Harper & Row.)

■ *Lateral Geniculate Nucleus*

The dorsal LGN is a layered structure (Fig. 9-20). The first two layers, which contain large neurons, are called the magnocellular layers. The other four layers are the parvocellular layers. There is a point-to-point projection from the retina to the LGN. The LGN thus has a retinotopic map. Cells that represent a particular retinal location are aligned along projection lines that can be drawn across the LGN (Fig. 9-20).

The projection from one eye is distributed to three of the layers of the LGN, to one of the magnocellular layers, and to two parvocellular layers. The contralateral eye projects to layers 1, 4, and 6; the ipsilateral eye projects to layers 2, 3, and 5. Another basis for the diversion of retinal input to different layers of the LGN depends on the subdivision of primate retinal ganglion cells into P and M cells. M cells innervate layers 1 and 2, whereas P cells supply layers 3 to 6. Furthermore, off-center P cells tend to end in layers 3 and 4 and on-center P cells in layers 5 and 6.

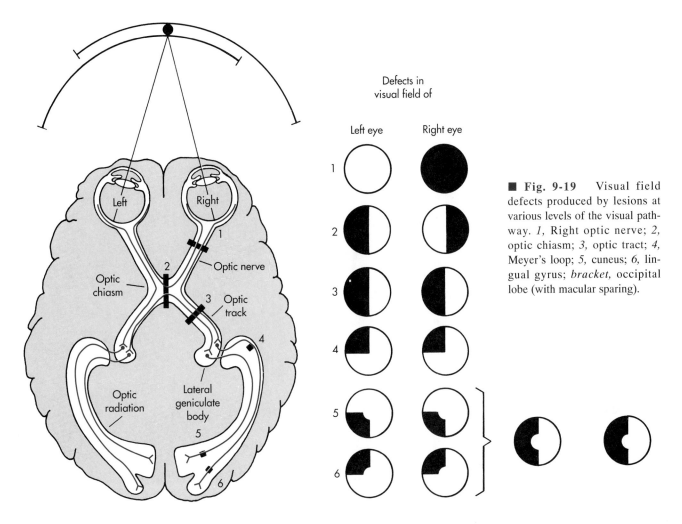

Defects in
visual field of

■ **Fig. 9-19** Visual field defects produced by lesions at various levels of the visual pathway. *1,* Right optic nerve; *2,* optic chiasm; *3,* optic tract; *4,* Meyer's loop; *5,* cuneus; *6,* lingual gyrus; *bracket,* occipital lobe (with macular sparing).

Most of the neurons in the LGN project to the striate cortex. However, about one quarter of the cells are interneurons that have an inhibitory function. Each LGN neuron receives an input from only a limited number of retinal ganglion cells. Consequently, LGN neurons have properties very similar to those of ganglion cells. For example, LGN neurons can be classified as P or M cells, and they have on-center or off-center receptive fields.

The LGN also receives input from the visual areas of the cerebral cortex, the thalamic reticular nucleus, and several nuclei of the brainstem reticular formation. The activity of LGN projection neurons is inhibited by interneurons both in the LGN and in the thalamic reticular nucleus. These cells use gamma-aminobutyric acid (GABA) as their inhibitory neurotransmitter. In addition, the activity of LGN neurons is influenced by brainstem neurons that use monoamine transmitters and by corticofugal pathways. These control systems serve to filter visual information and are likely to be important for selective attention.

■ *Striate Cortex*

The geniculostriate pathway ends chiefly in layer 4 of the striate cortex. A dense band of axons from the optic radi-

ation in layer 4 forms the **stripe of Gennari,** which accounts for the name of this part of the cerebral cortex. Axons that represent one eye or the other terminate alternately in patches known as **ocular dominance columns.** Cortical neurons in an ocular dominance column respond preferentially to input from the appropriate eye. Near the border between two ocular dominance columns, neurons respond about equally to inputs from the two eyes.

Like the LGN, the striate cortex contains a retinotopic map (actually, two interlaced retinotopic maps, one for each eye). The macula is represented by a region that is relatively large compared with that of the remainder of the retina (Fig. 9-21). The macular representation extends forward from the occipital pole for about one third of the length of the striate cortex.

The receptive fields of neurons in the striate cortex are more complex than those of LGN neurons. First, they may respond to stimulation of both eyes, although often the input from one eye dominates (see above). Second, some neurons in layer 4 that receive direct input from the LGN may be activated by stimulation of just one eye. Third, cortical neurons generally have **orientation selectivity;** i.e., they respond best when the stimulus is elongated, such as a bar or an edge, and oriented in a particular way with respect to the horizontal position (Fig. 9-22). Because neurons in a particular

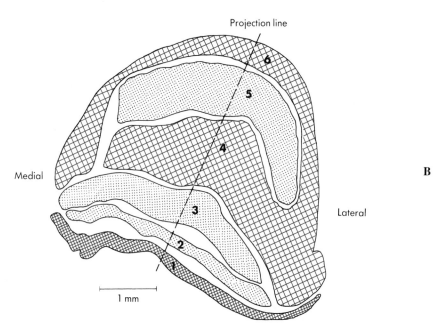

■ **Fig. 9-20** Section through the lateral geniculate nucleus (LGN) of a human infant. **A,** Micrograph of the Nissl-stained LGN. **B,** Drawing. The layers are numbered *1 to 6.* Cross-hatching indicates the layers innervated by the contralateral eye; the dots indicate the layers supplied by the ipsilateral eye. The projection line shows the location of cells in all the layers that map a point in the visual field. (**A** courtesy of T.L. Hickey and R.W. Guillery.)

zone of the cortex all tend to have the same orientation selectivity, they are considered to form an orientation column (Fig. 9-22). Cortical neurons may also display direction selectivity; i.e., they may respond when the stimulus is moved in one direction, but not when it is moved in the opposite direction.

Several theories have been proposed to account for these properties of neurons in the visual cortex. One theory holds that the patterns of convergence of neurons at different serial levels of the visual pathway cause the receptive fields to become progressively more complex. **Simple cells** have on- and off-zones in their receptive fields. However, the receptive fields are rectangular and

have an orientation selectivity. **Complex cells** reflect the convergent input of several simple cells. Their receptive fields also have an orientation preference but contain no distinct on- and off-zones, and many cells are particularly responsive to movement of the stimulus across the receptive field. **Hypercomplex cells** receive inputs from several complex cells and thus have even more elaborate receptive fields. However, this classification does not take into account the P- and M-cell pathways. Presumably, parallel P- and M-cell pathways contribute to the complexity of visual cortical organization. Cortical receptive field organization may depend on both serial and parallel processing.

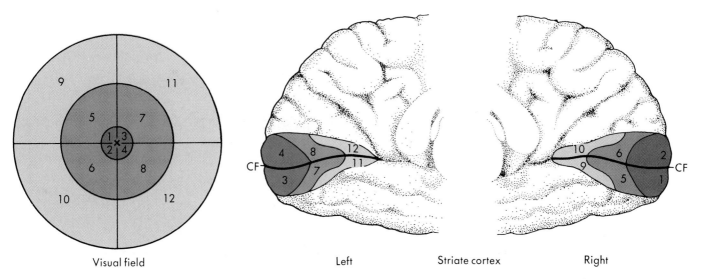

■ **Fig. 9-21**   The representation of different parts of the visual field *(left)* in the retinotopic map of the visual cortex is shown by the corresponding numbers.

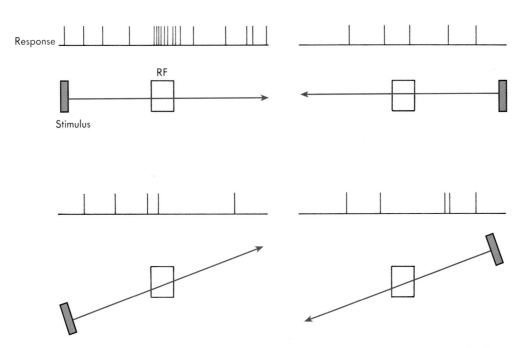

■ **Fig. 9-22**   Orientation and direction selectivity. The responses of a neuron in the visual cortex are shown for stimulus oriented vertically *(upper)* or obliquely *(lower)* and moved to the right or to the left *(arrows)*.

Stereopsis. **Stereopsis** is defined as binocular depth perception. It must be a cortical function, because it depends on convergent inputs from the two eyes. It appears to be caused by slight differences in the retinal images formed in the two eyes. Such disparities give different perspectives that lead to visual cues about depth. Stereopsis is useful only for relatively nearby objects. Depth cues are also available when a single eye is used.

Color vision. As already discussed, color vision may depend on the presence in the retina of cones of three different types, as well as on neurons in the visual pathway that show spectral opposition. Retinal ganglion cells, LGN neurons, and visual cortical neurons have been found that show spectral opponent properties (Fig. 9-23, *A*). These cells are the P cells. Other neurons, the M cells, respond to brightness but not to spectral opposition. The

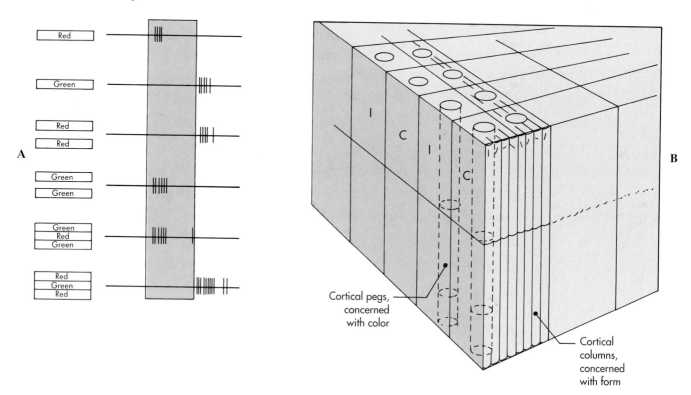

■ Fig. 9-23   A, Responses of a neuron in the striate cortex that responds to various combinations of red and green bars. The best response was to a red bar flanked by two green bars. **B,** Diagram of the columnar arrangement of the visual cortex. Ocular dominance columns are indicated by *I* (for ipsilateral) and *C* (for contralateral). Orientation columns are indicated by the short bars at various angles. The cortical pegs contain neurons like that of **A** with spectral opponent receptive fields.

spectral opponent neurons in the visual cortex are found in cortical "pegs" or "blobs." The relationship between the ocular dominance and orientation columns and the cortical color pegs is shown in Fig. 9-23, *B.*

■ *Superior Colliculus*

The **superior colliculus** is a layered structure in the midbrain (Fig. 9-24). The three most superficial layers are exclusively involved in visual processing, whereas the deeper layers receive multimodal inputs not only from the visual system but also from the somatosensory and auditory systems.

Neurons in the superficial layers of the superior colliculus receive a projection from retinal ganglion cells. The axons reach the superior colliculus through the brachium of the superior colliculus. The ganglion cells include both W and M cells (but not P cells) and are located chiefly in the contralateral nasal retina. Neurons in the superficial layer of the superior colliculus also receive a projection from the visual cortex, including the striate cortex. The cortical loop involves neurons activated by M cells. The superficial layer of the superior colliculus in turn projects to several thalamic nuclei (pulvinar, LGN) and is therefore indirectly connected with large areas of visual cortex.

The superior colliculus contains a retinotopic map. Collicular neurons are particularly sensitive to rapid stimulus motion in a particular direction. Most of the cells have binocular inputs, but they lack orientation selectivity.

Studies in cats demonstrate that the superior colliculus plays an important role in visual perception in these animals. Bilateral destruction of the striate cortex of cats impairs visual performance only slightly; some visual acuity is lost. The superior colliculus in cats may be particularly important for determining the location of objects in visual space. It is unclear how important "collicular vision" is in humans.

The deep layers of the superior colliculus receive connections from somatosensory and auditory pathways, as well as visual input from the superficial layers. Thus, the deep layers of the superior colliculus contain somatotopic and retinotopic maps, as well as a map of sound in space. Corresponding parts of these maps are overlaid. For example, an area that receives information about the contralateral visual field will also receive information about sounds that originate from the contralateral auditory space and about somatic stimuli applied to the contralateral surface of the body. In addition, the deep layers of the superior colliculus contain a motor map that functions to control eye and head position. For instance, activation of neurons in the superior colliculus by a visual

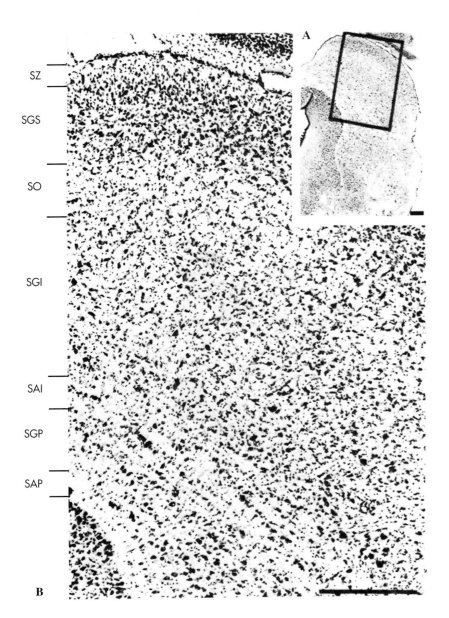

SZ
SGS
SO
SGI
SAI
SGP
SAP
A
B

■ **Fig. 9-24**   Coronal section through the superior colliculus in a primate. **A,** Low-power micrograph. **B,** Higher-power view of the region indicated by the box in **A.** *SZ,* Stratum zonale; *SGS,* st. griseum superficiale; *SO,* st. opticum; *SGI,* st. griseum intermedium; *SAI,* st. album intermedium; *SGP,* st. griseum profundum; *SAP,* st. album profundum. (Courtesy of D. Raczkowski.)

target causes movement of the eyes to center the visual target on the fovea. In this way, the superior colliculus is involved in reflex responses to the sudden appearance of a novel or threatening object in the visual field. Similarly, a sound or a sudden contact with the body will elicit appropriate eye and head movements to visualize the source of the stimulus. The descending pathways include connections to the oculomotor control system through tectoreticular connections and to the spinal cord through the tectospinal tract.

■ *Extrastriate Visual Cortex*

In animal studies, at least 25 different visual areas have been identified in the cerebral cortex in addition to the striate cortex. These extrastriate areas include several different parallel visual processing pathways. The P pathway originates with P cells and functions in the recognition of form and color. Some of the cortical structures in the P pathway include layer $4C_\beta$ of the striate cortex, area V4, and several areas in the inferotemporal region (Fig. 9-25). The processing of form includes recognition of complex visual patterns such as faces. Color information is processed separately from form. The M pathway originates with M cells and functions in motion detection and in the control of eye movements. Cortical structures in the M pathway include layers 4B and $4C_\alpha$ of the striate cortex, and areas MT (middle temporal) and MST (middle superior temporal) on the lateral aspect of the temporal lobe, as well as area 7a of the parietal lobe (Fig. 9-25). Both P and M pathways contribute to depth perception.

Lesions of the extrastriate visual cortex can produce various deficits. Bilateral lesions of the inferotemporal

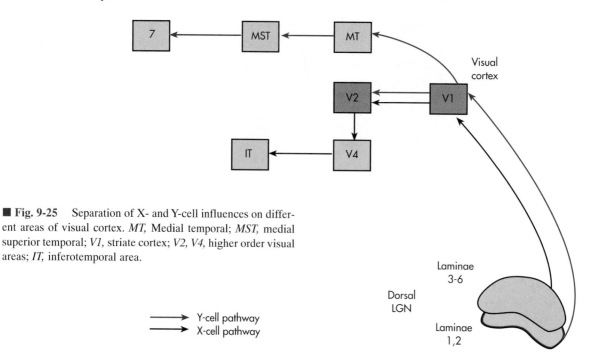

■ **Fig. 9-25** Separation of X- and Y-cell influences on different areas of visual cortex. *MT,* Medial temporal; *MST,* medial superior temporal; *V1,* striate cortex; *V2, V4,* higher order visual areas; *IT,* inferotemporal area.

cortex can result in cortical color blindness (**achromatopsia**) or in the inability to recognize faces, even of close members of the family (**prosopagnosia**). A lesion of area MT or MST can interfere with motion detection and with eye movements.

■ *Other Visual Pathways*

The visual pathways include connections to nuclei that serve functions other than vision. For example, a retinal projection to the suprachiasmatic nucleus of the hypothalamus controls circadian rhythmicity.

Another retinal projection is to the pretectum. This pathway activates parasympathetic preganglionic neurons in the **Edinger-Westphal nucleus,** which in turn causes pupillary constriction in the pupillary light reflex. The pretectal areas are interconnected through the posterior commissure, and thus the reflex causes both ipsilateral (direct) and contralateral (consensual) pupillary constriction.

■ *Summary*

1. The eye has three main layers. The fibrous layer includes the cornea and sclera; the vascular layer includes the choroid, iris, and ciliary body; the nervous layer is the retina.

2. The cornea is the most powerful refractive surface, but the lens has a variable power that allows images from near objects to be focused on the retina. Depth of field is adjusted by the iris. Stray light is absorbed by pigment.

3. The retina has 10 layers. The photoreceptor layer absorbs light. Photoreceptors synapse on retinal interneurons, which in turn synapse on each other and on ganglion cells. The latter project to the brain through the optic nerve.

4. The fovea is specialized for high resolution and color vision and contains only cones. The visual fixation point is imaged on the fovea.

5. The optic disc contains no photoreceptors and therefore is a blind spot.

6. Photoreceptors transduce visual signals and are hyperpolarized by light. Pathways through the retina involve relays by retinal interneurons. Bipolar pathways are more direct than amacrine ones. Horizontal cells mediate lateral inhibition. Bipolar cells and many ganglion cells have receptive fields with an on-center, off-surround or off-center, on-surround organization. Amacrine cells and some ganglion cells have large, diffuse receptive fields.

7. Many ganglion cells can be classified as P, M, or W cells. P cells with small receptive fields and tonic and linear responses signal fine detail and wavelength. M cells have nonlinear responses and signal motion. Most W cells are difficult to activate.

8. The axons of ganglion cells in the temporal retina project ipsilaterally; those in the nasal retina cross in the optic chiasm. Crossed axons end in layers 1, 4, and 6 of the lateral geniculate nucleus (LGN); uncrossed axons end in layers 2, 3, and 5. Layers 1 and 2, the magnocellular layers, receive M-cell projections; the other parvocellular layers receive P-cell projections.

9. The LGN projects to the striate cortex through the optic radiation. Some of the axons pass into the temporal

lobe in Meyer's loop. These axons carry visual information from the lower retinas and thus represent the contralateral upper visual field quadrants.

10. The LGN projection ends largely in layer 4 of the striate cortex. Information from one or the other eye predominates in ocular dominance columns. The striate cortex contains an orderly retinotopic map. Most striate cortical neurons respond best to bars or edges oriented in a particular way. Cells that prefer a particular stimulus orientation are grouped in orientation columns.

11. Stereopsis involves differences in the retinal images in the two eyes.

12. Color vision depends on wavelength discrimination, based on the three types of cone pigment and also on color opponent neurons.

13. The upper layers of the superior colliculus are involved in visual processing. The deep layers produce eye movements directed at visual targets that move into the field of vision or that are sources of somatosensory or auditory stimuli.

14. The many cortical extrastriate visual areas have different functions. Some in the inferotemporal cortex are influenced chiefly by P cells and function in form and color vision. Others in the middle temporal and parietal cortex are activated by M cells and function in motion detection and the control of eye movements.

■ *Self-Study Problems*

1. Given that the main refractive surface of the eye is the cornea, why is the refractive power of the lens so important?

2. What are some of the functions of the iris?

3. The excitatory amino acid glutamate is the neurotransmitter used at synapses between photoreceptor cells and bipolar neurons in the retina. How is it possible that glutamate depolarizes off-center bipolar cells and hyperpolarizes on-center bipolar cells?

4. What type of visual field defect would be caused by a lesion of the right lingual gyrus?

5. What deficits might be produced by a bilateral lesion of the inferotemporal region of the cerebral cortex?

■ *Bibliography*

Journal articles

Baylor D: How photons start vision, *Proc Natl Acad Sci USA* 93:560, 1996.

Curcio CA, Sloan KR, Kalina RE, Hendrickson AE: Human photoreceptor topography, *J Comp Neurol* 292:497, 1990.

Daw NW: The psychology and physiology of colour vision, *Trends Neurosci* 7:330, 1984.

Daw NW, Brunken WJ, Parkinson D: The function of synaptic transmitters in the retina, *Annu Rev Neurosci* 12:205, 1989.

Derrington AM, Lennie P: Spatial and temporal contrast sensitivities of neurones in lateral geniculate nucleus of macaque, *J Physiol (Lond)* 311:623, 1984.

DeYoe EA, Felleman DJ, Van Essen DC, McClendon E: Multiple processing streams in occipitotemporal visual cortex, *Nature* 371:151, 1994.

Felleman DJ, Van Essen DC: Distributed hierarchical processing in the primate cerebral cortex, *Cereb Cortex* 1:1, 1991.

Fitzpatrick D, Itoh K, Diamond IT: The laminar organization of the lateral geniculate body and the striate cortex in the squirrel monkey *(Saimiri sciureus), J Neurosci* 3:673, 1983.

Gilbert CD, Wiesel TN: Receptive field dynamics in adult primary visual cortex, *Nature* 356:150, 1992.

Land EH: The retinex theory of color vision, *Sci Am* 237:108, 1977.

Lee BB: Receptive field structure in the primate retina, *Vision Res* 36:631, 1996.

Livingstone MS, Nori S, Freeman DC, Hubel DH: Stereopsis and binocularity in the squirrel monkey, *Vision Res* 35:345, 1995.

Masland RH: Functional architecture of the retina, *Sci Am* 255:102, 1986.

Maunsell JH: The brain's visual world: representation of visual targets in cerebral cortex, *Science* 270:764, 1995.

Merigan WH, Maunsell JHR: How parallel are the primate visual pathways?, *Annu Rev Neurosci* 16:369, 1993.

Peng YW, Blackstone CD, Huganir RL, Yau KW: Distribution of glutamate receptor subtypes in the vertebrate retina, *Neuroscience* 66:483, 1995.

Schwartz EA: Phototransduction in vertebrate rods, *Annu Rev Neurosci* 8:339, 1985.

Stryer L: Cyclic GMP cascade of vision, *Annu Rev Neurosci* 9:87, 1986.

Tamamaki N, Uhlrich DJ, Sherman SM: Morphology of physiologically identified retinal X and Y axons in the cat's thalamus and midbrain as revealed by intraaxonal injection of biocytin, *J Comp Neurol* 354:583, 1995.

Tanaka K: Inferotemporal cortex and object vision, *Annu Rev Neurosci* 19:109, 1996.

Van Essen DC, Anderson CH, Felleman DJ: Information processing in the primate visual system: an integrated systems perspective, *Science* 255:419, 1992.

Books and monographs

Dowling JE: *The retina: an approachable part of the brain,* Cambridge, Mass, 1987, Belknap Press.

Hubel DH: *Eye, brain and vision,* New York, 1988, Freeman.

Kandel ER, Schwartz JH, Jessell TM: *Principles of neural science,* ed 3, New York, 1991, Elsevier.

Zeki S: *A vision of the brain,* Boston, 1993, Blackwell Scientific Publications.

The Auditory and Vestibular Systems

The peripheral parts of the auditory and vestibular systems share components of the bony and membranous labyrinths, use hair cells as mechanical transducers, and transmit information to the central nervous system (CNS) through the eighth cranial nerve. However, their CNS processing and sensory functions are quite distinct. The function of the auditory system is to transduce sound that allows us to recognize environmental cues and communicate with other organisms. The most complex auditory functions are those involved in language. The function of the vestibular system is to provide the CNS with information related to the position and movements of the head in space. The control of eye movements by the vestibular system is discussed in Chapter 13.

■ *Audition*

■ *Sound*

Sound is produced by waves of compression and decompression that are transmitted in air or in other elastic media such as water. Sound propagates at about 335 m/sec in air. The waves are associated with changes in pressure called sound pressure. The unit of sound pressure is N/m², but sound pressure is more commonly expressed as the **sound pressure level (SPL).** The unit of SPL is the **decibel (dB):**

$$SPL = 20 \log (P/P_R)$$

where P is the sound pressure and P_R is a reference pressure (either 0.0002 dyne/cm², the absolute threshold for human hearing, or 1 dyne/cm²).

Sound frequency is measured in cycles per second, or **Hertz (Hz).** Sound, however, is actually a mixture of pure tones. Each pure tone results from sinusoidal waves at a particular frequency and is characterized not only by its frequency but also by its amplitude and phase (Fig. 10-1). Thus, because most sounds are complex mixtures of pure tones, it is possible to break down the composition of a particular sound into a set of pure tones. This breakdown is done by **Fourier analysis.** Conversely, Fourier synthesis permits the construction of a sound by mixing pure

tones. Fig. 10-2 shows how a complex sound wave can be characterized by Fourier analysis to determine its frequency composition. The energy of this particular sound is concentrated at a frequency slightly greater than 100 Hz, or its fundamental frequency. A number of other frequencies (up to about 3000 Hz) are also present. **Noise** is a sound composed of many unrelated frequencies; **white noise** is a mixture of all audible frequencies.

The normal human ear is sensitive to pure tones with frequencies that range between about 20 and 20,000 Hz. The threshold for detection of a pure tone varies with its frequency (Fig. 10-3). The lowest thresholds for human hearing are for pure tones of about 1000 to 3000 Hz (Fig. 10-3). By definition, threshold at these frequencies is approximately 0 dB (reference pressure, 0.0002 dyne/cm²). A sound with an intensity 10 times greater would be 20 dB; one 100 times greater would be 40 dB.

According to this scale, speech has an intensity of about 65 dB. The main frequencies used in speech fall in the range of 300 to 3500 Hz. Sounds that exceed 100 dB can damage the peripheral auditory apparatus; those over 120 dB can cause pain. As people age, their ability to hear high frequencies declines, a condition called **presbycusis.**

■ *The Ear*

The peripheral auditory apparatus is the ear, which can be subdivided into the external ear, middle ear, and inner ear (Fig. 10-4).

External ear. The external ear includes the pinna, the external auditory meatus, and the auditory canal. The auditory canal contains glands that secrete **cerumen,** a waxy, protective substance. The pinna may help direct sounds into the auditory canal, at least in animals. The auditory canal transmits sound waves to the tympanic membrane. In humans, the auditory canal has a resonant frequency of about 3500 Hz and limits the frequencies that reach the tympanic membrane.

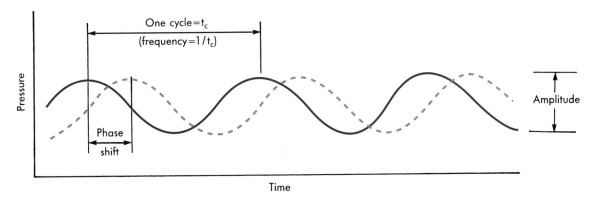

■ **Fig. 10-1** Two pure tones are shown by the solid and dashed lines. Frequency is determined from the wavelength as indicated. Amplitude is the peak-to-peak change in sound pressure. Both of the tones have the same frequency and amplitude, but they differ in phase.

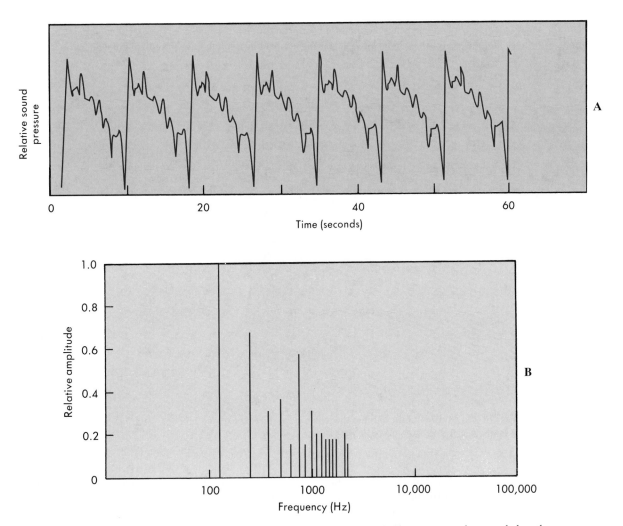

■ **Fig. 10-2** Fourier analysis of sound. **A,** A complex sound. The waves can be regarded as the sum of a number of pure tones. **B,** A Fourier spectrum indicating the component pure tones that make up the sound, as well as their relative strengths. (From Cornsweet TN: *Visual perception,* New York, 1970, Academic Press.)

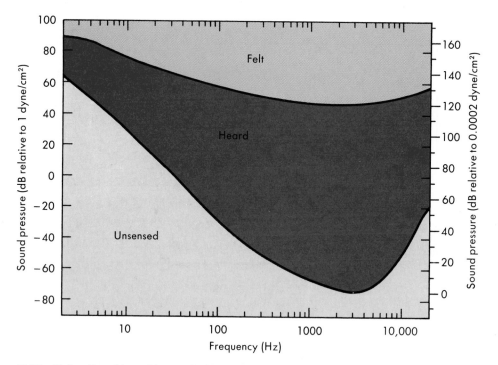

■ **Fig. 10-3**　Sound intensities required for hearing at different frequencies. The gray area is subthreshold for hearing. The dark-colored area is the normal range for audition. The light-colored area is the range at which sound is painful.

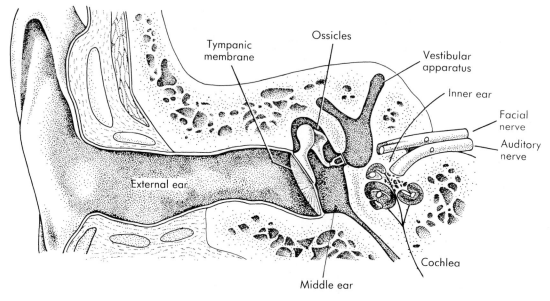

■ **Fig. 10-4**　Division of the ear into the external ear, middle ear, and inner ear. (Redrawn from von Bekesy G: *Sci Am* 197:66, 1957.)

Middle ear. The external ear is separated from the middle ear by the **tympanic membrane** (Fig. 10-5, *A*). The middle ear contains air. A chain of ossicles connects the tympanic membrane to the oval window, an opening into the inner ear. Adjacent to the oval window is the round window, another membrane-covered opening situated between the middle and inner ears (Fig. 10-

5, *B*). The ossicles include the **malleus,** the **incus,** and the **stapes.** The stapes has a footplate that inserts into the oval window. Beneath the oval window is a fluid-filled component of the **cochlea.** This component is called the **vestibule,** and it is continuous with a tubular structure known as the **scala vestibuli.** Inward movement of the tympanic membrane by a sound pressure

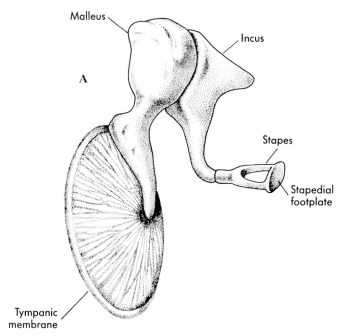

■ **Fig. 10-5**   **A,** Drawing of the tympanic membrane and the chain of ossicles. **B,** The way in which the movement of the stapedial footplate causes displacement of the round window because of fluid movements in the cochlea. (**A** redrawn from von Bekesy G: *Sci Am* 197:66, 1957; **B** redrawn from Kandel E, Schwartz JH: *Principles of neural science,* New York, 1981, Elsevier North-Holland.)

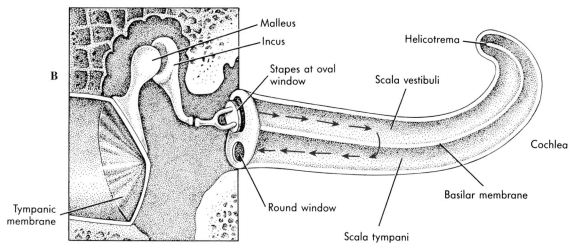

wave causes the chain of ossicles to push the footplate of the stapes into the oval window (Fig. 10-5, *B*). This movement of the stapes footplates in turn displaces the fluid within the scala vestibuli. The pressure wave that ensues within the fluid is transmitted through the **basilar membrane** of the cochlea to the **scala tympani** (see below) and causes the round window to bulge into the middle ear.

The tympanic membrane and the chain of ossicles serve as an impedance matching device. The ear must detect sound waves traveling in air, but the neural transduction mechanism depends on movements established in the fluid column within the cochlea. Thus, pressure waves in air must be converted into pressure waves in fluid. The acoustic impedance of water is much higher than that of air. Therefore, without a special device for impedance matching, most sound reaching the ear would simply be reflected. Impedance matching in the ear depends on (1) the ratio of the surface area of the tympanic membrane to that of the oval window and (2) the mechanical advantage of the lever system formed by the ossicle chain. The efficiency of the impedance match is sufficient to improve hearing by 10 to 20 dB.

The middle ear also serves other functions. Two muscles are found in the middle ear: the **tensor tympani** (supplied by the trigeminal nerve) and the **stapedius** (supplied by the facial nerve). These muscles attach, respectively, to the malleus and stapes. When they contract, they dampen movements of the ossicular chain and so decrease the sensitivity of the acoustic apparatus. This action can protect the acoustic apparatus against damaging sounds, such as vocalization, that can be anticipated. However, a sudden explosion can still damage the acoustic apparatus, because reflex contraction of the middle ear muscles does not occur quickly enough. The middle ear connects to the pharynx through the **eustachian tube.** Pressure differences between the external and middle ears are equalized through this passage. If fluid collects in the middle ear, such as during an infection, the eustachian tube may become blocked. The resultant pressure difference between the external and middle ears can produce pain by displacement of the tympanic membrane and, in extreme cases, by rupture of the tympanic membrane. Flying and diving can also cause pressure differences.

Inner ear. The inner ear includes the bony and membranous labyrinths. The cochlea and the vestibular apparatus are formed from these structures.

The cochlea is a spiral-shaped organ (Fig. 10-6). In humans, the spiral consists of $2^3/_4$ turns; it starts from a broad base and extends to a narrow apex. The cochlea forms from the rostral end of the bony and membranous labyrinths. The apex of the cochlea faces laterally (Fig. 10-6, *A*).

The bony labyrinth component of the cochlea includes several chambers. The space facing the oval window (Fig. 10-6, *B*) is called the vestibule. Continuous with the vestibule is the scala vestibuli, a spiral-shaped tube that extends to the apex of the cochlea. The scala vestibuli meets the scala tympani at the apex; they merge at the **helicotrema,** the connection between these two components of the bony labyrinth (Fig. 10-5). The scala tympani is another spiral-shaped tube that winds back down the cochlea to end at the round window (Figs. 10-5 and 10-6, *B*). The bony core of the cochlea around which the scalae turn is called the **modiolus.**

The membranous labyrinth component of the cochlea is the **scala media,** or **cochlear duct.** The cochlear duct is a membrane-bound spiral tube that extends 35 mm along the cochlea between the scala vestibuli and scala tympani. One wall of the scala media is formed by the basilar membrane, another by **Reissner's membrane,** and the third by the **stria vascularis** (Fig. 10-6, *C*).

The spaces within the cochlea are filled with fluid. The fluid in the scala vestibuli and scala tympani is **perilymph,** which closely resembles cerebrospinal fluid (CSF). The fluid in the scala media is **endolymph,** which differs considerably from CSF. Endolymph contains a high concentration of K^+ (about 145 mM) and a low concentration of Na^+ (about 2 mM); in this respect, it resembles intracellular fluid. Because endolymph has a positive potential (about +80 mV), a large potential gradient (about 140 mV) exists across the membranes of the hair cells found within the cochlea. (These hair cells, which are sensory receptors for sound, are discussed in more detail below.) Endolymph is secreted by the stria vascularis and is drained through the endolymphatic duct into the dural venous sinuses.

The neural apparatus responsible for transduction of sound is the **organ of Corti** (Fig. 10-6, *D*), which is located within the cochlear duct. It lies on the basilar membrane and consists of several components, including three rows of outer hair cells, a single row of inner hair cells, a gelatinous tectorial membrane, and a number of types of supporting cells. The organ of Corti in humans contains 15,000 outer and 3500 inner hair cells. A rigid scaffold is provided by the rods of Corti and the reticular lamina. Located at the apex of the hair cells are stereocilia, which can be described as nonmotile cilia. The stereocilia contact the tectorial membrane.

The organ of Corti is innervated by nerve fibers that belong to the cochlear division of the eighth cranial nerve. The 32,000 auditory afferent fibers in humans originate in sensory ganglion cells in the spiral ganglion, which is located within the modiolus. These nerve fibers penetrate the organ of Corti and terminate at the base of the hair cells (Figs. 10-6, *D*, and 10-7). Those going to the outer hair cells pass through the tunnel of Corti, an opening located below the rods of Corti.

About 90% of the fibers end on inner hair cells and the remainder on outer hair cells. Thus, in this arrangement several afferent fibers converge on each inner hair cell, whereas other afferent fibers diverge to supply many outer hair cells. In addition to afferent fibers, the organ of Corti is supplied by cochlear efferent fibers, which terminate on the outer hair cells and on the afferent fibers contacting the inner hair cells (Fig. 10-7). The cochlear efferent fibers originate in the superior olivary nucleus of the brainstem and are often called olivocochlear fibers. The efferent fibers that end on cochlear afferent fibers may be inhibitory and may help improve frequency discrimination.

The inner hair cells clearly provide most of the neural information about acoustic signals that the CNS uses for hearing. The function of the outer hair cells is less clear. The length of the outer hair cells is variable, suggesting that changes in outer hair cell length may affect the sensitivity or "tuning" of the inner hair cells. Cochlear efferent fibers may control outer hair cell length. Such a mechanism could conceivably influence the way the brain recognizes sound.

A common cause of deafness is the destruction of hair cells by loud sounds. Hair cells can be destroyed, for example, by exposure to industrial noise or by listening to high-intensity rock music. Typically, hair cells over certain parts of the cochlea are selectively damaged, and thus hearing may be lost over a discrete frequency range. Such a selective hearing loss can be diagnosed by **audiometry** (see below).

■ *Sound Transduction*

Sound waves are transduced by the organ of Corti in the following way. Sound waves that reach the ear cause the tympanic membrane to oscillate. These oscillations result

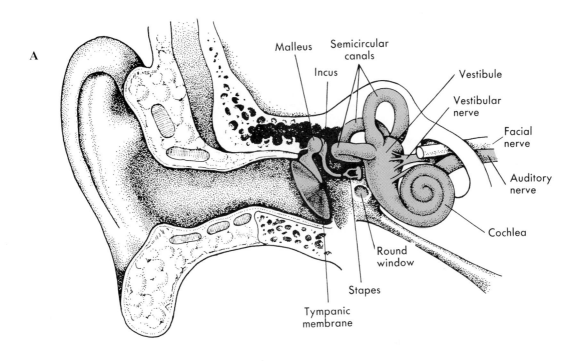

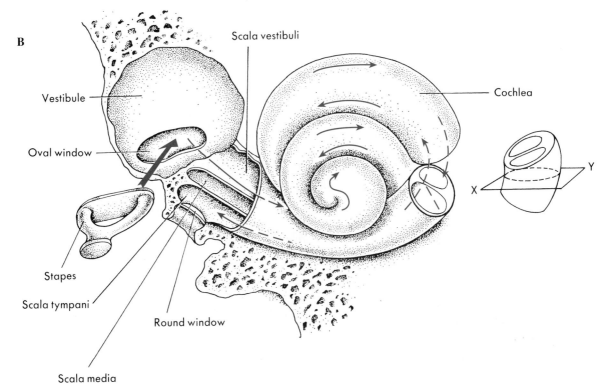

■ **Fig. 10-6**   Cochlear structure. **A,** The location of the right human cochlea in relation to the vestibular apparatus and middle and external ears. **B,** The relationships between the spaces within the cochlea. (**B** redrawn from Gulick WL: *Hearing: physiology and psychophysics,* New York, 1971, Oxford University Press; after Maloney.)

Continued

C

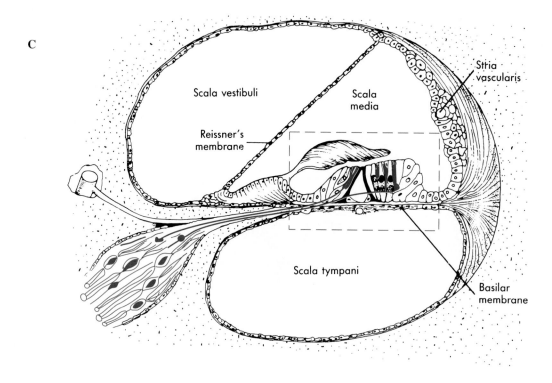

Scala vestibuli

Scala media

Stria vascularis

Reissner's membrane

Scala tympani

Basilar membrane

D

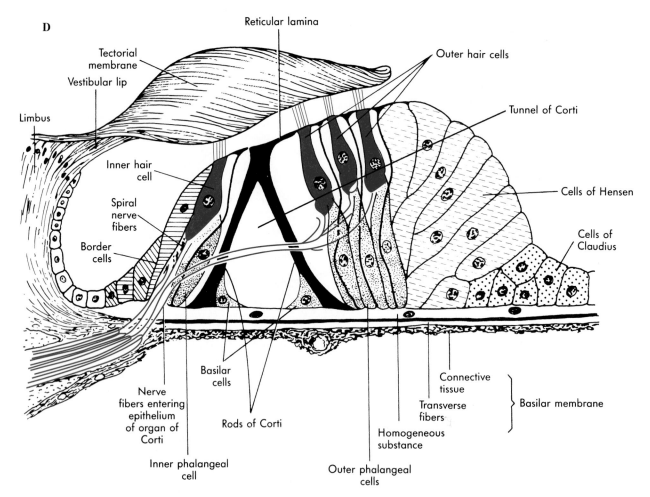

Reticular lamina

Tectorial membrane

Outer hair cells

Vestibular lip

Limbus

Tunnel of Corti

Inner hair cell

Cells of Hensen

Spiral nerve fibers

Cells of Claudius

Border cells

Nerve fibers entering epithelium of organ of Corti

Basilar cells

Rods of Corti

Inner phalangeal cell

Outer phalangeal cells

Homogeneous substance

Connective tissue

Transverse fibers

Basilar membrane

■ **Fig. 10-6, cont'd**   **C,** Drawing of a cross-section through the cochlea in the plane indicated by the inset to the right of **B. D,** Expanded view of the organ of Corti.

Inhibitory input from
ipsilateral VCN

Excitatory input from
contralateral VCN

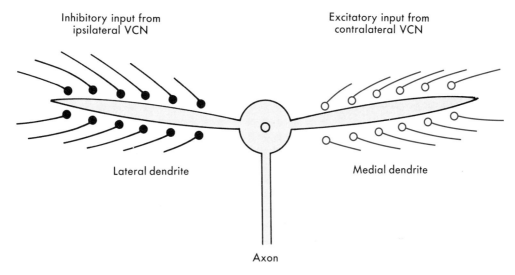

Lateral dendrite

Medial dendrite

Axon

■ **Fig. 10-13**   Diagram of the synaptic input to a neuron in the medial superior olivary nucleus. *VCN*, Ventral cochlear nucleus.

frequency modulation. Neurons in the primary auditory cortex form isofrequency columns (in which the neurons in the column have the same characteristic frequency) and alternating columns known as summation and suppression columns. Neurons in **summation columns** are more responsive to binaural than to monaural input. Neurons in **suppression columns** are less responsive to binaural than to monaural stimulation, and accordingly the response to one ear is dominant.

Bilateral lesions of the auditory cortex have little effect on the ability to distinguish the frequencies or intensity of different sounds, but the ability to localize sound and to understand speech is reduced. Unilateral lesions, however, have little effect, especially if the nondominant (for language) hemisphere is involved. Evidently, frequency discrimination depends on activity at lower levels of the auditory pathway, presumably the inferior colliculus.

■ *Deafness*

As already discussed, unilateral deafness is caused by damage to the peripheral auditory apparatus or to the cochlear nuclei, but not by CNS lesions. A discrete loss of hearing for particular frequencies can result from damage to a part of the organ of Corti (e.g., by exposure to intense sound, such as very loud rock music or industrial noise). The degree of deafness can be quantified for different frequencies by **audiometry.** In audiometry, each ear is presented with tones of dif-

ferent frequencies and intensities. An **audiogram** is plotted that shows the thresholds of each ear for representative frequencies of sound. Comparison with the audiogram of normal individuals shows the auditory deficit (in decibels). The pattern of deficit aids in the diagnosis of the cause of the hearing loss.

Two simple tests are often used clinically to distinguish the most important types of deafness, *conduction loss* and *sensorineural loss.* The **Weber test** is used to evaluate the presence of a conduction hearing loss. In this test, the base of a vibrating tuning fork is placed against the middle of the forehead and the subject is asked to localize the sound. Normally the sound is not localized to a particular ear. However, if the person has a conductive hearing loss (because of a punctured tympanic membrane, fluid in the middle ear, or loss of continuity of the ossicular chain), the sound is localized to the deaf ear because the sound is conducted to the cochlea through bone. Bone-conducted sound can activate the organ of Corti, although not as well as sound conducted normally through the tympanic membrane and ossicle chain. One reason why the sound in the Weber test is not localized to the normal ear may be that hearing in the normal ear is inhibited by the ambient sound level (**auditory masking).** In the Weber test the localization of sound to the ear deafened by a loss of the normal conduction mechanism can easily be demonstrated in normal subjects who are asked to place a finger in one ear to impair hearing in that ear. Conversely, in subjects with a sensorineural hearing loss (because of damage to the organ of Corti, cochlear nerve, or cochlear nuclei), sound is localized to the normal side. In the **Rinne test,** a vibrating tuning fork is placed against the mastoid process and the subject is asked to indicate when the sound dies out. The tuning fork is then held near the external auditory meatus. In normal subjects, the sound is again heard. If the conduction mechanism is damaged, the sound is not heard. Bone conduction in this case is better than air conduction. If the hearing loss is sensorineural, the sound is heard again.

■ *The Vestibular System*

The vestibular system detects angular and linear accelerations of the head. Signals from the vestibular system trigger head and eye movements to provide the retina with a stable visual image and to allow the body to make adjustments in posture to maintain balance. The following description of the vestibular system emphasizes the sensory aspects of vestibular function and introduces the central vestibular pathways. The role of the vestibular apparatus in motor control is discussed in Chapter 13.

■ *The Vestibular Apparatus*

Structure of the vestibular labyrinth. The vestibular apparatus, like the cochlea, consists of a component of the membranous labyrinth located within the bony labyrinth (Fig. 10-14). The vestibular apparatus on each side of the head is composed of three **semicircular ducts** and two **otolith organs**. These structures are surrounded by **perilymph** and contain **endolymph**. The semicircular ducts include the **horizontal, superior,** and **posterior ducts**. The otolith organs include the **utricle** and the **saccule**. A swelling called an **ampulla** is found on each semicircular duct. The semicircular ducts all connect with the utricle. The utricle joins the saccule through the **ductus reuniens**. The **endolymphatic duct** originates from the ductus reuniens and ends in the endolymphatic sac. The saccule has a connection with the cochlea through which endolymph produced by the stria vascularis of the cochlea can reach the vestibular apparatus.

The three semicircular ducts on one side of the head are matched with corresponding coplanar semicircular ducts on the other side. This arrangement allows the sensory epithelia in corresponding pairs of ducts on the two sides to sense movements of the head in all planes. Fig. 10-15 shows the orientation of the ducts on the two sides of the head; note that the cochlea is positioned rostrally to the vestibular apparatus and that the coil of the cochlea points laterally. The two horizontal ducts on each side of the head correspond, as do the superior ducts and the posterior ducts. An interesting feature of the horizontal ducts is that they are placed in the horizontal plane with respect to the horizon if the head is tilted down 30 degrees. The utricle is oriented nearly horizontally; the saccule is oriented vertically.

The ampulla of each of the semicircular ducts contains sensory epithelium. The sensory epithelium in a semicircular duct is called a **crista ampullaris** or **ampullary crest** (Fig. 10-16). An ampullary crest consists of a ridge in which vestibular hair cells are embedded. These hair cells are innervated by primary afferent fibers of the vestibular nerve, which is a subdivision of the eighth cranial nerve. Like cochlear cells, each vestibular hair cell contains a set of stereocilia on its apical surface. However, unlike cochlear hair cells, vestibular cells also contain a single **kinocilium**. The cilia on ampullary hair cells are embedded in a gelatinous structure called the **cupula**. The cupula crosses the ampulla and occludes its lumen completely. Movements of endolymph produced by angular accelerations of the head deflect the cupula and consequently bend the cilia on the hair cells. The cupula has the same specific gravity as the endolymph and thus is unaffected by linear acceleratory forces, such as that exerted by gravity.

The sensory epithelia of the otolith organs are called the **macula utriculi** and the **macula sacculi** (Fig. 10-17). Vestibular hair cells underlie each macula. As in the ampullary crests, the stereocilia and kinocilia of these hair cells are embedded in a gelatinous mass. However, the gelatinous mass in the macula contains numerous otoliths (small "stones") composed of calcium carbonate crystals. Together, the gelatinous mass and its otoliths are known as an **otolithic membrane.** The otoliths increase the specific gravity of the otolithic membrane to about twice that of the endolymph. Hence, the otolithic membrane tends to move when it is affected by a linear acceleration, such as that produced by gravity. Angular accelerations of the head do not affect the otolithic membranes, which do not protrude substantially into the lumen of the membranous labyrinth.

Innervation of sensory epithelia of vestibular apparatus. The cell bodies of the primary afferent fibers of the vestibular nerve are located in **Scarpa's ganglion.** As in the spiral ganglion, the neurons are bipolar, and their cell bodies, as well as axons, are myelinated. The vestibular nerve gives off separate branches to each of the sensory epithelia (Fig. 10-18). The vestibular nerve is accompanied by the cochlear and facial nerves in the internal auditory meatus of the skull.

Vestibular hair cells. Vestibular hair cells are of two types (Fig. 10-19). **Type I hair cells** are pear shaped, and they make synaptic contacts with chalice-like primary afferent terminals of vestibular afferent fibers. **Type II hair cells** are more rectangular, and they also synapse on vestibular afferent fibers. Vestibular efferent fibers synapse on the primary afferent fibers that synapse with type I hair cells. In contrast, the vestibular efferent fibers synapse directly on type II hair cells. These arrangements are similar to those of the cochlear afferent and efferent fibers on the inner and outer hair cells of the organ of Corti (Fig. 10-7). The efferent endings on type II hair cells may account for the tendency

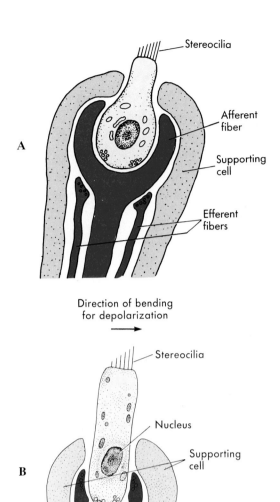

A

Direction of bending
for depolarization

B

Outer hair cell

■ **Fig. 10-7** Schematic drawing of inner **(A)** and outer **(B)** hair cell. The hair bundles extend into the tectorial membrane *(not shown)*. Efferent fibers *(light color)* from the olivocochlear bundle synapse on afferent fibers *(dark color)* that supply the inner hair cells **(A),** and they synapse directly on outer hair cells **(B).** Note that the hair bundles become gradually longer from left to right, which sets up an axis of polarization *(arrow).* Bending of the hairs in this direction depolarizes the hair cell; bending in the opposite direction hyperpolarizes the cell.

in fluid movements within the scala vestibuli and scala tympani (Fig. 10-5). Part of the hydraulic energy of these fluid movements is used to displace the basilar membrane, and with it the organ of Corti (Fig. 10-8). Owing to the shear forces set up by the relative displacements of the basilar membrane and the tectorial membrane, the stereocilia of the hair cells bend. When the stereocilia of a hair cell move toward the tallest cilium, the hair cell is depolarized; when the stereocilia bend in the opposite direction, the hair cell is hyperpolarized.

These changes in the membrane potential of the hair cells result from changes in cation conductance in membranes at the apical ends of the hair cells. The potential gradient that affects ion movement into the hair cells includes both the resting potential of the hair cells and the positive potential of the endolymph. As noted previously, the total gradient across the membrane of the hair cells is about 140 mV. *A change in membrane conductance in the apical membranes of the hair cells therefore results in a large current flow, which produces the receptor potential in these cells. This current flow can be recorded extracellularly as the* **cochlear microphonic potential,** *an oscillatory event that has the same frequency as the acoustic stimulus. The cochlear microphonic potential actually represents the sum of the receptor potentials of a number of hair cells.*

Hair cells, like retinal photoreceptors, release an excitatory neurotransmitter (probably glutamate or aspartate) when depolarized. The transmitter produces a generator potential, which excites the cochlear afferent nerve fibers with which the hair cell synapses. In summary, sound is transduced when oscillatory movements of the basilar membrane cause intermittent discharges of cochlear afferent nerve fibers. The activity of a large number of cochlear afferent fibers can be recorded extracellularly as a compound action potential.

However, most cochlear afferent fibers do *not* discharge in response to a particular sound frequency. One factor that influences which afferent fiber discharges is its location along the organ of Corti. The location of an afferent fiber is important because a given sound frequency causes different displacements of the basilar membrane at different locations along the organ of Corti (Fig. 10-9), in part because the width and tension along the basilar membrane differ. On the basis of these differences in width and tension, researchers originally concluded that different parts of the basilar membrane have different resonance frequencies. For example, the basilar membrane is about 100 μm wide at the base and 500 μm wide at the apex. It also has a higher tension at the base. Thus, the base was predicted to vibrate at higher frequencies than the apex, as do the shorter strings of musical instruments. However, experiments have shown that the basilar membrane moves as a whole in traveling waves (Fig. 10-9). Movements of the basilar membrane are maximal nearer the base of the cochlea at high-frequency tones and maximal nearer the apex at low-frequency tones. In effect, *the basilar membrane serves as a frequency analyzer; it distributes the stimulus along the organ of Corti so that different hair cells respond to different frequencies of sound. This observation forms the basis of the* **place theory** *of hearing.* In addition, hair cells located at different places along the organ of Corti are tuned to different frequencies because of differences in their stereocilia and in their biophysical properties. Because of these factors, the basilar membrane and organ of Corti have a so-called tonotopic map (Fig. 10-10).

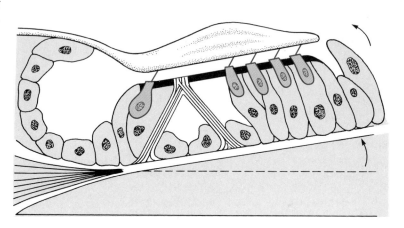

■ **Fig. 10-8**   A demonstration of how a movement of the basilar membrane will cause the stereocilia to bend because of shear forces produced by the relative displacement of the hair cells and the tectorial membrane.

Reticular lamina   Tectorial membrane

Basilar membrane

Rods of Corti   Hair cells

■ *Cochlear Nerve Fibers*

The activity of hair cells in the organ of Corti causes the primary afferent fibers traveling in the cochlear nerve to discharge. The cell bodies of these nerve fibers are located in the spiral ganglion; the peripheral processes end on hair cells, and the central processes terminate in the cochlear nuclei of the brainstem. Unlike most other primary afferent neurons, those of the eighth cranial nerve are bipolar cells. A myelin sheath surrounds both the cell bodies and the axons of these neurons.

Characteristic frequencies. A cochlear afferent fiber discharges maximally when stimulated by a particular sound frequency, called the **characteristic frequency** of that fiber. The characteristic frequency can be determined from a tuning curve for the fiber (Fig. 10-11). A **tuning curve** plots the threshold for activation of the nerve fiber by different sound frequencies. Typically, tuning curves are sharp near threshold but broad at high sound pressure levels. Both excitatory and inhibitory areas can be included in a tuning curve (Fig. 10-11, *A*). The sharpness of some tuning curves may reflect inhibitory processes.

Encoding. *The different features of an acoustic stimulus are encoded in the discharges of cochlear nerve fibers. Duration is signaled by the duration of neural activity; intensity is signaled both by the amount of neural activity and by the number of fibers that discharge.* For low-frequency sounds (up to 4000 Hz), the frequency is signaled by the tendency of an afferent fiber to discharge in phase with the stimulus (**phase locking**). Phase locking can occur for sounds with periods shorter than the absolutely refractory period, which limits neural discharges to rates lower than about 500 Hz. Therefore, if the tone is more than 500 Hz, a given fiber cannot discharge during each cycle. However, frequency information can be detected by the CNS from the activity of a population of afferent fibers, each of which discharges in phase with the stimulus. This observation forms the **frequency theory** of hearing. For high-frequency sounds, the place theory applies. The CNS interprets sounds that activate afferent fibers that supply hair cells near the base of the cochlea as being of high frequency. Thus, both the place and the frequency theories are required to explain the frequency coding of sound (**duplex theory**).

An important, although relatively uncommon, condition that can interrupt the function of cochlear nerve fibers is an **acoustic neurinoma,** a tumor of the Schwann cells of the eighth nerve. As the tumor

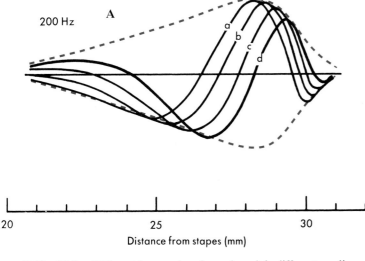

200 Hz

A

a
b
c
d

20   25   30

Distance from stapes (mm)

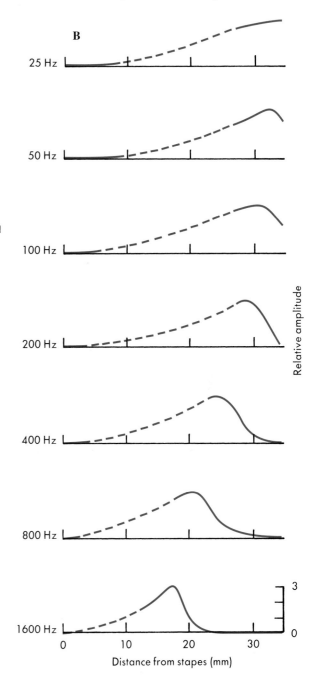

B

25 Hz

50 Hz

100 Hz

200 Hz

400 Hz

800 Hz

1600 Hz

Relative amplitude

3

0

0   10   20   30

Distance from stapes (mm)

■ **Fig. 10-9** Different frequencies of sound result in different amplitudes of displacement of the basilar membrane at different sites along the organ of Corti. **A,** A traveling wave produced in the basilar membrane by a sound of 200 Hz. The curves at *a, b, c,* and *d* represent the displacements of the basilar membrane at different times, and the dashed line is the envelope formed by the peaks of the wave at different times. The maximal deflection occurs at about 29 mm from the oval window. **B,** The envelopes of traveling waves produced by several frequencies of sound. Note that the maximal displacement varies with frequency and is closest to the oval window when the frequency is highest. (Redrawn from von Bekesy G: *Experiments in hearing,* New York, 1960, McGraw-Hill.)

grows, irritation of cochlear nerve fibers may cause a ringing sound in the affected ear **(tinnitus).** Eventually, conduction in the cochlear nerve fibers is blocked and the ear becomes deaf. The tumor may be operable while still small; therefore, early diagnosis is important. If the tumor is allowed to enlarge substantially, it can not only interrupt the entire eighth nerve and cause vestibular as well as auditory difficulties, but can also impinge on or distort neighboring cranial nerves (e.g., V, VII, IX, X) and produce cerebellar signs by compressing the cerebellar peduncles.

■ *Central Auditory Pathway*

The cochlear afferent fibers synapse in the most rostral part of the medulla on neurons of the dorsal and ventral cochlear nuclei (Fig. 10-12). These neurons give rise to axons that contribute to the central auditory pathways. Some of the axons cross to the contralateral side and ascend in the lateral lemniscus, the main ascending audi-

tory tract. Others connect with the ipsilateral or contralateral superior olivary nuclei. The superior olivary nuclei project through the ipsilateral and contralateral lateral lemnisci. Many of the auditory fibers cross in the trapezoid body, although some cross in the pontine tegmentum. The lateral lemniscus ends in the inferior colliculus. The two inferior colliculi are interconnected through the commissure of the inferior colliculus. Axons from neurons of the inferior colliculus ascend through the brachium of the inferior colliculus to terminate in the medial geniculate nucleus of the thalamus. The medial

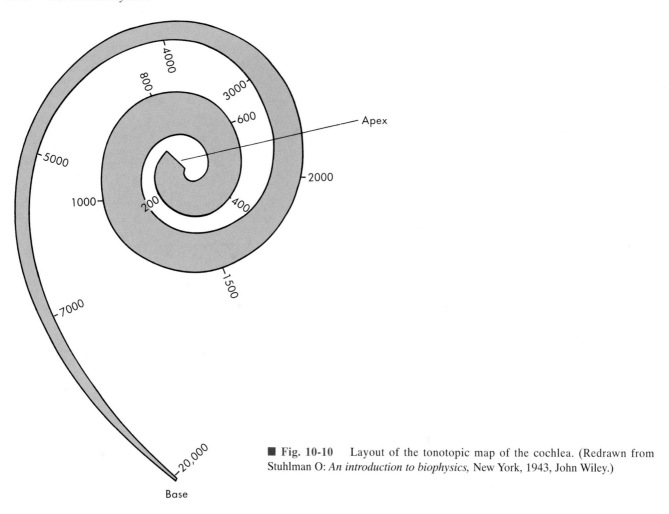

Apex

Base

■ **Fig. 10-10** Layout of the tonotopic map of the cochlea. (Redrawn from Stuhlman O: *An introduction to biophysics,* New York, 1943, John Wiley.)

geniculate nucleus gives rise to the auditory radiation, which ends in the auditory cortex, located in the transverse temporal gyrus in the temporal lobe. Projections from the auditory cortex also descend to the medial geniculate nucleus and inferior colliculus, and projections from the inferior colliculus descend to the superior olivary complex and cochlear nuclei.

A mixture of ascending auditory system fibers represents both ears at the level of the lateral lemniscus. Thus, the representation of auditory space is complex even at the brainstem level. Consequently, unilateral deafness may occur as a result of isolated lesions of the cochlear nuclei or more peripheral structures. Central lesions do not cause unilateral deafness, although they may interfere with sound localization or discrimination of tones.

Fig. 10-12 shows the distinction between core and belt regions of the inferior colliculus, medial geniculate nucleus, and auditory cortex. The **core regions** include the central nucleus of the inferior colliculus, the laminated part of the medial geniculate nucleus, and the primary auditory cortex (AI). The **belt regions** include the pericentral nucleus of the inferior colliculus; the nonlam-

inated ventral, dorsal, and magnocellular divisions of the medial geniculate nucleus; and nonprimary parts of the auditory cortex. The core regions may represent a more recently evolved component of the auditory system and may be responsible for frequency representation. The belt regions, on the other hand, receive not only auditory input but also a convergent input from the visual and somatosensory systems. Hence, the belt system may be involved in activities, such as speech, that require integration across several modalities.

■ *Functional Organization of the Central Auditory System*

Receptive fields and tonotopic maps. The responses of neurons in several structures that belong to the auditory system can be described by tuning curves (Fig. 10-11, *B*). By plotting the distribution of the characteristic frequencies of neurons within a nucleus or in the auditory cortex, a tonotopic map is revealed. Tonotopic maps have been found in the cochlear nuclei, superior olivary complex, inferior colliculus, medial geniculate nucleus, and auditory cortex. A given auditory structure may in fact contain several tonotopic maps.

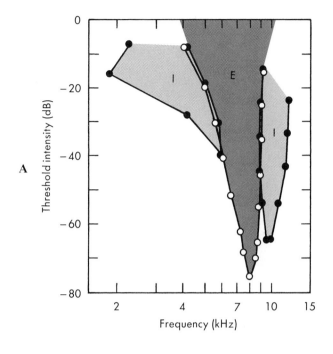

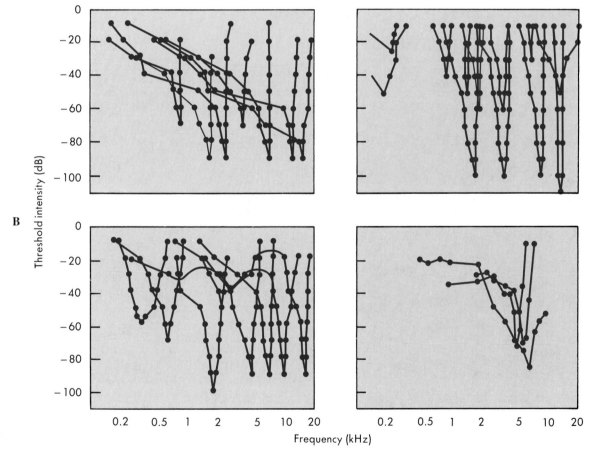

■ **Fig. 10-11** Tuning curves of neurons in the auditory system. Tuning curves can be considered as receptive field plots. **A,** A tuning curve with excitatory *(E)* and inhibitory *(I)* regions. **B,** Tuning curves for cochlear nerve fibers *(upper left),* neurons in the inferior colliculus *(upper right),* trapezoid body *(lower left),* and medial geniculate nucleus *(lower right).* (**A** redrawn from Arthur RM et al: *J Physiol (Lond)* 212:593, 1971; **B** redrawn from Katsui Y. In Rosenblith WA, editor: *Sensory communication,* Cambridge, Mass, 1961, MIT Press.)

Binaural interactions. Most auditory neurons at levels above the cochlear nuclei respond to stimulation of either ear (i.e., they have **binaural receptive fields**). Binaural receptive fields contribute to sound localization. A human can distinguish sounds originating from sources separated by as small an angle as 1 degree. *The auditory system uses certain clues to judge the origin of sounds. These clues include differences in the time (or phase) of sound arrival at the two ears and differences in sound intensity on the two sides of the head.*

These factors provide information about the location of a sound by influencing the activity of neurons in the

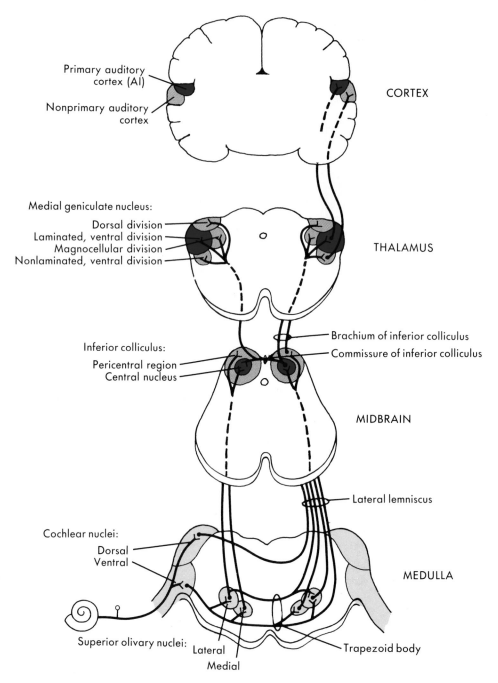

Primary auditory cortex (AI)
Nonprimary auditory cortex

CORTEX

Medial geniculate nucleus:
Dorsal division
Laminated, ventral division
Magnocellular division
Nonlaminated, ventral division

THALAMUS

Brachium of inferior colliculus
Commissure of inferior colliculus

Inferior colliculus:
Pericentral region
Central nucleus

MIDBRAIN

Lateral lemniscus

Cochlear nuclei:
Dorsal
Ventral

MEDULLA

Superior olivary nuclei: **Lateral**
Medial

Trapezoid body

■ **Fig. 10-12**   Central auditory pathway. Subdivision into core *(darker color)* and belt *(lighter color)* regions is shown for the inferior colliculus, medial geniculate nucleus, and auditory cortex.

superior olivary complex. For example, neurons in the medial superior olivary nucleus have medial and lateral dendrites. The synapses on the medial dendrites are largely excitatory and originate from the contralateral ventral cochlear nucleus (Fig. 10-13). Those on the lateral dendrites are mostly inhibitory and come from the ipsilateral ventral cochlear nucleus. Differences in the phase of the sound reaching the two ears affect the strength and timing of the excitation and inhibition reaching a particular medial olivary neuron. The activity of

that neuron can then provide information about sound localization. The lateral superior olivary nucleus uses differences in sound intensity reaching the two ears to provide information about the source of the sound.

Cortical organization. Serial features of the primary auditory cortex resemble those of other primary sensory-receiving areas. Not only are sensory maps, in this case tonotopic maps, present in the auditory cortex, but this cortical region also performs feature extractions. For example, some neurons are selective for the direction of

Inhibitory input from
ipsilateral VCN

Excitatory input from
contralateral VCN

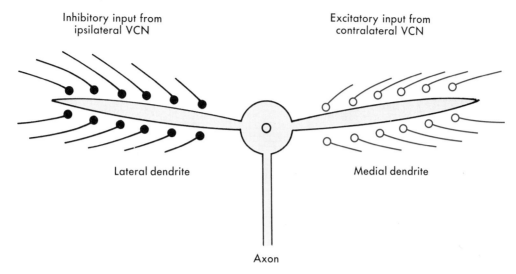

Lateral dendrite

Medial dendrite

Axon

■ **Fig. 10-13** Diagram of the synaptic input to a neuron in the medial superior olivary nucleus. *VCN,* Ventral cochlear nucleus.

frequency modulation. Neurons in the primary auditory cortex form isofrequency columns (in which the neurons in the column have the same characteristic frequency) and alternating columns known as summation and suppression columns. Neurons in **summation columns** are more responsive to binaural than to monaural input. Neurons in **suppression columns** are less responsive to binaural than to monaural stimulation, and accordingly the response to one ear is dominant.

Bilateral lesions of the auditory cortex have little effect on the ability to distinguish the frequencies or intensity of different sounds, but the ability to localize sound and to understand speech is reduced. Unilateral lesions, however, have little effect, especially if the nondominant (for language) hemisphere is involved. Evidently, frequency discrimination depends on activity at lower levels of the auditory pathway, presumably the inferior colliculus.

■ *Deafness*

As already discussed, unilateral deafness is caused by damage to the peripheral auditory apparatus or to the cochlear nuclei, but not by CNS lesions. A discrete loss of hearing for particular frequencies can result from damage to a part of the organ of Corti (e.g., by exposure to intense sound, such as very loud rock music or industrial noise). The degree of deafness can be quantified for different frequencies by **audiometry.** In audiometry, each ear is presented with tones of dif-

ferent frequencies and intensities. An **audiogram** is plotted that shows the thresholds of each ear for representative frequencies of sound. Comparison with the audiogram of normal individuals shows the auditory deficit (in decibels). The pattern of deficit aids in the diagnosis of the cause of the hearing loss.

Two simple tests are often used clinically to distinguish the most important types of deafness, *conduction loss* and *sensorineural loss.* The **Weber test** is used to evaluate the presence of a conduction hearing loss. In this test, the base of a vibrating tuning fork is placed against the middle of the forehead and the subject is asked to localize the sound. Normally the sound is not localized to a particular ear. However, if the person has a conductive hearing loss (because of a punctured tympanic membrane, fluid in the middle ear, or loss of continuity of the ossicular chain), the sound is localized to the deaf ear because the sound is conducted to the cochlea through bone. Bone-conducted sound can activate the organ of Corti, although not as well as sound conducted normally through the tympanic membrane and ossicle chain. One reason why the sound in the Weber test is not localized to the normal ear may be that hearing in the normal ear is inhibited by the ambient sound level (**auditory masking**). In the Weber test the localization of sound to the ear deafened by a loss of the normal conduction mechanism can easily be demonstrated in normal subjects who are asked to place a finger in one ear to impair hearing in that ear. Conversely, in subjects with a sensorineural hearing loss (because of damage to the organ of Corti, cochlear nerve, or cochlear nuclei), sound is localized to the normal side. In the **Rinne test,** a vibrating tuning fork is placed against the mastoid process and the subject is asked to indicate when the sound dies out. The tuning fork is then held near the external auditory meatus. In normal subjects, the sound is again heard. If the conduction mechanism is damaged, the sound is not heard. Bone conduction in this case is better than air conduction. If the hearing loss is sensorineural, the sound is heard again.

■ *The Vestibular System*

The vestibular system detects angular and linear accelerations of the head. Signals from the vestibular system trigger head and eye movements to provide the retina with a stable visual image and to allow the body to make adjustments in posture to maintain balance. The following description of the vestibular system emphasizes the sensory aspects of vestibular function and introduces the central vestibular pathways. The role of the vestibular apparatus in motor control is discussed in Chapter 13.

■ *The Vestibular Apparatus*

Structure of the vestibular labyrinth. The vestibular apparatus, like the cochlea, consists of a component of the membranous labyrinth located within the bony labyrinth (Fig. 10-14). The vestibular apparatus on each side of the head is composed of three **semicircular ducts** and two **otolith organs.** These structures are surrounded by **perilymph** and contain **endolymph.** The semicircular ducts include the **horizontal, superior,** and **posterior ducts.** The otolith organs include the **utricle** and the **saccule.** A swelling called an **ampulla** is found on each semicircular duct. The semicircular ducts all connect with the utricle. The utricle joins the saccule through the **ductus reuniens.** The **endolymphatic duct** originates from the ductus reuniens and ends in the endolymphatic sac. The saccule has a connection with the cochlea through which endolymph produced by the stria vascularis of the cochlea can reach the vestibular apparatus.

The three semicircular ducts on one side of the head are matched with corresponding coplanar semicircular ducts on the other side. This arrangement allows the sensory epithelia in corresponding pairs of ducts on the two sides to sense movements of the head in all planes. Fig. 10-15 shows the orientation of the ducts on the two sides of the head; note that the cochlea is positioned rostrally to the vestibular apparatus and that the coil of the cochlea points laterally. The two horizontal ducts on each side of the head correspond, as do the superior ducts and the posterior ducts. An interesting feature of the horizontal ducts is that they are placed in the horizontal plane with respect to the horizon if the head is tilted down 30 degrees. The utricle is oriented nearly horizontally; the saccule is oriented vertically.

The ampulla of each of the semicircular ducts contains sensory epithelium. The sensory epithelium in a semicircular duct is called a **crista ampullaris** or **ampullary crest** (Fig. 10-16). An ampullary crest consists of a ridge in which vestibular hair cells are embedded. These hair cells are innervated by primary afferent fibers of the vestibular nerve, which is a subdivision of the eighth cranial nerve. Like cochlear cells, each vestibular hair cell contains a set of stereocilia on its apical surface. However, unlike cochlear hair cells, vestibular cells also contain a single **kinocilium.** The cilia on ampullary hair cells are embedded in a gelatinous structure called the **cupula.** The cupula crosses the ampulla and occludes its lumen completely. Movements of endolymph produced by angular accelerations of the head deflect the cupula and consequently bend the cilia on the hair cells. The cupula has the same specific gravity as the endolymph and thus is unaffected by linear acceleratory forces, such as that exerted by gravity.

The sensory epithelia of the otolith organs are called the **macula utriculi** and the **macula sacculi** (Fig. 10-17). Vestibular hair cells underlie each macula. As in the ampullary crests, the stereocilia and kinocilia of these hair cells are embedded in a gelatinous mass. However, the gelatinous mass in the macula contains numerous otoliths (small "stones") composed of calcium carbonate crystals. Together, the gelatinous mass and its otoliths are known as an **otolithic membrane.** The otoliths increase the specific gravity of the otolithic membrane to about twice that of the endolymph. Hence, the otolithic membrane tends to move when it is affected by a linear acceleration, such as that produced by gravity. Angular accelerations of the head do not affect the otolithic membranes, which do not protrude substantially into the lumen of the membranous labyrinth.

Innervation of sensory epithelia of vestibular apparatus. The cell bodies of the primary afferent fibers of the vestibular nerve are located in **Scarpa's ganglion.** As in the spiral ganglion, the neurons are bipolar, and their cell bodies, as well as axons, are myelinated. The vestibular nerve gives off separate branches to each of the sensory epithelia (Fig. 10-18). The vestibular nerve is accompanied by the cochlear and facial nerves in the internal auditory meatus of the skull.

Vestibular hair cells. Vestibular hair cells are of two types (Fig. 10-19). **Type I hair cells** are pear shaped, and they make synaptic contacts with chalice-like primary afferent terminals of vestibular afferent fibers. **Type II hair cells** are more rectangular, and they also synapse on vestibular afferent fibers. Vestibular efferent fibers synapse on the primary afferent fibers that synapse with type I hair cells. In contrast, the vestibular efferent fibers synapse directly on type II hair cells. These arrangements are similar to those of the cochlear afferent and efferent fibers on the inner and outer hair cells of the organ of Corti (Fig. 10-7). The efferent endings on type II hair cells may account for the tendency

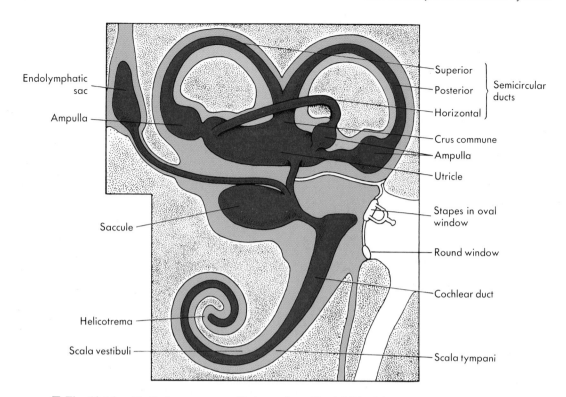

■ **Fig. 10-14** Vestibular apparatus. (Redrawn from Kandel ER, Schwartz JH: *Principles of neural science,* New York, 1981, Elsevier North-Holland.)

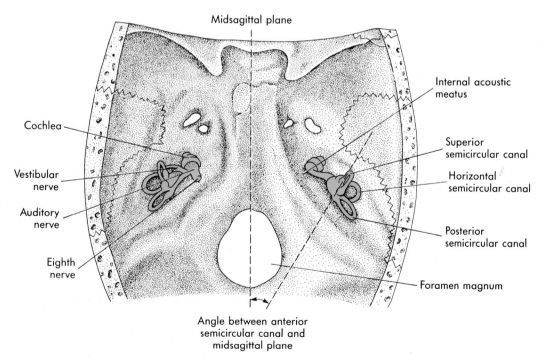

■ **Fig. 10-15** View of the base of the skull showing the orientation of structures of the inner ear. Coplanar pairs of semicircular ducts include the horizontal ducts, as well as the superior and contralateral posterior ducts. (Redrawn from Kandel ER, Schwartz JH: *Principles of neural science,* New York, 1981, Elsevier North-Holland.)

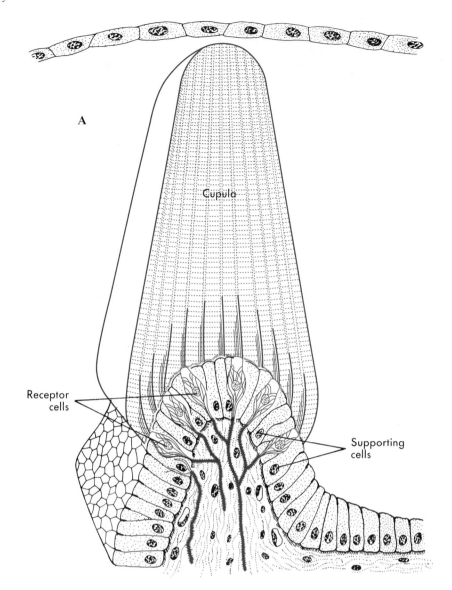

A

Cupula

Receptor cells

Supporting cells

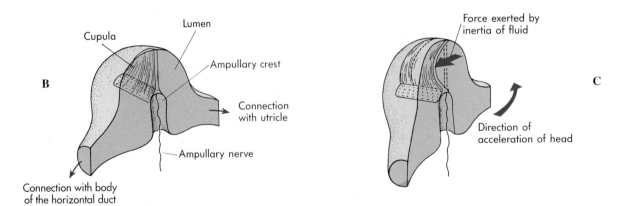

B

Cupula

Lumen

Ampullary crest

Connection with utricle

Ampullary nerve

Connection with body of the horizontal duct

C

Force exerted by inertia of fluid

Direction of acceleration of head

■ **Fig. 10-16** **A,** Drawing of an ampullary crest. The stereocilia and the kinocilium of each hair cell extend into the cupula. **B** and **C** show the distortion of the cupula that is produced when the head is rotated; **B** is before and **C** is during head rotation. (**A** redrawn from Wersäll J: *Acta Otolaryngol (Stockh)* suppl 162:1, 1956; **B** and **C** redrawn from Kandel ER, Schwartz JH, Jessell TM: *Principles of neural science,* ed 3, New York, 1991, Elsevier.)

■ **Fig. 10-17** Structure of the otolith organs. The saccule is shown in **A** and the utricle in **B.** (Redrawn from Lindeman HH: *Adv Otorhinolaryngol* 20:405, 1973.)

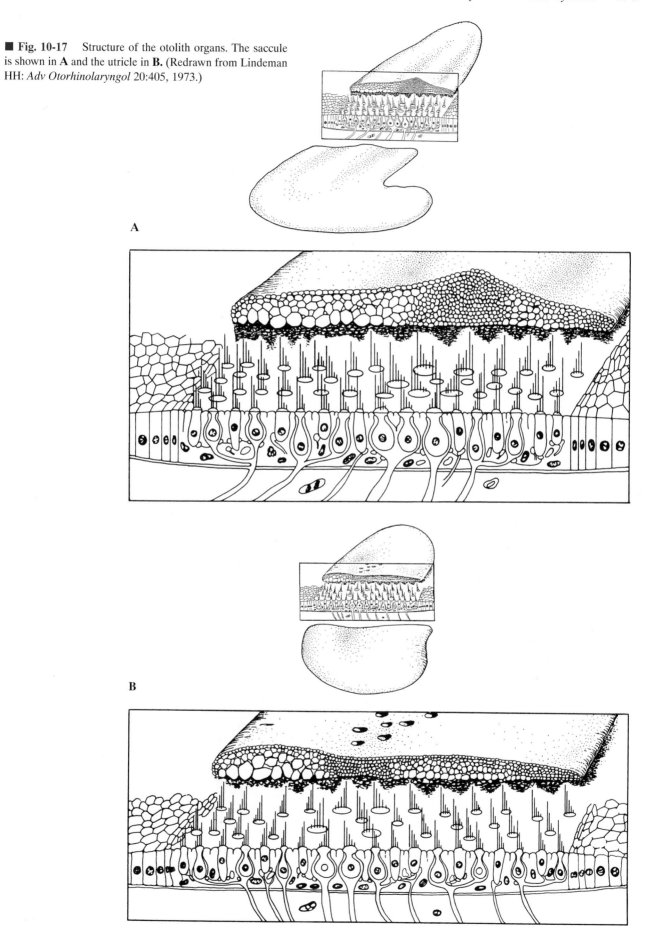

of the afferent fibers that receive synapses from these cells to discharge irregularly.

Vestibular transduction. Like cochlear hair cells, vestibular hair cells are functionally polarized. When the stereocilia are bent toward the longest cilium (in this case, the kinocilium), the conductance of the apical membrane increases for cations and the vestibular hair cell is depolarized (Fig. 10-20). Conversely, when the cilia are bent away from the kinocilium, the hair cell is hyperpolarized. The hair cell releases an excitatory neurotransmitter (either glutamate or aspartate) tonically, so that the afferent fiber on which it synapses has a resting discharge. When the hair cell is depolarized, more transmitter is released, and the discharge rate of the afferent fiber increases. Conversely, when the hair cell is hyperpolarized, less transmitter is released, and the firing rate of the afferent fiber slows or stops.

Semicircular ducts. So far, we have seen how the hair cells in the ampulla are triggered by movements of the head to sense sensory information for the brain. Actually, the movement of the cilia on the hair cells of the ampullary crests of the semicircular ducts, caused by angular accelerations of the head, triggers the hair cells and alters the release of neurotransmitter. These accelerations produce relative movements of the endolymph.

The inertia of the endolymph causes it to shift in relation to the fixed wall of the membranous labyrinth. This shift distorts the cupula and causes the cilia to bend. All the cilia in a given ampullary crest are oriented in the same direction. In the horizontal duct, the cilia are oriented toward the utricle; in the other ampulla, they are oriented away from the utricle.

The way in which an angular acceleration of the head affects the discharges of vestibular afferent fibers can be illustrated by the activity that originates from the horizontal ducts. Fig. 10-21 shows the horizontal ducts and utricle as seen from above. The hair cells in these ducts are polarized toward the utricle. Thus, movement of the cilia toward the utricle increases the discharge rates of the afferent fibers, whereas movement of the cilia away from the utricle reduces the discharge rate. In Fig. 10-21, the head is rotated to the left. This left-directed rotation causes the endolymph in the horizontal ducts to move to the right. This movement of endolymph bends the cilia on the hair cells of the ampulla of the left horizontal duct toward the utricle and those of the right duct away from the utricle. These effects on the cilia increase the firing rate in horizontal duct afferent fibers on the left and decrease the firing rate on the right.

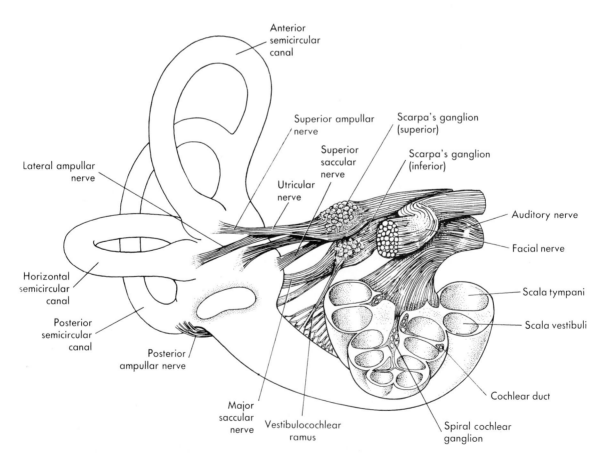

■ **Fig. 10-18** Innervation of the membranous labyrinth. (Redrawn from Best CH, Taylor NB: *Physiological basis of medical practice*, Baltimore, 1966, Williams & Wilkins.)

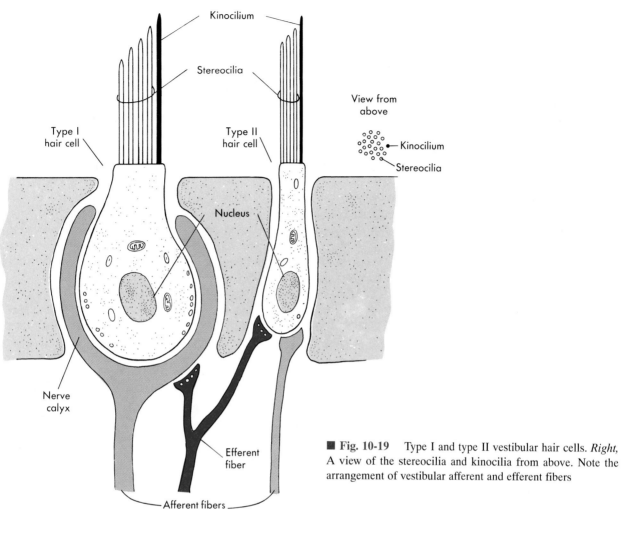

■ **Fig. 10-19** Type I and type II vestibular hair cells. *Right,* A view of the stereocilia and kinocilia from above. Note the arrangement of vestibular afferent and efferent fibers

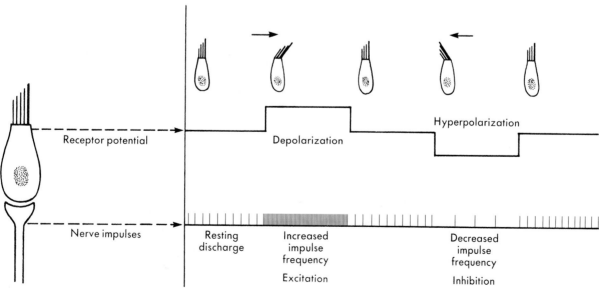

■ **Fig. 10-20** Functional polarization of vestibular hair cells. When the stereocilia are bent toward the kinocilium, the hair cell is depolarized and the afferent fiber is excited. When the stereocilia are bent away from the kinocilium, the hair cell is hyperpolarized and the afferent discharge slows or stops. (Redrawn from Kandel ER, Schwartz JH: *Principles of neural science,* New York, 1981, Elsevier North-Holland.)

Irritation of the vestibular labyrinth, as in **Meniere's disease,** can result in rhythmic conjugate deviations of the eyes, followed by quick return **saccades.** This condition is known as **nystagmus** (see Chapter 13). These eye movements are accompanied by a sense of **vertigo** and often **nausea.** The brain interprets a difference in input from the two vestibular systems in terms of head motion. Irritation (or destruction) of one labyrinth produces an asymmetry of input that results in the abnormal eye movements and associated psychological effects.

Otolith organs. The hair cells in the otolith organs, unlike those in the ampullary crests, are not all oriented in the same direction. Instead, they are oriented with respect to a ridge, called the **striola,** along the otolith organ (Fig. 10-22). In the utricle the hair cells on either side of the striola are polarized toward the striola, whereas in the saccule they are polarized away from the striola. Because the striola in each otolith organ is curved, the hair cells have diverse orientations. When the head is tilted so that gravity produces a different linear acceleration, the otolithic membranes shift and the

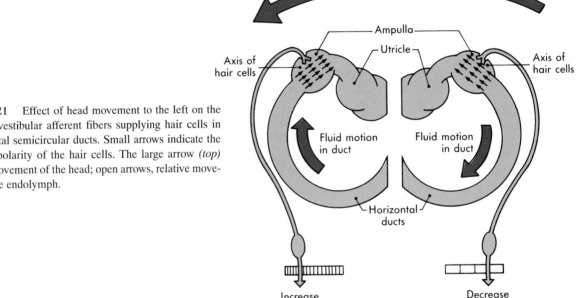

■ **Fig. 10-21** Effect of head movement to the left on the activity of vestibular afferent fibers supplying hair cells in the horizontal semicircular ducts. Small arrows indicate the functional polarity of the hair cells. The large arrow *(top)* indicates movement of the head; open arrows, relative movements of the endolymph.

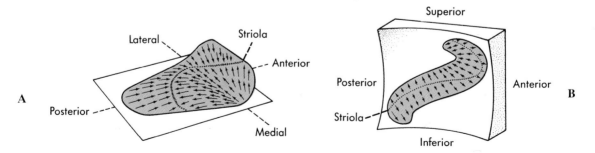

■ **Fig. 10-22** Functional polarization of hair cells in the otolith organs. **A,** The utricle. **B,** The saccule. The striola in each case is indicated by the dotted line. (Redrawn from Spoendlin HH. In Wolfson RJ, editor: *The vestibular system and its diseases,* Philadelphia, 1966, University of Pennsylvania Press.)

cilia of the hair cells bend in a new way. This bending of the hair cells changes the pattern of input from the otolith organs to the CNS. Similarly, a linear acceleration caused by other forces, such as might occur in a space launch or a free fall, will change the output from the otolith organs.

Central Vestibular Pathways

The vestibular afferent fibers project to the brainstem through the vestibular nerve. As mentioned earlier, the cell bodies of these afferent fibers are located in Scarpa's ganglion. The afferent fibers terminate in the vestibular nuclei, which are located in the rostral medulla and caudal pons (Fig. 10-23). The vestibular nuclei include the superior, lateral, medial, and inferior vestibular nuclei. Ampullary afferent fibers end preferentially in the superior, lateral, and medial vestibular nuclei, whereas otolithic afferent fibers end preferentially in the lateral and inferior nuclei. The afferent fibers also give off collaterals to the cerebel-

lum (Fig. 10-23, *right, upward-directed arrows*).

The vestibular nuclei give rise to a variety of projections, some of which are illustrated in Fig. 10-23, *left.* The superior and medial vestibular nuclei project through the medial longitudinal fasciculus to the oculomotor nuclei. Therefore, it is not surprising that the vestibular nuclei exert a powerful control over eye movements (the vestibulo-ocular reflex). The lateral and medial vestibular nuclei give rise to the lateral and medial vestibulospinal tracts. These pathways provide, respectively, for the activation of postural and neck muscles and thereby contribute to balance and to head movements (vestibulocollic reflex). Vestibular nuclei also project to the cerebellum, the reticular formation, and the contralateral vestibular complex (Fig. 10-23, *arrows extending leftward*), as well as to the thalamus. The latter mediate conscious sensations related to vestibular activity. The vestibular efferent fibers also originate from the vestibular nuclei.

Vestibular reflexes and clinical tests of vestibular function are described in Chapter 13.

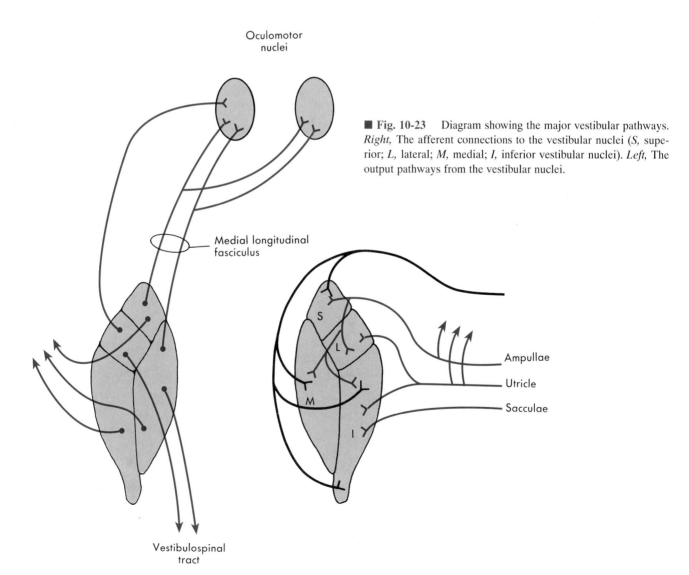

Oculomotor
nuclei

Medial longitudinal
fasciculus

S

L

M

I

Ampullae

Utricle

Sacculae

Vestibulospinal
tract

■ **Fig. 10-23**   Diagram showing the major vestibular pathways. *Right,* The afferent connections to the vestibular nuclei (*S,* superior; *L,* lateral; *M,* medial; *I,* inferior vestibular nuclei). *Left,* The output pathways from the vestibular nuclei.

■ *Summary*

1. Sound waves are combinations of pure tones, and the composition of a sound can be determined by Fourier analysis. A pure tone is characterized in terms of its amplitude, frequency, and phase.

2. The unit of sound pressure is the decibel. Hearing is most sensitive at about 3000 Hz.

3. The main parts of the ear are the external, middle, and inner ears. The external ear includes the pinna and auditory canal. The middle ear includes the tympanic membrane and a chain of ossicles that ends at the oval window. The middle ear is separated from the inner ear by the oval and round windows. The middle-ear apparatus serves as an impedance matching device for energy transfer between air and the fluid in the inner ear.

4. The inner ear contains the cochlea and vestibular apparatus. The cochlea has three main compartments: the scala vestibuli and scala tympani, which are parts of the bony labyrinth, and the scala media, which is part of the membranous labyrinth. The bony labyrinth contains perilymph; the membranous labyrinth contains endolymph.

5. The cochlear duct is bounded on one side by the basilar membrane, on which lies the organ of Corti, the sound transduction mechanism. Hair cells of the organ of Corti synapse with cochlear afferent fibers. They are also controlled by efferent fibers that originate in the superior olivary complex. When the basilar membrane oscillates, the stereocilia of the hair cells are subjected to shear forces at their contacts with the tectorial membrane. Bending of the stereocilia results in a membrane conductance change that causes neurotransmitter release and thus a generator potential in cochlear afferent fibers.

6. Hair cells near the base of the cochlea are best activated by high-frequency sounds and those near the apex by low-frequency sounds. A tonotopic organization is also found in central auditory structures, including the cochlear nuclei, superior olivary complex, inferior colliculus, medial geniculate nucleus, and primary auditory cortex.

7. Auditory processing in the central auditory pathway contributes to sound localization, frequency and intensity analysis, and speech recognition.

8. The vestibular apparatus is part of the membranous labyrinth and includes three semicircular ducts (horizontal, superior, and posterior) and two otolith organs (utricle and saccule) on each side of the head. These structures transduce angular (semicircular ducts) and linear (otolith organs) accelerations of the head.

9. The sensory epithelium, the crista ampullaris, of a semicircular duct is found in a dilation called the ampulla. Stereocilia and a single kinocilium extend from each hair cell into the cupula. Angular head movements displace the endolymph and distort the cupula, bending the cilia. If the stereocilia bend toward the kinocilium, the hair cell is depolarized, and the afferent fiber fires at an increased rate.

10. In the otolith organs, the cilia project into an otolithic membrane. Linear acceleration of the head displaces the otolithic membrane, which is sensitive to gravity because of the otoliths. The hair cells have various orientations, but displacements of the head are coded by the patterned input from the afferent fibers.

11. Central vestibular pathways include afferent connections to four vestibular nuclei and to the cerebellum. Vestibular nuclei project (a) in the medial longitudinal fasciculus to the oculomotor nuclei (to control eye position); (b) in the lateral vestibulospinal tract, which excites motor neurons to postural muscles (to control balance); and (c) in the medial vestibulospinal tract, which activates motor neurons to neck muscles (to control head position).

■ *Self-Study Problems*

1. What is a tonotopic map, and what are some structures that have such a map?

2. How is sound transduced?

3. How is sound encoded?

4. What is the neural mechanism for locating sounds in space?

5. What change in the firing rate of vestibular afferents from the left horizontal semicircular duct occurs when the head is rotated to the right?

■ *Bibliography*

Journal articles

Aitkin L, Park V: Audition and the auditory pathway of a vocal New World primate, the common marmoset, *Prog Neurobiol* 41:345, 1993.

Allen JB: Cochlear micromechanics—a physical model of transduction, *J Acoust Soc Am* 68:1660, 1981.

Allon N, Yeshurun Y: Functional organization of the medial geniculate body's subdivisions of the awake squirrel monkey, *Brain Res* 360:75, 1985.

Brownell WE, Bader CR, Bertrand D, de Ribaupierre Y: Evoked mechanical responses of isolated cochlear outer hair cells, *Science* 227:194, 1985.

Brugge JF, Reale RA, Hind JE: The structure of spatial receptive fields of neurons in primary auditory cortex of the cat, *J Neurosci* 16:4420, 1996.

Carleton SC, Carpenter MB: Afferent and efferent connections of the medial, inferior, and lateral vestibular nuclei, *Brain Res* 278:29, 1983.

Goldberg JM: The vestibular end organs: morphological and physiological diversity of afferents, *Curr Opin Neurobiol* 1:229, 1991.

Henderson D, Hamernik RP: Biological bases of noise-induced hearing loss, *Occup Med* 10:513, 1995.

Hudspeth AJ, Gillespie PG: Pulling springs to tune transduction: adaptation by hair cells, *Neuron* 12:1, 1994.

Imig TJ, Morel A: Organization of the thalamocortical auditory system in the cat, *Annu Rev Neurosci* 6:95, 1983.

Konishi M: Listening with two ears, *Sci Am* 268:66, 1993.

Lysakowski A, Minor LB, Fernandex C, Goldberg JM: Physiological identification of morphologically distinct afferent classes innervating the cristae ampullares of the squirrel monkey, *J Neurophysiol* 73:1270, 1995.

Masterton RB: Role of the central auditory system in hearing: the new direction, *Trends Neurosci* 15:280, 1992.

Moller MB: Audiological evaluation, *J Clin Neurophysiol* 11:309, 1994.

Books and monographs

Altschuler RA, Bobbin RP, Clopton BM, Hoffman DW: *Neurobiology of hearing: the central auditory system,* New York, 1991, Raven Press.

Altschuler RA, Bobbin RP, Hoffman DW: *Neurobiology of hearing: the cochlea,* New York, 1986, Raven Press.

Baloh RW, Honrubia V: *Clinical neurophysiology of the vestibular system,* Philadelphia, 1990, FA Davis.

Brodal A: *Neurological anatomy in relation to clinical medicine,* ed 3, New York, 1981, Oxford University Press.

Gelfand SA: *Hearing: an introduction to psychological and physiological acoustics,* New York, 1990, Marcel Dekker.

Wilson VJ, Melville JG: *Mammalian vestibular physiology,* New York, 1979, Plenum Press.

Yin TCT, Kuwada S: *Neuronal mechanisms of binaural interaction.* In Edelman GM, Cowan WM, editors: *Dynamic aspects of neocortical function,* New York, 1984, John Wiley.

Yost WA: *Fundamentals of hearing: an introduction,* San Diego, 1994, Academic Press.

CHAPTER

11

The Chemical Senses

The senses of **gustation** (taste) and **olfaction** (smell) depend on chemical stimuli that are present either in food and drink or in the air. In human evolution, these chemical senses may not have had the survival value of some of the other senses, but they contribute considerably to the quality of life and are important stimulants of digestion. In other animals, the chemical senses clearly had survival value and their activation evokes a number of social behaviors, including mating, territoriality, and feeding.

■ *Taste*

The stimuli we know as tastes are actually mixtures of four elementary taste qualities: salty, sweet, sour, and bitter. Taste stimuli that are particularly effective in eliciting these sensations include sodium chloride (NaCl), sucrose, hydrochloric acid, and quinine.

■ *Taste Receptors*

The sensation of taste depends on the activation of chemoreceptors located in taste buds. A **taste bud** consists of a group of 50 to 150 chemoreceptor cells, as well as supporting cells and basal cells (Fig. 11-1). The chemoreceptor cells synapse at their bases with primary afferent nerve fibers. The two types of chemoreceptor cells can be distinguished by differences in their synaptic vesicle content: one type has dense core vesicles, and the other, clear round vesicles. The apexes of these cells have microvilli that extend toward a taste pore.

Chemoreceptor cells live only about 10 days. They are constantly being replaced by new chemoreceptor cells that differentiate from basal cells located near the base of the taste bud.

Chemoreceptive molecules on the microvilli of chemoreceptor cells detect stimulatory molecules that diffuse into the taste pore from the overlying fluid layer. Part of this fluid originates from glands adjacent to the taste buds. A change in membrane conductance of a chemoreceptor cell leads to a receptor potential and to the

release of an excitatory neurotransmitter. The neurotransmitter evokes a generator potential in the primary afferent nerve fiber and causes a discharge that is transmitted to the central nervous system (CNS).

Coding for the four primary taste qualities is not based on complete selectivity of the chemoreceptors for the different qualities. Instead, a given chemoreceptor responds to stimuli that evoke several different taste qualities, although perhaps most vigorously to one. Recognition of taste quality appears to depend on the patterned input from a population of chemoreceptors. The intensity of the stimulus is reflected in the total amount of evoked activity.

■ *Distribution and Innervation of Taste Buds*

Taste buds are located on different types of taste papillae found on the tongue, palate, pharynx, and larynx (Fig. 11-2, *C*). The types of taste papillae include **fungiform** and **foliate papillae** on the anterior and lateral tongue and **circumvallate papillae** on the base of the tongue. The latter may contain several hundred taste buds; humans have a total of several thousand taste buds.

The sensitivity of the tongue for different taste qualities varies with the region of the tongue (Fig. 11-2, *A*). Sweet tastes are detected best at the tip of the tongue, salty and sour along the sides, and bitter at the base.

The taste buds are innervated by three cranial nerves, two of which are shown in Fig. 11-2, *B*. The **chorda tympani** branch of the facial nerve supplies taste buds on the anterior two thirds of the tongue, and the **glossopharyngeal** nerve supplies taste buds on the posterior one third of the tongue (Fig. 11-2, *B*). The **vagus** nerve supplies a few taste buds in the larynx and upper esophagus.

Taste is not evaluated in the routine neurologic examination. However, a detailed examination can include application of test substances to the anterior two thirds and the posterior third of the tongue on each side. The tongue must be kept protruded to prevent mixing of the

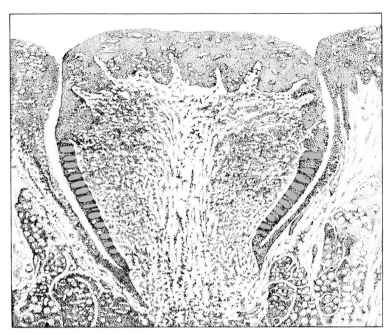

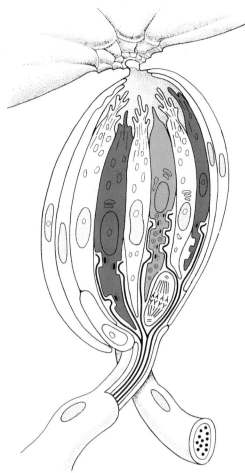

■ **Fig. 11-1**   Taste bud. The two types of chemoreceptor cells are shown in color and the supporting cells are uncolored. *Above,* A circumvallate papilla is shown with its taste buds indicated in color. *Right,* A taste bud is shown with the taste pore at the top and its innervation below. (Redrawn from Williams PL, Warwick R: *Functional neuroanatomy of man,* Philadelphia, 1975, WB Saunders.)

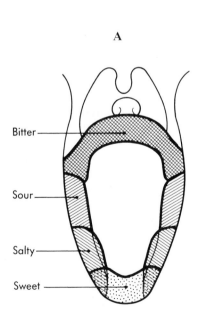

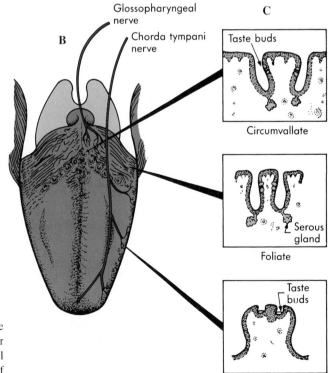

■ **Fig. 11-2**   **A,** Distribution of sensitivity for the four taste qualities. **B,** Innervation of the anterior two thirds and posterior one third of the tongue by the facial and glossopharyngeal nerves. **C,** The arrangement of taste buds in the three types of papillae.

test substances with saliva and subsequent redistribution to other areas of the tongue. Taste can also be tested by application of a galvanic current to the tongue. Taste sensation can be lost, for example, after damage to a cranial nerve that contains gustatory afferents.

■ *Central Pathways*

The cell bodies of taste fibers in cranial nerves VII, IX, and X are located in the geniculate, petrosal, and nodose ganglia, respectively (Fig. 11-3). The central processes of the afferent fibers enter the medulla, join the solitary tract, and synapse in the nucleus of the solitary tract (Fig. 11-3, *A*). In some animals, including several rodent species, the second-order taste neurons of the solitary nucleus project rostrally to the ipsilateral parabrachial nucleus. The parabrachial nucleus then projects to the small-celled (parvocellular) part of the **ventroposterior medial (VPM$_{pc}$)** nucleus of the thalamus (Fig. 11-3, *C*). In monkeys, the solitary nucleus projects directly to the VPM$_{pc}$ nucleus. The VPM$_{pc}$ nucleus is connected to two different gustatory areas of the cerebral cortex, one in the face area of the SI cortex and the other in the insula (Fig. 11-3, *D*). An unusual feature of the central gustatory pathway is that it is predominantly an uncrossed pathway (unlike the central somatosensory, visual, and auditory pathways, which are predominantly crossed).

■ *Olfaction*

The sense of smell is much better developed in other animals (**macrosmatic animals**) than in primates, including humans (**microsmatic animals**). The ability of dogs to track on the basis of odor is legendary, as is the use of **pheromones** by insects to attract mates. However, olfaction contributes to our emotional life, and odors can effectively call up memories.

■ *Olfactory Receptors*

Olfactory chemoreceptors are bipolar cells (Fig. 11-4). The apical surface of these chemoreceptor cells contains immobile cilia that detect odorants dissolved in the overlying mucous layer, and these cells give off an unmyelinated axon from the basal surface. This axon joins others in olfactory nerve filaments that penetrate the base of the skull through openings in the cribriform plate of the ethmoid bone. The olfactory nerves synaptically connect with the olfactory bulb, a CNS structure located at the base of the cranial cavity, just below the frontal lobe. The olfactory chemoreceptor cells are located in the olfactory mucosa, a specialized part of the nasopharynx with a total surface area on the two sides of about 10 cm^2 (Fig.

11-5). Humans have about 10^7 olfactory chemoreceptors. Like taste cells, olfactory chemoreceptors have a short lifespan (about 60 days), and are continuously replaced.

Odorant molecules are introduced to the olfactory mucosa by ventilatory air currents or from the oral cavity during feeding. Sniffing increases the influx of odorants. The odorants are temporarily bound in the mucus to an olfactory binding protein, which is secreted by a gland in the nasal cavity.

Odor has more primary qualities than does taste. There are at least six odor qualities: **floral, ethereal, musky, camphor, putrid,** and **pungent.** Natural stimuli with these odors are roses, pears, musk, eucalyptus, rotten eggs, and vinegar, respectively. The olfactory mucosa also contains somatosensory receptors of the trigeminal nerve. When performing clinical tests of olfaction, one must avoid activating these somatosensory receptors with noxious or thermal stimuli.

A few odorant molecules that reach an olfactory chemoreceptor cell produce a depolarizing receptor potential, which triggers a neural discharge. However, behavioral responses require the activation of a number of olfactory chemoreceptors. The receptor potential probably results from an increased conductance for Na$^+$. However, a G protein is also activated; therefore, a cascade of second messengers is also involved in olfactory transduction.

Olfactory coding resembles taste coding in that an individual olfactory chemoreceptor responds to more than one odorant class. Coding for a particular olfactory quality depends on the responses of many olfactory chemoreceptors, and the strength of the odorant is represented by the overall amount of afferent neural activity.

■ *Central Pathways*

The initial relay of the olfactory pathway is located in the olfactory bulb, which is a cortical structure. It contains three main cell types: **mitral cells, tufted cells,** and **interneurons (granule cells; periglomerular cells)** (Fig. 11-6). The dendrites of the mitral and tufted cells are long and branch to form the postsynaptic components of the olfactory glomeruli. The olfactory afferent fibers that reach the olfactory bulb from the olfactory mucosa ramify as they approach the olfactory glomeruli and then synapse on the dendrites of the mitral and tufted cells. Olfactory axons converge extensively onto mitral cell dendrites; as many as 1000 afferent fibers synapse on the dendrites of a single mitral cell. The granule and periglomerular cells are inhibitory interneurons. They form dendrodendritic reciprocal synapses with the dendrites of the mitral cells. Evidently, activity in a mitral cell depolarizes the inhibitory cells that synapse with it. An inhibitory neurotransmitter that acts back on the mitral cell is then released. The olfactory bulb has other inputs besides those formed by the olfactory nerves;

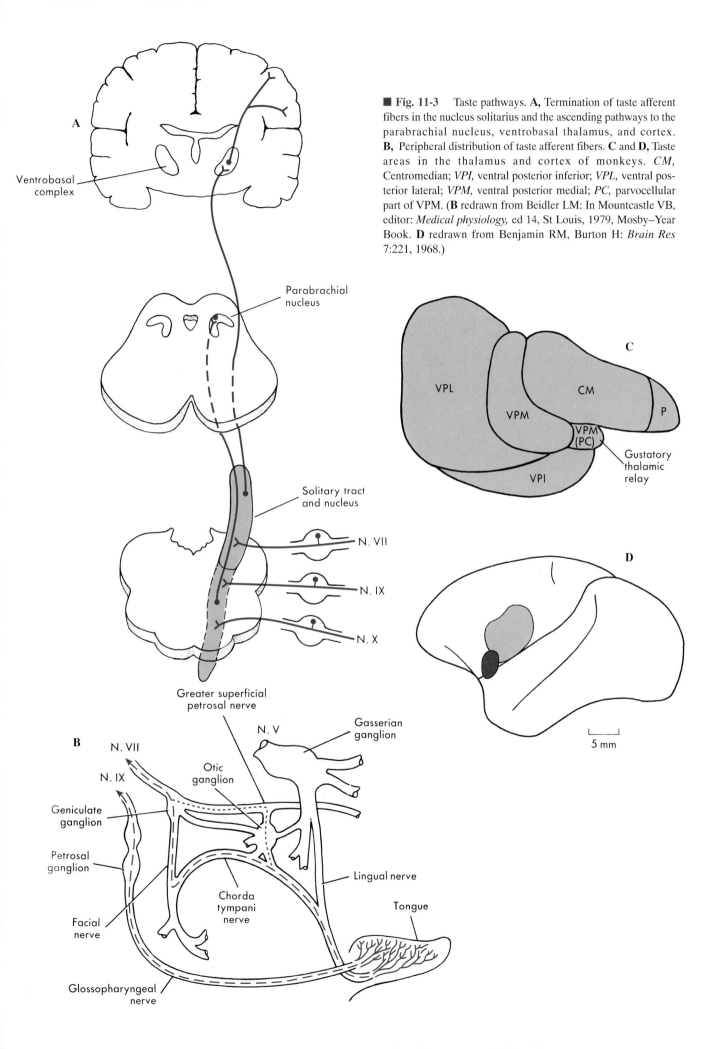

■ **Fig. 11-3** Taste pathways. **A,** Termination of taste afferent fibers in the nucleus solitarius and the ascending pathways to the parabrachial nucleus, ventrobasal thalamus, and cortex. **B,** Peripheral distribution of taste afferent fibers. **C** and **D,** Taste areas in the thalamus and cortex of monkeys. *CM,* Centromedian; *VPI,* ventral posterior inferior; *VPL,* ventral posterior lateral; *VPM,* ventral posterior medial; *PC,* parvocellular part of VPM. (**B** redrawn from Beidler LM: In Mountcastle VB, editor: *Medical physiology,* ed 14, St Louis, 1979, Mosby–Year Book. **D** redrawn from Benjamin RM, Burton H: *Brain Res* 7:221, 1968.)

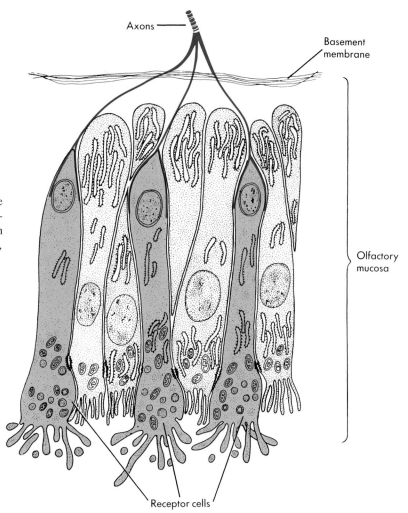

■ **Fig. 11-4** Olfactory chemoreceptors are shown in color and supporting cells are uncolored. (Redrawn from de Lorenzo AJD. In Zotterman Y, editor: *Olfaction and taste,* Elmsford, NY, 1963, Pergamon Press.)

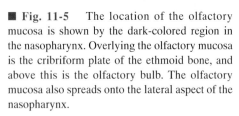

■ **Fig. 11-5** The location of the olfactory mucosa is shown by the dark-colored region in the nasopharynx. Overlying the olfactory mucosa is the cribriform plate of the ethmoid bone, and above this is the olfactory bulb. The olfactory mucosa also spreads onto the lateral aspect of the nasopharynx.

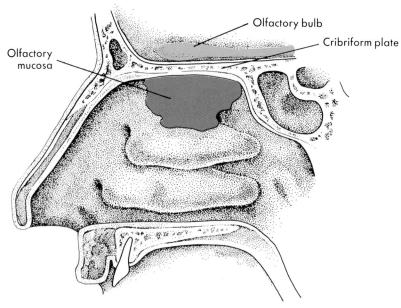

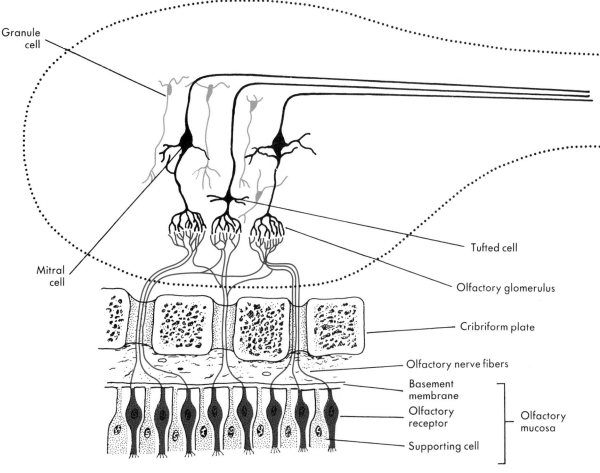

Granule cell

Mitral cell

Tufted cell

Olfactory glomerulus

Cribriform plate

Olfactory nerve fibers

Basement membrane

Olfactory receptor

Supporting cell

Olfactory mucosa

■ **Fig. 11-6** Drawing of a sagittal section through an olfactory bulb, showing the terminations of the olfactory chemoreceptor cells in the olfactory glomerulus and the intrinsic neurons of the olfactory bulb. The axons of the mitral and tufted cells are shown exiting in the olfactory tract to the right. (Redrawn from House EL, Pansky B: *A functional approach to neuroanatomy*, ed 2, New York, 1967, McGraw-Hill. Used with permission.)

these other inputs include a projection from the contralateral olfactory tract via the anterior commissure.

The axons of the mitral and tufted cells leave the olfactory bulb and enter the olfactory tract (Figs. 11-6 and 11-7). From here, the olfactory connections become highly complex. Within the olfactory tract is a nucleus called the **anterior olfactory nucleus.** Neurons in this structure receive synaptic connections from neurons of the olfactory bulb and project to the contralateral olfactory bulb through the anterior commissure. As the olfactory tract approaches the anterior perforated substance at the base of the brain, it splits into the lateral and medial olfactory striae. Axons of the lateral olfactory stria synapse in the primary olfactory receiving area, which includes the prepiriform cortex (and, in animals, the piriform lobe). The medial olfactory stria includes projections to the amygdaloid nucleus, as well as part of the cortex of the basal forebrain (Fig. 11-7).

Note that the olfactory pathway is the only sensory system that does not have an obligatory synaptic relay in the thalamus. The absence of this relay may reflect the phylogenetic primitiveness of the olfactory system. However, olfactory information does reach the mediodorsal nucleus of the thalamus and is then transmitted to the prefrontal and orbitofrontal cortex.

Olfaction is generally not examined in a routine neurologic examination. However, smell can be tested by having the patient inhale and identify an odorant. One nostril should be examined at a time while the other nostril is occluded. Strong odorants, such as ammonia, should be avoided, because they also activate trigeminal nerve fibers. Smell sensation can be lost (**anosmia**) after a basal skull fracture or after damage to one or both olfactory bulbs or tracts by a tumor (such as an **olfactory groove meningioma**). An aura of a disagreeable odor, often the smell of burning rubber, occurs during **uncinate fits,** which are epileptic seizures that originate in the region of the uncus.

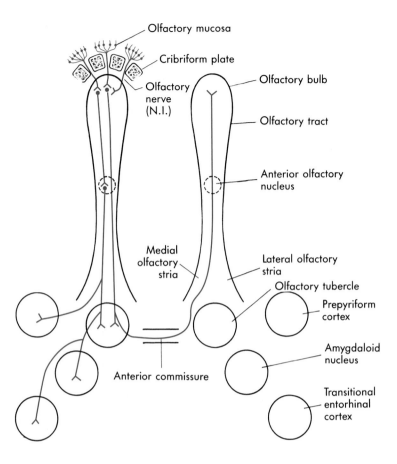

Fig. 11-7 Major olfactory pathways.

Summary

1. Taste buds detect gustatory stimuli. Populations of afferents are used to signal the four elementary qualities of taste: salty, sweet, sour, and bitter.

2. Taste buds are located on several kinds of papillae on the tongue and in the pharynx and larynx. Taste buds contain chemoreceptor cells arranged around a taste pore; these cells are innervated by taste afferent fibers of cranial nerves VII, IX, and X.

3. The afferent taste fibers synapse in the nucleus of the solitary tract. Higher pathways vary in different species. The parabrachial nucleus is included in rodents but not in primates. The thalamus gustatory nucleus is the small-celled part of the ventroposterior medial nucleus, and taste-receiving areas are located in the SI cortex and the insula.

4. Odors are detected by olfactory chemoreceptor cells in the olfactory mucosa. At least six elementary odor qualities are encoded by the population of olfactory afferent nerves.

5. The olfactory chemoreceptor cells project to the olfactory bulb, where they synapse in olfactory glomeruli on the dendrites of mitral and tufted cells. Local inhibitory dendrodendritic circuits are formed by the granule cells. The mitral and tufted cells project to the olfactory tract.

Self-Study Problems

1. How do the chemoreceptor cells of the gustatory and olfactory systems differ from primary somatovisceral afferent neurons?

2. How specific are the responses of taste and olfactory afferents to different chemical stimuli?

3. How do the patterns of central projections of the taste and olfactory pathways differ?

Bibliography

Journal articles

Anholt RRH: Molecular biology of olfaction, *Crit Rev Neurobiol* 7:1, 1993.

Axel R: The molecular logic of smell, *Sci Am* 273:154, 1995.

Bartoshuk LM, Beauchamp GK: Chemical senses, *Annu Rev Psychol* 45:419, 1994.

Gilbertson TA: The physiology of vertebrate taste reception, *Curr Opin Neurobiol* 3:532, 1993.

Hamilton RB, Norgren R: Central projections of gustatory nerves in the rat, *J Comp Neurol* 222:560, 1984.

Kinnamon SC: Taste transduction: a diversity of mechanisms, *Trends Neurosci* 11:491, 1988.

Lindemann B: Taste reception, *Physiol Rev* 76:718, 1996.

Mori K, Yoshihara Y: Molecular recognition and olfactory processing in the mammalian olfactory system, *Prog Neurobiol* 45:585, 1995.

Nef P: Early events in olfaction: diversity and spatial patterns of odorant receptors, *Receptors Channels* 1:259, 1993.

Ogawa H: Gustatory cortex of primates: anatomy and physiology, *Neurosci Res* 20:1, 1994.

Roper SD: The cell biology of vertebrate taste receptors, *Annu Rev Neurosci* 12:329, 1989.

Scott JW, Wellis DP, Riggott MJ, Buonviso N: Functional organization of the main olfactory bulb, *Micros Res Tech* 24:142, 1993.

Spector AC: Gustatory function in the parabrachial nuclei: implications from lesion studies in rats, *Rev Neurosci* 6:143, 1995.

Sullivan SL, Ressler KJ, Buck LB: Spatial patterning and information coding in the olfactory system, *Curr Opin Genet Dev* 5:516, 1995.

Torre V, Ashmore JF, Lamb TD, Menini A: Transduction and adaptation in sensory receptor cells, *J Neurosci* 15:7757, 1995.

Books and monographs

Brand JG et al, editors: *Chemical senses,* vol 1, *Receptor events and transduction in taste and olfaction,* New York, 1989, Marcel Dekker.

Finger TE, Silver WL, editors: *Neurobiology of taste and smell,* New York, 1987, John Wiley.

Getchell TV, Doty RL, Bartoshuk LM, Snow JB, editors: *Smell and taste in health and disease,* New York, 1991, Raven Press.

Kandel ER, Schwartz JH, Jessell TM: *Principles of neural science,* ed 3, New York, 1991, Elsevier.

Pfaff DW, editor: *Taste, olfaction, and the central nervous system,* New York, 1985, Rockefeller University Press.

Shepherd GM: *Neurobiology,* ed 2, New York, 1988, Oxford University Press.

Spinal Organization of Motor Function

Movements and posture depend on the coordinated contraction of muscles that operate around joints. Coordination of muscle contractions, in turn, depends on the amount and timing of the discharges of motor neurons to the appropriate muscles and the absence of discharges of motor neurons to inappropriate muscles. Thus, the motor system coordinates muscle actions through control of motor neuronal activity. Although motor control is in part under voluntary control, it occurs mainly by reflex action and subconscious mechanisms.

Spinal reflexes are important to motor activity. Many subconscious actions depend largely on simple reflexes that are triggered by the activation of sensory receptors. Activation of sensory receptors then excites interneurons and motor neurons in the spinal cord, and this excitation then triggers the contraction or relaxation of particular muscles. Spinal reflexes can be observed in **spinalized** individuals (i.e., individuals with spinal cord injuries that cause a complete functional transection of the spinal cord). Therefore, these reflexes do not depend on motor commands that originate in the brain and are conveyed to the spinal cord via descending motor pathways.

In addition, many of the motor acts that do originate from motor commands issued by the brain depend on spinal reflex circuitry for their implementation. Only a few of the descending pathways synapse directly on spinal cord motor neurons. Instead, most of the descending projections influence the activity of interneurons that are interposed in reflex circuits and thus alter ongoing spinal reflex activity.

This chapter describes a number of spinal cord reflex pathways. Motor pathways that descend from the brain are discussed in Chapter 13. The motor control systems of the brain are the topic of Chapter 14.

Spinal cord injury is common, especially in young males. Such injuries are caused by automobile collisions, sports accidents, war injuries, or gunshot wounds. Depending on the level and severity of the spinal cord injury, the individual affected may have **paraplegia** (paralysis of both lower extremities) or **quadriplegia** (paralysis of all four extremities). Much research has focused on ways to ameliorate spinal cord injury. Promising leads include (1) protection against secondary damage by administration of agents such as methylprednisolone shortly after the injury; (2) procedures to assist movement, such as electrical stimulation of muscle nerves of the lower extremities; and (3) treatments to encourage repair of the interrupted descending motor pathways.

In humans, an abrupt transection of the spinal cord results initially in a condition called **spinal shock,** which is characterized by a flaccid paralysis, areflexia, loss of autonomic function, and loss of all sensation below the level of the transection. In flaccid paralysis, the joint offers no resistance to passive movement when an examiner bends the joint. This absence of resistance results from the loss of muscle stretch reflexes, which normally cause muscle contractions that oppose changes in the position of the joint (see p 192). Spinal shock generally lasts 3 to 4 weeks. After spinal shock resolves, reflexes gradually return and then become hyperactive. The hyperactivity of spinal reflexes is demonstrated by greater resistance than normal when an examiner bends the joint. Voluntary movement and sensation never return, and the paralysis changes in character from flaccidity to spasticity. Furthermore, pathological reflexes appear (e.g., the **sign of Babinski**—see Chapter 13); muscle tone increases; and bowel and bladder functions return, but in altered form.

Hyperactivity affects both the muscle stretch reflexes and the flexion reflexes. Hyperactive stretch reflexes are associated not only with an increased resistance to passive stretch, but also often with **clonus** (an alternating contraction of agonist and antagonist muscles around a joint, such as the ankle, after an initial quick passive flexion of the joint). Hyperactive flexion reflexes in response to a noxious stimulus applied to a foot may include not only flexion of one or both lower extremities but also urination, defecation, and sweating. The posture is often one of maintained flexion of the lower extremities.

In animals, spinal transection produces similar changes, but the period of spinal shock is usually brief. Therefore, spinal reflexes can be studied in the absence of descending controls.

■ *Decerebration*

An experimental preparation that has been useful for the study of reflexes is the decerebrate preparation. Surgical decerebration is achieved by transecting the midbrain, often at an intercollicular level. Decerebrate animals no longer have sensation, and their motor control system is profoundly altered. Some descending pathways, such as those that originate in the cerebral cortex, are interrupted, whereas others, such as those that originate in the brainstem, remain intact. In fact, activity in some descending pathways becomes hyperactive because of a change in the balance of excitatory and inhibitory control systems. As a result, some spinal reflexes, such as the flexion reflex, are suppressed, whereas others, such as the stretch reflex, are exaggerated, a condition called **decerebrate rigidity.** Decerebrate rigidity causes decerebrate animals to maintain a posture that has been called **exaggerated standing.** Decerebrate preparations are thus ideal for the study of the stretch reflex as well as the inverse myotatic reflex (see p 194).

Human patients with brainstem damage may also develop a decerebrate state that has many of the same reflex features as animal preparations. The prognosis in such patients is poor when signs of decerebration appear.

■ *Sensory Receptors Responsible for Eliciting Spinal Reflexes*

As noted in the introduction to this chapter, activation of particular sensory receptors triggers simple reflexes that are largely responsible for many subconscious actions. Several important spinal reflexes are activated by muscle stretch receptors, including muscle spindles and Golgi tendon organs. These reflexes are the **muscle stretch reflex** (or **myotatic reflex**) and the **inverse myotatic reflex.** These reflexes are important for the maintenance of posture, and alteration in the activity of the circuits for these reflexes provides an important means by which descending pathways produce movements. Furthermore,

abnormalities in the stretch reflexes are prominent in disorders of the motor system. We have already seen how abnormalities in these reflexes contribute to the syndrome associated with complete spinal cord transection.

Another important reflex, the **flexion reflex,** is evoked by various sensory receptors in the skin, muscles, joints, and viscera. Afferents from the different receptors that are able to evoke a flexion reflex are often referred to as **flexion reflex afferents (FRAs)** (see later in this chapter.)

In the following sections, the muscle stretch receptors—muscle spindles and Golgi tendon organs—are discussed. These receptors are important both for spinal reflexes and for proprioception (see Chapter 8). Their structure and functional properties are described in detail here because a knowledge of their operation is useful for understanding the mechanisms that underlie the spinal reflexes.

■ *The Muscle Spindle*

The structure and function of muscle spindles are very complex. They are found in most skeletal muscles but are particularly concentrated in muscles that exert fine motor control (e.g., the small muscles of the hand). In large muscles, they are most abundant in those that are rich in slow twitch (type I) muscle fibers.

Structure of the muscle spindle. As its name implies, a **muscle spindle** (or neuromuscular spindle) is a spindle-shaped organ composed of a bundle of modified muscle fibers innervated by both sensory and motor axons (Fig. 12-1). The muscle spindle is about 100 μm in diameter and up to 10 mm long. The innervated part of the muscle spindle is encased in a connective tissue capsule. Within this capsule, fluid is contained within the so-called lymph space. The muscle spindle lies freely between regular muscle fibers. The distal ends of the spindle are attached to the connective tissue within the muscle (**endomysium**). The muscle spindles lie parallel to the regular muscle fibers. This arrangement has important functional implications, as is made clear below.

Muscle spindles contain modified muscle fibers called **intrafusal muscle fibers** to distinguish them from the regular or **extrafusal muscle fibers.** Individual intrafusal fibers are much narrower than extrafusal fibers and are too weak to contribute to muscle tension. Two types of intrafusal muscle fibers are found within muscle spindles: nuclear bag and nuclear chain fibers (Fig. 12-2). These names are derived from the arrangement of the nuclei in the two kinds of intrafusal fibers. **Nuclear bag fibers** are larger than nuclear chain fibers, and their nuclei are bunched together like a bag of oranges in the central region of the fiber. In **nuclear chain fibers,** the nuclei are arranged in a row.

Muscle spindles receive a complex innervation. The sensory supply includes a single **group Ia afferent** and a variable number of **group II afferent** fibers (Fig. 12-2).

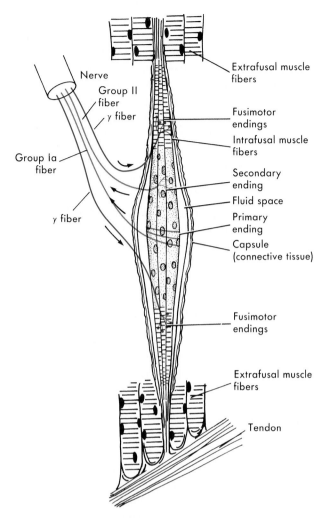

Fig. 12-1 Drawing of a muscle spindle. (Redrawn from Brodal A: *Neurological anatomy,* ed 3, New York, 1981, Oxford University Press.)

Group Ia fibers belong to the largest diameter class of sensory nerve fibers and conduct at 72 to 120 m/sec; group II fibers are intermediate in size and conduct at 36 to 72 m/sec (see Table 7-2). A group Ia afferent fiber forms a **primary ending,** which consists of a spiral-shaped terminal composed of branches of the group Ia fiber, on each of the intrafusal muscle fibers. Primary endings are found on both nuclear bag and nuclear chain fibers, a point that is functionally significant. The group II afferent fiber forms a **secondary ending,** which is found chiefly on nuclear chain fibers.

The motor supply to the muscle spindle consists of two types of γ motor axons (Fig. 12-2). **Dynamic γ motor axons** end on nuclear bag fibers. **Static γ motor axons** end on nuclear chain fibers. γ Motor axons are smaller in diameter than the α motor axons to extrafusal muscle. Hence they conduct more slowly (see Table 7-3).

Function of the muscle spindle. As the name **stretch receptor** implies, muscle spindles respond to muscle stretch. Fig. 12-3 shows the changes in the activity of an afferent fiber from a muscle spindle when the muscle spindle is both shortened (unloaded) by contraction of the extrafusal muscle fibers and lengthened by stretching the muscle. Contraction of the extrafusal muscle fibers causes the muscle spindle to shorten because of the parallel arrangement of the muscle spindle described earlier.

The activity of muscle spindle afferent fibers depends on the mechanical stretch of the afferent terminals on the intrafusal fibers. When the regular muscle fibers contract, the muscle spindle is shortened, the spacing between the coils of the afferent terminals is reduced, and the discharge rate of the afferent fiber decreases. Conversely, when the whole muscle is stretched, the muscle spindle is also stretched (because its ends are attached to the connective tissue framework of the muscle), and the elongation of the receptor terminals increases the discharge rate.

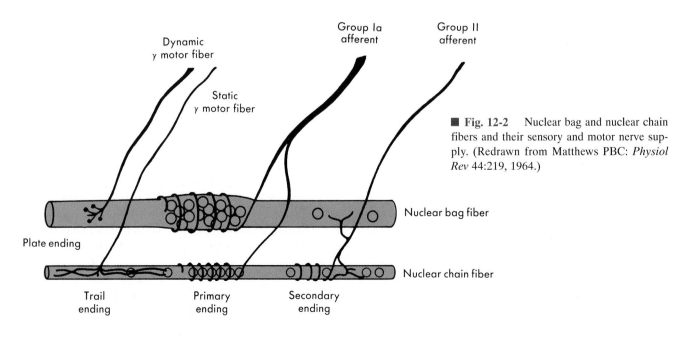

Fig. 12-2 Nuclear bag and nuclear chain fibers and their sensory and motor nerve supply. (Redrawn from Matthews PBC: *Physiol Rev* 44:219, 1964.)

The firing rates of both the group Ia fiber and the group II fiber are proportional to the length of the muscle spindle, as shown for both linear stretch (at the left in Fig. 12-4) and when the stretch is released (as shown at the right). This type of response is called the **static response** of muscle spindle afferent fibers. However, the primary and secondary endings of the afferent fibers respond differently to stretch. The primary ending is sensitive both to the amount of stretch and to its rate, whereas the secondary ending responds chiefly to the amount of stretch (Fig. 12-4). These differences in response can be seen in the behavior of the two endings.

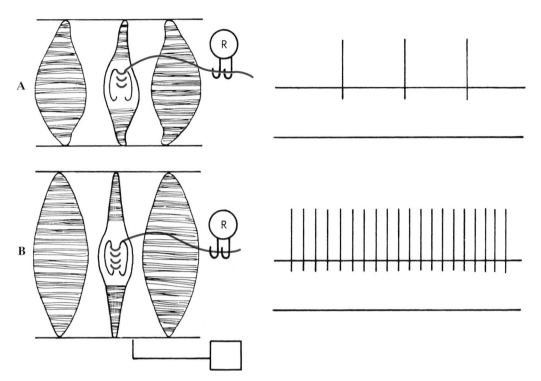

■ **Fig. 12-3** Changes in the discharge rate of a muscle spindle afferent fiber during muscle shortening (due to a contraction of the muscle) and during muscle lengthening (due to muscle stretch). During the contraction **A,** the muscle spindle is unloaded as a result of its parallel arrangement within the muscle. In **B,** the muscle spindle is stretched along with the muscle. *R* indicates the recording system. (Redrawn from Eyzaguirre C, Fidone SJ: *Physiology of the nervous system,* ed 2, Chicago, 1975, Mosby–Year Book; modified from Ruch TC, Patton HD: *Physiology and biophysics,* ed 19, Philadelphia, 1965, WB Saunders; and Hunt CC, Kuffler SW: *J Physiol* 113:298, 1951.)

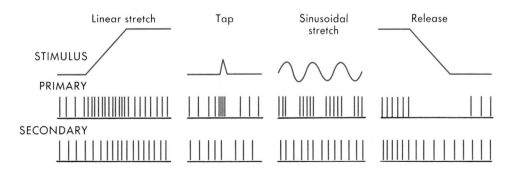

■ **Fig. 12-4** The responses of a primary ending and of a secondary ending to various types of changes in muscle length are shown to illustrate the difference in dynamic and static responsiveness of these endings. The waveforms at the top are the changes in muscle length. The vertical lines in the middle and bottom parts of the figure show the discharges of a primary and of a secondary ending. (Redrawn from Matthews PBC: *Physiol Rev* 44:219, 1964.)

The activity of the primary ending overshoots during muscle stretch, and the ending stops firing when the stretch is first released. These responses are called **dynamic responses** of the group Ia afferent fiber. The responses in the center of Fig. 12-4 are further examples of dynamic responses of the primary ending. Tapping the muscle or its tendon and sinusoidal stretch are much more effective in causing discharges of the primary than of the secondary ending.

These responses show that the primary endings signal both the length and the rate of change in length of the muscle, whereas the secondary endings signal only the length of the muscle. The mechanism for these differences between the behavior of primary and secondary endings appears to depend largely on the mechanical differences between the nuclear bag and nuclear chain fibers. As we maintained on p 188, both primary and secondary endings are found on nuclear bag and chain fibers, whereas secondary endings are found chiefly on nuclear chain fibers. Nuclear bag fibers lack contractile proteins in their equatorial regions because of the accumulation of nuclei in this region. Therefore, the nuclear bag fibers are readily stretched in their midregion. However, immediately after they are stretched, the equatorial region of nuclear bag fibers tends to return toward its original length as the polar regions lengthen. This phenomenon, called **creep,** is caused by the viscoelastic properties of these intrafusal fibers. The result is an overshoot in activity of the primary ending followed by a reduction in activity toward a new static level of firing.

In contrast to nuclear bag fibers, the length of the nuclear chain fibers more closely resembles that of the extrafusal muscle fibers because the nuclear chain fibers contain contractile proteins in their equatorial regions. Hence, they have more uniform viscoelastic properties throughout their length. Therefore, they do not display creep, and the secondary ending has only a static response.

Up to this point, we have described only how muscle spindles behave when the γ motor neurons are not active. However, the efferent innervation of muscle spindles is extremely important, because it determines the sensitivity of muscle spindles to stretch. For example, in Fig. 12-5, *A,* the activity of a muscle spindle afferent is shown during a steady stretch. As already discussed, when the extrafusal part of the muscle contracts (Fig. 12-5, *B*), the muscle spindle is unloaded, and the muscle spindle afferent may stop discharging. However, this effect of muscle spindle unloading can be counteracted if γ motor neurons

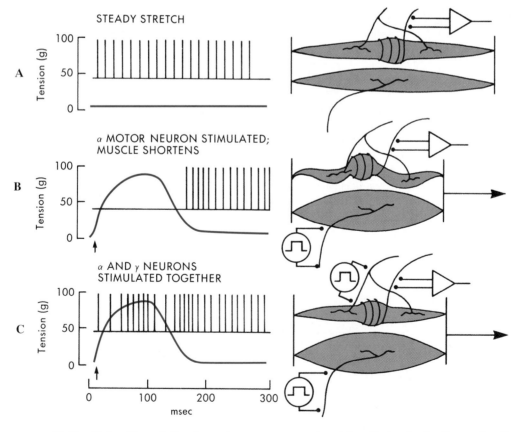

■ **Fig. 12-5**   The activity of γ motor axons can counteract the effects of unloading on the discharges of a muscle spindle afferent. **A,** The activity of a muscle spindle afferent is shown during steady stretch. **B,** The afferent stops firing when the extrafusal muscle fibers contract, owing to unloading of the muscle spindle. **C,** Activation of a γ motor neuron causes shortening of the muscle spindle, counteracting the effects of unloading. (Redrawn from Kuffler SW, Nicholls JG: *From neuron to brain,* Sunderland, Mass, 1976, Sinauer Associates.)

are stimulated. This stimulation causes the muscle spindle to shorten along with the extrafusal muscle fibers (Fig. 12-5, *C*). Actually, only the two polar regions of the muscle spindle contract; the equatorial region, where the nuclei are located, does not contract because it has little contractile protein. As a result, the equatorial region elongates, which stretches and excites the afferent terminals. This mechanism is very important in the normal operation of muscle spindles, because descending motor commands from the brain typically coactivate α and γ motor neurons and thus cause co-contraction of extrafusal and intrafusal muscle fibers (Fig. 12-6).

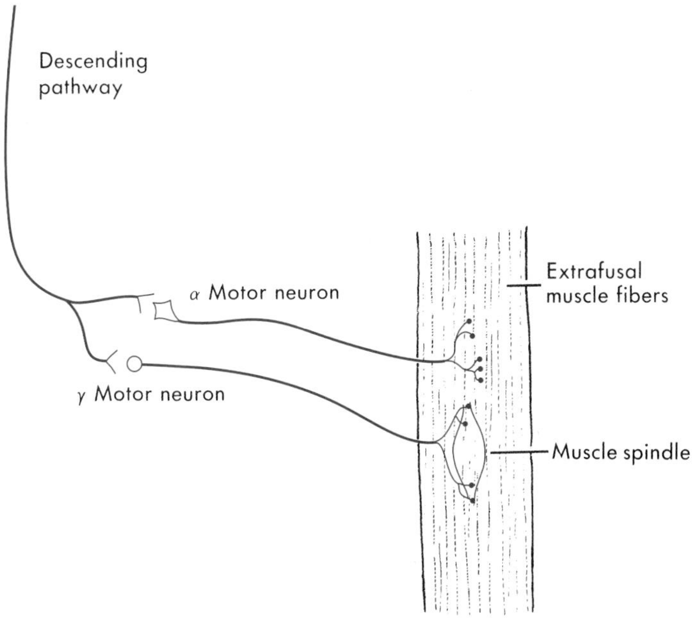

Another way in which afferent fibers influence reflex activity is through their interaction with nuclear bag fibers and nuclear chain fibers. As mentioned earlier, there are two types of γ motor neurons called dynamic and static γ motor neurons (Fig. 12-2). Dynamic γ motor axons end on nuclear bag fibers and static γ motor axons synapse on nuclear chain fibers. When a dynamic γ motor neuron is activated, the dynamic response of the group Ia afferent fiber is enhanced (Fig. 12-7, *D*). When a static γ motor neuron discharges, the static responses of both group Ia and II afferent fibers are enhanced (Fig. 12-7, *C*); at the same time, the dynamic response may be reduced. Different descending pathways can preferentially influence dynamic or static γ motor neurons and thereby alter the nature of reflex activity in the spinal cord.

■ *The Golgi Tendon Organ*

The other type of stretch receptor found in skeletal muscle is the Golgi tendon organ (Fig. 12-8). A **Golgi tendon organ** is formed from the terminals of a group Ib afferent fiber. The diameter of a Golgi tendon organ is about 100 μm and its length about 1 mm. The group Ib fiber has a large diameter and conducts in the same velocity range as the group Ia fiber (see Table 7-2). The terminals are wrapped about bundles of collagen fibers in the tendon of a muscle (or in tendinous inscriptions within the muscle). The sensory ending is arranged in series with the muscle, in contrast to the parallel arrangement of the muscle spindle.

Because of their arrangement in series with muscle, Golgi tendon organs can be activated either by muscle stretch or by contraction of the muscle (Fig. 12-9). However, muscle contraction is a more effective stimulus than muscle stretch. The actual stimulus is the force that

■ **Fig. 12-6**   Coactivation of an α and a γ motor neuron by a descending motor pathway.

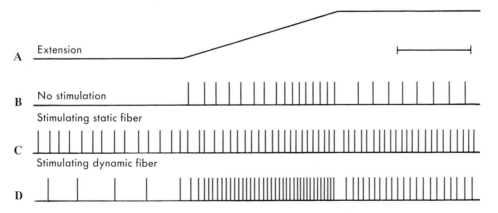

■ **Fig. 12-7**   Effects of static and dynamic γ motor neurons on the responses of a primary ending to muscle stretch. The upper trace is the time course of stretch (**A**). **B** shows the discharge of the group Ia fiber in the absence of γ motor neuron activity. In **C**, a static γ motor axon was stimulated, and in **D**, a dynamic γ motor axon was stimulated. (Redrawn from Crowe A, Matthews PBC: *J Physiol* 174:109, 1964.)

develops in the tendon that contains the Golgi tendon organ. Therefore, Golgi tendon organs signal force, unlike the muscle spindle, which signals muscle length and the rate of change in muscle length.

■ *Spinal Reflexes*

A reflex is defined as a simple, relatively stereotyped motor response to a specific type of stimulus. A **reflex arc** is the neuronal circuit responsible for a particular reflex. Typically, a reflex arc includes a set of sensory receptors of a particular kind that, when stimulated, elicit the reflex by exciting a set of interneurons and motor neurons (Fig. 12-10). Other interneurons and motor neu-

rons may also be inhibited, so that an appropriate pattern of muscle contractions occurs around one or more joints.

■ *The Myotatic or Stretch Reflex*

The stretch reflex is a key reflex in the maintenance of posture. In addition, changes in this reflex are involved in actions commanded by the brain, and pathological alterations are important signs of neurologic disease. This reflex actually has two forms: the phasic stretch reflex and the tonic stretch reflex. The **phasic stretch reflex** is elicited by primary endings of muscle spindles, whereas the **tonic stretch reflex** depends on both primary and secondary endings.

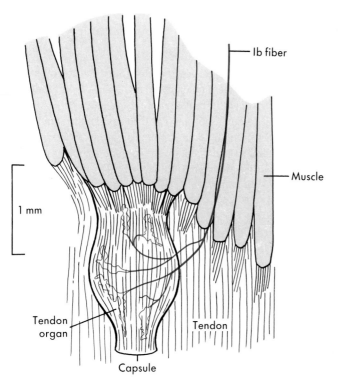

■ **Fig. 12-8**   Drawing of a Golgi tendon organ. (Redrawn from Barker D: *Muscle receptors,* Hong Kong, 1962, Hong Kong University Press.)

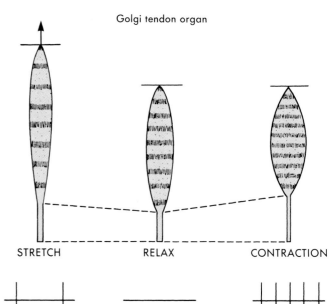

■ **Fig. 12-9**   Activation of a Golgi tendon organ by muscle stretch *(left)* or by contraction of the muscle *(right).* (Redrawn with permission from Eyzaguirre C, Fidone SJ: *Physiology of the nervous system,* ed 2, Chicago, 1975, Mosby–Year Book.)

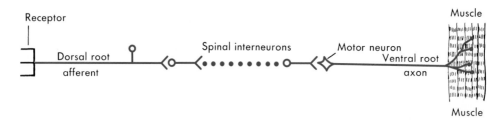

■ **Fig. 12-10**   Diagram of a reflex arc, including a sensory receptor, spinal interneurons, a motor neuron, and muscle.

The phasic stretch reflex. The reflex arc responsible for the phasic stretch reflex is shown in Fig. 12-11. A group Ia afferent fiber from a muscle spindle in the rectus femoris muscle branches as it enters the spinal cord. The branches enter the spinal cord gray matter. Some of the branches synapse directly (monosynaptically) on α motor neurons that supply the rectus femoris muscle (and its synergists, such as the vastus intermedius muscle), which extend the leg at the knee. The group Ia fiber and others like it produce a monosynaptic excitation of the α motor neuron. If the excitation is powerful enough, the motor neuron discharges and causes a contraction of the muscle.

Other branches of the group Ia fiber end on group Ia inhibitory interneurons, such as the one shown in black in Fig. 12-11. These inhibitory interneurons end on α motor neurons that innervate the hamstring muscles, including the semitendinosus muscle, which are antagonists and flex the knee. Activity in the Ia inhibitory interneurons inhibits the motor neurons to these antagonist muscles. A volley (stimulatory activity) in the group Ia afferent fibers from muscle spindles in the rectoris femoris muscle thus evokes both a quick contraction of this muscle and a concomitant relaxation of the hamstring muscles.

The organization of the stretch reflex arc guarantees that one set of α motor neurons is activated and the opposing set is inhibited. This arrangement is known as **reciprocal innervation.** Many reflexes have such a reciprocal innervation, but this type of innervation is not the only possible organization of a motor control system. In some instances, a motor command causes co-contraction of synergists and antagonists, for example, when a person makes a fist. The muscles that extend and flex the wrist contract and allow the wrist to resist motion.

A volley in group Ia afferent fibers is elicited when a physician taps the tendon of a muscle, such as the quadriceps, with a reflex hammer. The result is normally a brief muscular contraction that is quickly damped. When the excitability of the α motor neurons is altered pathologically, the phasic stretch reflex may be depressed or hyperexcitable. In the past, such a reflex was termed a **deep tendon reflex.** This term is a misnomer, however, because the receptors responsible for the reflex are in the muscle, not the tendon. The tendon only provides for a quick stretch of the muscle.

The tonic stretch reflex. The other type of stretch reflex, the tonic stretch reflex, is elicited by passively bending a joint. The reflex circuit is the same as that for the phasic stretch reflex (illustrated in Fig. 12-11), except that the receptors involved include both group Ia and group II afferent fibers from muscle spindles. Many group II fibers make monosynaptic excitatory connections with α motor neurons. Therefore, the tonic stretch reflex is largely a monosynaptic reflex, like the phasic stretch reflex. The tonic stretch reflex contributes to muscle tone, which is judged by the resistance that a joint offers to bending. However, its importance lies in its contribution to posture. When an individual stands, the joints of the leg must maintain a particular position to prevent falling. Any slight extension or flexion will elicit a tonic stretch reflex in the muscles required to oppose the movement, thus helping an individual stand upright. For example, if the knee of a soldier standing at attention begins to flex because of fatigue, the quadriceps muscle will be stretched, a tonic stretch reflex will be elicited, and the quadriceps will contract more, thereby opposing the flexion and restoring the posture.

γ Motor neurons and stretch reflexes. γ Motor neurons help set the sensitivity of the stretch reflexes. Muscle spindle afferent fibers have no direct influence on γ motor neurons. Motor neurons are affected polysynaptically only by the flexion reflex afferents at the spinal cord level and by descending commands. Thus, in many clinical disorders of motor control, the activity of γ motor neurons is inappropriate because of a change, for instance, in the activity of descending pathways. As already mentioned, spinal cord transection results initially in spinal shock, with a loss of the stretch reflexes. Spinal shock may be caused in part by the loss of descending excitation of γ motor neurons. When spinal shock eventually resolves, increased activity in γ motor neurons may underlie **spasticity,** in which phasic stretch reflexes are hyperactive, and **hypertonia,** in which tonic stretch reflexes are hyperactive.

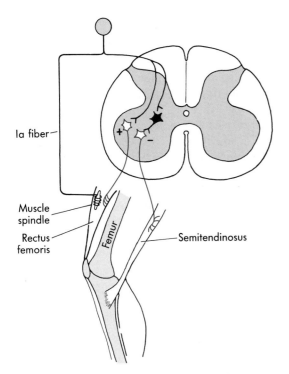

■ **Fig. 12-11**   Reflex arc of the stretch reflex. The interneuron shown in black is a group Ia inhibitory interneuron.

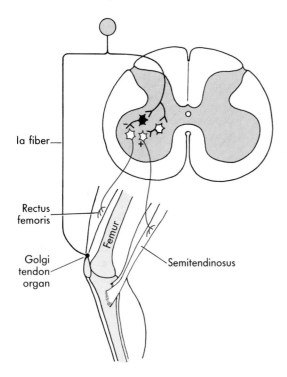

■ **Fig. 12-12**   Reflex arc of the inverse myotatic reflex. The interneurons include both excitatory *(clear)* and inhibitory *(black)* interneurons.

Testing with a reflex hammer is a common way for a physician to assess the level of excitability of spinal motor neurons. However, another approach is to stimulate the axons of group Ia fibers electrically and to examine changes in the reflex responses to a synchronous volley in muscle spindle afferent fibers. The reflex can be monitored objectively by **electromyography.** The monosynaptic reflex elicited by stimulating the tibial nerve at the popliteal fossa and recording from the triceps surae muscles is called an **H reflex** (for Hoffmann).

Inverse Myotatic Reflex

Activation of Golgi tendon organs has a reflex effect that seems to oppose the stretch reflex (it actually complements the stretch reflex, as discussed in the next paragraph). This reflex is called the **inverse myotatic reflex,** and its reflex arc is shown in Fig. 12-12. In this reflex, the receptor organs are Golgi tendon organs located in the rectus femoris muscle. The afferent fibers branch as they enter the spinal cord and end on interneurons. There are no monosynaptic connections to α motor neurons. Rather, the Golgi tendon organ pathway involves inhibitory interneurons that inhibit α motor neurons supplying the rectus femoris muscle and excitatory interneurons responsible for activating α motor neurons to the antagonistic hamstring muscles. Thus, the organization

of the inverse myotatic reflex is opposite to that of the stretch reflexes, which explains the name given to this reflex. However, the function of this reflex actually complements that of the stretch reflex. The Golgi tendon organs monitor force in the tendons that they supply. If, during maintained posture, such as standing at attention, the rectus femoris muscle begins to fatigue, the force in the patellar tendon will decline. The decline in force will reduce the activity of Golgi tendon organs in this tendon. Because these receptors normally inhibit the α motor neurons to the rectus femoris muscle, reduced activity of the Golgi tendon organs will enhance the excitability of the α motor neurons and increase the force. A coordinated reflex change will then occur, involving both muscle spindle and Golgi tendon organ afferent fibers, that causes a greater contraction of the rectus femoris muscle and maintenance of the posture.

When reflexes are hyperactive, it may be possible to demonstrate a **clasp-knife reflex.** When a joint is passively bent, resistance to the passive movement initially increases. However, if bending continues, the resistance suddenly decreases and the joint movement is readily completed. This change is caused by reflex inhibition. The clasp-knife reflex was once attributed to the activation of Golgi tendon organs, because these receptors were initially thought to have a high threshold to muscle stretch. However, it is now thought that the clasp-knife reflex is caused by activation of other high-threshold muscle receptors that supply the fascia around the muscle.

Flexion Reflexes

The afferent limb of flexion reflexes is furnished by a variety of sensory receptors called the **flexion reflex afferents (FRAs).** In flexion reflexes, afferent volleys (1) cause excitatory interneurons to activate α motor neurons that supply flexor muscles in the ipsilateral (same) limb and (2) cause inhibitory interneurons to prevent the activation of α motor neurons that supply the antagonistic extensor muscles (Fig. 12-13). This pattern of activity causes one or more joints to flex. In addition, commissural interneurons evoke the opposite pattern of activity in the contralateral (opposite) side of the spinal cord. This opposite pattern results in extension of the muscle, which is called the **crossed extension reflex.** The contralateral effect helps in maintaining balance.

There are several different types of flexion reflexes, although they produce similar patterns of muscle contraction. An important part of locomotion is the flexion phase, which involves a pattern of muscle contraction that can be regarded as a flexion reflex. This reflex is controlled predominantly by a neural circuit, called the **locomotor pattern generator,** in the spinal cord. However, afferent input can alter the locomotor pattern so that it can adapt to moment-by-moment changes in the terrain.

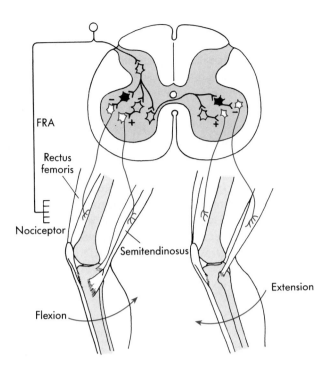

■ **Fig. 12-13** Reflex arc of the flexor reflex. Black interneurons are inhibitory and clear ones are excitatory. *FRA,* Flexion reflex afferent.

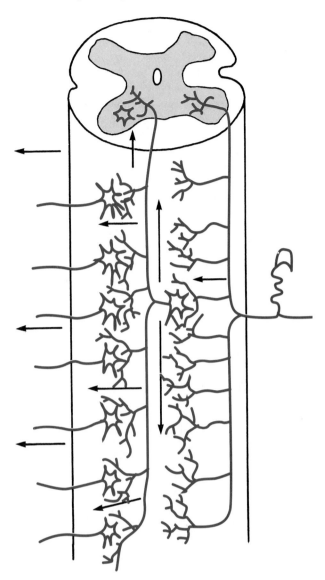

■ **Fig. 12-14** Drawing showing the divergence of the FRA pathways in the spinal cord. (Redrawn with permission from Eyzaguirre C, Fidone SJ: *Physiology of the nervous system,* ed 2, Chicago, 1975, Mosby–Year Book; slightly modified from Cajal SR: *Histologie du système nerveux,* Paris, 1909, Maloine.)

The most powerful flexion reflex is the **flexor withdrawal reflex.** This takes precedence over other reflexes, including those associated with locomotion, presumably because flexor withdrawal protects the limb from further damage. This reflex can readily be observed in a dog that holds a hurt paw away from the ground while walking. Nociceptors form the afferent limb of this reflex.

In the flexor withdrawal reflex, a strong noxious stimulus results in the withdrawal of the limb from the stimulus. In Fig. 12-13, the neural circuit of the flexion reflex is shown for neurons that affect only the knee joint. Actually, however, considerable divergence of the primary afferent and interneuronal pathways occurs in the flexion reflex (Fig. 12-14); in fact, all the major joints of a limb (e.g., hip, knee, ankle) may be involved in a strong flexor withdrawal reflex. The details of the operation of the flexor withdrawal reflex vary, depending on the nature and location of the stimulus. Fig. 12-15 shows differences in the amount of flexion at the hip, knee, and ankle that occur when different nerves of the hindlimb are stimulated electrically. This variability of the flexion reflex is called the **local sign.** Flexor withdrawal reflexes also occur in areas other than the limbs; for example, visceral disease may cause contractions of the muscles in the chest wall or abdomen, thereby decreasing the mobility of the trunk.

■ *Comparison of the Stretch and Flexion Reflexes*

The flexion reflexes have a number of properties that differ strikingly from those of the stretch reflex. These differences are listed in Table 12-1.

The stretch reflex is activated by stimulation of group Ia (and II) muscle spindle afferent fibers. It has a short latency because the excitation is monosynaptic. The afferent pathway shows some divergence because it affects all the α motor neurons that supply the muscle, plus some of those that supply synergistic muscles. In addition, the pathway activates inhibitory interneurons to antagonistic α motor neurons, an example of reciprocal innervation. The stretch reflex terminates when the afferent volley ceases, and it exerts a graded, specific, and discrete control over the muscles that operate across a joint, such as the knee or the ankle.

In contrast, the flexion reflex can be evoked by a variety of receptor types supplied by the FRAs. The latency is long, because the reflex arc is polysynaptic. Substantial divergence occurs in the reflex pathway, which may involve interneurons that influence α motor neurons supplying muscles at all the joints of a limb. In addition, the reflex can activate extensor motor neurons of the opposite limb. Thus, the flexion reflex involves double reciprocal innervation. The reflex is nonlinear. Weak stimuli have little or no effect, but when stimuli of a certain level of intensity are reached, a powerful flexor withdrawal reflex may be elicited that dominates other reflexes. The flexion may persist long after the stimulus ends, presumably because of afterdischarges of interneurons in the reflex arc.

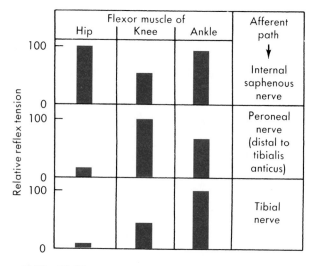

■ **Fig. 12-15**   Variations in the amount of flexion at the hip, knee, and ankle produced by electrical stimulation of nerves innervating different parts of the hindlimb. These variations are called the **local sign.** (Redrawn from Patton HD: *Reflex regulation of movement and posture.* In Ruch T, Patton HD, editors: *Physiology and biophysics,* vol IV, Philadelphia, 1982, WB Saunders.)

■ *Principles of Spinal Organization*

As discussed in relation to the stretch and especially the flexion reflex, divergence is an important aspect of reflex pathways (Fig. 12-14). Convergence is another important organizational feature of reflex arcs. **Convergence** is defined as the termination of several neurons on another neuron. For example, all the group Ia afferent fibers from the muscle spindles of a particular hindlimb muscle have convergent monosynaptic terminals on a given α motor neuron to that muscle. This convergent input accounts for the phenomenon of **spatial facilitation** in the stretch reflex. As we have noted, the flexion reflex, in contrast, displays considerable divergence. A variety of receptors are supplied in this arc, and different afferent inputs can trigger it (Fig. 12-15). This variability (the local sign) allows the reflex to withdraw the limb from a noxious stimulus. Only slight variations in the location of the stimulus may alter the nature of the withdrawal response.

An example of spatial facilitation is shown in Fig. 12-16. In this experiment, monosynaptic reflex is elicited by electrical stimulation of the group Ia fibers in each of two branches of a muscle nerve (Fig. 12-16, *A*). The reflex is characterized by recording the discharges of α motor axons from the appropriate ventral root. When muscle nerve branch A is stimulated, a small compound action potential is recorded as reflex A. Similarly, when muscle nerve branch B is stimulated, reflex B is recorded. These reflex discharges have a low electrical threshold because the group Ia fibers in the muscle nerve are large axons. Also, the latency of the reflex discharge is short, because the reflex pathway is monosynaptic and the conduction velocities of the afferent and motor axons are high.

Figure 12-16, *B* depicts the motor neurons contained within the motor nucleus. The medium-colored teardrop shapes enclose the α motor neurons that are activated when each muscle nerve branch is stimulated separately. Thus, two α motor neurons are activated when each muscle nerve branch is stimulated separately. When the two nerves are stimulated at the same time, a much larger reflex is recorded (see graph at right of Fig. 12-16, *B*). As the figure demonstrates, this reflex represents the discharges of seven α motor neurons. Thus, three additional α motor neurons (shown in the dark-colored teardrop) are

■ **Table 12-1**   Comparison of the stretch and flexion reflexes

	Stretch reflex	*Flexion reflex*
Afferent limb	Group Ia (and II) muscle spindle afferents	FRA
Latency	Short (monosynaptic)	Long (polysynaptic)
Divergence	Some	Widespread
Target muscle	Same and synergists of same side	Flexor muscles on same side; extensor muscles on opposite side
Reciprocal innervation	Yes	Yes (double)
Linearity	Linear	Nonlinear
Duration	Same as stimulus	May persist because of afterdischarges
Specificity	Specific to set of muscles	Less specific, involves many muscles

activated when the two muscle nerves are stimulated simultaneously.

The explanation for this spatial summation is that all the α motor neurons to the muscle are excited by either muscle afferent volley. However, when only one nerve is stimulated, the excitation is powerful enough to activate only two motor neurons. These motor neurons are located in the **discharge zone** (medium-colored area), whereas those that are excited, but not enough to reach threshold, are located in the **subliminal fringe** (lightly colored area). However, the combined excitation produced by simulta-

neous volleys in the two nerves reaches threshold in three additional motor neurons (facilitation zone), and a reflex discharge occurs in a total of seven motor neurons.

A similar effect could be elicited by repetitive stimulation of one of the muscle nerves, provided that the stimuli occur close enough together so that some of the excitatory effect of the first volley still persists after the second volley arrives. This effect is called **temporal summation.** Both spatial and temporal summation depend on the properties of the excitatory postsynaptic potentials evoked by the group Ia afferent fibers in α motor neurons (see Chapter 4).

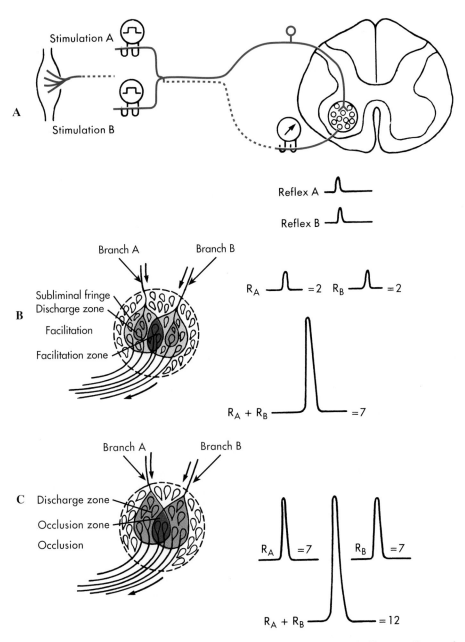

■ **Fig. 12-16** **A,** The arrangement for using electrically evoked afferent volleys and recordings from motor axons in a ventral root to study reflexes. **B,** An experiment in which combined stimulation of two muscle nerves resulted in spatial summation. In **C** the combined volleys caused occlusion. (Redrawn with permission from Eyzaguirre C, Fidone SJ: *Physiology of the nervous system,* ed 2, Chicago, 1975, Mosby–Year Book.)

The number of α motor neurons that supply each muscle is limited, and not all can be activated even by a large peripheral input. For these reasons, the availability of motor neurons for summation is limited. If a volley in one of the two muscle nerves of Fig. 12-16 reaches the motor nucleus at a time when the motor neurons are highly excitable, the reflex discharge will be relatively large (Fig. 12-16, *C*). A similar volley in the other muscle nerve might also produce a large reflex response. However, when the two muscle nerves are excited simultaneously, the reflex may be less than the sum of the two independently evoked reflexes. In this case, each muscle nerve activates seven α motor neurons, but the volleys in the two nerves together cause only twelve motor neurons to discharge. This phenomenon is called **occlusion.**

Reflex testing by the techniques described to demonstrate spatial and temporal summation and occlusion can also be used to demonstrate **inhibition.** A monosynaptic reflex discharge can be evoked (Fig. 12-16) by stimulating the group Ia afferent fibers in a muscle nerve. Evoking a monosynaptic reflex discharge in this way tests the reflex excitability of a population of α motor neurons. The discharges of either extensor or flexor α motor neurons can be recorded by choosing the proper muscle nerve to be stimulated. Other kinds of afferent fibers can also be stimulated. For example, stimulation of the group Ia afferent fibers in the nerve to the antagonist muscles produces **reciprocal inhibition.** If the small afferent fibers of a cutaneous nerve are stimulated to evoke a flexion reflex, the α motor neurons to extensor muscles are inhibited (and those to flexor muscles excited). Stimulation of a ventral root causes the excitation of inhibitory interneurons called **Renshaw cells** by way of the recurrent collaterals of α motor axons (Fig. 12-17). The Renshaw cells inhibit monosynaptic reflexes (and also group Ia inhibitory interneurons) and produce recurrent inhibition (or facilitation).

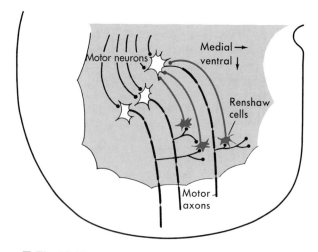

■ **Fig. 12-17**   Recurrent inhibitory pathway. (Redrawn from Eccles JC: *The physiology of synapses,* New York, 1964, Academic Press.)

Reflex testing of this kind has been used to determine the circuitry involved in the various reflexes described in this chapter. As mentioned earlier, similar reflex testing can be done in human subjects, using the H reflex as a test of the excitability of α motor neurons.

■ *Summary*

1. Transection of the spinal cord reveals the reflexes that depend only on spinal cord circuits. These include the stretch reflex and the flexion reflex.

2. Muscle spindles are complex sensory receptors found in muscle. They lie parallel to regular muscle fibers, and they contain nuclear bag and nuclear chain intrafusal muscle fibers. Group Ia afferent fibers form primary endings on nuclear bag and chain fibers, and group II fibers form secondary endings on nuclear chain fibers. Dynamic γ motor axons end on nuclear bag fibers and static γ motor axons on nuclear chain fibers.

3. Primary endings demonstrate both static and dynamic responses, which signal muscle length and rate of change in muscle length. Secondary endings demonstrate only static responses and signal only muscle length. γ Motor neurons cause muscle spindles to shorten, which prevents the unloading effect of muscle contraction.

4. Golgi tendon organs are located in the tendons of muscles and are arranged in series. They are supplied by group Ib afferent fibers and are excited both by stretch and by contraction of the muscle.

5. Reflexes are simple, stereotyped motor responses to a stimulus. A reflex arc includes the afferent fibers, interneurons, and motor neurons responsible for the reflex. The reflex arcs of many reflexes are located in the spinal cord or brainstem.

6. The stretch reflex includes (1) a monosynaptic excitatory pathway from group Ia (and II) muscle spindle afferent fibers to α motor neurons that supply the same and synergistic muscles and (2) a disynaptic inhibitory pathway to antagonistic motor neurons. Phasic stretch reflexes are triggered by the dynamic responses of group Ia fibers, and tonic stretch reflexes are triggered by the static responses of group Ia and II afferents.

7. The inverse myotatic reflex is evoked by Golgi tendon organs. Afferent volleys from a given muscle cause a disynaptic inhibition of α motor neurons to the same muscle, and they excite antagonist muscles. However, because Golgi tendon organs monitor force, their reflex action actually complements that of the stretch reflex.

8. The flexion reflex is evoked by volleys in flexion reflex afferent fibers that supply various receptors, including nociceptors. In the flexion reflex, ipsilateral flexor motor neurons are excited and extensor motor neu-

rons are inhibited through polysynaptic pathways. The opposite pattern may occur contralaterally. Locomotion has a flexion component. The flexor withdrawal reflex is another, more powerful, form of the flexion reflex. The flexor withdrawal reflex varies somewhat with the location of the stimulus (local sign).

9. Spinal reflexes can be studied by electrically stimulating the afferent fibers in nerves and recording volleys in α motor axons from ventral roots. Principles of reflex organization that are derived from such studies include spatial and temporal summation, occlusion, and various patterns of inhibition.

■ Self-Study Problems

1. After an acute, complete spinal cord transection, there is a period of spinal shock, and then a maintained state of altered spinal cord function. What changes are characteristic of chronic paraplegia?

2. Describe the innervation of the muscle spindle, and contrast the response properties of the two types of sensory endings and the actions of the two types of motor endings.

3. What do muscle spindles and Golgi tendon organs signal?

4. What are the phasic and tonic stretch reflexes, and how are these used clinically?

5. What is a flexion reflex?

■ Bibliography

Journal articles

Atkinson PP, Atkinson JL: Spinal shock, *Mayo Clin Proc* 71:384, 1996.

Banks RW: The motor innervation of mammalian muscle spindles, *Prog Neurobiol* 43:323, 1994.

Boyd IA: The isolated mammalian muscle spindle, *Trends Neurosci* 3:258, 1980.

Davidoff RA: Skeletal muscle tone and the misunderstood stretch reflex, *Neurology* 42:951, 1992.

Grillner S, Wallen P: Central pattern generators for locomotion, with special reference to vertebrates, *Annu Rev Neurosci* 8:233, 1985.

Rhoney DH, Luer MS, Hughes M, Hatton J: New pharmacologic approaches to acute spinal cord injury, *Pharmacotherapy* 16:382, 1996.

Sherrington CS: Flexion-reflex of the limb, crossed extension-reflex, and reflex stepping and standing, *J Physiol* 40:28, 1910.

Swett JE, Schoultz TW: Mechanical transduction in the Golgi tendon organ: a hypothesis, *Arch Ital Biol* 113:374, 1975.

Van Gijn J: The Babinski reflex, *Postgrad Med J* 71:645, 1995.

Books and monographs

Baldissera F, Hultborn H, Illert M: *Integration in spinal neuronal systems.* In Brooks VB, editor: *Handbook of physiology,* sect 1, *The nervous system,* vol II, *Motor control,* part 1, Bethesda, Md, 1981, American Physiological Society, p 509.

Binder MD, Mendell LM: *The segmental motor system,* New York, 1990, Oxford University Press.

Brooks VB: *The neural basis of motor control,* New York, 1986, Oxford University Press.

Houk JC, Rymer WZ: *Neural control of muscle length and tension.* In Brooks VB, editor: *Handbook of physiology,* sect 1, *The nervous system,* vol II, *Motor control,* part 1, Bethesda, Md, 1981, American Physiological Society, p 257.

Matthews PBC: *Muscle spindles: their messages and their fusimotor supply.* In Brooks VB, editor: *Handbook of physiology,* sect 1, *The nervous system,* vol II, *Motor control,* part 1, Bethesda, Md, 1981, American Physiological Society, p 189.

Sherrington CS: *The integrative action of the nervous system,* ed 2, New Haven, Conn, 1947, Yale University Press.

Stein RB, Lee RG: *Tremor and clonus.* In Brooks VB, editor: *Handbook of physiology,* sect 1, *The nervous system,* vol II, *Motor control,* part 1, Bethesda, Md, 1981, American Physiological Society, p 325.

Descending Pathways Involved in Motor Control

■ *Introduction: Topographic Organization of the Spinal Motor System and the Cranial Nerve Motor System*

As discussed in Chapter 7, spinal cord motor neurons are organized topographically in the ventral horn (see Fig. 7-11). Motor neurons that supply the axial musculature form a column of cells that extends the length of the spinal cord. In the cervical and lumbosacral enlargements, the cells are located in the most medial part of the ventral horn. Motor neurons that supply the limb muscles form columns that extend for one or two segments in the lateral part of the ventral horn in the cervical and lumbar enlargements. The motor neurons to the muscles of the distal limb are located most laterally, whereas those that innervate more proximal muscles are located more medially in the lateral ventral horn. Note that the α and γ motor neurons to a given muscle are found side by side in the same motor neuron column.

The interneurons that connect with the motor neurons in the enlargements are also topographically organized. In general, interneurons that supply the limb muscles are located mainly in the lateral parts of the deep dorsal horn and intermediate region, whereas those that supply the axial muscles are in the medial part of the ventral horn (Fig. 13-1). Because they receive synaptic connections from primary afferent fibers and from the axons of pathways that descend from the brain, many of these interneurons are found in spinal reflex arcs and in the descending motor control systems.

An important aspect of the interneuronal systems is that the laterally placed interneurons (those that supply the limb muscle) project ipsilaterally (i.e., on the same side) to motor neurons that supply the distal or the proximal limb muscles, whereas the medial motor neurons (those that supply axial muscles) project bilaterally (Fig. 13-1). This arrangement of the lateral interneurons allows

the limbs to be controlled independently. On the other hand, the bilateral arrangement of the medial motor neurons allows the axial muscles to provide postural support of the trunk and neck.

Fig. 13-2 shows some of the sites in the reflex circuitry that can be influenced by descending motor control pathways. Descending pathways can synapse on interneurons that cause presynaptic inhibition of primary afferent fibers or that participate in postsynaptic excitation or inhibition of other interneurons or of motor neurons. In addition, some descending pathways make direct excitatory connections to α or γ motor neurons.

A similar arrangement is found in cranial nerve motor nuclei. Most of the cranial nerve motor nuclei are similar to the axial motor nuclei of the spinal cord in that they supply muscles near the midline. For example, facial motor neurons that supply the corrugator muscle of the forehead and the orbicularis oculi muscles, which close the eyes, must operate bilaterally (e.g., the blink reflex causes both eyelids to close simultaneously). The head muscles, which function like the distal limb muscles, control facial expression and the tongue. The motor neurons that supply these muscles function independently. Thus, neurons in the facial motor nuclei that supply the lower face can elicit unilateral changes in facial expression, and hypoglossal motor neurons can move the tongue toward one side. The interneuronal systems in the brainstem are organized like those in the spinal cord to support these bilateral or unilateral motor activities.

■ *Classification of Descending Motor Pathways*

■ *Pyramidal versus Extrapyramidal Pathways*

Descending motor pathways have traditionally been subdivided into the pyramidal tract and the extrapyramidal pathways. This terminology reflects the important clini-

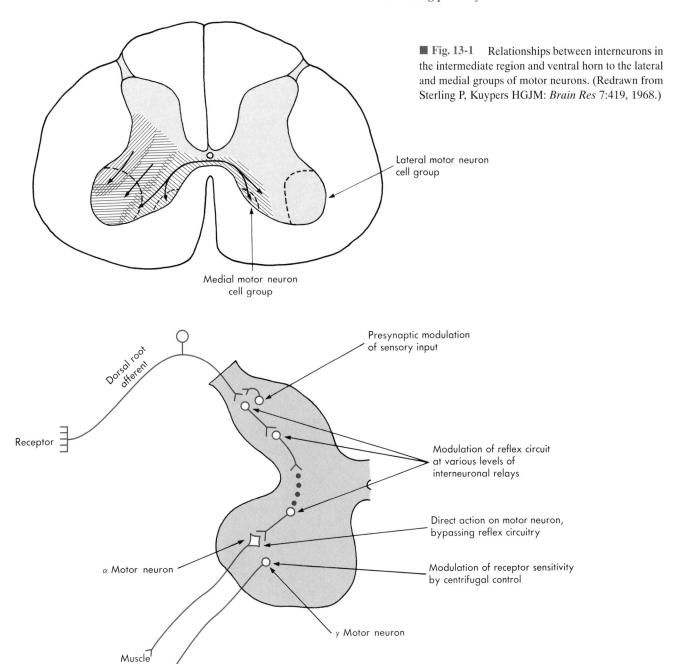

■ **Fig. 13-1** Relationships between interneurons in the intermediate region and ventral horn to the lateral and medial groups of motor neurons. (Redrawn from Sterling P, Kuypers HGJM: *Brain Res* 7:419, 1968.)

Lateral motor neuron cell group

Medial motor neuron cell group

Presynaptic modulation of sensory input

Dorsal root afferent

Receptor

Modulation of reflex circuit at various levels of interneuronal relays

Direct action on motor neuron, bypassing reflex circuitry

Modulation of receptor sensitivity by centrifugal control

α Motor neuron

γ Motor neuron

Muscle

Muscle spindle

■ **Fig. 13-2** Sites in a spinal reflex arc that are potential targets for descending motor control pathways.

cal dichotomy between pyramidal tract disease and extrapyramidal disease. In **pyramidal tract disease,** the corticospinal tract is interrupted. The signs of this disease were originally attributed to the loss of function of the pyramidal tract (so named because the corticospinal tract passes through the medullary pyramid). However, in many cases of pyramidal tract disease, the functions of other pathways are also altered, and pyramidal tract signs are not necessarily caused only by the loss of the corticospinal tract (see p 203).

The term **extrapyramidal** is even more problematic. The extrapyramidal tracts presumably include all descending motor pathways except the pyramidal tract. The term **extrapyramidal disease** generally signifies one of several diseases of the basal ganglia. However, the main motor pathway involved in basal ganglion diseases is the corticospinal tract (see Chapter 14). Other extrapyramidal motor pathways, such as the reticulospinal tract, play prominent roles in cerebellar and other motor disorders, as well as in basal ganglion disease. Because the basis of the pyramidal versus extrapyramidal classification system for the descending pathway is not clear, this classification is not used in this textbook.

■ *Lateral versus Medial Motor Systems*

Another way of classifying the motor pathways is based on their sites of termination in the spinal cord and on the consequent differences in their control of manipulation and posture. The **lateral pathways** are those that terminate directly on motor neurons or on the interneuronal groups in the lateral parts of the spinal cord gray matter

(Fig. 13-3). They excite motor neurons directly and influence reflex arcs that control the fine movements of the distal limbs as well as those that activate supporting musculature in the proximal limbs. The **medial pathways** end in the medial ventral horn on the medial group of interneurons (Fig. 13-3). These interneurons connect with motor neurons that control the axial musculature bilaterally and thereby contribute to balance and posture.

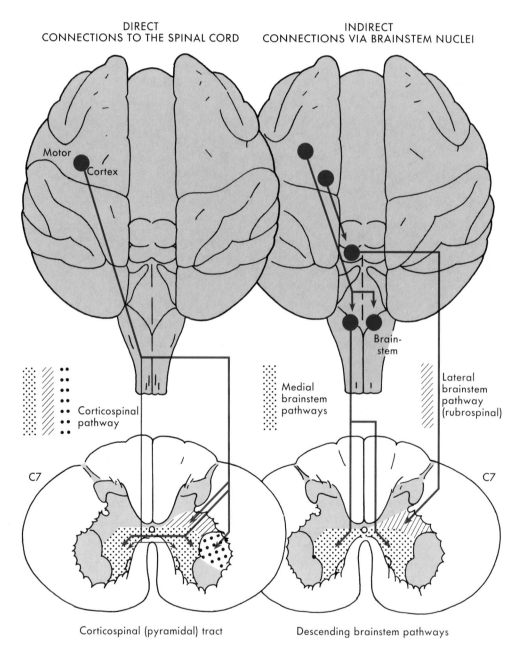

■ **Fig. 13-3**   Subdivision of the pathways descending from the cerebral cortex and brainstem to the spinal cord into a lateral and a medial system, based on the terminations of these pathways in the spinal cord gray matter. The lateral pathways end on motor neurons to distal muscles *(dots)* and interneurons projecting to these motor neurons *(hatched area)*. The medial pathways end on interneurons supplying motor neurons to the axial muscles *(stippled area)*. (Redrawn from Brinkman C: *Split-brain monkeys: cerebral control of contralateral and ipsilateral arm, hand, and finger movements*, doctoral dissertation, Rotterdam, The Netherlands, 1974, Erasmus University.)

They also contribute to the control of proximal limb muscles. In this textbook, we use the lateral/medial terminology to classify the descending motor pathways.

■ The Descending Motor Pathways

■ The Lateral System: Lateral Corticospinal Tract

The pathway that is most important for control of manipulative ability of the limbs in humans is the **lateral corticospinal tract** (Fig. 13-3). The ventral corticospinal tract belongs to the medial system (see p 205).

The **corticobulbar tract,** which projects to the cranial nerve motor nuclei, has subdivisions that are comparable with the lateral and ventral corticospinal tracts. One component of the corticobulbar tract ends in the part of the facial motor nucleus that innervates the muscles of facial expression in the lower face and in the hypoglossal nucleus that supplies the tongue muscles. This component of the corticobulbar tract is equivalent to the lateral corticospinal tract.

Organization of the lateral corticospinal and corticobulbar tracts. The corticospinal and corticobulbar tracts originate in a wide region of the cerebral cortex that includes the motor, premotor, and supplementary motor areas and the somatosensory cortex. The cells of origin of these tracts include both large and small pyramidal cells of layer V of the cortex and the giant pyramidal cells of Betz. Betz cells are a characteristic feature of the motor cortex.

In the most caudal region of the medulla, about 80% of the axons cross to the opposite side and then descend in the dorsal lateral funiculus as the lateral corticospinal tract. The remaining axons continue caudally in the ventral funiculus on the same side as the ventral corticospinal tract. The corticobulbar tract terminates in the brainstem at a level near target nuclei. Part of the corticobulbar tract ends contralaterally (i.e., on the opposite side) in the part of the facial nucleus that supplies muscles of the lower face and in the hypoglossal nucleus. This component of the corticobulbar tract is organized like the lateral corticospinal tract. The remainder of the corticobulbar tract ends bilaterally, and in this respect is organized like the ventral corticospinal tract.

Motor areas. The corticospinal projections from the motor and sensory areas of the cerebral cortex terminate in different parts of the spinal cord gray matter. The motor areas project to the intermediate region and ventral horn (Fig. 13-4), whereas the sensory areas project to the dorsal horn. Some motor area projections that descend in the lateral corticospinal tract terminate directly on motor neurons, while others terminate on interneurons of the lateral group (Fig. 13-4). The ventral corticospinal tract, on the other hand, ends bilaterally on the medial group of interneurons.

The motor cortex has a topographic organization that parallels that of the somatosensory cortex (Fig. 13-5, *A* and see also Fig. 8-11). The face is represented laterally, near the lateral fissure; the hand is represented more medially on the convexity of the cerebrum; and the lower extremity is represented largely on the medial aspect of the hemisphere. The figurine in the illustration is called a **motor homunculus.** The distortion of the various body parts in the homunculus indicates approximately how much of the cortex is devoted to their motor control.

The other cortical motor areas also contain somatotopic representations. Fig. 13-5, *B* shows the motor areas of the cerebral cortex of a monkey. The somatotopic map of the motor cortex is shown along the precentral gyrus. Note how closely this map resembles that of the human shown in Fig. 13-5, *A*. Other somatotopic maps exist in the SII cortex, which is located in the cortex of the roof of the lateral fissure (part of which is shown in Fig. 13-5, *B*), and in the supplementary motor cortex, which is located on the medial aspect of the hemisphere just rostral to the motor cortex. Note that the digital representation in monkeys (and presumably humans) is nearer to the central sulcus, whereas the proximal limbs are represented more rostrally. This arrangement is significant. Anatomic studies have shown that the caudal part of the precentral gyrus projects to the dorsolateral region of the ventral horn, which contains motor neurons that supply the distal musculature of the extremities. The rostral part of the precentral gyrus, however, projects to the intermediate region, which contains interneurons of the lateral group. Thus, the caudal part of the motor cortex can directly

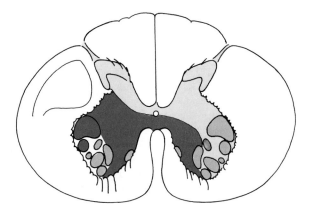

■ **Fig. 13-4** Region of termination of the part of the lateral and ventral corticospinal tracts that originates from the motor areas of the cerebral cortex. Part of the projection, that of the lateral corticospinal tract, is directly on motor neurons and part on the lateral interneurons. By contrast, the ventral corticospinal tract ends bilaterally on the medial interneurons. (Redrawn from Brinkman C: *Split-brain monkeys: cerebral control of contralateral and ipsilateral arm, hand, and finger movements,* doctoral dissertation, Rotterdam, The Netherlands, 1974, Erasmus University.)

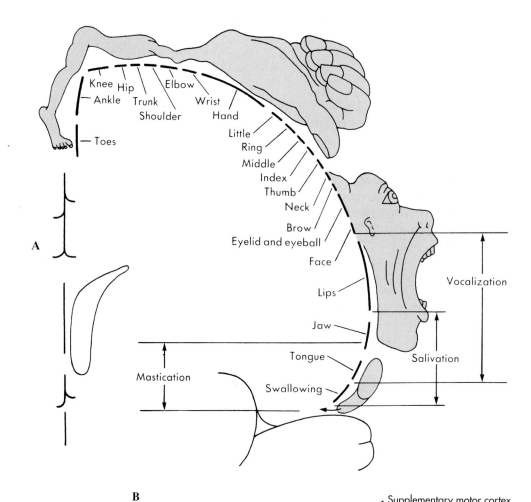

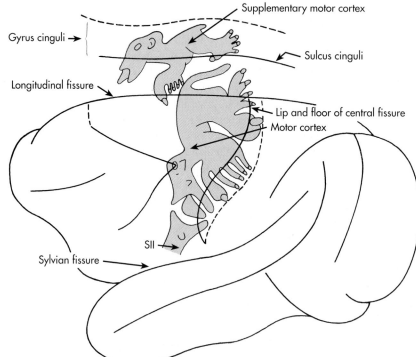

■ **Fig. 13-5**   Topographic organization of the motor cortex. **A,** The cortex is cut in a coronal section, and the somatotopic map of the body and face is shown as a "motor homunculus." The sizes of different body parts indicate the amount of cortex devoted to motor control of that part. **B,** The somatotopic organization of the motor cortex, supplementary motor cortex, and SII areas of the cerebral cortex of a monkey. (Redrawn from Eyzaguirre C, Fidone SJ: *Physiology of the nervous system,* ed 2, Chicago, 1975, Mosby–Year Book. **A** slightly modified from Penfield W, Rasmussen T: *The cerebral cortex of man,* New York, 1950, Macmillan; **B** slightly modified from Woolsey CN et al: *Res Publ Assoc Res Nerv Ment Dis* 30:238, 1952.)

influence the activity of motor neurons to the hand and digit muscles.

The motor cortex proper was first identified in electrical stimulation experiments. When an electrical stimulus is applied to the cerebral cortex, the lowest threshold points for a motor response are found to lie in the motor cortex. Such stimuli evoke discrete movements of distal muscles on the contralateral side. For example, when stimuli are applied in the face representation, the contralateral face moves; when the hand representation is stimulated, the contralateral hand moves.

The motor cortex has been explored in human patients undergoing surgery to remove scar tissue that had resulted in **posttraumatic epilepsy.** Often, resection of the scar cures the epilepsy. However, the surgeon must be careful not to damage normal areas of the motor cortex; such damage can paralyze the affected musculature.

The direct innervation of motor neurons by the lateral corticospinal tract can have important clinical consequences if this pathway is interrupted. The most important function lost after interruption of this pathway is fine control of the digits. Similarly, when the corticobulbar tract is interrupted, voluntary movements of the lower face and tongue are lost.

■ *The Medial System*

As already mentioned, the ventral corticospinal tract and much of the corticobulbar tract can be regarded as medial system pathways. These tracts end on the medial group of interneurons in the spinal cord and on equivalent medial system neurons in the brainstem. The axial muscles are controlled by these pathways. These muscles often contract bilaterally to provide postural support or some other bilateral function, such as chewing or wrinkling of the brow.

Other medial system pathways originate in the brainstem. Some of these pathways include the lateral and medial vestibulospinal tracts, the pontine and medullary reticulospinal tracts, and the tectospinal tract.

Lateral and medial vestibulospinal tracts. The lateral vestibulospinal tract originates from the lateral vestibular nucleus (Fig. 13-6, *A*). This nucleus has a somatotopic organization (Fig. 13-6, *B*). The lateral vestibulospinal tract descends ipsilaterally through the brainstem, then down the ventral funiculus of the spinal cord; it ends on interneurons of the medial group (Fig. 13-6, *A* and *C*). The lateral vestibulospinal tract excites motor neurons that supply proximal postural muscles. The sensory input to the lateral vestibular nucleus comes from both the semicircular ducts and the otolith organs in the ear. An important function of the lateral vestibulospinal tract is to assist with postural adjustments after

angular and linear accelerations of the head. In animals that have undergone decerebration (transection of the midbrain), the lateral vestibulospinal tract becomes hyperactive, presumably because of the loss of descending inhibitory controls. This hyperactivity is largely responsible for the extensor hypertonus seen in decerebrate animals.

The medial vestibulospinal tract originates from the medial vestibular nucleus (Fig. 13-7). It descends in the ventral funiculus of the spinal cord to cervical and midthoracic levels and ends on the medial group of interneurons (Fig. 13-6, *C*). The sensory input to the medial vestibular nucleus from the labyrinth comes chiefly from the semicircular ducts. This pathway thus mediates adjustments in head position in response to angular accelerations of the head.

The pontine and medullary reticulospinal tracts. The cells that give rise to the pontine reticulospinal tract are located in the medial pontine reticular formation. This tract descends in the ipsilateral ventral funiculus and ends on the medial group of interneurons (Fig. 13-8, *A*). Its function, like that of the lateral vestibulospinal tract, is to excite motor neurons to the proximal extensor muscles to support posture.

The medullary reticulospinal tracts arise from neurons of the medial medulla. The tracts descend bilaterally in the ventral lateral funiculus and end primarily on the medial group of interneurons, although some also end on lateral interneurons (Fig. 13-8, *B*). The function of the pathway is largely inhibitory. Some of the inhibitory connections end directly on motor neurons.

The tectospinal tract. The tectospinal tract originates in the deep layers of the superior colliculus (see Fig. 9-24). The axons cross to the contralateral side just below the periaqueductal gray matter, and they descend in the ventral funiculus of the spinal cord to terminate on the medial group of interneurons in the upper cervical spinal cord. The tectospinal tract regulates contralateral movements of the head in response to visual, auditory, and somatic stimuli.

■ *Monoaminergic Pathways*

In addition to the lateral and medial systems, less specifically organized systems descend from the brainstem to the spinal cord. These include several pathways that use monoamines as synaptic transmitters.

The locus caeruleus and the nucleus subcaeruleus are located in the upper pons and are composed of norepinephrine-containing neurons. These nuclei project widely to the spinal cord through the lateral funiculi, and they terminate on interneurons and motor neurons. The dominant effect of the pathway is inhibitory.

The raphe nuclei of the medulla give rise to several raphe-spinal projections to the spinal cord. Many of the raphe-spinal cells contain serotonin. Terminals on dorsal

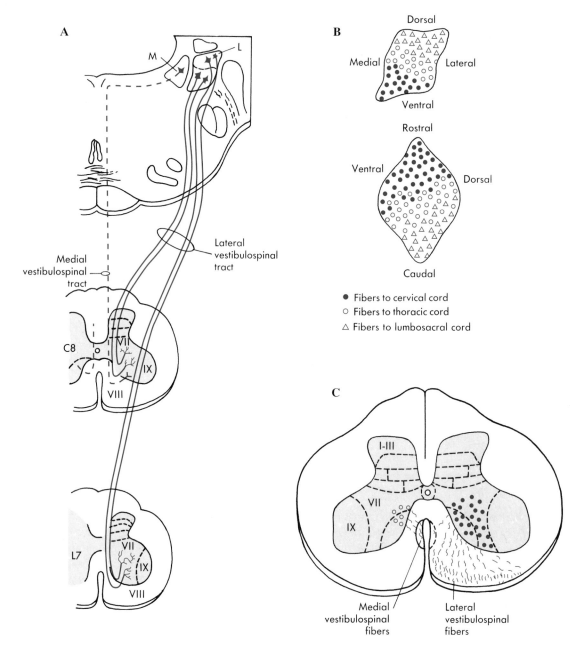

■ **Fig. 13-6**   Organization of the vestibulospinal tract of the cat. **A,** The projection from the lateral vestibulospinal tract. **B,** The somatotopic organization of the lateral vestibular nucleus. **C,** The zone of termination on the medial group of interneurons. The termination of the medial vestibulospinal tract is also shown. *M,* Medial; *L,* lateral. (Redrawn from Brodal A: *Neurological anatomy,* ed 3, New York, 1981, Oxford University Press.)

horn interneurons are inhibitory, whereas terminals on motor neurons are excitatory. The dorsal horn projection may inhibit nociceptive transmission, whereas the ventral horn projection may enhance motor activity.

In general, the monoaminergic pathways may alter the responsiveness of spinal cord circuits, including the reflex arcs. In this respect, they would cause widespread changes in excitability rather than produce discrete movements or specific changes in behavior.

A common cause of motor disorder in human patients is interruption of the corticospinal tract as it traverses the internal capsule; such interruptions occur in capsular strokes. The resultant disorder is often termed a **pyramidal tract syndrome** or **upper motor neuron disease.** The motor changes characteristic of this disorder include (1) increased phasic and tonic stretch reflexes (spasticity); (2) weakness, usually of the distal muscles, especially the finger muscles; (3) patho-

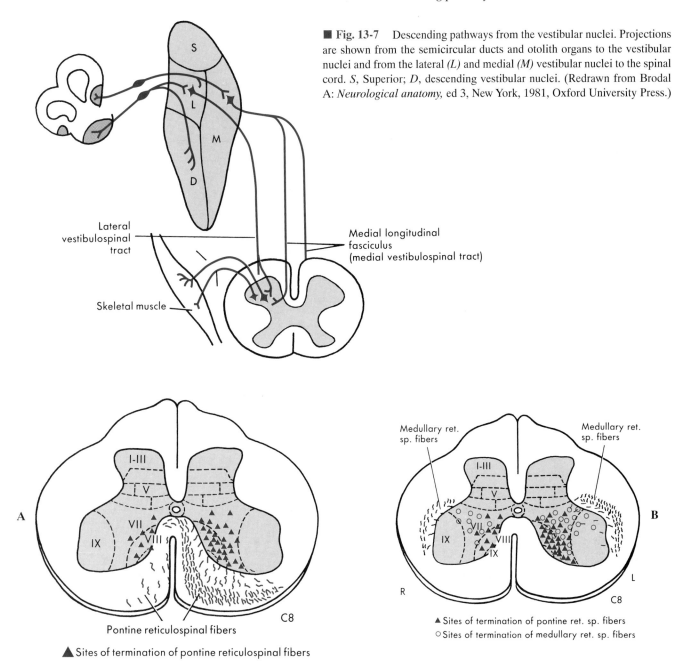

■ **Fig. 13-7** Descending pathways from the vestibular nuclei. Projections are shown from the semicircular ducts and otolith organs to the vestibular nuclei and from the lateral *(L)* and medial *(M)* vestibular nuclei to the spinal cord. *S,* Superior; *D,* descending vestibular nuclei. (Redrawn from Brodal A: *Neurological anatomy,* ed 3, New York, 1981, Oxford University Press.)

▲ Sites of termination of pontine reticulospinal fibers

▲ Sites of termination of pontine ret. sp. fibers
○ Sites of termination of medullary ret. sp. fibers

■ **Fig. 13-8** **A,** Course and terminations of the pontine reticulospinal tract. **B,** Course and terminations of the medullary reticulospinal tracts; the terminations of the pontine reticulospinal tract are also indicated. (Redrawn from Brodal A: *Neurological anatomy,* ed 3, New York, 1981, Oxford University Press.)

logical reflexes, including the **sign of Babinski** (dorsiflexion of the big toe and fanning of the other toes when the sole of the foot is stroked); and (4) a reduction in superficial reflexes, such as the abdominal and cremasteric reflexes. However, if only the corticospinal tract is interrupted, as can occur with a lesion of the medullary pyramid, most of these signs are absent. In this situation, the most prominent deficits are weakness of the distal muscles, especially of the fingers, and a positive sign of Babinski. Spasticity does not occur, but muscle tone decreases. Evidently,

spasticity depends on disordered function of the corticospinal tract and other pathways, such as the reticulospinal tracts.

The effects of interruption of the medial system pathways are quite different from those produced by corticospinal tract lesions. The main deficits of medial system interruption are an initial reduction in the tone of postural muscles and loss of righting reflexes (see p 208). Long-term effects include locomotion impairment and frequent falling. However, manual manipulation of objects is perfectly normal.

■ *Brainstem Control of Posture and Movement*

The importance of pathways that originate in the brainstem in motor control is evident from observations of the extensor hypertonus and the increased phasic stretch reflexes that occur in decerebrate animals (see Chapter 12). Particular brainstem systems have been identified that influence posture, locomotion, and eye movements.

■ *Postural Reflexes*

Several reflex mechanisms are evoked when the head is moved or the neck is bent. There are three types of postural reflexes: vestibular reflexes, tonic neck reflexes, and righting reflexes. The sensory receptors responsible for these reflexes include the vestibular apparatus, which is stimulated by head movements, and stretch receptors in the neck.

The **vestibular reflexes** constitute one class of postural reflexes. Rotation of the head activates sensory receptors of the semicircular ducts (see Chapter 10). In addition to eye movements (see p 209), the sensory input to the vestibular nuclei results in postural adjustments. These adjustments are mediated by commands transmitted to the spinal cord through the lateral and medial vestibulospinal tracts and the reticulospinal tracts. The lateral vestibulospinal tract activates extensor muscles that support posture. For instance, if the head is rotated to the left, the postural support is increased on the left side. This increased support prevents the subject from falling to the left as the head rotation continues. Any disease that eliminates labyrinthine function in the left ear will cause the affected person to tend to fall to the left. Conversely, any disease that irritates the left labyrinth will cause the affected person to tend to fall to the right. The medial vestibulospinal tract is responsible for contractions of neck muscles that oppose the induced movement **(vestibulocollic reflex).**

Tilting the head changes linear acceleration and activates the otolith organs of the vestibular apparatus. This activation can produce eye movements (see p 209) and postural adjustments. For example, tilting the head and body forward (without bending the neck and consequently without evoking the tonic neck reflexes) in a quadruped, such as a cat, results in extension of the forelimbs and flexion of the hindlimbs. The vestibular action tends to restore the body toward its original posture. Conversely, if the head and body are tilted backward (without bending the neck), the forelimbs flex and the hindlimbs extend. Otolithic organs also contribute to the **vestibular placing reaction.** If an animal, such as a cat, is dropped, stimulation of the utricles leads to extension of the forelimbs in preparation for landing.

The **tonic neck reflexes** are another type of positional reflex. These reflexes are activated by the muscle spindles found in the neck muscles. These muscles contain the largest concentration of muscle spindles of any muscle in the body. If the neck is bent (without tilting the head), the neck muscle spindles evoke the tonic neck reflexes without interference from the vestibular system. When the neck is extended relative to the body, the forelimbs extend and the hindlimbs flex (Fig. 13-9). The opposite effects occur when the neck is flexed. Note that these effects are the opposite of those evoked by the vestibular system. Furthermore, if the neck is bent to the left, the extensor muscles in the limbs on the left contract more and the flexor muscles in the limbs on the right side relax.

The third class of postural reflexes are the **righting reflexes.** These reflexes tend to restore an altered position of the head and body toward normal. The receptors responsible for righting reflexes include the vestibular apparatus, the neck stretch receptors, and mechanoreceptors of the body wall.

■ *Locomotion*

The spinal cord contains neural circuits that serve as a pattern generator for locomotion. There are actually several pattern generators, one for each limb involved in locomotion. These separate pattern generators permit independent movements of the limb. However, all these pattern generators are interconnected to ensure coordination of limb movements. The pattern generator for locomotion is an example of a biologic oscillator. Similar oscillators are responsible for such activities as scratching, chewing, and respiration.

The pattern generator for locomotion is normally activated by commands that descend from the brain. The **midbrain locomotor center** is thought to organize commands to initiate locomotion. Voluntary activity that originates in the motor cortex can trigger locomotion by the action of corticobulbar fibers on the midbrain locomotor center. The commands are relayed through the pontomedullary reticular formation via the reticulospinal tracts. Locomotion is also influenced by afferent activity. The afferent influence ensures that the pattern generator adapts to changes in the terrain as locomotion proceeds. Such changes may occur rapidly during running, and locomotion must then be adjusted to ensure proper coordination.

An important requirement for locomotion is adequate postural support. This support is normally provided by the postural muscles in response to activity in the reticulospinal tract. Immediately after transection of the spinal cord, postural activity is lost during spinal shock. In humans, locomotion is not recovered even after spinal shock resolves. However, some locomotion is possible in animals with spinal transection, especially if some postural support is provided by stimulation of afferent fibers or by pharmacologic activation of spinal cord interneuronal circuits.

■ *Control of Eye Position*

The position of the eyes is controlled by several neural systems. **Conjugate eye movements** (movements of both eyes in the same direction and amount) are controlled by the vestibulo-ocular reflex and by the optokinetic, saccadic, and pursuit movement systems. The eyes can also converge or diverge under the control of the vergence system.

Vestibulo-ocular reflex. The vestibulo-ocular reflex is designed to maintain a stable image on the retina during rapid head rotation. This reflex causes the eyes to move simultaneously in the direction opposite to, and in an amount equal to, head movement.

Optokinetic reflex. The optokinetic reflex is another means by which the nervous system compensates for head movements to maintain a visual target. This reflex maintains a stable image when head movements are slow, and the sensory input for the reflex is provided by the visual system. The optokinetic system can be activated by having a subject view a rotating drum painted with vertical stripes. A more familiar stimulus is provided by viewing telephone poles from a moving car.

Smooth pursuit. In contrast to the vestibulo-ocular and optokinetic reflexes, which allow the eyes to remain fixated on the visual target during head movements, the smooth pursuit system allows the eyes to remain fixated on a moving visual target even though the head may be still. Smooth pursuit occurs only when the stimulus is moving; it cannot result from a command.

The saccadic system. A **saccade** is a stereotyped rapid eye movement that allows a visual target to be cen-tered on the fovea of the retina. Saccades can be made voluntarily, or they can be a part of several reflexes. The velocity of a saccade is too rapid for visual processing. Hence, no visual feedback occurs during the movement. Saccades are corrected by smaller saccades that occur after the initial large change in eye position.

The vergence system. The vergence system allows the two eyes to converge or diverge, allowing fixation of the eyes on nearby or distant objects and on objects that approach or move away. During convergence movements, pupillary constriction and accommodation of the lens for near vision occur (see Chapter 9).

Neural circuit for the vestibulo-ocular reflex. Fig. 13-10 provides an overview of the neural pathways that make up the vestibulo-ocular reflex. The reflex is triggered by angular acceleration of the head, and the sensory receptors are located in the semicircular ducts (see Chapter 10). When the head is rotated to the left, for instance, the endolymph distorts the cupulas in the horizontal ducts. Activity in vestibular afferent fibers that supply the left horizontal duct increases, and activity in afferent fibers that supply the right duct decreases. The

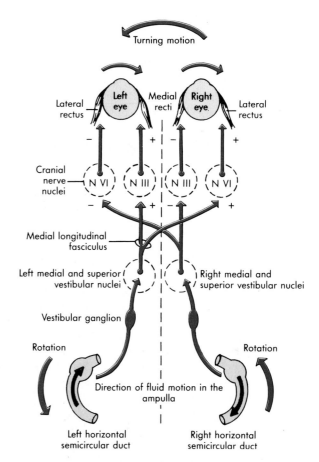

■ **Fig. 13-10** Neural circuit for the vestibulo-ocular reflex. The eyes, brainstem pathways, and horizontal semicircular ducts are viewed as from above. Rotation of the head to the left is indicated by the large arrows and the relative movement of endolymph to the right by the smaller arrows.

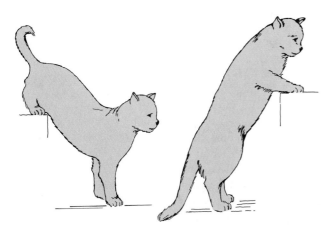

■ **Fig. 13-9** Effect of the tonic neck reflexes on limb position. The head is in a normal position in the cat, avoiding vestibular stimulation. Dorsiflexion of the neck causes extension of the forelimbs and flexion of the hindlimbs. Conversely, ventriflexion of the neck results in flexion of the forelimbs and extension of the hindlimbs. (Redrawn from Roberts TDM: *Neurophysiology of postural mechanisms,* London, 1979, Butterworth.)

afferent fibers project to the medial and superior vestibular nuclei. The increased activity in the vestibular nuclei on the left side activates ascending fibers (1) that project to the left oculomotor nucleus (through the medial longitudinal fasciculus) and excite medial rectus motor neurons and (2) that project to the right abducens nucleus and excite lateral rectus motor neurons. The reduced activity in the vestibular nuclei on the right side has the opposite effect on motor neurons to the right medial rectus and left lateral rectus. Reciprocal innervation also occurs in the ascending vestibular pathways; this innervation actively inhibits the motor neurons to antagonistic muscles.

As the head continues to rotate, the eyes reach the limit of their excursion. The eyes then perform a saccade in the same direction as the head rotation. They then fixate the visual target and again begin to rotate in the direction opposite to the head movement. Saccadic eye movements are so rapid that visual images are blurred, and therefore the visual process is minimally disrupted.

The alternation of slow and fast eye movements as the head turns is called **vestibular nystagmus.** This process is normal under these conditions of vestibular stimulation. However, vestibular nystagmus can also be produced by diseases that either reduce or increase vestibular afferent discharges. In such cases, the eye movements produce a sense that the environment is spinning, and the subject may report dizziness.

Another reflex that affects eye position and that originates with vestibular signals is **ocular counterrolling.** When the head is tilted, activation of the otolith organs rotates the eyes in the opposite direction. This movement tends to keep the retinal image aligned with the horizon.

When the labyrinth is irritated in one ear, as in **Meniere's disease,** or when a labyrinth is rendered nonfunctional, as may happen as a result of head trauma or disease of the labyrinth, the signals transmitted through the vestibulo-ocular reflex pathways from the two sides become unbalanced. Vestibular nystagmus can then result. For example, irritation of the labyrinth of the left ear can increase the discharges of afferents that supply the left horizontal semicircular duct. The signal produced resembles that normally produced when the head is rotated to the left; it causes a relative shift in endolymph toward the utricle and thus elicits a nystagmus with a slow phase to the right and fast phase to the left. The direction of nystagmus is named according to the fast movement; therefore, this nystagmus is "left-beating." Destruction of the labyrinth in the right ear produces similar effects as irritation of the left labyrinth.

Clinical testing of labyrinthine function is commonly done either by rotating the patient in a **Bárány chair** to activate the labyrinths in both ears or by introducing cold or warm water into the external auditory canal of one ear (caloric test). When a person is rotated in a Bárány chair, nystagmus develops during the rotation. The direction of the fast phase of the nystagmus should be in the same direction as the rotation. When the rotation of the chair is halted, nystagmus develops in the opposite direction (postrotatory nystagmus); if the person attempts to stand, he or she tends to fall and to feel dizzy.

The caloric test is more useful, because it can distinguish between malfunction of the labyrinths on the two sides. The head is bent backward about 60 degrees so that the two horizontal canals are essentially vertical. If warm water is introduced into the left ear, the endolymph in the left semicircular canal tends to rise as the specific gravity of the endolymph decreases, because of heating. As a result, the kinocilia of the left ampullary crest hair cells are deflected toward the utricle, the discharge of the afferents that supply this epithelium increases, and a nystagmus occurs with the fast phase toward the left. The nystagmus produces a sense that the environment is spinning to the right, and the subject tends to fall to the right. The opposite effects are produced if cold water if placed in the ear. A mnemonic expression that can help in remembering the direction of the nystagmus in the caloric test is COWS ("cold opposite, warm same"). In other words, cold water results in a fast phase of nystagmus toward the opposite side, and warm water causes a fast phase toward the same side.

■ *Gaze Centers*

In addition to the vestibular nuclei, brainstem centers for control of eye movement include the horizontal and vertical gaze centers. The **horizontal gaze center** consists of neurons in the reticular formation (paramedian pontine reticular formation) in the vicinity of the abducens nucleus. The **vertical gaze center** is located in the reticular formation of the midbrain.

The horizontal gaze center. Because the circuitry and operation of the horizontal gaze center are better understood than those of the vertical gaze center, the former are discussed here in detail. The horizontal gaze center controls both saccadic eye movements and smooth pursuit movements.

Fig. 13-11 is an overview of the neural circuitry by which the horizontal gaze center elicits conjugate eye movements, and Fig. 13-12 shows the activity of some of the types of neurons that form this circuitry. The right horizontal gaze center has excitatory connections with motor neurons in the ipsilateral abducens nucleus and with medial rectus motor neurons in the contralateral oculomotor nucleus. It also has inhibitory connections with the left horizontal gaze center via the reticular formation.

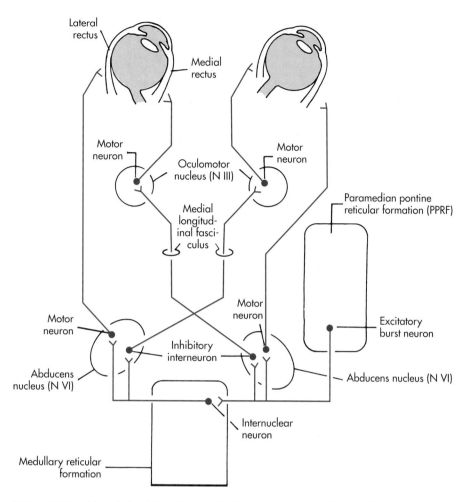

■ Fig. 13-11 Neural circuit by which the horizontal gaze center elicits conjugate eye movements. Excitation of burst neurons of the right horizontal gaze center causes activation of abducens motor neurons on the right and medial rectus motor neurons on the left. The ascending pathway to the oculomotor nucleus is through the medial longitudinal fasciculus. The left horizontal gaze center is simultaneously inhibited by way of the reticular formation.

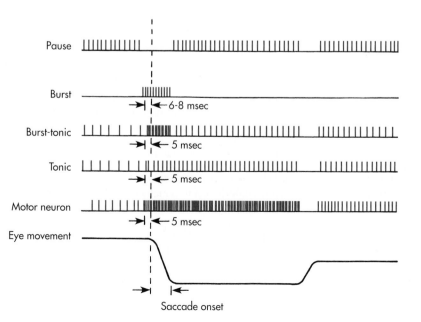

■ Fig. 13-12 Several types of neurons contribute to the circuitry by which the horizontal gaze center elicits conjugate eye movements. These include pause, burst, burst-tonic, and tonic neurons, in addition to motor neurons.

Burst neurons in one of the horizontal gaze centers may initiate saccadic eye movements (Fig. 13-12). At the same time, pause cells, which are inhibitory interneurons located in the nucleus of the dorsal raphe, stop the discharge of the contralateral burst cells. The activity of burst neurons and the inhibition of pause neurons are triggered by commands that originate elsewhere, such as the frontal eye field located in the premotor area of the contralateral frontal lobe or the superior colliculus (see Chapter 14). Tonic cells also participate in this center. Tonic cells discharge during smooth pursuit movements, and burst-tonic neurons fire both during saccades and during smooth pursuit movements. Presumably, the burst helps initiate the movement and the tonic activity maintains the new eye position. Tonic activity may arise as a consequence of activity in a neural integration circuit located in the nucleus prepositus hypoglossi, a nucleus found near the midline just rostral to the hypoglossal nucleus. Motor neurons to the eye muscles involved in a saccade show a burst-tonic form of discharge to initiate movement and then to maintain eye position.

A lesion of the brainstem that destroys one of the horizontal gaze centers tonically deviates the eyes toward the opposite side. This deviation is caused in part by the paralysis of the ipsilateral lateral rectus muscle, but also occurs because the tonic activity of the contralateral horizontal gaze center is no longer compensated for by the destroyed center. If the corticospinal tract is also interrupted on the same side, the limbs on the side of the body opposite to the lesion will be paralyzed.

The role of the cerebellum and the cerebral cortex in the control of eye movements is discussed in Chapter 14.

Superior colliculus. Neurons in the deep layers of the superior colliculus can trigger conjugate eye movements (saccades) that cause the eyes to target novel or threatening visual, auditory, or somatosensory stimuli. The superior colliculus sends impulses to the horizontal or vertical gaze centers to organize the conjugate eye movement.

■ *Summary*

1. Spinal cord motor neurons are organized topographically. Those in the lateral ventral horn supply the limb muscles, and those in the medial ventral horn supply the axial muscles. Lateral and medial groups of interneurons synapse on the respective lateral and medial groups of motor neurons.

2. Descending pathways can be subdivided into (1) a lateral system, which ends on motor neurons to limb muscles and on the lateral group of interneurons; and (2) a medial system, which ends on the medial group of interneurons.

3. The lateral system includes the lateral corticospinal tract and part of the corticobulbar tract. These pathways influence contralateral motor neurons that supply the musculature of the limbs, especially the digits, the muscles of the lower face, and the tongue.

4. The medial system includes the ventral corticospinal, lateral and medial vestibulospinal, pontine and medullary reticulospinal, and tectospinal tracts. These pathways mainly affect posture, and provide the motor background for movements of the limbs and digits.

5. Descending monoaminergic pathways affect the general level of excitability of spinal cord reflex circuits and ascending pathways.

6. Pathways that originate in the brainstem influence posture, locomotion, and eye movements. Postural reflexes include several vestibular reflexes (activation of extensor motor neurons as a result of head movements, the vestibulocollic reflex, the vestibular placing reaction, and ocular counterrolling), the tonic neck reflexes, and the righting reflexes.

7. Locomotion is triggered by commands relayed through the midbrain locomotor center. However, locomotor activity is organized by central pattern generators formed by spinal cord circuits and influenced by afferent input.

8. Conjugate eye movements are produced by several different control systems (vestibulo-ocular reflex, optokinetic reflex, smooth pursuit system, and saccadic system). Vergent eye movements are controlled by the vergence system.

9. The brainstem centers for control of eye movement include the vestibular nuclei, the horizontal and vertical gaze centers, and the superior colliculi.

■ *Self-Study Problems*

1. The descending motor control pathways can be divided into a lateral and a medial system. What are the main differences between these systems?

2. In humans, what are the consequences of interrupting the corticospinal and corticobulbar tracts and related descending motor pathways?

3. How is locomotion controlled?

4. What effect would you expect in a normal person during a caloric test in which cold water is introduced into the left ear?

5. A patient with a stroke cannot gaze conjugately to the left and has a spastic paralysis of the right arm and leg. What single lesion could explain the findings?

■ *Bibliography*

Journal articles

Armstrong DM: Review lecture: the supraspinal control of mammalian locomotion, *J Physiol* 405:1, 1988.

Buttner-Ennever JA: Patterns of connectivity in the vestibular nuclei, *Ann NY Acad Sci* 656:363, 1992.

Du Lac S, Raymond JL, Sejnowski TJ, Lisberger SG: Learning and memory in the vestibulo-ocular reflex, *Annu Rev Neurosci* 18:409, 1995.

Fuchs AF, Kaneko CRS, Scudder CA: Brainstem control of saccadic eye movements, *Annu Rev Neurosci* 8:307, 1985.

Grillner S, Wallen P: Central pattern generators for locomotion, with special reference to vertebrates, *Annu Rev Neurosci* 8:233, 1985.

Lisberger SG, Morris EJ, Tychsen L: Visual motion processing and sensory-motor integration for smooth pursuit eye movements, *Annu Rev Neurosci* 10:97, 1987.

Miles FA: The sensing of rotational and translational optic flow by the primate optokinetic system, *Rev Oculomot Res* 5:393, 1993.

Moschovakis AK, Highstein SM: The anatomy and physiology of primate neurons that control rapid eye movements, *Annu Rev Neurosci* 17:465, 1994.

O'Neill G: The caloric stimulus: mechanisms of heat transfer, *Br J Audiol* 29:87, 1995.

Pierrot-Deseilligny C et al: Cortical control of saccades, *Ann Neurol* 37:557, 1995.

Schall JD: Neural basis of saccade target selection, *Rev Neurosci* 6:63, 1995.

Sherrington CS: Decerebrate rigidity, and reflex coordination of movements, *J Physiol* 22:319, 1898.

Sparks DL: Translation of sensory signals into commands for control of saccadic eye movements: role of primate superior colliculus, *Physiol Rev* 66:118, 1986.

Wilson VJ: Vestibulospinal reflexes and the reticular formation, *Prog Brain Res* 97:211, 1993.

Wilson VJ et al: The vestibulocollic reflex, *J Vestib Res* 5:147, 1995.

Wurtz RH, Optican LM: Superior colliculus cell types and models of saccade generation, *Curr Opin Neurobiol* 4:857, 1994.

Books and monographs

Asanuma H: *The motor cortex,* New York, 1988, Raven Press.

Becker W: The neurobiology of saccadic eye movements, *Reviews of oculomotor research,* vol 3, Amsterdam, 1989, Elsevier.

Brodal A: *Neurological anatomy,* ed 3, New York, 1981, Oxford University Press.

DeJong RN: *The neurologic examination,* New York, 1979, Harper & Row.

Kandel ER, Schwartz JH, Jessell TM: *Principles of neural science,* New York, 1991, Elsevier.

Kuypers HGJM: *Anatomy of the descending pathways.* In Brooks VB, editor: *Handbook of physiology,* sect I, *The nervous system,* vol II, *Motor control,* part 1, Bethesda, Md, 1981, American Physiological Society.

Kuypers HGJM: *A new look at the organization of the motor system.* In Kuypers HGJM, Martin GF, editors: *Descending pathways to the spinal cord, Prog Brain Res* 57:390, 1982.

Phillips CB, Porter R: *Corticospinal neurones; their role in movement,* London, 1977, Academic Press.

Roberts TDM: *Neurophysiology of postural mechanisms,* London, 1979, Butterworth.

Wilson VJ, Melville Jones G: *Mammalian vestibular physiology,* New York, 1979, Plenum Press.

CHAPTER
14

Motor Control by the Cerebral Cortex, Cerebellum, and Basal Ganglia

In Chapter 12, emphasis was placed on reflexes, the simple, stereotyped motor acts that occur in response to specific stimuli. In this chapter the neural basis of voluntary movements is emphasized. Voluntary movements are often complex. They may vary when repeated and are often initiated as a result of cognitive processes rather than in response to an external stimulus.

The most important descending pathway for fine movements of the distal muscles, such as those that control the hand and fingers, is the lateral corticospinal tract. A portion of the corticobulbar tract is important for the control of facial and tongue movements. However, many other pathways are also engaged to activate more proximal and axial muscles, as described in Chapter 13.

Before any movement occurs, commands carried by descending motor pathways must first be organized in the brain. The target of the movement is identified by pooling sensory information in the posterior parietal cerebral cortex (Fig. 14-1). This information is then transmitted to the supplementary motor and premotor areas, where a motor plan is developed. The plan includes information about the specific muscles that need to be contracted, the strength of contraction, and the sequence of contraction. The motor plan is implemented by commands transmitted from the primary motor cortex through the descending pathways. Successful execution of these motor commands, however, depends on feedback provided to the motor cortex through the ascending pathways to the somatosensory cortex (Fig. 14-1, *B*), as well as through the visual pathway. During both the planning and execution stages of a movement, motor processing is also provided by two major motor control systems, the cerebellum (see p 219) and the basal ganglia (see p 227).

■ *Motor Control by the Cerebral Cortex*

■ *Cortical Motor Areas*

As discussed in Chapter 13, the primary motor areas in the cerebral cortex were originally mapped on the basis of experiments in which electrical stimuli applied to the cortex evoked discrete, contralateral movements. However, movements can also be evoked when other cortical areas are stimulated more intensely. On the basis of these stimulation studies, the deficits produced by lesions, anatomic experiments, electrophysiological recordings, and modern imaging studies in humans, several "motor" areas of the cerebral cortex have been recognized (Fig. 14-1). These areas include the primary motor cortex in the precentral gyrus, the premotor area just rostral to the cortex in the precentral gyrus, the secondary somatosensory cortex located in the roof of the lateral fissure (usually called SII), and the supplementary motor cortex on the medial aspect of the hemisphere. The frontal eye fields are located in a part of the premotor area just rostral to the face representation in the motor cortex.

Stimuli applied to the surface of the **primary motor cortex** evoke discrete contralateral (on the opposite side) movements that involve several muscles. However, microstimulation within the cortex with microelectrodes can elicit contractions of individual muscles. Mapping studies based on microstimulation reveal that the motor cortex consists of a mosaic of motor points related to particular muscles or sets of muscles. These points are called **cortical efferent zones,** which can be regarded as motor columns. They are organized somatotopically, and together they produce the motor homunculus (see Fig. 13-5).

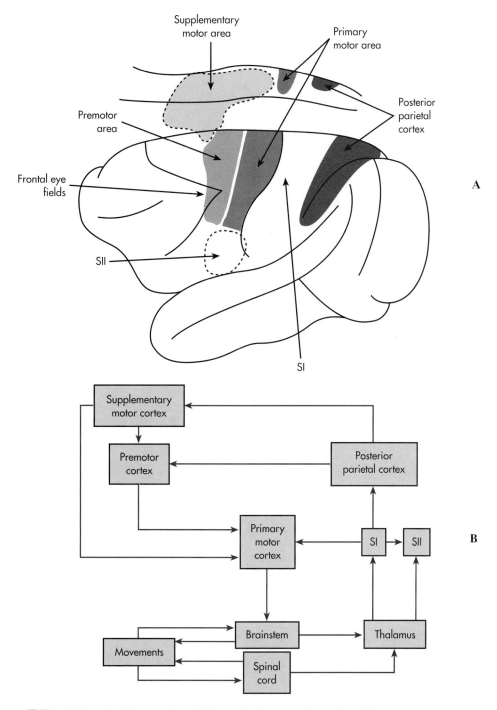

■ **Fig. 14-1** **A,** Motor regions of the cerebral cortex of a monkey. The motor cortex, premotor area, SII cortex, and supplementary motor cortex are indicated with different colors. The dashed lines around the secondary and supplementary cortex are meant to indicate that these areas are hidden from surface view. **B,** Flow diagram showing the sequence of activity in the voluntary motor and somatosensory feedback pathways. (**A** redrawn from Eyzaguirre C, Fidone SJ: *Physiology of the nervous system,* ed 2, Chicago, 1975, Mosby–Year Book.)

Stimulation of the **supplementary motor cortex** can produce vocalization or complex postural movements, such as a slow movement of the contralateral hand in an outward, backward, and upward direction. This hand movement is accompanied by a movement of the head and eyes toward the hand. The postural movements can be bilateral. Although stimulation can also evoke rhythmic movements from this area of the motor cortex, it can have the opposite result, namely, a temporary arrest of movement or speech. Removal of the supplementary motor cortex on one side produces slow movements of the contralateral extremities and a tendency to make forced grasping movements with the contralateral hand. Stimulation of the **premotor cortex** rarely causes movements unless a high stimulus intensity is used.

Stimulation of the **frontal eye fields** in one hemisphere causes a contralateral saccadic conjugate deviation of the eyes (see Chapter 13). Vertical saccades require bilateral stimulation of the frontal eye fields. Removal of the frontal eye field on one side transiently weakens the contralateral gaze, and in humans the eyes may deviate toward the side of the lesion. Memory-guided saccades are eliminated, but visually evoked saccades persist. However, bilateral lesions of the frontal eye fields and of the superior colliculi eliminate all saccadic eye movements.

A lesion of the frontal lobe, which can occur during a stroke, can prevent contralateral conjugate eye movements. Because the frontal eye fields on the contralateral side are intact, the eyes tend to deviate toward the side of the lesion. This impairment may be associated with a contralateral hemiplegia. This deficit pattern contrasts with that produced by a brainstem lesion that destroys the horizontal gaze center and also interrupts the corticospinal tract (see Chapter 13). A lesion of the horizontal gaze center on one side of the pons causes an inability to make conjugate eye movements toward the side of the lesion; the eyes will deviate toward the side contralateral to the lesion. If the corticospinal tract in the base of the pons is also interrupted, contralateral hemiplegia occurs.

■ *Connections of the Motor Regions of the Cortex*

The motor areas of the cortex receive input from a number of sources (Figs. 14-1 and 14-2). Ascending pathways that relay in the thalamus provide information about somatosensory events. This information can reach the motor cortex directly from the thalamus (from the ventral lateral [VL] nucleus) or indirectly by way of the SI somatosensory cortex. Both somatosensory and visual information is conveyed to the motor areas from the posterior parietal cortex. The frontal eye fields receive visual input from the occipital lobe (this connection is not shown in Fig. 14-1). The motor areas of the cortex also receive information through circuits that interconnect with the cerebellum and basal ganglia. In addition, the motor regions of the cortex are interconnected.

The output of the motor regions of the cortex to the spinal cord and brainstem is conducted through several descending pathways, which include not only direct projections through the corticospinal and corticobulbar tracts, but also indirect projections (by way of corticorubral and corticoreticular fibers) through the red nucleus and reticu-

lar formation. The motor regions also contribute to the cerebellar and basal ganglion circuits. The frontal eye fields project to the superior colliculus and also to the pontine and mesencephalic reticular formation.

■ *The Role of Premotor and Supplementary Motor Areas in Motor Programming*

The supplementary motor cortex is involved in motor programming and is active during both the planning and the execution stages of complex (but not simple) movements. Its actions are partly mediated by direct corticospinal connections, and partly by a relay to the primary motor cortex. Monitoring of the regional blood flow of the cerebral cortex during motor tasks shows that blood flow increases when the individual is merely thinking about a movement, as well as when the movement is actually executed. In contrast, the blood flow in the primary motor cortex increases only when the movement is executed. In addition to its role in motor planning, the supplementary motor cortex may assist in the coordination of posture and voluntary movements.

The premotor cortex receives a major input from the posterior parietal cortex, and its output chiefly influences the medial system of descending pathways. These connections suggest that this region of the cortex controls the axial muscles. Neurons in this area seem to discharge during the preparatory stages of a movement.

The posterior parietal cortex is often called the **parietal association cortex.** This region receives somatosensory, visual, vestibular, and auditory information from the primary sensory receiving areas. A lesion of the posterior parietal cortex in humans results in language disorders when the lesion is on the left side, but results in neglect of contralateral somatic or visual stimuli (**agnosia**) when the lesion is on the right side. Patients with right parietal lobe lesions have difficulty recognizing or drawing three-dimensional objects and recognizing spatial relationships (Fig. 14-3). Similar difficulties may be experienced by patients with lesions of the left parietal lobe, but these problems are masked by the language disorder.

Preparation for volitional movements requires several hundred milliseconds; the exact time depends on the difficulty of the task. Lesions of the premotor, supplementary motor, and posterior parietal areas can hamper the ability to prepare for voluntary movements. When such lesions are produced experimentally, the results resemble **apraxia,** which describes the failure of patients with frontal or parietal lobe lesions to perform complex movements despite retention of sensation and the ability to make simple movements.

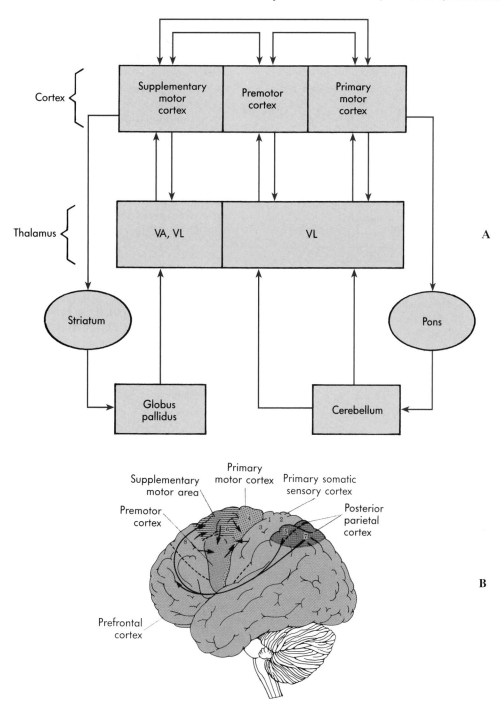

■ **Fig. 14-2** **A,** Some of the connections of the motor areas of the cortex with subcortical structures. *VA,* Ventral anterior thalamic nucleus; *VL,* ventral lateral thalamic nucleus. **B,** Some of the cortical projections involving the motor areas. Arrows indicate transmission in one direction, but there are also connections in the opposite direction. (Redrawn from Kandel ER, Schwartz JH, Jessell TM: *Principles of neural science,* ed 3, New York, 1991, Elsevier.)

■ *Activity of Individual Corticospinal Neurons*

The role of individual corticospinal neurons in the control of movements has been investigated in trained monkeys. In these experiments, discharges from these neurons are recorded in the primary motor cortex during the execution of a simple movement, such as wrist flexion,

that the monkey has previously learned (Fig. 14-4). The corticospinal neurons discharge before the onset of the movement, which suggests that these cells cause the movement. Furthermore, analysis of the electrical potentials from the appropriate muscle reveals that a particular corticospinal neuron excites a particular motor neuron monosynaptically. The discharges of corticospinal neurons appear to relate to the contractile force of the muscle that generates the movement or to the rate of change in force, rather than to the position of the joint.

Corticospinal neurons that influence more proximal muscles inhibit motor neurons to extensor muscles and

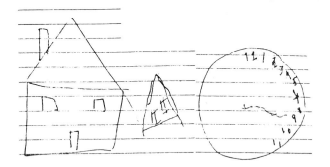

■ **Fig. 14-3** Drawing made by a patient 2 days after damage to the right parietal lobe. The drawing on the left was made by the physician to show a house. The drawing in the middle was made by the patient and was meant to copy the physician's drawing. The drawing of the clock with all the numbers on the right indicates neglect of the left extrapersonal space by the patient. (From Cotman CW, McGaugh JL: *Behavioral neuroscience,* New York, 1980, Academic Press.)

excite motor neurons to flexor muscles. Apparently, the corticospinal output in this case causes postural changes that support fine movements of the distal muscles. Other corticospinal neurons trigger fine movements through excitatory connections to motor neurons that supply the distal muscles.

A given corticospinal neuron may discharge before a movement occurs in any direction. However, a neuron tends to discharge most vigorously when the movement occurs in a preferred direction. Neurons in a motor column all evoke the same preferred direction of movement. Commands from a population of corticospinal neurons that evoke somewhat different preferred directions determine the actual direction of a movement.

■ *Sensory Feedback on Corticospinal Neurons*

As already emphasized, the corticospinal neurons of the primary motor cortex receive sensory information through the thalamus, as well as from sensory areas of the cerebral cortex. This information is used by the motor cortex to ensure that the movements it evokes are appropriate.

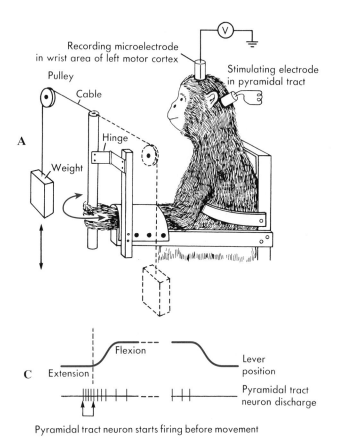

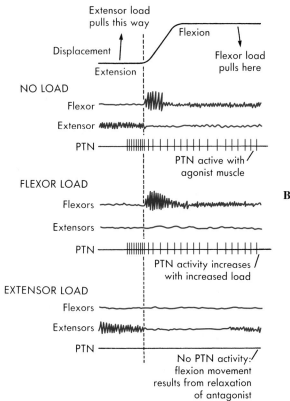

■ **Fig. 14-4** **A,** Experimental arrangement for recording from a corticospinal neuron during trained movements of the wrist. **B** and **C,** The cell discharges before the movement. With an extensor load (**B,** *lower trace*), the cell fails to discharge, indicating that it encodes force rather than displacement. *PTN,* Pyramidal tract neuron. (Redrawn from Kandel ER, Schwartz JH: *Principles of neural science,* New York, 1981, Elsevier Science.)

Fig. 14-5 shows how somatosensory information influences corticospinal neurons. Cutaneous receptors and proprioceptive receptors, such as muscle spindles, transmit information about the mechanical contact of a fingertip with a surface and the position of the finger joints via the ascending somatosensory pathways, such as the dorsal column–medial lemniscus system (see Chapter 8). The corticospinal neuron activates motor neurons that flex the finger. As the fingertip moves into contact with the surface, cutaneous receptors in the skin of the ventral surface of the fingertip discharge and thereby excite the corticospinal neuron through somatosensory projections. Muscle spindle afferent fibers activated by stretch of the flexor muscle as the finger contacts the surface also activate the corticospinal neuron. Thus, sensory feedback from both skin and muscle facilitates this activity of the corticospinal neuron and enhances the movement.

Another example of sensory feedback to the motor cortex is illustrated in Fig. 14-6. In this preparation, the corpus callosum and the optic chiasm of the monkey are surgically transected. As a result of this transection, visual information from either eye reaches only the ipsilateral (on the same side) cortex, and no information can be transmitted from one hemisphere to the other. The monkey's task is to remove a pellet of food from one of the wells on a board. This task requires fine movements

of the digits and thus involves corticospinal control that originates on the side of the brain contralateral to the hand used. When the right eye is open, the monkey can retrieve the food pellets with its left hand (Fig. 14-6, *A*). However, if the right eye is masked, the monkey can no longer retrieve the food with its left hand (Fig. 14-6, *B*), although it can with its right hand. This movement is possible because visual information that reaches the left hemisphere through the left eye influences corticospinal neurons in the left motor cortex, which in turn controls fine movements of the digits in the right hand (Fig. 14-7). The pathway that conveys the visual information to the motor cortex passes through the posterior parietal lobe.

■ *Motor Control by the Cerebellum*

■ *Overview of the Cerebellum's Role in Motor Control*

The cerebellum influences neither sensation nor muscle strength. However, it does help to regulate movements and posture, and it plays a key role in some forms of motor learning. The rate, range, force, and direction of movements are all influenced by the cerebellum. Therefore, damage to the cerebellum results in incoordination of movements.

The cerebellum helps regulate the vestibulo-ocular reflex, and it participates in the improvements in motor performances that result from practice of motor skills. It is therefore thought to be involved in motor learning.

The cerebellum exerts its motor control on a moment-by-moment basis. It uses sensory information from a variety of sources, most prominently from the proprioceptive system, to update its computations of body position, muscle length, and muscle tension. The cerebellum may be able to compare this sensory feedback with neural signals that are transmitted to the cerebellum from the motor areas of the cerebral cortex and that represent the desired motor act. Errors are corrected by output signals from the cerebellum to other components of the motor system.

■ *Cerebellar Organization*

The cerebellum ("little brain") is located in the posterior fossa of the cranium just below the occipital lobe, and it is connected to the brainstem. From the surface, only the cortex is visible. The cerebellar cortex is subdivided into three rostrocaudally arranged lobes: the anterior, posterior, and flocculonodular lobes (Fig. 14-8). The cerebellar lobes are separated by major fissures, the **primary fissure** and the **posterolateral fissure,** and each lobe is made up of one or more **lobules.** Each lobule of the cerebellar cortex is composed of a series of transverse folds, called **folia.**

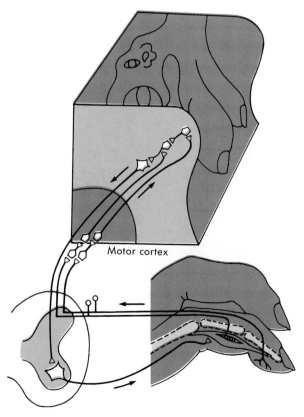

Motor cortex

■ Fig. 14-5 Sensory input to a corticospinal neuron that causes flexion of a digit. (Redrawn from Asanuma H: *Physiologist* 16:143, 1973.)

CONTRALATERAL EYE-HAND CONTROL   IPSILATERAL EYE-HAND CONTROL

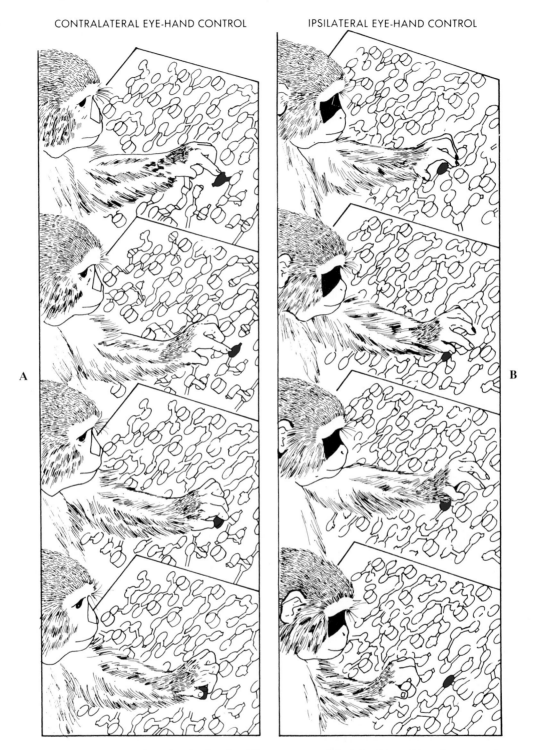

A

B

■ **Fig. 14-6** Drawings showing hand and finger movements by a monkey subjected to a complete commissurotomy. **A,** To retrieve a food pellet from a well, the monkey is able to use a precision grip involving hand and digit muscles. **B,** The task cannot be performed by the left hand when the right eye is masked. (Redrawn from Brinkman C: *Split-brain monkeys: cerebral control of contralateral and ipsilateral arm, hand, and finger movements,* doctoral dissertation, Rotterdam, The Netherlands, 1974, Erasmus University.)

Both the cerebellum and the cerebrum are cortical structures, and white matter is found in both of these parts of the brain beneath the cortex. When the cerebellum is sectioned, the white matter of the cerebellum can be seen beneath the cortex. Buried in the white matter are the deep cerebellar nuclei. The most lateral of these nuclei is the **dentate nucleus.** The other deep nuclei include the **emboliform, globose,** and **fastigial nuclei.**

Subdivisions of the Cerebellum

Phylogenetically, the cerebellum can be subdivided into the archicerebellum, paleocerebellum, and neocerebellum (Fig. 14-8). These subdivisions correspond to regions of the cerebellum that are dominated by vestibular input (the **vestibulocerebellum),** by spinal cord input (the **spinocerebellum),** and by indirect input from the cerebrum via the pontine nuclei (the **corticocerebellum).** The vestibulocerebellum consists chiefly of the flocculonodular lobe but also includes a small part of the vermis and intermediate cortex of the posterior lobe. The spinocerebellum is composed of most of the vermis and intermediate region. The corticocerebellum consists of the hemispheres.

Afferent Pathways of the Cerebellar Divisions

Vestibulocerebellum. The afferent pathways of the vestibulocerebellum include both direct projections of primary vestibular afferent fibers and also second-order projections from the vestibular nuclei, chiefly from the inferior nucleus (see Chapter 10). The vestibular afferent fibers enter the cerebellum through the ipsilateral inferior cerebellar peduncle. These fibers give off collaterals to the fastigial nuclei before they reach the flocculonodular lobe and parts of the posterior lobe. The vestibulocerebellum regulates eye movements, stance, and gait.

Spinocerebellum. The spinocerebellum has several somatotopic maps, one of which is located in the anterior lobe and another in the posterior lobe (Fig. 14-9). The trunk of the body is represented in the vermis and the extremities in the intermediate zone. The head is oriented toward the primary fissure in both of the somatotopic maps. Thus, the two maps are inverted with respect to each other. Visual and auditory information is received in the areas that represent the head. Stimulation of the cerebellar cortex results in movements of parts of the body that correspond to the sensory maps.

The ascending pathways that convey somatosensory information to the spinocerebellum include the dorsal and ventral spinocerebellar tracts from the lower extremities and trunk, and the cuneocerebellar and rostral spinocerebellar tracts from the upper extremities and trunk. The dorsal spinocerebellar tract originates from **Clarke's column,** a nucleus found in the thoracic and upper lumbar

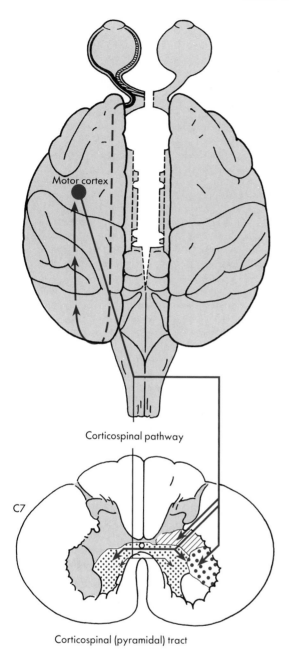

■ Fig. 14-7 Split-brain preparation, as in Fig. 14-6. Drawing above shows the relationship of pathways carrying visual information to the left hemisphere from the left eye to the corticospinal neurons on the left side that control hand and digit movement on the right. (Redrawn from Brinkman C: *Split-brain monkeys: cerebral control of contralateral and ipsilateral arm, hand, and finger movements,* doctoral dissertation, Rotterdam, The Netherlands, 1974, Erasmus University.)

In addition to this rostrocaudal organization, the cerebellum has a sagittal organization. At the midline of the cerebellum is the **vermis** (named for its segmented appearance, which resembles an earthworm). Extending laterally are the **hemispheres.** In the paravermal region, between the hemispheres and vermis, is the **intermediate region.**

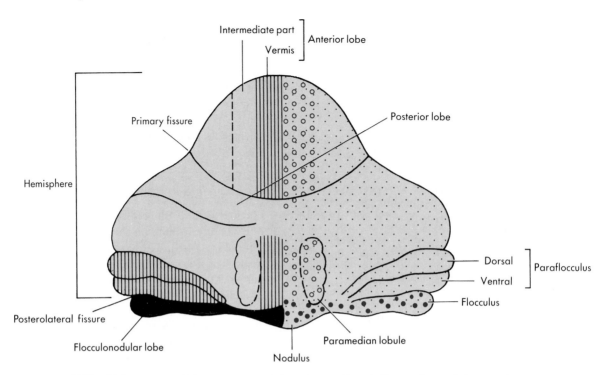

■ **Fig. 14-8**   The subdivision of the cerebellum into archicerebellum, paleocerebellum, and neo-cerebellum is shown by the black, hatched, and gray areas. Terminations of vestibulocerebellar fibers are indicated by the large dots, spinocerebellar fibers by the open circles, and pontocerebellar fibers by the small dots. (Redrawn from Brodal A: *Neurological anatomy,* ed 3, New York, 1981, Oxford University Press.)

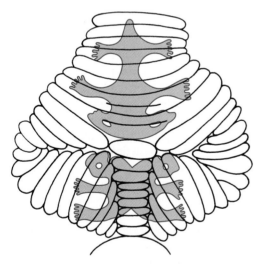

■ **Fig. 14-9**   Somatotopic maps in the spinocerebellum. (Redrawn from Snider R: The cerebellum, *Sci Am* 199:4, 1958.)

spinal cord. This nucleus receives input from muscle stretch receptors, and from cutaneous receptors through the dorsal funiculus. It projects its axons to the cerebellum by way of the ipsilateral dorsal lateral funiculus and the inferior cerebellar peduncle. These axons give off collaterals to the emboliform and globose nuclei en route to the cortical representations of the lower extremities and trunk.

The **cuneocerebellar tract** originates from the **lateral cuneate nucleus,** which is located in the caudal medulla just lateral to the main cuneate nucleus. The neurons of the lateral cuneate nucleus receive proprioceptive information and project to the cerebellum through the adjacent inferior cerebellar peduncle. As in the dorsal spinocerebellar tract, collaterals are provided to the emboliform and globose nuclei, and the projection ends in the forelimb and upper trunk representations. The dorsal and cuneocerebellar pathways provide discrete, current information to the cerebellum about limb position and muscle actions.

The ventral and rostral spinocerebellar tracts have a more complex organization, provide less discrete information than do the dorsal spinocerebellar and cuneocerebellar tracts, project bilaterally in the cerebellum, and operate under the control of descending systems. These tracts also indirectly project from the spinal cord to the cerebellum through relays in the dorsal column nucleus and in the lateral reticular nucleus of the medulla. The spinocerebellum regulates movements of the proximal limbs and trunk.

Corticocerebellum. The corticocerebellum regulates movements of the distal parts of the limbs and participates in motor planning. Wide areas of the cerebral cortex, including parts of the frontal, parietal, and temporal lobes, provide input to the corticocerebellum indirectly by connections to the pontine nuclei. The pontine nuclei also receive connections from the spinal cord and from

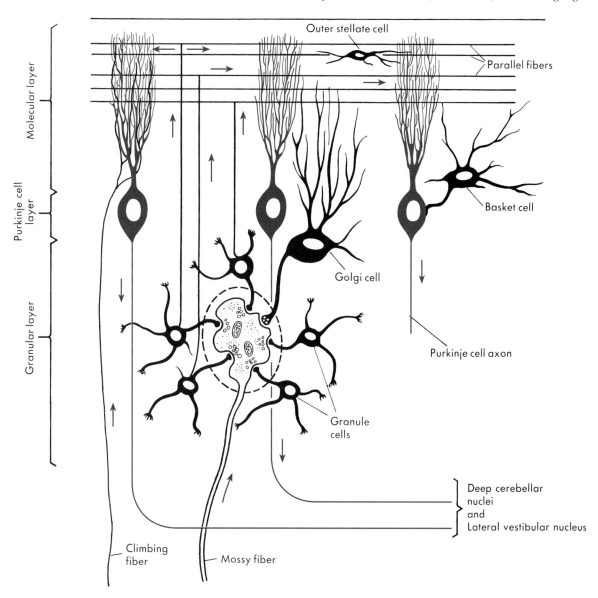

■ **Fig. 14-10**   Cerebellar cortex cut along the long axis of a folium. (Redrawn from Carpenter MB: *Human neuroanatomy,* ed 7, Baltimore, 1976, Williams & Wilkins; based on Gray EG: *J Anat* 95:345, 1961, and Eccles JC et al: *The cerebellum as a neurorial machine,* New York, 1967, Springer-Verlag.)

brainstem pathways. The pontocerebellar tract originates from the pontine nuclei, crosses the midline, and enters the cerebellum through the middle cerebellar peduncle. This tract gives off collaterals to the dentate nucleus on its way to the cortex of the cerebellar hemisphere.

■ *Inferior Olive*

The inferior olivary nucleus is a massive structure located in the rostral medulla. This nucleus receives input from the vestibular system, the spinal cord, and the cerebral cortex through a number of pathways. The cells of the inferior olivary nucleus give rise to the olivocerebellar tract, which crosses the midline and enters the cerebellum

through the contralateral inferior cerebellar peduncle. The axons are distributed to all parts of the cerebellum, and send collaterals to the deep cerebellar nuclei as well as to the cortex. Their terminals form special types of cerebellar afferent fibers called **climbing fibers;** in contrast, all the other cerebellar afferent pathways terminate in the cerebellar cortex as **mossy fibers** (see Fig. 14-10).

■ *Cerebellar Cortex*

Organization of the cerebellar cortex. The cerebellar cortex is organized in reference to its output cell, the **Purkinje cell.** The cell bodies of Purkinje cells form the middle of the three layers of the cerebellar cortex. The other two layers are the granular layer and the molecular layer (Fig. 14-10).

The granular layer is adjacent to the white matter and contains many interneurons, including **Golgi cells** and **granule cells;** these interneurons comprise about half the neurons in the brain. The mossy fibers in the cerebellar cortex form excitatory terminals on the dendrites of granule cells. A given granule cell receives convergent inputs from many mossy fibers. The terminal zones are called cerebellar glomeruli. The Golgi cells provide inhibitory projections to the glomeruli.

The axons of the granule cells ascend through the Purkinje cell layer to the molecular layer, where they bifurcate and form **parallel fibers.** The parallel fibers pass along the long axis of the folium and form excitatory synapses with the dendrites of the Purkinje and Golgi cells; they also form excitatory synapses with stellate and basket cells, which are the interneurons of the molecular layer. A given parallel fiber synapses with about 50 Purkinje cells, and a given Purkinje cell receives synapses from about 200,000 parallel fibers.

The stellate and basket cells of the molecular layer are inhibitory interneurons that synapse with Purkinje cells. The stellate cells form terminals on the dendrites of the Purkinje cells, and the basket cells form terminals on the cell bodies of the Purkinje cells. The basket cell projections to the Purkinje cells are oriented at right angles to the long axis of the folium. These basket cell axons are called **transverse fibers** (Fig. 14-11).

Activity of Purkinje cells in the cerebellar cortex. As mentioned, the Purkinje cells function as the output cells of the cerebellar cortex. They receive numerous excitatory synapses on their dendrites from the parallel fibers formed by the granule cells (Figs. 14-10 and 14-11). Each Purkinje cell also receives a powerful excitatory connection from a climbing fiber. The climbing fiber gives off numerous branches repeatedly as it ascends the dendritic tree and makes numerous active contacts with the Purkinje cell. Mossy fiber inputs to the cerebellar cortex cause a Purkinje cell to discharge single action potentials (**simple spikes),** whereas a single climbing fiber causes repetitive discharges of the

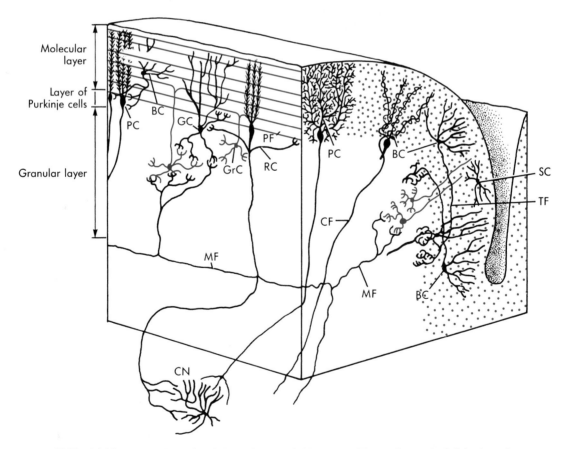

■ **Fig. 14-11**   Three-dimensional view of the cerebellar cortex. The cut face at the left is along the long axis of the folium; the cut face at the right is at right angles to the long axis. *PC,* Purkinje cell; *BC,* basket cell; *GC,* Golgi cell; *GrC,* granule cell; *PF,* parallel fiber; *RC,* recurrent collateral; *MF,* mossy fiber; *CF,* climbing fiber; *CN,* deep cerebellar nuclear cell; *SC,* stellate cell; *TF,* transverse fiber. (Redrawn from Fox CA: *The structure of the cerebellar cortex.* In Crosby EC, Humphrey TH, Lauer EW, editors: *Correlative anatomy of the nervous system,* New York, 1962, Macmillan.)

Purkinje cell (**complex spikes**) (Fig. 14-12). Because the climbing fibers generate complex spikes at a low frequency, they do not change the average firing rates of Purkinje cells. However, they probably do alter the responsiveness of Purkinje cells to mossy fiber inputs. These changes can be long-lasting and hence may play a role in motor learning (see p 226).

The Purkinje cell also receives inhibitory connections from the basket and stellate cells (Figs. 14-10 and 14-11). These connections produce inhibitory postsynaptic potentials in Purkinje cells (Fig. 14-12). The axon of the Purkinje cell descends through the granule layer and enters the cerebellar white matter (Fig. 14-11). Most Purkinje cell axons terminate in one of the deep cerebellar nuclei. However, some Purkinje cells in the vestibulocerebellum project from the cerebellum to the lateral vestibular nucleus. The discharge of the Purkinje cells inhibits the activity of neurons in the deep cerebellar nuclei and lateral vestibular nucleus. The inhibitory neurotransmitter used by Purkinje cells is gamma-aminobutyric acid (GABA).

Some of the circuits formed by the cerebellar afferent fibers, interneurons, and Purkinje cells are shown in Fig. 14-13. The mossy fiber pathway can activate granule cells and Purkinje cells, but it can also produce a feedforward inhibition of Purkinje cells through basket and stellate cells (Fig. 14-13, *A*). The climbing fiber pathway (Fig. 14-13, *B*) provides a powerful excitation of Purkinje cells. Mossy fiber inputs are regulated by inhibitory feedback from Golgi cells (Fig. 14-13, *C*).

Complicated interactions can occur between elements of the mossy fiber and climbing fiber pathways (Fig. 14-13, *D*).

It may seem paradoxical that the output of the cerebellar cortex is inhibitory. However, recall that all the input pathways to the cerebellum send collaterals to the deep cerebellar nuclei. It should not be surprising that the cells in the deep nuclei are very active. The role of the cerebellar cortex is to modulate this activity appropriately. Thus, the real output of the cerebellum is via the projections of the deep cerebellar nuclei.

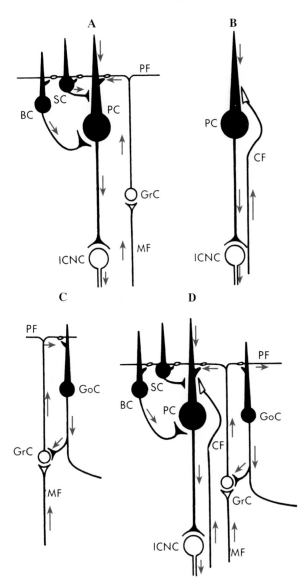

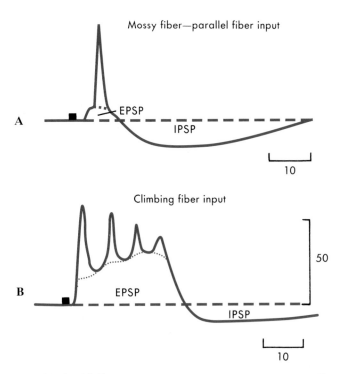

■ **Fig. 14-12**　Responses of a Purkinje cell to a mossy fiber input (**A**) and to a climbing fiber input (**B**). *EPSP,* Excitatory postsynaptic potential; *IPSP,* inhibitory postsynaptic potential.

■ **Fig. 14-13**　**A** to **D,** Neural circuits of the cerebellar cortex. Inhibitory neurons are black and excitatory ones clear. *PC,* Purkinje cell; *SC,* stellate cell; *BC,* basket cell; *PF,* parallel fiber; *GrC,* granule cell; *MF,* mossy fiber; *ICNC,* deep cerebellar nuclear cell; *CF,* climbing fiber; *GoC,* Golgi cell. (Redrawn from Eccles JC: *Nobel Symposium I: Muscular afferents and motor control,* New York, 1966, John Wiley.)

The role of cerebellar Purkinje cells in motor learning. As mentioned earlier, the climbing fibers may participate in motor learning by influencing the effectiveness of mossy fibers in exciting Purkinje cells. Evidence for this theory comes from experiments on the gain of the vestibulo-ocular reflex. The "gain" of a reflex describes the direction and amount of the response produced by that reflex. Normally, the gain of this reflex is one: when the head rotates to the left, the eyes will rotate by an equal angle, but in the opposite direction. However, if lenses are used to reverse the visual fields, the eye movements are reversed after a learning period. Thus, the reflex gain is reduced and finally changed in sign. This alteration in gain is prevented by a lesion of the vestibulocerebellum.

In monkeys, the frequency of complex spikes recorded from Purkinje cells initially increases as the animals learn to perform a new task. Once the task is learned, the frequency of complex spikes gradually decreases. The increased frequency of complex spikes is thought to cause changes in the efficacy of the synapses made by parallel fibers onto Purkinje cells. Such changes are believed to be the basis of motor learning. The mechanism for motor learning appears to be a form of long-term inhibition of the Purkinje cells.

■ *Projections of the Deep Cerebellar Nuclei*

The deep cerebellar nuclei receive topographically organized projections from the Purkinje cells of the different parasagittal zones of the cerebellum (Fig. 14-14).

Vestibulocerebellum and vermal spinocerebellum. Purkinje cells in the flocculonodular lobe and the remainder of the vermis project to the fastigial nucleus or directly to the lateral vestibular nucleus. The fastigial nucleus, in turn, projects to the lateral vestibular nucleus and to the pontine reticular formation. Thus, the output of these regions of the cerebellum influences axial and proximal limb muscles by way of the lateral vestibulospinal and pontine reticulospinal tracts, which belong to the medial motor projection system (see Chapter 13).

Intermediate spinocerebellum. The Purkinje cells of the paravermal region project to the emboliform and globose nuclei. These nuclei are connected with the contralateral red nucleus by fibers that leave the cerebellum in the superior cerebellar peduncle and then cross to the opposite side in the decussation of the brachium conjunctivum. This pathway allows the paravermal spinocerebellum to influence the discharges of neurons of the rubrospinal tract. The rubrospinal tract crosses at the midbrain level. Thus, the paravermal region on one side of the cerebellum influences motor activity ipsilaterally, because the cerebellar output crosses the midline, and the red nucleus output then recrosses. The rubrospinal tract controls movements of proximal muscles of the limbs and belongs to the lateral motor system.

Corticocerebellum. Purkinje cells of the cerebellar hemisphere project to the dentate nucleus. Neurons in the dentate nucleus project contralaterally through the superior cerebellar peduncle and the decussation of the brachium conjunctivum to the contralateral thalamus, and they end in the ventral lateral (VL) nucleus (Fig. 14-2). The thalamic neurons distribute their axons to the premotor and primary motor cortex, where they can influence the planning and initiation of voluntary movements. Like the spinocerebellum, the corticocerebellum on one side influences movements ipsilaterally because of its crossed connection with a contralaterally projecting motor output system, in this case the lateral corticospinal tract. The corticocerebellum affects distal muscles through the lateral corticospinal tract, which belongs to the lateral motor system. This system terminates in part directly on motor neurons to the distal muscles (see Chapter 13).

Damage to the cerebellum impairs motor function on the ipsilateral side of the body. The specific deficits that result depend on which functional component of the cerebellum is most affected. If the flocculonodular lobe is damaged, the motor disorders resemble those produced by a lesion of the vestibular apparatus; the disorders include difficulty in balance and gait and often nystagmus. If the vermis is affected, the motor disturbance affects the trunk, and if the intermediate region or hemisphere is involved, motor disorders occur in the limbs. The part of the limbs affected depends on the site of damage; hemispheric lesions affect the distal muscles more than do paravermal lesions.

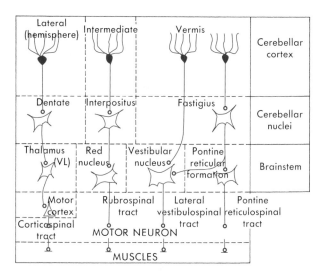

■ **Fig. 14-14** Cerebellar output. Inhibitory neurons are shown in solid color. (Redrawn from Bell CC, Dow RS: *Cerebellar circuitry.* In Schmitt FO et al, editors: *Neuroscience research summaries,* vol 2, Cambridge, Mass, 1967, MIT Press.)

Types of motor dysfunction in cerebellar disease include disorders of coordination, equilibrium, and muscle tone. Incoordination is called **ataxia.** It is often expressed as **dysmetria,** a condition in which errors in the direction and force of movements prevent a limb from being moved smoothly to a desired position. Ataxia may also be expressed as **dysdiadochokinesia,** in which repeated supinations and pronations of the arm are difficult to execute. When more complicated movements are attempted, **decomposition of movement** occurs, in which the movement is accomplished in a series of discrete steps, rather than as a smooth sequence. An **intention tremor** appears when the subject is asked to touch a target; the affected hand (or foot) develops a tremor that increases in magnitude as the target is approached. When equilibrium is disturbed, balance is difficult; the individual tends to fall toward the affected side and may walk with a wide-based stance. Speech may be slow and slurred, a defect called **scanning speech.** Muscle tone may be diminished (**hypotonia**). Hypotonia may be associated with a **pendular knee jerk;** when a phasic stretch reflex of the quadriceps muscle is elicited by striking the patellar tendon, the leg continues to swing back and forth because of the hypotonia, in contrast to the highly damped oscillation in a normal individual.

■ *Motor Control by Basal Ganglia*

The basal ganglia are the deep nuclei of the cerebrum. In association with other nuclei in the diencephalon and midbrain, the basal ganglia differ from the cerebellum in the way they regulate motor activity. Unlike the cerebellum, the basal ganglia do not receive an input from the spinal cord, but they do receive a direct input from the cerebral cortex. The main action of the basal ganglia is on the motor areas of the cortex by way of the thalamus. In addition to their role in motor control, the basal ganglia contribute to affective and cognitive functions. Lesions of the basal ganglia produce abnormal movements and posture.

■ *Organization of the Basal Ganglia and Related Nuclei*

The basal ganglia include the **caudate nucleus,** the **putamen,** and the **globus pallidus** (Fig. 14-15). Some authorities also include the **claustrum.** The term **corpus striatum** refers to these four structures, whereas the term **striatum** signifies only the caudate nucleus and putamen. These nuclei are separated by the anterior limb of the internal capsule; cellular bridges that exist between the nuclei give the structure a striated appearance. The globus pallidus has two parts, the external and the inter-

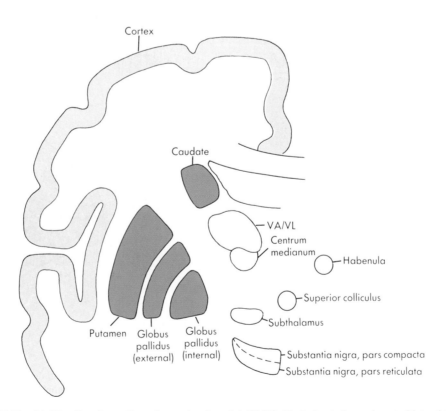

■ **Fig. 14-15**   Basal ganglia and associated nuclei. *VA/VL,* Ventral anterior and ventral lateral thalamic nuclei. (Redrawn from Brodal A: *Neurological anatomy,* ed 3, New York, 1981, Oxford University Press.)

nal segments, which are often referred to collectively as the **pallidum.** Together, the putamen and globus pallidus are often referred to as the **lentiform nucleus.**

Associated with the basal ganglia are several thalamic nuclei. These nuclei include the **ventral anterior (VA)** and **ventral lateral (VL) nuclei** and several components of the intralaminar complex, including the **centre median (CM)** nucleus. Other associated nuclei are the **subthalamic nucleus** of the diencephalon and the **substantia nigra** of the midbrain. The substantia nigra ("black substance") derives its name from its pigment content. Many of the neurons in this nucleus contain melanin, a byproduct of dopamine synthesis. The substantia nigra can be subdivided into a dorsal **pars compacta** and a ventral **pars reticulata.** The melanin-containing cells are located in the pars compacta.

■ *Connections and Operation of the Basal Ganglia*

Figs. 14-16 and 14-17 show the main connections of the basal ganglia. The circuitry of the basal ganglia is very complex and its operation is still unknown. The neurons of the striatum do not discharge before neurons in the motor cortex are activated by a sensory input. Hence, these neurons do not appear to be involved in the initiation of stimulus-triggered movements. However, the striatal neurons may be involved in internally generated motor commands.

All regions of the cerebral cortex project topographically to the striatum (caudate nucleus and putamen). An important component of the cortical input to the striatum originates in the motor cortex. The corticostriatal projection arises from neurons in layer V of the cortex and appears to use glutamate as its excitatory neurotransmitter. The striatum then influences neurons in the VA and VL nuclei of the thalamus by two pathways, direct and indirect (Fig. 14-18).

In the direct pathway, the striatum projects to the internal segment of the globus pallidus and to the pars reticulata of the substantia nigra (Fig. 14-18). This projection is inhibitory, and the transmitters include both GABA and substance P. The internal segment of the globus pallidus and the pars reticulata of the substantia nigra project to the VA and VL nuclei of the thalamus. The efferent fibers from the globus pallidus pass through the **ansa lenticularis** and the **fasciculus lenticularis.** These connections also use GABA and are inhibitory. The VA and

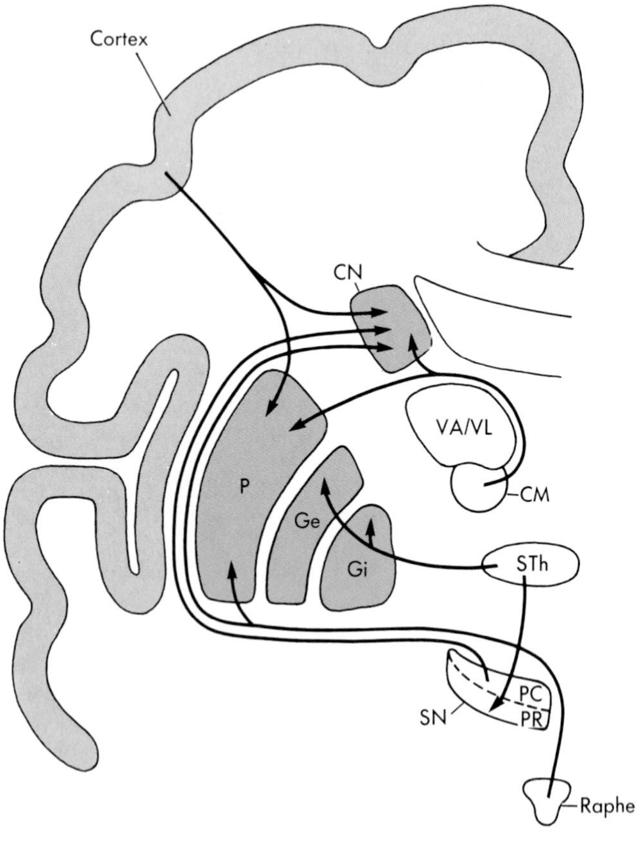

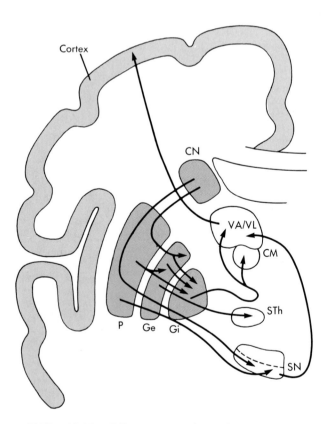

■ **Fig. 14-16**   Afferent pathways to the basal ganglia. *CN,* Caudate nucleus; *VA/VL,* ventral anterior and ventral lateral thalamic nuclei; *CM,* centre median; *STh,* subthalamic nucleus; *PC,* pars compacta; *PR,* pars reticulata; *SN,* substantia nigra; *Ge, Gi,* external and internal segments of globus pallidus; *P,* putamen. (Redrawn from Brodal A: *Neurological anatomy,* ed 3, New York, 1981, Oxford University Press.)

■ **Fig. 14-17**   Efferent connections of the basal ganglia, including intrinsic connections. *CN,* Caudate nucleus; *VA/VL,* ventral anterior and ventral lateral thalamic nuclei; *CM,* centre median; *STh,* subthalamic nucleus; *SN,* substantia nigra; *Ge, Gi,* external and internal segments of the globus pallidus; *P,* putamen. (Redrawn from Brodal A: *Neurological anatomy,* ed 3, New York, 1981, Oxford University Press.)

VL nuclei send excitatory connections to the prefrontal, premotor, and supplementary motor cortex. This input to the cortex influences motor planning, and also eventually affects the discharges of corticospinal and corticobulbar neurons. The pars reticulata also influences eye movements by a projection to the superior colliculus.

The direct pathway appears to function as follows. Neurons in the striatum have little background activity, and during movements they are activated by their inputs from the cortex and the intralaminar nuclei. In contrast, neurons in the internal segment of the globus pallidus have a high level of background activity. When the striatum is activated, its inhibitory projections to the globus pallidus slow the activity of pallidal neurons. However, the pallidal neurons themselves are inhibitory, and they normally provide a tonic inhibition of neurons in the VA and VL nuclei of the thalamus. Therefore, activation of the striatum disinhibits the neurons of the VA and VL nuclei, and such activation excites these neurons and their target neurons in the motor cortex.

The indirect pathway involves a connection from the striatum to the external segment of the globus pallidus, which projects to the subthalamic nucleus, which in turn projects back to the internal segment of the globus pallidus (Fig. 14-18). In this pathway, pallidal neurons in the external segment are inhibited by GABA and enkephalin released from striatal terminals in the globus pallidus. GABA and enkephalin disinhibit neurons of the subthalamic nucleus. The subthalamic neurons become more active because of the disinhibition, and they release glutamate in the internal segment of the globus pallidus. This transmitter excites neurons that project to the VA and VL thalamic nuclei. The pallidal action is inhibitory, and consequently the activity of the thalamic neurons decreases, as does that of the cortical neurons that they influence.

The direct and indirect pathways thus have opposing actions; an increase in the activity of either one of these pathways might lead to an imbalance in motor control. Such imbalances, which are typical of basal ganglion dis-

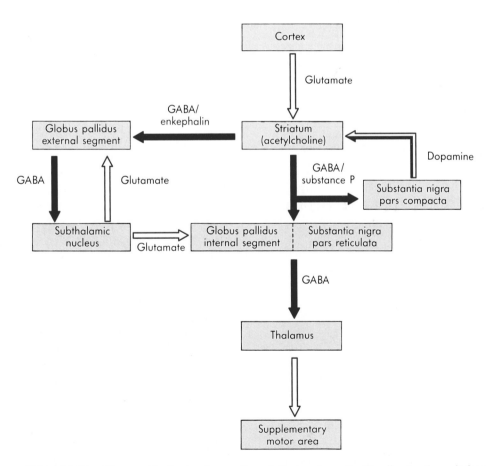

■ **Fig. 14-18** Direct and indirect pathways through the basal ganglia. The direct pathway is from the cortex to the striatum to the internal segment of the globus pallidus to the thalamus and back to the cortex. The indirect pathway is from the cortex to the striatum to the external segment of the globus pallidus to the subthalamic nucleus to the internal segment of the globus pallidus to the thalamus and back to the cortex. Solid color arrows show inhibitory connections; open arrows show excitatory connections. (Redrawn from Kandel ER, Schwartz JH, Jessell TM: *Principles of neural science*, ed 3, New York, 1991, Elsevier.)

eases, may be either an increase or a decrease in the motor output of the cortex.

Neurons in the pars compacta of the substantia nigra project to the striatum. Dopamine is the neurotransmitter used in this pathway; it appears to have an excitatory action on the direct pathway and an inhibitory action on the indirect pathway. Both actions facilitate activity in the cerebral cortex, and hence the projection from the substantia nigra to the striatum is important functionally.

■ Differences between the Basal Ganglion and Cerebellar Motor Loops

The organization of the motor loops that connect the basal ganglia and cerebellum with the motor regions of the cerebral cortex differs in several ways. The basal ganglia receive input from all areas of the cerebral cortex, whereas the input to the cerebellum from the cortex is more restricted. The output from the basal ganglia is also more widespread and reaches the prefrontal cortex, as well as all the premotor areas. The cerebellar circuit influences only the premotor and motor cortex. Finally, the basal ganglia do not receive somatosensory information from ascending pathways in the spinal cord, and they have few connections with the brainstem. In contrast, the cerebellum is the target of several somatosensory pathways, and it has rich connections with brainstem nuclei.

■ Subdivision of the Striatum into Striosomes and Matrix

On the basis of the associated neurotransmitters, the striatum has been subdivided into zones called **striosomes** and **matrix.** The cortical projections related to motor control end in the matrix area. The limbic system projects to the striosomes. The striosomes are thought to synapse in the pars compacta and influence the dopaminergic nigrostriatal pathway.

■ Role of the Basal Ganglia in Motor Control

The basal ganglia mainly influence the motor cortex. Therefore, the basal ganglia may have an important influence on the lateral system of motor pathways. Such an influence is consistent with some of the movement disorders observed in diseases of the basal ganglia. However, the basal ganglia also relate to the medial motor pathways, because diseases of the basal ganglia can affect the posture and tone of the proximal muscles.

The deficits seen in the various basal ganglion diseases include abnormal movements **(dyskinesias),** increases in muscle tone **(cogwheel rigidity),** and slowness in initiating movements **(bradykinesia).** Abnormal movements include **tremor, athetosis, chorea, ballism,** and **dystonia.** The tremor of basal ganglion disease is a "pill-rolling" tremor that occurs when the limb is at rest. **Athetosis** consists of slow, writhing movements of the distal parts of the limbs, whereas **chorea** is rapid, flicking movements of the extremities and facial muscles. **Ballism** is associated with violent, flailing movements of the limbs (ballistic movements). Finally, **dystonic movements** are slow truncal movements that distort body positions.

Parkinson's disease is a common disorder characterized by tremor, rigidity, and bradykinesia. This disease is caused by loss of neurons in the pars compacta of the substantia nigra and consequently a severe loss of dopamine in the striatum. Neurons of the locus caeruleus and the raphe nuclei, as well as of other monoaminergic nuclei, are also lost. Presumably, the loss of dopamine results in overactivity of the inhibitory pathway from the striatum to the globus pallidus and therefore a disinhibition of neurons in the VA and VL nuclei. The neurons in the VA and VL nuclei then activate neurons of the motor cortex and thus increase the discharges of motor neurons, including γ motor neurons.

Researchers studying Parkinson's disease have found that the disease can be mimicked in monkeys with a neurotoxin called 1-methyl-4-phenyl-1, 2, 3, 6-tetrahydropyridine (MPTP), which destroys dopamine-containing neurons. This discovery may help further our understanding of the abnormalities seen in Parkinsonism. Treatments for Parkinson's disease are currently aimed at replacing dopamine. For instance, before the dopaminergic neurons are completely lost, administration of L-dopa, a precursor of dopamine that can cross the blood-brain barrier, can relieve some of the motor disorders in Parkinson's disease. Currently, the possibility that dopamine-synthesizing neurons can be transplanted into the striatum is being explored.

Another basal ganglion disorder is **Huntington's disease,** which is the result of a genetic defect that involves an autosomal dominant gene on chromosome 4. The defect leads to the loss of GABA-ergic and cholinergic neurons of the striatum, and also to the degeneration of the cerebral cortex, with resultant dementia. Loss of inhibition of the globus pallidus presumably reduces the activity of neurons in the VA and VL nuclei. The reduction in activity of these neurons may cause the choreiform movements of Huntington's disease, although the exact mechanism is unclear.

Cerebral palsy is another common motor disorder associated with a lesion of the basal ganglia. In cerebral palsy, athetosis often occurs in association with lesions of both the striatum and globus pallidus. **Ballism** is produced by a partial lesion of the subthalamic nucleus. In all these disorders of the basal ganglia, the motor dysfunction is contralateral to the diseased component, because the main final output of the basal ganglia is mediated by the corticospinal tract.

Summary

1. Voluntary movements depend on interactions among motor areas of the cerebral cortex, the cerebellum, and the basal ganglia.

2. Motor areas of the cerebral cortex include (1) the primary motor cortex, which controls distal muscles of the extremities; (2) the premotor area, which helps control proximal and axial muscles; (3) the supplementary motor cortex, which participates in motor planning and in coordination; and (4) the frontal eye fields, which help initiate saccadic eye movements.

3. Individual corticospinal neurons discharge before voluntary contraction of related muscles is evident. The discharges are related to contractile force, rather than to joint position.

4. Cortical motor neurons receive feedback from the sensory systems by way of the somatosensory cortex and the posterior parietal lobe; this feedback helps correct motor commands.

5. The cerebellum influences the rate, range, force, and direction of movements. It also influences muscle tone and posture, as well as eye movements and balance. The cerebellum is involved in motor learning.

6. The vestibulocerebellum connects with the vestibular system and influences eye movements and balance by connections with the vestibulospinal and reticulospinal tracts.

7. The spinocerebellum receives input from spinal cord pathways. It controls (1) the axial musculature through the medial system of descending pathways and (2) the proximal limb muscles through the rubrospinal tract of the lateral system.

8. The corticocerebellum receives information from the cerebral cortex by way of the pontine nuclei. It controls the distal muscles of the limbs by connections to the motor cortex (via the thalamus) and lateral corticospinal tract. The corticocerebellum is also involved in motor planning.

9. Most of the input to the cerebellum is through pathways that end as mossy fibers. Mossy fibers evoke single action potentials called simple spikes in Purkinje cells. However, the inferior olive projections to the cerebellum end as climbing fibers. A climbing fiber produces repetitive discharges of a Purkinje cell. Complex spikes are thought to alter the effectiveness of simple spikes and to play a role in motor learning.

10. The basal ganglia include several deep telencephalic nuclei (including the caudate, putamen, and globus pallidus). They interact with the cerebral cortex, subthalamic nucleus, substantia nigra, and thalamus.

11. Activity transmitted from the cortex through the basal ganglia can either facilitate or inhibit thalamic neurons that project to motor areas of the cortex. The basal ganglia thus affect the output of the motor cortex.

12. Diseases of the cerebellum and basal ganglia affect motor behavior profoundly. The deficits caused by cerebellar and basal ganglia diseases can be understood on the basis of the interconnections of the cerebellum and basal ganglia with the lateral and medial motor systems.

Self-Study Problems

1. How do the roles of the premotor, supplementary motor, and primary motor cortices differ in the control of movements of skeletal muscles?

2. What is encoded by corticospinal neurons in the primary motor cortex?

3. What is the role of the cerebellum in motor control?

4. What are some of the roles of the basal ganglia in motor control?

5. What are the main motor system diseases that result from lesions affecting the functions of (1) the cerebellum and (2) the basal ganglia?

Bibliography
Journal articles

Alben RL, Young AB, Penney JB: The functional anatomy of basal ganglia disorders, *Trends Neurosci* 12:366, 1989.

Alexander GE, Crutcher MD: Functional architecture of basal ganglia circuits: neural substrates of parallel processing, *Trends Neurosci* 13:266, 1990.

Alexander GE, DeLong MR, Strick PL: Parallel organization of functionally segregated circuits linking basal ganglia and cortex, *Annu Rev Neurosci* 9:357, 1986.

Allen GL, Tsukahara N: Cerebrocerebellar communication systems, *Physiol Rev* 54:957, 1974.

Andersen RA: Encoding of intention and spatial location in the posterior parietal cortex, *Cereb Cortex* 5:457, 1995.

Cheney PD, Fetz EE: Functional classes of primate corticomotoneuronal cells and their relation to active force, *J Neurophysiol* 44:773, 1980.

DeLong MR: Primate models of movement disorders of basal ganglia origin, *Trends Neurosci* 13:281, 1990.

Donoghue JP, Sanes JN: Motor areas of the cerebral cortex, *J Clin Neurophysiol* 11:382, 1994.

Flaherty AW, Graybiel AM: Two input systems for body representations in the primate striatal matrix: experimental evidence in the squirrel monkey, *J Neurosci* 13:1120, 1993.

Gerfen CR: The neostriatal mosaic: multiple levels of compartmental organization in the basal ganglia, *Annu Rev Neurosci* 15:285, 1992.

Glickstein M, Yeo C: The cerebellum and motor learning, *J Cogn Neurosci* 2:69, 1990.

Goldman-Rakic PS, editor: Basal ganglia research, *Trends Neurosci* 13:241, 1990.

Holmes G: The cerebellum of man, *Brain* 62:1, 1939.

Horne MK, Butler EG: The role of the cerebello-thalamo-cortical pathway in skilled movement, *Prog Neurobiol* 46:199, 1995.

Kopin IJ: Parkinson's disease: past, present, and future, *Neuropsychopharmacology* 9:1, 1993.

Mountcastle VB, Atluri PP, Romo R: Selective output–discriminative signals in the motor cortex of waking monkeys, *Cereb Cortex* 2:277, 1992.

Parent A, Hazrati LN: Functional anatomy of the basal ganglia. I. The cortico-basal ganglia-thalamo-cortical loop, *Brain Res Rev* 20:91, 1995.

Parent A, Hazrati LN: Functional anatomy of the basal ganglia. II. The place of the subthalamic nucleus and external pallidum in basal ganglia circuitry, *Brain Res Rev* 20:128, 1995.

Riehle A, Requin J: Neuronal correlates of the specification of movement direction and force in four cortical areas of the monkey, *Behav Brain Res* 70:1, 1995.

Tanji J: The supplementary motor area in the cerebral cortex, *Neurosci Res* 19:251, 1994.

Thach WT, Goodkin HP, Keating JG: The cerebellum and the adaptive coordination of movement, *Annu Rev Neurosci* 15:403, 1992.

Vidal F, Bonnet M, Macar F: Programming the duration of a motor sequence: role of the primary and supplementary motor areas in man, *Exp Brain Res* 106:339, 1995.

Yurek DM, Sladek JR: Dopamine cell replacement: Parkinson's disease, *Annu Rev Neurosci* 13:415, 1990.

Books and monographs

Asanuma H: *The motor cortex,* New York, 1988, Raven Press.

Bloedel JR, Dichgans J, Precht W: *Cerebellar functions,* New York, 1985, Springer-Verlag.

Brodal A: *Neurological anatomy,* ed 3, New York, 1981, Oxford University Press.

Brooks VB: *The neural basis of motor control,* New York, 1986, Oxford University Press.

Brooks VB, editor: *Handbook of physiology,* sect 1, *The nervous system,* vol II, *Motor control,* part 2, Bethesda, MD, 1981, American Physiological Society.

Carpenter MB, Sutin J: *Human neuroanatomy,* ed 8, Baltimore, 1983, Williams & Wilkins.

Cotman CW, McGaugh JL: *Behavioral neuroscience,* New York, 1980, Academic Press.

DeJong RN: *The neurological examination,* ed 4, Hagerstown, Md, 1979, Harper & Row.

Ito M: *The cerebellum and motor control,* New York, 1984, Raven Press.

Kandel ER et al: *Principles of neural sciences,* ed 3, New York, 1991, Elsevier.

Phillips CG, Porter R: *Corticospinal neurones,* London, 1977, Academic Press.

CHAPTER

15

The Autonomic Nervous System and Its Central Control

The **autonomic nervous system** can be regarded as a part of the motor system. However, instead of skeletal muscle, the effectors of the autonomic nervous system are smooth muscle, cardiac muscle, and glands. Because the autonomic nervous system provides motor control of the viscera, it is sometimes called the **visceral motor system.** An older term for this system is the **vegetative nervous system.** This terminology is no longer used because it does not seem appropriate for a system that is important for all levels of activity, including aggressive behavior.

An important function of the autonomic nervous system is to assist the body in maintaining a constant internal environment **(homeostasis).** When internal stimuli signal that regulation of the body's environment is required, the central nervous system (CNS) and its autonomic outflow issue commands that lead to compensatory actions. For example, a sudden increase in systemic blood pressure activates the baroreceptors, which in turn adjust the autonomic nervous system and restore the blood pressure toward its previous level (see Chapter 28).

The autonomic nervous system also participates in appropriate coordinated responses to external stimuli. For example, the autonomic nervous system helps regulate pupil size in response to different intensities of ambient light. An extreme example of this regulation is the "fight-or-flight response" that occurs when a threat intensively activates the sympathetic nervous system. This activation causes a variety of responses. Adrenal hormones are released, the heart rate and blood pressure increase, bronchioles dilate, intestinal motility and secretion are inhibited, glucose metabolism increases, pupils dilate, hairs become erect owing to the action of piloerector muscles, cutaneous and splanchnic blood vessels constrict, and blood vessels in skeletal muscle dilate. However, the "fight-or-flight response" is an uncommon event; it does not represent the usual mode of operation of the sympathetic nervous system in daily life.

Accompanying the autonomic motor fibers in peripheral nerves are afferent fibers that originate from sensory receptors in the viscera. Many of these receptors trigger reflexes, but the activity of some receptors evokes sensory experiences, such as pain, hunger, thirst, nausea, and a sense of visceral distention. The chemical senses can also be considered visceral senses (see Chapter 11).

The term autonomic nervous system generally refers to the **sympathetic** and **parasympathetic nervous systems.** In this chapter, the **enteric nervous system** is also included as part of the autonomic nervous system, although it is sometimes considered a separate entity. In addition, because the autonomic nervous system is under CNS control, the central components of the autonomic nervous system are discussed in this chapter. This central component includes the hypothalamus and higher levels of the limbic system, which are associated with emotions and with many visceral behaviors (e.g., feeding, drinking, thermoregulation, reproduction, defense, and aggression) that have survival value.

■ Organization of the Autonomic Nervous System

The primary functional unit of the sympathetic and parasympathetic nervous systems is a two-neuron motor pathway, which consists of a preganglionic neuron, whose cell body is located in the CNS, and a postganglionic neuron, whose cell body is located in one of the autonomic ganglia. The enteric nervous system includes neurons and nerve fibers in the myenteric and submucosal plexuses, which are located in the wall of the gastrointestinal tract.

The sympathetic preganglionic neurons are located in the thoracic and upper lumbar segments of the spinal cord. For this reason, the sympathetic nervous system is sometimes referred to as the thoracolumbar division of the autonomic nervous system. In contrast, the parasympathetic preganglionic neurons are found in the brainstem and in the sacral spinal cord. Hence, this part of the autonomic nervous system is sometimes called the **craniosacral division.** Sympathetic postganglionic neurons are generally found in the paravertebral or the prevertebral ganglia, which are located at some distance from their target organs. Parasympathetic postganglionic neurons are found in parasympathetic ganglia near or actually within the walls of the target organs.

The control of the sympathetic and parasympathetic nervous systems of many organisms has often been described as antagonistic. This description is not entirely correct. It is more appropriate to consider these two parts of the autonomic control system as working in a coordinated way—sometimes acting reciprocally and sometimes synergistically—to regulate visceral function. Furthermore, not all visceral structures are innervated by both systems. For example, the smooth muscles and

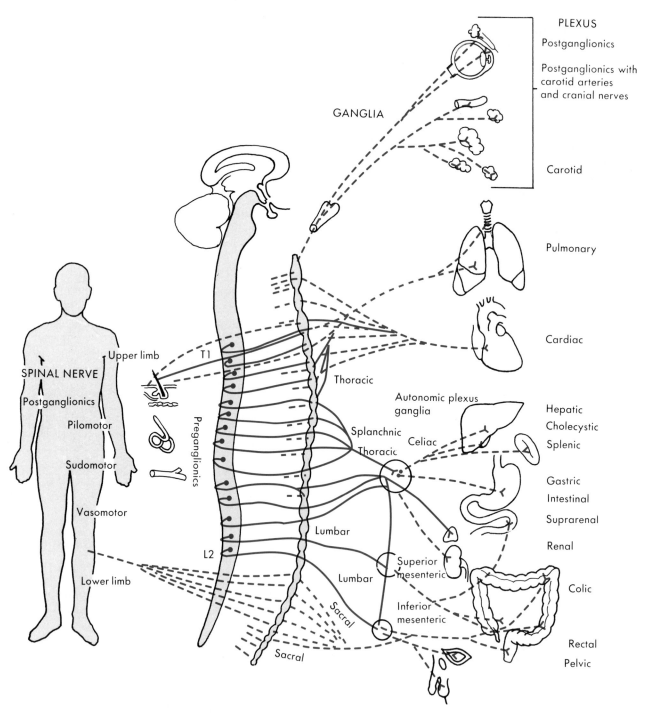

■ **Fig. 15-1**   Sympathetic nervous system and its distribution. (Redrawn from Bhagat BD, Young PA, Biggerstaff DE: *Fundamentals of visceral innervation,* Springfield, Ill, 1977, Charles C Thomas.)

glands in the skin and most of the blood vessels in the body receive only sympathetic innervation; only a small fraction of the blood vessels have parasympathetic innervation. The parasympathetic nervous system does not innervate the body wall but only structures in the head and the thoracic, abdominal, and pelvic cavities.

The Sympathetic Nervous System

Sympathetic preganglionic neurons are concentrated in the **intermediolateral cell column** in the thoracic and upper lumbar segments of the spinal cord (Figs. 15-1 and 15-2). Some neurons may also be found in the C8 segment. In addition to the **intermediolateral cell column,** groups of sympathetic preganglionic neurons are found in other locations, including the lateral funiculus, the intermediate region, and the part of lamina X dorsal to the central canal.

The axons of the preganglionic neurons are often small, myelinated nerve fibers known as B fibers. However, some axons are unmyelinated C fibers. They leave the spinal cord in the ventral root and enter the paravertebral ganglion at the same segmental level through a white communicating ramus. White rami are found only from T1 to L2. The preganglionic axons may synapse on postganglionic neurons in this ganglion, or they may pass through the ganglion and enter either the sympathetic chain or a splanchnic nerve (Fig. 15-2).

Preganglionic axons in the paravertebral sympathetic chain of ganglia may travel rostrally or caudally to a nearby or distant paravertebral ganglion and then synapse. If the synapse is in a paravertebral ganglion, the postganglionic axon often passes through a gray communicating ramus to enter a spinal nerve. Each of the 31 pairs of spinal nerves has a gray ramus. Postganglionic axons are distributed through the peripheral nerves to effectors, such as piloerector muscles, blood vessels, and sweat glands, located in the skin, muscle, and joints. Postganglionic axons are generally unmyelinated (C fibers), although some exceptions exist. The distinction between white and gray rami is based on the relative content of myelinated and unmyelinated axons in these rami.

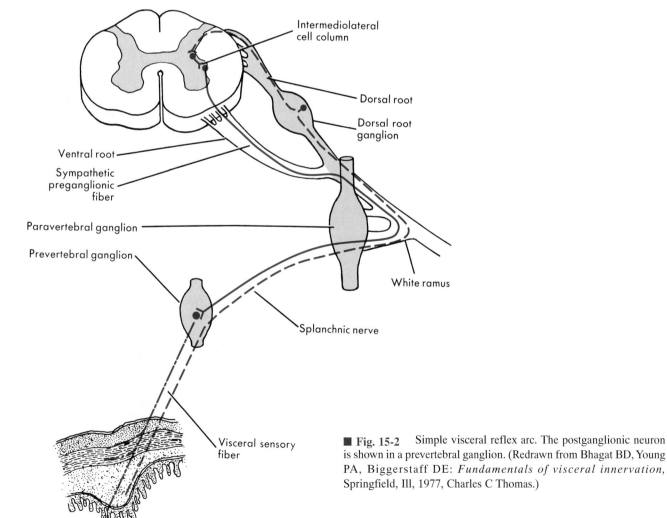

Intermediolateral cell column

Dorsal root

Dorsal root ganglion

Ventral root

Sympathetic preganglionic fiber

Paravertebral ganglion

Prevertebral ganglion

White ramus

Splanchnic nerve

Visceral sensory fiber

■ **Fig. 15-2**   Simple visceral reflex arc. The postganglionic neuron is shown in a prevertebral ganglion. (Redrawn from Bhagat BD, Young PA, Biggerstaff DE: *Fundamentals of visceral innervation,* Springfield, Ill, 1977, Charles C Thomas.)

Preganglionic axons in a splanchnic nerve often travel to a prevertebral ganglion and synapse, or they may pass through the ganglion and an autonomic plexus and end in a more distant ganglion. Some preganglionic axons pass through a splanchnic nerve and end directly on cells of the adrenal medulla.

The sympathetic chain extends from cervical to coccygeal levels of the spinal cord. This arrangement serves as a distribution system, enabling preganglionic neurons, which are limited to thoracic and upper lumbar segments, to activate postganglionic neurons that innervate all body segments. However, there are fewer paravertebral ganglia than there are spinal segments, because some of the segmental ganglia fuse during development. For example, the superior cervical sympathetic ganglion represents the fused ganglia of C1 to C4; the middle cervical sympathetic ganglion is the fused ganglia of C5 and C6; and the inferior cervical sympathetic ganglion is the combination of the ganglia at C7 and C8. The term **stellate ganglion** refers to a fusion of the inferior cervical sympathetic ganglion with the ganglion of T1. The superior cervical sympathetic ganglion provides postganglionic innervation to the head and neck, and the middle cervical and stellate ganglia innervate the heart, lungs, and bronchi.

Generally, the sympathetic preganglionic neurons are distributed to ipsilateral (on the same side) ganglia and thus control autonomic function on the same side of the body. One important exception is that the sympathetic innervation of the intestine and of the pelvic viscera is bilateral. As with motor neurons to skeletal muscle, sympathetic preganglionic neurons that control a particular organ are spread over several segments. For example, the sympathetic preganglionic neurons that control sympathetic functions in the head and neck region are distributed in C8 to T5, whereas those that control the adrenal gland are located in T4 to T12.

The Parasympathetic Nervous System

The parasympathetic postganglionic neurons are located in several cranial nerve nuclei in the brainstem, as well as in the intermediate region of the S3 and S4 segments of the sacral spinal cord (Fig. 15-3). The cranial nerve nuclei that contain parasympathetic preganglionic neurons are the **Edinger-Westphal nucleus** (cranial nerve III), the **superior** (cranial nerve VII) and **inferior** (cranial nerve IX) **salivatory nuclei,** and the **dorsal motor nucleus** and **nucleus ambiguus** (cranial nerve X). Postganglionic parasympathetic cells are located in cranial ganglia, including the ciliary ganglion (preganglionic input is from the Edinger-Westphal nucleus), the pterygopalatine and submandibular ganglia (input from the superior salivatory nucleus), and the otic ganglion (input from the inferior salivatory nucleus). The ciliary ganglion innervates the pupillary sphincter and ciliary muscles in the eye. The pterygopalatine ganglion sup-

plies the lacrimal gland, as well as glands in the nasal and oral pharynx. The submandibular ganglion projects to the submandibular and sublingual salivary glands and glands in the oral cavity. The otic ganglion innervates the parotid salivary gland and glands in the mouth.

Other parasympathetic postganglionic neurons are located near or in the walls of visceral organs in the thoracic, abdominal, and pelvic cavities. Neurons of the enteric plexus include cells that can also be considered parasympathetic postganglionic neurons. These cells receive input from the vagus or pelvic nerves. The vagus nerves innervate the heart, lungs, bronchi, liver, and pancreas and all of the gastrointestinal tract from the esophagus to the splenic flexure of the colon. The remainder of the colon and rectum, as well as the urinary bladder and reproductive organs, is supplied by sacral parasympathetic preganglionic neurons that distribute through the pelvic nerves to postganglionic neurons in the pelvic ganglia.

The parasympathetic preganglionic neurons that project to the viscera of the thorax and part of the abdomen are located in the dorsal motor nucleus of the vagus and the nucleus ambiguus. The dorsal motor nucleus is largely **secretomotor** (it activates glands), whereas the nucleus ambiguus is **visceromotor** (it modifies the activity of cardiac muscle). The dorsal motor nucleus supplies visceral organs in the neck (pharynx, larynx), thoracic cavity (trachea, bronchi, lungs, heart, esophagus), and abdominal cavity (including much of the gastrointestinal tract, liver, and pancreas). Electrical stimulation of the dorsal motor nucleus causes gastric acid secretion, as well as secretion of insulin and glucagon by the pancreas. Although projections to the heart have been described, their function is uncertain. The nucleus ambiguus contains two groups of neurons: (1) a dorsal group that activates striated muscle in the soft palate, pharynx, larynx, and esophagus (branchiomotor) and (2) a ventrolateral group that innervates and slows the heart (see also Chapter 24).

Visceral Afferent Fibers

The visceral motor fibers in the autonomic nerves are accompanied by visceral afferent fibers. Most of these afferent fibers supply information that originates from sensory receptors in the viscera. The activity of these sensory receptors never reaches the level of consciousness. Instead, these afferent fibers form the afferent limb of reflex arcs. Both viscerovisceral and viscerosomatic reflexes are elicited by these afferent fibers. Visceral reflexes operate at a subconscious level, and they are very important for homeostatic regulation and adjustment to external stimuli.

The fast-acting neurotransmitters released by visceral afferent fibers are not well documented, although many of these neurons may release an excitatory amino acid transmitter, such as glutamate. However, visceral afferent

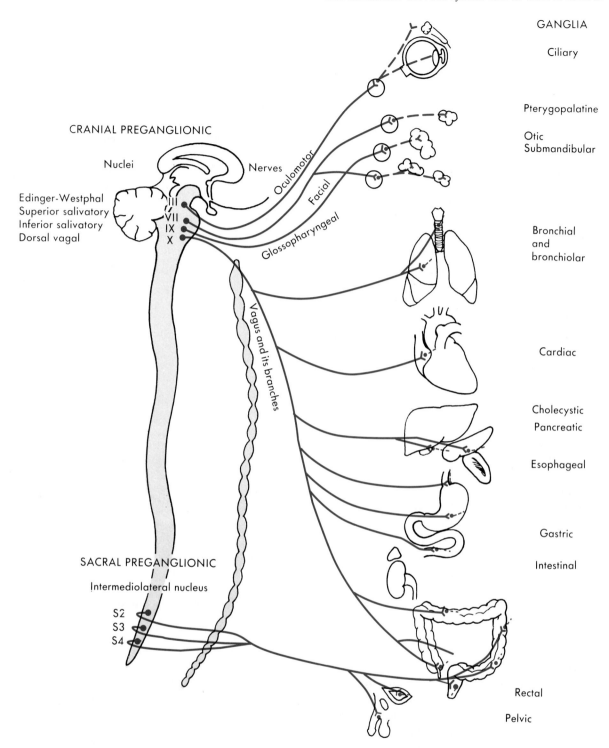

■ Fig. 15-3 Parasympathetic nervous system. (Redrawn from Bhagat BD, Young PA, Biggerstaff DE: *Fundamentals of visceral innervation,* Springfield, Ill, 1977, Charles C Thomas.)

fibers do contain many neuropeptides, or combinations of these, including angiotensin II, arginine-vasopressin, bombesin, calcitonin gene–related peptide, cholecystokinin, galanin, substance P, enkephalin, oxytocin, somatostatin, and vasoactive intestinal polypeptide.

Visceral afferent fibers that mediate sensation include nociceptors that travel in sympathetic nerves, such as the splanchnic nerves. Visceral pain is caused by excessive distention of hollow viscera, contraction against an obstruction, or ischemia. The origin of visceral pain is often difficult to identify because of its diffuse nature and its tendency to be referred to somatic structures (see Chapter 8). Visceral nociceptors in sympathetic nerves reach the spinal cord via the sympathetic chain, white rami, and dorsal roots. The terminals of the nociceptive afferent fibers distribute widely in the superficial dorsal horn and also in laminae V and X. They activate not only local interneurons, which participate in reflex arcs, but also projection cells, which include spinothalamic tract cells that signal pain to the brain.

A major visceral nociceptive pathway from the pelvis involves a relay in the lumbosacral spinal cord onto postsynaptic dorsal column neurons that project to the nucleus gracilis. Visceral nociceptive signals are then transmitted to the ventral posterior lateral nucleus of the thalamus and presumably from there to the cerebral cortex. Interruption of this pathway accounts for the beneficial effects of surgically induced lesions of the dorsal column at a lower thoracic level to relieve pain produced by cancers of the pelvic organs.

Other visceral afferent fibers travel in parasympathetic nerves. These fibers are generally involved in reflexes rather than in sensation (except for the taste afferent fibers; see Chapter 11). For example, the baroreceptor afferent fibers that innervate the carotid sinus are in the glossopharyngeal nerve. They enter the brainstem and pass through the solitary tract to terminate in the nucleus of that solitary tract. These neurons connect with interneurons in the brainstem reticular formation. These interneurons, in turn, project to the autonomic preganglionic neurons that control heart rate and blood pressure (see Chapter 28).

The nucleus of the solitary tract receives information from all visceral organs, except those in the pelvis. It is subdivided into several areas that receive information from specific visceral organs.

■ *The Enteric Nervous System*

The enteric nervous system, which is located in the walls of the gastrointestinal tract, contains about 100 million neurons. The enteric nervous system is subdivided into the myenteric plexus, which lies between the longitudinal and circular muscle layers of the gut, and the submucosal plexus, which lies in the submucosa of the gut. The neurons of the myenteric plexus control gastrointestinal motility (see Chapter 37), whereas those in the submucosal plexus regulate body fluid homeostasis (see Chapter 38).

The types of neurons found in the myenteric plexus include not only excitatory and inhibitory motor neurons (which can be considered as parasympathetic postganglionic neurons) but also interneurons and primary afferent neurons. The afferent neurons supply mechanoreceptors within the wall of the gastrointestinal tract. These mechanoreceptors form the afferent limb of reflex arcs within the enteric plexus. Local excitatory and inhibitory interneurons process these reflexes, and the output is sent through the motor neurons to the smooth muscle cells. *Excitatory motor neurons release acetylcholine and substance P; inhibitory motor neurons release dynorphin and vasoactive intestinal polypeptide.* The circuitry of the enteric plexus is so extensive that it can coordinate the movements of an intestine that has been completely removed from the body. However, normal function requires innervation by the autonomic preganglionic neurons and regulation by the CNS.

Activity in the enteric nervous system is modulated by the sympathetic nervous system. *Sympathetic postganglionic neurons that contain norepinephrine inhibit intestinal motility, those that contain norepinephrine and neuropeptide Y regulate blood flow, and those that contain norepinephrine and somatostatin control intestinal secretion.* Feedback is provided by intestinofugal neurons that project back from the myenteric plexus to the sympathetic ganglia.

The submucosal plexus regulates ion and water transport across the intestinal epithelium and glandular secretion. It also communicates with the myenteric plexus to ensure coordination of the functions of the two components of the enteric nervous system. The neurons and neural circuits of the submucosal plexus are not as well understood as are those of the myenteric plexus, but many of the neurons release neuropeptides, and the neural networks are well organized.

■ *Autonomic Ganglia*

The main type of neuron found in autonomic ganglia is the postganglionic neuron. These cells receive synaptic connections from preganglionic neurons, and they project to autonomic effector cells. However, many autonomic ganglia also contain interneurons. These interneurons process some information within the autonomic ganglia; the enteric plexus can be regarded as an elaborate example of this kind of processing. One type of interneuron found in some autonomic ganglia contains a high concentration of catecholamines. Hence, these interneurons have been called **small, intensely fluorescent (SIF) cells.** The SIF cells are believed to be inhibitory.

■ *Neurotransmitters*

■ *Neurotransmitters in Autonomic Ganglia*

The classic neurotransmitter of autonomic ganglia, whether sympathetic or parasympathetic, is acetylcholine. The two classes of acetylcholine receptors in autonomic ganglia are **nicotinic** and **muscarinic receptors,** so named because of their responses to the plant alkaloids, **nicotine** and **muscarine.** Nicotinic acetylcholine receptors can be blocked by such agents as **curare** or **hexamethonium,** and muscarinic receptors can be blocked by **atropine.** Nicotinic receptors in autonomic ganglia differ somewhat from those on skeletal muscle cells.

Nicotinic and muscarinic receptors both mediate excitatory postsynaptic potentials, but at different rates. Stimulation of preganglionic neurons elicits a fast excitatory postsynaptic potential (EPSP), followed by a slow EPSP. The fast EPSP results from activation of nicotinic receptors, which cause the opening of ion channels. The slow EPSP is mediated by muscarinic receptors that inhibit the **M current,** a current produced by a potassium conductance.

Neurons in autonomic ganglia also release neuropeptides that act as neuromodulators. Besides acetylcholine, sympathetic preganglionic neurons may release enkephalin, substance P, luteinizing hormone–releasing hormone, neurotensin, or somatostatin.

Catecholamines, such as norepinephrine or dopamine, serve as the neurotransmitters of the SIF cells in autonomic ganglia.

■ *Neurotransmitters between Postganglionic Neurons and Autonomic Effectors*

Sympathetic postganglionic neurons. Sympathetic postganglionic neurons typically release norepinephrine, which excites some effector cells but inhibits other effector cells. The receptors on the target cells may be either α- or β-adrenergic receptors. These receptors are further subdivided into α_1, α_2, β_1, and β_2 receptors. The distribution of these types of receptors, and the actions that they mediate when activated by sympathetic postganglionic neurons, are listed for various target organs in Table 15-1.

α_1 Receptors are located postsynaptically, but α_2 receptors may be either presynaptic or postsynaptic. Receptors located presynaptically are generally called **autoreceptors;** they usually inhibit transmitter release. The effects of agents that excite α_1 or α_2 receptors can be distinguished by using antagonists to block these receptors specifically. For example, prazosin is a selective α_1 antagonist, and yohimbine is a selective α_2 antagonist. The effects of α_1 receptors are mediated by activation of the inositol trisphosphate–diacylglycerol second messenger system (see Chapter 5). On the other hand, α_2 receptors decrease the rate of synthesis of cyclic AMP through an action on a G protein.

β Receptors are subdivided into β_1 and β_2 receptors on the basis of the ability of antagonists to block them. The proteins that make up the two types of β receptors are similar, with seven membrane-spanning regions connected by intracellular and extracellular domains (see Chapter 5). Agonist drugs that work on β receptors activate a G protein, which stimulates adenylyl cyclase to increase the cyclic AMP concentration. This action is terminated by the build-up of guanosine diphosphate.

Receptors can also be antagonized by the action of α_2 receptors.

β Receptors can also be antagonized by the action of α_2 receptors. The number of β receptors can be regulated. If the β receptors are exposed to agonists, they can be desensitized by phosphorylation. Their numbers can also be decreased if they become internalized. β Receptors can also increase in number (up-regulation), for example, by denervation. The number of α receptors is also regulated.

In addition to releasing norepinephrine, sympathetic postganglionic neurons release neuropeptides, such as somatostatin or neuropeptide Y. For example, cells that release both norepinephrine and somatostatin supply the mucosa of the gastrointestinal tract, and cells that release both norepinephrine and neuropeptide Y innervate blood vessels in the gut and the limb. Another chemical mediator in sympathetic postganglionic neurons is adenosine triphosphate (ATP).

The endocrine cells of the adrenal medulla are similar in many respects to sympathetic postganglionic neurons (see also Chapter 51). They receive input from sympathetic preganglionic neurons, are excited by acetylcholine, and release catecholamines. However, the cells of the adrenal medulla differ from sympathetic postganglionic neurons in that they release catecholamines into the circulation rather than synaptically. Also, the main catecholamine released is epinephrine, not norepinephrine (in humans 80% of the catecholamine released by the adrenal medulla is epinephrine, and 20% is norepinephrine).

Some sympathetic postganglionic neurons release acetylcholine rather than norepinephrine as their neurotransmitter. For example, sympathetic postganglionic neurons that innervate eccrine sweat glands are cholinergic. The acetylcholine receptors are muscarinic and are therefore blocked by atropine. Similarly, some blood vessels are innervated by cholinergic sympathetic postganglionic neurons. In addition to releasing acetylcholine, the postganglionic neurons that supply the sweat glands also release neuropeptides, including calcitonin gene–related peptide and vasoactive intestinal polypeptide.

Parasympathetic postganglionic neurons. The neurotransmitter used by parasympathetic postganglionic neurons is acetylcholine. The effects of these neurons on various target organs are listed in Table 15-1. Parasympathetic postganglionic actions are mediated by muscarinic receptors. On the basis of binding studies, the action of selective antagonists, and molecular cloning, several types of muscarinic receptors have now been discovered. At least two types of muscarinic receptors, M_1 and M_2, can be distinguished on the basis of the action of the antagonist pirenzepine. M_1 receptors have a high affinity for pirenzepine, and their activation enhances the secretion of gastric acid. M_2 receptors have a low affinity for pirenzepine, and their activation slows the heart. A subtype of the M_2 receptor activates glands such as the lacrimal and submaxillary glands.

■ **Table 15-1**   Responses of effector organs to autonomic nerve impulses

Effector organs	Receptor type	Adrenergic impulses,[1] responses[2]	Cholinergic impulses,[1] responses[2]
Eye	α		
Radial muscle, iris		Contraction (mydriasis) ++	—
Sphincter muscle, iris		—	Contraction (miosis) +++
Ciliary muscle	β	Relaxation for far vision +	Contraction for near vision +++
Heart			
SA node	β_1	Increase in heart rate ++	Decrease in heart rate; vagal arrest +++
Atria	β_1	Increase in contractility and conduction velocity ++	Decrease in contractility, and (usually) increase in conduction velocity ++
AV node	β_1	Increase in automaticity and conduction velocity ++	Decrease in conduction velocity; AV block +++
His-Purkinje system	β_1	Increase in automaticity and conduction velocity +++	Little effect
Ventricles	β_1	Increase in contractility, conduction velocity, automaticity, and rate of idioventricular pacemakers +++	Slight decrease in contractility
Arterioles			
Coronary	α, β_2	Constriction +; dilation[3] ++	Dilation±
Skin and mucosa	α	Constriction +++	Dilation[4]
Skeletal muscle	α, β_2	Constriction ++; dilation[3,5] ++	Dilation[6] +
Cerebral	α	Constriction (slight)	Dilation[4]
Pulmonary	α, β_2	Constriction +; dilation[3]	Dilation[4]
Abdominal viscera, renal	α, β_2	Constriction +++; dilation[5] +	—
Salivary glands	α	Constriction +++	Dilation ++
Veins (systemic)	α, β_2	Constriction ++; dilation ++	—
Lung			
Bronchial muscle	β_2	Relaxation +	Contraction ++
Bronchial glands	?	Inhibition (?)	Stimulation +++
Stomach			
Motility and tone	α_2, β_2	Decrease (usually)[7] +	Increase +++
Sphincters	α	Contraction (usually) +	Relaxation (usually) +
Secretion		Inhibition (?)	Stimulation +++
Intestine			
Motility and tone	α_2, β_2	Decrease[7] +	Increase +++
Sphincters	α	Contraction (usually) +	Relaxation (usually) +
Secretion		Inhibition (?)	Stimulation ++
Gallbladder and ducts		Relaxation +	Contraction +
Kidney	β_2	Renin secretion ++	—
Urinary bladder			
Detrusor	β	Relaxation (usually) +	Contraction +++
Trigone and sphincter	α	Contraction ++	Relaxation ++
Ureter			
Motility and tone	α	Increase (usually)	Increase (?)
Uterus	α, β_2	Pregnant: contraction (α); nonpregnant: relaxation (β)	Variable[8]
Sex organs, male	α	Ejaculation +++	Erection +++
Skin			
Pilomotor muscles	α	Contraction ++	—
Sweat glands	α	Localized secretion[9] +	Generalized secretion +++
Spleen capsule	α, β_2	Contraction +++; relaxation +	—
Adrenal medulla		—	Secretion of epinephrine and norepinephrine
Liver	α, β_2	Glycogenolysis, gluconeogenesis[10] +++	Glycogen synthesis +
Pancreas			
Acini	α	Decreased secretion +	Secretion ++
Islets (β cells)	α	Decreased secretion +++	—
	β_2	Increased secretion +	—
Fat cells	α, β_1	Lipolysis[10] +++	—
Salivary glands	α	Potassium and water secretion +	Potassium and water secretion +++
	β	Amylase secretion +	—
Lacrimal glands		—	Secretion +++
Nasopharyngeal glands		—	Secretion ++
Pineal gland	β	Melatonin synthesis	—

See footnotes on p 241.

Muscarinic receptors, like adrenergic receptors, have diverse actions. Some of their effects are mediated by specific second messenger systems. For example, cardiac M_2 muscarinic receptors may act by way of the inositol trisphosphate (IP_3) system, and they may also inhibit adenylyl cyclase and thus cAMP synthesis. Muscarinic receptors aiso open or close ion channels, particularly K^+ or Ca^{++} channels. This action on ion channels is likely to occur through activation of G proteins. A third action of muscarinic receptors is to relax vascular smooth muscle by an effect on endothelial cells, which produce endothelium-derived relaxing factor (EDRF). It has recently been shown that EDRF is actually nitric oxide, a gas released when arginine is converted to citrulline by nitric oxide synthase (see Chapter 28). Nitric oxide relaxes vascular smooth muscle by stimulating guanylate cyclase and thereby increasing levels of cGMP, which in turn activates a cGMP-dependent protein kinase (see Chapter 5).

The number of muscarinic receptors is regulated, and exposure to muscarinic agonists decreases the number of receptors by internalization of the receptors.

■ *Central Control of Autonomic Function*

The discharges of autonomic preganglionic neurons are controlled by pathways that synapse on autonomic preganglionic neurons. The pathways that influence autonomic activity include spinal cord or brainstem reflex pathways and also descending control systems that originate at higher levels of the nervous system, such as the hypothalamus.

■ *Examples of Autonomic Control of Particular Organs*

The autonomic control of different target organs depends on local reflex circuitry and on signals from various parts of the CNS (Table 15-1).

Pupil. The sphincter and dilator muscles of the iris determine the size of the pupil. Activation of the sympathetic innervation of the eye dilates the pupil (**mydriasis**), which occurs during emotional excitement and also in response to painful stimulation. The neurotransmitter at the sympathetic postganglionic synapses is norepinephrine, which acts at α receptors.

Sympathetic control of the pupil is sometimes affected by disease. For example, interruption of the sympathetic innervation of the head and neck results in **Horner's syndrome.** This syndrome is characterized by pupillary constriction, partial ptosis caused by paralysis of the superior tarsal muscle, loss of sweating on the face, vasodilation of facial skin, and withdrawal of the eye into the orbit (**enophthalmos**). Horner's syndrome can be produced by a lesion that (1) destroys the sympathetic preganglionic neurons in the upper thoracic spinal cord, (2) interrupts the cervical sympathetic chain, or (3) damages the lower brainstem in the region of the reticular formation through which pathways descend to the spinal cord to activate sympathetic preganglionic neurons.

The parasympathetic nervous system exerts an action on pupillary size opposite to that of the sympathetic nervous system. The sympathetic system elicits pupillary dilation, while the parasympathetic system constricts the pupil (**meiosis**). The main neurotransmitter at the postganglionic parasympathetic synapse is acetylcholine, which acts on muscarinic receptors. However, peptides may also serve as neuromodulators for some neurons.

Pupil size is reduced by the pupillary light reflex and during accommodation for near vision. In the **pupillary light reflex,** light that strikes the retina is processed by retinal circuits that excite W-type retinal ganglion cells (see Chapter 9). These cells are light sensitive. The axons of some of the W cells project through the optic nerve and tract to the pretectal area, where they synapse in the olivary pretectal nucleus. This nucleus contains neurons

■ **Table 15-1 footnotes**

From Goodman LS, Gilman A: *The pharmacological basis of therapeutics,* ed 6, New York, 1980, Macmillan.
[1]A long dash signifies no known functional innervation.
[2]Responses are designated 1+ to 3+ to provide an approximate indication of the importance of adrenergic and cholinergic nerve activity in the control of the various organs and functions listed.
[3]Dilation predominates *in situ* owing to metabolic autoregulatory phenomena.
[4]Cholinergic vasodilation at these sites is of questionable physiological significance.
[5]Over the usual concentration range of physiologically released, circulating epinephrine, β-receptor response (vasodilation) predominates in blood vessels of skeletal muscle and liver, and α-receptor response (vasoconstriction) in blood vessels of other abdominal viscera. The renal and mesenteric vessels also contain specific dopaminergic receptors, activation of which causes dilation, but their physiological significance has not been established.
[6]Sympathetic cholinergic system causes vasodilatation in skeletal muscle, but this is not involved in most physiological responses.
[7]It has been proposed that adrenergic fibers terminate at inhibitory β receptors on smooth muscle fibers and at inhibitory α receptors on parasympathetic cholinergic (excitatory) ganglion cells of Auerbach's plexus.
[8]Depends on stage of menstrual cycle, amount of circulating estrogen and progesterone, and other factors.
[9]Palms of hands and some other sites ("adrenergic sweating").
[10]There is significant variation among species in the type of receptor that mediates certain metabolic responses.

that are also light sensitive. Activity of the light-detection neurons of the olivary pretectal nucleus causes pupillary constriction by means of bilateral connections with parasympathetic preganglionic neurons in the Edinger-Westphal nuclei. The reflex results in contraction of the pupillary sphincter muscle.

In the **accommodation response,** information from M cells of the retina is transmitted to the striate cortex through the geniculostriate visual pathway (see Chapter 9). The stimulus that triggers accommodation is thought to be a blurred retinal image and disparity of the image between the two eyes. After the information is processed in the visual cortex, signals are transmitted directly or indirectly to the middle temporal cortex, where they activate neurons in the visual area known as MT. MT neurons transmit signals to the midbrain that activate parasympathetic preganglionic neurons in the Edinger-Westphal nuclei bilaterally, which results in pupillary constriction. At the same time, signals are transmitted to the ciliary muscle, causing it to contract. This ciliary muscle contraction allows the lens to round up and increase its refractile power.

The pupillary light reflex is sometimes absent in patients with syphilis that affects the CNS (i.e., in tabes dorsalis). Although the pupil fails to respond to light, it has a normal accommodation response. This condition is known as the **Argyll Robertson pupil.** The exact mechanism is controversial, but one explanation is that the brachium of the superior colliculus is interrupted, as are the fibers in the brachium that pass from the optic tract to the pretectal area. Thus, although the input to the olivary pretectal nucleus is interrupted, the optic tract connection to the lateral geniculate nucleus is intact.

Urinary bladder. The urinary bladder is controlled by reflex pathways in the spinal cord and also by a supraspinal center (Fig. 15-4). The sympathetic innervation originates from preganglionic sympathetic neurons in the upper lumbar segments of the spinal cord. Postganglionic sympathetic axons act to inhibit the smooth muscle (**detrusor muscle**) throughout the body of the bladder, and act to excite the smooth muscle of the trigone region and of the internal urethral sphincter. The detrusor muscle is tonically inhibited during filling of the bladder, and this prevents urine from being voided. The inhibition of the detrusor muscle is mediated by the action of norepinephrine on β receptors, whereas the excitation of the trigone and internal urethral sphincter is elicited by the action of norepinephrine on α receptors.

The external sphincter of the urethra also helps prevent voiding. This sphincter is a striated muscle and it is innervated by motor axons in the pudendal nerves, which are somatic nerves. The motor neurons are located in **Onuf's nucleus,** in the ventral horn of the sacral spinal cord.

The parasympathetic preganglionic neurons that control the bladder are located in the sacral spinal cord (S2 and S3 or S3 and S4 segments). These cholinergic neurons project through the pelvic nerves and are distributed to ganglia in the pelvic plexus and in the bladder wall. Postganglionic parasympathetic neurons in the bladder wall innervate the detrusor muscle, as well as the trigone and sphincter. The parasympathetic activity contracts the detrusor muscle and relaxes the trigone and sphincter. These actions result in **micturition,** or urination. Some of the postganglionic neurons are cholinergic and others purinergic (they release ATP).

Micturition is normally controlled by the **micturition reflex** (Fig. 15-4). Mechanoreceptors in the bladder wall are excited by both stretch and contraction of the muscles in the bladder wall. Thus, as urine accumulates and distends the bladder, the mechanoreceptors begin to discharge. The pressure in the urinary bladder is low during filling (5 to 10 cm H_2O), but it increases abruptly when micturition begins. Micturition can be triggered either by a reflex or voluntarily. In reflex micturition, bladder afferent fibers excite neurons that project to the brainstem

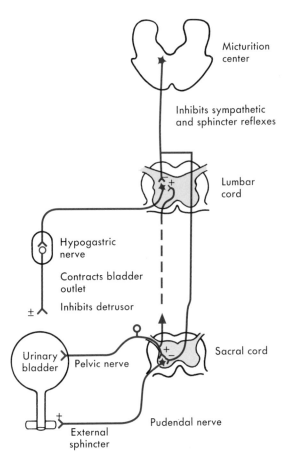

■ **Fig. 15-4**   Pathway for the reflexes that control the urinary bladder. (Redrawn from de Groat WC, Booth AM: *Autonomic systems to bladder and sex organs.* In Dyck PJ et al, editors: *Peripheral neuropathy,* ed 2, Philadelphia, 1984, WB Saunders.)

and activate the micturition center in the rostral pons **(Barrington's center).** The ascending projections also inhibit sympathetic preganglionic neurons that prevent voiding. When a sufficient level of activity occurs in this ascending pathway, micturition is triggered by the micturition center. Commands reach the sacral spinal cord through a reticulospinal pathway. Activity in the sympathetic projection to the bladder is inhibited and the parasympathetic projections to the bladder are activated. Contraction of the muscle in the wall of the bladder causes a vigorous discharge of the mechanoreceptors that supply the bladder wall and thereby further activate the supraspinal loop. The normal result is complete emptying of the bladder.

A spinal reflex pathway also exists for micturition. This pathway is operational in the newborn infant. However, with maturation, the supraspinal control pathways take on a dominant role in triggering micturition. After spinal cord injury, human adults lose bladder control during the period of spinal shock (urinary incontinence). As the spinal cord recovers from spinal shock, some degree of bladder function is recovered because of an enhancement of the spinal cord micturition reflex. However, the bladder has an increased muscle tone and fails to empty completely. These circumstances frequently lead to urinary infections.

■ *Autonomic Centers in the Brain*

An autonomic center consists of a local network of neurons that respond to inputs from a particular source and that influence distant neurons by way of long efferent pathways. The **micturition center** is the autonomic center in the pons that regulates micturition. Many other autonomic centers with diverse functions are also located in the brain. Vasomotor and vasodilator centers are in the medulla, and respiratory centers are in the medulla and pons. Perhaps the greatest concentration of autonomic centers is found in the hypothalamus.

The hypothalamus. The hypothalamus is a part of the diencephalon. Some of the nuclei of the hypothalamus are shown in Figs. 15-5 and 15-6. In the rostrocaudal dimension, the hypothalamus can be subdivided into three regions: **suprachiasmatic, tuberal,** and **mammillary regions.** Some important nuclei of the hypothalamus include the **supraoptic, paraventricular, tuberal,** and **mammillary nuclei.** Continuing anteriorly from the hypothalamus are telencephalic structures, the preoptic region and septum. Both the preoptic and septal regions help regulate autonomic function. Important fiber tracts that course through the hypothalamus are the **fornix,** the **medial forebrain bundle,** and the **mammillothalamic tract.** The fornix is used as a landmark to divide the hypothalamus into the medial and the lateral hypothalamus. Some of the connections of the hypothalamus are shown in Fig. 15-7.

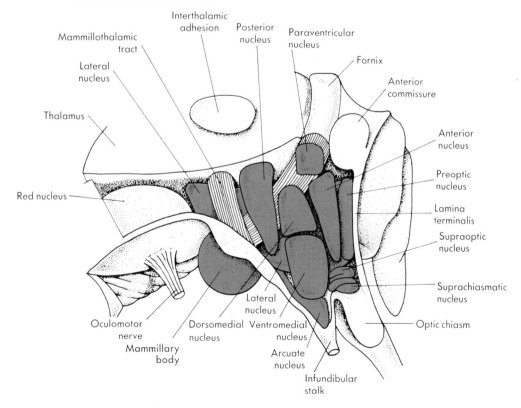

■ **Fig. 15-5** Main nuclei of the hypothalamus seen in a view from the third ventricle. (Redrawn from Nauta WJH, Haymaker W: *The hypothalamus,* Springfield, Ill, 1969, Charles C Thomas.)

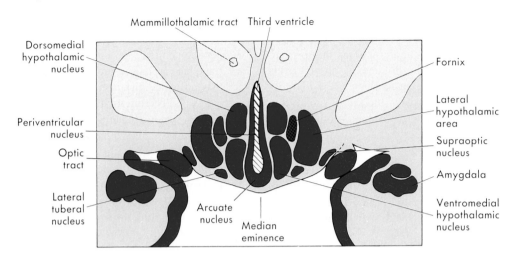

■ **Fig. 15-6**   Nuclei of the hypothalamus as seen in a frontal section. The fornix is a fiber bundle that divides the hypothalamus into lateral and medial regions. (From Kandel ER, Schwartz JH: *Principles of neural science,* ed 2, New York, 1985, Elsevier.)

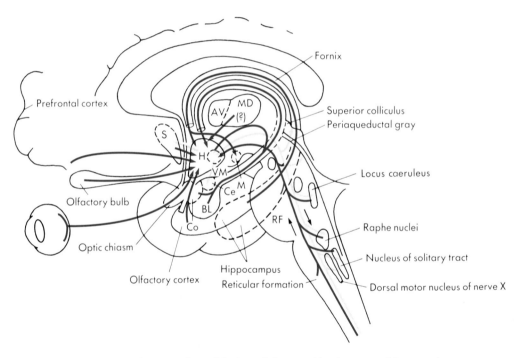

■ **Fig. 15-7**   The main connections of the hypothalamus with other parts of the central nervous system. *AV,* Anterior ventral nucleus of thalamus; *BL,* basal lateral amygdala; *Ce,* central nucleus of the amygdala; *Co,* cortical amygdala; *H,* hypothalamus; *M,* mammillary body; *MD,* mediodorsal nucleus of thalamus; *RF,* reticular formation; *S,* septum; *VM,* ventromedial hypothalamic nucleus. (Redrawn from Brodal A: *Neurological anatomy,* ed 3, London, 1981, Oxford University Press. Reprinted by permission.)

The hypothalamus has many functions, and its control of autonomic function is emphasized here. See Chapter 49 for a discussion of hypothalamic control of endocrine function.

***Temperature regulation.* Homeothermic animals** are those able to regulate their body temperature. When the environmental temperature decreases, the body adjusts by reducing heat loss and by increasing heat production. Conversely, when the temperature rises, the body increases its heat loss and reduces heat production.

Information about the external temperature is provided by thermoreceptors in the skin (and probably other organs, such as muscle). Internal temperature is monitored by central thermoreceptive neurons in the anterior hypothalamus. The central thermoreceptors monitor the temperature of the blood. The system acts as a servomechanism (a control system that uses negative feedback to operate another system) with a set point at normal body temperature. Error signals, which represent a deviation from the set point, evoke responses that tend to restore body temperature toward the set point. These responses are mediated by the autonomic, somatic, and endocrine systems.

Cooling causes shivering, which consists of asynchronous muscle contractions that increase heat production. Increases in thyroid gland activity and in sympathetic neural activity tend to increase heat production metabolically. Heat loss is reduced by piloerection and by cutaneous vasoconstriction. Piloerection is effective in animals with fur but not in humans; in the latter, the result is goose bumps.

Warming the body causes changes in the opposite direction. The activity of the thyroid gland diminishes, which leads to reduced metabolic activity and less heat production. Heat loss is increased by sweating and cutaneous vasodilation.

The hypothalamus serves as the temperature servomechanism. The heat loss responses just discussed are organized by the heat loss center, which is composed of neurons located in the preoptic region and anterior hypothalamus. As might be expected, lesions here prevent sweating and cutaneous vasodilation, and they cause **hyperthermia** when the individual is placed in a warm environment. Conversely, electrical stimulation of the heat loss center causes cutaneous vasodilation and inhibits shivering. Heat conservation responses are organized by neurons in the posterior hypothalamus, which form a heat production and conservation center. Lesions in the area dorsolateral to the mammillary body eliminate heat production and conservation and can cause **hypothermia** when the subject is in a cold environment. Electrical stimulation in this region of the brain evokes shivering.

Thermoregulatory responses are also produced when the hypothalamus is locally warmed or cooled. These responses reflect the presence of central thermoreceptive neurons in the hypothalamus.

In fever, the set point for body temperature is elevated, which can be caused by the release of a pyrogen by microorganisms. The pyrogen changes the set point, leading to increased heat production by means of shivering and to heat conservation by means of cutaneous vasoconstriction.

Regulation of food intake. Food intake is also regulated by a servomechanism. However, the set point is affected by many factors. Sensory signals that help regulate food intake operate both on a short-term basis to control ingestion and on a long-term basis to control body weight. Glucoreceptors in the hypothalamus sense the level of blood glucose and use this information to control food intake. Their main action occurs when blood glucose levels decrease. Opioid peptides and pancreatic polypeptide stimulate food intake; cholecystokinin inhibits food intake. Insulin and adrenal glucocorticoids also affect food intake (see also Chapters 46, 47, and 51).

Lesions of the lateral hypothalamus suppress food intake (**aphagia**), which can cause starvation and death. Electrical stimulation in the lateral hypothalamus stimulates the subject to eat. These observations suggest that the lateral hypothalamus contains a **feeding center.** Converse effects are produced by manipulations of the ventromedial nucleus of the hypothalamus. A lesion here causes hyperphagia, an increased food intake that can result in obesity, whereas electrical stimulation stops feeding behavior. This area of the hypothalamus is known as the **satiety center.** The feeding and satiety centers operate reciprocally.

Further work is needed to clarify the role of other parts of the nervous system in feeding behavior. Some structures that are involved are shown in Fig. 15-8.

Regulation of water intake. Water intake also depends on a servomechanism. Fluid intake is influenced by blood osmolality and volume (Fig. 15-9).

With water deprivation the extracellular fluid becomes hyperosmotic, which in turn causes intracellular fluid to become hyperosmotic. The brain contains neurons that serve as osmoreceptors, which detect increases in the osmotic pressure of the extracellular fluid (see also Chapters 42 and 49). The osmoreceptors appear to be located in the organum vasculosum of the lamina terminalis, which is a circumventricular organ. Circumventricular organs surround the cerebral ventricles and lack a blood-brain barrier. The subfornical organ and the organum vasculosum are involved in thirst. The area postrema serves as a chemosensitive zone that triggers vomiting.

Water deprivation also causes a decrease in blood volume, which is sensed by receptors in the low-pressure side of the vasculature, including the right atrium (see also Chapter 42). In addition, decreased blood volume triggers the release of renin by the kidney. Renin breaks down angiotensinogen into angiotensin I, which is then hydrolyzed to angiotensin II (see Chapter 42). This peptide stimulates drinking by an action on angiotensin II receptors in another of the circumventricular organs, the subfornical organ. Angiotensin II also causes vasoconstriction and release of aldosterone and antidiuretic hormone (ADH).

Insufficient water intake is usually a greater problem than excess water intake. When more water is taken in than is required, it is easily eliminated by inhibition of the release of ADH from neurons in the supraoptic nucleus at their terminals in the posterior pituitary gland (see Chapters 42 and 49). As already mentioned, signals that inhibit ADH release include increased blood volume and decreased osmolality of the extracellular fluid. Other areas of the hypothalamus, particularly the preoptic region and lateral hypothalamus, help regulate water intake, as do several structures outside the hypothalamus.

Other autonomic control structures. Several regions of the forebrain other than the hypothalamus also play a role in autonomic control. These include the central nucleus of the amygdala and the bed nucleus of the stria terminalis, as well as various areas of the cerebral cortex. Information reaches these higher centers from viscera through an ascending system that involves the nucleus of the solitary tract, the parabrachial nucleus, the periaqueductal gray, and the hypothalamus. Descending pathways that help control autonomic activity originate from such structures as the paraventricular nucleus of the hypothalamus, the A5 noradrenergic cell group, the rostral ventrolateral medulla, and the raphe nuclei and adjacent structures of the ventromedial medulla.

■ Neural Influences on the Immune System

Environmental stress can cause immunosuppression, in which the number of helper T cells and the activity of natural killer cells are reduced. Immunosuppression can even be the result of classical conditioning. One mechanism for such an effect involves the release of corticotropin-releasing factor (CRF) from the hypothalamus. CRF releases the adrenocorticotropic hormone (ACTH) from the pituitary gland; ACTH release stimulates the

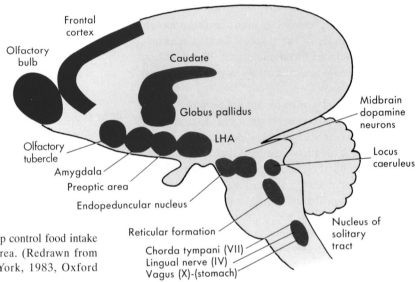

■ **Fig. 15-8** Structures thought to help control food intake in rats. *LHA,* Lateral hypothalamic area. (Redrawn from Shepherd GM: *Neurobiology,* New York, 1983, Oxford University Press.)

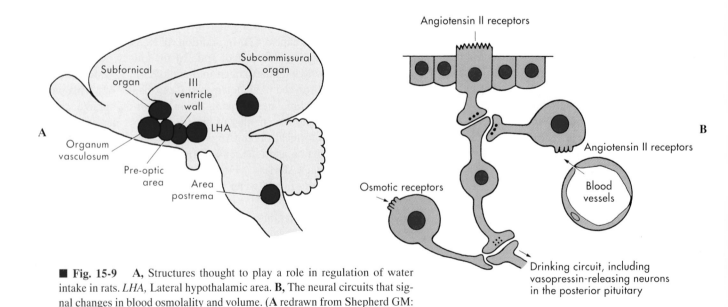

■ **Fig. 15-9** **A,** Structures thought to play a role in regulation of water intake in rats. *LHA,* Lateral hypothalamic area. **B,** The neural circuits that signal changes in blood osmolality and volume. (**A** redrawn from Shepherd GM: *Neurobiology,* New York, 1983, Oxford University Press.)

secretion of adrenal corticosteroids, which cause immunosuppression (see Chapter 51). Other mechanisms include direct neural actions on lymphoid tissues. The immune system also may influence neural activity.

■ Emotional Behavior

The limbic system helps to control emotional behavior, in part by an influence on the hypothalamus. The limbic lobe is phylogenetically the oldest part of the cerebral cortex. A circuit that connects the limbic lobe with the hypothalamus (the Papez circuit) may regulate emotional behavior. The neural components of this circuit constitute the limbic system (Fig. 15-10).

The Papez circuit connects many areas of the neocortex to the hypothalamus. Information passes from the cingulate gyrus to the entorhinal cortex and hippocampus, and from there to the mammillary bodies in the hypothalamus. The mammillothalamic tract then connects the hypothalamus with the anterior thalamic nuclei, which project back to the cingulate gyrus. Other structures included in the limbic system circuitry are the amygdala and the bed nucleus of the stria terminalis.

Bilateral temporal lobe lesions can produce the **Klüver-Bucy syndrome,** which is characterized by loss of the ability to detect and recognize the meaning of objects from visual cues (**visual agnosia**), a tendency to examine objects orally, attention to irrelevant stimuli, hypersexuality, change in dietary habits, and decreased emotionality. The components of this syndrome can be attributed to damage to different parts of the neocortex and limbic cortex. For instance, the changes in emotional behavior are largely the result of lesions of the amygdala, whereas the visual agnosia is caused by damage to visual areas in the temporal neocortex.

■ Summary

1. The autonomic nervous system is a motor system that controls smooth muscle, cardiac muscle, and glands. It helps maintain homeostasis and coordinates responses to external stimuli. Its components are the sympathetic, parasympathetic, and enteric nervous systems.

2. Autonomic motor pathways involve preganglionic and postganglionic neurons. Preganglionic neurons reside in the CNS, whereas postganglionic neurons lie in peripheral ganglia.

3. Sympathetic preganglionic neurons are located in the thoracolumbar region of the spinal cord, and sympathetic postganglionic neurons are located in paravertebral and prevertebral ganglia.

4. Parasympathetic preganglionic neurons are located in cranial nerve nuclei or in the sacral spinal cord, and parasympathetic postganglionic neurons reside in ganglia located in or near the target organs.

5. Visceral afferent fibers supply sensory receptors in the viscera. Some have a sensory function, such as visceral pain and taste, but most activate reflexes.

6. The enteric nervous system includes the myenteric and submucosal plexuses in the wall of the gastrointestinal tract. The myenteric plexus regulates motility, and the submucosal plexus regulates ion and water transport and secretion. The neural circuitry of the enteric plexuses permits coordinated activity in the isolated intestine, but normal function depends on intact autonomic control.

7. Neurotransmitters at the synapses of preganglionic neurons in autonomic ganglia include acetylcholine (acting at both nicotinic and muscarinic receptors) and a number of neuropeptides. Interneurons release catecholamines. Sympathetic postganglionic neurons generally release norepinephrine (acting at α_1, α_2, β_1, or β_2 adrenergic receptors) as their neurotransmitter, although neuropeptides are also released. Sympathetic postganglionic neurons that supply sweat glands release acetylcholine. Parasympathetic postganglionic neurons release acetylcholine (acting on M_1 or M_2 muscarinic receptors).

8. The pupil is controlled reciprocally by the sympathetic and parasympathetic nervous systems. Sympathetic activity causes pupillary dilation (mydriasis); parasympathetic activity causes pupillary constriction (meiosis). The sympathetic pathway can be activated by excitement or

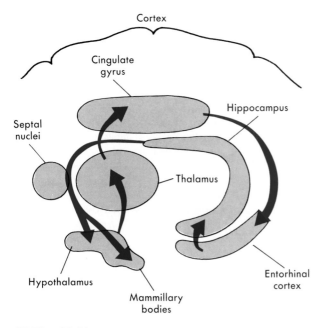

■ Fig. 15-10   The Papez circuit. (From Groves PM, Schlesinger K: *Introduction to biological psychology,* ed 2, Dubuque, Iowa, 1982, William C Brown. All rights reserved. Reprinted by permission.)

pain. Parasympathetic pathways are involved in the pupillary light reflex and in accommodation.

9. Emptying of the urinary bladder depends on parasympathetic outflow during the micturition reflex. Sympathetic constriction of the external sphincter of the urethra prevents voiding. The micturition reflex is triggered by stretch receptors and is controlled in normal adults by a micturition center in the pons.

10. The hypothalamus contains several centers that control autonomic and other activity. These include the heat loss and heat production and conservation centers, the feeding and satiety centers, and centers that regulate fluid intake.

11. Information about visceral activities reaches other autonomic control centers outside the hypothalamus. A number of descending pathways control visceral function through activation of the autonomic nervous system.

12. The limbic system consists of several cortical and other structures. It controls emotional behavior, in part by activation of the autonomic nervous system.

■ *Self-Study Problems*

1. Do the sympathetic and parasympathetic nervous systems always serve antagonistic functions?

2. What are the functions of visceral afferent fibers?

3. Describe the micturition reflex in the normal adult.

4. What is the Klüver-Bucy syndrome?

■ *Bibliography*

Journal articles

Andersson B: Regulation of water intake, *Physiol Rev* 58:482, 1978.

Benarroch EE: Neuropeptides in the sympathetic system: presence, plasticity, modulation, and implications, *Ann Neurol* 36:6, 1994.

Burnstock G: The changing face of autonomic neurotransmission, *Acta Physiol Scand* 126:67, 1986.

Bylund DB, Prichard DC: Characterization of α_1- and α_2-adrenergic receptors, *Int Rev Neurobiol* 243:343, 1983.

Cabanac M: Temperature regulation, *Annu Rev Physiol* 37:415, 1975.

Gershon MD: The enteric nervous system, *Annu Rev Neurosci* 4:227, 1981.

Greenwood B, Davison JS: The relationship between gastrointestinal motility and secretion, *Am J Physiol* 252:G1, 1987.

Johnson AK, Cunningham JT: Brain mechanisms and drinking: the role of lamina terminalis–associated systems in extracellular thirst, *Kidney Int* 32:S35, 1987.

Kalia M: Brain stem localization of vagal preganglionic neurons, *J Auton Nerv Syst* 3:451, 1981.

Kötter R, Meyer N: The limbic system: a review of its empirical foundation, *Behav Brain Res* 52:105, 1992.

Lundberg JM, Hokfelt T: Multiple coexistence of peptides and classical transmitters in peripheral autonomic and sensory neurons—functional and pharmacological implications, *Prog Brain Res* 68:241, 1986.

Moncada S, Radomski MW, Palmer RM: Endothelium-derived relaxing factor. Identification as nitric oxide and role in the control of vascular tone and platelet function, *Biochem Pharmacol* 37:2495, 1988.

Nathanson NM: Molecular properties of the muscarinic acetylcholine receptor, *Annu Rev Neurosci* 10:195, 1987.

Papez JW: A proposed mechanism of emotion, *Arch Neurol Psychiat* 38:725, 1937.

Petras JM, Faden AI: The origin of sympathetic preganglionic neurons in the dog, *Brain Res* 144:3563, 1978.

Sandner G et al: What brain structures are active during emotions? Effects of brain stimulation elicited aversion on c-fos immunoreactivity and behavior, *Behav Brain Res* 58:9, 1993.

Smith OA, DeVito JL: Central neural integration for the control of autonomic responses associated with emotion, *Annu Rev Neurosci* 7:43, 1984.

Books and monographs

Appenzeller O: *The autonomic nervous system,* ed 4, Amsterdam, 1990, Elsevier.

Bannister R, Mathias CJ, editors: *Autonomic failure. A textbook of clinical disorders of the autonomic nervous system,* ed 3, Oxford, 1992, Oxford University Press.

Björklund A et al, editors: *Handbook of chemical neuroanatomy,* vol 6, *The peripheral nervous system,* Amsterdam, 1988, Elsevier.

Brodal A: *Neurological anatomy,* ed 3, New York, 1981, Oxford University Press.

Cannon WB: *The wisdom of the body,* ed 2, New York, 1939, WW Norton.

Furness JB, Costa M: *The enteric nervous system,* Edinburgh, 1987, Churchill Livingstone.

Gabella G: *Structure of the autonomic nervous system,* New York, 1976, John Wiley.

Gross PM: *Circumventricular organs and body fluids,* vols I–III, Boca Raton, Fla, 1987, CRC Press.

Jänig J, Hicks MS, editors: *Reflex sympathetic dystrophy: a reappraisal,* Seattle, 1996, International Association for the Study of Pain (IASDP) Press.

Johnson LR, editor: *Physiology of the gastrointestinal tract,* ed 2, New York, 1987, Raven Press.

Kalivas PW, Barnes CD, editors: *Limbic motor circuits and neuropsychiatry,* Boca Raton, Fla, 1993, CRC Press.

Karczmar AG et al: *Autonomic and enteric ganglia: transmission and its pharmacology,* New York, 1986, Plenum Press.

Loewy AD, Spyer KM, editors: *Central regulation of autonomic functions,* New York, 1990, Oxford University Press.

Low PA, editor: *Clinical autonomic disorders. Evaluation and management,* Boston, 1992, Little, Brown.

Pick J: *The autonomic nervous system: morphological, comparative, clinical and surgical aspects,* Philadelphia, 1970, JB Lippincott.

Schmidt RF, Thews G: *Human physiology,* Heidelberg, 1983, Springer-Verlag.

Torrens M, Morrison JFB: *The physiology of the lower urinary tract,* Berlin, 1987, Springer-Verlag.

The Cerebral Cortex and Higher Functions of the Nervous System

Interactions between different parts of the cerebral cortex and between the cerebral cortex and other parts of the brain are responsible for the higher functions that characterize humans. The neural basis for some of these higher functions is discussed in this chapter.

■ *The Cerebral Cortex*

The cerebral cortex in humans occupies a volume of about 600 cm³ and a surface area of 2500 cm². The surface of the cortex is highly convoluted and is folded into ridges, known as **gyri.** Gyri are separated by grooves, called **sulci** (if shallow) or **fissures** (if deep). This folding increases the surface area of the cortex. From the surface, much of the cortex cannot be seen because of the presence of this folding (see Fig. 6-2).

The cerebral cortex can be divided into the left and right hemispheres. The cerebral cortex can also be subdivided into a number of lobes, including the **frontal, parietal, temporal,** and **occipital lobes.** These lobes are named for the overlying bones of the skull (see Fig. 6-2). The frontal and parietal lobes are separated by the central sulcus; they are separated from the temporal lobe by the lateral fissure. The occipital and parietal lobes are separated (on the medial surface of the hemisphere) by the parieto-occipital fissure. Buried within the lateral fissure is another lobe, the **insula.** The **limbic lobe** is formed by the cortex on the medial aspect of the hemisphere that borders on the brainstem. Part of the limbic lobe, the **hippocampal formation,** is folded into the temporal lobe and cannot be seen from the surface of the brain (Fig. 16-1). At the base of the brain can be seen an area of **olfactory cortex,** which includes the olfactory tubercle in the anterior perforated substance and the prepiriform lobe (see Chapter 11).

Activity in the cerebral cortex in the two hemispheres is coordinated by interconnections through the cerebral commissures. The bulk of the neocortex on the two sides

of the cortex is connected through the massive **corpus callosum** (see Fig. 6-3). Parts of the temporal lobes connect through the anterior commissure, and the hippocampal formations on the two sides communicate through the hippocampal commissure (which is formed between the fornices on the two sides as they pass under the corpus callosum).

■ *Functions of the Lobes of the Cerebral Cortex*

Although it has been disputed in the past, it is now clear that specific functions can be associated with the different lobes of the cerebral hemispheres.

Frontal lobe. One of the main general functions of the **frontal lobe** is motor behavior. As discussed in Chapter 14, the motor, premotor, and supplementary motor areas are located in the frontal lobe, as is the frontal eye field. These areas are responsible for the planning and executing of voluntary motor acts. In addition, the **motor speech area (Broca's area)** is located in the inferior frontal gyrus in the hemisphere that is dominant for language (almost always the left hemisphere; see the following discussion). In addition, the prefrontal cortex in the rostral part of the frontal lobe plays a major role in personality and emotional behavior.

Bilateral lesions of this part of the brain may be produced either by disease or by a surgically induced frontal lobotomy. These lesions produce deficits in attention, difficulty in problem solving, and inappropriate social behavior. Aggressive behavior is also reduced, and the motivational-affective component of pain is lost, although pain sensation remains. Frontal lobotomies are rarely performed today, because improved drug therapies have become available for mental illness and for chronic pain.

Parietal lobe. The **parietal lobe** contains the **somatosensory cortex** and the adjacent **parietal association cortex** (see Chapter 8). This lobe is involved in the

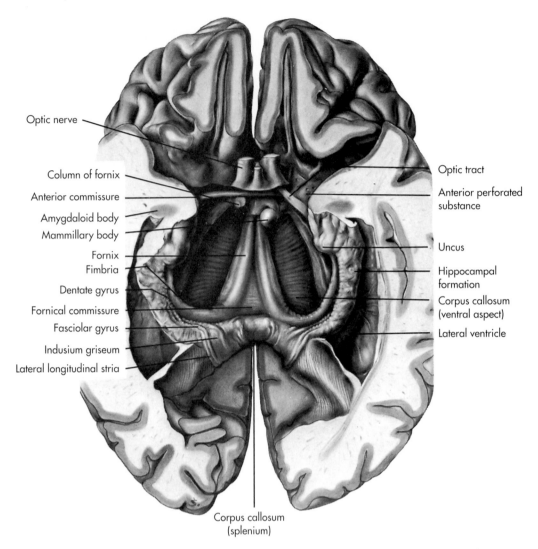

Optic nerve

Column of fornix
Anterior commissure
Amygdaloid body
Mammillary body
Fornix
Fimbria
Dentate gyrus
Fornical commissure
Fasciolar gyrus
Indusium griseum
Lateral longitudinal stria

Optic tract
Anterior perforated
substance
Uncus
Hippocampal
formation
Corpus callosum
(ventral aspect)
Lateral ventricle

Corpus callosum
(splenium)

■ **Fig. 16-1**   View of the base of the brain after dissection to reveal the hippocampal formation and related structures from below. (From Mettler FA: *Neuroanatomy,* St Louis, 1948, Mosby–Year Book.)

processing and perception of somatosensory information. Connections with the frontal lobe allow somatosensory information to affect voluntary motor activity. Visual information from the occipital lobe reaches the parietal association cortex and also the frontal lobe, and it assists in visual guidance of voluntary movements. Somatosensory information can also be transferred to the language centers, such as Wernicke's area, in the dominant language hemisphere (see the following discussion). The parietal lobe in the nondominant hemisphere is involved in spatial analysis, as shown by the effects of lesions (see Chapters 8 and 14).

Occipital lobe. *The primary function of the occipital lobe is visual processing and perception* (see Chapter 9). Occipital eye fields affect eye movements, and a projection to the midbrain assists in the control of convergent eye movements, pupillary constriction, and accommodation, all of which occur when the eyes adjust for near vision.

Temporal lobe. The **temporal lobe** performs many different functions. One of these is hearing, which depends on the processing and perception of information related to sounds (see Chapter 10). Another function is the processing of vestibular information. Several visual areas have been discovered in the temporal lobe; hence, this lobe functions in higher-order visual processing (see Chapter 9). For example, the inferior temporal gyrus is involved in the recognition of faces. In addition, Meyer's loop, which forms part of the optic radiation, passes through the temporal lobe. Therefore, temporal lobe lesions can damage this part of the optic radiation. Similarly, some of Wernicke's area lies in the posterior region of the temporal lobe (see the following); damage to the temporal lobe in the dominant hemisphere can therefore cause language disorders.

The medial temporal lobe belongs to the limbic system, which participates in emotional behavior and the autonomic nervous system (see Chapter 15). The hippocampal formation is thought to be involved in learning and memory (see below).

The functions of the different lobes of the cerebral cortex have been defined both from the effects of lesions produced by disease or by surgical interventions to treat disease in humans, and from experiments on animals. In another approach, the physical manifestations of **epileptic seizures** have been correlated with the brain locations that give rise to the seizures **(epileptic seizure foci).** For example, epileptic foci in the motor cortex cause movements on the contralateral side; the exact movements relate to the somatotopic location of the seizure focus. Seizures that originate in the somatosensory cortex cause an **epileptic aura,** in which a sensation is experienced. Similarly, seizures that start in the visual cortex cause a visual aura (scintillations, colors); those in the auditory cortex, an auditory aura (humming, buzzing, ringing); and those in the vestibular cortex, a feeling of spinning. Complex behaviors result from seizures that originate in the temporal lobe; in addition, a malodorous aura may be perceived if the olfactory cortex is involved **(uncinate fit).**

■ *Neocortical Layering and Subdivisions*

The cerebral cortex can be subdivided phylogenetically into the **archicortex** (or allocortex), **paleocortex** (or juxta-allocortex), and **neocortex** (also called isocortex). In humans, 90% of the cortex is neocortex.

The different phylogenetic subdivisions of the cerebral cortex are distinguished on the basis of their layering pattern (Fig. 16-2). The neocortex is generally characterized by the presence of six cortical layers. On the other hand, the archicortex has only three layers, and the paleocortex has four to five layers.

Cell types in neocortex. A number of different cell types are present in the neocortex. The most abundant cell types are the **pyramidal cells, stellate cells** (various types of nonpyramidal cells), and **fusiform cells** (Fig. 16-2). Pyramidal cells have a large triangular cell body, a long apical dendrite, and several basal dendrites. These cells are the main cortical efferent cells. The axon emerges from the cell body opposite the apical dendrite, and it projects into the subcortical white matter. The axon may give off collateral branches as it descends through the cortex. Pyramidal cells use an excitatory amino acid (such as glutamate or aspartate) as their neurotransmitter. **Stellate cells,** often called **granule cells,** are interneurons. They have a small cell body and numerous branched dendrites. Some are excitatory interneurons; these cells are abundant in layer IV of the cortex (see above). Their axons ascend toward the supragranular layers. Other stellate cells are inhibitory

interneurons that use gamma-aminobutyric acid (GABA) as their neurotransmitter. **Fusiform cells** are less common. The cell body is elongated, and it gives off dendrites from either end. These cells are oriented vertically to the cortical surface.

Cytoarchitecture of cortical layers. Each of the six layers of the neocortex has a characteristic cellular content (Fig. 16-2). Layer I (molecular layer) has few neuronal cell bodies; instead, it contains mostly axon terminals and synapses on dendrites. Layer II (external granular layer) contains mostly stellate cells, although some pyramidal cells are found in this layer. Layer III (external pyramidal layer) consists mostly of small pyramidal cells. Layer IV (internal granular layer) includes mostly stellate cells, including spiny stellate cells. Layer V (internal pyramidal layer) is dominated by large pyramidal cells. Layer VI (multiform layer) contains pyramidal, fusiform, and other types of cells.

Myeloarchitecture of cortical layers. The cortex contains concentrations of myelinated axons that are oriented either horizontally or vertically. Prominent horizontal sheets of axons can be found in layers I, IV, and V (Fig. 16-2). Axon sheets in layers IV and V are called the outer and inner lines of Baillarger. In the visual cortex, a particularly prominent outer line of Baillarger, known as the stripe of Gennari, gives this part of the cortex the name *striate* cortex. Vertical collections of axons, formed by cortical afferent and efferent fibers, cross the lower layers of the cortex (Fig. 16-2). These vertical collections of afferent and efferent fibers, and the cortical neurons with which they connect, are presumed to be the morphologic basis of cortical columns (see Chapters 8 to 10 and 14).

Cortical afferent and efferent fibers. The cortical afferent fibers tend to synapse in particular cortical layers; the site depends on where these fibers originate. Similarly, cortical efferent fibers that originate from particular layers project to particular destinations.

Thalamocortical afferent fibers from thalamic nuclei that have specific cortical projections end chiefly in layers III, IV, and VI. Neurons in other thalamic nuclei project diffusely and terminate in layers I and VI.

Several nonthalamic, diffusely projecting nuclei (including the basal nucleus of Meynert, the locus caeruleus, and the dorsal raphe nucleus) project to all cortical layers. These projections modulate cortical activity globally, perhaps in conjunction with changes in state (e.g., sleep or waking). The neurotransmitter in the basal nucleus of Meynert is acetylcholine; in the locus caeruleus, norepinephrine; and in the dorsal raphe nucleus, serotonin.

The cortical efferent fibers originate largely from pyramidal cells. Pyramidal cells of layers II and III project to other cortical areas, either ipsilaterally (on the same side) or contralaterally (on the opposite side). Pyramidal cells of layer V project in many descending pathways and have synaptic targets in the spinal cord, brainstem, red nucleus, and striatum. They also project to thalamic nuclei that provide diffuse projections back to the cortex. Pyramidal cells of layer VI form corticothalamic projections to thalamic nuclei with specific cortical projections. Reciprocal thalamocortical and corticothalamic interconnections are likely to make important contributions to the **electroencephalogram (EEG)** (see below).

Regional variations in neocortical structure. On the basis of differences in the cytoarchitecture, a number of subdivisions of the neocortex can be recognized. Most of the cortex is constructed of six readily distinguishable layers.

The **agranular cortex** of motor areas contains relatively few nonpyramidal cells; the lack of nonpyramidal cells is the basis for the name of this cortex. Instead, pyramidal cells predominate. This kind of cortex appears to specialize in output cells, and thus the presence of this type of cortex in the motor and premotor areas is not surprising.

Another type of cortex also has a relatively small number of pyramidal cells and is dominated by nonpyramidal cells. This type of cortex is called **granular cortex** (or **koniocortex,** for "dustlike"). Evidently, it is specialized for processing afferent input. Therefore, the presence of this kind of cortex in the primary sensory receiving areas, the somatosensory cortex (SI), the primary auditory cortex, and the primary visual (striate) cortex is reasonable.

Most of the other regions of cortex show less dramatic variations. These areas have six well-demarcated layers.

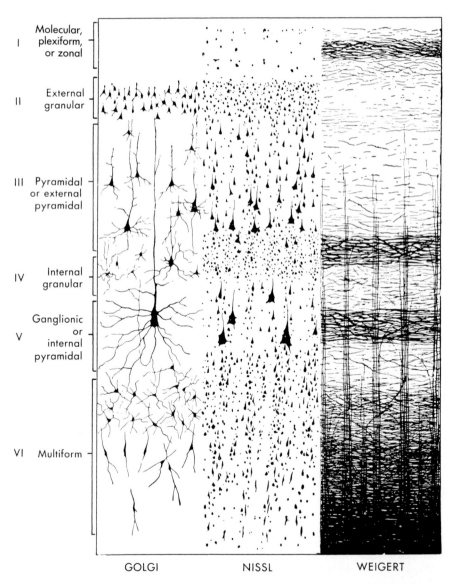

■ Fig. 16-2   Lamination of the neocortex. Neurons in the different layers are demonstrated by the Golgi stain *(left column)* and the Nissl stain *(middle column),* while myelinated fibers are shown by the myelin sheath stain *(right column).* The layers are numbered at the left. (From Brodal A: *Neurological anatomy,* ed 3, London, 1981, Oxford University Press.)

Another subdivision of the cerebral cortex was performed by Brodmann (Fig. 16-3). On the basis of an extensive cytoarchitectural analysis, Brodmann divided the cortex into 47 discrete areas. Important areas include: Brodmann's areas 3, 1, and 2, which form the SI cortex; area 4, the primary motor cortex; area 6, the premotor cortex; areas 41 and 42, the primary auditory cortex; and area 17, the primary visual cortex (striate cortex). Detailed studies have confirmed that the Brodmann areas are in fact distinctly different, with respect to both their interconnections and their functions.

■ *Allocortex*

About 10% of the human cerebral cortex is archicortex and paleocortex. The archicortex has a three-layered structure; the paleocortex has four to five layers. The paleocortex is located at the border between the archicortex and neocortex.

Hippocampal formation. The hippocampal formation forms part of the archicortex. In humans, it is folded into the temporal lobe and can be viewed only when the brain is dissected (Fig. 16-1). The hippocampal formation consists of several parts, including the hippocampus (Ammon's horn or cornu Ammonis), the dentate gyrus, and the subiculum. These components are well demarcated in a cross-section through the hippocampal formation (Fig. 16-4).

The hippocampus has three layers: molecular, pyramidal cell, and polymorphic. These resemble layers I, V, and VI in the neocortex. The folding of the hippocampus imparts an inverted appearance, because the white matter is located at the surface of the lateral ventricle (Fig.

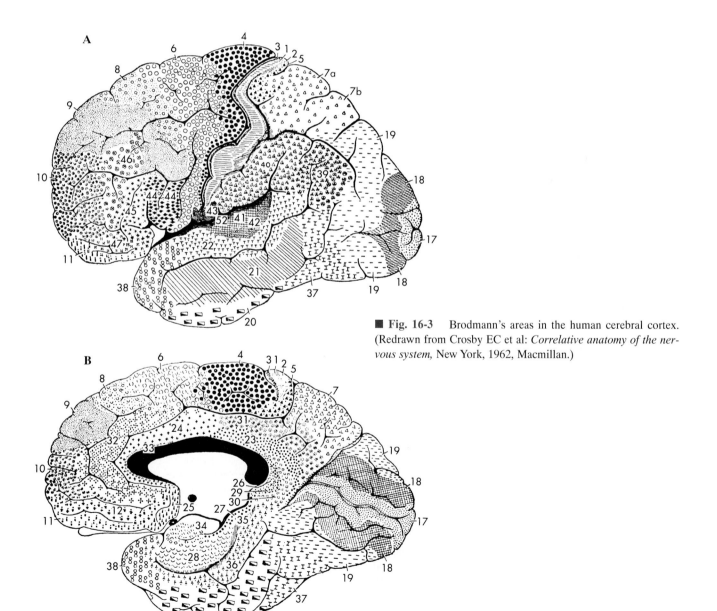

■ **Fig. 16-3** Brodmann's areas in the human cerebral cortex. (Redrawn from Crosby EC et al: *Correlative anatomy of the nervous system,* New York, 1962, Macmillan.)

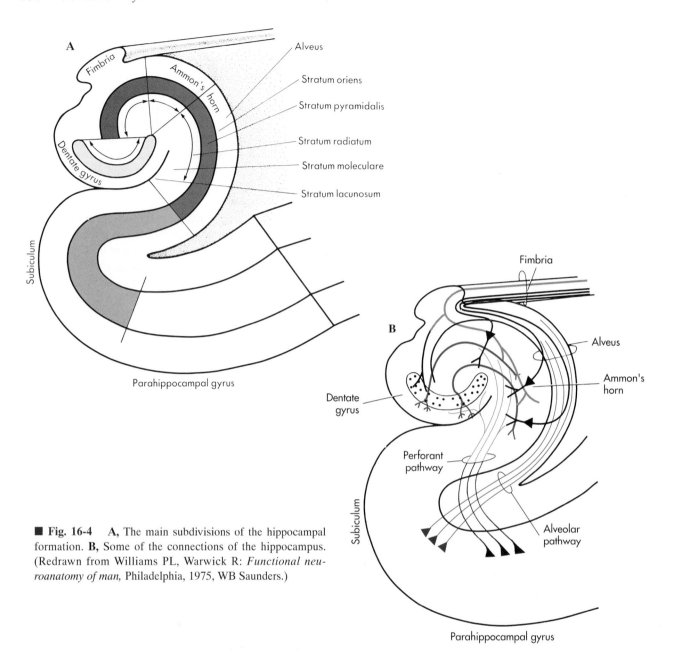

■ **Fig. 16-4** **A,** The main subdivisions of the hippocampal formation. **B,** Some of the connections of the hippocampus. (Redrawn from Williams PL, Warwick R: *Functional neuroanatomy of man,* Philadelphia, 1975, WB Saunders.)

16-4). The white matter covering the hippocampus is called the *alveus,* which contains hippocampal afferent and efferent fibers. The axons in the alveus continue into a nerve fiber bundle called the *fimbria;* the fimbria is continuous with the fornix.

The dentate gyrus is also a three-layered cortex. However, its middle layer is the granule cell layer instead of the pyramidal layer. The axons of the granule cells do not leave the hippocampal formation. Instead, they project to Ammon's horn.

The hippocampal formation receives its main neural input from the entorhinal cortex of the parahippocampal gyrus through two main projections, the **perforant path** and the **alvear path** (Fig. 16-4, *B*). Important, generally reciprocal, connections are formed between pyramidal cells of the hippocampus and (a) the septal nuclei and

mammillary body by way of the fornix, and (b) the contralateral hippocampal formation by way of the fornix and the hippocampal commissure. The granule cell layer of the dentate gyrus also projects to the hippocampus.

■ *Higher Functions of the Nervous System*

■ *The Electroencephalogram*

An **electroencephalogram (EEG)** is a recording of the rhythmic electrical activity that can be made from the cerebral cortex via electrodes placed on the skull. In an **electrocorticogram,** electrical activity of the cortex is recorded via electrodes placed on the surface of the brain.

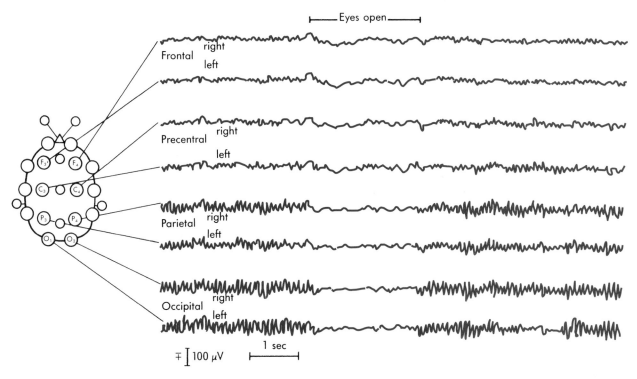

■ **Fig. 16-5**   Electroencephalogram (EEG) in a normal, resting, awake human. The recordings were made from eight channels at the same time. The electrode positions are indicated. When the eyes were opened, the alpha rhythm was blocked. (From Schmidt RF, editor: *Fundamentals of neurophysiology,* ed 2, New York, 1978, Springer-Verlag.)

In human studies, the EEG is recorded from a grid of standard recording sites. Thus, EEGs can be recorded from approximately the same sites at different times from one individual or from analogous sites in different subjects (Fig. 16-5). The EEG is an important diagnostic tool in clinical neurology and is particularly useful in patients with epilepsy.

The normal EEG consists of waves of various frequencies. The dominant frequencies depend on several factors, including the state of wakefulness, the age of the subject, the location of the recording electrodes, and the absence or presence of drugs or disease. When a normal awake adult is relaxed with eyes closed, the dominant frequencies of the EEG recorded over the parietal and occipital lobes are about 8 to 13 Hz; this is called the **alpha rhythm** (see Fig. 16-5). If the subject is asked to open his or her eyes, the EEG becomes less synchronized and the dominant frequency increases to 13 to 30 Hz, which is called the **beta rhythm.** The **delta** (0.5 to 4 Hz) and **theta** (4 to 7 Hz) **rhythms** are observed during sleep (see the following discussion) (Fig. 16-6).

The EEG waves are derived from alternating excitatory and inhibitory synaptic potentials that occur in cortical neurons as a result of thalamocortical and other input. The potentials are produced chiefly by extracellular currents that flow vertically across the cortex during the generation of synaptic potentials in the pyramidal cells. The extracellular currents associated with action potentials are too small, fast, and asynchronous to be recorded with EEG electrodes.

Although a brief EEG wave is sometimes referred to as a *spike,* this term does not refer to action potentials. The potentials recorded from an EEG are relatively large (around 100 μV). These large potentials reflect the organization of the many pyramidal cells, which are arranged with their apical dendrites aligned in parallel to form a dipole sheet. One pole of this sheet is oriented toward the cortical surface and the other toward the subcortical white matter. Note that the sign of an EEG wave does not in itself indicate whether pyramidal cells are being excited or inhibited. For instance, a negative EEG potential may be generated at the surface of the skull (or cortex) by excitation of apical dendrites or by inhibition near the somas. Conversely, a positive EEG wave can be produced by inhibition of the apical dendrites or by excitation near the somas.

■ *Evoked Potentials*

An EEG change, called a **cortical evoked potential,** can be elicited by a stimulus. A cortical evoked potential is best recorded from the part of the skull located over the cortical area being stimulated. For example, a visual stimulus results in an evoked potential that can be recorded best over the occipital bone, whereas a

Drowsy (8 to 12 cps) alpha waves

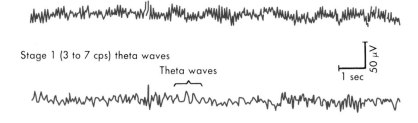

Stage 1 (3 to 7 cps) theta waves

Theta waves

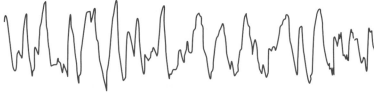

Stage 2 (12 to 14 cps) sleep spindles and K complexes

Sleep spindle   K complex →

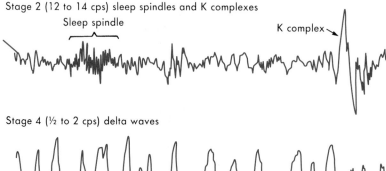

■ Fig. 16-6 EEG during drowsiness and stages 1, 2, and 4 of slow wave (non–rapid eye movement [non-REM]) sleep and in REM sleep. (Modified from Shepherd GM: *Neurobiology,* London, 1983, Oxford University Press.)

Stage 4 (½ to 2 cps) delta waves

REM sleep—low voltage, fast

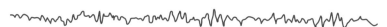

somatosensory evoked potential is recorded most effectively near the junction of the frontal and parietal bones. Evoked potentials reflect the synaptic potentials that occur in large numbers of cortical neurons. They may also reflect activity in subcortical structures.

Evoked potentials are small compared with the size of the EEG waves. However, their apparent size can be enhanced by a process called **signal averaging.** In this process, the stimulation is repeated and EEGs are recorded during each trial. With repeated stimulation, the evoked potential occurs at a fixed interval after the stimulus on each trial. However, the EEG may show a positive or a negative deflection on different trials during the time of occurrence of the evoked potential. In signal averaging, the evoked potentials are averaged electronically. The EEG waves average out, whereas the evoked potentials sum.

Evoked potentials are used clinically to assess the integrity of a sensory pathway, at least to the level of the primary sensory receiving area. These potentials can be recorded in comatose individuals, as well as in infants too young to permit a sensory examination.

The initial parts of the auditory evoked potential actually reflect activity in the brainstem; therefore, this evoked potential can be used to assess the function of brainstem structures.

■ *Sleep-Wake Cycle*

Sleep and wakefulness are among the many functions of the body that show **circadian** (about 1 day) periodicity. The sleep-wake cycle has an endogenous periodicity of about 25 hours, but it normally becomes entrained to the day-night cycle. However, the entrainment can be disrupted when the subject is isolated from the environment or shifts time zones (jet lag).

Characteristic changes in the EEG can be correlated with the changes in behavioral state during the sleep-wake cycle. **Beta-wave** activity dominates in the awake, aroused individual (Fig. 16-5). During the awake state, the EEG is said to be **desynchronized;** it displays low-voltage, high-frequency activity. In relaxed individuals with eyes closed, the EEG is dominated by **alpha waves** (Figs. 16-5 and 16-6). As the person falls asleep, he or she passes sequentially through four stages of **slow-wave** sleep (called stages 1 through 4) over a period of 30 to 45 minutes (Fig. 16-6). In stage 1, alpha waves are interspersed with lower-frequency waves (3 to 7 Hz) called **theta waves.** In stage 2, the EEG slows further, but the slow-wave activity is interrupted by **sleep spindles,** which are bursts of activity at 12 to 14 Hz, and by large **K complexes** (large, slow potentials). Stage 3 sleep is associated with **delta waves,** which occur at frequencies of 0.5 to 2 Hz, and with occasional sleep spindles. Stage 4 is characterized by delta waves.

During slow-wave sleep the muscles of the body relax, but the posture is adjusted intermittently. The heart rate and blood pressure decrease and gastrointestinal motility increases. The ease with which individuals can be awakened decreases progressively as they pass through these sleep stages. As they awaken, they pass through the sleep stages in reverse order.

About every 90 minutes, slow-wave sleep changes to a different form of sleep, called **rapid eye movement (REM)** sleep. In REM sleep, the EEG again becomes desynchronized. The low-voltage, fast activity of REM sleep resembles that seen in the EEG from an aroused subject (Fig. 16-6, *bottom trace*). The similarity of the EEG to that of an awake individual and the difficulty in awakening the person have suggested the term **paradoxical sleep** for this type of sleep. Muscle tone is completely lost, but phasic contractions occur in a number of muscles, most notably the eye muscles. The resultant rapid eye movements are the basis of the name for this type of sleep. Many autonomic changes also take place. Temperature regulation is lost, and meiosis occurs. Penile erection may also occur during this type of sleep. Heart rate, blood pressure, and respiration change intermittently. Several episodes of REM sleep occur each night. Although it is difficult to arouse a person from REM sleep, internal arousal is common. Most dreams occur during REM sleep.

The proportion of slow-wave (non-REM) to REM sleep varies with age. Newborn children spend about half of their sleep time in REM sleep, whereas the elderly have little REM sleep. About 20% to 25% of the sleep of young adults is REM sleep.

The purpose of sleep is still unclear. However, it must have a high value, because so much of life is spent in sleep and because lack of sleep can be debilitating. Medically important disorders of the sleep-wake cycle include **insomnia, bedwetting, sleepwalking, sleep apnea,** and **narcolepsy.**

The mechanism of sleep is incompletely understood. Stimulation in the brainstem reticular formation in a large region known as the **reticular activating system** causes arousal and low-voltage, fast EEG activity. Sleep was once thought to be caused by a reduced level of activity in the reticular activating system. However, substantial data, including the observations that anesthesia of the lower brainstem results in arousal, and that stimulation in the medulla near the nucleus of the solitary tract can induce sleep, suggest that sleep is an active process. Neurotransmitters may also be involved in the sleep mechanism. On the basis of these findings, investigators have tried to relate sleep mechanisms to brainstem networks that use these neurotransmitters. Investigators have found that manipulations of the levels of serotonin, norepinephrine, and acetylcholine in the brain can affect the sleep-wake cycle.

The source of circadian periodicity in the brain appears to be the suprachiasmatic nucleus of the hypothalamus. This nucleus receives projections from the retina, and its neurons seem to form a biological clock. Destruction of the suprachiasmatic nucleus disrupts a number of biological rhythms, including the sleep-wake cycle.

The EEG becomes abnormal under a variety of pathological circumstances. For example, during coma, the EEG is dominated by delta activity. **Brain death** is defined by a sustained, flat EEG reading.

Epilepsy commonly causes EEG abnormalities. There are several forms of epilepsy, and examples of EEG patterns from some of these variants are shown in Fig. 16-7. Epileptic seizures can be either partial or generalized.

One form of partial seizures originates in the motor cortex and results in localized contractions of contralateral muscles. The contractions may then spread to other muscles; the spread follows the somatotopic sequence of the motor cortex (see Fig. 13-5). Complex partial seizures (which may occur in **psychomotor epilepsy**) originate in the limbic lobe and result in illusions and semipurposeful motor activity. During and between focal seizures, the EEG may reveal spikes (Fig. 16-7, *C* and *D*).

Generalized seizures involve wide areas of the brain and loss of consciousness. Two major types of generalized seizures are **petit mal** and **grand mal.** In petit mal epilepsy, consciousness is lost transiently and the EEG displays spike and wave activity (Fig. 16-7, *B*). In **grand mal seizures,** consciousness is lost for a longer period, and the individual may fall to the ground if he or she is standing when the seizure starts. The seizure begins with a generalized increase in muscle tone **(tonic phase),** followed by a series of jerky movements **(clonic phase).** The bowel and bladder may be evacuated. The EEG shows widely distributed seizure activity (Fig. 16-7, *A*).

EEG spikes that occur between full-blown seizures are called **interictal spikes.** Similar events can be studied experimentally. These spikes arise from abrupt, long-lasting depolarizations, called **depolarization shifts,** which trigger repetitive action potentials in cortical neurons. These depolarization shifts may reflect several changes in epileptic foci. Such

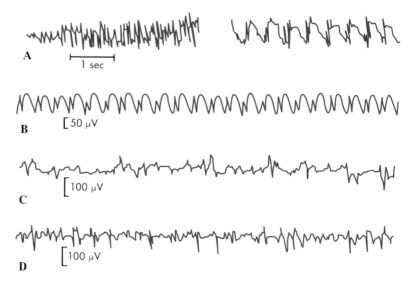

■ **Fig. 16-7** EEG abnormalities in several forms of epilepsy. **A,** EEG during the tonic *(left)* and clonic *(right)* phases of a grand mal seizure. **B,** Spike and wave components of a petit mal seizure. **C,** EEG in temporal lobe epilepsy. **D,** A focal seizure. (Redrawn from Eyzaguirre C, Fidone SJ: *Physiology of the nervous system,* ed 2, Chicago, 1975, Mosby–Year Book.)

changes include regenerative Ca⁺⁺-mediated dendritic action potentials in cortical neurons and a reduction in inhibitory interactions in cortical circuits. Electrical field potentials and the release of K⁺ and excitatory amino acids from hyperactive neurons may also contribute to the increased cortical excitability seen in depolarization shifts.

Cerebral Dominance and Language

In most people, the left cerebral hemisphere is the **dominant hemisphere** with respect to language. This dominance has been demonstrated (1) by the effects of lesions of the left hemisphere, which may produce deficits in language function **(aphasia);** and (2) by the transient aphasia (inability to speak or write) that results when a short-acting anesthetic is introduced into the left carotid artery. Lesions of the right hemisphere and the injection of anesthetic into the right carotid artery do not usually affect language substantially. The right hemisphere is dominant for functions other than language. For example, left-handedness reflects a motor dominance of the right hemisphere. However, in most left-handed people, the left hemisphere is still dominant for language. Differences in the size of an area called the **planum temporale,** which is located in the floor of the lateral fissure, correlate with language dominance. The left planum temporale is usually larger than that of the right hemisphere.

Several areas in the left hemisphere are involved in language. **Wernicke's area** is a large region centered in the posterior part of the superior temporal gyrus near the auditory cortex. Another important language area, **Broca's area,** is located in the posterior part of the inferior frontal gyrus, close to the face representa-

tion of the motor cortex. Damage to Wernicke's area results in **sensory aphasia,** in which the person has difficulty understanding spoken or written language; however, speech production remains fluent. Conversely, a lesion of Broca's area causes **motor aphasia.** Individuals with motor aphasia have difficulty speaking and writing, although they can understand language relatively well.

A person with sensory aphasia may not have auditory or visual impairment, and a person with motor aphasia may have normal motor control of the muscles responsible for speech or writing. Thus, aphasia does not depend on an alteration in sensation or in the motor system; rather, it is a deficit in the reception or planning of language expression. However, lesions in the dominant hemisphere may be large enough to result in mixed forms of aphasia, as well as in sensory changes or paralysis of some of the muscles used to express language.

Interhemispheric Transfer

The two cerebral hemispheres can function relatively independently, as in the case of language function. However, information must be transferred between the hemispheres, in order to coordinate activity on the two sides of the body. In other words, each hemisphere must know what the other is doing. Much of the information transferred between the two hemispheres is transmitted through the corpus callosum, although some is transmitted through other commissures (e.g., anterior commissure, midbrain commissures).

An experiment that shows the importance of the corpus callosum for interhemispheric transfer of information is illustrated in Fig. 16-8. An animal with an intact optic chiasm and corpus callosum and with the left eye closed learns a visual discrimination task (Fig. 16-8, *A*). The information is transmitted to both hemispheres through the bilateral connections made by the optic chiasm or through the corpus callosum, or both. When the animal is tested with the left eye open and the right eye closed (Fig. 16-8, *center*), the task can still be performed, because both hemispheres have learned the task. If the optic chiasm is transected before the animal is trained, the result is the same (Fig. 16-8, *B*). Therefore, information is presumably transferred between the two hemispheres through the corpus callosum. This finding can be confirmed by cutting both the optic chiasm and corpus callosum before training (Fig. 16-8, *C*). Now the information is not transferred, and each hemisphere must learn the task independently.

A similar experiment has been done in human subjects who have had a surgical transection of the corpus callosum to prevent the interhemispheric spread of epilepsy (Fig. 16-9). The optic chiasm remained intact. Directing visual information to one or the other hemisphere was possible by having the subject fix his or her vision on a point on a screen. A picture of an object was then projected to one side of the fixation point. Visual information about the picture reached only the contralateral hemisphere. An opening beneath the screen allowed the patient to manipulate objects that could not be seen. The objects included those shown in the projected pictures. Normal individuals would be able to locate the correct object with either hand. However, the patients with a transected corpus callosum could locate the correct object only with the hand ipsilateral to the projected image (contralateral to the hemisphere that received the visual information). The visual information must have had access to the motor areas of the cortex for the hand to explore and recognize the correct object. With the corpus callosum cut, the visual and motor areas are interconnected only on the same side of the brain.

Another test involved asking the subject to identify verbally what object was seen in the picture. The patient would make a correct verbal response to a picture that was projected to the right of the fixation point so that the visual information reached only the left (language-dominant) hemisphere. However, the patient could not verbally identify a picture that was presented to the left hemifield because the visual information reached only the right hemisphere.

Similar observations can be made in patients with a transected corpus callosum when different forms of stimuli are used. For example, when such patients are given a verbal command to raise the right arm, they can do so without difficulty. The language centers in the left hemisphere send signals to the motor areas on the same side, and these signals produce the movement of the right arm. However, the patients cannot respond to a command to raise the left arm. The language areas on the left side cannot influence the motor areas on the right unless the corpus callosum is intact. The result is a type of apraxia (inability to control voluntary movement).

Somatosensory stimuli applied to the right side of the body can be described by patients with a transected corpus callosum. However, these patients cannot describe the same stimuli applied to the left side of the body. Again, information that reaches the right somatosensory areas of the cortex cannot reach the language centers if the corpus callosum has been cut.

The functional capabilities of the two hemispheres can be compared by exploring the performance of individuals with a transected corpus callosum. For example, such patients solve three-dimensional puzzles better with the right than with the left hemisphere; this finding suggests that the right hemisphere specializes in spatial tasks. Other functions that seem to be associated with the right rather than the left hemisphere are facial expression, body language, and speech intonations. The corpus callosum promotes coordination between the two hemispheres, which can also be shown in patients with a transected corpus callosum. These patients lack coordination. When they are dressing, for example, one hand may button a shirt while the other tries to unbutton it.

A striking conclusion of experiments on these patients is that the two hemispheres can operate quite independently when they are no longer interconnected. However, one hemisphere can express itself with language, whereas the other communicates only nonverbally.

■ *Learning and Memory*

Major functions of the higher levels of the nervous system are learning and memory. *Learning is a neural mechanism by which the individual changes his or her behavior as the result of experience. Memory refers to the storage mechanism for what is learned.*

Types of learning. The two broad classes of learning are **nonassociative** and **associative learning.** Nonassociative learning does not depend on a particular relationship between what is learned and some other stimulus. For example, in a type of nonassociative learning called **habituation,** a repeated stimulus causes a response that gradually diminishes. The response presumably diminishes because the individual learns that the stimulus is not important. A familiar example is the change in attention that typically occurs when a new clock is presented to a subject. At first the ticking noise may be annoying and may cause some difficulty in sleeping. However, after several nights the clock is no longer noticed. Unfortunately, the response to the clock's morning alarm may be diminished.

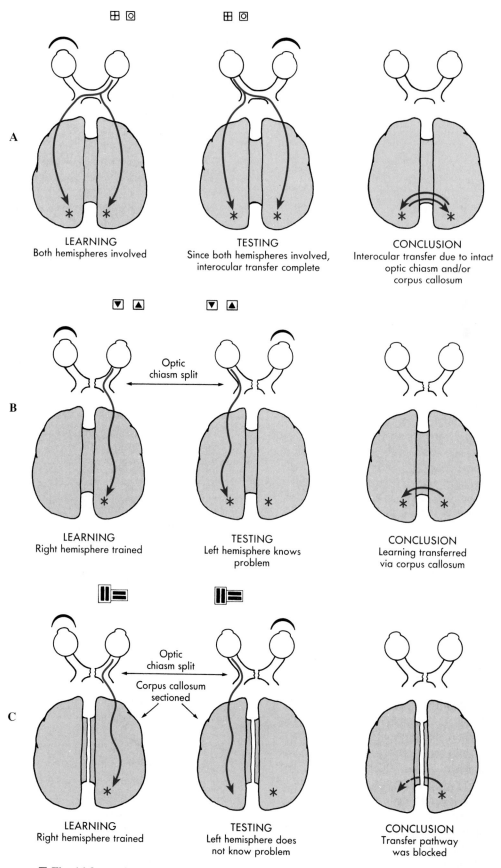

■ **Fig. 16-8**   Role of the corpus callosum in the interhemispheric transfer of visual information. **A,** Learning involves one eye. The discrimination depends on distinguishing between a cross and a circle. **B,** Discrimination is between triangles oriented with the apex up or down. **C,** Discrimination is between vertical and horizontal bars.

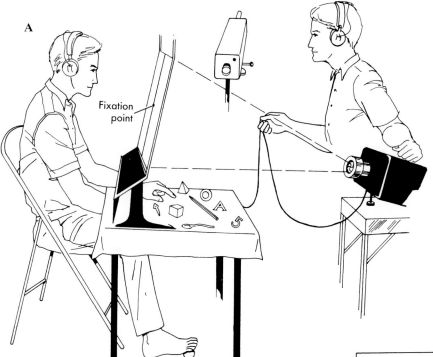

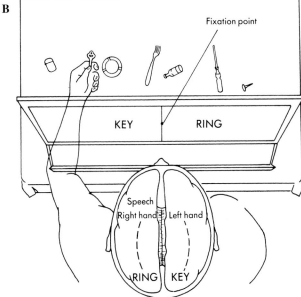

■ **Fig. 16-9** Tests in a patient with a transected corpus callosum. **A,** The patient fixes on a point on a rear projection screen, and pictures are projected to either side of the fixation point. The hand can palpate objects that correspond to the projected pictures, but these cannot be seen. **B,** Response by the left hand to a picture of a key in the left field of view. However, the verbal response is that the patient sees a picture of a ring. (Redrawn from Sperry RW. In Schmitt FO, Worden FG, editors: *The neurosciences: third study program*, Cambridge, Mass, 1974, MIT Press.)

Another type of nonassociative learning is **sensitization.** In sensitization, a strong and consequently threatening stimulus results in a greater probability of a response to later similar stimuli. When the stimulus is first given, the response may be minimal. However, with repetition, the response increases. For example, a spanking can lead to a greater likelihood that a child will obey a parent's admonition. Thus, in sensitization, learning occurs in a direction opposite to that seen in habituation, presumably so that the behavior becomes directed toward escape from the stimulus.

Associative learning occurs when the learning process involves some relationship between stimuli. In **classical conditioning,** a temporal association is made

between a neutral conditioned stimulus and an unconditioned stimulus that elicits an unlearned response. An example of classical conditioning is the behavior of dogs in Pavlov's experiments on conditioned reflexes. For example, food presented to a hungry dog elicits an unconditioned response, salivation. If a bell is rung just before the food is presented, the dog learns to associate the bell with the food. Eventually, ringing the bell alone causes salivation. If the combination of conditioned (food) and unconditioned (the bell) stimuli is repeated, and the timing relationship is maintained, the association between these stimuli is learned, at which point the conditioned stimulus alone will elicit the unlearned response (salivation). Of course, if the food fails to appear consistently when the bell is rung, the conditioned response fades away, a process called **extinction.**

Another form of associative learning is **instrumental** or **operant conditioning.** In this process, when the response to a stimulus is reinforced, the probability of the response changes. The reinforcement can be either positive or negative. An example of positive reinforcement is giving a fish to a porpoise for jumping out of the water through a hoop. An example of negative reinforcement would be sending a child to his or her room for misbehaving. With positive reinforcement the response probability increases; with negative reinforcement the probability decreases.

Experiments on the mechanisms of learning. The neural circuitry involved in learning in mammals is complex; hence, it has been difficult to study these mechanisms. An alternative approach has been to examine the cellular basis of learning in the simpler nervous systems of invertebrates, such as the marine mollusk Aplysia. By isolating a connection between a single sensory neuron and a motor neuron responsible for a particular motor response, modeling habituation, sensitization, and even conditioning has been possible.

These experiments have shown that the presynaptic endings of the sensory neuron can change the amount of neurotransmitter released (Fig. 16-10) during learning. For example, during short-term habituation, the amount of transmitter released in successive responses gradually diminishes. The change involves an alteration in the Ca^{++} current that triggers neurotransmitter release. The cause of this change is that repeated action potentials lead to a reduction in the number of available Ca^{++} channels. Long-term habituation can also be produced. In this case, the number of synaptic endings and active zones in the remaining terminals decreases.

On the other hand, in short-term sensitization, an interneuron may release serotonin onto the presynaptic terminal, and the serotonin may stimulate adenylyl cyclase and the build-up of cAMP intracellularly. This increase in intracellular cAMP, in turn, causes phosphorylation of K^+ channels, a decrease in K^+ current, and broadening of the presynaptic action potential. Broadened action potentials cause more transmitter to be released, which increases synaptic efficacy and leads to a larger response. More transmitter is also mobilized. In long-term sensitization, the numbers of synaptic terminals and active zones formed by the presynaptic neurons increase, and the dendrites of the postsynaptic neurons expand. Similar kinds of events may also occur in associative learning.

Long-term potentiation. Another model of learning is provided by a synaptic phenomenon called **long-term potentiation (LTP).** LTP has been studied most intensively in slices of the hippocampus in vitro. However, LTP has also been described in the neocortex and in other parts of the nervous system. Repetitive activation of an afferent pathway to the hippocampus or of one of the intrinsic connections increases the responses of the pyramidal cells. The increased responses (the LTP) last for hours in vitro (and even days to weeks in vivo). The forms of LTP differ, depending on the particular synaptic system. The mechanism of the enhanced synaptic efficacy seems to involve both presynaptic and postsynaptic events. The neurotransmitters involved in LTP include excitatory amino acids that act on N-methyl-D-aspartate (NMDA) receptors, which evoke a resultant postsynaptic influx of Ca^{++} ions. Second messenger pathways (including G proteins, Ca^{++}/calmodulin–dependent protein kinase II, protein kinase G, and protein kinase C) are also involved, and these kinases cause protein phosphoryla-

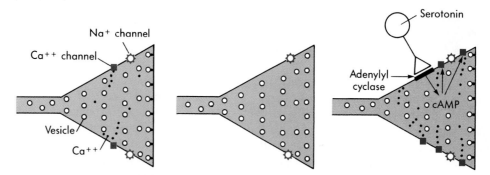

■ **Fig. 16-10**   Aplysia model of short-term habituation and sensitization. *Left,* A synapse in the control state. Invasion of the action potential into the ending causes Na^+ influx through Na^+ channels, resulting in the opening of Ca^{++} channels and transmitter release. *Middle,* Repeated activity has reduced the number of available Ca^{++} channels and thus decreased transmitter release. *Right,* Repeated strong stimulation activates a serotonergic interneuron, which releases serotonin onto the terminal, causing an increase in cAMP, a reduction in K^+ channel opening, and spike broadening. The broadened spikes cause increased transmitter release. (Redrawn from Kandel ER, Schwartz JH: *Principles of neural science,* New York, 1981, Elsevier–North Holland.)

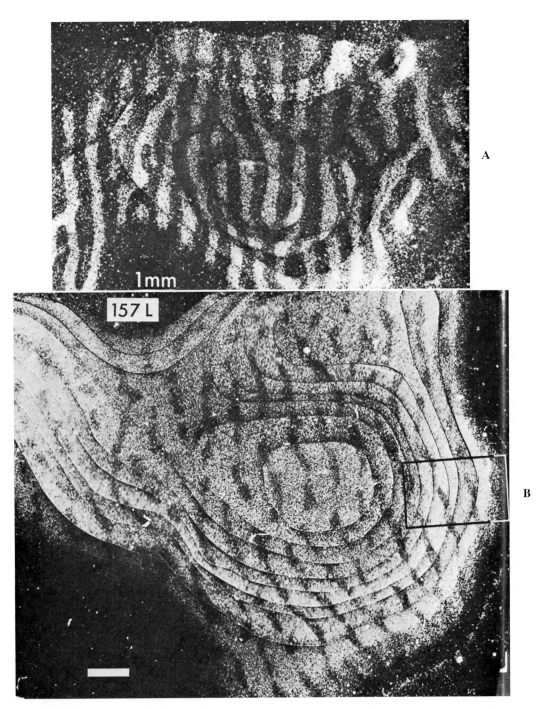

■ **Fig. 16-11**   Plasticity in the visual pathway as a result of sensory deprivation during development. The ocular dominance columns are demonstrated by autoradiography after injection of a radioactive tracer into one eye. The tracer is transported to the lateral geniculate nucleus and then transneurally transported to the striate cortex. The cortex is labeled in bands that alternate with unlabeled bands whose input is from the uninjected eye. **A,** Normal pattern; **B,** Changed pattern in an animal raised with monocular visual deprivation. The injection was into the nondeprived eye, and the ocular dominance columns for this eye were clearly expanded. In other experiments, it could be shown that the ocular dominance columns for the deprived eye contracted. (**A** from Hubel DH, Wiesel TN: Functional architecture of macaque monkey visual cortex, *Proc R Soc Lond B* 198:1, 1977; **B** from LeVay S, Hubel DH, Wiesel TN: The development of ocular dominance columns in normal and visually deprived monkeys, *J Comp Neurol* 191:1, 1980.)

tion and changes in the responsiveness of neurotransmitter receptors. A retrograde messenger, perhaps nitric oxide (or carbon monoxide), may be released from postsynaptic neurons to act on presynaptic endings in such a way as to enhance transmitter release. Immediate-early genes are also activated during LTP. Hence, changes in gene expression may also be involved.

In some cases, LTP is associative. In associative LTP, a weak synaptic input is strengthened when it is temporally associated with a stronger input. In other cases, LTP is nonassociative. The hypothesis that LTP is involved in at least some aspects of memory is reasonable.

Another form of synaptic remodeling is **long-term depression (LTD).** LTD has been studied most extensively in the cerebellum, but it also occurs in the hippocampus and in other regions of the central nervous system (CNS). Some of the same factors, such as Ca^{++} influx and activation of signal transduction mechanisms, may account for the induction of LTD, just as for LTP.

Memory. With regard to the stages of memory storage, a distinction between **short-term memory** and **long-term memory** is useful. Recent events appear to be stored in **short-term memory** by ongoing neural activity, because short-term memory persists for only minutes. Short-term memory is used, for instance, to remember a telephone number after calling the operator. **Long-term memory** can be subdivided into an intermediate form, which can be disrupted, and a long-lasting form, which is difficult to disrupt. Memory loss can be caused by a disruption of memory per se, or it can be a result of interference with the mechanism for recovering information from memory. Long-term memory may involve structural changes in the nervous system, because this form of memory can remain intact even after events that disrupt short-term memory.

The temporal lobes appear to be particularly important for memory, because bilateral removal of the hippocampal formation severely and permanently disrupts recent memory. Short- and long-term memories are unaffected, but new long-term memories can no longer be stored.

Neural plasticity. Damage to the nervous system can induce remodeling of neural pathways and thereby alter behavior. Such remodeling is said to reflect the **plasticity** of the nervous system. The CNS is much more plastic than was once believed. For example, the development of neural connections may be altered by certain interventions, such as by lesions of the brain or by sensory deprivation. Plasticity is greatest in the developing brain, but some degree of plasticity remains in the adult brain.

The capability for developmental plasticity may change for some neural systems at a time referred to as the **critical period.** For example, it may be possible to alter the connections formed in the visual pathways during their development, but only up to a particular developmental period. In visually deprived animals, the visual connections may be abnormal (Fig. 16-11). However,

visual deprivation that occurs after several postnatal months does not result in abnormal connections, and neither does restoration of vision after this time repair the abnormal connections in previously visually deprived animals. The plastic changes seen in such experiments may reflect a competition between fibers for synaptic connections with postsynaptic neurons in the developing nervous system. If a developing neural pathway "loses" in such a competition, the result may be a neurologic deficit in the adult.

A consequence of visual deprivation during development of the visual pathways may be **amblyopia** of the deprived eye. Amblyopia is reduced visual capacity, and it can occur, for example, in children with strabismus (cross-eye) because of a relative weakness of one of the extraocular muscles. Similar effects can be produced by a cataract or by uncorrected myopia.

Plastic changes can also occur after injury to the brain in adults. Sprouting of new axons does occur in the damaged CNS. However, the sprouts do not necessarily restore normal function, and many neural pathways do not appear to sprout. Additional knowledge concerning neural plasticity in the adult nervous system is vital if medical therapy is to be improved for many diseases of the nervous system and after neural trauma.

■ *Summary*

1. The cerebral cortex can be subdivided into lobes, based on the pattern of gyri and sulci. Each lobe has special functions, as shown by the effects of lesions or seizures.

2. The cerebral cortex can be subdivided into neocortex, archicortex, and paleocortex. The neocortex typically has six layers, whereas the other types of cortex have fewer layers.

3. The neocortex contains a number of cell types, including pyramidal cells, which serve as the output cells, and several kinds of interneurons. The pyramidal cells release an excitatory amino acid neurotransmitter, whereas the inhibitory interneurons are GABA-ergic.

4. Specific thalamocortical afferent fibers terminate in the middle layers and layer VI; diffuse thalamocortical afferent fibers synapse in layers I and VI. Cortical efferent fibers from layers II and III project to other areas of the cortex; those from layer V project to many subcortical targets, including the spinal cord, brainstem, and striatum, as well as to diffuse thalamic nuclei; and layer VI distributes to the appropriate specific thalamic nucleus.

5. The cortical structure varies in different regions. Agranular (type 1) cortex is found in the motor areas, whereas granular cortex (koniocortex; type 5 cortex)

occurs in the primary sensory receiving areas. Several types of homotypical cortex are found elsewhere in the neocortex. Brodmann's areas reflect these variations of cortical structure and correlate with functionally discrete areas. The archicortex has three layers, as typified by the hippocampus and dentate gyrus of the hippocampal formation.

6. The electroencephalogram (EEG) varies with the state of the sleep-wake cycle, disease, and other factors. EEG rhythms include alpha, beta, theta, and delta waves. The EEG reflects synaptic activity of pyramidal cells. Cortical evoked potentials are stimulus-triggered changes in the EEG and are useful clinical tests of sensory transmission.

7. Sleep can be divided into slow-wave and rapid eye movement (REM) forms. Slow-wave sleep progresses through stages 1 to 4, each with a characteristic EEG pattern. Most dreams occur during REM sleep. Sleep is produced actively by a brainstem mechanism, and its circadian rhythmicity is controlled by the suprachiasmatic nucleus.

8. The EEG helps in the recognition of the various forms of epilepsy. Seizures are associated with depolarization shifts in pyramidal cells. Such shifts are caused by dendritic Ca^{++} spikes and a reduction in inhibitory processing.

9. The left cerebral hemisphere is dominant for language in most individuals. Wernicke's area is responsible for the understanding of language and Broca's area for its expression.

10. Information is transferred between the two hemispheres through the corpus callosum. This structure coordinates the two sides of the brain. The right hemisphere dominates the left in spatial tasks, facial expression, body language, and speech intonation.

11. Learning includes nonassociative and associative forms. Two kinds of nonassociative learning are habituation and sensitization. Associative learning includes classical and operant conditioning. Short-term changes in learning include changes in synaptic efficacy; long-term changes involve alterations in the number of synapses.

12. Long-term potentiation is mediated by an increased synaptic efficacy that lasts hours to weeks and that involves both presynaptic and postsynaptic changes.

13. Memory includes short-term (minutes), recent, and long-term storage processes and a retrieval mechanism. The hippocampal formation is important for recent memory.

14. Damage may alter neural pathways during early development of the nervous system. These alterations may become permanent after a critical period, and they may result in neurologic deficits in adults.

■ *Self-Study Problems*

1. What are the functions of the main lobes of the cerebrum?

2. How is the EEG recorded and what do the oscillations mean?

3. How can an evoked potential be detected, considering the large variability of individual responses and the fact that each individual response is small compared with the size of the EEG?

4. Distinguish between REM and non-REM sleep.

5. Distinguish between motor and sensory aphasia.

■ *Bibliography*

Journal articles

Artola A, Singer W: Long-term depression of excitatory synaptic transmission and its relationship to long-term potentiation, *Trends Neurosci* 16:480, 1993.

Bekklers JM, Stevens CF: Presynaptic mechanism for long-term potentiation in the hippocampus, *Nature* 346:724, 1990.

Ben-Ari Y, Anikksztejn L, Bregestovski P: Protein kinase C modulation of NMDA currents: an important link for LTP induction, *Trends Neurosci* 15:333, 1992.

Benowitz LI, et al: Hemispheric specialization in nonverbal communication, *Cortex* 19:5, 1983.

Damaasio AR, Geschwind N: The neural basis of language, *Annu Rev Neurosci* 7:127, 1984.

Dichter MA, Ayala GF: Cellular mechanisms of epilepsy: a status report, *Science* 237:157, 1987.

Dragunow M: A role for immediate-early transcription factors in learning and memory, *Behav Genet* 26:293, 1996.

Geschwind N: Specializations of the human brain, *Sci Am* 241:180, 1979.

Hawkins RD, Zhuo M, Arancio O: Nitric oxide and carbon monoxide as possible retrograde messengers in hippocampal long-term potentiation, *J Neurobiol* 25:652, 1994.

Lisman J: The CaM kinase II hypothesis for the storage of synaptic memory, *Trends Neurosci* 17:406, 1994.

Milner B: Some cognitive effects of frontal-lobe lesions in man, *Phil Trans R Soc Lond B* 298:211, 1982.

Prince DA: Neurophysiology of epilepsy, *Annu Rev Neurosci* 1:395, 1978.

Rosenwasser AM: Behavioral neurobiology of circadian pacemakers: a comparative perspective, *Prog Psychobiol Physiol Psychol* 13:155, 1988.

Sperry RW: Mental unity following surgical disconnection of the cerebral hemispheres, *Harvey Lect* 62:293, 1964.

Voronin LL: Quantal analysis of hippocampal long-term potentiation, *Rev Neurosci* 5:141, 1994.

Books and monographs

Andersen RA: *Inferior parietal lobe function in spatial perception and visuomotor integration.* In Plum F, editor: *Handbook of physiology,* sect 1, *The nervous system,* vol 6, *Higher functions of the brain,* part 2, Bethesda, Md, 1987, American Physiological Society.

Benson DF: *Aphasia, alexia, and agraphia,* New York, 1979, Churchill Livingstone.

Bergamini L, Bergamasco B: *Cortical evoked potentials in man,* Springfield, Ill, 1967, Charles C Thomas.

Dudai Y: *The neurobiology of memory: concepts, findings, trends,* Oxford, 1989, Oxford University Press.

Fulton JF: *Frontal lobotomy and affective behavior: a neurophysiological analysis,* New York, 1951, Norton.

Fuster JM: *The prefrontal cortex: anatomy, physiology, and neuropsychology of the frontal lobe,* ed 2, New York, 1989, Raven Press.

Gazzaniga MS, LeDoux JE: *The integrated mind,* New York, 1978, Plenum Press.

Kandel ER et al: *Principles of neural science,* ed 3, New York, 1991, Elsevier.

Kryger MH, Roth T, Dement WC, editors: *Principles and practice of sleep medicine,* Philadelphia, 1989, WB Saunders.

Pavlov IP: *Lectures on conditioned reflexes,* New York, 1928, International Publishers (Translated by W.H. Gantt).

Penfield W, Jasper H: *Epilepsy and the functional anatomy of the human brain,* Boston, 1954, Little, Brown.

Peters A, Jones EG, editors: *Cerebral cortex,* vol 1, *Cellular components of the cerebral cortex,* New York, 1984, Plenum Press.

Peters A, Jones EG, editors: *Cerebral cortex,* vol 2, *Functional properties of cortical cells,* New York, 1984, Plenum Press.

Squire LR: *Memory and brain,* New York, 1987, Oxford University Press.

Steriade M, McCarley RW: *Brainstem control of wakefulness and sleep,* New York, 1990, Plenum Press.

MUSCLE

Richard A. Murphy

Contractile Mechanism of Muscle Cells

Traditionally, muscles have been classified according to their anatomy (striated versus smooth muscle). Another way muscles are classified is according to their innervation. Thus, voluntary muscles under conscious control are distinguished from involuntary muscles under the control of the autonomic nervous system. However, the properties of different muscle cells are more readily understood in terms of their functional roles. *In this classification, the basic distinction is between muscle cells attached to the skeleton and those located in the walls of hollow organs* (Table 17-1).

Muscle cells attached to the skeleton are striated and under voluntary control. They are often very long and bridge the attachment points of the muscle to the skeleton. This arrangement allows the cells to function independently. The total force produced by a muscle reflects the sum of the forces generated by its active cells. The musculoskeletal system is arranged so that most gravitational loads are borne by the skeleton and ligaments. Skeletal muscle cells are normally relaxed and are usually recruited to generate force and movement.

In contrast to muscle cells attached to the skeleton, muscle cells in the walls of hollow organs cannot function independently. The walls of hollow organs contain a continuous sheet of muscle in which muscle cells are mechanically linked in series like the links in a chain. All the cells must bear the same force and contract uniformly. Changes in pressure are transmitted throughout hollow organs, and contraction of some cells necessarily alters the load on the others.

Muscle cells in hollow organs (typically involuntary and smooth) have two functional roles. Like skeletal muscle cells, they generate force and movement and they also maintain organ dimensions against applied loads. For example, vascular smooth muscle must bear the load imposed by the blood pressure to regulate blood flow. The contractile and regulatory systems of smooth muscle cells are more complex than those of skeletal muscle; the complexity allows them to carry out load-bearing functions economically. Cardiac muscle (see Chapter 23) is distinctive because it has properties of both skeletal and hollow organ muscle. Cardiac muscle forms a hollow organ and contracts as a unit, but it also has the cellular structure and high-power output of skeletal muscle.

This chapter describes the cellular and molecular processes of muscle cell contraction. The basic apparatus for conversion of chemical energy into mechanical energy (**chemomechanical transduction**) in the form of force development or movement is considered first in a discussion of skeletal muscle cells. Chapter 18 is devoted to integrated tissue function and the capacity of skeletal muscles to adapt to changing requirements. Smooth muscle cells found in the various organs have distinctive features not found in skeletal muscles, and these features are discussed in Chapter 19. Specific information about the function of smooth muscle and its innervation can be found in the chapters describing the vascular, airway, gastrointestinal, and other organ systems.

■ *Structure of the Contractile Apparatus in Skeletal Muscle*

■ *Myofibrils*

A skeletal muscle is composed of bundles of extremely large, multinucleated cells up to 80 μm in diameter and sometimes many centimeters long (Fig. 17-1). These cells, like those in cardiac muscle, exhibit a striking banding pattern responsible for their classification as **striated muscles.** The striations arise from a highly organized arrangement of subcellular structures. There are few instances in biology in which ultrastructure provides such a clear basis for understanding cell function as it does in striated muscle. Careful study of Figs. 17-1, 17-2, and 17-3 is important to this understanding. The electron micrograph in Fig. 17-1, *B* reveals bundles of fila-

■ **Table 17-1** Muscle classification

Type	Skeletal	Cardiac	Smooth
Location (typical)	Attached to skeleton	Heart	Hollow organs
Anatomy	Striated	Striated	Nonstriated
Neural control	Voluntary	Involuntary	Involuntary
Output	High power	High power	Low power
Typical activity	Normally relaxed	Pump (repetitive)	Normally contracting (variable)

ments, called **myofibrils,** running along the axis of the cell. The gross striation pattern of the cell results from a repeating pattern in the myofibrils (Fig. 17-2).

The banding pattern evident in skeletal muscle arises from two sets of filaments in the myofibrils. Their organization is most clearly seen in a diagram that exaggerates their cross-sectional dimensions (Fig. 17-3). The dark striations constitute a region that contains a lattice of **thick filaments.** A second lattice consists of **thin filaments** attached to a transverse, darkly stained structure that is part of the force-transmitting cytoskeleton. The thin filaments interdigitate with the thick filaments. *The thick and thin filament arrays form the contractile system, and the repeating unit of thick and thin filament arrays in each myofibril is the basic contractile unit, called a* **sarcomere.** Cross-sections of the myofibril reveal the relationship between thin and thick filaments (Fig. 17-3). The thin filaments form a hexagonal array around each thick filament. Each thin filament is equidistant from three thick filaments. Thus, in vertebrate striated muscle, there are two thin filaments for every thick filament in each half of a sarcomere.

■ *The Cytoskeleton*

The expression of external force by a muscle cell is dependent on an internal cellular **cytoskeleton.** This cytoskeleton links the thick and thin filaments into the precise myofibrillar geometry (Fig. 17-3) and thus forms a scaffold for the contractile proteins. Transverse cytoskeletal elements couple the two filament lattices within a sarcomere, and also include **intermediate filaments** that link the sarcomeres of adjacent myofibrils. The principal longitudinal elements of the cytoskeleton are two giant proteins: **titin** and **nebulin.**

Individual titin molecules bridge transverse cytoskeletal elements from the center of the thick filament lattice to the end of the sarcomere. Most of a titin molecule is part of a thick filament, where it may serve as a template for filament formation. The remainder is a highly elastic

domain whose length changes with that of the sarcomere. Each thin filament in skeletal muscle has a single long nebulin molecule, which is thought to act as a ruler that sets thin filament lengths at 1.05 μm. Nebulin appears to be absent in cardiac and smooth muscle, where thin filament lengths are more variable.

■ *Thin Filaments*

Composition and structure. Thin filaments are ubiquitous constituents of all nucleated cells and are a dominant feature in muscle. All thin filaments contain two major proteins, **actin** and **tropomyosin.** Actin is a globular protein with a molecular weight of 43,000 daltons. It polymerizes under conditions that exist in the cytoplasm to form twisted, two-stranded filaments (Fig. 17-4). Tropomyosin is a rod-shaped molecule composed of two separate polypeptide chains. The individual polypeptides have a basic α-helical structure, and the two helical peptides are wound around each other to form a supercoil. Molecules with this structure are long, rigid, and insoluble. The rod-shaped molecules of tropomyosin stretch along each strand of the thin filament. Each tropomyosin molecule is associated with six or seven globular actin molecules in one strand.

Other proteins are associated with the thin filaments. Some, such as nebulin, are cytoskeletal. Others are involved in regulation of the interaction of actin with the thick filament. In striated muscle, the regulatory protein is **troponin,** which is bound to tropomyosin (Fig. 17-4). Regulatory proteins differ among major muscle types and are discussed in Chapters 18 and 19.

Lattice organization and polarity. Thin filaments are anchored at the end of the sarcomere (called the **Z disk**) in striated muscle and are polar. Thus, thin filaments on each side of the Z disk "point" in opposite directions. In cross-section, the thin filaments can be seen to form a hexagonal lattice around each thick filament in striated muscles (Fig. 17-3).

■ *Thick Filaments*

A very large protein (about 470,000 daltons), **myosin,** aggregates to form the thick filaments. Small amounts of other proteins are present, including a single core titin molecule in each half of the thick filament. The myosin molecule consists of six different polypeptides: one pair of large heavy chains and two pairs of light chains. Each heavy chain consists of a rodlike heavy chain tail with an α-helical structure; the two heavy chains are twisted around each other to form a supercoil. At the end of each heavy chain is a globular tertiary structure. Thus, each myosin molecule has two "heads" (Fig. 17-5, *A*). One polypeptide of each pair of light chains is associated with the molecule.

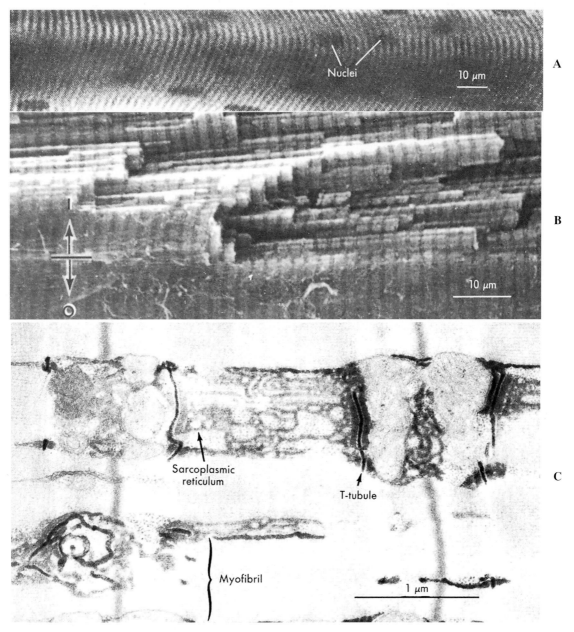

■ **Fig. 17-1** **A,** Segment of a single cell from human gastrocnemius muscle. Cross-striations of alternating dark and light bands are visible along with nuclei located peripherally. **B,** Scanning electron micrograph of a skeletal muscle cell shows the cell surface *(O)* and interior *(I)* with tightly packed myofibrils. **C,** Electron micrograph of a longitudinal section through a mouse skeletal muscle cell. The tissue is stained to show the internal membrane system of the sarcoplasmic reticulum as a very dark network of interconnecting tubules. Invaginations of the cell membranes (T tubules) are visible as dark elements extending into the cell at the level of the junction between the dark and light bands. (**A** from Leeson CR, Leeson TS: *Histology,* ed 3, Philadelphia, 1976, WB Saunders; **B** from Sawada H, Ishikawa H, Yamada E: *Tissue Cell* 10:183, 1978; **C** courtesy of Dr. Michael S. Forbes.)

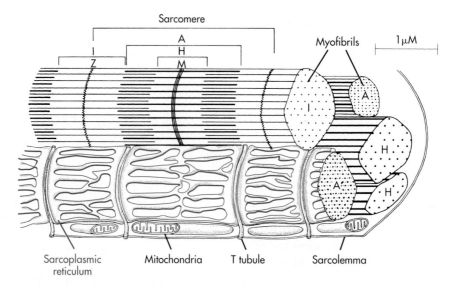

■ **Fig. 17-2**   Drawing illustrating the three-dimensional relationships between membrane elements and the filament lattice. (Redrawn from Leeson CR, Leeson TS: *Histology,* ed 3, Philadelphia, 1976, WB Saunders.)

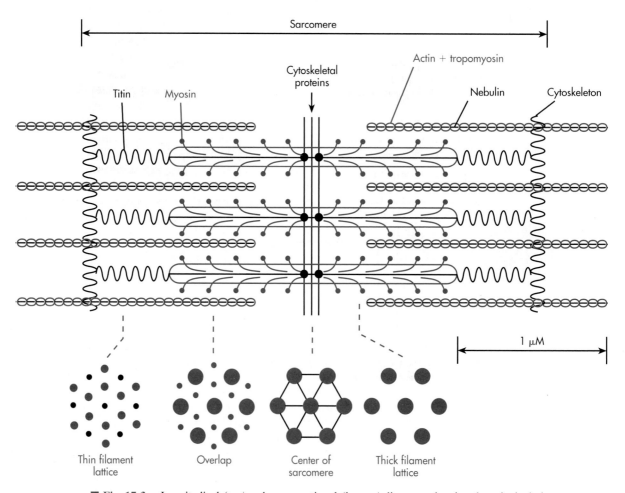

■ **Fig. 17-3**   Longitudinal *(top)* and cross-sectional *(bottom)* diagrams showing the principal elements of the sarcomeric cytoskeleton *(black)* and the thick and thin filaments *(color)* forming the contractile apparatus.

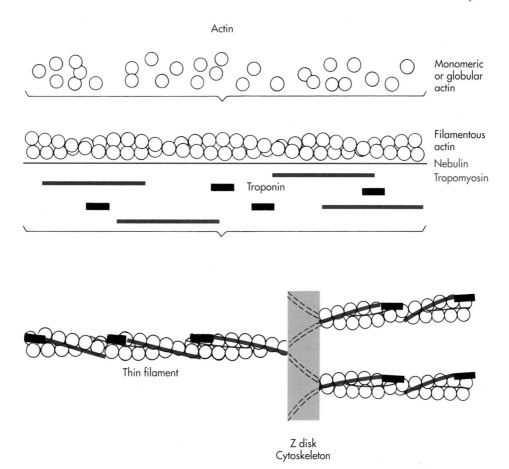

■ Fig. 17-4 Composition and structure of thin filaments in muscle. Globular actin monomers *(top)* polymerize into a two-stranded helical filament along with a molecule of nebulin *(thin, color)* that determines the thin filament length in skeletal muscle. The thin filament structure is completed with the addition of stiff, rod-shaped tropomyosin molecules *(color)*. Troponin *(black rectangles)* is a regulatory protein bound to the tropomyosin component of the thin filament in vertebrate striated muscles *(bottom)*. For clarity the tropomyosin-troponin complexes associated with only one strand of the actin helix are illustrated. Thin filaments are anchored to cytoskeletal Z disks in striated muscles. Filaments on each side of a Z disk have opposite polarities.

When the myosin molecule is exposed to a proteolytic enzyme, such as trypsin or papain, it is cleaved into one long and one short rod segment and two globular fragments. The cleavage points shown in Fig. 17-5, *A* indicate flexible regions that serve as hinges for the molecule.

In the cytoplasm of a striated muscle cell, myosin molecules aggregate to form thick filaments. The tails of the myosin molecules associate to form the thick filament backbone. The remainder of the myosin molecule, which consists of the globular heads and the "arm" portion between the hinges, projects laterally from the thick filament (Fig. 17-6, *B*). These projections are visible in electron micrographs and are termed **cross-bridges,** because they can link adjacent thick and thin filaments (Fig. 17-5, *B*). Thick filament formation begins with the end-to-end association of the tails of the myosin molecules (Fig. 17-6, *A*). The central portion of the thick filament lacks cross-

bridge projections and the cross-bridges in each half of the filament are oriented in the opposite direction. The cross-bridges project in groups of three from the thick filament (Fig. 17-6, *B*). Successive crowns of cross-bridges are rotated. Thick filaments in striated muscle are 1.6 μm long and contain an estimated 300 to 400 cross-bridges.

The **muscular dystrophies** constitute a group of genetically determined diseases that typically occur in childhood. These diseases are characterized by progressive muscle degeneration and weakness, followed by loss of heart and lung function that frequently results in early death. The genes involved in these diseases code for a group of proteins that form the dystrophin-glycoprotein complex. It is thought that this complex couples thin filaments in the cytoplasmic cytoskeleton across the membrane with proteins in the extracellular matrix. Some of these proteins are intracellular, while others are extracellular. Deficiencies in expression of the proteins in the dystrophin-glycoprotein complex cause these diseases, although the function of the complex remains conjectural.

■ *Cross-bridge Interactions with the Thin Filament*

■ *Cross-bridge Properties*

Each cross-bridge consists of two identical globular myosin heads that exhibit a remarkable set of properties. Most studies suggest that the two heads act largely independently in the reactions discussed in this section. However, the behavior of one head may be influenced by reactions that involve the other **(cooperativity).** The properties of the myosin head depend on the intact glob-ular portion of the heavy chain and the two associated light chains.

Myosin can catalyze the hydrolysis of adenosine triphosphate (ATP) to produce adenosine diphosphate (ADP) and inorganic phosphate (P_i). However, the ATPase activity of myosin is inhibited by the high magnesium concentrations that exist in cells. Myosin can also bind to actin to form an **actomyosin** complex that has high ATPase activity in muscle cells. *The interaction between actin and myosin, associated with ATP hydrolysis, represents the fundamental chemomechanical transduction process in which chemical energy is converted into mechanical energy by the intact muscle cell.*

The splitting of ATP by actomyosin is a complex cycle involving many steps. The most important steps are illustrated in Fig. 17-7, *A.* In a relaxed muscle, regulatory systems prevent actin-myosin interactions (Fig. 17-7, *A*). This inhibition is overcome on stimulation by Ca^{++} ions. This regulatory process is considered in Chapter 18. In the presence of ATP, ADP and P_i are bound to each myosin head, and the myosin heads exhibit a high affin-

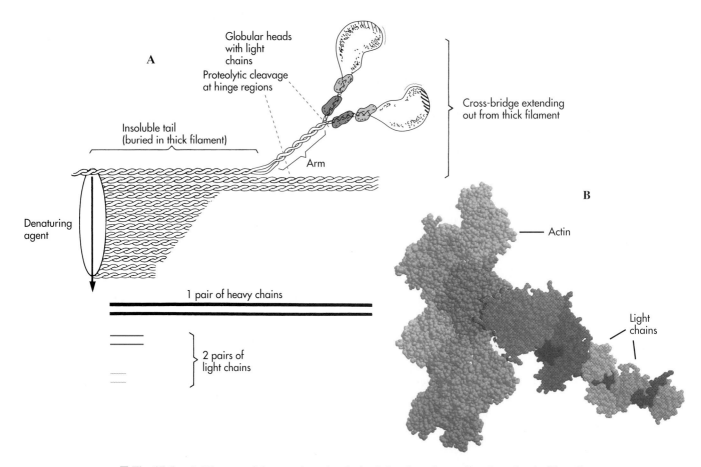

■ **Fig. 17-5** **A,** Diagram of the myosin molecule *(top)* showing a long tail and two heads. The tail regions of many myosin molecules associate in the cytoplasm to form a thick filament with the heads projecting from the surface. The individual myosin molecule can be dissociated into three pairs of polypeptides by denaturing agents *(bottom).* The molecule can also be cleaved by proteolytic enzymes (at sites shown by the dashed lines) into two rod-shaped fragments plus one pair of globular fragments. **B,** Space-filling model showing how one myosin head containing light chains *(color)* binds to actin in a thin filament *(gray).* (**B** courtesy of Ivan Rayment, University of Wisconsin.)

ity for actin. The ADP and P_i are released after the myosin heads bind to actin and undergo a conformational change (Fig. 17-7). The release of ADP and P_i allows an ATP molecule to bind to myosin, and the affinity of myosin for actin (as A—M) is greatly reduced. The dissociation of myosin and actin is followed by the hydrolysis of the bound ATP, but the products (ADP and P_i) remain bound to myosin in the succeeding step. The energy released by the hydrolysis of ATP is stored in the myosin molecule, which is now in a high-energy state with its high affinity for actin renewed.

In otherwise healthy young individuals, a common cause of sudden cardiac death is **hypertrophic cardiomyopathy.** This inherited cardiac disease is characterized by enlargement of the muscle cells in the ventricle of the heart. The disease varies clinically, but it is the result of one of many mutations in the genes that encode the myosin heavy or light chains (Fig. 17-5, *B*). The abnormal changes in the myosin heavy chains associated with the cardiomyopathies cluster in four regions of the myosin head. These regions are important in chemomechanical transduction. Impaired contractile function at the cross-bridge level is the apparent stimulus for the heart's adaptation to maintain adequate cardiac output through growth (hypertrophy) of the muscle cells.

■ *The Cross-bridge Cycle and Contraction*

The cycle associated with ATP hydrolysis by isolated actomyosin releases the energy in ATP without any conversion into mechanical work. Chemomechanical transduction involves conformational changes in the cross-bridges, changes that lead to filament movements that produce shortening and force development (Fig. 17-7).

In a resting muscle, cross-bridges are not attached to the thin actin filaments, and they are oriented perpendicularly to the myosin filament. When a muscle is stimulated, a rise in the myoplasmic Ca^{++} concentration produces changes in the myofilament structure and allows the cross-bridge to bind to the thin filament (considered in the section on control mechanisms; step 1 in Fig. 17-7, *A*). The hinge regions of the cross-bridge permit the myosin head to swing toward the thin filament. Cross-bridge attachment occurs because of the high affinity of the cross-bridge–ADP-P_i complex for actin. *Cross-bridges preferentially assume a conformation that minimizes their free energy.* The preferred conformation for attachment to the thin filament corresponds to a 90-degree orientation with respect to the filaments (Fig. 17-7, *B*). The chemical structure of the myosin head alters during step 2, when ADP and P_i are released. The decrease in the free energy of the resultant actomyosin (AM) complex occurs only when its conformation

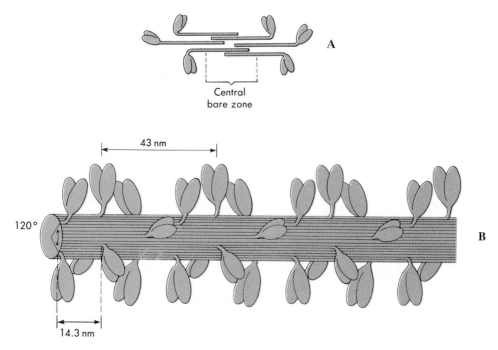

■ **Fig. 17-6** Proposed structure of the thick filament. **A,** Initiation of filament. Filament formation begins with an end-to-end association of the tails of myosin molecules. **B,** Segment of filament. "Crowns" of three cross-bridges project at intervals of 14.3 nm along the thick filament, and successive crowns are rotated. The result is a thick filament with rows of cross-bridges projecting toward the surrounding lattice of thin filaments. The core titin molecule is not illustrated. (Redrawn from Murray JM, Weber A: *Sci Am* 230:58, 1974.)

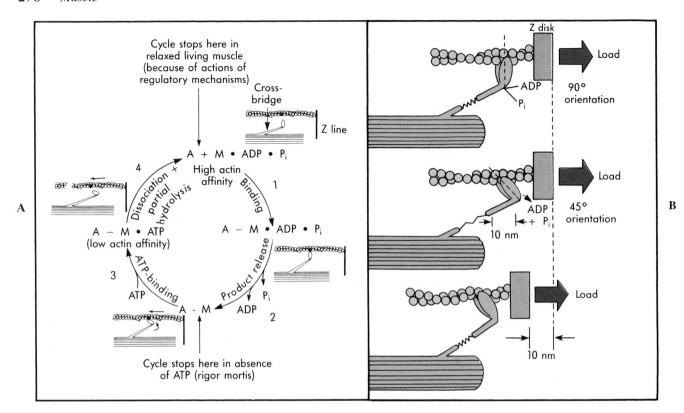

■ Fig. 17-7   A, Mechanism of adenosine triphosphate *(ATP)* hydrolysis by actomyosin and the major steps in the cross-bridge cycle that produces contraction. Actin in the thin filament *(A)* and the myosin cross-bridge projecting from the thick filament *(M)* interact cyclically. This interaction involves a number of steps during which ATP is hydrolyzed, and the energy released is harnessed to induce conformational changes in the cross-bridge. Each cycle causes the thick and thin filaments to interdigitate by about 10 nm. **B,** The preferred or minimal free energy conformation of the cross-bridge with bound adenosine diphosphate *(ADP)* and inorganic phosphate *(P$_i$)* is 90 degrees *(top)*. This changes to 45 degrees after the release of ADP and P$_i$ *(middle)*. The transition from 90 degrees to 45 degrees generates a force on the thin filament represented by the stretched spring *(middle)* that causes the sarcomere to shorten *(bottom)*. (From Berne RM, Levy MN, editors: *Principles of physiology,* St Louis, 1990, Mosby–Year Book.)

changes from 90 to 45 degrees. *Part of the free energy made available from ATP hydrolysis is captured in this conformational change, which minimizes the free energy and thereby generates a force that causes the thick and thin filaments to interdigitate.* The AM complex has a high affinity for ATP, and the binding of ATP induces cross-bridge detachment (Fig. 17-7, step 3). Partial ATP hydrolysis to regenerate the cross-bridge–ADP-P$_i$ complex raises the free energy, and the 90-degree conformation is again favored (step 4).

The force output of single cross-bridges has been measured and is the same in all types of muscles. The resultant movement of a thin filament past a thick filament is only about 10^{-9} m, and the force generated is 3 to 5×10^{-12} newtons (defined in Table 17-2). The way in which enormous numbers of such cycles are coupled to generate muscular contraction is considered in the following section. The cycle continues until the cross-bridges are detached from the thin filaments by control systems (which remove Ca^{++} from the myoplasm and produce relaxation) or until the supply of ATP is exhausted.

■ Table 17-2   Basic mechanical variables in muscle contraction

Parameter (symbol)	Units	Definition
Force (F)	Newton (n)	
Length (L)	Meter (m)	
Time (T)	Second (sec)	
Derived variables		
Velocity (V)	m/sec	Change in length/ change in time
Work (W)	n·m = joules	Force times distance
Power (P)	n·m/sec = watts	Work/time
Stress (S)	n/m^2	Force/cross-section area

Adapted from Berne RM, Levy MN, editors: *Principles of physiology,* St Louis, 1990, Mosby–Year Book.

ATP depletion is an abnormal condition in muscle cells, and it arrests the cross-bridge cycle by the formation of permanent AM complexes (Fig. 17-7, *A*). Death leads to muscular rigidity (rigor mortis) when ATP depletion causes permanent cross-bridge attachment.

■ *Biophysics of the Contractile System*

Quantitative estimates of the mechanical output of muscles have provided important information about the mechanism of chemomechanical transduction and its control. The measurement of muscle contraction also provides a way of assessing the effects of neurotransmitters, drugs, and hormones and of quantifying pathological changes. The important mechanical variables in muscle are force and length (Table 17-2). The basic approach in muscle mechanics is to control one of these variables and measure the other as a function of time.

■ *Force-Length Relationships and the Sliding-Filament Mechanism*

The sliding-filament model describes the movement of thick and thin filaments in a sarcomere during muscle contraction. According to this model, the thick and thin filaments do not shorten; rather, they increase their overlap. In the following section, the way in which muscle cells generate force as a result of the increased overlap of the thick and thin filaments is explained.

Force generation depends on the length of the muscle. In Fig. 17-8, the points on the curves are determined experimentally under conditions in which the length of the muscle is fixed, and the maximal force is measured during a contraction. Such a contraction at constant length is termed **isometric.** Force varies with the size of the muscle, and it is best expressed as a **stress** (force/cross-sectional area of the muscle) to allow comparisons among muscles. A relaxed muscle is elastic, and it requires a force to stretch it to a longer length. The resultant **passive force-length** or **stress-length relationship** reflects the properties of connective tissue in intact muscles. Individual muscle cells are much more elastic than muscle bundles, and their relaxed stress-length properties reflect the elasticity of the cytoskeleton. The stress increases when a muscle is stimulated to contract isometrically. The difference between the stress-length curves for contracting and relaxed muscles is the **active stress-length relationship** that characterizes the contractile system (Fig. 17-8, *B* and *C*).

Correlating the structural and mechanical relationships in muscle reveals that active stress is proportional to the overlap between thick and thin filaments in a sarcomere (Fig. 17-8, *C*). As the muscle is stretched beyond the length (L_o) at which maximal active force (F_o) is developed, active stress decreases linearly with the decrease in overlap between thick and thin filaments. We can conclude from this observation that *stress is proportional to the number of cross-bridges that can interact with the thin filaments in each half-sarcomere.* Force declines at sarcomere lengths less than L_o. The decline in force is partially a result of disturbances in the filament lattice geometry, as diagrammed in Fig. 17-8, *C,* when thick filaments collide

with Z disks and thin filaments overlap. However, when muscle lengths are short, the control mechanisms for the contractile machinery become less sensitive to the stimulus, and partial inactivation contributes to the low stress at short lengths. Slight variations in sarcomere lengths in whole muscles obscure the inflection points detected in the stress-length curves for sarcomeres (compare Fig. 17-8, *B* and *C*).

Enormous forces can be placed on tendons by large muscles such as the gastrocnemius. The greatest stress on a tendon occurs upon gravitational loading of a contracting muscle. Injuries may occur as the result of a fall or sudden stretch, which subjects a contracting muscle to an abrupt, large increase in stress. Rupture of an Achilles tendon represents such an injury.

Because the lengths of the thick and thin filaments and their packing density are similar in striated muscles from different vertebrates, they all generate similar maximal stresses at L_o. *The maximal stress is about $3 \times 10^5 \ n/m^2$ (or up to 3 kg/cm^2) of cell cross-sectional area.*

■ *Velocity-Stress Relationships and the Contraction Cycle*

Another basic relationship that characterizes the output of a muscle can be obtained when the load or stress on a muscle is held constant and the shortening velocity is measured. A contraction at constant load is termed **isotonic.** *Shortening velocity is determined by the load on the muscle, as illustrated by the hyperbolic velocity-stress curve shown in Fig. 17-9. Muscles lift a heavy load slowly, shorten rapidly when lightly loaded, and exhibit their maximal shortening velocity (V_o) with no load.* Figs. 17-9 and 17-10 also show that a contracting muscle can withstand (briefly) a heavier stress when forcibly stretched than it can develop isometrically. The strength of the cross-bridge attachment to the thin filament is greater than the force generated by movement at the cross-bridge. Consequently, *muscles can bear a load about 1.6 times F_o before the cross-bridge attachment is mechanically broken and rapid lengthening occurs.*

The contractile system operates most efficiently (i.e., has the greatest mechanical work output for the chemical energy used) with optimal loading. This efficiency is illustrated by the power-stress curve. **Power,** or work/time, is simply the product of force and velocity, and power can be calculated by multiplying these variables at any point on the velocity-force curve (Fig. 17-9). Maximal power is obtained with a load of about 30% of the maximal force that can be developed. A muscle contracting isometrically does no work (force × distance = 0), nor does a muscle shortening with no load. The mechanical efficiency (work performed/ATP consumed) of such contractions is necessarily zero. Inefficient contractions are often physiologi-

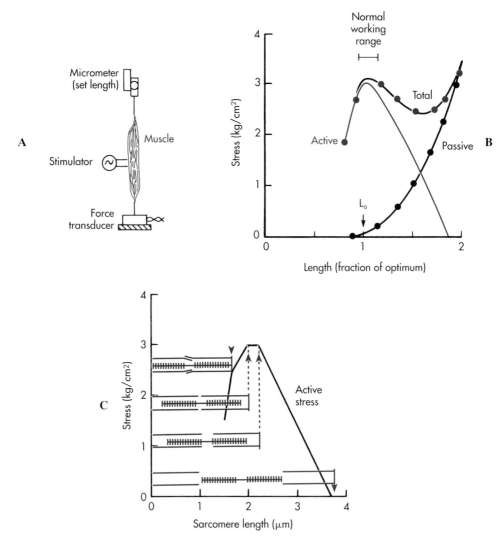

■ **Fig. 17-8** Stress-length relationships in isometrically contracting muscle. **A,** Schematic diagram of experimental apparatus in which the tissue is attached to a micrometer to set the length and a transducer to measure force. Force is normalized as a stress, to allow comparisons of muscles of differing size (i.e., force/cross-sectional area of the muscle cells). Values of stress at different lengths are obtained in the relaxed muscle *(black dots)* and in the maximally stimulated muscle *(colored dots)* and plotted as shown in **B.** Three stress-length curves are shown for skeletal muscle: (1) the passive stress exerted as a function of the length of the relaxed muscle, (2) the total stress exerted by the maximally stimulated muscle (passive + active), and (3) the active stress-length curve for the contractile machinery obtained as the difference between the total and passive stresses at any length *(colored curve).* All muscles have an inherent maximal force-generating capacity, which is obtained at the optimal length (L_o). **C,** Precise studies of the stress-length behavior of the sarcomeres in single skeletal muscle cells reveal the dependence of stress on the overlap of thick and thin filaments. Diagrams of four sarcomeres at lengths where the slope of the stress-length curve changes show how filament interactions and active stress depend on sarcomere length. (Data from Gordon AM, Huxley AF, Julian FJ: *J Physiol (Lond)* 184:170, 1966.)

cally important when either high-speed or maximal force is appropriate. The optimal **efficiency** of the contractile system in converting chemical energy into mechanical work is about 40% to 45%. The remaining energy is converted to heat, which can raise the temperature of working muscles by several degrees.

If a sarcomere is to shorten more than 10 nm during a single cross-bridge cycle, each cross-bridge must detach and then reattach at a new site on the thin filament closer to the Z line. The cross-bridges must cycle asynchronously to maintain a constant force and permit continuous shortening.

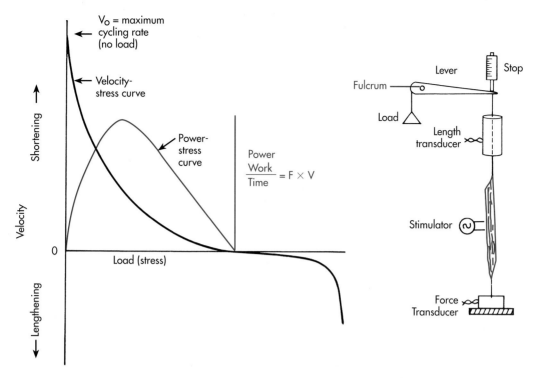

■ Fig. 17-9   The dependence of shortening velocity on the load (stress) on an isometrically contracting muscle. Shortening velocity may be measured using a lever system, which permits a muscle to shorten against a constant load. Velocity (= Δ length / Δ time) is measured using a length transducer. The velocity-load curve is constructed from points obtained in a series of contractions against different loads. (The initial length in these experiments is at L_o, and only a slight shortening is permitted.) If the load placed on the muscle is greater than the load that the active cross-bridges can bear, the muscle will lengthen. Consequently, the velocity-load curve can be extended to describe this situation. The power output of a muscle *(colored curve)* is the mechanical work (force times distance shortened) per unit of time and can be calculated as the product of load times shortening velocity.

Shortening velocities in a muscle depend on several factors. First, the velocity varies with the number of sarcomeres in a muscle cell. Total shortening and shortening velocity are the sum of the movements of thin filaments past thick filaments times the number of half-sarcomeres in the cell. To allow comparisons between different muscles, velocities can be calculated in terms of micrometers per second per half-sarcomere. However, it is more common to normalize shortening velocities by reporting values in terms of optimal muscle lengths (L_o) per second, which accounts for the number of sarcomeres in a cell. The velocity also depends on the load on the muscle; the velocity-stress relationship shows that cross-bridge cycling rates fall as the stress on the cross-bridges increases. This effect can be understood by referring to Fig. 17-10. The conformational change in the cross-bridge, which causes shortening between attachment and detachment, is opposed by the load. Heavier loads increase the average time for the conformational change to occur and to allow a new cycle to take place. An unloaded cross-bridge can cycle at a maximal rate, indicated by V_o. This maximal rate depends only on the mo-

lecular properties of the myosin isoform synthesized within a striated muscle cell. The direct proportionality between the ATPase activity of myosin isolated from a cell and the V_o for that cell illustrates this molecular diversity, which is responsible for physiological differences in the speed of contraction of muscle cells from different sources.

■ *Summary*

1. The basic contractile unit of a striated muscle cell is the sarcomere, which consists of a centrally located array of thick filaments that interdigitate with thin filaments attached to the cytoskeleton at each end of the sarcomere (the Z lines). Myofibrils contain many sarcomeres in series, and muscle cells contain large numbers of myofibrils in parallel.

2. Thin filaments consist of polymers of actin, tropomyosin and nebulin, plus the Ca^{++}-binding regulatory protein troponin in vertebrate striated muscle. Thick filaments consist mainly of myosin and titin. The "head"

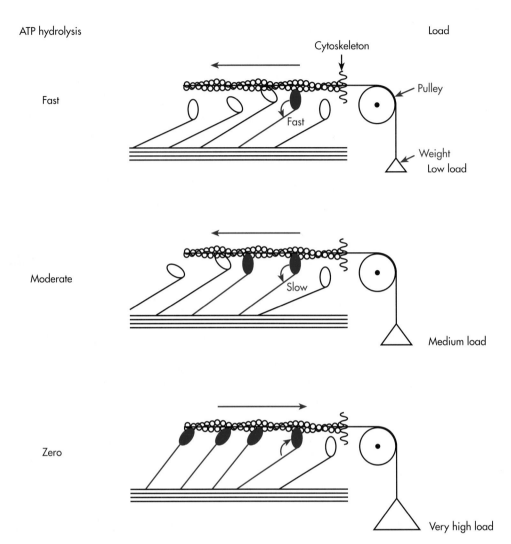

■ **Fig. 17-10** Effect of load on cross-bridge cycling. At low loads *(top),* shortening requires few cross-bridges in an attached, force-generating or force-bearing state *(color).* The transition from 90 to 45 degrees and detachment occurs rapidly at low loads and many cross-bridges are detached. At higher loads *(center)* the 90- to 45-degree transition occurs more slowly and more time is spent in a force-generating conformation. An imposed load greater than the cross-bridges can develop is resisted *(bottom).* The attached high-energy cross-bridges with their bound ADP and P_i are strained by the load from 90 to 135 degrees in the lengthening muscle before the linkage to the thin filament ruptures. The ADP and P_i are never released and the cross-bridge has a high affinity for actin, so it immediately reattaches without ATP hydrolysis. Most of the cross-bridges are attached so that large imposed loads can be resisted.

regions of individual myosin molecules project laterally from the filament. These projections, called cross-bridges, contain the actin- and ATP-binding sites.

3. A high free energy state of the cross-bridges occurs after ATP binding and hydrolysis to form the myosin–ADP-P_i complex, which has a high affinity for actin. Rapid attachment to the thin filaments in a preferred 90-degree conformation follows. Subsequent release of bound P_i and ADP leads to a complex whose free energy is minimized after a conformational change to 45 degrees. This conformational change produces a force on the thin filament and movement toward the center of the sarcomere. ATP binding reduces the affinity of myosin for actin, and the cross-bridges detach from the thin filament. ATP hydrolysis regenerates the myosin–ADP-P_i complex in a 90-degree conformation to complete the cross-bridge cycle.

4. Force generation is a function of the number of cross-bridges that can interact with the thin filaments. Force/cross-sectional area (or stress) reaches a very high value because of the mechanical coupling of the forces generated by enormous numbers of cross-bridges.

5. The velocity-load relationship shows that muscles shorten more slowly as the load is increased in isotonic contractions. Power output is maximized at moderate loads at which 40% to 45% of the free energy of ATP hydrolysis is converted into mechanical work.

6. Contracting muscles often lengthen when opposing forces are very high. Stresses on muscle, tendons, or skeleton can be very high under such conditions, because cross-bridges can transiently bear loads that are about 1.6-fold higher than they develop isometrically.

7. Velocity depends on the number of sarcomeres in a muscle cell. Sarcomere-shortening velocities are a function of cross-bridge cycling rates and load. Maximal cycling rates at zero load are determined by the isoform of myosin expressed in a cell.

■ *Self-Study Problems*

1. Compare the force-generating capacities and maximal shortening velocities of hypothetical muscles consisting of (1) one cell with 50 sarcomeres vs. (2) two cells with 25 sarcomeres each.

2. Mammals have a number of genes that code for different actin isoforms. The various genes are expressed in different types of muscle. Nevertheless, actin is one of the most highly conserved proteins known. What factors might explain this pattern in actin diversity?

3. What are the key elements that make force generation by cross-bridge cycling possible?

■ *Bibliography*

Journal articles

Bandman E: Contractile protein isoforms in muscle development, *Dev Biol* 154:273, 1992.

Burton K: Myosin step size: estimates from motility assays and shortening muscle, *J Muscle Res Cell Motil* 13:590, 1992.

Cooke R: The actomyosin engine, *FASEB J* 9:636, 1995.

Dos Remedios CG, Moens PDJ: Actin and the actomyosin interface: a review, *Biochim Biophys Acta Bio-Energetics* 1228:99, 1995.

Eisenberg E, Hill TL: Muscle contraction and free energy transduction in biological systems, *Science* 227:999, 1985.

Epstein HF, Fischman DA: Molecular analysis of protein assembly in muscle development, *Science* 251:1039, 1991.

Homsher E, Millar NC: Caged compounds and striated muscle contraction, *Annu Rev Physiol* 52:875, 1990.

Ishijima A et al: Multiple- and single-molecule analysis of the actomyosin motor by nanometer-piconewton manipulation with a microneedle: unitary steps and forces, *Biophysical J* 70:383, 1996.

Josephson RK: Contraction dynamics and power output of skeletal muscle, *Annu Rev Physiol* 55:527, 1993.

Obinata T: Contractile proteins and myofibrillogenesis, *Int Rev Cytol* 143:153, 1993.

Peters SE: Structure and function in vertebrate skeletal muscle, *Am Zool* 29:221, 1989.

Rayment I et al: Structure of the actin-myosin complex and its implications for muscle contraction, *Science* 261:58, 1993.

Rayment I et al: Three-dimensional structure of myosin subfragment-1: a molecular motor, *Science* 261:50, 1993.

Schoenberg M: Equilibrium muscle crossbridge behavior: the interaction of myosin crossbridges with actin, *Adv Biophys* 29:55, 1993.

Seow CY, Ford LE: Shortening velocity and power output of skinned muscle fibers from mammals having a 25,000-fold range of body mass, *J Gen Physiol* 97:541, 1991.

Small JV, Fürst DO, Thornell L-E: The cytoskeletal lattice of muscle cells, *Eur J Biochem* 208:559, 1992.

Trinick J: Titin and nebulin: protein rulers in muscle, *Trends Biochem Sci* 19:405, 1994.

Warshaw DM: The in vitro motility assay: a window into the myosin molecular motor, *News Physiol Sci* 11:1, 1996.

Books and monographs

Hochachka PW: *Muscles as molecular and metabolic machines,* Boca Raton, Fla, 1994, CRC Press.

Huxley A: *Reflections on muscle,* Princeton, NJ, 1980, Princeton University Press.

Kreis T, Vale R, editors: *Guidebook to the cytoskeletal and motor proteins,* Oxford, 1993, Oxford University Press.

Peachey LD, Adrian RH, editors: *Handbook of physiology,* sect 10, *Skeletal muscle,* Bethesda, Md, 1983, American Physiological Society.

Pollack GH: *Muscles and molecules: uncovering the principles of biological motion,* Seattle, Wash, 1990, Ebner & Sons.

Squire JM: *Molecular mechanisms in muscular contraction,* Boca Raton, Fla, 1990, CRC Press.

Skeletal Muscle Physiology

Contraction of skeletal muscles is voluntary and controlled by the motor pathways in the central nervous system (CNS) (see Chapters 12 to 14). Each mammalian muscle cell is innervated by one branch of a motor nerve. The process of neuromuscular transmission, whereby an action potential in the motor nerve elicits an action potential in the muscle cell plasma membrane (the sarcolemma), is described in Chapter 4. Here the focus is on the control of skeletal muscle at the cellular and tissue levels. The control mechanisms discussed include (1) the generation of a transient increase in the myoplasmic Ca^{++} concentration, which is triggered by signal transduction at the sarcolemma and which constitutes the intracellular messenger that triggers cross-bridge cycling; (2) regulation of the output of a muscle by coordinating the mechanical responses of many muscle cells; (3) matching of energy consumption to adenosine triphosphate (ATP) production; and (4) adaptive changes in muscle associated with growth and use. *The overall process by which depolarization of the sarcolemma causes Ca^{++} release into the myoplasm and the subsequent binding of Ca^{++} to regulatory sites to initiate cross-bridge cycling is termed* **excitation-contraction coupling** *(E-C coupling).*

■ *Cross-bridge Regulation by Ca^{++} and Troponin*

■ *The Role of Troponin in Cross-bridge Regulation*

The thin actin filaments of vertebrate skeletal and cardiac muscles contain **troponin,** a regulatory protein. One molecule of troponin is bound to one end of each tropomyosin molecule (Fig. 18-1 and see Fig. 17-4). Troponin binds up to four Ca^{++} ions in a cooperative manner so that either all or none of the binding sites are usually occupied by Ca^{++}. In the presence of micromolecular concentrations of Ca^{++}, the binding sites on troponin are occupied, and this causes a change in the conformation of the thin filament (Fig. 18-1). *Ca^{++} binding to troponin acts as a switch that allows cross-bridges to attach to the thin filament and cycle.*

In vertebrate skeletal and cardiac muscle, the contraction-relaxation cycle involves five steps: (1) action potentials in the sarcolemma cause the myoplasmic Ca^{++} to rise above 0.1 μM, (2) binding of Ca^{++} to troponin changes the thin filament conformation, (3) cross-bridges attach and cycle, (4) cessation of stimulation is followed by Ca^{++} removal from the myoplasm and dissociation of Ca^{++} from troponin, and (5) the thin filament returns to a configuration in which further cross-bridge cycles are inhibited.

The binding of Ca^{++} ions to troponin exhibits a steep response curve. This signifies that even relatively small changes in Ca^{++} produce large changes in the number of active cross-bridges and force development (Fig. 18-1). Each cross-bridge cycle is associated with ATP hydrolysis; therefore, myofibrillar ATPase activity is also proportional to the Ca^{++} concentration.

■ *Regulation of the Cellular Ca^{++} Concentration*

The myoplasmic Ca^{++} concentration in relaxed muscle is very low (< 0.1 μM). This resting Ca^{++} concentration is maintained by active transport mechanisms against very large concentration gradients. *Contraction is initiated by release of Ca^{++} into the myoplasm, and relaxation follows Ca^{++} removal.* Four anatomically and functionally distinct membrane elements are involved in the regulation of the cellular Ca^{++} concentration: (1) the **motor end-plate,** where neuromuscular transmission occurs (see Chapter 4); (2) the sarcolemma, where the action potential is propagated away from the endplate (see Chapter 3); (3) the **transverse** or **T-tubular system,** which conducts the action potential from the sarcolemma inward to the myofibrils (Fig. 18-2); and (4) the **sarcoplasmic reticulum,** an intracellular membrane system that constitutes a storage compartment for Ca^{++} (Fig. 18-3 and see Figs. 17-1 and 17-2).

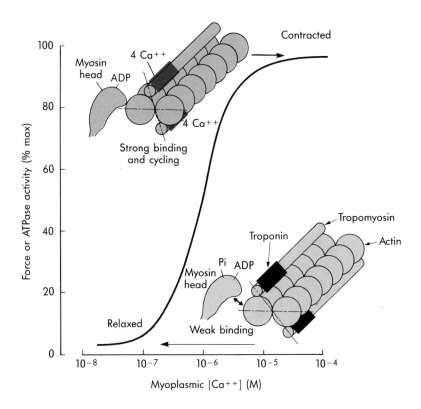

■ **Fig. 18-1** Regulation of the cross-bridge cycle by Ca++. Ca++ activates contraction by binding to troponin in striated muscle. Troponin is associated with tropomyosin as a 1:1 complex in the thin filament (here shown with the strands untwisted for clarity). A conformational change occurs in all the proteins in the illustrated segment of the thin filament when Ca++ binds to troponin (*color*). This change allows attachment of the myosin heads and cross-bridge cycling. (Redrawn from Hartshorne DJ. In Lapedes DN, editor: *Yearbook of science and technology,* New York, 1976, McGraw-Hill.)

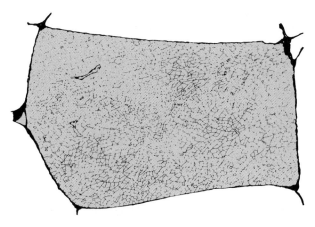

■ **Fig. 18-2** The T-tubular system in a skeletal muscle, reconstructed from high-voltage electron micrographs of serial transverse sections. The extensive network of T tubules across the fiber has many openings to the extracellular space. (From Peachey LD, Eisenberg BR: Reproduced from the *Biophysical Journal,* 22:145, 1978, by permission of the Biophysical Society.)

Structure of the T-tubular system and the sarcoplasmic reticulum. The sarcolemma separates the extracellular space from the **myoplasm,** the intracellular space that contains the contractile apparatus. Small transverse tubules (T tubules) open to the extracellular space at the sarcolemma and form a network in the interior of the cell. This T-tubule network surrounds the myofibrils and forms a grid across the cell near the ends of the thick filaments in each sarcomere of mammalian striated muscles (Fig. 18-2 and see Fig. 17-2). Despite the extent of T-tubule development, the volume of this system constitutes only 0.1% to 0.5% of the cell volume. Action potentials are propagated from the sarcolemma down the T tubule into the interior of the cell. The T tubules are closely associated with the fenestrated sheath of sarcoplasmic reticular membranes that surrounds the myofibrils (Fig. 18-3 and see Figs. 17-1, *C* and 17-2). This sheath or compartment consists of repeating units with (1) expanded elements that surround the T tubules and (2) narrower elements that run along the myofibrils.

Regulation of the Ca++ concentration by the sarcoplasmic reticulum. The sarcoplasmic reticulum occupies about 1% to 5% of the volume of mammalian skeletal muscle cells. This intracellular structure contains large amounts of calcium. The sarcoplasmic reticular membrane is highly specialized. Its protein component consists almost entirely of transport pumps in the vicinity of the myofibrils and of Ca++ channels adjacent to the T-tubular membranes. The pumps have a higher affinity for Ca++ than does troponin. Through the action of this active transport system, 2 mol of Ca++ are sequestered in the sarcoplasmic reticulum for each mole of ATP hydrolyzed. These pumps maintain the low resting myoplasmic Ca++ concentration.

When an action potential is transmitted along the sarcolemma, Ca++ is released from the sarcoplasmic reticulum into the myoplasm. This mechanism involves (1) a brief depolarization of T-tubular membranes during the

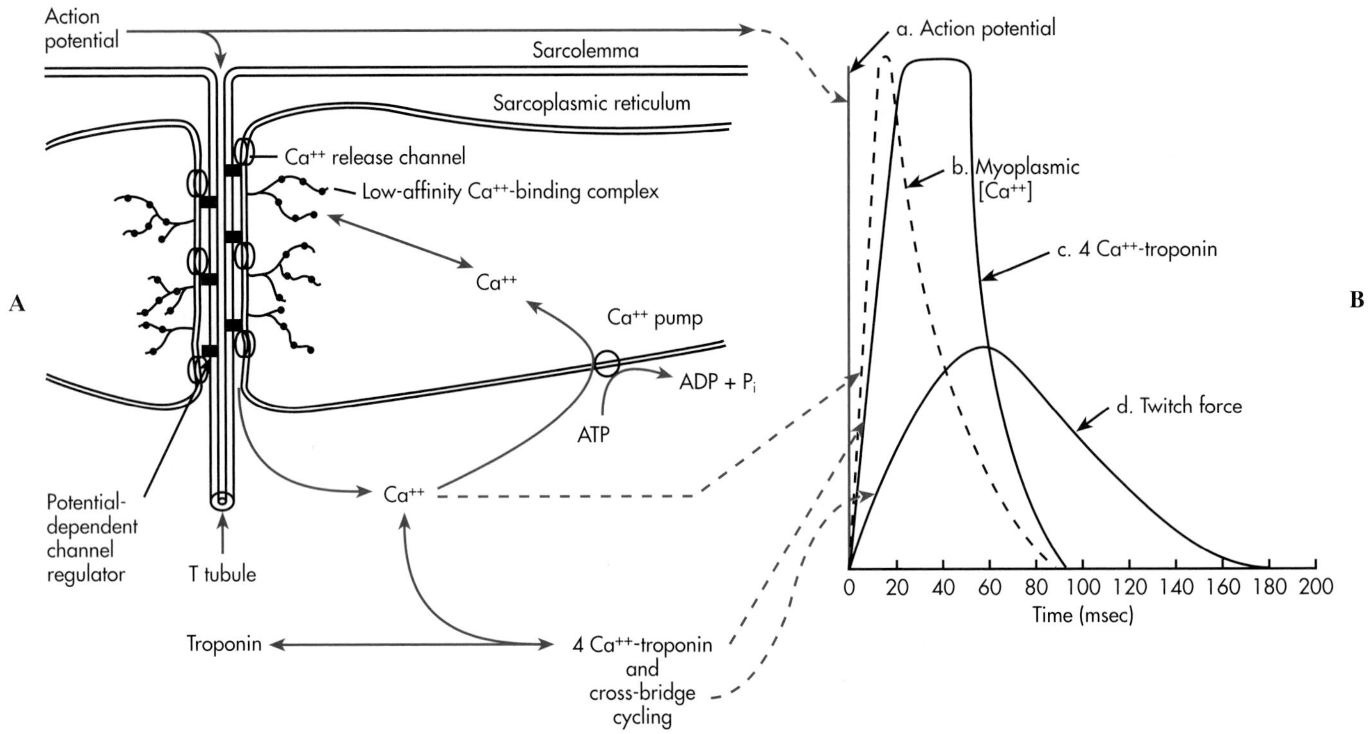

■ **Fig. 18-3**   **A,** Membranes and proteins involved in the regulation of myoplasmic Ca^{++} in skeletal muscle. Action potentials propagating along the sarcolemma (**B,** *a*) depolarize T-tubular membranes containing voltage-sensitive elements that regulate the opening of Ca^{++} channels in the adjacent membranes of the sarcoplasmic reticulum. A pulse of Ca^{++} ions (**B,** *b*) diffuses out of the sarcoplasmic reticulum into the myoplasm while the channel is open. In the myoplasm, the Ca^{++} can bind to troponin (**B,** *c*) and initiate cross-bridge cycling (**B,** *d*) or to Ca^{++} pumps that return it to the sarcoplasmic reticulum where most Ca^{++} ions reversibly associate with low-affinity Ca^{++}-binding proteins.

action potential, (2) opening of the Ca^{++} channels in the closely apposed sarcoplasmic reticulum membrane, and (3) release of a pulse of Ca^{++} into the myoplasm (Fig. 18-3). Most of the released Ca^{++} binds to troponin to initiate contraction. However, the increased myoplasmic Ca^{++} concentration also activates sarcoplasmic reticulum pumps that rapidly restore the resting state, unless another action potential is elicited.

The interior of the sarcoplasmic reticulum also contains a low-affinity, high-capacity Ca^{++}-binding protein complex (Fig. 18-3, *A*). This complex loosely binds Ca^{++} and thus reduces the sarcoplasmic reticular concentration of Ca^{++} from about 20 mM (if all the Ca^{++} were free) to about 0.5 mM. As a result of this binding, the Ca^{++} transport pump must act against a reduced concentration gradient.

Muscle generates considerable heat during contraction, and shivering is a mechanism by which cross-bridge cycling is used to generate heat. However, muscle cells may also play a role in maintaining body temperature without contractile activity in a process called **nonshivering thermogenesis.** Heat production is most dramatic in specialized muscle cells called *heater cells,* which have few myofilaments and high numbers of mitochondria and sarcoplasmic reticulum membranes. Best known in billfish, these cells generate heat by the release and reuptake of Ca^{++} from the sarcoplasmic reticulum. Ca^{++} pumping uses ATP produced by high rates of oxidative phosphorylation. The importance of heat generation by Ca^{++} cycling in noncontracting skeletal muscle of mammals is uncertain, but it is the mechanism of a genetic disease called **malignant hyperthermia.** Affected individuals have a mutant form of the Ca^{++}-release channel of the sarcoplasmic reticulum. Abnormal release of Ca^{++} is typically triggered during surgery by certain anesthetic agents, and results in elevated myoplasmic Ca^{++} and rapid cycling of Ca^{++} between the myoplasm and the sarcoplasmic reticulum. This elevated Ca^{++} pumping and the associated contractions lead to a rapid and often lethal rise in body temperature.

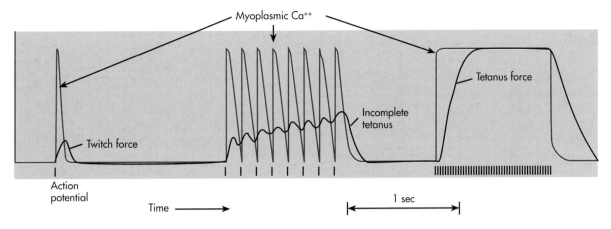

■ **Fig. 18-4** The force of contraction can be graded by repetitive stimulation that keeps myoplasmic Ca⁺⁺ elevated in an incomplete or a complete tetanus. Individual stimuli eliciting action potentials are indicated by short vertical lines.

Excitation-contraction coupling in skeletal muscle. Ca⁺⁺ release from the sarcoplasmic reticulum depends on the magnitude of the membrane potential. The threshold potential (called the *mechanical threshold*) for opening of the Ca⁺⁺ channels in the sarcoplasmic reticulum is about −50 mV.

Action potentials in skeletal muscle cells are quite uniform. Hence, the electrical signal for muscle activation is constant, and it leads to the release of a reproducible pulse of Ca⁺⁺ (Fig. 18-4). A single action potential may release a sufficient amount of Ca⁺⁺ to fully activate the contractile machinery in skeletal muscles. However, Ca⁺⁺ is very rapidly pumped back into the sarcoplasmic reticulum before the muscle has time to develop its maximal force (Fig. 18-3). *The resultant submaximal response to a single action potential is termed a* **twitch.** *Repetitive action potentials cause summation of twitches, which produces a partial or complete* **tetanus,** *as the Ca⁺⁺ pulses are added together to maintain saturating Ca⁺⁺ concentrations for troponin in the myoplasm* (Fig. 18-4).

■ *Energy Use and Supply*

Muscular contraction demands a constant supply of ATP at a rate proportional to consumption. In this section, the ATP requirements for various types of contractions (muscle energetics) are considered. The ways in which cells can provide adequate ATP are then reviewed. Finally, the matching of ATP production and use is described for particular fiber types.

Muscle cells are specialized for specific contractile activities, and a knowledge of fiber types is needed to understand many physiological aspects of muscle function in the body. Muscle makes up about 45% to 50% of total body mass. Thus, the enormous increase in energy expenditure during sustained exercise dictates many of

the functional characteristics of the cardiovascular and respiratory systems.

■ *Energetics of Muscle*

ATP consumption or metabolism in relaxed muscle is associated with basal cellular activities, such as maintaining ion gradients and synthesizing and degrading cellular constituents. This **resting metabolism** in striated muscles represents only a small fraction of the maximal ATP use associated with contraction. The energy requirements for activation, associated with action potentials and Ca⁺⁺ release into the myoplasm, are also comparatively small.

Every cycle of each of the enormous number of cross-bridges in a muscle cell requires one ATP molecule (see Fig. 17-7). One of the factors on which cycling rates in skeletal muscle depend is the load on the muscle (see Fig. 17-9). Shortening velocities and cross-bridge cycling rates are maximal when the load on a muscle is zero. These maximal rates are determined by the structure of the myosin molecule expressed in a muscle cell (myosin isoforms) and are associated with maximal rates of ATP consumption. As the load on a muscle is increased, cross-bridge cycling and ATP consumption rates decrease (see Fig. 17-10). In an isometric contraction in which no shortening or work occurs, ATP consumption rates remain elevated as some cross-bridges detach and reattach at the same point on the thin filament. The economy (the ATP cost) of force maintenance in isometric contractions, where no work is done, is very poor in striated muscle. Forcible stretching of a contracting muscle reduces ATP consumption rates further as the work is done *on* the muscle rather than *by* the muscle. Cross-bridges attach, are broken, and reattach, but no ATP is hydrolyzed as the myosin remains in the high-energy myosin-ADP-Pᵢ state throughout the process (see Fig. 17-10).

■ *Muscle Metabolism*

Muscle shares the same ATP-generating mechanisms that are found in all nucleated cells (Fig. 18-5), although the relative importance of the different mechanisms varies in different muscle cell types.

1. **Direct phosphorylation** of adenosine diphosphate (ADP) to regenerate ATP from creatine phosphate is an extremely rapid reaction. This pathway usually functions as a buffer to maintain the normal myoplasmic ATP levels of 3 to 5 mM at the beginning of contraction, while other systems for regenerating ATP are being turned on. Myoplasmic creatine phosphate concentrations are about 20 mM, which is sufficient to provide the energy for only a few twitches. In the second direct phosphorylation reaction, adenylyl kinase (often termed *myokinase in muscle*) transfers a phosphate group from one ADP to another to form ATP and adenosine monophosphate (AMP). This reaction plays an important regulatory role in glycolysis (*colored arrows,* Fig. 18-5).

2. **Glycolysis** is very rapid and readily meets the ATP demands of the fastest muscle cells. Consequently, glycolysis is important in cells of this type and in all muscle cells when the oxygen supply is inadequate. However, this pathway has a net yield of only 2 mol of ATP per mol of glucose (or 3 mol if the glucose is derived from cell glycogen), and thus it is inefficient. In the presence of oxygen, pyruvate is converted to CO_2 instead of lactate (aerobic glycolysis), and the net yield of ATP is improved threefold. ATP production by glycolysis may also be limited by the cellular stores of glycogen, which can be rapidly depleted.

3. **Oxidative phosphorylation** of fatty acids is the primary source of energy in muscles that are frequently

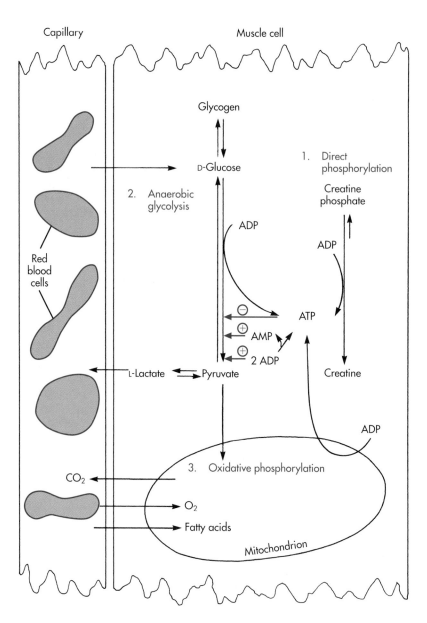

■ Fig. 18-5   Metabolic pathways in muscle. ATP is supplied via direct phosphorylation of ADP (1), glycolysis (2) and oxidative phosphorylation (3).

active. Not only is oxidative phosphorylation efficient (36 mol ATP/mol glucose), but it can operate continuously when circulation is adequate. However, oxidative phosphorylation is a slow process. It cannot meet the maximal ATP consumption rates of rapidly contracting skeletal muscle fibers unless a major portion of the fibers consists of mitochondria that are close to a capillary.

■ Matching of ATP Production and Consumption

One of the two isoenzymatic forms of myosin characteristic of skeletal muscle cells has a higher rate of ATP hydrolysis than the other. Muscle cells in which this "fast" myosin is synthesized have greater shortening velocities. Using appropriate histochemical methods, thin sections can be cut from frozen muscles and incubated with ATP under conditions in which only the slow myosin isoform is enzymatically active. The phosphate released is trapped on the section and "stains" the slow fibers. Fig. 18-6, *A* illustrates how fast fibers (types IIA and IIB) and slow fibers (type I) are typically intermixed in most mammalian skeletal muscles. Table 18-1 provides a summary of the fiber types and the nomenclature in general use.

Other histochemical reactions can be applied to serial sections cut from the same muscle to estimate the activities of enzymes in the oxidative (Fig. 18-6, *B*) and glycolytic (Fig. 18-6, *C*) metabolic pathways. The metabolic capacities of muscle fibers vary considerably. However, in most fast (type II) fibers, the activities of glycolytic enzymes are high and the activities of oxidative enzymes are low. These characteristics are confirmed by observations of only a few mitochondria in electron micrographs of fast fibers. Fast fibers with rapid contraction velocities have a much more extensive sarcoplasmic reticulum than do slow fibers, and have high pumping rates that can quickly activate and inactivate the contractile machinery. *Because the ATP consumption rates in the myofibrils and sarcoplasmic reticulum of fast fibers can readily be matched by glycolysis, a metabolism based mainly on glycolysis is appropriate, provided that the fibers are recruited only occasionally and briefly.*

A fiber of small diameter and with very high mitochondrial and capillary densities could synthesize ATP oxidatively at rates that characterize the fast myosin isoenzyme. Some fast fibers with high glycolytic *and* oxidative capacities are found in mammals (these fibers are uncommon in humans). These fibers belong to the subclassification of fast type IIA fibers shown in Table 18-1.

Slow type I fibers can meet relatively modest metabolic demands with oxidative phosphorylation. The muscle cells or tissues that contain mostly type I (or type IIA) fibers contain compounds associated with oxygen binding (e.g., hemoglobin, myoglobin, cytochromes). Because these compounds are red, types I and IIA fibers are sometimes called **red fibers.**

Cardiac muscle resembles slow skeletal muscle in expressing myosin isoenzymes with moderate ATPase activities. As might be expected, this continuously active cardiac muscle is almost entirely oxidative and is highly sensitive to interruptions in its blood supply.

The oxidation of fatty acids provides most of the ATP used by the muscles in the body. However, all muscles are also capable of using other substrates, such as carbohydrates, certain amino acids, and ketone bodies.

■ Musculoskeletal Relationships

Individual muscle cells are encased in a connective tissue layer called the **endomysium.** Groups of skeletal muscle cells form **fascicles** that are bounded by another connective tissue layer called the **perimysium.** These fascicles are grouped into the definitive muscle, which is covered by a third connective tissue layer called the **epimysium.** The three connective tissue layers are composed mainly of elastin and collagen fibrils. An estimated 250 million cells are found in the more than 400 skeletal muscles in humans. Each of these muscles exerts specific forces or movements via tendons that are usually attached to the skeleton.

■ **Table 18-1** Basic classification of skeletal muscle fiber types

	Type I: slow oxidative (red)	Type IIB: fast glycolytic (white)	Type IIA*: fast oxidative (red)
Myosin isoenzyme (ATPase rate)	Slow	Fast	Fast
Sarcoplasmic reticular Ca++ pumping capacity	Moderate	High	High
Diameter (diffusion distance)	Moderate	Large	Small
Oxidative capacity: mitochondrial content, capillary density, myoglobin	High	Low	Very high
Glycolytic capacity	Moderate	High	High

*Comparatively infrequent in humans and other primates. In the text a simple designation of type II fiber refers to a fast-glycolytic (type IIB) fiber.

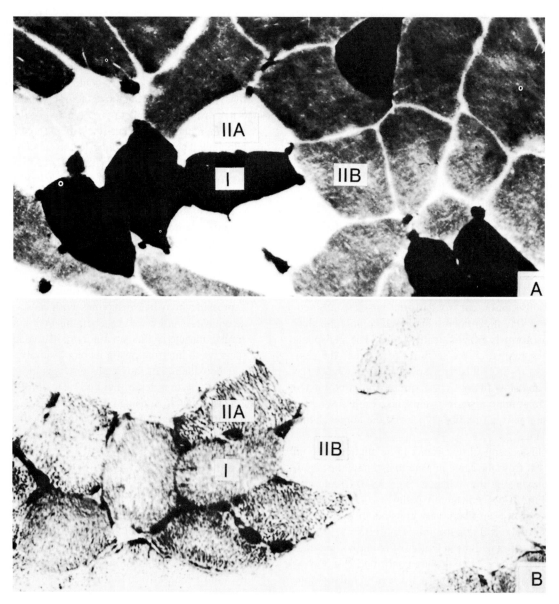

■ **Fig. 18-6**   Histochemical staining of cross-sections of the feline semitendinosus skeletal muscle. **A,** Staining for the ATPase activity of the slow myosin isoenzyme of type I fibers. Type IIB fibers stain more than type IIA fibers in this species, and the myosins in these two types of fast fibers may differ. **B,** Staining for succinic dehydrogenase activity, an enzyme associated with oxidative phosphorylation.

The strength of a muscle depends on the numbers and sizes of the muscle's cells and on their anatomic arrangement. *Increasing the diameter of a muscle fiber by synthesis of new myofibrils* **(hypertrophy)** *and/or the formation of more muscle cells* **(hyperplasia)** *will increase the force-generating capacity* (Fig. 18-7). The force generating capacity remains unchanged if the length of the cells is increased by adding more sarcomeres in series, without increasing the cross-sectional area of the cells. However, *the absolute velocity of contraction and the total shortening capacity of the cell increase with the addition of more sarcomeres* (Fig. 18-7).

The force and velocity of muscle contraction depend not only on the number of sarcomeres and myofibrils in the muscle cells, but also on the orientation of the cells within the tissue. Measurements of intact muscles directly reflect cellular properties only when the cells are arranged in parallel with each other and also parallel to the axes of the tendons that transmit the force (Fig. 18-8). This parallel arrangement maximizes shortening capacity and velocity for a muscle. However, force-generating capacity can be enhanced at the expense of shortening capacity and velocity by arrangements that place the muscle fibers at an angle to the tendons. Examples of

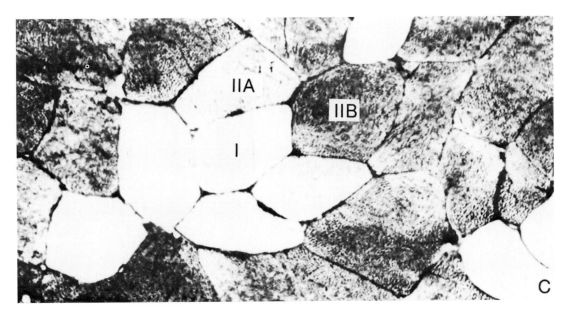

■ **Fig. 18-6, cont'd**　**C,** PAS stain indicating glycolytic capacity. Three distinct fiber types can be differentiated in these serial sections: slow oxidative or type I, fast glycolytic or type IIB, and fast oxidative (and glycolytic) or type IIA fibers. (× 450.) (From Hoppeler H et al: *Respir Physiol* 44:94, 1981.)

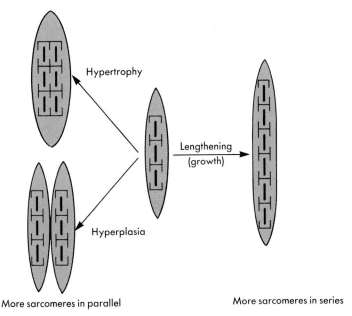

■ **Fig. 18-7**　Effects of growth on the mechanical output of a muscle cell. Growth may consist of adding new myofibrils (depicted as a series of model sarcomeres) within a cell (hypertrophy), formation of new cells (hyperplasia), or adding more sarcomeres in series as the muscle cells lengthen along with skeletal growth. The effects of the illustrated cell growth on the absolute force (newtons), shortening velocity (m/sec), and shortening capacity (m) of the muscle are summarized at the bottom of the figure.

such pennate (feather-like) arrangements are illustrated in Fig. 18-8.

Some skeletal muscles, including those that surround the mouth and anus, serve as sphincters. Striated muscles are also found in the upper portions of the esophagus, and these are active during swallowing. Others may be attached to the skin. However, most skeletal muscles are attached to the skeleton. The attachments are made by **tendons** or flattened sheets, called **aponeuroses,** both of which contain the highly inextensible protein **collagen.** A muscle is usually named in terms of its **origin** at the proximal or relatively fixed point and its insertion on the bone that is moved (the distinction between origin and insertion is sometimes arbitrary). A muscle bridges one or, more frequently, two joints. Consequently, the contraction of an individual muscle can move more than one bone.

Specific coordinated movements require the actions of two or more muscles. **Synergists** are muscles that act together; **antagonists** are muscles that oppose each other. **Kinesiology** is the study of the interactions of groups of muscles. Electromyographic techniques have been used to reveal the complex nature of coordinated muscle movements. In one such technique, the summed electrical activity of a muscle is detected from electrodes placed on the overlying skin. Another technique can detect the activity of a single muscle cell by means of needle electrodes inserted into the muscle. These techniques reveal that a specific movement may involve contractions of antagonistic muscles and may not involve contractions of some synergistic muscles. The activity patterns are often unpredictable and can be determined only by direct recordings. In general, the interactions of the muscles

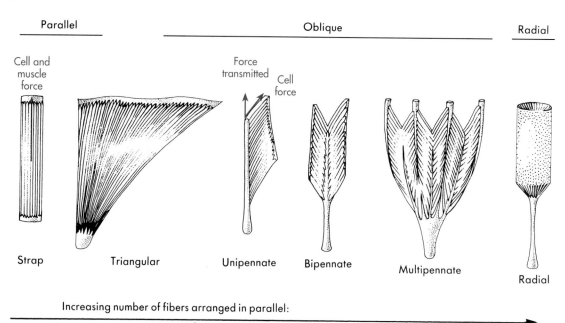

Parallel   Oblique   Radial

Cell and muscle force

Force transmitted

Cell force

Strap   Triangular   Unipennate   Bipennate   Multipennate   Radial

Increasing number of fibers arranged in parallel:

↑ Force-generating capacity, ↓ shortening velocity and capacity

■ **Fig. 18-8**   Some arrangements of skeletal muscle fibers. The force generated by all the individual cells is fully transmitted to the skeleton in only a few straplike muscles. The cells in most muscles are arranged at an angle to the axis of the muscle. This allows more fibers to be attached to a tendon and increases the total force-generating capacity. However, not all the force generated by each cell is usefully transmitted to the tendon with an oblique geometry, and the overall shortening velocity and shortening capacity of the muscle are less than that of the individual cells. (Redrawn from *Gray's Anatomy*, ed 35 (British), Philadelphia, 1973, WB Saunders.)

serve not only to move a specific bone, but also to fix or stabilize another bone or joint.

Activities (such as hiking or particularly downhill running) in which contracting muscles are stretched and lengthened too vigorously are followed by more pain and stiffness than are comparable efforts such as cycling. The resultant dull, aching pain develops slowly and reaches its peak within 24 to 48 hours. The pain is associated with a reduced range of motion, stiffness, and weakness of the affected muscles. The prime factors that cause the pain are swelling and inflammation that result from injury to muscle cells, most commonly near the myotendinous junction. Fast type II motor units are more affected than are type I motor units, because the maximal forces are highest in large cells, where the loads imposed are some 60% greater than the maximal force the cells can develop. Recovery is slow and depends on regeneration of the injured sarcomeres.

The bones act as lever systems with significant mechanical consequences. As illustrated in Fig. 18-9, when the forearm is perpendicular to the upper arm, the biceps muscle of a person holding a 20-kg load must develop an isometric force of 140 kg. Another consequence of the skeletal lever system is that slight shorten-

ing of the muscles can evoke large movements of the limbs (Fig. 18-9). Consequently, sarcomere lengths remain close to their optimum for force development in most movements (see Fig. 17-8).

■ *Coordination of Muscular Activity*
■ *Motor Nerves and Motor Units*

The cell bodies of the motor nerves (α motor axons) are located in the ventral horn of the spinal cord (Fig. 18-10). The axons exit via the ventral roots and reach the muscle through mixed peripheral nerves. The motor nerves branch in the muscle, with each branch innervating a single muscle cell in mammals. The specialized cholinergic synapse that forms the neuromuscular junction, and the neuromuscular transmission process that generates an action potential in the muscle fiber, are described in Chapter 4. A **motor unit** consists of the motor nerve and all the muscle fibers innervated by that nerve. *The motor unit (and not the individual muscle cell) is the functional contractile unit, because all the muscle cells within a motor unit contract synchronously when the motor nerve fires.* The muscle cells of a motor unit are not segregated anatomically into distinct groups, and considerable intermixture of cells occurs among neighboring motor units.

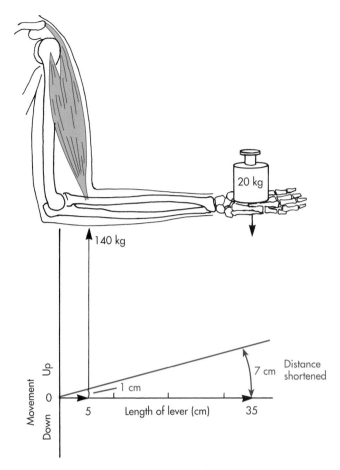

■ **Fig. 18-9**   Example of the musculoskeletal lever system. The biceps muscle operates at a 7:1 mechanical disadvantage in this situation and must generate high forces to support a weight on the hand. However, little shortening of the biceps muscle is required to produce large displacements of the hand. (Redrawn from Guyton AC: *Textbook of medical physiology,* ed 6, Philadelphia, 1981, WB Saunders.)

Skeletal muscle cells are rarely the primary cells involved in diseases that affect motor function. Most of the pathological changes associated with these diseases involve the motor pathways of the nervous system or neuromuscular transmission. The resultant functional denervation is followed by atrophy and eventual degeneration of muscle cells. A previously common infectious disease, **poliomyelitis,** destroys motor axons. Other diseases may involve immune system dysfunction. **Myasthenia gravis** is a progressive autoimmune disease in which antibodies against an individual's own acetylcholine receptors in the motor endplate are produced. The resultant weakness caused by blockade of neuromuscular transmission can be symptomatically treated with inhibitors of acetylcholinesterase, which enables high concentrations of acetylcholine to build up in the endplate clefts. Neuromuscular diseases are fatal

if they block transmission in the diaphragm and other respiratory muscles.

Motor units display considerable specialization. Some consist of only two or three muscle fibers, while others contain over 1000 cells in large muscles. The cell bodies and axons of the motor nerve increase in size with the number of muscle fibers in the unit. This relationship is understandable in terms of the metabolic requirements for synthesis and release of acetylcholine. A distinction between slow oxidative (type I) and fast glycolytic (type II) muscle fibers is shown in Table 18-1. This classification also applies to motor units, because all the fibers in one motor unit are of the same type (Table 18-2). The smaller motor units normally consist of type I cells (Table 18-2, Fig. 18-10). Note that only the contraction velocity or myosin ATPase activity clearly distinguishes the fiber types. These two characteristics reflect the presence of different myosin isoforms in the cells. Metabolic differences arise from different cellular contents of mitochondria, for example, and the glycolytic or oxidative capacity may vary considerably between motor units of the same type.

The inputs to the motor nerves are both excitatory and inhibitory (described in Chapters 12 to 14). The inputs to the motor neurons come from (1) neurons from the brain; (2) neurons originating in the spinal cord; and (3) neurons from a variety of receptors within a muscle, from its antagonists and synergists, and from the same group of contralateral muscles (Fig. 18-10). A motor neuron fires when the sum of the excitatory and inhibitory inputs depolarizes the cell to its critical membrane potential.

■ *Recruitment of Motor Units*

The functional importance of the variations among motor units can be illustrated by considering how the motor units in a muscle are progressively recruited in graded contractions. Increasing excitatory or decreasing inhibitory input to the motor neuron pool in the ventral horn of the spinal cord will depolarize the cell bodies. However, a given level of excitatory input will produce more depolarization of the smallest neurons because of their smaller membrane areas. Thus, the first axons to fire are those of the smallest motor units. The conduction velocity of the action potential will be relatively low because axons of small diameter transmit action potentials at a slower rate than axons of larger diameters (see Chapter 3). The total force developed by the muscle will therefore be small, because only a few cells of moderate diameter are present in these units.

Fig. 18-11 shows the basic relationships between motor unit recruitment and total force generated by a muscle. In the far left column, "31" indicates the number of small motor units (those that consist mostly of type I fibers) among those sampled in the muscle that devel-

■ **Fig. 18-10**   The motor unit and some inputs. Large and small motor units are mixed within a single muscle. An example of each is illustrated in a pair of contralateral muscles. The motor unit contracts in response to an action potential in the motor axon. Contraction is elicited when the sum of the inputs from synapses on the cell body depolarizes the motor neuron to its critical firing potential.

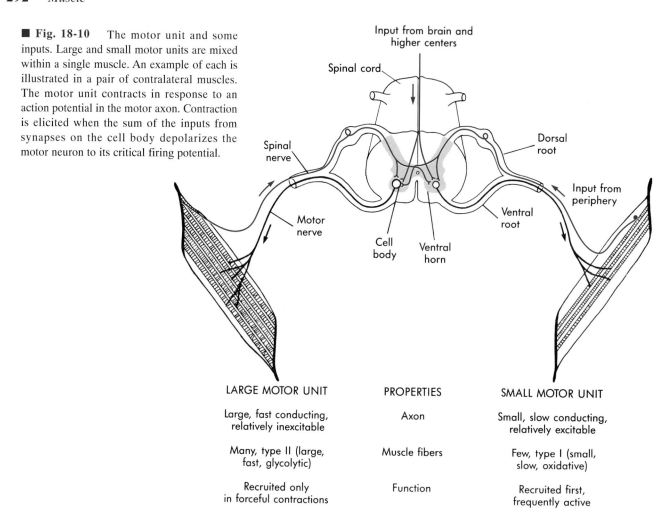

LARGE MOTOR UNIT	PROPERTIES	SMALL MOTOR UNIT
Large, fast conducting, relatively inexcitable	Axon	Small, slow conducting, relatively excitable
Many, type II (large, fast, glycolytic)	Muscle fibers	Few, type I (small, slow, oxidative)
Recruited only in forceful contractions	Function	Recruited first, frequently active

■ **Table 18-2**   Properties of motor units

	Motor unit classification	
Characteristics	*Type I*	*Type II*
Properties of nerve		
Cell diameter	Small	Large
Conduction velocity	Fast	Very fast
Excitability	High	Low
Properties of muscle cells		
Number of fibers	Few	Many
Fiber diameter	Moderate	Large
Force of unit	Low	High
Metabolic profile	Oxidative	Glycolytic
Contraction velocity	Moderate	Fast
Fatigability	Low	High

oped up to 10 g force (average, 5 g) when tetanized. If all 31 motor units fired together, the total force generated would be about 0.15 kg, if we assume an average force of 5 g/unit. The important point here is that *these small motor units are recruited first, and they remain active as long as any part of the muscle is contracting. Many such small motor units permit fine gradations of movement.*

When the excitatory input increases, somewhat larger axons fire. In the sample depicted in Fig. 18-11, fewer motor units could generate between 10- and 20-g force, but their summed contributions to the total force in the muscle are comparable, that is, 10 units × 15 g (average force) = 0.15 kg, as shown by the height of the colored column. The total force generated by the muscle with the increased level of excitatory input is now the sum of 31 units (with an average force of 5 g) plus 10 units (with an average force of 15 g). The total force thus equals 0.31 kg. A smooth gradation in contractile force is still maintained because the percentage increase in force produced by a larger motor unit remains small when added to the force already being generated. Fig. 18-11 shows that smaller numbers of larger motor units are successively recruited until all motor units are contracting. Some evidence indicates that the largest motor units are so inexcitable that most persons cannot recruit them voluntarily. Recruitment of such large, inexcitable motor units may account for the exceptional displays of strength exhibited by people under stress when increased excitatory activity occurs in the CNS.

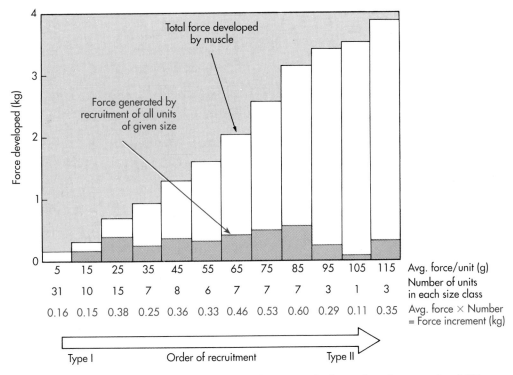

Avg. force/unit (g)	5	15	25	35	45	55	65	75	85	95	105	115
Number of units in each size class	31	10	15	7	8	6	7	7	7	3	1	3
Avg. force × Number = Force increment (kg)	0.16	0.15	0.38	0.25	0.36	0.33	0.46	0.53	0.60	0.29	0.11	0.35

Type I   Order of recruitment   Type II

■ **Fig. 18-11**   Relationships between the size of a motor unit, the number of motor units of different size classes in a muscle, the contributions of each class of motor units to force development *(colored numbers),* and the order of recruitment of motor units of different sizes. See text for further explanations. (Data from Henneman E, Olson CB: *J Neurophysiol* 28:581, 1965.)

The pattern of increasing force illustrated in Fig. 18-11 is a consequence of recruitment by the **size principle.** Recruitment by size and the simultaneous increase in firing rates, which allows each unit to increase its force by tetanization, are responsible for gradations in contractile force. Because the larger motor units are also faster, whole muscle contraction velocities can be increased by recruiting more motor units. Recruiting more units also contributes to the increase in contraction velocity by reducing the effective load on each muscle cell; the diminished load allows faster cross-bridge cycling rates.

The size principle also explains the metabolic profile pattern of the motor units. *Highly oxidative units are those that are used most. Maximal efforts, in which fast motor units are also recruited, cannot be sustained because of the rapid depletion of glycogen.* This intracellular source of energy is needed to supply the glycolytic pathway, which allows the high rates of ATP consumption to be met.

■ *Tone in Skeletal Muscle*

The skeletal system supports the body mass efficiently when posture is normal. The amount of energy expended for the muscular contraction required to maintain a standing posture is remarkably small. However, muscles normally exhibit some level of contractile activity. Isolated, unstimulated muscles are "relaxed" and flaccid, but even "relaxed" muscles in the body are comparatively firm. This firmness, or **tone,** is caused by low levels of contractile activity in some of the motor units that are driven by reflex arcs from receptors in the muscles; muscle tone can be abolished by sectioning the dorsal root. Tone in skeletal muscles should be distinguished from "tone" in smooth muscles (see Chapter 19).

■ *Fatigue*

Remarkably little is known about the factors responsible for muscle fatigue. Fatigue may potentially occur at any of the points involved in muscle contraction, from the brain to the muscle cells, as well as in the cardiovascular and respiratory systems that maintain energy supplies.

Cellular fatigue. Fatigue of motor units can be assessed experimentally by recording the maximal stress maintained during prolonged contraction or during a series of brief tetani elicited by direct stimulation of the motor nerve to the muscle. During the latter type of stimulation, the oxygen supply to the muscle is adequate when the circulation is intact. Tetanic stress decays rapidly to a level that can be maintained for long periods (Fig. 18-12). This decay represents the rapid

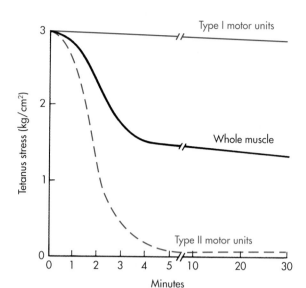

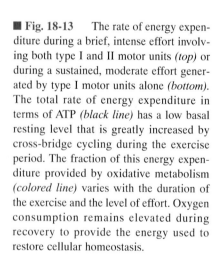

■ Fig. 18-12   Fatigue of a skeletal muscle in which half of the cross-sectional area is composed of slow, oxidative type I motor units and the other half of fast, glycolytic type II motor units. The muscle was briefly tetanized once every second by stimulation of its motor nerve in situ. With this regimen, type II motor units exhibit rapid cellular fatigue and failure to contract, whereas type I motor units maintain almost normal contractile responses.

and almost total failure of the fast motor units. The decline in tetanic stress is paralleled by glycogen and creatine phosphate depletion and by lactic acid production, which suggests that ATP depletion leads to the failure of contraction. However, the decline in stress occurs when the ATP pool is not greatly reduced, and the muscle fibers do not go into rigor. Slow motor units, which can meet the energy demands of this stimulus regimen, do not exhibit significant fatigue for many hours. Evidently, some factor associated with energy metabolism can inhibit contraction, but this factor has not been clearly identified. Some evidence suggests that **neuromuscular fatigue** in the largest fast motor units is caused by the limited ability of the motor nerve to synthesize and release acetylcholine.

General fatigue. Most persons tire and cease exercise long before the motor unit fatigue of the type illustrated in Fig. 18-12 occurs. *General physical fatigue may be defined as a homeostatic disturbance produced by work. The basis for the perceived discomfort (or even pain) probably involves many factors.* These factors may include decrease in plasma glucose levels and accumulation of metabolites. Motor system function in the CNS is not impaired. Highly motivated and trained athletes can withstand the discomfort of the fatigue and will exercise to the point at which some motor unit

■ Fig. 18-13   The rate of energy expenditure during a brief, intense effort involving both type I and II motor units *(top)* or during a sustained, moderate effort generated by type I motor units alone *(bottom).* The total rate of energy expenditure in terms of ATP *(black line)* has a low basal resting level that is greatly increased by cross-bridge cycling during the exercise period. The fraction of this energy expenditure provided by oxidative metabolism *(colored line)* varies with the duration of the exercise and the level of effort. Oxygen consumption remains elevated during recovery to provide the energy used to restore cellular homeostasis.

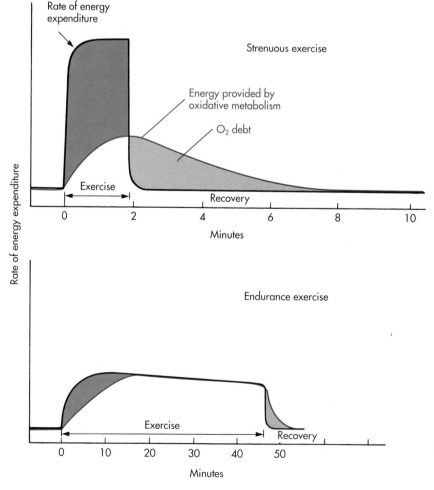

fatigue occurs. Part of the enhanced performance observed after training involves motivational factors.

Recovery. Muscle metabolism, blood flow, and oxygen uptake remain elevated for some time after exercise (see also Chapter 31). **Oxygen debt** (Fig. 18-13) is the excess amount of oxygen consumed over that required for resting metabolism when energy use by the contractile system has stopped. Some oxygen debt occurs even with low levels of exercise, because slow oxidative motor units consume considerable ATP (derived from creatine phosphate or glycolysis) before oxidative metabolism can increase ATP production to meet steady-state requirements. The oxygen debt is much greater with strenuous exercise, when fast glycolytic motor units are used. The oxygen debt is approximately equal to the energy consumed during exercise minus that supplied by oxidative metabolism (i.e., the dark- and light-colored areas in Fig. 18-13 are roughly equal). The additional oxygen used during recovery from exercise represents the energy requirements for restoring normal cellular metabolite levels.

■ *Trophic Responses of Skeletal Muscle*

Trophic factors are those factors responsible for long-term development and maintenance of the specific characteristics of a tissue. *Skeletal muscle exhibits considerable plasticity (ability to modify the phenotype or properties of its cells),* as shown by a variety of experimental studies.

■ *Growth and Development*

Skeletal muscle fibers differentiate before they are innervated (neuromuscular junctions may be formed well after birth). Before innervation, the muscle fibers physiologically resemble slow type I cells. Acetylcholine receptors are distributed throughout the sarcolemma of these uninnervated cells and are supersensitive to that neurotransmitter. An endplate is formed when the first growing nerve terminal establishes contact with a muscle cell. The cell forms no further association with nerves, and the receptors to acetylcholine become concentrated in the endplate membranes. Cells innervated by a small motor neuron form slow oxidative motor units. Fibers innervated by large motor nerves develop all the characteristics of fast type II motor units. Thus, innervation produces major cellular changes, including the synthesis of the fast and slow myosin isoforms, which replace embryonic or neonatal variants.

An increase in muscle strength and size occurs during maturation. As the skeleton grows, so must the muscle cells lengthen. Lengthening is accomplished by formation of additional sarcomeres at the ends of the muscle cells, a process that is reversible. For example, the length of a cell decreases when terminal sarcomeres are elimi-

nated, which can occur when a limb is immobilized with the muscle in a shortened position, or when an improperly set fracture leads to a shortened limb segment. *The gradual increase in strength and diameter of a muscle during growth is achieved mainly by hypertrophy (Fig. 18-7). Skeletal muscles have a limited ability to form new fibers (hyperplasia) by differentiation of satellite cells that are present in the tissues.* Injured cell segments that contain nuclei can grow and fuse with other segments to regenerate a cell. However, major cellular destruction leads to replacement with scar tissue. Overall, the structure of skeletal muscle cells adjusts remarkably to the demands of the organism.

Space flight exposes astronauts to a microgravity environment that mechanically unloads their muscles. This unloading leads to a rapid loss of muscle mass and weakness. Antigravity muscles that frequently contract to support the body typically have a high number of slow oxidative motor units. These type I motor units atrophy the most rapidly, and the ability to generate tetanic force is impaired. Maximal shortening velocities increase in muscles that consist mainly of slow motor units. The increase in velocity is correlated with the expression of the fast myosin isoform; infrequent recruitment in the microgravity environment may explain this change. An important aspect of space medicine is the design of exercise programs that minimize such phenotypic changes during prolonged space flight.

■ *Denervation, Reinnervation, and Cross-Innervation*

Various studies have shown the importance of innervation to the skeletal muscle phenotype (Fig. 18-14). If the motor nerve is cut, muscle **fasciculation** occurs. Fasciculation describes small, irregular contractions caused by the release of acetylcholine from the terminals of the degenerating distal portion of the axon. Several days after denervation, muscle **fibrillation** begins. Fibrillation is characterized by spontaneous, repetitive contractions. At this time, the cholinergic receptors have spread out over the entire cell membrane (in effect reverting to their preinnervation embryonic arrangement). The muscle fibrillations reflect supersensitivity to acetylcholine. Muscles also **atrophy,** with a decrease in the size of the muscle and of its cells. Atrophy is progressive in humans, with degeneration of some cells 3 or 4 months after denervation. Most of the muscle fibers are replaced by fat and connective tissue after 1 to 2 years. These changes can be reversed if reinnervation occurs within a few months. Reinnervation is normally achieved by growth of the peripheral stump of the motor nerve axons along the old nerve sheath.

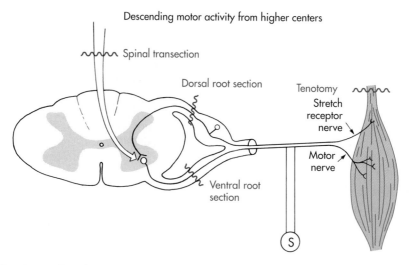

Descending motor activity from higher centers

Spinal transection

Dorsal root section

Tenotomy
Stretch
receptor
nerve

Motor
nerve

Ventral root
section

S

■ **Fig. 18-14**   Experimental or pathological situations that modify the phenotype of skeletal muscles. Normal contractile activity in the muscle can be abolished by ventral root section that cuts the motor nerves (peripheral denervation). In a muscle with normal innervation, contractile activity can be increased by pacemakers *(S)* implanted on the motor nerves. Activity can be decreased by blocking excitatory pathways from higher centers (spinal transection) or by interrupting the reflex arcs that modify muscle activity through dorsal root section. If the muscle tendon is severed (tenotomy), stretch receptors within the tendon and muscle become inactive. Tenotomy also decreases excitatory input to the motor nerves.

Reinnervation of a formerly fast type II fiber by a small motor axon causes that cell to redifferentiate into a slow type I fiber, and vice versa. Such observations suggest that large and small motor nerves differ qualitatively, and that the nerves have specific "trophic" effects on the muscle fibers. Although nerve terminals do release substances in addition to the primary neurotransmitter at synapses, an alternative explanation of the trophic effects of innervation is probably correct. Simply put, *it is the frequency of contraction that determines fiber development and phenotype.* Electrical stimulation via electrodes implanted in the muscle can lessen denervation atrophy. More strikingly, chronic low-frequency stimulation of fast motor units (by a pacemaker with electrodes placed on their motor nerves) causes fast motor units to be converted to slow units. Some conversion toward a typical fast-fiber phenotype can occur when the frequency of contraction in slow units is greatly decreased by reducing the excitatory input in the ventral horn. The excitatory input can be reduced by sectioning the appropriate spinal or dorsal root or by severing the tendon, which functionally inactivates peripheral mechanoreceptors (Fig. 18-14).

The reason why frequency of contraction could determine fiber development and phenotype involves gene expression and protein synthesis. Fibers that undergo frequent contractile activity form many mitochondria and synthesize the slow isoform of myosin. Fibers innervated by large, inexcitable axons contract infrequently. Such relatively inactive fibers typically form few mitochondria and have large concentrations of glycolytic enzymes. The fast isoform of myosin is synthesized in such cells.

■ *Response to Exercise*

Exercise physiologists identify three categories of training regimens and responses (Table 18-3): learning, endurance, and strength training. In practice, most athletic endeavors involve elements of all three. The learning aspect of training involves motivational factors as well as neuromuscular coordination. This aspect of training does not involve adaptive changes in the muscle fibers per se. However, motor skills can persist for years without regular training, unlike the responses of muscle cells to exercise.

All healthy persons can maintain some level of continuous muscular activity that is supported by oxidative metabolism. This level can be greatly increased by a regular exercise regimen that is sufficient to induce adaptive responses. *The adaptive response of skeletal muscle fibers to endurance exercise is mainly the result of an increase in the oxidative metabolic capacity of the motor units involved.* This demand places an increased load on the cardiovascular and respiratory systems and increases the capacity of the heart and respiratory muscles. The latter effects are responsible for the principal health benefits associated with endurance exercise.

Muscle strength can be increased by regular massive efforts that involve most motor units. Such efforts recruit fast glycolytic motor units as well as slow oxidative motor units and are brief. The blood supply may be interrupted as tissue pressures rise above the intravascular pressures during maximal contractions. The reduced blood flow further limits the duration of the contraction. *Regular maximal strength exercise, such as weight lift-*

■ **Table 18-3** Effects of exercise

Type of training	Example	Major adaptive response
Learning/coordination	Typing	Increased rate and accuracy of motor skills (central nervous system)
Endurance (submaximal, sustained efforts)	Marathon running	Increased oxidative capacity in all involved motor units with limited cellular hypertrophy
Strength (brief, maximal efforts)	Weight lifting	Hypertrophy and enhanced glycolytic capacity of motor units employed

ing, induces synthesis of more myofibrils and hypertrophy of the active muscle cells. The increased stress also induces growth of tendons and bones.

Most studies indicate that the effects of exercise on muscle are quantitative. Endurance exercise does not cause fast motor units to become slow, with the synthesis of the slow myosin isoenzyme, nor do maximal muscular efforts produce a shift from slow to fast motor units. However, experiments that involve cross-innervation and other techniques show that such shifts are possible. Nevertheless, any practical exercise regimen, when superimposed on normal daily activities, probably does not change the pattern of activation of motor units sufficiently to shift the myosin isoform expression. Two additional factors that affect the motor unit phenotype and athletic performance are hormones and genetic make-up.

Steroid hormones influence muscle growth. Testosterone is a major factor responsible for the greater muscle mass in males, because it has anabolic or myotrophic actions as well as androgenic (masculinization) effects (see Chapters 51 and 52). A variety of synthetic molecules, designated as anabolic steroids, have been designed to enhance muscle growth while minimizing the androgenic actions. These drugs are widely used by body builders and athletes in sports in which strength is important. The doses are typically ten- to fifty-fold greater than might be prescribed therapeutically in individuals with impaired hormone production. Unfortunately, none of these compounds lack androgenic effects. Hence, at the doses used, they induce serious hormone disturbances, including a depression of testosterone production. A major issue is whether these drugs do in fact increase athletic performance in individuals with normal circulating levels of testosterone. After some four decades of use, the scientific facts remain uncertain, and most experimental studies in animals have not documented significant effects on muscle development. Reports in humans remain controversial. Proponents claim increases in strength that provide the edge in world-class performance. Critics argue that these increases are largely placebo effects associated with expectations and motivational factors, and they contend that the side effects are dangerous. The public debate on abuse of anabolic steroids has led to their designation as controlled substances, along with opiates, amphetamines, and barbiturates.

■ *Summary*

1. Excitation-contraction coupling involves (1) binding of acetylcholine (which is released from the motor nerve) to receptors in the endplate membrane—this receptor interaction increases the endplate conductance and generates an action potential that propagates in both directions along the muscle cell; (2) mobilization of Ca^{++}; (3) a thin filament conformational change caused by the allosteric binding of Ca^{++}; and (4) cross-bridge attachment and cycling.

2. The sarcoplasmic reticulum that surrounds each myofibril contains a pool of Ca^{++} that is mobilized when the action potential propagated along the sarcolemma depolarizes transverse tubules. This depolarization briefly opens Ca^{++} channels in the opposing sarcoplasmic reticulum membrane. A transient increase in the myoplasmic Ca^{++} concentration follows the action potential.

3. The binding of four Ca^{++} ions to troponin induces the conformational change in the thin filament that enables cross-bridges to bind and cycle. Cycling continues until the myoplasmic Ca^{++} is returned to its low resting concentration by active transport into the sarcoplasmic reticulum. Ca^{++} dissociates from troponin, the thin filament is "switched off," and relaxation ensues. The mechanical response to a single action potential is a twitch.

4. Sufficient Ca^{++} is released by an action potential to activate all the thin filaments. The force of a twitch is much less than the maximum that can be developed because the release of Ca^{++} is too brief to allow generation of the maximal force.

5. The force of contraction is graded in a skeletal muscle cell by increasing the frequency of action potentials, and thereby maintaining the thin filaments in a state of prolonged cross-bridge cycling (tetanus). In a skeletal muscle, force is also increased by the recruitment of

more motor units. Changing filament overlap has minimal effects in most skeletal muscles because the skeleton constrains changes in lengths to values near the optimum for force development.

6. Skeletal muscles have a high power output when they shorten, and they consume ATP at a rapid rate. The ATP cost is minimized by the efficient conversion of chemical to mechanical energy. ATP consumption is lower during isometric contractions, but considerable cycling still occurs. Consequently, the economy of force maintenance is poor in isometric contractions. The high free energy of the myosin–ADP-P_i complex is never released when a contracting muscle is stretched. The transformation of an attached cross-bridge from a 90-degree to a 45-degree conformation cannot occur when sarcomeres are lengthening: therefore, no ATP is consumed by cross-bridge cycling.

7. Contraction requires ATP production to be matched by ATP consumption in a muscle cell. ATP production by oxidative phosphorylation can match ATP consumption in slow muscle fibers that are phenotypically red as a result of the iron in molecules that bind oxygen (hemoglobin, myoglobin, cytochromes).

8. Fast fibers are recruited only during maximal efforts, because their high rates of ATP consumption are typically matched by glycolysis. Depletion of the cellular stores of glycogen and other factors lead to rapid fatigue.

9. Motor nerves branch in a muscle and may form neuromuscular junctions with hundreds of muscle cells. Such groupings are termed motor units because firing of the nerve causes all the cells in the unit to contract simultaneously. The smaller motor units in a muscle are recruited first because of the high excitability of their motor nerve; therefore, these units are most frequently active. All the muscle fibers in such units are slow, oxidative cells that are most suited for sustained activity.

10. Skeletal muscle cells atrophy after denervation, and they depend on the activity of their motor nerves for maintenance of the differentiated phenotype. Reinnervation by axon growth along the original nerve sheath can reverse these changes. Reinnervation of the muscle cell by an excitable motor nerve may result in a phenotypic shift from a fast to a slow fiber. Skeletal muscle has a limited capacity to replace cells lost as a result of trauma or disease.

11. Skeletal muscle exhibits considerable phenotypic plasticity. Normal growth is associated with cellular hypertrophy caused by the addition of more myofibrils and more sarcomeres at the ends of the cell to match skeletal growth. Strength training induces cellular hypertrophy, whereas endurance training increases the oxidative capacity of all involved motor units. Training regimens are not sufficient to alter fiber type or the expression of myosin isoforms.

■ *Self-Study Problems*

1. List in sequence the events involved in excitation-contraction coupling in skeletal muscle contraction and relaxation, and underscore all the membranes involved.

2. Why does force continue to rise during a twitch for some time after the myoplasmic Ca^{++} has fallen well below its peak concentration?

3. What are the distinguishing characteristics of slow type I motor units?

4. How is the force generated by a skeletal muscle varied?

■ *Bibliography*

Journal articles

Block BA: Thermogenesis in muscle, *Annu Rev Physiol* 56:535, 1994.

Booth FW, Thomason DB: Molecular and cellular adaptation of muscle in response to exercise: perspectives of various models, *Physiol Rev* 71:541, 1991.

Cooke R: The actomyosin engine, *FASEB J* 9:636, 1995.

Cope TC, Pinter MJ: The size principle: still working after all these years, *News Physiol Sci* 10:280, 1995.

Fitts RH: Cellular mechanisms of muscle fatigue, *Physiol Rev* 74:49, 1994.

Florini JR: Hormonal control of muscle growth, *Muscle Nerve* 10:577, 1987.

Josephson RK: Contraction dynamics and power output of skeletal muscle, *Annu Rev Physiol* 55:527, 1993.

Krier J, Adams T: Properties of sphincteric striated muscle, *News Physiol Sci* 5:263, 1990.

Pozzan T, Rizzuto R, Volpe P, Meldolesi J: Molecular and cellular physiology of intracellular calcium stores, *Physiol Rev* 74:595, 1994.

Rios E, Pizarro G: Voltage sensor of excitation-contraction coupling in skeletal muscle, *Physiol Rev* 71:849, 1991.

Schiaffino S, Reggiani C: Molecular diversity of myofibrillar proteins: gene regulation and functional significance, *Physiol Rev* 76:371, 1996.

Schneider MF: Control of calcium release in functioning skeletal muscle fibers, *Annu Rev Physiol* 56:463, 1994.

Books and monographs

Bagshaw CR: *Muscle contraction,* London, 1993, Chapman & Hall.

Hochachka PW: *Muscles as molecular and metabolic machines,* Boca Raton, Fla, 1994, CRC Press.

Lieber RL: *Skeletal muscle structure and function: implications for rehabilitation and sports medicine,* Baltimore, 1994, Williams & Wilkins.

McMahon TA: *Muscles, reflexes, and locomotion,* Princeton, NJ, 1984, Princeton University Press.

Netter FH: *The CIBA collection of medical illustrations,* vol 8, *Musculoskeletal system,* West Caldwell, NJ, 1987, CIBA-Geigy.

Peachey LD, Adrian RH, editors: *Handbook of physiology*, sect 10, *Skeletal muscle,* Bethesda, Md, 1983, American Physiological Society.

Rowel LB, Shepherd JT, editors: *Handbook of physiology*, sect 12, *Exercise: regulation and integration of multiple systems*, Bethesda, Md, 1996, American Physiological Society.

Rüegg JC: *Calcium in muscle contraction,* ed 2, Berlin, 1992, Springer-Verlag.

Woledge RC et al: *Energetic aspects of muscle contraction*, London, 1985, Academic Press.

Smooth Muscle

Muscle plays important roles in the function of most organs. Nonstriated (or smooth) muscle cells are a major component of the airways, vasculature, alimentary canal, urogenital tract, and other systems. *Smooth muscle must develop force or shorten to provide motility or to alter the dimensions of an organ. However, in the absence of a skeleton, smooth muscle must also be capable of economical sustained or tonic contractions to maintain organ dimensions against imposed loads. For example, the blood vessels must be able to withstand the blood pressure. In hollow organs, smooth muscle cells are mechanically coupled like links in a chain in hollow organs, and all the cells must respond in a highly coordinated fashion.* In keeping with all of these requirements, smooth muscle is structurally and functionally diverse.

To understand the many differences between smooth and skeletal muscle, consider the complications imposed by smooth muscle's lack of skeletal attachment:

1. Cellular responses are coordinated by complex neural and hormonal control systems that act on the smooth muscle cells. The action of these systems requires extensive communication between the smooth muscle cells.
2. The fibrillar contractile apparatus and its force-transmitting cytoskeleton must be able to operate in nonlinear configurations and over a greater range of lengths than striated muscle cells.
3. Adenosine triphosphate (ATP) consumption must be minimized in those smooth muscle cells that typically are continuously active.

■ *Overview of Smooth Muscle*

■ *Types of Smooth Muscle*

Many attempts have been made to classify smooth muscle into general categories. Although it can be classified according to specific characteristics (e.g., structure, electrophysiology, innervation), smooth muscle is too diverse to allow rigorous generalizations. A useful functional dis-

tinction is whether the smooth muscle cells in an organ contract rhythmically or intermittently or whether they are continuously active. Examples of the former are found in the gastrointestinal and urogenital systems (Fig. 19-1). The cells in the walls of these organs are called **phasic** smooth muscle. In contrast, smooth muscle located in the sphincters at the ends of these organs are continuously contracted, like the muscle in the walls of blood vessels and airways. These cells are called **tonic** smooth muscle. Typically, phasic smooth muscles contract in response to action potentials that propagate from cell to cell. In contrast, **tone** (continuous partial activation) is not associated with action potentials, although it is proportional to the membrane potential. Both types of contraction are based on common molecular mechanisms for contraction and its control, and all smooth muscle cells appear to be capable of both phasic and tonic behavior.

■ *Structure of Smooth Muscle Cells*

Smooth muscle cells typically form layers around hollow organs. The simplest structure is tubular; this structure is found in blood vessels or airways (Fig. 19-2, *A*). In most vessels, the smooth muscle cells are arranged circumferentially, so that contraction reduces the diameter of the tube. This contraction increases the resistance to the flow of blood or air but has little effect on the length of the organ. Smooth muscle cell organization is more complex in the gastrointestinal tract, whose role is to mix and propel the contents. Layers of smooth muscle in both circumferential and longitudinal orientations provide the mechanical actions (Fig. 19-2, *B*). Coordination between the layers depends on a complex system of autonomic nerves linked by plexuses; these plexuses are characteristically located between the two muscle layers (see Chapter 37).

The smooth muscle in the walls of sacular structures, such as the urinary bladder or rectum, allows the organ to increase in size with the accumulation of urine or feces under little pressure. The varied arrangement of cells in the walls of these organs contributes to their ability to reduce the internal volume almost to zero during urination or defecation. Smooth muscle cells in hollow organs occur in a spectrum of forms, depending on their function and the mechanical loads (Fig. 19-2, *C*). However, in all hollow organs, the smooth muscle is separated from the contents of the organ by other cellular elements, which may be as simple as the vascular endothelium or as complex as the mucosa of the digestive tract. The walls of hollow organs also contain large amounts of connective tissue that bear an increasing share of the wall stress as the organ volume increases.

The following sections describe the structural components that enable smooth muscle to set or alter hollow organ volumes. *These include the contractile and regulatory proteins, force-transmitting systems (cellular cytoskeleton and linkages between cells and to the extracellular matrix), and membrane systems that transduce extracellular signals into changes in the myoplasmic* Ca^{++} *concentration.*

Cell-to-cell contacts. The variety of specialized contacts that exist between involuntary muscle cells serve two functions: mechanical linkage and communication. In contrast to skeletal muscle cells, which are normally attached at either end to a tendon, smooth (and cardiac) muscle cells are connected to each other. Because smooth muscle cells are anatomically arranged in series, they must not only be mechanically linked, but must also be activated simultaneously and to the same degree. This mechanical and functional linkage is crucial to smooth muscle function. If such linkages did not exist, contraction in one region would simply stretch another region without a substantial decrease in radius or increase in pressure. The mechanical connections are provided by attachments to sheaths of connective tissue and by specific junctions between muscle cells.

Several types of junctions are found in smooth muscle (Fig. 19-3, *A*). One junction is the **gap junction,** in which

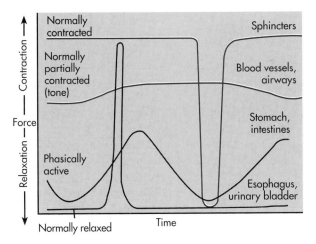

■ Fig. 19-1 Some contractile activity patterns exhibited by smooth muscles. Tonic smooth muscles are normally contracted and generate a variable steady-state force *(color).* Examples are sphincters, blood vessels, and airways. Phasic smooth muscles commonly exhibit rhythmic contractions (gastrointestinal tract) but may contract intermittently in physiological activities under voluntary control (voiding, swallowing) *(black).*

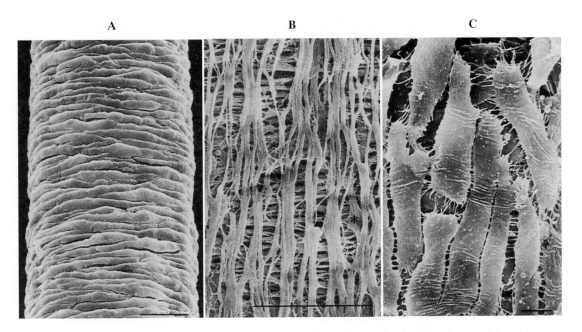

■ Fig. 19-2 Scanning electron micrographs of smooth muscle. **A,** Muscular arteriole with fusiform cells in a circular orientation (bar: 20 μm). **B,** Superimposed images of circular *(below)* and longitudinal *(above)* layers of intestinal smooth muscle sandwiching neural components of the myenteric plexus *(asterisks)* (bar: 50 μm). **C,** Rectangular smooth muscle cells with thin projections to adjacent cells in a small testicular duct (bar: 5 μm). (From Uehara Y et al. In Motta PM, editor: *Ultrastructure of smooth muscle,* Norwell, Mass, 1990, Kluwer Academic.)

adjacent plasma membranes are separated by only 2 or 3 nm. Gap junctions are of particular importance in forming low-resistance pathways. Gap junctions also allow chemical communication by diffusion of low-molecular-weight compounds. In certain tissues, such as the outer longitudinal layer of smooth muscle in the intestine, large numbers of such junctions exist. Action potentials are readily propagated from cell to cell through such tissues. Other junctions are also presumed to carry out similar mechanical functions (Fig. 19-3, *A*).

Cells and membranes. Embryonic smooth muscle cells do not fuse, and each differentiated cell has a single, centrally located nucleus (Figs. 19-2 and 19-4). Although dwarfed by skeletal muscle cells, smooth muscle cells are

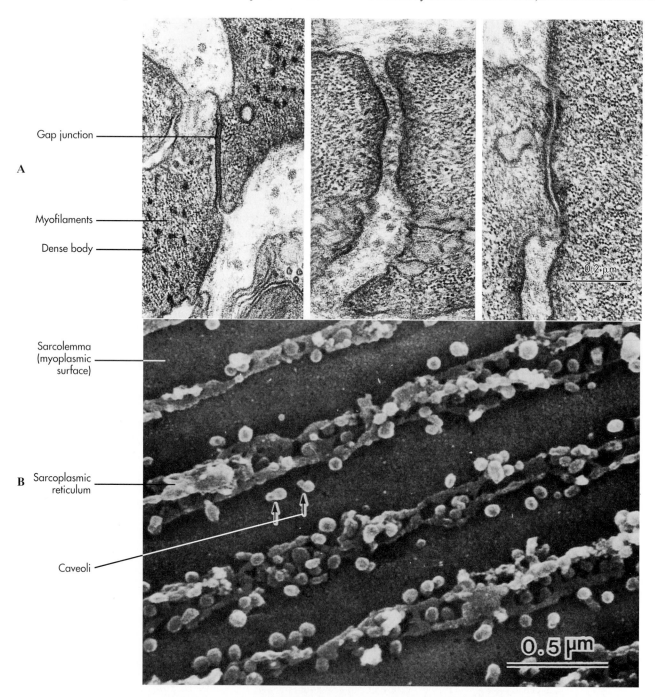

■ **Fig. 19-3**   Junctions and membranes in smooth muscle. **A,** Transmission electron micrograph of junctions between intestinal smooth muscle cells. **B,** Scanning electron micrograph of the inner surface of the sarcolemma of an intestinal smooth muscle cell. Longitudinal rows of caveoli project into the myoplasm *(small, light-colored spheres)* surrounded by darker elements of the tubular sarcoplasmic reticulum. The attachments of thin filaments to the sarcolemma between the rows of membrane elements were removed during specimen preparation. (**A** from Gabella G and **B** from Inoué T. In Motta PM, editor: *Ultrastructure of smooth muscle,* Norwell, Mass, 1990, Kluwer Academic.)

large: they are typically 40 to 600 μm long at their optimal lengths for force generation. These cells are 2 to 10 μm in diameter at the level of the nucleus, and most taper toward their ends. Contracting cells become quite distorted as a result of forces exerted on the cell by attachments to other cells or to the extracellular matrix (Fig. 19-4), and cross-sections of these cells are often very irregular.

Smooth muscle cells lack T tubules, the tiny invaginations of the sarcolemma that provide electrical links to the sarcoplasmic reticulum of skeletal muscle. However, the sarcolemma has longitudinal rows of tiny saclike inpocketings called **caveoli** (Fig. 19-3). Caveoli increase the large surface-to-volume ratio of the cells, but their functional role is uncertain.

The average diameter of most smooth muscle cells is not much greater than that of a striated muscle myofibril. The sarcolemma, rather than an elaborate sarcoplasmic reticulum, surrounds the myofilaments of smooth muscle cells. *Ca^{++} diffuses into the cell through channels in the*

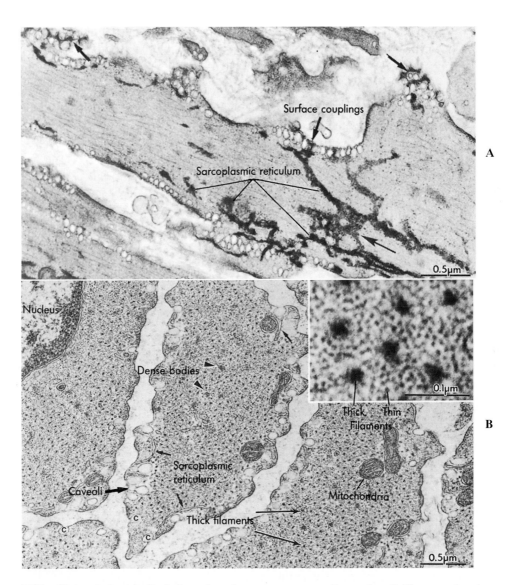

■ **Fig. 19-4**　**A,** Longitudinal view of a pulmonary artery smooth muscle cell. The sarcoplasmic reticulum is stained with osmium ferricyanide and appears to form a continuous network throughout the cell consisting of tubules, fenestrated sheets *(long arrows),* and surface couplings at the cell membrane *(short arrows).* **B,** Transverse section of a bundle of venous smooth muscle cells illustrating the regular spacing of thick filaments *(long arrows)* and the relatively large number of surrounding thin (actin) filaments *(inset).* Dense bodies *(arrowheads)* are sites of attachment for the thin actin filaments and equivalent to the Z disks of striated muscles. Elements of sarcoplasmic reticulum *(short arrows)* occur at the periphery of these cells. (From Somlyo AP, Somlyo AV: *Smooth muscle structure and function.* In Fozzard HA et al, editors: *The heart and cardiovascular system,* ed 2, New York, 1992, Raven Press.)

sarcolemma during activation, and the extracellular fluid contains an important Ca⁺⁺ pool for regulation of contraction. However, smooth muscle has a sarcoplasmic reticulum that also contains an intracellular Ca^{++} pool (Figs. 19-3, *B* and 19-4). This Ca^{++} pool can be mobilized when stimulatory neurotransmitters, hormones, or drugs bind to receptors on the sarcolemma. The amount of sarcoplasmic reticulum in smooth muscle cells varies (2% to 6% of cell volume) and can approximate that of skeletal muscle. Chemical signals link the sarcolemma and the sarcoplasmic reticulum.

Smooth muscle cells contain a prominent rough endoplasmic reticulum and Golgi apparatus, which are located centrally at each end of the nucleus. These structures reflect significant protein synthetic and secretory functions. The scattered mitochondria (Fig. 19-4) are sufficient for oxidative phosphorylation to generate the increased ATP consumed during contraction.

The fibrillar contractile apparatus. Thick and thin filaments of muscle cells are about 10,000 times longer than their diameter and are tightly packed. Therefore, the probability of observing an intact filament by electron microscopy is extremely low. The thick and thin filaments of skeletal muscle are easy to localize because of their precise transverse alignment, which appears as striations. Not all the cytoskeletal and contractile filaments in smooth muscle are in uniform transverse alignment, and striations are absent. The lack of striation does not imply a lack of order but the need for improved three-dimensional imaging technologies to detect the precise organization of thick and thin filaments in contractile units that are analogous to sarcomeres.

Cell cytoskeleton. The cytoskeleton in muscle cells serves as attachment points for the thin filaments and permits force transmission to the ends of the cell. The contractile apparatus in smooth muscle is not organized into myofibrils, and Z disks are lacking. The functional equivalents of the Z disks in smooth muscle cells are ellipsoidal **dense bodies** in the myoplasm and **dense areas** that form bands along the sarcolemma (Figs. 19-4 and 19-5). These structures serve as attachment points for the thin filaments and contain α-actinin, a protein also found in the Z disks of striated muscle. **Intermediate filaments** with diameters between those of thin filaments (7 nm) and thick filaments (15 nm) are prominent in smooth muscle. These filaments link the dense bodies and areas into a cytoskeletal network (Fig. 19-5). The intermediate filaments consist of protein polymers of **desmin** or **vimentin.**

Myofilaments. Little is known about how the contractile apparatus of smooth muscle cells is organized into a contractile unit that is functionally equivalent to a sarcomere. Fig. 19-5 synthesizes some information about myofilament and cytoskeletal arrangements; important details are lacking about the structures of the thick and thin filaments and their overlap at various points on the force-length relationship.

The thin filaments of smooth muscle have the same actin and tropomyosin composition and structure as skeletal muscle (see Fig. 17-4). However, the thin filaments lack troponin and nebulin, and they contain two proteins not found in striated muscle: **caldesmon** and **calponin.** The precise roles of these proteins are unknown, but they do not appear to be fundamental to cross-bridge cycling. The cellular contents of actin and tropomyosin in smooth muscle are about twice that of striated muscle. Most of the myoplasm is filled with thin filaments that are approximately aligned along the long axis of the cell. The thin filaments exhibit the same polarity with respect to their attachments as those in striated muscle. In contrast, the myosin content of smooth muscle is only one fourth that of striated muscle. Small groups of three to five thick filaments are aligned and are surrounded by many thin filaments. These groups of thick filaments with interdigitating thin filaments connected to dense bodies or areas (Fig. 19-5) may be the equivalent of the sarcomere.

The contractile apparatus of adjacent cells is mechanically coupled by the links between membrane-dense areas (Fig. 19-5). This coupling reflects the fact that smooth muscle cells are not functionally independent contractile units.

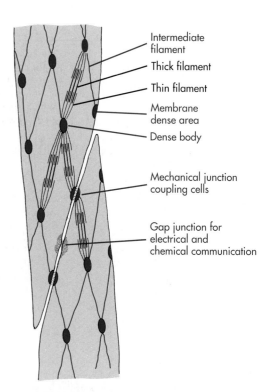

Intermediate filament

Thick filament

Thin filament

Membrane dense area

Dense body

Mechanical junction coupling cells

Gap junction for electrical and chemical communication

■ **Fig. 19-5**   Apparent organization of the cytoskeleton *(color)* and myofilaments in smooth muscles. Small contractile elements functionally equivalent to a sarcomere presumably underlie the similarities in mechanics between smooth and skeletal muscles. Linkages consisting of specialized junctions or interstitial fibrillar material functionally couple the contractile apparatus of adjacent cells.

■ Control Systems of Smooth Muscle Cells

■ Neuromuscular Relationships

Neural control of contraction in involuntary muscle is more complex than in skeletal muscle. Three factors must be considered: *(1) the types of innervation and neurotransmitters, (2) the proximity of the nerves to the muscle cells, and (3) the type and distribution of the receptors for neurotransmitters in the muscle cell membranes* (Fig. 19-6).

The types of innervation found in smooth muscle can be divided into three categories. **Extrinsic innervation** is derived from axons of the autonomic nervous system. In arteries, for example, extrinsic innervation is in large part limited to sympathetic nerves. However, both sympathetic and parasympathetic innervation are commonly present in other tissues. **Intrinsic nerves** contained in plexuses may occur within the smooth muscle tissue, particularly in the gastrointestinal tract. Finally, **afferent sensory neurons** that mediate various reflexes are found in the plexuses. The innervation of the gastrointestinal

tract alone is larger than the total motor system for all the skeletal muscles. At the other end of the spectrum, a few smooth muscle tissues have no innervation.

Neuromuscular junctions and neuromuscular transmission in involuntary muscle are functionally comparable with skeletal muscle. Both types of muscle exhibit presynaptic transmitter release, diffusion across the "junction," and combination with a postsynaptic receptor. However, elaborate neuromuscular contacts at axon terminals are not found in smooth muscle. Autonomic nerves that supply smooth muscle have a series of swollen areas or varicosities that are spaced at intervals along the axon. These varicosities contain the vesicles that contain the neurotransmitters (Fig. 19-6). Each varicosity functions as a neuromuscular junction, although the adjacent muscle membranes exhibit little specialization. In tissues with a rich neural regulation, a gap of about 6 to 20 nm is found between the varicosities and the muscle cell membrane. The average gap is about 80 to 120 nm, and occasionally considerably more in tissues in which neural control is less extensive.

The neurotransmitters that are released in smooth muscle contraction and their presynaptic and postsynaptic

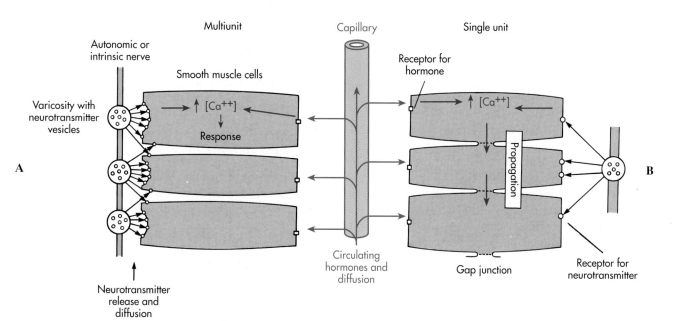

A **B**

■ **Fig. 19-6** Control systems of smooth muscle. Contraction (or inhibition of contraction) of smooth muscles can be initiated by (1) intrinsic activity of pacemaker cells, (2) neurally released transmitters, or (3) circulating or locally generated hormones or signaling molecules. The combination of a neurotransmitter, hormone, or drug with specific receptors activates contraction by increasing cell Ca^{++}. The response of the cells depends on the concentration of the transmitters or hormones at the cell membrane and the nature of the receptors present. Hormone concentrations depend on diffusion distance, release, reuptake, and catabolism. Consequently, cells lacking close neuromuscular contacts will have a limited response to neural activity unless they are electrically coupled so that depolarization is transmitted from cell to cell. **A,** Multiunit smooth muscles resemble striated muscles in that there is no electrical coupling, and neural regulation is important. **B,** Single-unit smooth muscles are like cardiac muscle, and electrical activity is propagated throughout the tissue. Most smooth muscles probably lie between the two ends of the single-unit–multiunit spectrum.

effects are highly variable. Marked individuality of the responses of different tissues that contain involuntary muscle is achieved by differences in their innervation, the types of transmitter released, and the nature of the receptors for each transmitter.

The enteric nervous system controls many aspects of gastrointestinal function, including motility. It contains more neurons than does the spinal cord, and it contains every class of neurotransmitter found in the brain. In effect, the enteric nervous system serves as a brain for the gut, with the central nervous system only fine-tuning motor function. Some children are born without enteric nerves in the distal portions of the colon. In this tissue, intrinsic innervation is essential for smooth muscle contraction and motility. Severe constipation and a distended abdomen are symptoms of this disorder, called **Hirschsprung's disease.** This condition was lethal until surgical treatments were developed to remove the uninnervated sections. The absence of nerves is caused by mutant genes that disrupt the signals necessary for the embryonic nerves to migrate to the colon.

■ *Relationships with Other Cell Types*

Contractile function in smooth muscle can be modulated by cells other than nerves. For example, specialized junctional regions can be observed between the membranes of the smooth muscle cells and the endothelial cells that line blood vessels. The actions of some circulating hormones or drugs can be mediated by the endothelial cells. For example, circulating acetylcholine, acting on endothelial cell receptors, produces arterial smooth muscle relaxation. Nitric oxide (NO) has been identified as the signal released from endothelial cells that mediates vasodilation. Acetylcholine causes contraction when it binds directly with cholinergic receptors in the arterial smooth muscle cell membrane.

Another example of a local control mechanism for vascular smooth muscle contraction is the formation of adenosine as a consequence of the increased metabolism during contraction of skeletal muscle. Adenosine diffuses from the skeletal muscle cells to receptors on the vascular smooth muscle cells of the arteries, and induces smooth muscle relaxation and vasodilation. The result is an increase in blood flow to the contracting skeletal muscle cells.

■ *Patterns of Function*

Involuntary muscle groups can be divided into **multiunit** and **single-unit** tissues (Fig. 19-6). Multiunit tissues are those in which each cell is not extensively coupled with other muscle cells through gap junctions. Contraction of multiunit smooth muscle is primarily controlled by extrinsic innervation or hormonal diffusion. Skeletal muscles exemplify this pattern, which is also typical of a few smooth muscles (e.g., those in the vas deferens and iris). However, all smooth muscle cells that are anatomically arranged in series must be part of the same functional contractile unit, although many nerves may be involved. Single-unit tissues (Fig. 19-6, *B*) are exemplified by the heart and by a number of smooth muscles that undergo rhythmical contractile activity. All the cells in single-unit tissues are electrically coupled through cell-to-cell junctions. Single-unit tissues can maintain fairly normal contractile activity without extrinsic innervation. The activity pattern in denervated single-unit muscles is caused by **pacemaker cells** and **intrinsic reflex pathways.**

Note that this distinction between single-unit and multiunit tissues is oversimplified. In reality, *most smooth muscles are controlled and coordinated by a combination of neural elements, by some degree of coupling, and by locally produced activators or inhibitors.* One generalization that can be made is that tonic muscles that maintain more or less continuous levels of tone (such as arterioles and sphincters [Fig. 19-1]) approach the multiunit end of the spectrum. Characteristically, such tissues do not exhibit action potentials when stimulated. Tissues that undergo phasic (rhythmical) activity, such as peristalsis, usually generate action potentials that are propagated from cell to cell. Such tissues more fully meet the criteria characterizing single-unit muscles.

■ *Contraction of Smooth Muscle*

The evidence that the sliding filament–cross-bridge mechanism underlies contraction largely rests on similarities in the mechanics of smooth and striated muscles.

■ *The Force-Length Relationship*

Smooth muscles contain large amounts of connective tissue, which is composed of extensible **elastin** fibrils and inextensible **collagen** fibrils. Because this extracellular matrix can withstand high distending forces or loads, it is responsible for the passive force-length curve measured in relaxed tissues. This ability of the matrix also limits organ volume. The active force developed on stimulation depends on tissue length. *When lengths are normalized to* L_o *(the optimal length for force development), the force-length curves for smooth and skeletal muscle are very similar* (see Fig. 17-8, *B*). This similarity provides strong support for a sliding filament mechanism in smooth muscle. The force-length curves of the two muscle types differ quantitatively, however. Smooth muscle cells often shorten more in vivo than do striated muscle cells. Smooth muscles are characteristically only partially activated, and the peak isometric forces attained vary with the stimulus. Smooth muscles can generate active stresses comparable with striated muscle. However, smooth muscle contains only about one fourth of the myosin (and thus cross-bridge) content of striated muscles. This discrepancy between myosin content of smooth and skeletal muscle does not imply that cross-bridges in smooth muscle have a greater force-generating capacity. However, active cross-bridges in smooth muscle are much more likely to be in the attached, force-generating configuration because of their slow cycling kinetics.

■ *Velocity-Stress Relationships and the Cross-bridge Cycle*

Smooth and striated muscles both exhibit a hyperbolic dependence of shortening velocity on load, and they have an optimal power output at a load of 0.3 F_o. Both have the ability to bear (transiently) applied loads greater than the developed active stress (see Fig. 17-9). Contraction velocities are far slower in smooth muscle than in striated muscle. One factor that underlies these slow velocities is that myosin isoforms in smooth muscle cells have low ATPase activity.

Skeletal muscle cells have a unique velocity-stress curve (see Fig. 17-9) in which shortening velocities are determined only by load and the myosin isoform. In contrast, both forces and shortening velocities, which reflect the numbers of cycling cross-bridges and their cycling rates, vary in smooth muscles. These variations can be observed experimentally. When activation of smooth muscle is altered, for example, by different frequencies of nerve stimulation or changing hormone concentrations (Fig. 19-7, *B*), a "family" of velocity-stress curves can be derived. *These results imply that both cross-bridge cycling rates and the number of active cross-bridges in smooth muscle are regulated in some way, in marked contrast to striated muscle. This difference in the output of a similar myosin motor is conferred by a regulatory system that depends on the phosphorylation of cross-bridges, which in turn depends on the amount of Ca^{++} in the myoplasm.* The steady-state dependence of shortening velocity at zero load or stress on Ca^{++}-dependent cross-bridge phosphorylation is illustrated in Fig. 19-7, *C* and *D*. The mechanisms for this Ca^{++}-dependent phosphorylation are considered below.

A description of the contractions of smooth muscle cells in terms of force-length or velocity-force relationships allows comparison with striated muscle cells and assessment of contractile system properties but is not directly applicable to the mechanics of hollow organs. Pressure-volume relationships are often used to describe organ function (described in Chapters 26 and 29).

■ *Calcium and Cross-bridge Regulation*

As in striated muscle, *contraction in smooth muscle depends on an increase in the myoplasmic Ca^{++} concentration. However, smooth muscles lack troponin, and Ca^{++} regulates cross-bridge attachment and cycling indirectly.* Two aspects of regulation are considered here. The first aspect whereby Ca^{++} regulates cross-bridge interactions with the thin filament is discussed in this section. The second concerns the mechanisms that regulate the myoplasmic Ca^{++} concentration in response to inputs to the cell membrane. This aspect is discussed in the next section.

Regulation of cross-bridge attachment. In skeletal or cardiac muscle, activation involves the release of Ca^{++} from the sarcoplasmic reticulum, binding to troponin, and a conformational change in the thin filament that allows cross-bridge attachment and cycling (see Figs. 17-7 and 18-1). However, purified smooth muscle myosin cannot interact with thin filaments even in the presence of Ca^{++}. Rather, cross-bridge attachment in smooth muscle is dependent on phosphorylation in which an inorganic phosphate group derived from ATP hydrolysis is covalently attached to a specific site on the myosin regulatory light chain that is part of the cross-bridge (see Fig. 17-5). Phosphorylation is an enzymatic reaction and is initiated when a specific kinase, **myosin kinase,** is activated by an increase in the myoplasmic Ca^{++} concentration. Myosin kinase is activated by association with a Ca^{++}-binding protein, **calmodulin.** *In smooth muscle, activation involves signals to the cell membrane systems to increase Ca^{++}, occupation of the four high-affinity binding sites on calmodulin, binding of the resultant $4Ca^{++}$-calmodulin complex to myosin kinase, and transfer of a phosphate from ATP to the cross-bridge* (Fig. 19-8). The phosphorylated cross-bridge can then attach to the thin filament and cycle.

The kinetics of cross-bridge cycling are comparatively slow in smooth muscle. However, they involve the same reactions as in skeletal muscle (see Fig. 17-7) and they result in the same force (3 to 5×10^{-12} newtons) and shortening (about 10^{-9} m) per cycle. Cycling continues with hydrolysis of one ATP per cycle until the myoplasmic Ca^{++} concentration falls, the kinase becomes inactive, and the cross-bridges are dephosphorylated by **myosin phosphatase** (Fig. 19-8).

Regulation of contraction by phosphorylation. The scheme depicted in Fig. 19-8 implies that proportional changes in cross-bridge phosphorylation and force should follow changes in the myoplasmic Ca^{++} concentration. Such changes are observed after brief periods of stimulation (Fig. 19-9, *A*). However, initial Ca^{++} levels are not sustained during tonic contractions, in which both the Ca^{++} concentration and cross-bridge phosphorylation values decrease (Fig. 19-9, *B*). Nevertheless, force may slowly increase to high sustained values. Smooth muscle can slowly develop near-maximal force when only 20%

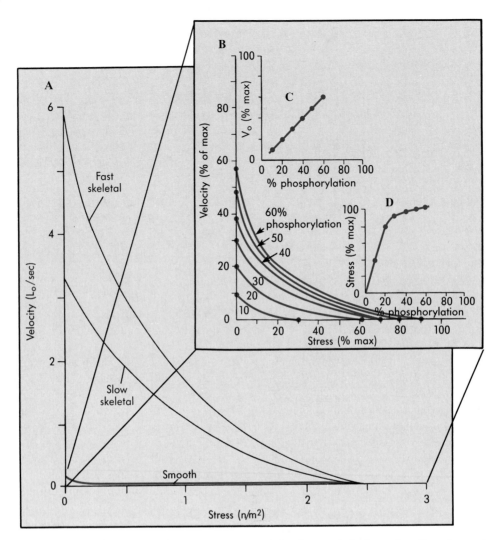

■ **Fig. 19-7** **A,** Velocity-stress curves for fast and slow human skeletal muscle cells and smooth muscle. **B,** Smooth muscles have variable velocity-stress relationships that are determined by the level of Ca++-stimulated cross-bridge phosphorylation. **C,** Maximal shortening velocities with no load (intercepts on the ordinate in **B**) are directly dependent on cross-bridge phosphorylation. **D,** Active stress (abscissa intercepts in **B**) rises rapidly with phosphorylation, and near maximal stress may be generated with only 20% to 30% of the cross-bridges in the phosphorylated state. (From Berne RM, Levy MN, editors: *Principles of physiology,* St Louis, 1990, Mosby–Year Book.)

to 30% of the cross-bridges are phosphorylated (Fig. 19-7, *D*). Higher levels of phosphorylation increase cross-bridge cycling rates, however, as manifested in shortening velocities (Fig. 19-7, *C*) and ATP consumption. This ability of smooth muscle to sustain high force with reduced cross-bridge cycling rates during tonic contractions allows for the economical maintenance of organ dimensions. This contributes to the remarkably low rates of ATP consumption by smooth muscles. However, it does imply that the regulatory scheme depicted in Fig. 19-8 is incomplete, because a sizable fraction of the cross-bridges that contribute to the force is dephosphorylated in intact smooth muscle.

The simplest hypothesis that can explain the behavior illustrated in Figs. 19-7 and 19-9 is shown in Fig. 19-10. *Both free and attached cross-bridges are substrates for myosin kinase and phosphatase. Thus covalent regulation doubles the number of potential cross-bridge states. Phosphorylation is a prerequisite for cross-bridge attachment, but a variety of pathways may be followed during the resultant cycle.* The most rapid pathway is for the cross-bridge to remain phosphorylated (traversing the four colored states in Fig. 19-10). However, an attached cross-bridge may be dephosphorylated. Dephosphorylation of attached cross-bridges will lead to a slower average cycling rate,

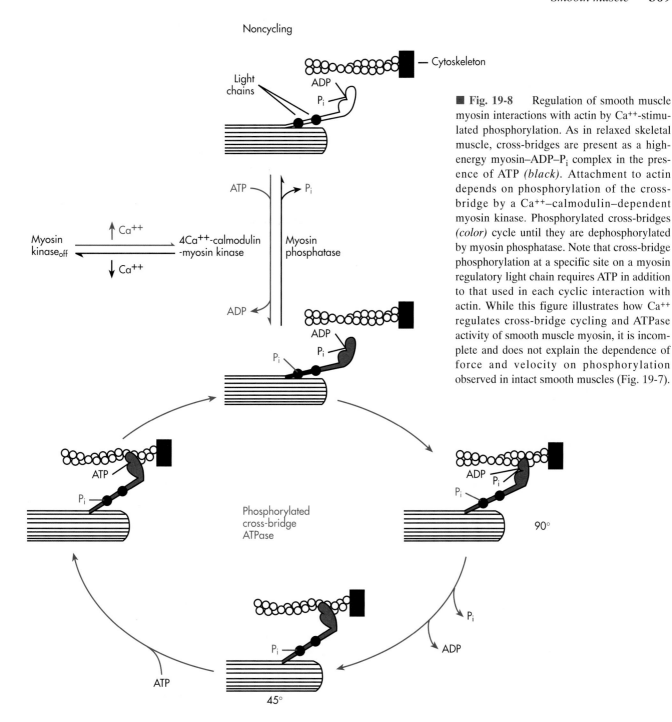

Noncycling

Light chains

Cytoskeleton

ADP

P_i

ATP — P_i

Myosin kinase$_{off}$ $\rightleftharpoons$ $\uparrow$ Ca^{++} / $\downarrow$ Ca^{++} — 4Ca^{++}-calmodulin -myosin kinase

Myosin phosphatase

ADP

ADP

P_i

P_i

ATP

P_i

Phosphorylated cross-bridge ATPase

ADP P_i

P_i

90°

P_i

ADP

ATP

P_i

45°

■ **Fig. 19-8** Regulation of smooth muscle myosin interactions with actin by Ca^{++}-stimulated phosphorylation. As in relaxed skeletal muscle, cross-bridges are present as a high-energy myosin–ADP–P_i complex in the presence of ATP *(black)*. Attachment to actin depends on phosphorylation of the cross-bridge by a Ca^{++}–calmodulin–dependent myosin kinase. Phosphorylated cross-bridges *(color)* cycle until they are dephosphorylated by myosin phosphatase. Note that cross-bridge phosphorylation at a specific site on a myosin regulatory light chain requires ATP in addition to that used in each cyclic interaction with actin. While this figure illustrates how Ca^{++} regulates cross-bridge cycling and ATPase activity of smooth muscle myosin, it is incomplete and does not explain the dependence of force and velocity on phosphorylation observed in intact smooth muscles (Fig. 19-7).

because cross-bridge detachment is slower plus the cross-bridge must be rephosphorylated before another cycle can begin. *When cell Ca^{++} concentrations are high, most of the cross-bridges will be phosphorylated (the myosin kinase:phosphatase activity ratio is high) and shortening velocities or rates of force development will be relatively high. When Ca^{++} concentrations fall during sustained contractions (Fig. 19-9), the likelihood that a cross-bridge will be dephosphorylated and spend more time in an attached, force-generating con-formation will increase.* Note, however, that a low rate of Ca^{++}-stimulated phosphorylation is essential for any contraction. The muscle will relax if Ca^{++} falls below the concentration required for binding to calmodulin and activation of myosin light chain kinase (about 0.1 μM). Under some experimental conditions, the sensitivity of cross-bridge phosphorylation to Ca^{++} can be altered. Further research may implicate other mechanisms in modulating the responses of smooth muscle to various stimuli.

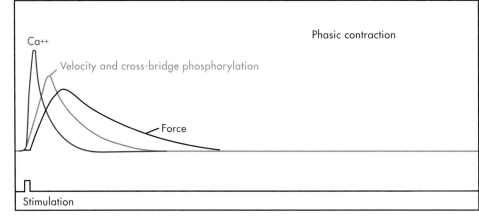

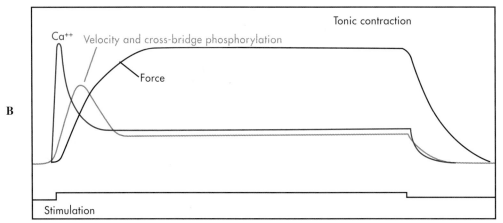

■ **Fig. 19-9**   Time course of events in cross-bridge activation and contraction in smooth muscle. **A,** A brief period of stimulation is associated with Ca++ mobilization followed by cross-bridge phosphorylation and cycling to produce a brief phasic, twitchlike contraction. **B,** In a sustained tonic contraction produced by prolonged stimulation, the Ca++ and phosphorylation levels typically fall from an initial peak (allowing rapid force development). Force (tone) is maintained at reduced Ca++, and phosphorylation with lower cross-bridge cycling rates manifested by lower shortening velocities and ATP consumption.

Inappropriate contraction of smooth muscle is associated with many pathological situations. One example is a sustained vasospasm of a cerebral artery that develops several hours after a **subarachnoid hemorrhage.** The delay is attributed to the time required for extravascular red cell hemolysis to release oxyhemoglobin and possibly other vasoactive compounds. Free radicals raise the myoplasmic Ca++ concentration in the arterial smooth muscle cells. The rise in Ca++ levels activates myosin kinase, which leads to cross-bridge phosphorylation and contraction. The vasoconstriction deprives areas of the brain of oxygen and may lead to permanent injury or death. For a few days the cerebral artery remains sensitive to vasoactive agents, and vasodilators may restore flow. Subsequently, the smooth muscle cells cease to respond, and they lose contractile proteins and secrete extracellular collagen. The lumen remains constricted as a result of structural and mechanical changes that do not involve active contraction.

Energetics and metabolism. As in skeletal muscle, cross-bridge cycling in smooth muscle increases ATP consumption (black ATP→ADP + P$_i$ in Fig. 19-10). Energy expenditure is minimal during imposed stretches, low during isometric contractions, and somewhat larger during shortening. However, the energetics of smooth muscle are quantitatively very different from striated muscle, for two reasons. First, smooth muscle myosin has a very slow detachment rate, even when phosphorylated. The second reason is the further slowing of cycling rates caused by decreases in Ca++-dependent phosphorylation rates. Because detachment is the rate-limiting step in cross-bridge cycling, almost all active cross-bridges will be generating force in smooth muscle, whereas many will

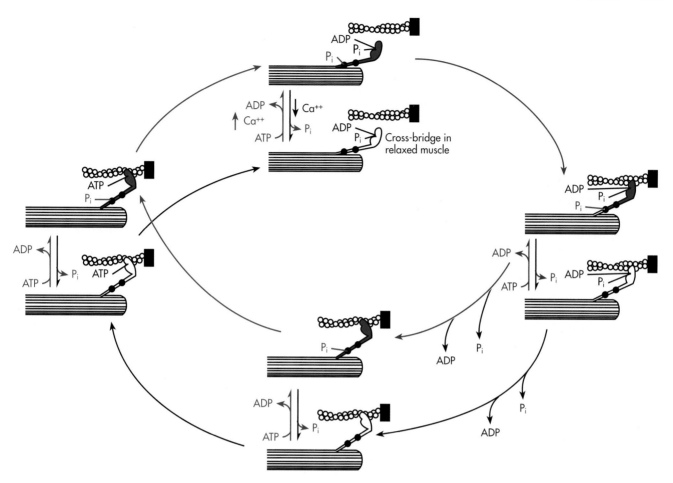

■ Fig. 19-10   Covalent regulation allows eight cross-bridge states in smooth muscle. The four dephosphorylated states are the same as in skeletal muscle *(black)*. However, phosphorylation *(vertical colored arrows)*
is obligatory for attachment. Phosphorylated cross-bridges *(color)* cycle comparatively rapidly.
Dephosphorylation of a cross-bridge during a cycle by a constitutively active myosin phosphatase *(vertical
black arrows)* slows cycling rates. Ca⁺⁺ regulates cross-bridge cycling by determining phosphorylation rates.
Note that ATP is required for both regulation *(vertical arrows)* and cycling *(curved arrows)*.

be in the detached portions of the cycle in skeletal muscle.
The result is high forces with low rates of ATP consumption in smooth muscle because of cross-bridge cycling.

Both smooth and striated muscle require energy for the
ion pumping associated with maintenance of membrane
potentials and Ca⁺⁺ sequestration. However, smooth
muscle has an additional cost associated with regulation.
ATP consumption for cross-bridge phosphorylation *(vertical arrows* in Fig. 19-10) may approach that used for
cross-bridge cycling. This ATP consumption lowers the
efficiency of smooth muscle (mechanical work/ATP
hydrolyzed). Nevertheless, sustained, isometric contractions are important for muscles in hollow organs where
the efficiency is zero (no work is done). Under such conditions, some smooth muscles can sustain the same force
as a skeletal muscle while using 300-fold less ATP. *The
savings in ATP consumption by cross-bridge cycling
greatly exceed the additional ATP cost of covalent regulation in a muscle with no physiological requirements for
rapid shortening.*

The metabolic needs of smooth muscle during contraction are readily met by oxidative phosphorylation
because consumption rates are low. Fatigue does not
occur unless the circulation is blocked. Aerobic glycolysis with lactate production normally supports membrane
ion pumps even when oxygen is plentiful.

■ *Regulation of Myoplasmic Ca⁺⁺ Concentration*

The mechanisms that couple activation to contraction
in smooth muscle involve two Ca⁺⁺ pools: one in the
sarcolemma and one in the sarcoplasmic reticulum.
The sarcolemma regulates Ca⁺⁺ influx and efflux from
the extracellular Ca⁺⁺ pool (the extracellular fluid).
The sarcoplasmic reticulum membranes determine
Ca⁺⁺ movements between the myoplasm and the intracellular pool.

Several factors explain the presence of numerous
mechanisms that interact to determine the myoplasmic

Ca⁺⁺: (1) smooth muscles are functionally diverse and must be able to generate various types of mechanical activity; (2) the activity of mechanically linked cells must be coordinated while enabling discrete responses of individual tissues; and (3) covalent regulation requires precise control of the myoplasmic Ca⁺⁺ concentration, which allows regulation of myosin phosphorylation. In contrast, the myoplasmic Ca⁺⁺ concentration is not regulated in skeletal muscles because the action potential–induced release of Ca⁺⁺ from the sarcoplasmic reticulum fully activates the contractile apparatus. The principal mechanisms that govern the myoplasmic Ca⁺⁺ concentration in smooth muscle cells are illustrated in Fig. 19-11.

The sarcoplasmic reticulum. The role of the sarcoplasmic reticulum, with its intracellular Ca⁺⁺ pool, is comparable with skeletal muscle. Activation opens Ca⁺⁺ channels, and the myoplasmic Ca⁺⁺ concentration rapidly increases. However, this release is not linked to voltage sensors, but to binding of a second messenger, **inositol 1,4,5-trisphosphate (IP₃),** to receptors in the sarcoplasmic reticulum. IP₃ is generated by a stimulus that acts on sarcolemmal receptors that are coupled via a guanine nucleotide binding protein **(G protein)** to activate **phospholipase C.** Phospholipase C hydrolyzes

phosphatidyl inositol bisphosphate (PIP₂), and IP₃ is one of the products of the reaction. This complex process may permit a graded Ca⁺⁺ release from the sarcoplasmic reticulum and enable many different neurotransmitters and hormones to mobilize Ca⁺⁺ from the sarcoplasmic reticulum. Refilling of the sarcoplasmic reticulum with Ca⁺⁺ depends on the extracellular concentration of Ca⁺⁺, but the details of this process remain uncertain.

The sarcolemma. Smooth muscles have effective methods that lower Ca⁺⁺ concentrations from the initial peaks that follow a stimulus. Reduction in the Ca⁺⁺ concentration is achieved by pumping Ca⁺⁺ out of the cell by active transport through the sarcolemma and by a passive exchange coupled to the influx of 3 Na⁺ ions (Fig. 19-11).

Sustained contraction of smooth muscle is totally dependent on the extracellular Ca⁺⁺ pool. The steady-state myoplasmic Ca⁺⁺, and thus cross-bridge phosphorylation, is regulated by the sum of the stimulus-dependent processes that govern Ca⁺⁺ exchange with the extracellular pool. Although not shown in Fig. 19-11, the inputs to the cell membrane can also be inhibitory. These inhibitory inputs cause a lowering of the myoplasmic Ca⁺⁺ concentration and induce relaxation or a reduction in tone.

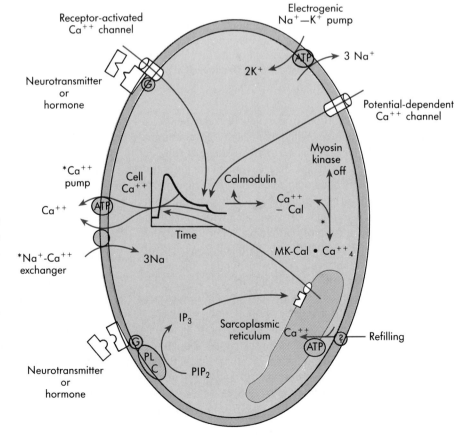

■ **Fig. 19-11** Principal mechanisms determining the myoplasmic Ca⁺⁺ concentration in smooth muscle. Ca⁺⁺ release from the sarcoplasmic reticulum is a rapid initial event in activation, whereas the sarcolemma is involved in the subsequent stimulus-dependent regulation of cell Ca⁺⁺. The sarcolemma integrates many simultaneous excitatory and inhibitory inputs to govern the cellular response. Higher-order regulatory mechanisms can alter the activity of various pumps, exchangers, or enzymes (the asterisks designate well-established instances). *G,* Guanine nucleotide binding proteins; *ATP,* process requires ATP hydrolysis; *PL C,* phospholipase C; *PIP₂,* phosphatidyl inositol bisphosphate; *IP₃,* inositol 1,4,5-trisphosphate.

Two categories of Ca⁺⁺ channels are present in the sarcolemma: **receptor-activated** and **potential-dependent** channels (Fig. 19-11). The conductance of receptor-activated Ca⁺⁺ channels is linked to receptor occupancy. Binding of neurotransmitters or hormones can induce contractions with very little change in membrane potential (this process is called **pharmacomechanical coupling** [Fig. 19-12, *D*]). Such channels can also be linked by G proteins to receptors that bind inhibitory neurotransmitters or hormones.

An important component of the membrane potential in smooth muscle cells arises from a Donnan potential, based on the differential permeabilities of Na⁺ and K⁺ ions, as in skeletal muscle. However, the pump that transports these ions across the smooth muscle membrane is electrogenic and expels 3 Na⁺ ions in exchange for 2 K⁺ ions (Fig. 19-11). One positive charge is removed from the cell for each cycle of the pump, and the membrane potential thus becomes more negative.

The conductance of K⁺ channels in the sarcolemma is also regulated by receptor-mediated mechanisms. Agents that decrease the K⁺ permeability of the membrane cause the membrane potential to become less negative. A less negative membrane potential can increase force, because the sarcolemma contains potential-dependent Ca⁺⁺ channels whose summed conductance increases with depolarization (Fig. 19-11). Thus, (1) action potentials, (2) graded depolarization caused by slowing of Na⁺-K⁺ exchange or a reduced K⁺ channel permeability, or (3) depolarization propagated via gap junctions from adjacent cells all increase Ca⁺⁺ influx and force. Fig. 19-12 illustrates some common relationships between membrane potential and contractile force.

Other second messengers and relaxation. A variety of drugs and hormones relax smooth muscles by increasing the cellular concentrations of cyclic adenosine monophosphate (cAMP) or cyclic guanosine monophosphate (cGMP). Nitric oxide (NO) is an inhibitory signal

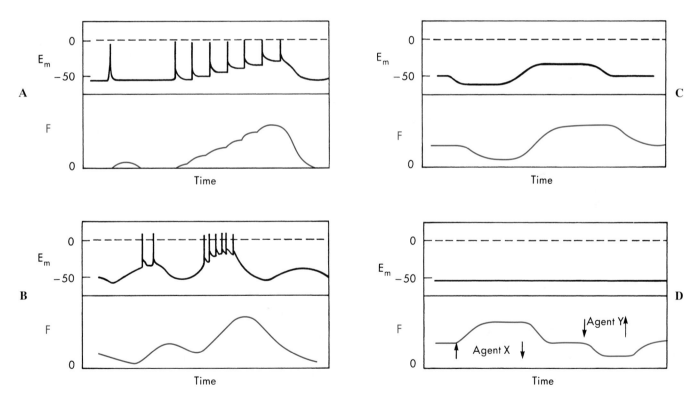

■ **Fig. 19-12**   Relationships between membrane potential *(E_m)* and force generation *(F)* characteristic of different types of smooth muscle. **A,** Action potentials may be generated and lead to a twitch or larger summed mechanical responses. Action potentials are characteristic of single-unit smooth muscles (many visceral). Gap junctions permit the spread of action potentials throughout the tissue. **B,** Rhythmical activity produced by slow waves that trigger action potentials. The contractions are usually associated with a burst of action potentials. Slow oscillations in membrane potential usually reflect the activity of electrogenic pumps in the cell membrane. **C,** Tonic contractile activity may be related to the value of the membrane potential in the absence of action potentials. Graded changes in E_m are common in multiunit smooth muscles (e.g., vascular), where action potentials are not generated and propagated from cell to cell. **D,** Pharmacomechanical coupling; changes in force produced by the addition or removal *(arrows)* of drugs or hormones that have no significant effect on the membrane potential.

produced by nerves and vascular endothelial cells that relaxes smooth muscle by increasing cGMP. The protein kinases activated by these second messengers can phosphorylate a variety of enzymes and modify their activities. Relaxation can result from enhanced Ca^{++} extrusion or sequestration, presumably by phosphorylation of Ca^{++} pumps. Alternatively, hyperpolarization will reduce Ca^{++} influx and cross-bridge phosphorylation, and thereby result in a decline in force and a slowing of cross-bridge cycling rates.

■ *Functional Adaptations of Smooth Muscle*

■ *Neurotrophic Relationships*

Unlike skeletal muscles, *involuntary muscles depend in part on their extrinsic innervation for maintenance of their phenotype and normal function.* This lack of total

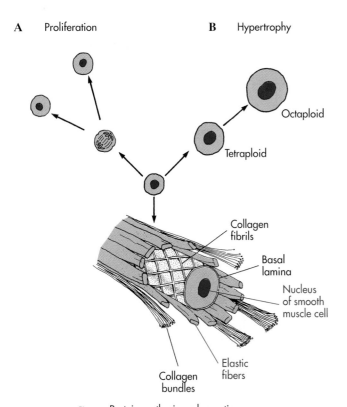

A   Proliferation   B   Hypertrophy

Octaploid

Tetraploid

Collagen fibrils

Basal lamina

Nucleus of smooth muscle cell

Collagen bundles

Elastic fibers

C   Protein synthesis and secretion

■ **Fig. 19-13**   Smooth muscle cells carry out many activities. **A,** They retain the capacity to divide during normal growth or in certain pathological responses such as formation of atherosclerotic plaques. **B,** Cells may also hypertrophy in response to increased loads. Chromosomal replication, not followed by cell division, yields cells with a greater content of contractile proteins. **C,** Smooth muscle cells also synthesize and secrete the constituents of the extracellular matrix.

dependence on extrinsic innervation may be related to the fact that smooth muscles can maintain contractile activity by other mechanisms when they are denervated. However, supersensitivity to neurotransmitters occurs in smooth muscle after denervation.

■ *Development and Hypertrophy*

During development and growth, the number of smooth muscle cells increases (**hyperplasia**) (Fig. 19-13). Smooth muscle tissue mass also increases if an organ is subjected to a sustained increase in mechanical work. This increase in mass is called compensatory **hypertrophy.** A striking example occurs in the arterial media in hypertension. The increased mechanical load on the muscle cells appears to be the common factor that induces hypertrophy in involuntary muscles. Tissue hypertrophy is sometimes caused by cellular hypertrophy. Chromosomal replication can result in significant numbers of polyploid muscle cells. The polyploid cells contain multiple sets of the normal number of chromosomes. They synthesize more contractile proteins and thus increase in size (Fig. 19-13).

The myometrium, which is the smooth muscle component of the uterus, undergoes hypertrophy as parturition (birth) approaches. Hormones play an important role in this response. The smooth muscle is quiescent during pregnancy (when the hormone progesterone predominates), and few gap junctions that electrically couple the smooth muscle cells are present. At term, under the dominant influence of estrogen, the myometrium undergoes marked hypertrophy. Large numbers of gap junctions form just before birth and convert the myometrium into a single-unit tissue to coordinate contraction during parturition.

Although involuntary muscles are involved in the physiological adjustments to exercise, sustained changes in the mechanical loading that induce cellular adaptations are usually the result of a pathological condition (e.g., hypertension). A fairly common example in men is urinary bladder hypertrophy caused by benign or cancerous **enlargement of the prostate gland,** which obstructs the bladder outlet. The clinical result is difficulty in micturition, distention of the bladder, and impaired emptying. The ability of the bladder smooth muscle to contract and develop stress is diminished. The reasons for these changes remain unexplained, but they involve phenotypic modulation of the smooth muscle cells with altered contractile protein isoform expression and gross anatomic distortion of the bladder wall. Neuromuscular changes also affect myoplasmic Ca^{++} mobilization and cross-bridge phosphorylation. Fortunately, normal structure and function are usually restored after the obstruction is alleviated.

■ *Synthetic and Secretory Functions*

The growth and development of tissues that contain smooth muscles are associated with increases in the connective tissue matrix. Smooth muscle cells can synthesize and secrete the materials that make up this matrix. These components include collagen, elastin, and proteoglycans (Fig. 19-13). The synthetic and secretory capacities are evident when smooth muscle cells with extensive contractile filament arrays are isolated and placed in tissue culture. The cells rapidly lose thick myosin filaments and much of the thin filament lattice. Their places are filled by a greatly expanded rough endoplasmic reticulum and Golgi apparatus (cellular structures associated with protein synthesis and secretion). The phenotypically altered cells multiply and lay down connective tissues in the culture plate. This process is reversible, and some degree of redifferentiation with formation of thick filaments occurs after cell replication ceases. The determinants of the smooth muscle cell phenotype are largely unknown, but hormones and growth factors in the blood, as well as the mechanical loads on the cells, are implicated in the control of phenotypic modulation.

Atherosclerosis is a disease characterized by lesions located in the endothelium of blood vessels. The lesions are induced by disorders such as hypertension, diabetes, and smoking that injure the endothelium. By diminishing blood flow and thereby oxygen supply to such vital organs as the heart or brain, the lesions are responsible for more morbidity and mortality than any other cause in developed countries. Three formed elements (monocytes, T lymphocytes, and platelets) that circulate in the bloodstream act on the vascular endothelium. There, they generate chemotactic factors and mitogens that modify the structure of the surrounding smooth muscle cells. The latter lose most of their thick and thin filaments, and develop an extensive rough endoplasmic reticulum and Golgi complex. These cells migrate to the subendothelial space (the arterial intima), proliferate, and participate in formation of the fatty lesions or the fibrous plaques that characterize atherosclerosis.

■ *Summary*

1. Smooth muscle in hollow organs has two roles: (1) to develop force or shorten like skeletal muscle and (2) to contract tonically to maintain organ dimensions against imposed loads.

2. Smooth muscle cells are linked by a variety of junctions that serve both mechanical and communication roles. These linkages are essential in cells that must contract uniformly.

3. Smooth muscle cells have a high ratio of surface area to volume, and the sarcolemma plays an active role in Ca^{++} exchange between the extracellular fluid and the myoplasm. The sarcoplasmic reticulum contains an intracellular Ca^{++} pool that can be mobilized to transiently increase the myoplasmic concentration of Ca^{++}.

4. Smooth muscles contain contractile units that consist of small groups of thick myosin filaments that interdigitate with large numbers of thin filaments attached to Z-disk equivalents, termed dense bodies or membrane-dense areas. No striations are evident.

5. The extracellular control systems include (1) extrinsic and intrinsic nerves that release a variety of transmitters that may be excitatory or inhibitory, (2) circulating hormones, (3) locally generated signaling substances, (4) junctions with other smooth muscle cells that allow electrical or chemical communication, and (5) junctions with other cell types that mediate signals.

6. Contraction is caused by a sliding filament–cross-bridge mechanism. The stress-length relationships, hyperbolic velocity-load relationships, power output curves, and the ability to resist imposed loads are comparable with those of skeletal muscle. Shortening velocities and ATP consumption rates are very low in smooth muscle, in keeping with expression of a myosin isoform with low activity. Uniquely, smooth muscles have variable velocity-stress relationships that reflect regulation of both the numbers of active cross-bridges (determining force) and their average cycling rates for a given load (determining velocity).

7. The response to sustained or tonic stimulation is a rapid contraction (for this muscle type) followed by sustained force maintenance with reduced cross-bridge cycling rates and ATP consumption. This behavior is advantageous for muscles that may need to withstand continuous external forces, such as blood vessels that must be able to withstand blood pressure.

8. Smooth muscle lacks troponin, and a covalent mechanism regulates cross-bridge cycling. Phosphorylation of cross-bridges by a Ca^{++}-dependent myosin kinase is necessary for attachment to the thin filament. Dephosphorylation of an attached cross-bridge slows its cycling rates. Higher myoplasmic Ca^{++} concentrations increase the ratio of myosin kinase to myosin phosphatase activities, with the result that more of the cross-bridges remain phosphorylated throughout a cycle. Shortening velocities are thus proportionally increased.

9. Cross-bridge phosphorylation accounts for a significant fraction of the total ATP consumption of smooth muscle and contributes to a low efficiency. This disadvantage is more than offset by the savings in ATP consumption during tonic contractions, in which the economy is very high. Smooth muscle can consume less than $1/300^{th}$ of the ATP to maintain the same force as striated muscle.

10. Covalent regulation requires precise control of the myoplasmic Ca^{++} concentration that determines myosin kinase activity. This requirement and the ability to generate varied patterns of contractile activity underlie complex mechanisms that regulate cell Ca^{++}. In the sarcolemma, these mechanisms include (1) receptor-activated Ca^{++} channels, (2) membrane potential gated Ca^{++} channels, (3) Ca^{++} pumps, (4) electrogenic Na^+-K^+ pumps, and (5) Na^+-Ca^{++} exchangers.

11. The Ca^{++} channels in the sarcoplasmic reticulum open in response to a chemical rather than an electrical signal. Neurotransmitters or hormones that act via receptors in the sarcolemma can activate phospholipase C, followed by generation of the second messenger, inositol 1,4,5-trisphosphate (IP_3). IP_3 then binds to receptors on the sarcoplasmic reticulum.

12. The relationships between membrane potential and contractile activity range from action potentials that elicit small "twitches" that can be summed to tonic responses that are correlated with slow changes in membrane potential and are unaccompanied by action potentials. Neurotransmitters can alter force with no evident change in membrane potential (pharmacomechanical coupling).

13. Smooth muscle is also a synthetic and secretory cell with a major role in the formation of the extensive extracellular matrix that surrounds and links the cells. Cellular hypertrophy occurs in response to physiological needs, and smooth muscle cells retain the potential to divide.

■ *Self-Study Problems*

1. What evidence supports a sliding filament–crossbridge mechanism of contraction in smooth muscle?

2. What are the general factors that explain the extraordinary functional diversity among smooth muscles from various organs?

3. List the steps that link an increase in myoplasmic Ca^{++} to contraction in smooth muscle.

4. What factors determine relaxation in smooth muscle?

5. What determines the rate of contraction in smooth muscles?

■ *Bibliography*

Journal articles

Berridge MJ: Inositol trisphosphate and calcium signaling, *Nature* 361:315, 1993.

Carl A, Lee HK, Sanders KM: Regulation of ion channels in smooth muscles by calcium, *Am J Physiol* 271 (*Cell Physiol* 40):C9, 1996.

Chen Q, van Breemen C: Function of smooth muscle sarcoplasmic reticulum, *Adv Second Messenger Phosphoprotein Res* 26:335, 1992.

Christ GJ et al: Gap junctions in vascular tissues, *Circ Res* 79:631, 1996.

Huizinga JD et al: Intercellular communication in smooth muscle, *Experientia* 48:932, 1992.

Lincoln TM, Cornwell TL: Towards an understanding of the mechanism of action of cyclic AMP and cyclic GMP in smooth muscle relaxation, *Blood Vessels* 28:129, 1991.

Mecham RP, Stenmark KR, Parks WC: Connective tissue production by vascular smooth muscle in development and disease, *Chest* 99 (suppl):43S, 1991.

Missiaen L et al: Calcium ion homeostasis in smooth muscle, *Pharmacol Ther* 56:191, 1992.

Murphy RA: What is special about smooth muscle? The significance of covalent crossbridge regulation, *FASEB J* 8:311, 1994.

Owens GK: Regulation of differentiation of vascular smooth muscle cells, *Physiol Rev* 75:487, 1995.

Raeymaekers L, Wuytack F: Ca^{2+} pumps in smooth muscle cells, *J Muscle Res Cell Motil* 14:141, 1993.

Sanders KM: Ionic mechanisms of electrical rhythmicity in gastrointestinal smooth muscles, *Annu Rev Physiol* 54:439, 1992.

Somlyo AP, Somlyo AV: Signal transduction and regulation in smooth muscle, *Nature* 372:231, 1994.

Trybus KM: Regulation of smooth muscle myosin, *Cell Motil Cytoskeleton* 18:81, 1991.

Books and monographs

Bárány M, editor: *Biochemistry of smooth muscle contraction,* San Diego, Calif, 1996, Academic Press.

Moreland RS, editor: *Regulation of smooth muscle contraction,* New York, 1991, Plenum.

Motta PM, editor: *Ultrastructure of smooth muscle,* Lancaster, England, 1990, Kluwer Academic.

Sperelakis N, Wood JD: *Frontiers in smooth muscle research* (Prog in Clin Biol Res 327), New York, 1990, Wiley-Liss.

Wood JD, editor: *Handbook of physiology: the gastrointestinal system,* section 6, vol I, Motility and circulation, Bethesda, Md, 1989, American Physiological Society.

THE CARDIOVASCULAR SYSTEM

Robert M. Berne

Matthew N. Levy

Blood and Hemostasis

■ *Blood*

Blood performs many functions in the body. The main function of the circulating blood is to carry oxygen and nutrients to the tissues and to remove carbon dioxide and waste products from the tissues. In addition, blood transports other substances (e.g., hormones) from their sites of production to their sites of action and white blood cells and platelets to where they are needed. Blood also aids in the distribution of water, solutes, and heat and thus contributes to **homeostasis,** the maintenance of a constant internal body environment.

Blood consists of red blood cells, white blood cells, and platelets suspended in a complex solution **(plasma)** of gases, salts, proteins, carbohydrates, and lipids. The circulating blood volume accounts for about 7% of body weight. Approximately 55% of the blood is plasma; the protein content is 7 g/dl (about 4 g/dl of albumin and 3 g/dl of plasma globulins).

■ *Blood Components*

Erythrocytes. The erythrocytes (red blood cells) are flexible, biconcave disks that transport oxygen to the body tissues (Fig. 20-1). Erythrocytes are unusual in that they lack a nucleus. The average erythrocyte is 7 μm in diameter. Erythrocytes arise from stem cells in the bone marrow. During maturation, they lose their nuclei before entering the circulation, where their average lifespan is 120 days. Approximately 5 million erythrocytes are present per microliter of blood.

The main protein in erythrocytes is hemoglobin (about 15 g/dl of blood). Hemoglobin consists of **heme,** an iron-containing tetrapyrrole, linked to **globin,** a protein composed of four polypeptide chains (two α and two β in the normal adult). The iron moiety of hemoglobin binds loosely and reversibly to oxygen to form **oxyhemoglobin.** The affinity of hemoglobin for oxygen is affected by pH, temperature, and 2,3-diphosphoglycerate concentration. These factors facilitate O_2 uptake in the lungs and its release in the tissues (see Chapter 35). Changes in the

polypeptide subunits of globin can also affect the affinity of hemoglobin for O_2. For example, fetal hemoglobin has two γ chains instead of two β chains, which increases its affinity for O_2. Changes in the polypeptide subunits of globin can also result in disease states, such as **sickle cell anemia** and **thalassemia.**

The number of circulating red cells remains fairly constant under normal conditions. The production of erythrocytes **(erythropoiesis)** is regulated by the glycoprotein **erythropoietin,** which is secreted mainly by the kidneys. Erythropoietin regulates erythrocyte production by accelerating the differentiation of stem cells in the bone marrow.

Anemia and chronic hypoxia (e.g., as a result of living at high altitudes) stimulate erythrocyte production and can produce **polycythemia,** an increased number of red blood cells. When the hypoxic stimulus is removed in subjects with altitude polycythemia, the high red blood cell concentration in the blood inhibits erythropoiesis. The red blood cell count is also greatly increased in **polycythemia vera,** a disease of unknown cause. The elevated erythrocyte concentration in this disease can increase blood viscosity, the point where flow to vital tissues becomes impaired (see Chapter 25).

Leukocytes. Normally about 4000 to 10,000 leukocytes (white blood cells) are present per microliter of blood. The leukocytes include **granulocytes** (65%), **lymphocytes** (30%), and **monocytes** (5%). Of the granulocytes, about 95% are **neutrophils,** 4% **eosinophils,** and 1% **basophils.** During fetal development, white blood cells arise from primitive stem cells in the bone marrow (Fig. 20-1). After birth, granulocytes and monocytes continue to be produced in the bone marrow, whereas lymphocytes are produced in lymph nodes, spleen, and thymus.

The granulocytes and monocytes are motile, nucleated cells that contain **lysosomes,** which in turn contain enzymes capable of digesting foreign material, such as microorganisms, damaged cells, and cellular debris. Thus, the leukocytes constitute a major defense mechanism against infections. Microorganisms or the products of cell destruction release **chemotactic substances** that attract granulocytes and monocytes. When the migrating leukocytes reach the foreign agents, they engulf them (**phagocytosis**) and then destroy them by the action of enzymes that form **oxygen-derived free radicals** and **hydrogen peroxide.**

Lymphocytes vary in size and have large nuclei. Most lymphocytes lack cytoplasmic granules (Fig. 20-1). The two main types are **B lymphocytes,** which are responsible for humoral immunity, and **T lymphocytes,** which are responsible for cell-mediated immunity. When stimulated by an **antigen** (a foreign protein on the surface of a microorganism or allergen), the B lymphocytes are transformed into **plasma cells,** which synthesize and release antibodies (gamma globulin). Antibodies are carried by the bloodstream to the site of infection, where they "tag" foreign invaders for destruction by other components of the immune system.

The main T lymphocytes are cytotoxic and are responsible for long-term protection against some viruses, bacteria, and cancer cells. They are also responsible for the rejection of transplanted organs.

Other T lymphocytes are **helper T cells,** which activate B cells, and **suppressor T cells,** which inhibit B-cell activity. Special B and T lymphocytes, called **memory cells,** "remember" specific antigens. These cells can quickly generate an immune response when subsequently exposed to the same antigen.

Protection against several infectious diseases has been achieved by injection of the appropriate antigen. Also, **vaccines** have been developed for certain diseases that involve injection of killed or attenuated organisms (antigens) into suitable hosts (horses, sheep). Vaccines work by stimulating the production of specific antibodies against a particular microorganism.

Platelets. Platelets are small (3-μm) nuclear cell fragments of **megakaryocytes.** The megakaryocytes reside in the bone marrow. When mature, they break up into platelets, which enter the circulation. The platelets are important in hemostasis, as discussed later in this chapter.

■ *Blood Groups*

In humans, there are four principal blood groups, designated O, A, B, and AB. These blood groups differ in the types of antigens that are present on the erythrocytes. Persons with type A blood have A antigens; those with type B, B antigens; those with type AB, both A and B antigens; and those with type O, neither antigen. In addition, the plasma of group O blood contains antibodies to A, B, and AB. Group A plasma contains antibodies to B antigens, and group B plasma contains antibodies to A antigens. Group AB plasma has no antibodies to O, A, or B antigens. In blood transfusions, cross-matching is necessary to prevent agglutination of donor red cells by antibodies in the plasma of the recipient. Because plasma of groups A, B, and AB has no antibodies to group O erythrocytes, people with group O blood are called **universal donors.** Conversely, persons with AB blood are called **universal recipients,** because their plasma has no antibodies to antigens of the other three groups.

In addition to the ABO blood grouping, there are **Rh (Rhesus factor)-positive** and **RH-negative groups.**

An Rh-negative person can develop antibodies to Rh-positive red blood cells if exposed to Rh-positive blood. For example, during pregnancy, a mother who is Rh negative can make antibodies for Rh-positive cells if the fetus is Rh positive (inherited from the father). Rh-positive red cells from the fetus can enter the maternal bloodstream at the time of placental sep-

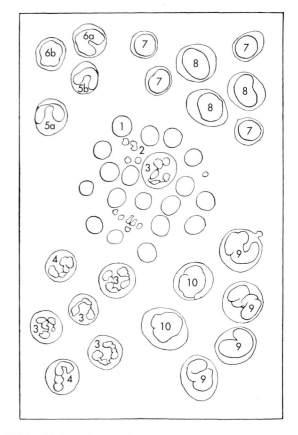

■ **Fig. 20-1**   The morphology of blood cells. *1,* Normal red cells; *2,* platelets; *3,* neutrophils; *4,* neutrophil, band form; *5a,* eosinophil, two lobes; *5b,* eosinophil, band form; *6a,* basophil, band form; *6b,* metamyelocyte, basophilic; *7,* lymphocyte, small; *8,* lymphocyte, large; *9,* monocyte, mature; *10,* monocyte, young. (From Daland GA: *A color atlas of morphologic hematology,* Cambridge, Mass, 1951, Harvard University Press.)

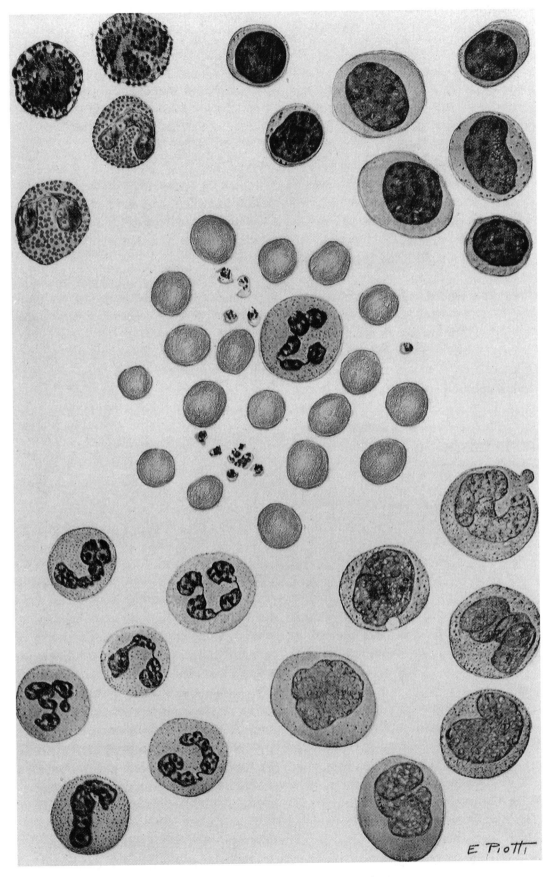

■ **Fig. 20-1, cont'd**   For legend see opposite page.

aration and induce Rh-positive antibodies in the mother's plasma. The Rh-positive antibodies from the mother can also reach the fetus via the placenta, and agglutinate and hemolyze fetal red cells (**erythroblastosis fetalis,** a hemolytic disease of the newborn). Red blood cell destruction can also occur in Rh-negative individuals who have previously been transfused with Rh-positive blood and have developed Rh antibodies. If these individuals are given a subsequent transfusion of Rh-positive blood, the transfused red blood cells will be destroyed by the Rh antibodies in their plasma.

■ *Hemostasis*

Hemostasis is defined as the arrest of bleeding. When blood vessels are damaged bleeding occurs. *Three processes then act to stem the flow of blood: vasoconstriction, platelet aggregation, and blood coagulation.*

■ *Vasoconstriction*

Physical injury to a blood vessel elicits a contractile response (**vasoconstriction**) of the vascular smooth muscle and thus a narrowing of the vessel. Vasoconstriction in severed arterioles or small arteries can completely close the lumen of the vessel and stop the flow of blood. The contraction of the vascular smooth muscle is probably caused by direct mechanical stimulation by the penetrating object, as well as by mechanical stimulation of the perivascular nerves.

■ *Platelet Aggregation*

Damage to the endothelium of a blood vessel causes platelets to adhere to the site of injury. The adherent platelets release **adenosine diphosphate** and **thromboxane A$_2$**, which cause additional platelets to adhere. The aggregation of platelets may continue in this manner until

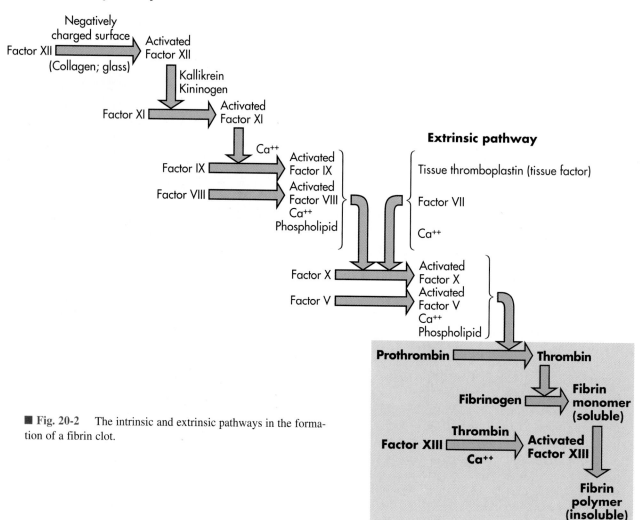

■ **Fig. 20-2**   The intrinsic and extrinsic pathways in the formation of a fibrin clot.

some of the small blood vessels become blocked by the mass of aggregated platelets. Platelets are prevented from aggregating along the length of the normal vessel by the antiaggregation action of **prostacyclin.** This substance is released from the normal endothelial cells in the adjacent, uninjured part of the vessel. Platelets also release **serotonin (5-hydroxytryptamine),** which enhances vasoconstriction, as well as **thromboplastin,** which hastens blood coagulation.

Bleeding is an important clinical problem and trauma is the most common cause of bleeding. Gastrointestinal bleeding can also occur and cause severe anemia or even cardiovascular shock, and occult blood in the stools can be the first sign of cancer of the bowel or peptic ulcer.

When the platelet count is low, as in **thrombolytopenic purpura,** tiny hemorrhages **(petechiae)** or larger hemorrhages **(ecchymoses)** may appear in the skin and mucous membranes.

Bleeding occurs into the tissues (especially joints) in **hemophilia,** a hereditary disease. The disease occurs only in males, but the genetic abnormality is carried by females.

■ *Blood Coagulation*

Blood clotting is a complex process consisting of sequential activation of various factors that are present in an inactive state in the blood. The cascade of reactions in which one activated factor activates another is depicted in Fig. 20-2. Several of the factors are synthesized in the liver, as is vitamin K, which is essential for synthesis of these liver-derived clotting factors.

The key step in blood clotting is the conversion of fibrinogen to fibrin by thrombin. The clot formed by this reaction consists of a dense network of fibrin strands in which blood cells and plasma are trapped (Fig. 20-3). The two blood coagulation pathways, the **extrinsic** and the **intrinsic pathways,** converge on the activation of factor X, which catalyzes the cleavage of prothrombin to thrombin (Fig. 20-2). Blood clotting via the extrinsic pathway is initiated by tissue damage and the release of tissue thromboplastin. Blood clotting via the intrinsic pathway is initiated by exposure of the blood to a damaged endothelium or a negatively charged surface. When the endothelium of blood vessels is damaged, blood comes into contact with collagen. Outside the body, clotting can occur when blood comes into contact with negatively charged surfaces, such as glass. If blood is carefully drawn into a syringe coated with silicone, clotting is greatly delayed.

After a clot is formed, the actin and myosin of the platelets trapped in the fibrin mesh interact in a manner similar to that in muscle. The resultant contraction pulls the fibrin strands toward the platelets, and thereby extrudes the **serum** (plasma without fibrinogen) and

shrinks the clot. This process is called **clot retraction.** The function of clot retraction is not clear, but it may serve to approximate the edges of severed small blood vessels.

Several cofactors are required for blood coagulation (Fig. 20-2); the most important is calcium. If the calcium ions in blood are removed or bound, coagulation will not occur.

Clot lysis. Blood clots may be liquefied **(fibrinolysis)** by a proteolytic enzyme called **plasmin.** Normal blood contains **plasminogen,** an inactive precursor of plasmin. Activators of the conversion of plasminogen to plasmin are found in tissues, plasma, and urine **(urokinase).**

Exogenous plasminogen activators, such as **streptokinase** and **tissue plasminogen activator (tPA),** are used clinically to dissolve intravascular clots. This treatment is used especially to dissolve clots in the coronary arteries of patients with **acute myocardial infarction** (damage to the heart muscle, most frequently caused by a clot in a major coronary artery).

Anticoagulants. Blood coagulation can be prevented in vitro by the addition of citrate or oxalate, which removes the calcium ions from solution. For rapid in vivo anticoagulation, **heparin,** a sulfated polysaccharide produced by mast cells, is injected intravenously.

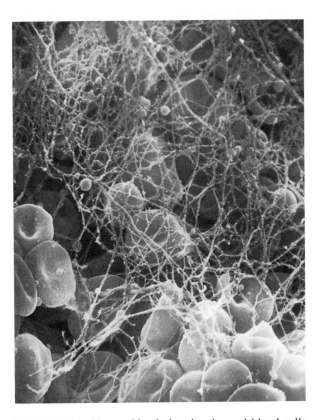

■ **Fig. 20-3** Human blood clot showing red blood cells immobilized within a network of fibrin threads. The small spheres are platelets. Scanning electron micrograph ($\times$ 9000). (From Shelly WB: *JAMA* 249:3089, 1983.)

Heparin is used in artificial perfusion circuits during open heart surgery and for prevention of intravascular clot extension. For prolonged anticoagulation, **dicumarol** is used. This drug inhibits the synthesis of vitamin K–dependent factors and is used in treating such conditions as **thrombophlebitis** (inflammation of a vein associated with an intravascular blood clot).

■ Summary

1. Blood consists of red blood cells (erythrocytes), white blood cells (leukocytes and lymphocytes), and platelets, which are suspended in a solution containing salts, proteins, carbohydrates, and lipids.

2. There are four major blood groups, O, A, B, and AB. Type O blood can be given to persons in any of the blood groups because the plasma of all the blood groups lacks antibodies to group O erythrocytes. Hence, people with type O blood are referred to as universal donors. People with AB blood are referred to as universal recipients because their plasma lacks antibodies to erythrocytes of all the blood groups. In addition to O, A, B, and AB blood groups, there are Rh-positive and Rh-negative blood groups.

3. A cascade of reactions that constitute the intrinsic and extrinsic pathways is involved in blood coagulation. The final steps where the two pathways join are (a) the conversion of prothrombin to thrombin and (b) the conversion of fibrinogen to fibrin, a reaction catalyzed by thrombin.

4. Blood clots may be liquefied by plasmin, a proteolytic enzyme whose formation from plasminogen is catalyzed by tissue activators or by exogenous activators (e.g., streptokinase, tissue plasminogen activator [tPA]).

■ Self-Study Problems

1. After a small cut of the tip of a finger, what mechanisms act to stop the flow of blood?

2. What constitutes a universal blood donor and a universal blood recipient? What happens when blood from a universal recipient is infused into the vein of a universal donor?

■ Bibliography

Journal articles

Hyun BH, editor: Diagnostic hematology, *Hematol Oncol Clin North Am* 8:598, 1994.

Jackson CM, Nemerson Y: Blood coagulation, *Annu Rev Biochem* 49:765, 1980.

Ross JM, McIntire LV: Molecular mechanisms of mural thrombosis under dynamic flow conditions, *News Physiol Sci* 10:117, 1995.

Shattil SJ, Bennet JS: Platelets and their membranes in hemostasis: physiology and pathophysiology, *Ann Intern Med* 94:108, 1981.

Books and monographs

Babior BM, Stossel TP: *Hematology: a pathophysiological approach,* New York, 1984, Churchill Livingstone.

Eastham RD: *Clinical haematology,* ed 6, Bristol, 1984, John Wright/PSG.

Erslev AJ, Gabuzda TG: *Pathophysiology of blood,* ed 3, Philadelphia, 1985, WB Saunders.

Ogston D: *The physiology of hemostasis,* Cambridge, 1983, Harvard University Press.

Ratnoff OD, Forbes CD, editors: *Disorders of hemostasis,* Orlando, Fla, 1984, Grune & Stratton, Inc.

CHAPTER
21

The Circuitry

The circulatory, endocrine, and nervous systems constitute the principal coordinating and integrating systems of the body. The nervous system facilitates communications and the endocrine glands regulate certain body functions. The circulatory system serves to transport and distribute essential substances to the tissues and to remove byproducts of metabolism. The circulatory system also participates in homeostatic mechanisms such as regulation of body temperature, fluid maintenance, and adjustments of oxygen and nutrient supply in different physiological states.

The cardiovascular system that accomplishes these tasks is composed of a pump (the heart), a series of distributing and collecting tubes (the blood vessels), and an extensive system of thin vessels that permit rapid exchange between the tissues and the vascular channels (the capillaries). In this section, we discuss the function of these components of the vascular system and their control mechanisms (with their checks and balances). By altering the flow of blood to tissues, these control mechanisms are able to meet the changing requirements of different tissues in response to a variety of physiological and pathological conditions.

The function of the parts of the circulatory system is discussed in detail in subsequent chapters. This chapter provides a general, functional overview of the circulatory system.

■ *The Heart*

The heart consists of two pumps in series: one pump propels blood through the lungs for exchange of oxygen and carbon dioxide (the **pulmonary circulation**) and the other pump propels blood to all other tissues of the body (the **systemic circulation**). The flow of blood through the heart is one-way (unidirectional). Unidirectional flow through the heart is achieved by the appropriate arrangement of flap valves. Although the cardiac output is intermittent, continuous flow to the body tissues (periphery) occurs by distention of the aorta and its branches during ventricular contraction (**systole**) and by elastic recoil of the walls of the large arteries with forward propulsion of the blood during ventricular relaxation (**diastole).**

■ *Blood Vessels*

Blood moves rapidly through the aorta and its arterial branches. These branches narrow and their walls become thinner as they approach the periphery. They also change histologically. The aorta is a predominantly elastic structure, but the peripheral arteries become more muscular until at the arterioles the muscular layer predominates (Fig. 21-1).

In the large arteries, frictional resistance is relatively small and pressures are only slightly less than in the aorta. The small arteries, on the other hand, offer moderate resistance to blood flow. This resistance reaches a maximal level in the arterioles, which are sometimes referred to as the stopcocks of the vascular system. Hence, *the pressure drop is greatest across the terminal segment of the small arteries and the arterioles* (Fig. 21-2). Adjustment in the degree of contraction of the circular muscle of these small vessels permits regulation of tissue blood flow and aids in the control of arterial blood pressure.

In addition to the reduction in pressure along the arterioles, there is a change from a pulsatile to a steady blood flow (Fig. 21-3). *The pulsatile arterial blood flow, caused by the intermittent ejection of blood from the heart, is damped at the capillary level by a combination of two factors: distensibility of the large arteries and frictional resistance in the small arteries and arterioles.*

In a patient with hyperthyroidism (**Graves' disease**), the basal metabolism is elevated and is often associated with arteriolar vasodilation. This reduction in arteriolar resistance diminishes the damping effect on the pulsatile arterial pressure and is manifested as pulsatile flow in the capillaries, as observed in the finger nailbed of patients with this ailment.

Many capillaries arise from each arteriole. The total cross-sectional area of the capillary bed is very large, despite the fact that the cross-sectional area of each capillary is less than that of each arteriole. As a result, blood flow velocity becomes quite slow in the capillaries, analogous to the decrease in velocity of flow (Fig. 21-3) in the wide regions of a river. Because capillaries consist of short tubes with walls that are only one cell thick and because flow velocity is low, conditions in the capillaries are ideal for the exchange of diffusible substances between blood and tissue.

On its return to the heart from the capillaries, blood passes through venules and then through veins of increasing size. Pressure within these vessels progressively decreases until the blood reaches the right atrium (Fig. 21-2). Near the heart, the number of veins decreases, the thickness and composition of the vein walls change (Fig. 21-1), the total cross-sectional area of the venous chan-

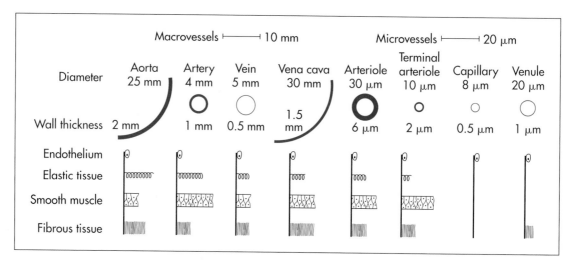

■ Fig. 21-1 Internal diameter, wall thickness, and relative amounts of the principal components of the vessel walls of the various blood vessels that compose the circulatory system. Cross-sections of the vessels are not drawn to scale because of the huge range from aorta and venae cavae to capillary. (Redrawn from Burton AC: *Physiol Rev* 34:619, 1954.)

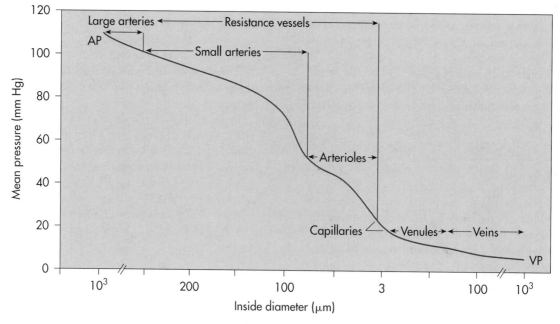

■ Fig. 21-2 Pressure drop across the vascular system in the hamster cheek pouch. *AP*, Mean arterial pressure; *VP*, venous pressure. (Redrawn from David MJ et al: *Am J Physiol* 250:H291, 1986.)

nels diminishes, and the **velocity of blood flow** increases (Fig. 21-3). Note that the velocity of blood flow and the cross-sectional area at each level of the vasculature are essentially mirror images (Fig. 21-3).

Data from a 20-kg dog (Table 21-1) indicate that between the aorta and the capillaries the number of vessels increases about 3 billion-fold, and the total cross-sectional area increases about 500-fold. The volume of blood in the systemic vascular system is greatest in the veins and venules (67%). Only 5% of total blood volume exists in the capillaries, and 11% of total blood volume is found in the aorta, arteries, and arterioles. In contrast, blood volume in the pulmonary vascular bed is about equally divided among the arterial, capillary, and venous vessels. The cross-sectional area of the venae cavae is larger than that of the aorta. Therefore, the velocity of flow is slower in the venae cavae than that in the aorta (Fig. 21-3).

■ *The Cardiac Cycle*

Blood entering the right ventricle via the right atrium is pumped through the pulmonary arterial system at a mean pressure about one seventh that in the systemic arteries. The blood then passes through the lung capillaries, where carbon dioxide in the blood is released and oxygen is taken up. The oxygen-rich blood returns via the pulmonary veins to the left atrium, where it is pumped from the ventricle to the periphery, thus completing the cycle.

In the normal, intact circulation, the total volume of blood is constant, and an increase in the volume of blood in one area must be accompanied by a decrease in another. However, the distribution of the circulating blood to the different regions of the body is determined by the output of the left ventricle and by the contractile state of the resistance vessels (arterioles) of these regions.

■ **Table 21-1**   Vascular dimensions in a 20-kg dog

Vessels	*No.*	*Total cross-sectional area (cm²)*	*Total blood volume (%)*
Systemic			
Aorta	1	2.8 ⎤	
Arteries	40-110,000	40 ⎬	11
Arterioles	2.8×10^6	55 ⎦	
Capillaries	2.7×10^9	1357	5
Venules	1×10^7	785 ⎤	
Veins	660,000-110	631 ⎬	67
Venae cavae	2	3.1 ⎦	
Pulmonary			
Arteries and arterioles	$1\text{-}1.5 \times 10^6$	137	3
Capillaries	2.7×10^9	1357	4
Venules and veins	$1 \times 10^6\text{-}4$	210	5
Heart			
Atria	2 ⎤		
Ventricles	2 ⎦		5

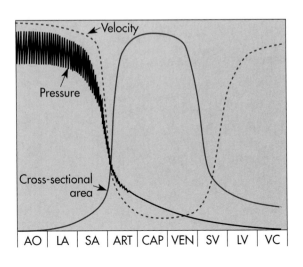

■ **Fig. 21-3**   Phasic pressure, velocity of flow, and cross-sectional area of the systemic circulation. *The important features are the inverse relationship between velocity and cross- sectional area, the major pressure drop across the small arteries and arterioles, and the maximal cross-sectional area and minimal flow rate in the capillaries. AO, Aorta; LA, large arteries; SA, small arteries; ART, arterioles; CAP, capillaries; VEN, venules; SV, small veins; LV, large veins; VC, venae cavae.*

The circulatory system is composed of conduits arranged in series and in parallel (Fig. 21-4). This arrangement, which is discussed in subsequent chapters, has important implications in terms of resistance, flow, and pressure in the blood vessels.

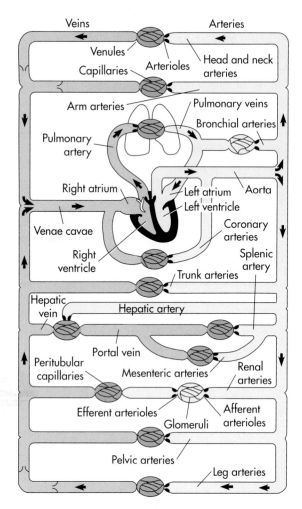

■ **Fig. 21-4**   Schematic diagram of the parallel and series arrangement of the vessels composing the circulatory system. The capillary beds are represented by thin lines connecting the arteries *(on the right)* with the veins *(on the left)*. The crescent-shaped thickenings proximal to the capillary beds represent the arterioles (resistance vessels). (Redrawn from Green HD: In Glasser O, editor: *Medical physics,* vol 1, Chicago, 1944, Mosby–Year Book.)

■ *Summary*

1. The circulatory system consists of a pump (the heart), a series of distributing and collecting tubes (blood vessels), and an extensive system of thin vessels that permit rapid exchange of substances between the tissues and blood.

2. The greatest resistance to blood flow, and hence the greatest pressure drop, in the arterial system occurs at the level of the small arteries and the arterioles.

3. Pulsatile pressure is progressively damped by the elasticity of the arteriolar walls and the frictional resistance of the small arteries and arterioles, so that capillary blood flow is essentially nonpulsatile.

4. Velocity of blood flow is inversely related to the cross-sectional area at any point along the vascular system.

5. Most of the blood in the systemic vascular bed is located in the venous side of the circulation.

■ *Self-Study Problems*

1. What physical characteristics of arterioles enable them to maintain arterial blood pressure and to adjust the distribution of blood flow?

2. Why does most of the blood in the systemic circulation reside in the veins and venules?

3. Where in the systemic circulation is velocity of blood flow fastest and where is it slowest? Why?

4. Why is flow pulsatile in the systemic arterial system but nonpulsatile in the capillaries and venous systems?

Electrical Activity of the Heart

Two centuries ago, Galvani and Volta demonstrated that electrical phenomena were involved in the spontaneous contractions of the heart. In 1855, Kölliker and Müller found that when they placed the nerve of an innervated skeletal muscle preparation in contact with the surface of a beating frog's heart, the skeletal muscle twitched with each cardiac contraction. The researchers concluded that the spontaneous excitation of the heart had generated sufficient electrical activity to excite the motor nerve fibers and stimulate the skeletal muscle.

The electrical events that normally take place in the heart initiate cardiac contraction. Disorders in electrical activity can induce serious and sometimes lethal disturbances in the cardiac rhythm.

■ *Transmembrane Potentials*

To investigate the electrical behavior of single cardiac cells, researchers insert a microelectrode into the interior of the cell. The microelectrode is attached to a galvanometer, a device that measures the strength of an electrical current. The potential changes recorded from a typical ventricular muscle fiber are illustrated in Fig. 22-1, *A*. When two electrodes are placed in an electrolyte solution near a strip of quiescent cardiac muscle, no potential difference (point *a*) is measurable between the two electrodes. At point *b*, when one of the electrodes is inserted into the interior of a cardiac muscle fiber (Fig. 22-1), the galvanometer immediately records a potential difference (V_m) across the cell membrane. The potential of the interior of the cell is about 90 mV lower than that of the surrounding medium. This electronegativity of the interior of the resting cell with respect to the exterior is also characteristic of skeletal and smooth muscle, nerves, and most cells within the body (see also Chapter 2).

At point *c*, the ventricular cell is excited by an electronic stimulator, and the cell membrane rapidly depolarizes. During depolarization, the potential difference is actually reversed, such that the potential of the interior of the cell exceeds that of the exterior by about 20 mV. The

rapid **upstroke** of the action potential is designated **phase 0.** The upstroke is followed immediately by a brief period of partial, **early repolarization (phase 1),** and then by a **plateau (phase 2)** that persists for about 0.1 to 0.2 second. The membrane then repolarizes **(phase 3)** until the resting state of polarization **(phase 4)** is again attained (at point *e*). **Final repolarization** (phase 3) develops more slowly than does depolarization (phase 0).

The relationships between the electrical events in the cardiac muscle and actual contraction of the cardiac muscle are shown in Fig. 22-2. Rapid depolarization (phase 0) occurs before force develops, and completion of repolarization coincides approximately with peak force. The relaxation of the muscle takes place mainly during phase 4 of the action potential. The duration of contraction parallels the duration of the action potential.

■ *Principal Types of Cardiac Action Potentials*

Two main types of action potentials take place in the heart and are shown in Fig. 22-1. One type, the **fast response,** occurs in normal atrial and ventricular myocytes and the specialized conducting fibers (**Purkinje** fibers of the heart). The other type of action potential, the **slow response,** occurs in the **sinoatrial (SA) node,** the natural pacemaker region of the heart, and in the **atrioventricular (AV) node,** the specialized tissue that conducts the cardiac impulse from atria to ventricles.

Fast responses may change to slow responses under certain pathological conditions. For example, in coronary artery disease, a region of cardiac muscle is deprived of its normal blood supply. As a result, the K^+ concentration in the interstitial fluid that surrounds the affected muscle cells rises because K^+ is lost from the inadequately perfused (or **ischemic**) cells. The action potentials in some of these cells may then be converted from fast to slow responses. An experimental conversion from a fast to a slow response is illustrated in Fig. 22-14.

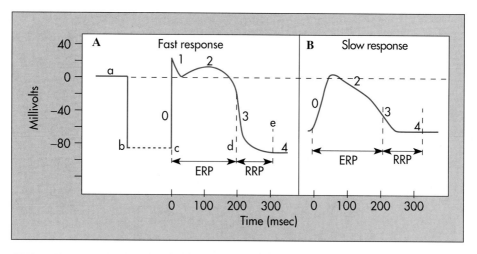

■ **Fig. 22-1** Changes in transmembrane potential recorded from a fast-response and a slow-response cardiac fiber in isolated cardiac tissue immersed in an electrolyte solution. **A,** At time *a* the microelectrode was in the solution surrounding the cardiac fiber. At time *b* the microelectrode entered the fiber. At time *c* an action potential was initiated in the impaled fiber. Time *c* to *d* represents the effective refractory period (*ERP*), and time *d* to *e* represents the relative refractory period (*RRP*). **B,** An action potential recorded from a slow-response cardiac fiber. Note that, compared with the fast-response fiber, the resting potential of the slow fiber is less negative, the upstroke (phase *0*) of the action potential is less steep, the amplitude of the action potential is smaller, phase *1* is absent, and the relative refractory period (*RRP*) extends well into phase *4* after the fiber has fully repolarized.

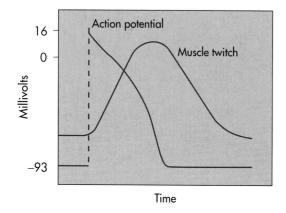

■ **Fig. 22-2** Time relationships between the developed force and the changes in transmembrane potential in a thin strip of ventricular muscle. (Redrawn from Kavaler F, Fisher VJ, Stuckey JH: *Bull N Y Acad Med* 41:592, 1965.)

As shown in Fig. 22-1, not only is the resting membrane potential (phase 4) of the fast response considerably more negative than that of the slow response, but the slope of the upstroke (phase 0), the amplitude of the action potential, and the extent of the overshoot of the fast response are greater than in the slow response. The amplitude of the action potential and the steepness of the upstroke are important determinants of how fast the action potential is propagated. In slow-response cardiac tissue, the action potential is propagated more slowly than in fast-response cardiac tissue. In addition, the conduction is more likely to be blocked in slow-response cardiac tissue than in fast-response tissue. Slow conduc-

tion and a tendency toward conduction block increase the likelihood of some rhythm disturbances.

■ *Ionic Basis of the Resting Potential*

The various phases of the cardiac action potential are associated with changes in the permeability of the cell membrane, mainly to sodium, potassium, and calcium ions. Changes in cell membrane permeability alter the movement of these ions across the membrane. The permeability of the membrane to a given ion, its transmembrane concentration difference, and the transmembrane electrical potential difference define the net quantity of the ion that will diffuse across the membrane. Changes in permeability are accomplished by the opening and closing of ion channels that are specific for the individual ions.

As with all other cells in the body (see also Chapter 2), the concentration of potassium ions inside a cardiac muscle cell ($[K^+]_i$) is far greater than the concentration outside the cell ($[K^+]_o$) (Fig. 22-3). The reverse concentration gradient exists for sodium and calcium ions. Estimates of the extracellular and intracellular concentrations of Na^+, K^+, and Ca^{++} and the equilibrium potentials (this term is defined later in this chapter) for these ions are compiled in Table 22-1.

The resting cell membrane is relatively permeable to K^+ but much less so to Na^+ and Ca^{++}. Hence, K^+ tends to diffuse from the inside to the outside of the cell in the direction of the K^+ concentration gradient, as shown on the right side of the cell in Fig. 22-3.

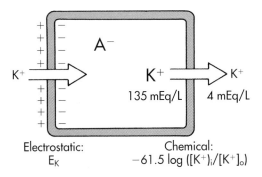

Electrostatic:
E_K

Chemical:
$-61.5 \log ([K^+]_i/[K^+]_o)$

■ **Fig. 22-3** The balance of chemical and electrostatic forces acting on a resting cardiac cell membrane. The estimations are based on a 34:1 ratio of the intracellular to extracellular K⁺ concentrations and the existence of a nondiffusible anion (A^-) inside, but not outside, the cell.

■ **Table 22-1** Intracellular and extracellular ion concentrations and equilibrium potentials in cardiac muscle cells

Ion	Extracellular concentrations (mM)	Intracellular concentrations (mM)*	Equilibrium potential (mV)
Na⁺	145	10	70
K⁺	4	135	−94
Ca⁺⁺	2	10^{-4}	132

Modified from Ten Eick RE, Baumgarten CM, Singer DH: *Prog Cardiovasc Dis* 24:157, 1981.

*The intracellular concentrations are estimates of the free concentrations in the cytoplasm

Any flux of K⁺ that occurs during phase 4 takes place mainly through specific **K⁺ channels.** Several types of K⁺ channels exist in cardiac cell membranes. Some of these channels are regulated (i.e., they open and close) according to the transmembrane potential, whereas others are regulated by a chemical signal (e.g., the extracellular acetylcholine concentration). One of the specific K⁺ channels through which K⁺ passes during phase 4 is a voltage-regulated channel that conducts the **inwardly rectifying K⁺ current.** This current is symbolized i_{K1}, and is discussed in more detail later (Fig. 22-8). For now, it is only necessary to know how this current is established. Many of the anions (labeled A^-), such as the proteins, inside the cell, are not free to diffuse out with the K⁺ (Fig. 22-3). Therefore, the K⁺ diffuses out of the cell and leaves the impermeant A^- behind. The deficiency of cations then causes the interior of the cell to become electronegative (see also Chapter 2). As a result, the positively charged K⁺ ions are attracted to the interior of the cell by the negative potential that exists there, as shown on the left side of the cell in Fig. 22-3.

Therefore, two opposing forces are involved in the movement of K⁺ across the cell membrane. A chemical force, based on the concentration gradient, results in net outward diffusion of K⁺. The counterforce is based on electrostatic differences between the interior and exterior

of the cell. If the system came into equilibrium, the chemical and the electrostatic forces would be equal. As explained in Chapter 2, this equilibrium is expressed by the **Nernst equation** for potassium:

$$E_K = 61.5 \log([K^+]_i/[K^+]_o)$$

The right-hand term represents the chemical potential difference, and the left-hand term, E_K, represents the electrostatic potential difference that would exist across the cell membrane if K⁺ were the only diffusible ion. E_K is called the **potassium equilibrium potential.**

When the measured concentrations of $[K^+]_i$ and $[K^+]_o$ for mammalian myocardial cells are substituted into the Nernst equation, the calculated value of E_K equals about −95 mV (Table 22-1). This value is close to, but slightly more negative than, the resting potential actually measured in myocardial cells. Therefore, the potential that tends to drive K⁺ out of the resting cell is small. The actual resting potential is slightly less negative than the predicted potential because the cell membrane is slightly permeable to other ions, notably to Na⁺. The balance of the forces acting on Na⁺ is opposite to the balance of forces acting on K⁺ in resting cardiac cells. The intracellular Na⁺ concentration, $[Na^+]_i$, is much lower than the extracellular concentration, $[Na^+]_o$. The sodium equilibrium potential, E_{Na}, expressed by the Nernst equation, is about 70 mV (Table 22-1).

At equilibrium, therefore, an electrostatic force of about 70 mV, oriented with the inside of the cell more positive than the outside, is necessary to counterbalance the chemical potential for Na⁺. However, as we have seen, the actual resting membrane potential of myocytes is about −90 mV. Hence, both chemical and electrostatic forces act to pull extracellular Na⁺ into the cell. The influx of Na⁺ through the membrane is small, however, because the membrane of the resting cell is not very permeable to Na⁺. Nevertheless, this small inward current of Na⁺ is sufficient to cause the potential (V_m) on the inside of the resting cell membrane to be slightly less negative than the value (E_K) predicted by the Nernst equation for K⁺ (Fig. 22-4).

The dependence of V_m on the conductances and on the intracellular and extracellular concentrations of K⁺, Na⁺, and other ions is described by the **chord conductance equation,** as explained in Chapter 2. This equation reveals that relative—not absolute—membrane conductances to Na⁺ and K⁺ determine the resting potential. In the resting cardiac cell, the conductance (g_K) to K⁺ is about 100 times greater than the conductance (g_{Na}) to Na⁺. Therefore, the chord conductance equation reduces essentially to the Nernst equation for K⁺. Because g_{Na} is so small in the resting cell, changes in external Na⁺ concentration do not significantly affect V_m (Fig. 22-5).

When the ratio $[K^+]_i/[K^+]_o$ is decreased experimentally by raising $[K^+]_o$ in a suspension of myocytes, the measured value of V_m approximates the value of E_K predicted by the Nernst equation (Fig. 22-4). For extracellular K⁺

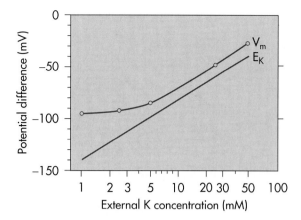

■ **Fig. 22-4**   Transmembrane potential (V_m) of a cardiac muscle fiber varies inversely with the potassium concentration of the external medium. The straight line (E_K) represents the change in transmembrane potential predicted by the Nernst equation for potassium. (Redrawn from Page E: *Circulation* 26:582, 1962, with permission of the American Heart Association.)

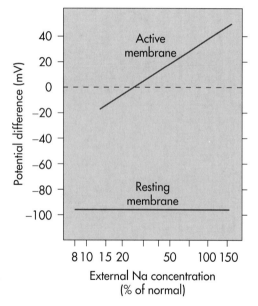

■ **Fig. 22-5**   Concentration of sodium in the external medium is a critical determinant of the amplitude of the action potential in cardiac muscle (*upper line*) but it has very little influence on the resting membrane potential (*lower line*). (Redrawn from Weidmann S: *Elektrophysiologie der Herzmuskelfaser,* Bern, 1956, Verlag Hans Huber.)

concentrations greater than about 5 mM, the measured values correspond closely with the predicted values. The measured levels are only slightly less than those predicted by the Nernst equation because g_K is so much greater than g_{Na}. However, for values of $[K^+]_o$ below about 5 mM, g_K decreases as $[K^+]_o$ is diminished. As g_K decreases, the effect of g_{Na} on the transmembrane potential becomes relatively more significant, as predicted by the chord conductance equation. This change in g_K accounts for the greater deviation of the measured V_m from the value predicted by the Nernst equation for K^+ at low levels of $[K^+]_o$.

■ *Ionic Basis of the Fast Response*

■ *Phase 0: Genesis of the Upstroke*

Any stimulus that abruptly changes the resting membrane potential to a critical value (called the **threshold**) results in an action potential. The characteristics of fast response action potentials are shown in Fig. 22-1, *A*. The rapid depolarization (phase 0) is related almost exclusively to the influx of Na^+ into the myocyte due to a sudden increase in g_{Na}. The **amplitude** of the action potential (the potential change during phase 0) varies linearly with the logarithm of $[Na^+]_o$, as shown in Fig. 22-5. When $[Na^+]_o$ is reduced from its normal value of about 140 mM to about 20 mM, the cell is no longer excitable.

The physical and chemical forces responsible for these transmembrane movements of Na^+ are diagrammed in Fig. 22-6. When the resting membrane potential, V_m, is suddenly changed to the threshold level of about −65 mV, the properties of the cell membrane change dramatically. Na^+ enters the myocyte through specific **fast Na^+ channels** that exist in the membrane (see also Chapter 3). These channels can be blocked by the puffer fish toxin, **tetrodotoxin.** Also, many of the drugs used to treat certain cardiac rhythm disturbances **(cardiac arrhythmias)** act by blocking these fast Na^+ channels.

The manner in which Na^+ moves through these fast channels suggests that the flux is controlled by two types of **gates** in each channel. One of these, the **m gate,** tends to open the channel as V_m becomes less negative. This is therefore called an **activation gate.** The other gate, the **h gate,** tends to close the channel as V_m becomes less negative and hence is called an **inactivation gate.** The "m" and "h" designations were originally employed by Hodgkin and Huxley in their mathematical model of impulse conduction in nerve fibers.

As we have seen, the V_m of a resting cell is about −90 mV. The m gates are closed and the h gates are wide open, as shown in Fig. 22-6, *A*. Because the concentration of Na^+ outside the cell is greater than the Na^+ concentration inside the cell, the interior of the cell is electrically negative with respect to the exterior. Hence, both chemical and electrostatic forces are oriented to draw Na^+ into the cell.

The electrostatic force in Fig. 22-6, *A,* is a potential difference of 90 mV, and it is represented by the white arrow. The chemical force, based on the difference in Na^+ concentration between the outside and inside of the cell, is represented by the black arrow. For a Na^+ concentration difference of about 130 mM, a potential difference of 60 mV (with the inside more positive than outside) is necessary to counterbalance the chemical, or diffusional, force, according to the Nernst equation for Na^+. Therefore, the net chemical force that favors the inward movement of Na^+ in Fig. 22-6 (*black arrows*) is equivalent to a potential difference of 60 mV. In the resting cell, the total electrochemical force that favors the inward movement of Na^+ is 150 mV (*A*). The m gates are closed,

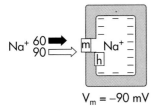

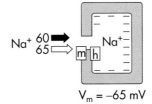

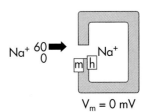

A, During phase 4, the chemical (60 mV) and electrostatic (90 mV) forces favor influx of Na⁺ from the extracellular space. Influx is negligible, however, because the activation *(m)* gates are closed.

B, If V_m is brought to about −65 V, the *m* gates begin to swing open, and Na⁺ begins to enter the cell. This reduces the negative charge inside the cell, and thereby opens still more Na⁺ channels, which accelerates the influx of Na⁺. The change in V_m also initiates the closure of inactivation *(h)* gates, which operate more slowly than the *m* gates.

C, The rapid influx of Na⁺ sharply decreases the negativity of V_m. As V_m approaches 0, the electrostatic force attracting Na⁺ into the cell is neutralized. Na⁺ continues to enter the cell, however, because of the substantial concentration gradient, and V_m begins to become positive.

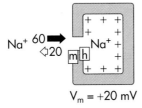

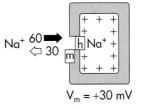

D, When V_m is positive by about 20 mV, Na⁺ continues to enter the cell, because the diffusional forces (60 mV) exceed the opposing electrostatic forces (20 mV). The influx of Na⁺ is slow, however, because the net driving force is small, and many of the inactivation gates have already closed.

E, When V_m reaches about 30 mV, the *h* gates have now all closed, and Na⁺ influx ceases. The *h* gates remain closed until the first half of repolarization, and thus the cell is absolutely refractory during this entire period. During the second half of repolarization, the *m* and *h* gates approach the state represented by panel A, and thus the cell is relatively refractory.

■ **Fig. 22-6**　The gating of a sodium channel in a cardiac cell membrane during phase 4 (**A**) and during various stages of the action potential upstroke (**B** to **E**). The positions of the *m* and *h* gates in the fast Na⁺ channels are shown at the various levels of V_m. The electrostatic forces are represented by the white arrows and the chemical (diffusional) forces by the black arrows.

however, and the conductance of the resting cell membrane to Na⁺ is low. Therefore, in resting state, virtually no Na⁺ moves into the cell.

Any stimulus that makes V_m less negative tends to open the m gates, and thereby tends to activate the fast Na⁺ channels. The precise potential required to open the m gates and thus activate the Na⁺ channels varies somewhat from one channel to another in the cell membrane. As V_m becomes progressively less negative, more and more m gates swing open, and the influx of Na⁺ accelerates (Fig. 22-6, *B*). The entry of Na⁺ into the interior of the cell neutralizes some of the negative charges within the cell, and thereby makes V_m still less negative. The consequent change in V_m then opens more m gates and augments the inward Na⁺ current. This process is called **regenerative.** As V_m approaches about −65 mV, the remaining m gates rapidly swing open in the fast Na⁺ channels until virtually all the m gates are open (Fig. 22-6, *B*).

The rapid opening of the m gates in the fast Na⁺ channels is responsible for the large and abrupt increase in Na⁺ conductance (g_Na) that occurs in phase 0 (the upstroke) of

the action potential (Fig. 22-7). The rapid influx of Na⁺ accounts for the steepness of the upstroke of the action potential. The maximal rate of change of V_m varies from 100 to 200 V/sec in myocardial cells and from 500 to 1000 V/sec in Purkinje fibers. Although Na⁺ that enters the cell during one action potential alters V_m by more than 100 mV, the actual quantity of Na⁺ that enters the cell is so small that the resultant change in the intracellular Na⁺ concentration cannot be measured. Hence, the chemical force remains virtually constant, and only the electrostatic force changes throughout the action potential. In Fig. 22-6, note that the lengths of the black arrows remain constant (denoting a chemical force of 60 mV), while the white arrows change in magnitude and direction.

As Na⁺ rushes into the cardiac cell during phase 0, the negative charges inside the cell are neutralized, and V_m becomes progressively less negative. When V_m falls to zero (Fig. 22-6, *C*), an electrostatic force no longer exists to pull Na⁺ into the cell. As long as the fast Na⁺ channels are open, however, Na⁺ continues to enter the cell because of the large concentration gradient. This continuation of

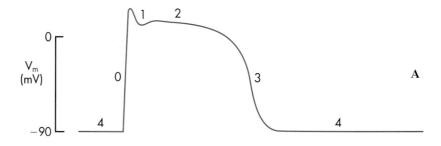

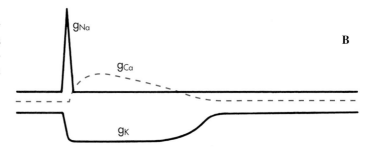

■ **Fig. 22-7** Changes in the conductances of Na^+ (g_{Na}), Ca^{++} (g_{Ca}), and K^+ (g_K) during the various phases of the action potential (**A**) of a fast-response cardiac cell. The conductance diagram (**B**) shows directional changes only.

the inward Na^+ current causes the inside of the cell to become positively charged (Fig. 22-6, *D*). This reversal of the membrane polarity is the so-called **overshoot** of the cardiac action potential. Such a reversal of the electrostatic gradient would, of course, tend to repel the entry of additional Na^+ (Fig. 22-6, *D*). However, as long as the inwardly directed chemical forces exceed the outwardly directed electrostatic forces, the net flux of Na^+ is directed inward, although the rate at which Na^+ enters the cell diminishes.

The inward Na^+ current finally stops when the h (inactivation) gates close (Fig. 22-6, *E*). Like the activity of the m gates, the activity of the h gates is governed by the value of V_m. However, the m gates open very rapidly (in about 0.1 msec), whereas the closure the h gates requires a few milliseconds. Phase 0 is finally terminated when all of the h gates have closed, thereby inactivating the fast Na^+ channels. The closure of the h gates so soon after the opening of the m gates accounts for the quick return of g_{Na} from its maximum to its resting value (Fig. 22-7).

The h gates then remain closed until the cell has partially repolarized during phase 3 (at about time *d* in Fig. 22-1, *A*). From time *c* to time *d* the cell is in its **effective refractory period** and will not respond to further excitation. This mechanism prevents a sustained, tetanic contraction of cardiac muscle. *Tetanic contraction of the ventricular myocytes would retard ventricular relaxation and therefore interfere with the normal intermittent pumping action of the heart.*

About midway through phase 3 (time *d* in Fig. 22-1, *A*), the m and h gates in some of the fast Na^+ channels have resumed the states shown in Fig. 22-6, *A*. Such channels are said to have **recovered from inactivation.** The cell can begin to respond (but weakly at first) to further excitation (Fig. 22-15). Throughout the remainder of phase 3 the cell completes its recovery from inactivation. By time *e* in Fig. 22-1, *A*, the h gates have reopened and the m

gates have reclosed in all the fast Na^+ channels; that is, they have resumed the status depicted in Fig. 22-6, *A*.

■ *Phase 1: Genesis of Early Repolarization*

In many cardiac cells that have a prominent plateau, phase 1 constitutes an early, brief period of limited repolarization. In Fig. 22-1, this brief repolarization is represented by a notch between the end of the upstroke and the beginning of the plateau. Repolarization occurs briefly owing to the activation of a **transient outward current** (i_{to}), carried mainly by K^+. Activation of K^+ channels during phase 1 causes a brief efflux of K^+ from the cell, because the interior of the cell is positively charged and because the internal K^+ concentration greatly exceeds the external K^+ concentration (Fig. 22-8). As a result of this transient efflux of positively charged ions, the cell is briefly and partially repolarized (phase 1).

The phase 1 notch is prominent in ventricular Purkinje fibers (Fig. 22-13) and in myocytes located in the epicardial and midmyocardial regions of the ventricular wall (Fig. 22-9). However, the notch is negligible in myocytes from the endocardial region (Fig. 22-9). The cycle length of depolarization also appears to affect phase 1. When the basic cycle length at which the epicardial and midmyocardial fibers are depolarized is increased from 300 to 8000 msec, the phase 1 notch becomes more pronounced and the action potential duration is increased substantially. The same increase in basic cycle length in endocardial fibers has no effect on phase 1 and only a small effect on the action potential duration (Fig. 22-9). In the presence of 4-aminopyridine, which blocks the K^+ channels that carry i_{to}, the phase 1 notch becomes much less prominent in the action potentials recorded from the epicardial and midmyocardial regions of the ventricles.

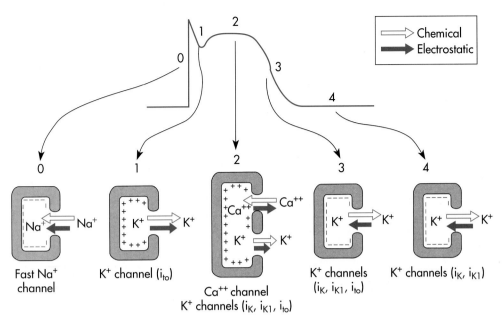

■ **Fig. 22-8**   The principal ionic currents and channels that generate the various phases of the action potential in a cardiac cell. Phase 0: The chemical and electrostatic forces both favor the entry of Na^+ into the cell through fast Na^+ channels to generate the upstroke. Phase 1: The chemical and electrostatic forces both favor the efflux of K^+ through i_{to} channels to generate early, partial repolarization. Phase 2: During the plateau, the net influx of Ca^{++} through Ca^{++} channels is balanced by the efflux of K^+ through i_K, i_{K1}, and i_{to} channels. Phase 3: The chemical forces that favor the efflux of K^+ through i_K, i_{K1}, and i_{to} channels predominate over the electrostatic forces that favor the influx of K^+ through these same channels. Phase 4: The chemical forces that favor the efflux of K^+ through i_K and i_{K1} channels exceed very slightly the electrostatic forces that favor the influx of K^+ through these same channels.

■ *Phase 2: Genesis of the Plateau*

During the plateau of the action potential, Ca^{++} enters the myocardial cells through **calcium channels,** which activate and inactivate much more slowly than do the fast Na^+ channels. During the flat portion of phase 2 (Fig. 22-8), this influx of positive charge carried by Ca^{++} is counterbalanced by the efflux of positive charge carried by K^+. K^+ exits through channels that conduct mainly the i_{to}, i_K, and i_{K1} currents. The i_{to} current is responsible for phase 1, as described previously, but it is not completely inactivated until after phase 2 has expired. The i_K and i_{K1} currents are described later in this chapter.

Ca^{++} conductance during the plateau. The Ca^{++} channels are voltage-regulated channels that are activated as V_m becomes progressively less negative during the upstroke of the action potential. Various types of Ca^{++} channels have been identified in cardiac tissues (see Chapter 3), but this discussion concentrates on the predominant channel, the so-called L-type Ca^{++} channel. Some of the important characteristics of this channel are illustrated in Fig. 22-10, which also shows the Ca^{++} currents generated by voltage-clamping an isolated atrial myocyte. Note that when V_m is suddenly increased to +30 mV from a holding potential of −30 mV, an inward Ca^{++} current is activated. Note also that after the inward Ca^{++} current reaches its maximal value (in the downward direction), it returns to zero only very gradually (i.e., the channel inactivates very slowly). Thus, because the current that passes through these channels is long-lasting, the channels are designated "L-type."

Opening of the Ca^{++} channels is reflected by an increase in Ca^{++} conductance (g_{Ca}) immediately after the upstroke of the action potential (Fig. 22-7). At the beginning of the action potential, the intracellular Ca^{++} concentration is much less than the extracellular concentration (Table 22-1). Consequently, the increase in g_{Ca} promotes an influx of Ca^{++} into the cell throughout the plateau. *This influx of Ca during the plateau is involved in excitation-contraction coupling,* as described in Chapters 17 and 23.

Various factors, such as neurotransmitters and drugs, may substantially influence g_{Ca}. The adrenergic neurotransmitter **norepinephrine,** the β-adrenergic receptor agonist **isoproterenol,** and various other **catecholamines** may enhance Ca^{++} conductance, whereas the parasympathetic neurotransmitter **acetylcholine** may decrease Ca^{++} conductance. The enhancement of Ca^{++} conductance by catecholamines is probably the principal mechanism by which they enhance cardiac muscle contractility.

To enhance Ca^{++} conductance, catecholamines first interact with β-**adrenergic receptors** in the cardiac cell membrane. This interaction stimulates the membrane-bound enzyme **adenylyl cyclase,** which raises the intracellular concentration of **cyclic adenosine monophosphate (cAMP)** (see also Chapter 5). The rise in the level of cAMP enhances the activation of the L-type Ca^{++} channels in the cell membrane (Fig. 22-10) and thus augments the influx of Ca^{++} into the cells from the interstitial fluid. Conversely, acetylcholine interacts with **muscarinic receptors** in the cell membrane to inhibit adenylyl cyclase. In this way, acetylcholine antagonizes the activation of Ca^{++} channels, and thereby diminishes g_{Ca}.

The **Ca^{++} channel antagonists** are substances that block Ca^{++} channels. Examples include the drugs **verapamil** and **diltiazem.** These drugs decrease g_{Ca}, thereby impeding the influx of Ca^{++} into myocardial cells. The Ca^{++} channel antagonists decrease the duration of the action potential plateau and diminish the strength of the cardiac contraction (Fig. 22-11). Paradoxically, although Ca^{++} channel antagonists have a depressant effect on the contractile strength of the heart, these agents are used widely in the treatment of **congestive heart failure,** a common clinical condition in which the contractile performance of the heart is already compromised. As a result, the heart is unable to generate enough blood flow to meet the needs of the tissues. The Ca^{++} channel antagonists weaken the cardiac contraction and depress the contraction of the vascular smooth muscle, thereby inducing generalized vasodilation. This diminished vascular resistance reduces the counterforce (**afterload**) that opposes the propulsion of blood from the ventricles into the arterial system, as explained in Chapters 25 and 26. Hence, vasodilator drugs, such as the Ca^{++} channel antagonists, are often referred to as **afterload-reducing drugs.** This ability to diminish the counterforce leads to a more adequate cardiac output, despite the direct cardiac depressant effect of these drugs.

K^+ conductance during the plateau. During the plateau of the action potential, the concentration gradient for K^+ across the cell membrane is virtually the same as it is during phase 4, but V_m is positive. Therefore, both the chemical and the electrostatic forces favor the efflux of K^+ from the cell (Fig. 22-8). If g_K were the same dur-

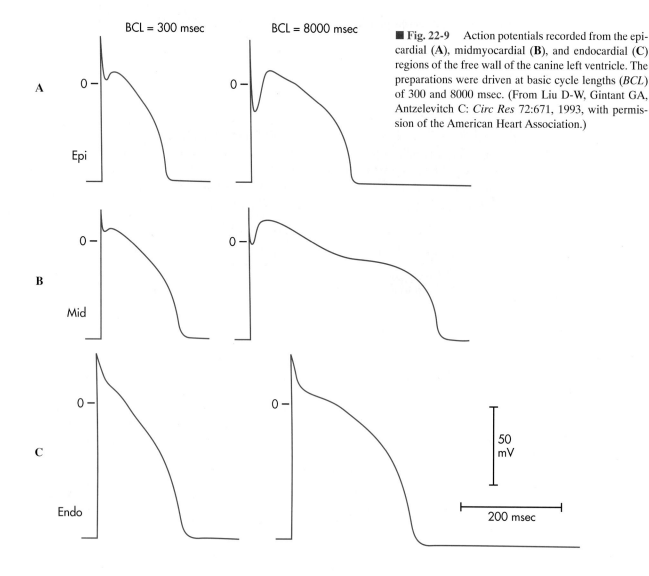

■ **Fig. 22-9** Action potentials recorded from the epicardial (**A**), midmyocardial (**B**), and endocardial (**C**) regions of the free wall of the canine left ventricle. The preparations were driven at basic cycle lengths (*BCL*) of 300 and 8000 msec. (From Liu D-W, Gintant GA, Antzelevitch C: *Circ Res* 72:671, 1993, with permission of the American Heart Association.)

ing the plateau as it is during phase 4, the efflux of K⁺ during phase 2 would greatly exceed the influx of Ca⁺⁺, and a sustained plateau could not be achieved. However as V_m approaches and then attains positive values near the peak of the action potential upstroke, g_K suddenly decreases (Fig. 22-7). *The diminished K⁺ current associated with the reduction in g_K prevents an excessive loss of K⁺ from the cell during the plateau.*

This reduction in g_K at both positive and low negative values of V_m is called **inward rectification.** Inward rectification is a characteristic of several K⁺ currents, including the i_{K1} current. The current-voltage relationship of the K⁺ channels that conduct i_{K1} has been determined by voltage-clamping cardiac cells (Fig. 22-12). Note that for the cell depicted in the figure, the current-voltage curve intersects the voltage axis at a V_m of about

−70 mV. The absence of ionic current flow at the point of intersection indicates that the electrostatic forces are equal to the chemical (diffusional) forces (Fig. 22-3) at this potential. In this ventricular cell preparation, therefore, the Nernst equilibrium potential (E_K) for K⁺ is −70 mV. This value reflects the ratio of intracellular to extracellular K⁺ concentration that prevails in this particular experimental preparation.

When the membrane potential is clamped at levels negative to −70 mV in this same isolated cardiac cell (Fig. 22-12), the electrostatic forces exceed the chemical forces and an inward K⁺ current is induced (as denoted by the negative values of K⁺ current over this range of voltages). Note also that for V_m more negative than −70 mV, the curve has a steep slope, even at the point of intersection (at which $V_m = E_K$). Thus when V_m equals or is negative to E_K, a small change in V_m induces a substantial change in K⁺ current; that is, g_K is large. During phase 4, the V_m of a myocardial cell is slightly less negative than E_K (Fig. 22-4). The substantial g_K that prevails during phase 4 of the cardiac action potential (Fig. 22-7) is accounted for mainly by the i_{K1} channels.

When the transmembrane potential is clamped at levels less negative than −70 mV (Fig. 22-12), the chemical forces exceed the electrostatic forces. Therefore, the net K⁺ currents are directed outward (as denoted by the corresponding positive values of K⁺ current). Note that for V_m values less negative than −70 mV the curve is relatively flat, and for V_m values less negative than about −30 mV the K⁺ current is virtually zero. Thus, at V_m values that prevail during the action potential plateau, the efflux of K⁺ through the i_{K1} channels is negligible. Conversely, as we have seen, the inwardly directed K⁺ current is sub-

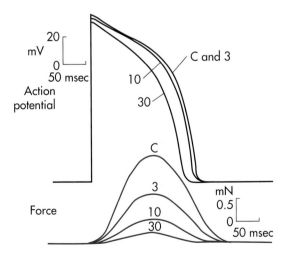

■ Fig. 22-10 Effect of isoproterenol on the Ca⁺⁺ current conducted by L-type Ca⁺⁺ channels in voltage-clamped, canine atrial myocytes when the potential was changed from −30 to +30 mV. (Redrawn from Bean BP: *J Gen Physiol* 86:1, 1985.)

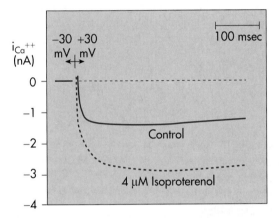

■ Fig. 22-11 Effects of diltiazem, a Ca⁺⁺ channel antagonist, on the action potentials (in millivolts) and isometric contractile forces (in millinewtons) recorded from an isolated papillary muscle of a guinea pig. The tracings were recorded under control conditions *(C)* and in the presence of diltiazem, in concentrations of 3, 10, and 30 μmol/L. (Redrawn from Hirth C, Borchard U, Hafner D: *J Mol Cell Cardiol* 15:799, 1983.)

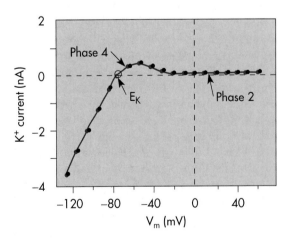

■ Fig. 22-12 Inwardly rectified K⁺ currents recorded from a rabbit ventricular myocyte when the potential was changed from a holding potential of −80 mV to various test potentials. Positive values along the vertical axis represent outward currents; negative values represent inward currents. The V_m coordinate of the point *(open circle)* at which the curve intersects the X axis is the reversal potential; it denotes the Nernst equilibrium potential, at which point the chemical and electrostatic forces are equal. (Redrawn from Giles WR, Imaizumi Y: *J Physiol (Lond)* 405:123, 1988.)

stantial for those values of V_m that prevail during phase 4. Thus, the i_{K1} current is **inwardly rectified.**

The characteristics of another K^+ channel, the **delayed rectifier (i_K)** channel, also contribute to the low g_K that prevails during the plateau. These K^+ channels are closed during phase 4, but they are activated by the potentials that prevail toward the end of phase 0. However, activation proceeds very slowly during the plateau. Hence, activation of these channels tends to increase g_K very gradually during phase 2. Thus, these channels play only a minor role during phase 2, but they do contribute to the process of final repolarization (phase 3), as described below.

The action potential plateau persists as long as the efflux of charge carried mainly by K^+ is balanced by the influx of charge carried mainly by Ca^{++}. The effects of altering this balance are demonstrated by the action of the calcium channel antagonist diltiazem in an isolated papillary muscle preparation. Fig. 22-11 shows that with increasing concentrations of diltiazem, the voltage of the plateau becomes progressively less positive and the duration of the plateau diminishes. Similarly, administration of certain K^+ channel antagonists prolongs the plateau substantially.

■ *Phase 3: Genesis of Final Repolarization*

The process of final repolarization (phase 3) starts at the end of phase 2, when the efflux of K^+ from the cardiac cell begins to exceed the influx of Ca^{++}. As we have noted, at least three outward K^+ currents (i_{to}, i_K, and i_{K1}) contribute to the final repolarization (phase 3) of the cardiac cell (Fig. 22-8).

The transient outward (i_{to}) and the delayed rectifier (i_K) currents help initiate repolarization. These currents are therefore important determinants of the duration of the plateau. For example, the plateau duration is substantially less in atrial than in ventricular myocytes (Fig. 22-19). Electrophysiological experiments reveal that the intensity of the outward K^+ current during the plateau is greater in atrial than in ventricular myocytes. When the outward K^+ current exceeds the inward Ca^{++} current, repolarization begins. Hence, the greater the K^+ current during phase 2, the earlier repolarization begins. The greater density of the K^+ current in atrial than in ventricular myocytes accounts for the shorter action potentials in atrial than in ventricular myocytes.

The action potential duration in ventricular myocytes varies considerably with the locations of these myocytes in the ventricular walls (Fig. 22-9). The delayed rectifier (i_K) current appears to account for these differences. In endocardial myocytes, where the action potential duration is least, the intensity of i_K is greatest. The converse applies to the midmyocardial myocytes. The intensity of i_K and the action potential duration are intermediate for the epicardial myocytes.

The inwardly rectified K^+ current, i_{K1}, does not participate in the initiation of repolarization, because the conduc-

tance of these channels is very small at the range of V_m values that prevail during the plateau. However, *the i_{K1} channels do contribute substantially to the rate of repolarization once phase 3 has been initiated.* As the net efflux of cations causes V_m to become increasingly negative during phase 3, the conductance of the channels that carry the i_{K1} current progressively increases. In Fig. 22-12, the hump in the flat portion of the current-voltage curve reflects the increase in i_{K1} conductance as V_m changes from about -20 to about -60 mV. Thus, as V_m passes through this range of values positive to the Nernst equilibrium potential (open circle in Fig. 22-12), the outward K^+ current increases and thereby accelerates repolarization.

■ *Phase 4: Restoration of Ionic Concentrations*

The excess Na^+ that enters the cell rapidly during phase 0 and more slowly throughout the cardiac cycle is eliminated by the action of the enzyme Na^+,K^+-ATPase. This enzyme ejects 3 Na^+ in exchange for 2 K^+ that had exited from the cell mainly during phases 2 and 3. Similarly, most of the excess Ca^{++} that had entered the cell mainly during phase 2 is eliminated principally by a Na^+/Ca^{++} exchanger, which exchanges 3 Na^+ for 1 Ca^{++}. However, some of the Ca^{++} is eliminated by an ATP-driven Ca^{++} pump (Fig. 23-5).

■ *Ionic Basis of the Slow Response*

Fast-response action potentials (Fig. 22-1, *A*) consist of four principal components: an upstroke (phase 0); an early, partial repolarization (phase 1); a plateau (phase 2); and a final repolarization (phase 3). However, in the slow response (Fig. 22-1, *B*), the upstroke is much less steep, early repolarization (phase 1) is absent, the plateau is less prolonged and not as flat, and the transition from the plateau to the final repolarization is less distinct.

Blocking fast Na^+ channels with tetrodotoxin in a fast-response fiber can generate slow responses under appropriate conditions. The Purkinje fiber action potentials shown in Fig. 22-13 clearly exhibit the two response types. In the control tracing (*A*), the typical fast-response action potential displays a prominent notch, which separates the upstroke from the plateau. In action potentials *B* to *E*, progressively larger quantities of tetrodotoxin are added to the bathing solution to produce a graded blockade of the fast Na^+ channels. Fig. 22-13 shows that the upstroke and notch become progressively less prominent in action potentials *B* to *D*. In action potential *E*, the notch has disappeared and the upstroke is very gradual; the action potential resembles a typical slow response.

Certain cells in the heart, notably those in the SA and AV nodes, are normally slow-response fibers. In such fibers, depolarization is achieved mainly by the influx of Ca^{++} through the Ca^{++} channels. Repolarization is accomplished in these fibers by the inactivation of the

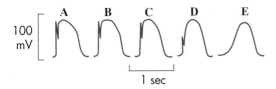

100 mV

A B C D E

1 sec

■ Fig. 22-13 Effect of tetrodotoxin on the action potentials recorded in a calf Purkinje fiber perfused with a solution containing epinephrine and K^+ (10.8 mM). The concentration of tetrodotoxin was 0 M in **A**, 3×10^{-8} M in **B**, 3×10^{-7} M in **C**, and 3×10^{-6} M in **D** and **E**; **E** was recorded later than **D**. (Redrawn from Carmeliet E, Vereecke J: *Pflugers Arch* 313:300, 1969.)

Ca^{++} channels and by the increased K^+ conductance through the i_{K1} and i_K channels (Fig. 22-8).

■ *Conduction in Cardiac Fibers*

Now that we have seen how an action potential is generated, let us turn to how an action potential is conducted in a cardiac fiber. An action potential traveling down a cardiac muscle fiber is propagated by local circuit currents, much as it does in nerve and skeletal muscle fibers (see Chapter 3). The characteristics of conduction differ in fast- and slow-response fibers.

■ *Conduction of the Fast Response*

In fast-response fibers, the fast Na^+ channels are activated when the transmembrane potential of one region of the fiber suddenly changes from a resting value of about -90 mV to the threshold value of about -70 mV. The inward Na^+ current then rapidly depolarizes the cell at that site. This portion of the fiber becomes part of the depolarized zone, and the border is displaced accordingly. The same process then begins at the new border. This process is repeated again and again, and the border moves continuously down the fiber as a wave of depolarization (see Fig. 3-11).

The conduction velocity along the fiber varies directly with the amplitude of the action potential and the rate of change of potential (dV_m/dt) during phase 0. The amplitude of the action potential equals the difference in potential between the fully depolarized and the fully polarized regions of the cell interior. The magnitude of the local currents is proportional to this potential difference (see Chapter 3). Because these local currents shift the potential of the resting zone toward the threshold value, they act as the local stimuli that depolarize the adjacent resting portion of the fiber to its threshold potential. *The greater the potential difference between the depolarized and polarized regions (i.e., the greater the amplitude of the action potential), the more effective are the local stimuli in depolarizing adjacent parts of the membrane and the more rapidly is the wave of depolarization propagated down the fiber.*

The rate of change of potential (dV_m/dt) during phase 0 is also an important determinant of the conduction velocity. If the active portion of the fiber depolarizes gradually, the local currents between the resting region and the neighboring depolarizing region are small. The resting region adjacent to the active zone is depolarized gradually, and consequently more time is required for each new section of the fiber to reach threshold.

The level of the resting membrane potential is also an important determinant of conduction velocity. This factor operates by influencing the amplitude of the action potential and the slope of the upstroke. The transmembrane potential just prior to depolarization may vary for the following reasons: (1) the external K^+ concentration has changed (Fig. 22-4); (2) in cardiac fibers that are intrinsically automatic, V_m becomes progressively less negative during phase 4 (Fig. 22-19, *B*); and (3) if the cell is excited prematurely, the cell membrane has not repolarized fully from the preceding excitation (Fig. 22-15). In general, the less negative the level of V_m, the less is the velocity of impulse propagation, regardless of the reason for the change in V_m.

The V_m level affects conduction velocity because the inactivation, or h, gates (Fig. 22-6) in the fast Na^+ channels are voltage dependent. The less negative the V_m, the greater is the number of h gates that tend to close. During the normal process of excitation, depolarization proceeds so rapidly during phase 0 that the comparatively slow h gates do not close until the end of that phase. However, if partial depolarization is produced by a more gradual process, such as by an elevation of the level of external K^+, the gates have ample time to close and thereby inactivate some of the Na^+ channels. When the cell is partially depolarized, many of the Na^+ channels are already inactivated; thus, only a fraction of the Na^+ channels is available to conduct the inward Na^+ current during phase 0.

Fig. 22-14 shows the results of an experiment in which the resting V_m of a bundle of Purkinje fibers is closed by altering the value of $[K^+]_o$. When $[K^+]_o$ is 3 mM (*A* and *F*), the resting V_m is -82 mV and the slope of phase 0 is steep. At the end of phase 0, the overshoot attains a value of 30 mV. Hence, the amplitude of the action potential is 112 mV. The tissue is stimulated at some distance from the impaled cell, and the stimulus artifact (*St*) appears as a diphasic deflection just before phase 0. The distance from this artifact to the beginning of phase 0 is inversely proportional to the conduction velocity.

When $[K^+]_o$ is increased gradually to 16 mM (*B* to *E*), the resting V_m becomes progressively less negative. At the same time, the amplitudes and durations of the action potentials and the steepness of the upstrokes all diminish. As a consequence, the conduction velocity diminishes progressively. At $[K^+]_o$ levels of 14 and 16 mM (*D* and *E*), the resting V_m attains levels sufficient to inactivate all the fast Na^+ channels. The action potentials in panels *D* and *E* are characteristic slow responses.

Most of the experimentally induced changes in transmembrane potential shown in Fig. 22-14 also take place in patients with **coronary artery disease.** When blood flow to a region of the myocardium is diminished, the supply of oxygen and metabolic substrates delivered to the ischemic tissues is insufficient. The Na⁺, K⁺-ATPase in the membrane of the cardiac myocytes requires considerable metabolic energy to maintain the normal transmembrane exchanges of Na⁺ and K⁺. When blood flow is inadequate, the activity of the Na⁺, K⁺-ATPase is impaired, and the ischemic myocytes gain excess Na⁺ while losing K⁺ to the surrounding interstitial space. Consequently, the K⁺ concentration in the extracellular fluid surrounding the ischemic myocytes is elevated, and therefore the myocytes are affected by the elevated K⁺ concentration in much the same way as is the myocyte depicted in Fig. 22-14. Such changes may disturb cardiac rhythm and conduction critically.

Conduction of the Slow Response

Local circuits (see Fig. 3-11) are also responsible for propagation of the slow response. However, the characteristics of the conduction process differ quantitatively from those of the fast response. The threshold potential is about −40 mV for the slow response, and conduction is much slower than for the fast response. The conduction velocities of the slow responses in the SA and AV nodes are about 0.02 to 0.1 m/sec. The fast-response conduction velocities are about 0.3 to 1 m/sec for myocardial cells and 1 to 4 m/sec for the specialized conducting (Purkinje) fibers in the ventricles. Slow responses are more likely to be blocked than are fast responses. Also, fast-response fibers can respond at repetition rates that are much greater than the repetition rates of slow-response fibers.

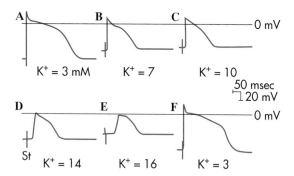

■ **Fig. 22-14** Effect of changes in external potassium concentration on the transmembrane action potentials recorded from a Purkinje fiber. The stimulus artifact (St) appears as a biphasic spike to the left of the upstroke of the action potential. The horizontal lines near the peaks of the action potentials denote 0 mV. (From Myerburg RJ, Lazzara R. In Fisch E, editor: *Complex electrocardiography,* Philadelphia, 1973, FA Davis.)

Cardiac Excitability

Owing to the rapid development of artificial pacemakers and other electrical devices for correcting serious cardiac rhythm disturbances, detailed knowledge of cardiac excitability is essential. The excitability characteristics of cardiac cells differ considerably, depending on whether the action potentials are fast or slow responses.

Fast Response

Once the fast response has been initiated, the depolarized cell is no longer excitable until the cell is partially repolarized (Fig. 22-1, *A*). The interval from the beginning of the action potential until the fiber is able to conduct another action potential is called the **effective refractory period.** In the fast response, this period extends from the beginning of phase 0 to a point in phase 3 where repolarization has reached about −50 mV (time *c* to time *d* in Fig. 22-1, *A*). At about this value of V_m, the electrochemical m and h gates for many of the fast Na channels have been reset.

However, the cardiac fiber is not fully excitable until it has been completely repolarized (time *e* in Fig. 22-1, *A*). Before complete repolarization (period *d* to *e* in the figure), an action potential may be evoked only when the stimulus is stronger than a stimulus that could elicit a response during phase 4. Period *d* to *e* is called the **relative refractory period.**

When a fast response is evoked during the relative refractory period of a previous excitation, its characteristics vary with the membrane potential that exists at the time of stimulation (Fig. 22-15). The later in the relative refractory period the fiber is stimulated, the greater is the increase in the amplitude of the response and in the slope of the upstroke. Presumably, the number of fast Na⁺ channels that have recovered from inactivation increases as repolarization proceeds during phase 3. As a consequence of the greater amplitude and upstroke slope of the evoked response, the propagation velocity also increases the later in the relative refractory period that the fiber is stimulated. Once the fiber is fully repolarized, the response is constant no matter what time in phase 4 the stimulus is applied.

In a patient who has occasional **premature depolarizations** (Fig. 22-39), the timing of these early beats may determine their clinical consequence. If they occur late in the relative refractory period of the preceding depolarization, or after full repolarization, the premature depolarization is probably inconsequential. However, if the premature depolarizations originate early in the relative refractory period, conduction of the premature impulse from the site of origin will be slow, and hence reentry is more likely to occur. If that reentry is irregular (i.e., if **fibrillation** ensues), the consequence may be very grave (Fig. 22-41).

■ *Slow Response*

In slow-response fibers, the relative refractory period frequently extends well beyond phase 3 (Fig. 22-1, *B*). Even after the cell has completely repolarized, it may be difficult to evoke a propagated response for some time. This characteristic of slow-response fibers is called **postrepolarization refractoriness.**

Action potentials evoked early in the relative refractory period are small and the upstrokes are not very steep (Fig. 22-16). The amplitudes and upstroke slopes progressively improve as action potentials are elicited later in the relative refractory period. The recovery of full excitability is much slower than in the fast response. Impulses that arrive early in the relative refractory period are conducted much more slowly than those that arrive late in that period. The lengthy refractory periods also lead to conduction blocks. Even when slow responses recur at a low repetition rate, the fiber may be able to conduct only a fraction of those impulses; for example, only alternate impulses may be propagated (Fig. 22-38, *B*).

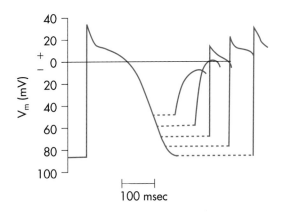

■ **Fig. 22-15**   The changes in action potential amplitude and upstroke slope as action potentials are initiated at different stages of the relative refractory period of the preceding excitation. (Redrawn from Rosen MR, Wit AL, Hoffman BF: *Am Heart J* 88:380, 1974.)

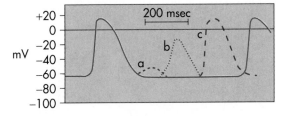

■ **Fig. 22-16**   Effects of excitation at various times after the initiation of an action potential in a slow-response fiber. In this fiber, excitation very late in phase 3 (or early in phase 4) induces a small, nonpropagated (local) response *(a)*. Later in phase 4, a propagated response *(b)* can be elicited, but its amplitude is small and the upstroke is not very steep; this response is conducted very slowly. Still later in phase 4, full excitability is regained, and the response *(c)* displays normal characteristics. (Modified from Singer DH et al: *Prog Cardiovasc Dis* 24:97, 1981.)

■ *Effects of Cycle Length*

Changes in cycle length alter the duration of action potentials in cardiac cells (Figs. 22-9 and 22-17) and thus change their refractory periods. Consequently, changes in cycle length are often important factors in the initiation or termination of certain arrhythmias (irregular heat rhythms). The changes in action potential durations produced by stepwise reductions in cycle length from 2000 to 200 msec in a Purkinje fiber are shown in Fig. 22-17. Note that as the cycle length diminishes, the action potential duration decreases. The direct correlation between action potential duration and cycle length is mediated by changes in g_K that involve at least two types of K$^+$ channels, namely, those that conduct the delayed rectifier K$^+$ current, i_K, and those that conduct the transient outward K$^+$ current, i_{to}.

The i_K current is activated at values of V_m near zero, but the current activates slowly and remains activated for hundreds of milliseconds. The i_K current also inactivates very slowly. Consequently, as the basic cycle length diminishes, each action potential tends to occur earlier in the inactivation period of the i_K current of the preceding action potential. Therefore, the shorter the basic cycle length, the greater is the outward K$^+$ current during phase 2, and hence the shorter the duration of the action potential.

The i_{to} current also influences the relationship between cycle length and action potential duration. The i_{to} current is also activated at near zero potentials, and its magnitude varies inversely with the cardiac cycle length. Therefore, as cycle length decreases, the resultant increase in the outward K$^+$ current shortens the plateau. The relative

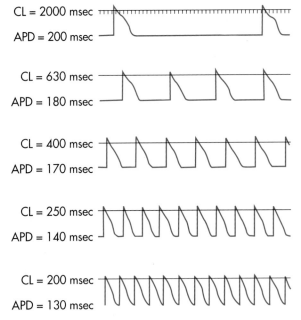

■ **Fig. 22-17**   Effect of changes in cycle length *(CL)* on the action potential duration *(APD)* of canine Purkinje fibers. (Modified from Singer D, Ten Eick RE: *Am J Cardiol* 28:381, 1971.)

contributions of i_K and of i_{to} to the relationship between action potential duration and cardiac cycle length vary from species to species.

■ *Natural Excitation of the Heart*

The nervous system controls various aspects of cardiac behavior, such as the heart rate and the strength of each contraction. However, cardiac function does not require an intact innervation. Indeed, a cardiac transplant patient, whose heart is completely denervated, can adapt well to stressful situations. The ability of the denervated, transplanted heart to function and adapt to changing conditions lies in certain intrinsic properties of cardiac tissue, especially its automaticity.

The properties of **automaticity** *(the ability to initiate its own beat) and* **rhythmicity** *(the regularity of such pacemaking activity) allow the heart to beat even when it is completely removed from the body.* If the coronary vasculature of an excised heart is artificially perfused with blood or an oxygenated electrolyte solution, rhythmic cardiac contractions persist for many hours. At least some cells in the atria and ventricles can initiate beats; such cells mainly reside in the nodal tissues or specialized conducting fibers of the heart.

The region of the mammalian heart that ordinarily generates impulses at the greatest frequency is the **sinoatrial (SA) node;** it is the main **pacemaker** of the heart. Detailed mapping of the electrical potentials on the surface of the right atrium reveals that two or three sites of automaticity, located 1 or 2 cm from the SA node itself, serve along with the SA node as an **atrial pacemaker complex.** At times, all of these loci initiate impulses simultaneously. At other times, the site of earliest excitation shifts from locus to locus, depending on certain conditions, such as the level of autonomic neural activity.

Regions of the heart other than the SA node may initiate beats under special circumstances. Such sites are called **ectopic foci,** or **ectopic pacemakers.** Ectopic foci may become pacemakers when (1) their own rhythmicity becomes enhanced, (2) the rhythmicity of the higher-order pacemakers becomes depressed, or (3) all conduction pathways between the ectopic focus and those regions with greater rhythmicity become blocked. Ectopic pacemakers may act as a safety mechanism when normal pacemaking centers fail. However, if an ectopic center fires while the normal pacemaking center still functions, the ectopic activity may induce either sporadic rhythm disturbances, such as **premature depolarizations** (Fig. 22-39), or continuous rhythm disturbances, such as **paroxysmal tachycardias** (Fig. 22-40).

When the SA node or other components of the atrial pacemaker complex are excised or destroyed, pacemaker cells in the AV junction usually take over the pacemaker function for the entire heart. After some time, which may vary from minutes to days, automatic cells in the atria usually become dominant. Purkinje fibers in the specialized conduction system of the ventricles also display automaticity. Characteristically, these fibers fire at a very slow rate. When the AV junction cannot conduct cardiac impulses from the atria to the ventricles (Fig. 22-38, *C*), these **idioventricular pacemakers** in the Purkinje fiber network initiate the ventricular contractions, but at a frequency of only 30 to 40 beats/min.

■ *Sinoatrial Node*

In humans, the SA node is about 8 mm long and 2 mm thick and lies posteriorly in the groove at the junction between the superior vena cava and the right atrium (Fig. 22-18). The sinus node artery runs lengthwise through the center of the node. The SA node contains two principal types of cells: (1) small, round cells, which have few organelles and myofibrils; and (2) slender, elongated cells, which are intermediate in appearance between the round and "ordinary" atrial myocardial cells. The round cells are probably the pacemaker cells, whereas the slender, elongated cells probably conduct the impulses within the node and to the nodal margins.

A typical transmembrane action potential recorded from a cell in the SA node is depicted in Fig. 22-19, *B*. Compared with the transmembrane potential recorded from a ventricular myocardial cell (Fig. 22-19, *A*), the resting potential of the SA node cell is usually less negative, the upstroke of the action potential (phase 0) is less steep, a plateau is not sustained, and repolarization (phase 3) is more gradual. These attributes are all characteristic of the slow response. Again, as in cells that exhibit the slow response, tetrodotoxin has no influence on the SA nodal action potential. Thus, the upstroke of the action potential is not produced by an inward current of Na^+ through fast channels.

The transmembrane potential during phase 4 is much less negative in SA (and AV) nodal automatic cells than in atrial or ventricular myocytes because the i_{K1} (inward

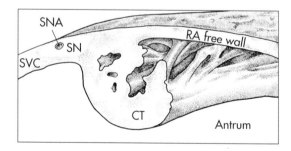

■ **Fig. 22-18** Location of the sinoatrial (SA) node near the junction between the superior vena cava (*SVC*) and the right atrium (*RA*). *SN,* SA node; *SNA,* sinoatrial artery; *CT,* crista terminalis. (Redrawn from James TN: *Am J Cardiol* 40:965, 1977.)

rectifying) type of K⁺ channel is sparse in the nodal cells. Therefore, the ratio of g_K to g_{Na} during phase 4 is much less in the nodal cells than in the myocytes. Hence, during phase 4, V_m deviates much more from the K⁺ equilibrium potential (E_K) in nodal cells than it does in myocytes.

However, the principal feature of a pacemaker fiber that distinguishes it from the other fibers we have discussed resides in phase 4. In nonautomatic cells, the potential remains constant during this phase, whereas *a pacemaker fiber is characterized by a slow diastolic depolarization throughout phase 4.* Depolarization proceeds at a steady rate until a threshold is attained, triggering an action potential.

The discharge frequency of pacemaker cells may be varied by a change in (1) the rate of depolarization during phase 4, (2) the maximal negativity during phase 4, or (3) the threshold potential (Fig. 22-20). When the rate of slow diastolic depolarization is increased (from *b* to *a* in Fig. 22-20, *A*), the threshold potential is attained earlier, and the heart rate increases. A rise in the threshold potential (from TP-1 to TP-2 in Fig. 22-20, *B*) delays the onset

of phase 0 (from time *b* to time *c*), and the heart rate is reduced accordingly. Similarly, when the maximal negative potential is increased (from *a* to *d* in Fig. 22-20, *B*), more time is required to reach threshold TP-2 when the slope of phase 4 remains unchanged, and the heart rate therefore diminishes.

Ordinarily, the frequency of pacemaker firing is controlled by the activity of both divisions of the autonomic nervous system. Increased sympathetic nervous activity, through the release of norepinephrine, raises the heart rate principally by increasing the slope of the slow diastolic depolarization. This mechanism of increasing heart rate occurs during physical exertion, anxiety, or certain illnesses, such as **febrile infectious diseases.**

Increased vagal activity, through the release of acetylcholine, diminishes the heart rate by hyperpolarizing the pacemaker cell membrane and reducing the slope of the slow diastolic depolarization (Fig. 22-21). These mechanisms of decreasing heart rate occur when vagal activity is predominant. An extreme example is **vasovagal syncope,** a brief period of lightheadedness or loss of consciousness caused by an intense burst of vagal activity. This type of syncope is a reflex response to pain or certain psychological stimuli.

Changes in autonomic neural activity usually do not change heart rate by altering the threshold level of V_m that initiates the firing of a nodal pacemaker cell. However, certain antiarrhythmic drugs, such as **quinidine** and **procainamide,** do raise the threshold potential of the automatic cells to less negative values.

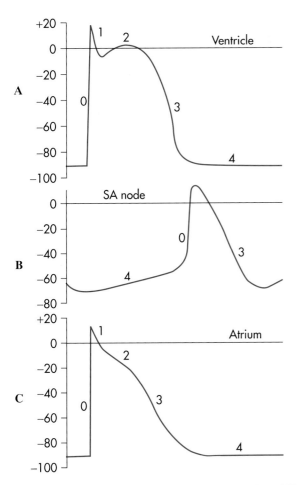

■ **Fig. 22-19** Typical action potentials (in millivolts) recorded from cells in the ventricle (**A**), SA node (**B**), and atrium (**C**). Sweep velocity in **B** is one half that in **A** or **C**. (From Hoffman BF, Cranefield PF: *Electrophysiology of the heart,* New York, 1960, McGraw-Hill.)

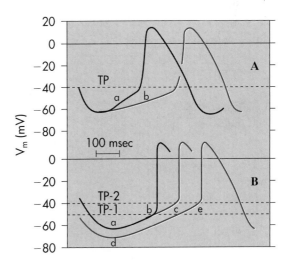

■ **Fig. 22-20** Mechanisms involved in the changes in frequency of pacemaker firing. In **A,** a reduction in the slope (from *a* to *b*) of slow diastolic depolarization diminishes the firing frequency. In **B,** an increase in the threshold potential (from *TP-1* to *TP-2*) or an increase in the magnitude of the resting potential (from *a* to *d*) also diminishes the firing frequency. (Redrawn from Hoffman BF, Cranefield PF: *Electrophysiology of the heart,* New York, 1960, McGraw-Hill.)

Ionic basis of automaticity. Several ionic currents contribute to the slow diastolic depolarization that characteristically occurs in the automatic cells in the heart. In the pacemaker cells of the SA node, at least three ionic currents mediate the slow diastolic depolarization: (1) an inward current, i_f, induced by hyperpolarization; (2) an inward Ca^{++} current, i_{Ca}; and (3) an outward K^+ current, i_K (Fig. 22-22).

The inward current, i_f, is activated near the end of repolarization. This "funny" current is carried mainly by Na^+ through specific channels that differ from the fast Na^+ channels. The current was dubbed "funny" because its discoverers had not expected to detect an inward Na^+ current in pacemaker cells after completion of repolarization. This current is activated as the membrane potential becomes more negative than about -50 mV. The more negative the membrane potential at this time, the greater is the activation of the i_f current.

The second current responsible for diastolic depolarization is the Ca^{++} current, i_{Ca}. This current is activated toward the end of phase 4, as the transmembrane potential reaches a value of about -55 mV (Fig. 22-22). Once the Ca^{++} channels are activated, influx of Ca^{++} into the cell increases. This influx accelerates the rate of diastolic depolarization, which then leads to the upstroke of the action potential. A decrease in the external Ca^{++} concentration (Fig. 22-23) or the addition of calcium channel antagonists (Fig. 22-24) diminishes the amplitude of the action potential and the slope of the slow diastolic depolarization in SA node cells.

The progressive diastolic depolarization mediated by the two inward currents, i_f and i_{Ca}, is opposed by an outward current, the delayed rectifier K^+ current, i_K. This efflux of K^+ tends to repolarize the cell after the upstroke of the action potential. K^+ continues to move out well beyond the time of maximal repolarization, but it diminishes throughout phase 4 (Fig. 22-22). As the current

diminishes, its opposition to the depolarizing effects of the two inward currents (i_{Ca} and i_f) also gradually decreases.

The ionic basis for automaticity in the AV node pacemaker cells resembles that in the SA node cells. Similar mechanisms also account for automaticity in ventricular Purkinje fibers, except that the Ca^{++} current is not involved. In other words, the slow diastolic depolarization is mediated principally by the imbalance between the effects of the hyperpolarization-induced inward current, i_f, and the gradually diminishing outward K^+ current, i_K.

The autonomic neurotransmitters affect automaticity by altering the ionic currents across the cell membranes. The adrenergic transmitters increase all three currents involved in SA nodal automaticity. To increase the slope of diastolic depolarization, the augmentations of i_f and

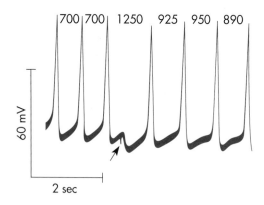

■ **Fig. 22-21** Effect of a brief vagal stimulus *(arrow)* on the transmembrane potential recorded from an SA node pacemaker cell in an isolated cat atrium preparation. The cardiac cycle lengths, in milliseconds, are denoted by the numbers at the top of the figure. (Modified from Jalife J, Moe GK: *Circ Res* 45:595, 1979, with permission of the American Heart Association.)

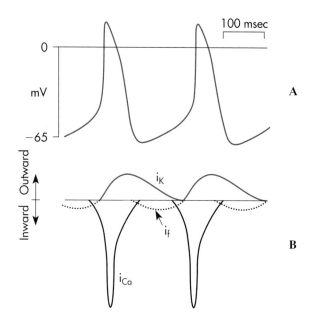

■ **Fig. 22-22** The transmembrane potential changes (**A**) that occur in SA node cells are produced by three principal currents (**B**): (1) an inward Ca^{++} current, i_{Ca}; (2) a hyperpolarization-induced inward current, i_f; and (3) an outward K^+ current, i_K.

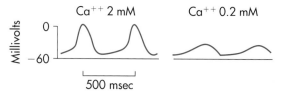

■ **Fig. 22-23** Transmembrane action potentials recorded from an SA node pacemaker cell in an isolated rabbit atrium preparation. The concentration of Ca^{++} in the bath was reduced from 2 mM to 0.2 mM. (Modified from Kohlhardt M, Figulla HR, Tripathi O: *Basic Res Cardiol* 71:17, 1976.)

i_{Ca} by the adrenergic transmitters must exceed the enhancement of i_K.

The hyperpolarization (Fig. 22-21) induced by the acetylcholine released at the vagus endings in the heart is achieved by an increase in g_K. This change in conductance is mediated through activation of specific K^+ channels, the **acetylcholine-regulated K^+** channels. Acetylcholine also depresses the i_f and i_{Ca} currents. The autonomic neural effects on cardiac cells are described in greater detail in Chapter 24.

Overdrive suppression. The automaticity of pacemaker cells diminishes after a period of excitation at a high frequency. This phenomenon is known as **overdrive suppression.** Because the intrinsic rhythmicity of the SA node is greater than that of the other latent pacemaking sites in the heart, the firing of the SA node tends to suppress the automaticity in the other loci.

> If an ectopic focus in one of the atria suddenly began to fire at a high rate (e.g., 150 impulses/min) in an individual with a normal heart rate of 70 beats/min, the ectopic site would become the pacemaker for the entire heart. When that rapid ectopic focus suddenly stopped firing, the SA node might remain briefly quiescent because of overdrive suppression. The interval from the end of the period of overdrive until the SA node resumes firing is called the **sinus node recovery time.** In patients with **sick sinus syndrome,** the sinus node recovery time is prolonged. The resultant period of **asystole** (absence of a heartbeat) may cause the patient to lose consciousness.

Overdrive suppression results from the activity of the membrane pump, Na^+, K^+-ATPase, which extrudes 3 Na^+ from the cell in exchange for 2 K^+. Normally, a certain amount of Na^+ enters the cardiac cell during each depolarization. The more frequently the cell is depolarized, therefore, the more Na^+ enters the cell per minute. At high excitation frequencies, the activity of the Na^+, K^+-ATPase increases to extrude this larger amount of Na^+ from the cell interior. Because the amount of Na^+ extruded by the pump exceeds the amount of K^+ that enters the cell, the activity of the Na^+, K^+-ATPase hyperpolarizes the cell. Therefore, the slow diastolic depolarization requires more time to reach the firing threshold,

as shown in Fig. 22-20, *B.* Furthermore, when the overdrive suddenly ceases, the activity of the Na^+, K^+-ATPase does not slow down instantaneously but temporarily remains overactive. This excessive extrusion of Na^+ opposes the gradual depolarization of the pacemaker cell during phase 4, and thereby suppresses the cell's intrinsic automaticity transiently.

■ *Atrial Conduction*

From the SA node, the cardiac impulse spreads radially throughout the right atrium (Fig. 22-25) along ordinary atrial myocardial fibers, at a conduction velocity of approximately 1 m/sec. A special pathway, the anterior interatrial myocardial band (or Bachmann's bundle), conducts the impulse from the SA node directly to the left atrium. The wave of excitation that proceeds inferiorly through the right atrium ultimately reaches the AV node, which is normally the sole route of entry of the cardiac impulse to the ventricles.

The configuration of the atrial transmembrane potential is depicted in Fig. 22-19, *C.* Compared with the potential recorded from a typical ventricular fiber (Fig. 22-19, *A*), the atrial plateau (phase 2) is briefer and less developed, and repolarization (phase 3) is slower. The action potential duration in atrial myocytes is shorter than that in ventricular myocytes because the efflux of K^+ is greater during the plateau in atrial myocytes than in ventricular myocytes.

■ *Atrioventricular Conduction*

The atrial excitation wave reaches the ventricles via the AV node. In adult humans, this node is approximately 22 mm long, 10 mm wide, and 3 mm thick. The node is situated posteriorly on the right side of the interatrial septum near the ostium of the coronary sinus. The AV node contains the same two cell types as the SA node, but the round cells in the AV node are less abundant and the elongated cells predominate.

The AV node is made up of three functional regions: (1) the AN region, the transitional zone between the atrium and the remainder of the node; (2) the N region,

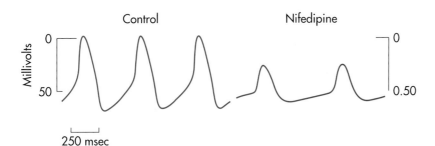

■ **Fig. 22-24** Effects of nifedipine (5.6×10^{-7} M), a Ca^{++} channel antagonist, on the transmembrane potentials recorded from an SA node cell in a rabbit. (From Ning W, Wit AL: *Am Heart J* 106:345, 1983.)

the midportion of the AV node; and (3) the NH region, the zone in which nodal fibers gradually merge with the bundle of His, which is the upper portion of the specialized conducting system for the ventricles. Normally, the AV node and bundle of His are the only pathways along which the cardiac impulse travels from atria to ventricles.

Some people have accessory AV pathways. Because these pathways often serve as a part of a reentry loop (Fig. 22-30), they can be associated with serious cardiac rhythm disturbances. **Wolff-Parkinson-White syndrome,** a congenital disturbance, is the most common clinical disorder in which a bypass tract of myocardial fibers serves as an accessory pathway between atria and ventricles. Ordinarily, the syndrome causes no functional abnormality. The disturbance is easily detected in the electrocardiogram (ECG) because a portion of the ventricular myocardium is excited via the bypass tract before the remainder of the ventricular myocardium is excited via the AV node and His-Purkinje system. This preexcitation can be seen as a bizarre configuration in the ventricular (QRS) complex of the ECG. Occasionally, however, a reentry loop develops in which the atrial impulse travels to the ventricles via one of the two AV pathways (AV node or bypass tract), and then back to the atria through the other of the two pathways. Continuous circling around the loop leads to a very rapid rhythm **(supraventricular tachycardia).** This rapid rhythm may be incapacitating because it may not allow sufficient time for ventricular filling. Transient block of the AV node by injecting adenosine intravenously or by increasing vagal activity reflexly (by pressing on the neck over the carotid sinus region) usually abolishes the tachycardia and restores a normal sinus rhythm.

Several features of AV conduction are of physiological and clinical significance. The principal delay in the passage of the impulse from the atria to the ventricles occurs in the AN and N regions of the AV node. The conduction velocity is actually less in the N region than in the AN region. However, the path length is substantially greater in the AN than in the N region. The conduction times through the AN and N zones account for the delay between the start of the **P wave** (the electrical manifestation of the spread of atrial excitation) and the **QRS complex** (spread of ventricular excitation) on an ECG (Fig. 22-33). *Functionally, the delay between atrial and ventricular excitation permits optimal ventricular filling during atrial contraction.*

In the N region, slow-response action potentials prevail. The resting potential is about -60 mV, the upstroke velocity is low (about 5 V/sec), and the conduction velocity is about 0.05 m/sec. Tetrodotoxin, which blocks the fast Na^+ channels, has virtually no effect on the action potentials in this region (or on any other slow-response fibers). Conversely, Ca^{++} channel antagonists decrease the amplitude and duration of the action potentials (Fig. 22-26) and depress AV conduction. The shapes of the action potentials in the AN region are intermediate between those in the N region and atria. Similarly, the action potentials in the NH region are transitional between those in the N region and bundle of His.

Like other slow-response action potentials, the relative refractory period of cells in the N region extends well beyond the period of complete repolarization; that is, these cells display postrepolarization refractoriness (Fig. 22-16). As the time between successive atrial depolarizations is decreased, conduction through the AV junction slows (Fig. 22-27). An abnormal prolongation of the AV conduction time is called **first-degree AV block** (Fig.

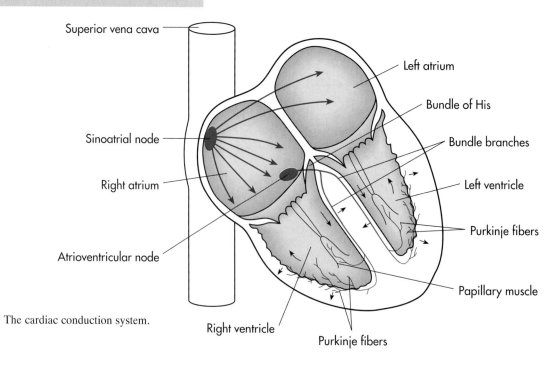

■ **Fig. 22-25** The cardiac conduction system.

22-38, *A*). Most of the prolongation of AV conduction induced by a decrease in atrial cycle length takes place in the N region of the AV node.

Impulses tend to be blocked in the AV node at stimulation frequencies that are easily conducted in other regions of the heart. If the atria are depolarized at a high repetition rate, only a fraction (e.g., one half) of the atrial impulses might be conducted through the AV junction to the ventricles. The conduction pattern in which only a fraction of the atrial impulses are conducted to the ventricles is called **second-degree AV block** (Fig. 22-38, *B*). This type of block may protect the ventricles from excessive contraction frequencies, wherein the filling time between contractions might be inadequate.

Retrograde conduction can occur through the AV node. However, the propagation time is significantly longer and the impulse is blocked at lower repetition rates when the impulse is conducted in the retrograde instead of in the antegrade direction. Finally the AV node is a common site for reentry; the underlying mechanisms are explained on p 349.

The autonomic nervous system regulates AV conduction. Weak vagal activity may simply prolong the AV conduction time. Thus, for any given atrial cycle length, the atrium to His (A-H) or atrium to ventricle (A-V) conduction time will be prolonged by vagal stimulation (Fig. 22-27). Stronger vagal activity may cause some or all of the impulses arriving from the atria to be blocked in the node. The conduction pattern in which none of the atrial impulses reach the ventricles is called **third-degree,** or **complete, AV block** (Fig. 22-38, *C*). The vagally induced delay or absence of conduction through the A-V junction occurs mainly in the N region of the node.

Acetylcholine released by the vagal nerve fibers hyperpolarizes the conducting fibers in the N region (Fig. 22-28). The greater the hyperpolarization at the time of arrival of the atrial impulse, the more impaired is the AV conduction. In the experiment shown in Fig. 22-28, vagus nerve fibers are stimulated intensely (at *St*) shortly before the second atrial depolarization *(A₂)*. That atrial impulse arrives at the AV node cell when its cell membrane is maximally hyperpolarized in response to the vagal stimulus. The absence of a corresponding depolarization of the bundle of His shows that the vagal stimulus prevents the conduction of the second atrial impulse through the AV node. Only a small, nonpropagated response to the second atrial impulse is evident in the recording from the conducting fiber.

The cardiac sympathetic nerves, on the other hand, facilitate AV conduction. They decrease the AV conduction

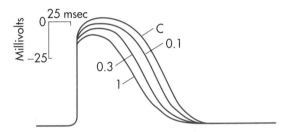

■ **Fig. 22-26** Transmembrane potentials recorded from a rabbit atrioventricular (AV) node cell under control conditions *(C)* and in the presence of the calcium channel antagonist diltiazem, in concentrations of 0.1, 0.3, and 1 μmol/L. (Redrawn from Hirth C, Borchard U, Hafner D: *J Mol Cell Cardiol* 15:799, 1983.)

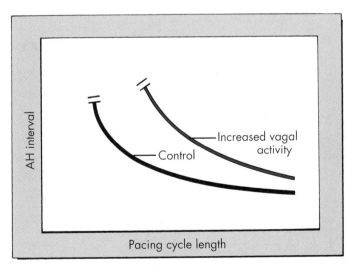

■ **Fig. 22-27** Changes in atrium-His *(AH)* intervals induced by pacing the atria at various cycle lengths in a group of human subjects under control conditions and during a reflexly induced increase in vagal activity produced by the intravenous infusion of phenylephrine. (Redrawn from Page RL et al: *Circ Res,* 68:1614, 1991, with permission of the American Heart Association.)

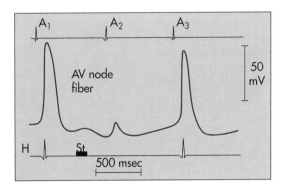

■ **Fig. 22-28** Effects of a brief vagal stimulus *(St)* on the transmembrane potential recorded from an AV nodal fiber from a rabbit. Note that shortly after vagal stimulation, the membrane of the fiber was hyperpolarized. The atrial excitation *(A₂)* that arrived at the AV node when the cell was hyperpolarized failed to be conducted, as denoted by the absence of a depolarization in the His electrogram *(H).* The atrial excitations that preceded *(A₁)* and followed *(A₃)* excitation A₂ were conducted to the His bundle region. (Redrawn from Mazgalev T et al: *Am J Physiol* 251:H631, 1986.)

time and enhance the rhythmicity of the latent pacemakers in the AV junction. The norepinephrine released at the sympathetic nerve terminals increases the amplitude and slope of the upstroke of the AV nodal action potentials, principally in the AN and N regions of the node.

■ *Ventricular Conduction*

The bundle of His passes subendocardially down the right side of the interventricular septum for about 1 cm and then divides into the right and left **bundle branches** (Figs. 22-25 and 22-29). The right bundle branch, which is a direct continuation of the bundle of His, proceeds down the right side of the interventricular septum. The left bundle branch, which is considerably thicker than the right, arises almost perpendicularly from the bundle of His and perforates the interventricular septum. On the subendocardial surface of the left side of the interventricular septum, the left bundle branch splits into a thin anterior division and a thick posterior division.

Impulse conduction in the right or left bundle branch or in either division of the left bundle branch may be impaired. Conduction blocks may develop in one or more of these conduction pathways as a consequence of **coronary artery disease** or degenerative processes associated with aging, and they give rise to characteristic ECG patterns. Block of either of the main bundle

branches is known as right or left **bundle branch block.** Block of either division of the left bundle branch is called left anterior or left posterior **hemiblock.**

The right bundle branch and the two divisions of the left bundle branch ultimately subdivide into a complex network of conducting fibers, called **Purkinje fibers,** which spread out over the subendocardial surfaces of both ventricles. In certain mammalian species, such as cattle, the Purkinje fiber network is arranged in discrete, encapsulated bundles (Fig. 22-29).

Purkinje fibers have abundant, linearly arranged sarcomeres, as do myocytes. However, the T-tubular system is absent in the Purkinje fibers of many species, although it is well developed in the myocytes. Purkinje fibers are the broadest cells in the heart: they are 70 to 80 μm in diameter, compared with diameters of 10 to 15 μm for ventricular myocytes. Partly because of their large diameter, conduction velocity (1 to 4 m/sec) in the Purkinje fibers exceeds that of any other fiber type within the heart. The increased conduction velocity permits a rapid activation of the entire endocardial surface of the ventricles.

The action potentials recorded from Purkinje fibers resemble those of ordinary ventricular myocardial fibers (Figs. 22-9 and 22-19, *A*). In general, phase 1 is prominent in Purkinje fiber action potentials (Fig. 22-13) and the duration of the plateau (phase 2) is intermediate between those of epicardial and midmyocardial myocytes (Fig. 22-9).

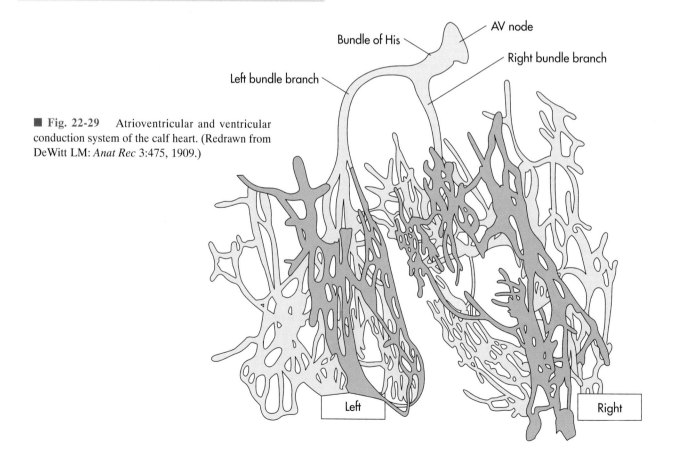

■ **Fig. 22-29** Atrioventricular and ventricular conduction system of the calf heart. (Redrawn from DeWitt LM: *Anat Rec* 3:475, 1909.)

AV node

Bundle of His

Right bundle branch

Left bundle branch

Left

Right

Because of the long refractory period of Purkinje fiber action potentials, many premature excitations of the atria are conducted through the AV junction but are blocked by the Purkinje fibers. Blockage of these atrial excitations prevents premature contraction of the ventricles. This function of protecting the ventricles against the effects of premature atrial depolarizations is especially pronounced at slow heart rates, because the action potential duration, and hence the effective refractory period of the Purkinje fibers, varies inversely with the heart rate (Fig. 22-17). At slow heart rates, the effective refractory period of the Purkinje fibers is especially prolonged; as the heart rate increases, the refractory period diminishes. Similar directional changes in the refractory period occur also in ventricular myocytes in response to changes in rate (Fig. 22-9). However, in the AV node, the effective refractory period does not change appreciably over the normal range of heart rates, and it actually increases at very rapid heart rates (Fig. 22-27). Therefore, *when the atrium is excited at high repetition rates, it is the AV node that protects the ventricles from these excessively high frequencies.*

The first portions of the ventricles to be excited by impulses arriving from the AV node are the interventricular septum (except the basal portion) and the papillary muscles. The wave of activation spreads into the substance of the septum from both its left and right endocardial surfaces. Early contraction of the septum tends to make it more rigid and allows it to serve as an anchor point for the contraction of the remaining ventricular myocardium. Also, early contraction of the papillary muscles prevents eversion of the AV valves during ventricular systole.

The endocardial surfaces of both ventricles are activated rapidly, but the wave of excitation spreads from endocardium to epicardium at a slower velocity (about 0.3 to 0.4 m/sec). Because the right ventricular wall is appreciably thinner than the left, the epicardial surface of the right ventricle is activated earlier than that of the left ventricle. Also, apical and central epicardial regions of both ventricles are activated somewhat earlier than their respective basal regions. The last portions of the ventricles to be excited are the posterior basal epicardial regions and a small zone in the basal portion of the interventricular septum.

■ *Reentry*

Under certain conditions, a cardiac impulse may reexcite some myocardial region through which it had passed previously. This phenomenon, known as **reentry,** is responsible for many clinical **arrhythmias** (disturbances of cardiac rhythm). The reentry may be **ordered** or **random.** In the ordered variety the impulse traverses a fixed anatomic path, whereas in the random type the path continues to change.

The conditions necessary for reentry are illustrated in Fig. 22-30. In each of the four panels a single bundle *(S)* of cardiac fibers splits into a left *(L)* and right *(R)* branch. A connecting bundle *(C)* runs between the two branches. Normally the impulse moving down bundle *S* is conducted along the *L* and *R* branches (panel *A*). As the impulse reaches connecting link *C*, it enters from both sides and becomes extinguished at the point of collision. The impulse from the left side cannot proceed farther because the tissue beyond is absolutely refractory; it has just been depolarized from the other direction. The impulse also cannot pass through bundle *C* from the right, for the same reason.

Panel *B* shows that the impulse cannot complete the circuit if antegrade block exists in the *L* and *R* branches of the fiber bundle. Furthermore, if bidirectional block exists at any point in the loop (e.g., branch *R* in panel *C*), the impulse also cannot reenter.

A necessary condition for reentry is that at some point in the loop the impulse can pass in one direction but not in the other . This phenomenon is called **unidirectional block.** As shown in panel *D*, the impulse may travel down branch *L* normally and become blocked in the antegrade direction in branch *R*. The impulse that was conducted down branch *L* and through the connecting branch *C* may be able to penetrate the depressed region in branch *R* from the retrograde direction, even though the antegrade impulse had been blocked previously at this same site. Why is the antegrade impulse blocked but not the retrograde impulse? The reason is that the antegrade impulse arrives at the depressed region in branch *R* earlier than the retrograde impulse, because the retrograde impulse traverses a longer path. Therefore, the antegrade

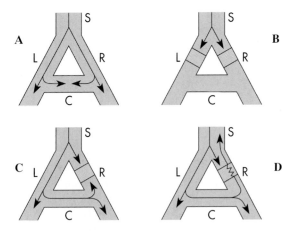

■ **Fig. 22-30** The role of unidirectional block in reentry. In **A,** an excitation wave traveling down a single bundle *(S)* of fibers continues down the left *(L)* and right *(R)* branches. The depolarization wave enters the connecting branch *(C)* from both ends and is extinguished at the zone of collision. In **B,** the wave is blocked in the *L* and *R* branches. In **C,** bidirectional block exists in branch *R*. In **D,** unidirectional block exists in branch *R*. The antegrade impulse is blocked, but the retrograde impulse is conducted through and reenters bundle *S*.

impulse may be blocked simply because it arrives at the depressed region during its effective refractory period. If the retrograde impulse is delayed sufficiently, the refractory period may have ended and the impulse can be conducted back into bundle *S*.

Although unidirectional block is a necessary condition for reentry, it alone cannot cause reentry. *For reentry to occur, the effective refractory period of the reentered region must be shorter than the propagation time around the loop.* In panel *D*, if the tissue just beyond the depressed zone in branch *R* is still refractory from the antegrade depolarization, the retrograde impulse will not be conducted into branch *S*. Therefore the conditions that promote reentry are those that prolong conduction time or shorten effective refractory period.

The functional components of the reentry loops responsible for specific arrhythmias in intact hearts are diverse. Some loops are large and involve entire specialized conduction bundles, whereas others are microscopic. The loop may include myocardial fibers, specialized conducting fibers, nodal cells, and junctional tissues in almost any conceivable arrangement. Also, cardiac cells in the loop may be normal or deranged.

■ *Triggered Activity*

Triggered activity is so named because it is always coupled to a preceding action potential. Because reentrant activity is also coupled to a preceding action potential, the arrhythmias induced by triggered activity are usually difficult to distinguish from those induced by reentry. Triggered activity is caused by **afterdepolarizations.** Two types of afterdepolarizations are recognized: **early (EAD)** and **delayed (DAD).** EADs appear at the end of the plateau (phase 2) or about midway through repolarization (phase 3), whereas DADs occur near the very end of repolarization or just after full repolarization (phase 4).

Early afterdepolarizations. EADs tend to appear near the end of the action potential plateau or during repolarization, but before the cell has fully repolarized. They are more likely to occur when the prevailing heart rate is slow; a rapid heart rate suppresses EADs. In the experiment shown in Fig. 22-31, EADs are induced by cesium in an isolated Purkinje fiber preparation. No afterdepolarizations are evident when the preparation is driven at a cycle length of 2 seconds. When the cycle length is increased to 4 seconds, however, EADs appear. Most of the EADs are subthreshold *(first two arrows)*, but one of the EADs reaches threshold and triggers an action potential. When the cycle length is increased to 6 seconds, each driven action potential generates an EAD that triggers a second action potential. Furthermore, when the cycle length is increased to 10 seconds, each driven action potential triggers a salvo of four or five additional action potentials.

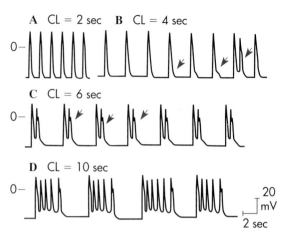

■ **Fig. 22-31** Effect of pacing at different cycle lengths *(CL)* on cesium-induced early afterdepolarizations (EADs) in a canine Purkinje fiber. **A,** EADs not evident. **B,** EADs first appear *(arrows)*. Third EAD reaches threshold and triggers an action potential *(third arrow)*. **C,** EADs that appear after each driven depolarization trigger an action potential. **D,** Triggered action potentials occur in salvos. (Modified from Damiano BP, Rosen M: *Circulation* 69:1013, 1984, with permission of the American Heart Association.)

EADs are more likely to occur in cardiac cells with prolonged action potentials than in cells with shorter action potentials. For example, EADs can be induced more readily in myocytes from the midmyocardial region of the ventricular walls than in myocytes from the endocardial or epicardial regions, owing to the disparity in these cells' action potential durations (Fig. 22-9). Furthermore, EADs may be produced experimentally by interventions that prolong the action potential. As we have seen, in the experiment shown in Fig. 22-31, EADs are more prevalent as the basic cycle length is increased. Such increases in basic cycle length do, of course, prolong the action potential (Fig. 22-17), and this prolongation undoubtedly contributes to the generation of the EADs. Certain antiarrhythmic drugs, such as **quinidine,** act to prolong the action potential. Consequently, these drugs increase the likelihood that EADs may occur. Hence, *antiarrhythmic drugs are also frequently proarrhythmic.*

The direct correlation between a cell's action potential duration and its susceptibility to EADs is probably related to the time required for the Ca^{++} channels in the cell membranes to recover from inactivation. When action potentials are sufficiently prolonged, those Ca^{++} channels that were activated at the beginning of the plateau have sufficient time to recover from inactivation and thus may be reactivated before the cell fully repolarizes. This secondary activation could then trigger an early afterdepolarization.

Delayed afterdepolarizations. In contrast to EADs, DADs are more likely to occur when the heart rate is high. The most important characteristics of DADs are shown in Fig. 22-32. In the experiment depicted in this

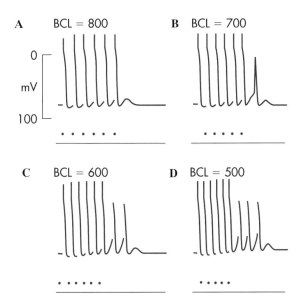

A BCL = 800   B BCL = 700

0
mV
100

C BCL = 600   D BCL = 500

■ **Fig. 22-32**   Transmembrane action potentials recorded from isolated canine Purkinje fibers. Acetylstrophanthidin, a digitalis-like agent, was added to the bath, and sequences of six driven beats (denoted by the dots) were produced at basic cycle lengths *(BCL)* of 800, 700, 600, and 500 msec. Note that delayed afterpotentials occurred after the driven beats, and that these afterpotentials reached threshold after the last driven beat in panels **B** to **D**. (From Ferrier GR, Saunders JH, Mendez C: *Circ Res* 32:600, 1973, with permission of the American Heart Association.)

figure, transmembrane potentials are recorded from Purkinje fibers exposed to a high concentration of acetylstrophanthidin, a digitalis-like substance. In the absence of any driving stimuli, these fibers are quiescent.

In each panel of Fig. 22-32, a sequence of six driven depolarizations is induced at a specific basic cycle length. When the cycle length is 800 msec (*A*), the last driven depolarization is followed by a brief, partial depolarization (DAD) that does not reach threshold. Once that afterdepolarization subsides, the transmembrane potential remains constant until another driving stimulus is given. The upstroke of a DAD can be detected after each of the first five driven depolarizations.

When the basic cycle length is reduced to 700 msec (*B*), the DAD that followed the last driven beat does reach threshold, and a nondriven depolarization (or extrasystole) ensues. This extrasystole is itself followed by an afterpotential that is subthreshold. Reducing the basic cycle length to 600 msec (*C*) also evokes an extrasystole after the last driven depolarization. The afterpotential that follows the extrasystole does reach threshold, however, and a second extrasystole occurs. When the six driven depolarizations are separated by intervals of 500 msec (*D*), a sequence of three extrasystoles follows. Slightly shorter basic cycle lengths or slightly greater concentrations of acetylstrophanthidin evoke a long sequence of nondriven beats; such a sequence resembles a paroxysmal tachycardia (Fig. 22-40).

DADs are associated with elevated intracellular Ca^{++} concentrations. The amplitudes of the DADs are increased by interventions that raise intracellular Ca^{++} concentrations. Such interventions include increasing the extracellular Ca^{++} concentration and administering toxic amounts of digitalis glycosides. The elevated levels of intracellular Ca^{++} provoke the oscillatory release of Ca^{++} from the sarcoplasmic reticulum. Hence, in myocardial cells, DADs are accompanied by small, rhythmic changes in developed force. The high intracellular Ca^{++} concentrations also activate certain membrane channels that permit the passage of Na^+ and K^+. The net flux of these cations constitutes a **transient inward current, i_{ti}**, that is at least partly responsible for the afterdepolarization of the cell membrane. The elevated intracellular Ca^{++} concentration may also activate Na^+, Ca^{++} exchange (see Chapter 1). This electrogenic exchanger, which pumps 3 Na^+ into the cell for each Ca^{++} it ejects, also creates a net inward current of cations that contributes to the DAD.

■ *Electrocardiography*

The ECG enables the physician to infer the course of the cardiac impulse by recording the variations in electrical potential at various loci on the surface of the body. By analyzing the details of these fluctuations of electrical potential, the physician gains valuable insight into (1) the anatomic orientation of the heart; (2) the relative sizes of its chambers; (3) various disturbances of rhythm and conduction; (4) the extent, location, and progress of ischemic damage to the myocardium; (5) the effects of altered electrolyte concentrations; and (6) the influence of certain drugs (notably digitalis, antiarrhythmic agents, and Ca^{++} channel antagonists). Because electrocardiography is an extensive and complex discipline, only elementary principles are considered in this section.

■ *Scalar Electrocardiography*

In electrocardiography a **lead** is the electrical connection from the patient's skin to the recording device (electrocardiograph). The leads are connected to a galvanometer (a device that measures the strength of an electrical current) within the electrocardiograph. The systems of leads used to record routine ECGs are oriented in certain planes of the body. The diverse electromotive forces that exist in the heart at any moment can be represented by a three-dimensional **vector** (a quantity with magnitude and direction). A system of recording leads oriented in a given plane detects only the projection of the three-dimensional vector on that plane. The potential difference between two recording electrodes represents the projection of the vector on the line between the two leads. Components of vectors projected on such lines are not vectors but **scalar quantities** (having magnitude, but not direction). Hence, a recording of changes of the differences of potential between two points on the surface of the skin over time is called a scalar ECG.

The scalar ECG detects changes over time of the electrical potential between some point on the surface of the skin and an indifferent electrode, or between pairs of points on the skin surface. The cardiac impulse progresses through the heart in a complex, three-dimensional pattern. Hence, the precise configuration of the ECG varies from individual to individual, and in any given individual the pattern varies with the anatomic location of the leads. The graphic display of the electrical impulse recorded by an ECG is called a **tracing.**

In general, a tracing consists of P, QRS, and T waves (Fig. 22-33). The PR interval (or more precisely, the PQ interval) is a measure of the time from the onset of atrial activation to the onset of ventricular activation; it normally ranges from 0.12 to 0.20 second. A considerable fraction of this time involves passage of the impulse through the AV conduction system. *Pathological prolongations of the PR interval are associated with disturbances of AV conduction, which may be produced by inflammatory, circulatory, pharmacologic, or nervous mechanisms.*

The configuration and amplitude of the QRS complex vary considerably among individuals. The duration is usually between 0.06 and 0.10 second. An abnormally prolonged QRS complex may indicate a block in the normal conduction pathways through the ventricles (such as a block of the left or right bundle branch). During the ST interval, the entire ventricular myocardium is depolarized. Therefore, the ST segment normally lies on the **isoelectric line.** *Any appreciable deviation of the ST segment from the isoelectric line may indicate ischemic damage of the myocardium.* The QT interval is sometimes referred to as the period of "electrical systole" of the ventricles; the QT interval is closely correlated with the

mean action potential duration of the ventricular myocytes. The QT interval duration is about 0.4 second, but it varies inversely with heart rate, mainly because the myocardial cell action potential duration varies inversely with heart rate (Fig. 22-17).

In most leads, the T wave is deflected in the same direction from the isoelectric line as is the major component of the QRS complex, although biphasic or oppositely directed T waves are perfectly normal in certain leads. When the T wave and QRS complex deviate in the same direction from the isoelectric line, it indicates that the repolarization process proceeds in a direction counter to the depolarization process. *T waves that are abnormal either in direction or in amplitude may indicate myocardial damage, electrolyte disturbances, or cardiac hypertrophy.*

■ *Standard Limb Leads*

The original ECG lead system was devised by Einthoven. In his lead system, the vector sum of all cardiac electrical activity at any moment is called the **resultant cardiac vector.** This directional electrical force is considered to lie in the center of an equilateral triangle whose apices are located in the left and right shoulders and the pubic region (Fig. 22-34). This triangle, called Einthoven's triangle, is oriented in the frontal plane of the body. Hence, only the projection of the resultant cardiac vector on the frontal plane is detected by this system of leads. For convenience, the electrodes are connected to the right and left forearms rather than to the corresponding shoulders, because the arms represent simple extensions of the leads from the shoulders. Similarly, the leg represents an extension of the lead system from the pubis, and thus the third electrode is usually connected to an ankle (usually the left one).

Certain conventions dictate the manner in which these standard limb leads are connected to the galvanometer. Lead I records the potential difference between the left arm *(LA)* and the right arm *(RA)*. The galvanometer connections are such that when the potential at *LA* (V_{LA}) exceeds the potential at *RA* (V_{RA}), the galvanometer stylus is deflected upward from the isoelectric line. In Figs. 22-34 and 22-35, this arrangement of the galvanometer connections for lead I is designated by a (+) at *LA* and by a (−) at *RA*. Lead II records the potential difference between *RA* and *LL* (left leg), and the stylus is deflected upward when V_{LL} exceeds V_{RA}. Finally, lead III registers the potential difference between *LA* and *LL*, and the stylus is deflected upward when V_{LL} exceeds V_{LA}. These galvanometer connections were arbitrarily chosen so that the QRS complexes are upright in all three standard limb leads in most normal individuals.

Let the frontal projection of the resultant cardiac vector at some moment be represented by an arrow (tail negative, head positive), as in Fig. 22-34. The potential dif-

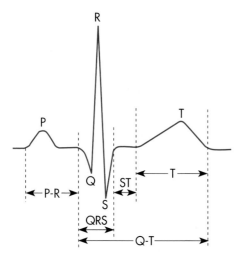

■ **Fig. 22-33** The important deflections and intervals of a typical scalar electrocardiogram.

ference, $V_{LA} - V_{RA}$, recorded in lead I is represented by the component of the vector projected along the horizontal line between *LA* and *RA*, also shown in Fig. 22-34. If the vector makes an angle, Θ, of 60 degrees with the horizontal line (as in Fig. 22-35, *A*), the magnitude of the potential recorded by lead I equals the vector magnitude times cosine 60 degrees. The deflection recorded in lead I is upward because the positive arrowhead lies closer to *LA* than to *RA*. The deflection in lead II is also upright because the arrowhead lies closer to *LL* than to *RA*. The magnitude of the lead II deflection is greater than that in lead I because in this example the direction of the vector parallels that of lead II; therefore, the magnitude of the projection on lead II exceeds that on lead I. Similarly, in lead III, the deflection is upright and its magnitude equals that in lead I.

If the vector in Fig. 22-35, *A* is the result of electrical events that occur during the peak of the QRS complex, the orientation of this vector is said to represent the **mean electrical axis** of the heart in the frontal plane. The positive direction of this axis is taken in the clockwise direction from the horizontal plane (contrary to the usual mathematical convention). In normal individuals, the average mean electrical axis is approximately + 60

degrees (as in Fig. 22-35, *A*). Therefore, the QRS complexes are usually upright in all three leads and largest in lead II.

Changes in the mean electrical axis may occur if the anatomic position of the heart is altered or in certain cardiovascular disturbances that alter the relative mass of the right and left ventricles. For example, the axis tends to shift toward the left (more horizontal) in short, stocky individuals and toward the right (more vertical) in tall, thin persons. Also, in left or right **ventricular hypertrophy** (increased myocardial mass of either ventricle), the axis shifts toward the hypertrophied side.

If the mean electrical axis shifts substantially to the right (as in Fig. 22-35, *B*, where Θ = 120 degrees), the projections of the QRS complexes on the standard leads change considerably. In this case, the largest upright deflection is in lead III, and the deflection in lead I is inverted because the arrowhead is closer to *RA* than to *LA*. When the axis shifts to the left (Fig. 22-35, *C*, where Θ = 0 degrees), the largest upright deflection is in lead I, and the QRS complex in lead III is inverted.

In addition to limb leads I, II, and III, other limb leads that are also oriented in the frontal plane are routinely recorded in patients. The axes of such **unipolar limb leads** form angles of + 90, −30, and −150 degrees with

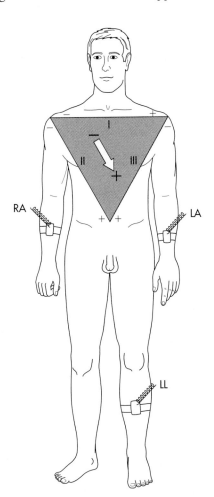

■ Fig. 22-34 Einthoven triangle, illustrating the galvanometer connections for standard limb leads I, II, and III.

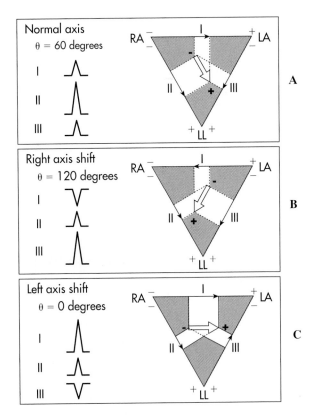

■ Fig. 22-35 Magnitude and direction of the QRS complexes in limb leads I, II, and III, when the mean electrical axis (Θ) is 60 degrees **(A)**, 120 degrees **(B)**, and 0 degrees **(C).**

the horizontal axis. Furthermore, the **precordial leads** are also recorded to determine the projections of the cardiac vector on the sagittal and transverse planes of the body. These precordial leads are recorded from six selected points on the anterior and lateral surfaces of the chest in the vicinity of the heart. The unipolar and precordial lead systems are described in all textbooks on electrocardiography and are not considered further here.

■ *Arrhythmias*

Cardiac arrhythmias reflect disturbances of either **impulse initiation** or **impulse propagation.** Disturbances of impulse initiation include those that arise from the SA node and those that originate from various ectopic foci. The principal disturbances of impulse propagation are conduction blocks and reentrant rhythms.

■ *Altered Sinoatrial Rhythms*

Earlier in this chapter, mechanisms that vary the firing frequency of cardiac pacemaker cells were described (Fig. 22-20). Changes in the SA nodal firing rate are usually produced by the cardiac autonomic nerves. Examples of ECGs of **sinus tachycardia** and **sinus bradycardia** are shown in Fig. 22-36. The P, QRS, and T deflections are all normal, but the cardiac cycle duration (the PP interval) is altered. Characteristically, in response to sinus bradycardia or tachycardia development, cardiac frequency changes gradually, and several beats are required to attain its new steady-state value. ECG evidence of respiratory cardiac arrhythmia is common and manifests as a rhythmic variation in the PP interval at the respiratory frequency (Fig. 24-10).

■ *Atrioventricular Conduction Blocks*

Various physiological, pharmacologic, and pathological processes can impede impulse transmission through the AV conduction tissue. The site of block can be localized more precisely by recording the **His bundle electrogram** (Fig. 22-37). To obtain such tracings, an electrode catheter is introduced into a peripheral vein and threaded centrally until the electrode lies in the AV junctional region. When the electrode is properly positioned, a distinct deflection (*H* in Fig. 22-37) is registered as the cardiac impulse passes through the bundle of His. The time intervals required for propagation from the atrium to the bundle of His (A-H interval) and from the bundle of His to the ventricles (H-V interval) may be measured accurately. Abnormal prolongation of the former or latter interval indicates block above or below the bundle of His, respectively.

Three degrees of AV block can be distinguished, as shown in Fig. 22-38. **First-degree AV block** is characterized by a prolonged P-R interval. In Fig. 22-38, *A*, the PR interval is 0.28 second; an interval greater than 0.20 second is abnormal. In most cases of first-degree block, the A-H interval is prolonged and the H-V interval is normal. Hence, the delay in a first-degree AV block is located above the His bundle (i.e., in the AV node).

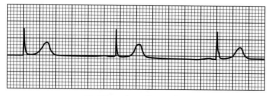

A, Normal sinus rhythm.

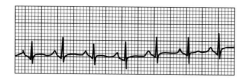

B, Sinus tachycardia.

C, Sinus bradycardia.

■ **Fig. 22-36** **A to C,** Sinoatrial rhythms.

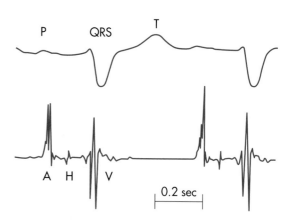

■ **Fig. 22-37** His bundle electrogram (*lower tracing,* retouched) and lead II of the scalar electrocardiogram (*upper tracing*). The deflection, *H,* which represents the impulse conduction over the bundle of His, is clearly visible between the atrial *(A)* and the ventricular *(V)* deflections. The conduction time from the atria to the bundle of His is denoted by the A-H interval; that from the bundle of His to the ventricles, by the H-V interval. (Courtesy of Dr. J. Edelstein.)

In **second-degree AV block,** all QRS complexes are preceded by P waves, but not all P waves are followed by QRS complexes. The ratio of P waves to QRS complexes is usually the ratio of two small integers (such as 2:1, 3:1, or 3:2). Fig. 22-38, *B* illustrates a typical 2:1 block. The site of block may be located above or below the His bundle. A block below the bundle is usually more serious than one above the bundle, because the former is more likely to evolve into a third-degree block. An artificial pacemaker is frequently implanted when the block is below the bundle.

Third-degree AV block is often referred to as **complete heart block** because the impulse is completely unable to traverse the AV conduction pathway from atria to ventricles. The most common sites of complete block are distal to the bundle of His. In complete heart block, the atrial and ventricular rhythms are entirely independent, as shown in Fig. 22-38, *C.* Because of the slow ventricular rhythm (32 beats/min in this example), the distribution of blood flow to the body is often inadequate, especially during muscular activity. Third-degree block is often associated with **syncope** (pronounced lightheadedness), which is caused principally by insufficient cerebral blood flow. Third-degree block is one of the most common conditions that require artificial pacemakers.

■ *Premature Depolarizations*

Premature depolarizations occur occasionally in most normal individuals, but they arise more commonly under certain abnormal conditions. They may originate in the atria, AV junction, or ventricles. One type of premature depolarization follows a normally conducted depolarization after a constant time interval (the **coupling interval**). If the normal depolarization is suppressed in some way (e.g., by vagal stimulation), the premature depolarization is also abolished. Such premature depolarizations are called **coupled extrasystoles,** or simply **extrasystoles,** and they probably reflect a reentry phenomenon (Fig. 22-30). A second type of premature depolarization occurs as the result of enhanced automaticity in some ectopic focus. This ectopic center may fire regularly, and a zone of tissue that conducts unidirectionally may protect this center from being depolarized by the normal cardiac impulse. If this premature depolarization occurs at a regular interval or at an integer multiple of that interval, the disturbance is called **parasystole.**

A **premature atrial depolarization** is shown in Fig. 22-39, *A.* In the tracing, the normal interval between beats is 0.89 second (heart rate, 68 beats/min). The premature atrial depolarization (second P wave in the figure) follows the preceding P wave by only 0.56 second. The

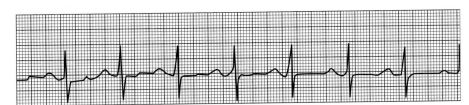

A, First-degree AV block.

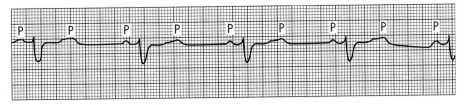

B, Second-degree AV block (2:1).

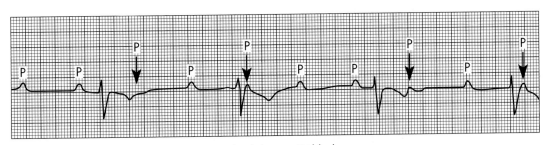

C, Third-degree AV block.

■ **Fig. 22-38** AV blocks. **A,** First-degree block; PR interval is 0.28 second. **B,** Second-degree block (2:1). **C,** Third-degree block; note the dissociation between the P waves and the QRS complexes.

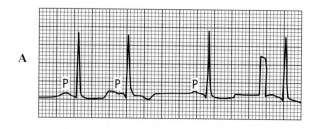

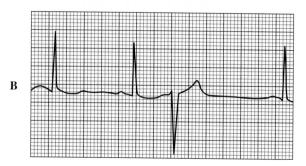

■ **Fig. 22-39**   A premature atrial depolarization (**A**) and a premature ventricular depolarization (**B**). The premature atrial depolarization (the second beat in the top tracing) is characterized by an inverted P wave and normal QRS and T waves. The interval after the premature depolarization is not much longer than the usual interval between beats. The brief rectangular deflection just before the last depolarization is a standardization signal. The premature ventricular depolarization is characterized by bizarre QRS and T waves and is followed by a compensatory pause.

configuration of the premature P wave differs from the configuration of the other, normal P waves because the course of atrial excitation, which originates at some ectopic focus in the atrium, differs from the normal spread of excitation, which originates at the SA node. The configuration of the QRS complex of the premature depolarization is usually normal because the ventricular excitation spreads over the usual pathways.

A **premature ventricular depolarization** appears in Fig. 22-39, *B*. Because the premature excitation originates at some ectopic focus in the ventricles, the impulse propagation is abnormal and the configurations of the QRS and T waves are entirely different from the normal deflections. The premature QRS complex follows the preceding normal QRS complex by only 0.47 second. The interval after the premature excitation is 1.28 seconds, which is considerably longer than the normal interval between beats (0.89 second). The interval (1.75 seconds) from the QRS complex just before the premature excitation to the QRS complex just after it is virtually equal to the duration of two normal cardiac cycles (0.89 + 0.89 = 1.78 seconds).

The prolonged interval that usually follows a premature ventricular depolarization is called a **compensatory pause.** This pause occurs because the ectopic ventricular impulse does not disturb the natural rhythm of the SA

node, either because the ectopic ventricular impulse is not conducted retrograde through the AV conduction system or because the SA node had already fired at its natural interval before the ectopic impulse could have reached it and depolarized it prematurely. Likewise, the SA nodal impulse generated just before or after the ventricular extrasystole usually does not affect the ventricle, because the AV junction and perhaps also the ventricles are still refractory from the premature excitation. In Fig. 22-39, *B*, the P wave associated with the extrasystole occurs synchronously with the T wave of the premature ventricular depolarization, and therefore it cannot easily be identified in the tracing.

■ *Ectopic Tachycardias*

In contrast to the gradual rate changes that characterize sinus tachycardia, tachycardias that originate from an ectopic focus typically begin and end abruptly. Hence, such ectopic tachycardias are usually called **paroxysmal tachycardias.** Episodes of paroxysmal tachycardia may persist for only a few beats or for many hours or days, and episodes often recur. Paroxysmal tachycardias may result from (1) the rapid firing of an ectopic pacemaker, (2) triggered activity secondary to afterpotentials that reach threshold, or (3) an impulse that circles a reentry loop repetitively.

Paroxysmal tachycardias that originate in the atria or in the AV junctional tissues (Fig. 22-40, *A*) are usually indistinguishable, and therefore both are included in the term **paroxysmal supraventricular tachycardia.** In this tachycardia, the impulse often circles a reentry loop that includes atrial and AV junctional tissue. The QRS complexes are often normal, because ventricular activation proceeds over the usual pathways.

As its name implies, **paroxysmal ventricular tachycardia** originates from an ectopic focus in the ventricles. The ECG is characterized by repeated, bizarre QRS complexes that reflect the abnormal intraventricular impulse conduction (Fig. 22-40, *B*). Paroxysmal ventricular tachycardia is much more ominous than supraventricular tachycardia, because the former is frequently a precursor of ventricular fibrillation, a lethal arrhythmia described in the next section.

■ *Fibrillation*

Under certain conditions, cardiac muscle undergoes an irregular type of contraction that is entirely ineffectual in propelling blood. Such an arrhythmia is termed **fibrillation,** and the disturbance may involve either the atria or the ventricles. Fibrillation probably represents a reentry phenomenon, in which the reentry loop fragments into multiple, irregular circuits.

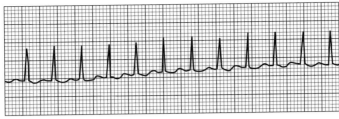

A, Supraventricular tachycardia.

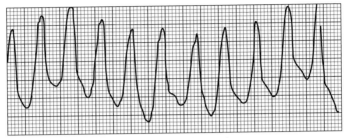

B, Ventricular tachycardia.

■ **Fig. 22-40**   **A** and **B,** Paroxysmal tachycardias.

The ECG changes in **atrial fibrillation** are shown in Fig. 22-41, *A*. This arrhythmia occurs in various types of chronic heart disease. The atria do not contract and relax sequentially during each cardiac cycle, and thus they do not contribute to ventricular filling. Instead, the atria undergo a continuous, uncoordinated, rippling motion. P waves do not appear in the ECG; they are replaced by continuous irregular fluctuations of potential, called **f waves.** The AV node is activated at intervals that may vary considerably from cycle to cycle. Hence, no constant interval occurs between successive QRS complexes or between successive ventricular contractions. Because the strength of ventricular contraction depends on the interval between beats (as explained on p 390), the volume and rhythm of the pulse are irregular. In many patients, the atrial reentry loop and the pattern of AV conduction are more regular than they are in atrial fibrillation. The rhythm is then referred to as **atrial flutter.**

Atrial fibrillation and flutter are not life threatening; some people with these disturbances can even perform full activity. **Ventricular fibrillation,** on the other hand, leads to loss of consciousness within a few seconds. The irregular, continuous, uncoordinated twitchings of the ventricular muscle fibers pump no blood. Death ensues unless immediate effective resuscitation is achieved or unless the rhythm spontaneously reverts to normal, which rarely occurs. Ventricular fibrillation may supervene when the entire ventricle, or some portion of it, is deprived of its normal blood supply. It may also occur as a result of electrocution or in response to certain drugs and anesthetics. In the ECG

(Fig. 22-41, *B*), irregular fluctuations of potential are manifested.

Ventricular fibrillation is often initiated when a premature impulse arrives during the **vulnerable period,** which coincides with the downslope of the T wave of the ECG. During this period, the excitability of the cardiac cells varies spatially. Some fibers are still in their effective refractory periods; others have almost fully recovered their excitability; and still others are able to conduct impulses but only at very slow conduction velocities. Consequently, the action potentials are propagated over the chambers in many irregular wavelets that travel along circuitous paths and at various conduction velocities. As a region of cardiac cells becomes excitable again, it is ultimately reentered by one of the wave fronts traveling around the chamber. Hence, the process is self-sustaining.

Atrial fibrillation may be changed to a normal sinus rhythm by drugs that prolong the refractory period. As the cardiac impulse completes the reentry loop, it may then encounter the myocardial fibers that are no longer excitable. However, dramatic therapy is required in ventricular fibrillation. Conversion to a normal sinus rhythm is accomplished by means of a strong electrical current that places the entire myocardium briefly in a refractory state. Techniques have been developed to safely administer the current through the intact chest wall. In successful cases, the SA node again takes over the normal pacemaker function for the entire heart. When atrial defibrillation does not respond adequately to drugs, electrical defibrillation may also be used to correct this condition.

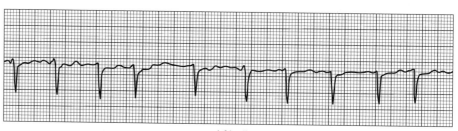

A, Atrial fibrillation.

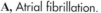

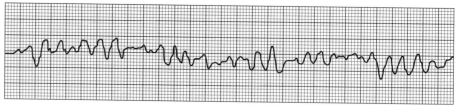

B, Ventricular fibrillation.

■ **Fig. 22-41**   Atrial and ventricular fibrillation.

■ *Summary*

1. The transmembrane action potentials that can be recorded from cardiac myocytes contain the following five phases:

Phase 0: The action potential upstroke is produced when a suprathreshold stimulus rapidly depolarizes the membrane by activating the fast Na^+ channels.

Phase 1: The notch is an early partial repolarization that is achieved by the efflux of K^+ through transmembrane channels that conduct the transient outward current, i_{to}.

Phase 2: The plateau represents a balance between the influx of Ca^{++} through transmembrane Ca^{++} channels and the efflux of K^+ through several types of K^+ channels.

Phase 3: Final repolarization is initiated when the efflux of K^+ exceeds the influx of Ca^{++}. The resultant partial repolarization rapidly increases the K^+ conductance and rapidly restores full repolarization.

Phase 4: The resting potential of the fully repolarized cell is determined mainly by conductance of the cell membrane to K^+ through i_{K1} channels.

2. Fast-response action potentials are recorded from atrial and ventricular myocardial fibers and from ventricular specialized conducting (Purkinje) fibers. The action potential is characterized by a large amplitude, a steep upstroke, and a relatively long plateau.

3. The effective refractory period of fast-response fibers begins at the upstroke of the action potential and persists until midway through phase 3. The fiber is relatively refractory during the remainder of phase 3, and it regains full excitability when it is fully repolarized (phase 4).

4. Slow-response action potentials are recorded from normal SA and AV nodal cells and from abnormal myocardial cells that have been partially depolarized. The action potential is characterized by a less negative resting potential, a smaller amplitude, a less steep upstroke, and a shorter plateau than is the fast-response action potential. The upstroke is produced by the activation of Ca^{++} channels.

5. Slow-response fibers become absolutely refractory at the beginning of the upstroke, and partial excitability may not be regained until very late in phase 3 or until after the fiber is fully repolarized.

6. Automaticity is characteristic of certain cells in the SA and AV nodes and in the ventricular specialized conducting system. Slow depolarization of the membrane during phase 4 is the hallmark of automaticity.

7. Normally the SA node initiates the impulse that induces cardiac contraction. This impulse is propagated from the SA node to the atrial tissues and ultimately reaches the AV node. After a delay in the AV node, the cardiac impulse is propagated throughout the ventricles.

8. Ectopic foci in the atrium, AV node, or His-Purkinje system may initiate propagated cardiac impulses if the normal pacemaker cells in the SA node are suppressed or if the rhythmicity of the ectopic automatic cells is abnormally enhanced.

9. Under certain abnormal conditions, afterdepolarizations may appear early in phase 3 of a normally initiated beat, or the afterdepolarizations may be delayed until near the end of phase 3 or the beginning of phase 4. Such afterdepolarizations may themselves trigger propagated impulses. Early afterdepolarizations are more likely to occur when the basic cycle length of the initiating beats is very long and when the cardiac action potentials are abnormally prolonged. Delayed afterdepolarizations are more likely to occur when the basic cycle length of the initiating beats is short and when the cardiac cells are overloaded with Ca^{++}.

10. Simple conduction block is the retardation or failure of impulse propagation in a cardiac fiber.

11. A cardiac impulse may traverse a loop of cardiac fibers and reenter previously excited tissue when the impulse is conducted slowly around the loop, and when the impulse is blocked unidirectionally in some section of the loop.

12. The electrocardiogram (ECG), which is recorded from the surface of the body, traces the conduction of the cardiac impulse throughout the heart.

13. The ECG may be used to detect and analyze certain cardiac arrhythmias, such as altered sinoatrial rhythms, AV conduction blocks, premature depolarizations, ectopic tachycardias, and atrial and ventricular fibrillation.

■ *Self-Study Problems*

1. What major movements of ions account for each phase of the action potential of a typical fast-response myocardial cell?

2. Why is the cardiac action potential propagated more slowly in an AV node cell than in an atrial or ventricular myocyte?

3. By what pathways does a cardiac impulse that originates in the SA node arrive in the ventricular myocardium?

4. What electrophysiological conditions lead to reentry?

5. What electrocardiographic changes occur in first-, second-, and third-degree AV block?

■ *Bibliography*
Journal articles

Antzelevitch C, Sicouri S: Clinical relevance of cardiac arrhythmias generated by afterdepolarization: role of M cells in the generation of U waves, triggered activity and torsade de pointes, *J Am Coll Cardiol* 23:259, 1994.

Balke CW et al: Biophysics and physiology of cardiac calcium channels, *Circulation* 87:VII-49, 1993.

Beaumont J et al: A model study of changes in excitability of ventricular muscle cells: inhibition, facilitation, and hysteresis, *Am J Physiol* 268:H1181, 1995.

Billette J, Nattel S: Dynamic behavior of the atrioventricular node: a functional model of interaction between recovery, facilitation, and fatigue, *J Cardiovasc Electrophysiol* 5:90, 1994.

Delmar M: Role of potassium currents on cell excitability in cardiac ventricular myocytes, *J Cardiovasc Electrophysiol* 3:474, 1993.

Demir SS, Clark JW, Murphey CR, Giles WR: A mathematical model of a rabbit sinoatrial node cell, *Am J Physiol* 266:C832, 1994.

DiFrancesco D: Pacemaker mechanisms in cardiac tissue, *Annu Rev Physiol* 55:455, 1993.

Grant AO: Evolving concepts of cardiac sodium channel function, *J Cardiovasc Electrophysiol* 1:53, 1990.

Irisawa H, Brown HF, Giles W: Cardiac pacemaking in the sinoatrial node, *Physiol Rev* 73:197, 1993.

January CT, Shorofsky S: Early afterdepolarizations: newer insights into cellular mechanisms, *J Cardiovasc Electrophysiol* 1:161, 1990.

Levy MN: Role of calcium in arrhythmogenesis, *Circulation* 80:IV-23, 1989.

Liu D-W, Gintant GA, Antzelevitch C: Ionic bases for electrophysiological distinctions among epicardial, midmyocardial, and endocardial myocytes from the free wall of the canine left ventricle, *Circ Res* 72:671, 1993.

Meijler FL, Janse MJ: Morphology and electrophysiology of the mammalian atrioventricular node, *Physiol Rev* 68:608, 1988.

Nichols CG et al: Inward rectification and implications for cardiac excitability, *Circ Res* 78:1, 1996.

Reiter M: Calcium mobilization and cardiac inotropic mechanisms, *Pharmacol Rev* 40:189, 1988.

Rosen MR: Links between basic and clinical cardiac electrophysiology, *Circulation* 77:251, 1988.

Schuessler RB, Boineau JP, Bromberg BI: Origin of the sinus impulse, *J Cardiovasc Electrophysiol* 7:263, 1996.

Sicouri S, Antzelevitch C: Electrophysiologic characteristics of M cells in the canine left ventricular free wall, *J Cardiovasc Electrophysiol* 6:591, 1995.

Spach MS, Josephson ME: Initiating reentry: the role of nonuniform anisotrophy in small circuits, *J Cardiovasc Electrophysiol* 5:182, 1994.

Waldo AL, Wit AL: Mechanisms of cardiac arrhythmias, *Lancet* 341:1189, 1993.

Books and monographs

Armour JA, Ardell JL: *Neurocardiology,* New York, 1994, Oxford University Press.

Cranefield PF, Aronson RS: *Cardiac arrhythmias: the role of triggered activity and other mechanisms,* Mt. Kisco, NY, 1988, Futura Publishing.

Dangman KH, Miura DS: *Electrophysiology and pharmacology of the heart: a clinical guide,* New York, 1991, Marcel Dekker.

Fozzard HA et al: *Heart and cardiovascular system. Scientific foundations,* New York, 1991, Raven Press.

Hille B: *Ionic channels of excitable membranes,* ed 2, Sunderland, Mass, 1991, Sinauer Associates.

Langer GA, editor: *Calcium and the heart,* New York, 1990, Raven Press.

Levy MN, Schwartz PJ: *Vagal control of the heart: experimental basis and clinical implications,* Armonk, NY, 1994, Futura Publishing.

Mazgalev T, Dreifus LS, Michelson EL: *Electrophysiology of the sinoatrial and atrioventricular nodes,* New York, 1988, Alan R Liss.

Sperelakis N: *Physiology and pathophysiology of the heart,* ed 3, Boston, 1995, Kluwer Academic.

Spooner PM et al: *Ion channels in the cardiovascular system: function and dysfunction,* Armonk, NY, 1994, Futura Publishing.

Wit AL, Janse MJ: *Ventricular arrhythmias of ischemia and infarction: electrophysiological mechanisms,* Armonk, NY, 1993, Futura Publishing.

Zipes DP, Jalife J: *Cardiac electrophysiology: from cell to bedside,* ed 2, Philadelphia, 1995, WB Saunders.

CHAPTER

23

The Cardiac Pump

It is nearly impossible to contemplate the pumping action of the heart without being struck by its simplicity of design, its wide range of activity and functional capacity, and the staggering amount of work it performs over an individual's lifetime. A useful way to understand how the heart accomplishes its important task is to consider the relationships between the structure and function of its components.

■ *Structure of the Heart in Relation to Function*

■ *The Myocardial Cell*

A number of important morphologic and functional differences exist between myocardial and skeletal muscle cells. Despite these differences, the contractile elements within the two types of cells are actually quite similar. Each skeletal and cardiac muscle cell is composed of **sarcomeres** (from Z line to Z line) containing thick filaments and thin filaments. Thick filaments are composed of myosin (in the band), while thin filaments contain actin. The thin filaments extend from the point at which they are anchored to the Z line (through the I band) to interdigitate with the thick filaments. As in skeletal muscle, shortening of cardiac muscle filaments occurs by the sliding filament mechanism. Actin filaments slide along adjacent myosin filaments by cycling of the intervening cross-bridges and thereby bring the Z lines closer together (see Chapter 17).

Skeletal and cardiac muscle also show similar length-force relationships. The developed force is maximal when the muscle begins its contractions at resting sarcomere lengths of 2 to 2.4 μm. At this resting length, there is optimal overlap of thick and thin filaments, and the number of cross-bridge attachments is maximal. Stretch of the myocardium and increases in load enhance the affinity of troponin C for Ca^{++}. It is still not known how an increase in sarcomere length increases the sensitivity of the myofilaments to calcium. One explanation is that the thick and thin filaments are brought closer to each other as the diameter of the muscle fiber narrows during stretch. When sarcomeres are stretched beyond the optimal length, the developed force of cardiac muscle drops to less than maximal value owing to less overlap of the filaments and hence less cycling of the cross-bridges. At resting sarcomere lengths shorter than optimal value, the thin filaments overlap, which diminishes contractile force.

In general, the fiber length-force relationship for the papillary muscle also holds true for fibers in the intact heart. This relationship may be expressed graphically, as in Fig. 23-1, by substituting ventricular systolic pressure for force, and end-diastolic ventricular volume for myocardial resting fiber (and hence sarcomere) length. The lower curve in Fig. 23-1 represents the increment in pressure produced by each increment in volume when the heart is in diastole. The upper curve represents the peak pressure developed by the ventricle during systole at each degree of filling, and illustrates the **Frank-Starling relationship** (also called *Starling's law of the heart*) of initial myocardial fiber length (or initial volume) to force (or pressure) development by the ventricle.

Note that the pressure-volume curve in diastole is initially quite flat, which indicates that large increases in volume can be accommodated with only small increases in pressure. In contrast, systolic pressure development is considerable at the lower filling pressures. However, the ventricle becomes much less distensible with greater filling, as evidenced by the sharp rise of the diastolic curve at large intraventricular volumes. In the normal intact heart, peak force may be attained at a filling pressure of about 12 mm Hg. At this intraventricular diastolic pressure, which is about the upper limit observed in the normal heart, the sarcomere length is 2.2 μm. However, developed force peaks at filling pressures as high as 30 mm Hg in the isolated heart. At even higher diastolic pressures (>50 mm Hg), the sarcomere length is not greater than 2.6 μm. This ability to resist stretch of the myocardium at high filling pressures probably resides in the noncontractile constituents of the heart tissue (connective tissue) and may serve as a safety factor against overloading of the heart in diastole. Usually, ventricular diastolic pressure is about 0 to 7 mm Hg, and the average

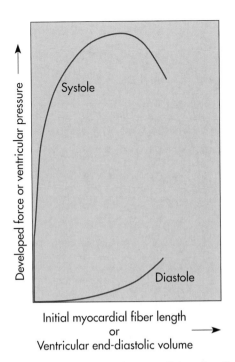

Developed force or ventricular pressure

Systole

Diastole

Initial myocardial fiber length
or
Ventricular end-diastolic volume

■ **Fig. 23-1** Relationship of myocardial resting fiber length (sarcomere length) or end-diastolic volume to developed force or peak systolic ventricular pressure during ventricular contraction in the intact dog heart. (Redrawn from Patterson SW, Piper H, Starling EH: *J Physiol* 48:465, 1914.)

diastolic sarcomere length is about 2.2 μm. Thus, *the normal heart operates on the ascending portion of the Frank-Starling curve* depicted in Fig. 23-1.

If the heart becomes greatly distended with blood during diastole, as may occur in **cardiac failure,** it functions less efficiently. More energy is required (greater wall tension) for the distended heart to eject the same volume of blood per beat than for the normal undilated heart. The less efficient pumping of the distended heart is an example of Laplace's law (see p 431), which states that the tension in the wall of a vessel (in this case the ventricles) equals the transmural pressure (pressure across the wall, or distending pressure) times the radius of the vessel or chamber. The Laplace relationship applies to infinitely thin-walled vessels but can be applied to the heart if correction is made for wall thickness. The equation is τ = Pr/w where τ = wall stress, P = transmural pressure, r = radius, and w = wall thickness.

■ *The Cardiac Pump*

Functional anatomy of cardiac muscle. A striking difference between the appearance of the cardiac and skeletal muscle is the presence of what appears to be a syncytium in cardiac muscle with branching intercon-

necting fibers (Figs. 23-2 and 23-3). A syncytium is a multinucleated, protoplasmic mass of cells. However, the myocardium is not a true anatomic syncytium because the myocardial fibers are indeed separated from each other. Laterally, the myocardial fibers are separated from adjacent fibers by their respective sarcolemmas, and the end of each fiber is separated from its neighbor by dense structures, **intercalated disks,** that are continuous with the sarcolemma (Figs. 23-2 to 23-4). Nevertheless, *cardiac muscle functions as a syncytium;* that is, a stimulus applied to any one part of the cardiac muscle results in the contraction of the entire muscle. A wave of depolarization followed by contraction of the entire myocardium (an *all-or-none response*) occurs when a suprathreshold stimulus is applied to any one focus.

As the wave of excitation approaches the end of a cardiac cell, the spread of excitation to the next cell depends on the level of the electrical conductance of the boundary between the two cells. **Gap junctions (nexi)** with high conductances are present in the intercalated disks between adjacent cells (Figs. 23-2 to 23-4). These gap junctions, which facilitate the conduction of the cardiac impulse from one cell to the next, are made up of **connexons,** hexagonal structures that connect the cytosol of adjacent cells. Each connexon consists of six polypeptides that surround a core channel approximately 1.6 to 2.0 mm wide. Each channel thus serves as a low-resistance pathway for cell-to-cell conductance (see Chapter 4).

Impulse conduction in cardiac tissues progresses more rapidly in a direction parallel to the long axes of the constituent fibers than in a direction perpendicular to the long axes of those fibers. Gap junctions exist in the borders between myocardial fibers that are in contact with each other longitudinally; they are sparse or absent in the borders between myocardial fibers that lie side by side.

Another difference between cardiac and fast skeletal muscle fibers is in the number of mitochondria (**sarcosomes**) in the two tissues. Fast skeletal muscle is called on for relatively short periods of repetitive or sustained contraction, and can metabolize anaerobically and build up a substantial oxygen debt. Fast skeletal muscle fibers contain relatively few mitochondria. In contrast, cardiac muscle contracts repetitively for a lifetime and requires a continuous supply of oxygen. Cardiac muscle is therefore very rich in mitochondria (Figs. 23-2 to 23-4). The large number of mitochondria—which contain the enzymes necessary for oxidative phosphorylation—allows for the rapid oxidation of substrates with the synthesis of adenosine triphosphate (ATP) that sustains the myocardial energy requirements.

To provide adequate oxygen and substrate for its metabolic machinery, the myocardium is also endowed with a rich capillary supply, about one capillary per fiber. Thus, diffusion distances are short, and oxygen, carbon dioxide, substrates, and waste material can move rapidly between the myocardial cell and capillary. A structure called the **transverse (T) tubular system** within

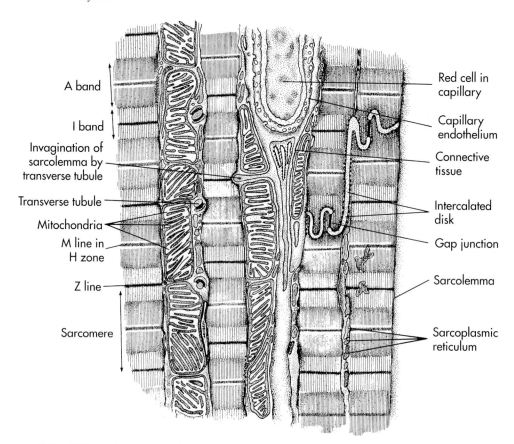

A band

I band

Invagination of
sarcolemma by
transverse tubule

Transverse tubule

Mitochondria

M line in
H zone

Z line

Sarcomere

Red cell in
capillary

Capillary
endothelium

Connective
tissue

Intercalated
disk

Gap junction

Sarcolemma

Sarcoplasmic
reticulum

■ **Fig. 23-2** Diagram of an electron micrograph of cardiac muscle showing large numbers of mitochondria and the intercalated disks with nexi (gap junction), transverse tubules, and longitudinal tubules.

myocardial cells participates in this exchange of substances between the capillary blood and the myocardial cells. In electron micrographs of myocardium, the T-tubular system appears as deep invaginations of the sarcolemma into the fiber at the Z lines (Figs. 23-2 to 23-4). The lumina of these T tubules are continuous with the bulk interstitial fluid, and they play a key role in excitation-contraction coupling.

In mammalian ventricular cells, adjacent T tubules are interconnected by longitudinally running or axial tubules, thus forming an extensively interconnected lattice of "intracellular" tubules (Fig. 23-4). This T-tubule system is open to the interstitial fluid, is lined with a basement membrane continuous with that of the surface sarcolemma, and contains micropinocytotic vesicles. Thus, in ventricular cells, the T-tubular system provides the myofibrils and mitochondria with ready access to the interstitial fluid. The T-tubular system is absent or poorly developed in atrial cells of many mammalian hearts.

A network of **sarcoplasmic reticulum** (Fig. 23-4), consisting of small-diameter sarcotubules, is also present surrounding the myofibrils. These sarcotubules are believed to be "closed," because colloidal tracer particles (2 to 10 nm in diameter) do not enter them. They do not contain basement membrane. Flattened elements of the sarcoplasmic reticulum are often found in close proximity to the T-tubular system, as well as to the surface sarcolemma, forming **diads.**

Excitation-contraction coupling. The earliest studies on isolated hearts perfused with isotonic saline solutions indicated that optimal concentrations of Na^+, K^+, and Ca^{++} are necessary for cardiac muscle contraction. Without Na^+, the heart is not excitable and will not beat, because the action potential depends on extracellular Na ions. In contrast, the resting membrane potential is independent of the Na ion gradient across the membrane (see Fig. 22-5). Under normal conditions, the extracellular K^+ concentration is about 4 mM. A reduction in extracellular K^+ has little effect on myocardial excitation and contraction. However, increases in extracellular K^+, if great enough, produce depolarization, loss of excitability of the myocardial cells, and cardiac arrest in diastole. *Ca^{++} is also essential for cardiac contraction.* Removal of Ca^{++} from the extracellular fluid results in decreased contractile force and eventual arrest in diastole. Conversely, an increase in extracellular Ca^{++} enhances contractile force, and very high Ca^{++} concentrations induce cardiac arrest in systole (rigor). *The free intracellular Ca^{++} is the agent responsible for the contractile state of the myocardium.*

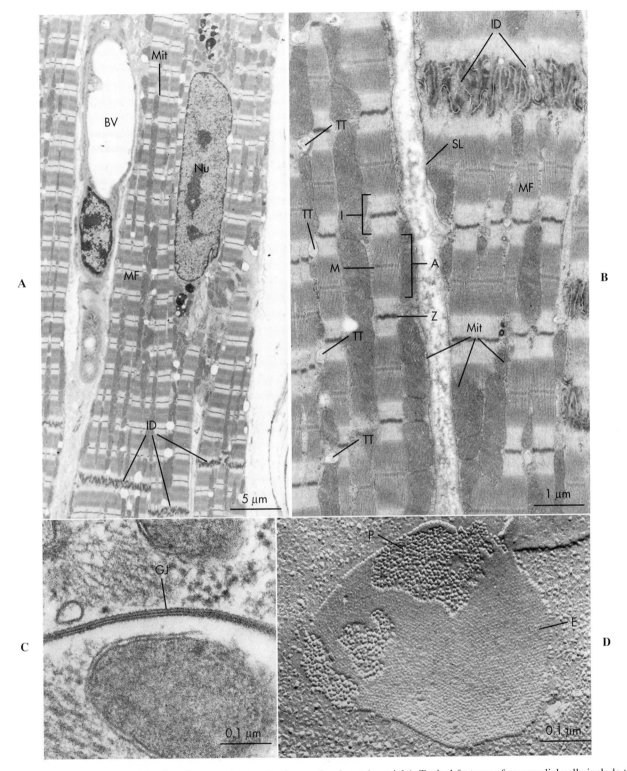

■ **Fig. 23-3** **A,** Low-magnification electron micrograph of a monkey heart (ventricle). Typical features of myocardial cells include the elongated nucleus *(Nu),* striated myofibrils *(MF)* with columns of mitochondria *(Mit)* between the myofibrils, and intercellular junctions (intercalated disks, *ID*). A blood vessel *(BV)* is located between two myocardial cells. **B,** Medium-magnification electron micrograph of monkey ventricular cells showing details of the ultrastructure. The sarcolemma *(SL)* is the boundary of the muscle cells and is thrown into multiple folds where the cells meet at the intercalated disk region *(ID).* The prominent myofibrils *(MF)* show distinct banding patterns, including the A band *(A),* dark Z lines *(Z),* I band regions *(I),* and M lines *(M)* at the center of each sarcomere unit. Mitochondria *(Mit)* occur either in rows between myofibrils or in masses just underneath the sarcolemma. Regularly spaced transverse tubules *(TT)* appear at the Z-line levels of the myofibrils. **C,** High-magnification electron micrograph of a specialized intercellular junction between two myocardial cells of the mouse. Called a gap junction *(GJ)* or nexus, this attachment consists of very close apposition of the sarcolemmal membranes of the two cells and appears in thin section to consist of seven layers. **D,** Freeze-fracture replica of mouse myocardial gap junction, showing distinct arrays of characteristic intramembranous particles. Large particles *(P)* belong to the inner half of the sarcolemma of one myocardial cell, whereas the "pitted" membrane face *(E)* is formed by the outer half of the sarcolemma of the cell above.

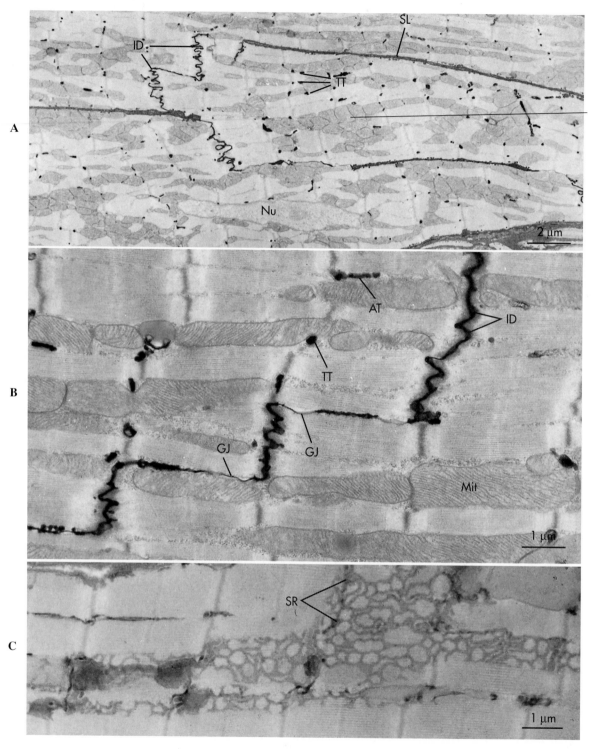

■ **Fig. 23-4**   **A,** Low-magnification electron micrograph of the right ventricular wall of a mouse heart. Tissue was fixed in a phosphate-buffered glutaraldehyde solution and postfixed in ferro-cyanide-reduced osmium tetroxide. This procedure has resulted in the deposition of electron-opaque precipitate in the extracellular space, thus outlining the sarcolemmal borders *(SL)* of the muscle cells and delineating the intercalated disks *(ID)* and transverse tubules *(TT)*. *Nu,* Nucleus of the myocardial cell. **B,** Mouse cardiac muscle in longitudinal section, treated as in **A.** The path of the extracellular space is traced through the intercalated disk region *(ID),* and sarcolemmal invaginations that are oriented transverse to the cell axis (transverse tubules, *TT)* or parallel to it (axial tubules, *AT)* are clearly identified. Gap junctions *(GJ)* are associated with the intercalated disk. Mitochondria are large and elongated and lie between the myofibrils. **C,** Mouse cardiac muscle. Tissue was treated with ferrocyanide-reduced osmium tetroxide to identify the internal membrane system (sarcoplasmic reticulum, *SR).* Specific staining of the SR reveals its architecture as a complex network of small-diameter tubules that are closely associated with the myofibrils and mitochondria.

Excitation of cardiac muscle starts when a wave of excitation spreads rapidly along the myocardial sarcolemma from cell to cell via gap junctions. Excitation also spreads into the interior of the cells via the T tubules (Figs. 23-2 to 23-4), which invaginate the cardiac fibers at the Z lines. Electrical stimulation at the Z line or the application of ionized Ca to the Z lines in the skinned (sarcolemma removed) cardiac fiber elicits a localized contraction of adjacent myofibrils. During the plateau (phase 2) of the action potential, Ca^{++} permeability of the sarcolemma increases. Ca^{++} flows down its electrochemical gradient and enters the cell through Ca^{++} channels in the sarcolemma and in the invaginations of the sarcolemma, the T tubules (see also Chapters 18 and 22).

Opening of the Ca^{++} channels is believed to be caused by phosphorylation of the channel proteins by a cyclic adenosine monophosphate (cAMP)–dependent protein kinase. The primary source of extracellular Ca^{++} is the interstitial fluid (10^{-3} M Ca^{++}). Some Ca^{++} may also be bound to the sarcolemma and to the **glycocalyx,** a mucopolysaccharide that covers the sarcolemma. The amount of calcium that enters the cell interior from the extracellular space is not sufficient to induce contraction

of the myofibrils. Instead, it acts as a trigger (**trigger Ca^{++}**) to release Ca^{++} from the sarcoplasmic reticulum (where the intracellular Ca^{++} is stored) (Fig. 23-5). The concentration of free Ca^{++} in the cytoplasm increases from a resting level of about 10^{-7} M to levels of 10^{-6} to 10^{-5} M during excitation. This Ca^{++} then binds to the protein troponin C. The Ca^{++}-troponin complex interacts with tropomyosin to unblock active sites between the actin and myosin filaments. This unblocking action allows cross-bridge cycling and hence contraction of the myofibrils (see Chapter 18).

Mechanisms that raise the cytosolic Ca^{++} concentration increase the developed force, and those that lower the cystolic Ca^{++} concentration decrease the developed force. For example, catecholamines increase the movement of Ca^{++} into the cell by phosphorylation of the channels via a cAMP-dependent protein kinase (see also Chapters 18 and 22). In addition, catecholamines, like other agonists, enhance myocardial contractile force by increasing the sensitivity of the contractile machinery to Ca^{++}. Increasing the extracellular concentration of Ca^{++} or decreasing the Na^+ gradient across the sarcolemma also results in an increase in the cytosolic concentration of Ca^{++}.

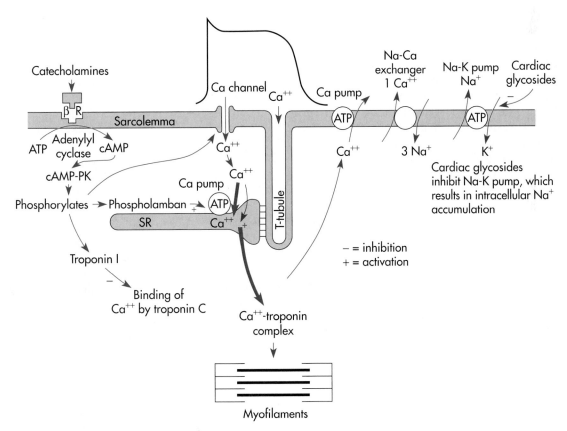

■ **Fig. 23-5**   Schematic diagram of the movements of calcium in excitation-contraction coupling in cardiac muscle. The influx of Ca^{++} from the interstitial fluid during excitation triggers the release of Ca^{++} from the saroplasmic reticulum *(SR)*. The free cytosolic Ca^{++} activates contraction of the myofilaments (systole). Relaxation (diastole) occurs as a result of uptake of Ca^{++} by the sarcoplasmic reticulum, by extrusion of intracellular Ca^{++} by Na^+-Ca^{++} exchange, and to a limited degree by the Ca pump. *βR,* Beta-adrenergic receptor; *cAMP,* cyclic adenosine monophosphate; *cAMP-PK,* cyclic AMP–dependent protein kinase.

The sodium gradient can be reduced by increasing the intracellular concentration of Na^+ or decreasing the extracellular concentration of Na^+. Cardiac glycosides increase intracellular Na^+ concentration by "poisoning" the Na^+, K^+-ATPase, which results in an accumulation of Na^+ in the cells. The elevated cytosolic Na^+ reverses the direction of the Na,Ca exchanger so that less Ca^{++} is removed from the cell. A lowered extracellular Na^+ concentration causes less Na^+ to enter the cell, and hence less exchange of Na^+ for Ca^{++} (Fig. 23-5).

Developed tension is diminished by a reduction in extracellular Ca^{++} concentration, by an increase in the Na^+ gradient across the sarcolemma, or by administration of a Ca^{++} channel antagonist (channel blocker) that prevents Ca^{++} from entering the myocardial cell (see Fig. 22-11).

A patient in **heart failure** with a dilated heart, low cardiac output, fluid retention, high venous pressure, an enlarged liver, and peripheral edema is often treated with digitalis and a diuretic. The digitalis increases cardiomyocyte intracellular calcium, thereby enhancing contractile force. The diuretic reduces extracellular fluid volume, thereby lessening the volume load (preload) on the heart and reducing venous pressure, liver congestion, and edema.

At the end of systole, the Ca^{++} influx stops, and the sarcoplasmic reticulum is no longer stimulated to release Ca^{++}. In fact, the sarcoplasmic reticulum avidly takes up Ca^{++} by means of an ATP-energized calcium pump. This pump is stimulated by **phospholamban** after the phospholamban is phosphorylated by cAMP-dependent protein kinase. In addition, phosphorylation of troponin I inhibits the Ca^{++} binding to troponin C. This process permits tropomyosin to again block the sites for interaction between the actin and myosin filaments, and relaxation (diastole) occurs (see also Chapters 17 and 18).

Cardiac contraction and relaxation are both accelerated by catecholamines and adenylyl cyclase activation. The resultant increase in cAMP activates the cAMP-dependent protein kinase, which phosphorylates the Ca channel in the sarcolemma. These events cause more Ca^{++} to move into the cell, thereby accelerating contraction. However, these events also accelerate *relaxation* by phosphorylating phospholamban, which enhances Ca^{++} uptake by the sarcoplasmic reticulum, and by phosphorylating troponin I, which inhibits the Ca^{++} binding of troponin C. Thus, the phosphorylations by cAMP-dependent protein kinase serve to increase both the speed of contraction *and* the speed of relaxation.

Mitochondria also take up and release Ca^{++}, but the process is too slow to have an impact on normal excitation-contraction coupling. Only at very high intracellular Ca^{++} levels (pathological states) do the mitochondria take up a significant amount of Ca^{++}.

The Ca^{++} that enters the cell to initiate contraction must be removed during diastole. The removal is primarily accomplished by the exchange of 3 Na^+ for 1 Ca^{++} (Fig. 23-5). Ca^{++} is also removed from the cell by an electrogenic pump that uses ATP to transport Ca^{++} across the sarcolemma (Fig. 23-5).

Myocardial contractile machinery and contractility. The sequence of events that occur during the contraction of a preloaded and afterloaded papillary muscle is shown in Fig. 23-6. In Fig. 23-6, *A*, the muscle is relaxed and bears no weight. For the intact left ventricle,* this situation is analogous to the point in the cardiac cycle when the ventricle has relaxed after ejection, the aortic valve is closed, and the mitral valve is about to open (the end of isovolumic relaxation—see p 373 and Fig. 23-10). In Fig. 23-6, *B*, the resting muscle is stretched by a preload, which in the intact heart represents the end of filling of the left ventricle during ventricular diastole (in other words, it represents the **end-diastolic volume**). In Fig. 23-6, *C*, the resting muscle is still stretched by the preload, but a supported afterload has been added without allowing the muscle to be stretched further. In the intact heart, this situation is analogous to the point in the cardiac cycle when ventricular contraction has started and the mitral valve has closed, but the aortic valve has not yet opened because the ventricle has not developed enough intraventricular pressure to open it (isovolumic contraction phase—see p 372 and Fig. 23-10). In Fig. 23-6, *D*, the ventricle has contracted and lifted the afterload. In the intact heart, this situation represents left ventricular ejection into the aorta. During ejection, the afterload is represented by aortic and intraventricular pressures, which are virtually equal to each other.

The preload can be increased by greater filling of the left ventricle during diastole (Fig. 23-1). At lower end-diastolic volumes, incremental increases in filling pressure during diastole elicit a greater systolic pressure during the subsequent contraction. Systolic pressure increases until a maximal systolic pressure is reached at the optimal preload (Fig. 23-1). If diastolic filling continues beyond this point, no further increase in developed pressure will occur. At very high filling pressures, peak pressure development in systole is reduced.

At a constant preload, a higher systolic pressure can be reached during ventricular contractions by raising the afterload (e.g., increasing aortic pressure by restricting the runoff of blood to the periphery during diastole). Incremental increases in afterload produce progressively higher peak systolic pressures (Fig. 23-7). If the afterload increases continue, the afterload becomes so great that the ventricle can no longer generate enough force to open the aortic valve (Fig. 23-7). At this point, ventricular sys-

---

*The left ventricle has been chosen because it supplies the entire body except the lungs, and thus faces the larger afterload. However, the principles of preload and afterload apply equally well to the right ventricle.

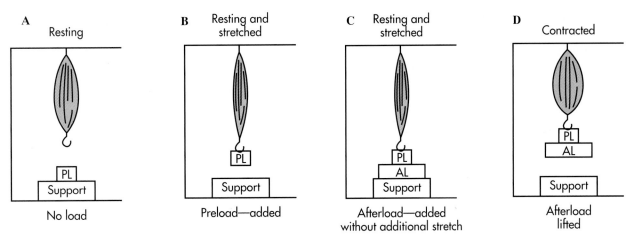

A Resting

B Resting and stretched

C Resting and stretched

D Contracted

No load

Preload—added

Afterload—added without additional stretch

Afterload lifted

■ **Fig. 23-6** Preload and afterload in a papillary muscle. **A,** Resting stage—in the intact heart just before opening of the AV valves. **B,** Preload—in the intact heart at the end of ventricular filling. **C,** Supported preload plus afterload—in the intact heart just before opening of the aortic valve. **D,** Lifting preload plus afterload—in the intact heart ventricular ejection with a decrease in ventricular volume. *PL,* Preload; *AL,* afterload; *PL + AL* = total load.

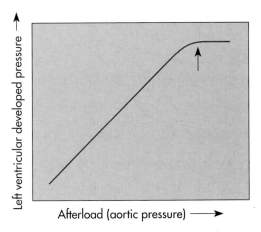

■ **Fig. 23-7** Effect of increasing afterload on developed pressure at constant preload. At the arrow, maximal developed pressure is reached. Further increments in afterload prevent opening of the aortic valve.

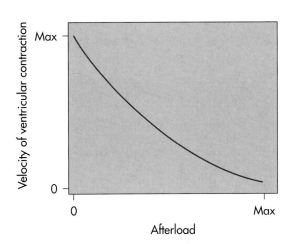

■ **Fig. 23-8** Effect of increasing afterload on the velocity of contraction at constant preload.

tole is totally isometric; there is no ejection of blood, and thus no change in volume of the ventricle during systole. The maximal pressure developed by the left ventricle under these conditions is the maximal isometric force the ventricle is capable of generating at a given preload. At preloads below the optimal filling volume, an increase in preload can yield a greater maximal isometric force (Fig. 23-1).

Force and velocity are functions of the intracellular concentration of free calcium ions. At a constant velocity, force equals the afterload during shortening of the muscle with contraction. *Force and velocity are inversely related. With no load, the velocity of the muscle contraction is maximal, whereas with a maximal load (when contraction can no longer shorten the muscle), velocity is zero* (Fig. 23-8).

Preloads and afterloads depend on certain characteristics of the vascular system and the behavior of the heart. With respect to the vasculature, the degree of venomotor tone and peripheral resistance influence preload and afterload. With respect to the heart, a change in rate or stroke volume can also alter preload and afterload. Hence, cardiac and vascular factors interact to produce effects on preload and afterload (see Chapter 29 for a full explanation).

In contrast to the normal heart, strips of papillary muscle from the terminally failing human heart show no increase in developed force with increases in preload.

If the phospholamban gene is ablated in mice, myocardial contractility is enhanced, as evidenced by increased work at a given preload, afterload, and heart rate, and by a greater dP/dt (see below).

Contractility represents the performance of the heart at a given preload and afterload. Contractility is defined as *the change in peak isometric force (isovolumic pressure) at a given initial fiber length (end-diastolic volume)*. Contractility can be augmented with certain drugs, such as norepinephrine or digitalis, and with an increase in contraction frequency (**tachycardia**). The increase in contractility (**positive inotropic effect**) produced by any of these interventions is reflected by incremental increases in developed force and velocity of contraction.

In rare instances, patients have accidentally received excessive doses of epinephrine subcutaneously for severe asthmatic attacks. The patients develop marked tachycardia and increases in myocardial contractility, cardiac output, and total peripheral resistance. The result is dangerously high blood pressure. Treatment consists of a tourniquet on the injected limb, with intermittent brief releases of the tourniquet, and the use of adrenergic blocking drugs.

Indices of contractility. A reasonable index of myocardial contractility can be obtained from the contour of ventricular pressure curves (Fig. 23-9). A hypodynamic heart is characterized by an elevated end-diastolic pressure, a slowly rising ventricular pressure, and a somewhat reduced ejection phase (curve *C*, Fig. 23-9). A hyperdynamic heart (such as a heart stimulated by norepinephrine) shows reduced end-diastolic pressure, fast-rising ventricular pressure, and a brief ejection phase (curve *B*, Fig. 23-9). The slope of the ascending limb of the ventricular pressure curve indicates the maximal rate of force development by the ventricle (maximal rate of change in pressure with time—maximal dP/dt, as illustrated by the tangents to the steepest portion of the ascending limbs of the ventricular pressure curves in Fig. 23-9). The slope is maximal during the isovolumic phase of systole (Fig. 23-10). At any given degree of ventricular filling, the slope provides an index of the initial contraction velocity, and hence of contractility.

A similar indication of the contractile state of the myocardium can be obtained from the velocity of blood flow that initially occurs in the ascending aorta during the cardiac cycle (the initial slope of the aortic flow curve) (Fig. 23-10). Also, the **ejection fraction,** which is the ratio of the volume of blood ejected from the left ventricle per beat (**stroke volume**) to the volume of blood in the left ventricle at the end of diastole (end-diastolic volume), is widely used clinically as an index of contractility. Other measurements (or combinations of measurements) that reflect the magnitude or velocity of the ventricular contraction have been used to assess the contractile state of the cardiac muscle. No index is

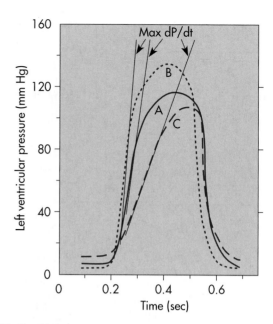

■ **Fig. 23-9**   Left ventricular pressure curves with tangents drawn to the steepest portions of the ascending limbs to indicate maximal dP/dt values. *A,* Control; *B,* hyperdynamic heart, as with norepinephrine administration; *C,* hypodynamic heart, as in cardiac failure.

entirely satisfactory at present, which undoubtedly accounts for the several indices currently in use.

Cardiac chambers. The atria are thin-walled, low-pressure chambers that function more as large-reservoir conduits of blood for their respective ventricles than as important pumps for the forward propulsion of blood. The ventricles were once thought to be composed of bands of muscle. However, it now appears that they are formed by a continuum of muscle fibers that originate from the fibrous skeleton at the base of the heart (chiefly around the aortic orifice). These fibers sweep toward the heart apex at the epicardial surface. They pass toward the endocardium and gradually undergo a 180-degree change in direction to lie parallel to the epicardial fibers and form the endocardium and papillary muscles (Fig. 23-11). At the apex of the heart, the fibers twist and turn inward to form papillary muscles. At the base of the heart and around the valve orifices, they form a thick, powerful muscle that not only decreases ventricular circumference for ejection of blood, but also narrows the atrioventricular (AV) valve orifices as an aid to valve closure. Ventricular ejection is also accomplished by a decrease in the longitudinal axis as the heart begins to narrow toward the base. The earlier contraction of the apical part of the ventricles, coupled with approximation of the ventricular walls, propels the blood toward the outflow tracts. The right ventricle, which develops a mean pressure about one seventh of that developed by the left ventricle, is considerably thinner than the left.

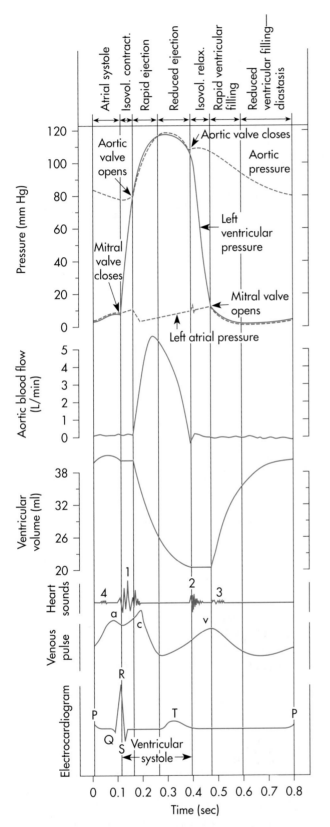

Fig. 23-10 Left atrial, aortic, and left ventricular pressure pulses correlated in time with aortic flow, ventricular volume, heart sounds, venous pulse, and the electrocardiogram for a complete cardiac cycle in the dog.

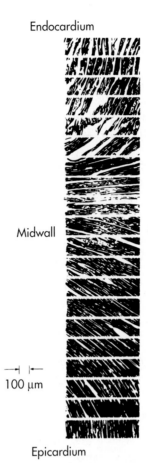

Endocardium

Midwall

100 μm

Epicardium

Fig. 23-11 Sequence of photomicrographs showing fiber angles in successive sections taken from the middle of the free wall of the left ventricle from a heart in systole. The sections are parallel to the epicardial plane. The fiber angle is 90 degrees at the endocardium, running through 0 degrees at the midwall to −90 degrees at the epicardium. (From Streeter DD Jr et al: *Circ Res* 24:339, 1969, with permission of the American Heart Association.)

Cardiac valves. The cardiac valves consist of thin flaps of flexible, tough, endothelium-covered fibrous tissue (valve leaflets) that is firmly attached at the base to the fibrous valve rings. Movements of the valve leaflets are essentially passive, and the orientation of the cardiac valves is responsible for unidirectional flow of blood through the heart. There are two types of valves in the heart: the **atrioventricular** and the **semilunar valves** (Figs. 23-12 and 23-13).

Atrioventricular valves. The AV valve located between the right atrium and the right ventricle is made up of three cusps (**tricuspid valve**), whereas that between the left atrium and the left ventricle has two cusps (**mitral valve**). The total area of the cusps of each AV valve is approximately twice that of the respective AV orifice, so that considerable overlap of the leaflets occurs in the closed position (Figs. 23-12 and 23-13). Attached to the free edges of these valves are fine, strong ligaments (**chordae**

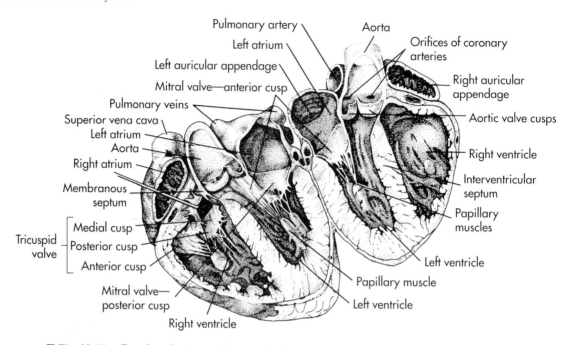

Pulmonary artery
Aorta
Orifices of coronary arteries
Left atrium
Left auricular appendage
Right auricular appendage
Mitral valve—anterior cusp
Pulmonary veins
Aortic valve cusps
Superior vena cava
Left atrium
Aorta
Right ventricle
Right atrium
Interventricular septum
Membranous septum
Papillary muscles
Tricuspid valve
Medial cusp
Posterior cusp
Anterior cusp
Left ventricle
Mitral valve— posterior cusp
Papillary muscle
Right ventricle
Left ventricle

■ **Fig. 23-12** Drawing of a heart split perpendicular to the interventricular septum to illustrate the anatomic relationships of the leaflets of the atrioventricular and aortic valves.

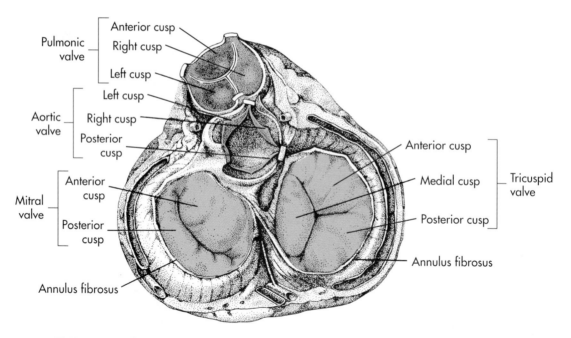

Pulmonic valve
Anterior cusp
Right cusp
Left cusp
Aortic valve
Left cusp
Right cusp
Posterior cusp
Anterior cusp
Medial cusp
Tricuspid valve
Mitral valve
Anterior cusp
Posterior cusp
Posterior cusp
Annulus fibrosus
Annulus fibrosus

■ **Fig. 23-13** Four cardiac valves as viewed from the base of the heart. Note how the leaflets overlap in the closed valves.

tendineae), which arise from the powerful papillary muscles of the respective ventricles and prevent the valves from becoming everted during ventricular systole.

In the normal heart, the valve leaflets remain relatively close together during ventricular filling and thus provide a funnel for the transfer of blood from atrium to ventricle. The partial approximation of the valve surfaces during diastole is caused by eddy currents behind the leaflets and also by some tension on the free edges of the valves.

This tension is exerted by the chordae tendineae and papillary muscles that are stretched by the filling ventricle.

Movements of the mitral valve leaflets throughout the cardiac cycle are shown in an **echocardiogram** (Fig. 23-14). Echocardiography consists of sending short pulses of high-frequency sound waves (ultrasound) through the chest tissues and the heart and recording the echoes reflected from the various structures. The timing and pattern of the reflected waves provide such information as

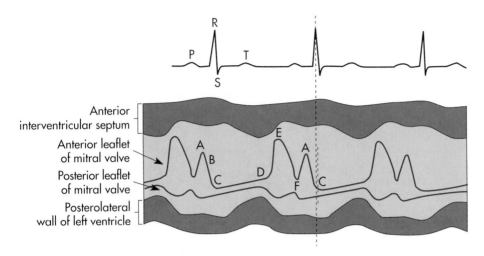

Anterior
interventricular septum

Anterior leaflet
of mitral valve

Posterior leaflet
of mitral valve

Posterolateral
wall of left ventricle

■ **Fig. 23-14** Drawing made from an echocardiogram showing movements of the mitral valve leaflets (particularly the anterior leaflet) and the changes in the diameter of the left ventricular cavity and the thickness of the left ventricular walls during cardiac cycles in a normal person. D to C, Ventricular diastole; C to D, ventricular systole; D to E, rapid filling; E to F, reduced filling (diastasis); F to A, atrial contraction. The mitral valve closes at C and opens at D. Simultaneously recorded electrocardiogram at top.

the diameter of the heart, the ventricular wall thickness, and the magnitude and direction of the movements of various components of the heart.

In Fig. 23-14, the echocardiogram is positioned to depict movement of the anterior leaflet of the mitral valve. The posterior leaflet moves in a pattern that is a mirror image of the anterior leaflet, but in the projection shown in Fig. 23-14 its movements appear to be much smaller. At point *D*, the mitral valve opens, and during rapid filling *(D to E)* the anterior leaflet moves toward the ventricular septum. During the reduced filling phase *(E to F)*, the valve leaflets float toward each other, but the valve does not close. The ventricular filling contributed by atrial contraction *(F to A)* forces the leaflets apart, followed by a second approximation of the leaflets *(A to C)*. At point *C* the valve is closed by ventricular contraction. The valve leaflets, which bulge toward the atrium, stay pressed together during ventricular systole *(C to D)*.

Semilunar valves. The semilunar valves located between the right ventricle and the pulmonary artery and between the left ventricle and the aorta consist of three cuplike cusps attached to the valve rings (Figs. 23-12 and 23-13). At the end of the reduced ejection phase of ventricular systole, blood flow briefly reverses toward the ventricles (shown as a negative flow in the phasic aortic flow curve in Fig. 23-10). This reversal of blood flow snaps the cusps together and prevents regurgitation of blood into the ventricles. During ventricular systole, the cusps do not lie back against the walls of the pulmonary artery and aorta, but instead float in the bloodstream at a point approximately midway between the vessel walls and their closed position. Behind the semilunar valves are small outpocketings of the pulmonary artery and aorta **(sinuses of Valsalva),** where eddy currents develop that tend to keep the valve cusps away from the vessel walls. In addition, the orifices of the right and left coronary arteries are behind the right and the left cusps, respectively, of the aortic valve. Were it

not for the presence of the sinuses of Valsalva and the eddy currents developed therein, the coronary ostia could be blocked by the valve cusps.

The pericardium. The pericardium is an epithelialized fibrous sac. It closely invests the entire heart and the cardiac portion of the great vessels and is reflected onto the cardiac surface as the epicardium. The sac normally contains a small amount of fluid, which provides lubrication for the continuous movement of the enclosed heart. The distensibility of the pericardium is small, so that it strongly resists a large, rapid increase in cardiac size. Because of this characteristic, the pericardium plays a role in preventing sudden overdistention of the chambers of the heart. However, in congenital absence of the pericardium or after its surgical removal, cardiac function still remains within physiological limits. Nevertheless, with the pericardium intact, an increase in diastolic pressure in one ventricle increases the pressure and decreases the compliance of the other ventricle.

Heart sounds. Four sounds are usually produced by the heart, but only two are ordinarily audible through a stethoscope. With electronic amplification, the less intense sounds can be detected and recorded graphically as a **phonocardiogram.** This means of registering faint heart sounds helps to delineate the precise timing of the heart sounds relative to other events in the cardiac cycle.

The first heart sound is initiated at the onset of ventricular systole (Fig. 23-10) and consists of a series of vibrations of mixed, unrelated, low frequencies (a noise). It is the loudest and longest of the heart sounds, has a crescendo-decrescendo quality, and is heard best over the apical region of the heart. The tricuspid valve sounds are heard best in the fifth intercostal space just to the left of the sternum; the mitral sounds are heard best in the fifth intercostal space at the cardiac apex.

The first heart sound is chiefly caused by oscillation of blood in the ventricular chambers and vibration of the chamber walls. The vibrations are engendered in part by the abrupt rise of ventricular pressure with acceleration of blood back toward the atria. However, the main cause of the first heart sound is the sudden tension and recoil of the AV valves and adjacent structures with deceleration of the blood as the AV valves close. The vibrations of the ventricles and the contained blood are transmitted through surrounding tissues and reach the chest wall (where they may be heard or recorded). The intensity of the first sound is a function of the force of ventricular contraction and of the distance between the valve leaflets. The first sound is loudest when the leaflets are farthest apart, as occurs when the interval between atrial and ventricular systoles is prolonged (AV valve leaflets float apart) or when ventricular systole immediately follows atrial systole.

The second heart sound, which occurs with the abrupt closure of the semilunar valves (Fig. 23-10), is composed of higher-frequency vibrations (higher pitch), is of shorter duration and lower intensity, and has a more snapping quality than the first heart sound. Semilunar valve closure initiates oscillations of the columns of blood and the tensed vessel walls by the stretch and recoil of the closed valve. The portion of the second sound caused by closure of the pulmonic valve is heard best in the second thoracic interspace just to the left of the sternum, whereas that caused by closure of the aortic valve is heard best in the same intercostal space but to the right of the sternum. Conditions that cause the semilunar valves to close more rapidly than usual, such as increases in pulmonary artery or aortic pressure (e.g., pulmonary or systemic hypertension), increase the intensity of the second heart sound. The aortic valve sound is usually louder than the pulmonic, but in cases of pulmonary hypertension the reverse is true.

A normal phonocardiogram taken simultaneously with an electrocardiogram (ECG) is illustrated in Fig. 23-15. The first sound starts just beyond the peak of the R waves. Note that this sound is composed of irregular waves and is of greater intensity and duration than the second sound, which appears at the end of the T wave. A third and fourth heart sound do not appear on this record.

The third heart sound is sometimes heard in children with thin chest walls or in patients with left ventricular failure. It consists of a few low-intensity, low-frequency vibrations heard best in the region of the apex. The vibrations occur in early diastole and are caused by abrupt cessation of ventricular distention and deceleration of blood entering the ventricles.

In overloaded hearts, as in congestive heart failure, when the ventricular volume is very large and the ventricular walls are stretched to the point where distensibility abruptly decreases, a third heart sound may be heard. A third heart sound in patients with heart disease is usually a grave sign.

A fourth, or atrial, sound consists of a few low-frequency oscillations. This sound is occasionally heard

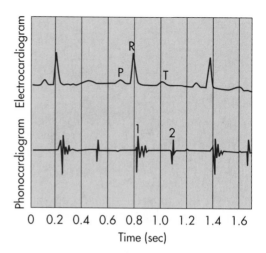

■ **Fig. 23-15**   Phonocardiogram illustrating the first and second heart sounds and their relationship to the P, R, and T waves of the electrocardiogram. Time lines = 0.04 second.

in normal individuals. It is caused by oscillation of blood and cardiac chambers created by atrial contraction (Fig. 23-10).

Because the onset and termination of right and left ventricular systoles are not precisely synchronous, differences in the time of vibration of the two AV valves or two semilunar valves can sometimes be detected with the stethoscope. Asynchrony of valve vibrations, which may sometimes indicate abnormal cardiac function, is heard as a **split sound** over the apex of the heart for the AV valves and over the base for the semilunar valves.

Mitral insufficiency and **mitral stenosis** produce, respectively, systolic and diastolic murmurs heard best at the cardiac apex. **Aortic insufficiency** and **aortic stenosis,** on the other hand, produce, respectively, diastolic and systolic murmurs heard best in the second intercostal space just to the right of the sternum. The characteristics of the murmur serve as an important guide in the diagnosis of valvular disease.

When the third and fourth (atrial) sounds are accentuated, as occurs in certain abnormal conditions, triplets of sounds may occur, resembling the sound of a galloping horse. These **gallop rhythms** are essentially of two types: **presystolic gallop** caused by accentuation of the atrial sound, and **protodiastolic gallop** caused by accentuation of the third heart sound.

■ *The Cardiac Cycle*

■ *Ventricular Systole*

Isovolumic contraction.   The onset of ventricular contraction coincides with the peak of the R wave on an ECG and the initial vibration of the first heart sound. It is indicated on the ventricular pressure curve as the earliest rise in ventricular pressure after atrial contraction.

The time between the start of ventricular systole and the opening of the semilunar valves (when ventricular pressure rises abruptly) is called **isovolumic** (literally, "same volume") **contraction.** This term is appropriate because ventricular volume remains constant during this brief period (Fig. 23-10).

The increment in ventricular pressure during isovolumic contraction is transmitted across the closed valves. Isovolumic contraction has also been referred to as isometric contraction ("isometric" describes a contraction of a muscle that produces increased tension at a constant length). However, some cardiac muscle fibers shorten and others lengthen, as evidenced by changes in ventricular shape; it is therefore not a true isometric contraction.

Ejection. Opening of the semilunar valves marks the onset of the ventricular ejection phase, which may be subdivided into an earlier, shorter phase **(rapid ejection)** and a later, longer phase **(reduced ejection).** The rapid ejection phase is distinguished from the reduced ejection phase by three factors: (1) the sharp rise in ventricular and aortic pressures that terminates at the peak ventricular and aortic pressures, (2) a more abrupt decrease in ventricular volume, and (3) a greater aortic blood flow (Fig. 23-10). The sharp decrease in the left atrial pressure curve at the onset of ejection results from the descent of the base of the heart and stretch of the atria. During the reduced ejection period, runoff of blood from the aorta to the periphery exceeds ventricular output, and therefore aortic pressure declines. Throughout ventricular systole, the blood returning to the atria produces a progressive increase in atrial pressure.

Note that during the first third of the ejection period, left ventricular pressure slightly exceeds aortic pressure and blood flow into the aorta accelerates (continues to increase), whereas during the last two thirds of ventricular ejection the reverse holds true. This reversal of the ventricular-aortic pressure gradient in the presence of continued flow of blood from the left ventricle to the aorta (caused by the momentum of the forward blood flow) is the result of storage of potential energy in the stretched arterial walls. This stored potential energy decelerates blood flow into the aorta. The peak of the flow curve coincides with the point at which the left ventricular pressure curve intersects the aortic pressure curve during ejection. Thereafter, flow decelerates (continues to decrease) because the pressure gradient has been reversed.

In right ventricular ejection, a shortening of the free wall of the right ventricle (descent of the tricuspid valve ring) occurs in addition to lateral compression of the chamber. However, with left ventricular ejection, very little shortening of the base-to-apex axis occurs, and ejection is accomplished chiefly by compression of the left ventricular chamber.

The effect of ventricular systole on left ventricular diameter is shown in an echocardiogram (Fig. 23-14). During ventricular systole (Fig. 23-14, *C* to *D*), the sep-

tum and the free wall of the left ventricle become thicker and move closer to each other.

Fig. 23-10 shows a tracing of a venous pulse curve taken from a jugular vein. The *c* wave in this tracing is caused by the impact of the common carotid artery with the adjacent jugular vein and to some extent by the abrupt closure of the tricuspid valve in early ventricular systole. Note that except for the *c* wave, the venous pulse closely follows the atrial pressure curve.

At the end of ejection, a volume of blood approximately equal to that ejected during systole remains in the ventricular cavities. This **residual volume** is fairly constant in normal hearts. However, the residual volume is smaller with increased heart rate or reduced outflow resistance and larger when the opposite conditions prevail.

An increase in myocardial contractility, as produced by catecholamines or by digitalis in a patient with a depressed heart, may decrease residual volume and increase stroke volume and ejection fraction. With severely hypodynamic and dilated hearts, as in **heart failure,** the residual volume can become many times greater than the stroke volume.

In addition to serving as a small adjustable blood reservoir, the residual volume, to a limited degree, allows for transient disparities between the outputs of the two ventricles.

■ *Ventricular Diastole*

Isovolumic relaxation. Closure of the aortic valve produces the characteristic **incisura (notch)** on the descending limb of the aortic pressure curve and the second heart sound (with some vibrations evident on the atrial pressure curve), and it marks the end of ventricular systole. The period between closure of the semilunar valves and opening of the AV valves is termed **isovolumic relaxation.** It is characterized by a precipitous fall in ventricular pressure without a change in ventricular volume.

Rapid filling phase. The major part of ventricular filling occurs immediately on opening of the AV valves. At this point the blood that had returned to the atria during the previous ventricular systole is abruptly released into the relaxing ventricles. This period of ventricular filling is called the **rapid filling phase.** In Fig. 23-10 the onset of the rapid filling phase is indicated by the decrease in left ventricular pressure below left atrial pressure. This pressure reversal results in the opening of the mitral valve. The rapid flow of blood from atria to relaxing ventricles produces a decrease in atrial and ventricular pressures and a sharp increase in ventricular volume.

Elastic recoil of the previous ventricular contraction may help draw blood into the relaxing ventricle when residual volume is small, especially when ventricular contractility is enhanced (such as when catecholamines are administered). However, this mechanism probably does not contribute to ventricular filling under most normal conditions.

Diastasis. The rapid filling phase is followed by a phase of slow filling called **diastasis.** During diastasis, blood returning from the periphery flows into the right ventricle, and blood from the lungs flows into the left ventricle. This small, slow addition to ventricular filling is indicated by a gradual rise in atrial, ventricular, and venous pressures and in ventricular volume (Fig. 23-10).

Atrial systole. The onset of atrial systole occurs soon after the beginning of the P wave of the ECG (curve of atrial depolarization). The transfer of blood from atrium to ventricle made by the peristalsis-like wave of atrial contraction completes the period of ventricular filling. Atrial systole is responsible for the small increases in atrial, ventricular, and venous pressures, as well as in ventricular volume shown in Fig. 23-10. Throughout ventricular diastole, atrial pressure barely exceeds ventricular pressure. This small pressure difference indicates that the pathway through the open AV valves during ventricular filling has low resistance.

Because there are no valves at the junctions of the venae cavae and right atrium or of the pulmonary veins and left atrium, atrial contraction can force blood in both directions. Actually, little blood is pumped back into the venous tributaries during the brief atrial contraction, mainly because of the inertia of the inflowing blood.

Atrial contraction is not essential for ventricular filling, as can be observed in atrial fibrillation or complete heart block. In atrial fibrillation, the atrial myofibers contract in an uncoordinated fashion and therefore cannot pump blood into the ventricles. In complete heart block, the atria and ventricles beat independently of each other. However, ventricular filling can be normal with these two arrhythmias.

The contribution of atrial contraction to ventricular filling is governed to a great extent by the heart rate and position of the AV valves. At slow heart rates, filling practically ceases toward the end of diastasis, and atrial contraction contributes little additional filling. During tachycardia, however, diastasis is abbreviated and the atrial contribution can become substantial, especially if the atrial contraction occurs immediately after the rapid filling phase, when the AV pressure gradient is maximal. Should tachycardia become so great that the rapid filling phase is encroached on, atrial contraction assumes great importance in rapidly propelling blood into the ventricle during this brief period of the cardiac cycle. Of course, if the period of ventricular relaxation is so brief that filling is seriously impaired, even atrial contraction cannot provide adequate ventricular filling. The consequent reduction in cardiac output may result in syncope (fainting). Obviously, if atrial contraction occurs simultaneously

with ventricular contraction, no atrial contribution to ventricular filling can occur.

Pressure-volume relationship. The changes in left ventricular pressure and volume throughout the cardiac cycle are summarized in Fig. 23-16. Time is not considered in this **pressure-volume loop.** Diastolic filling starts at *A* and terminates at *C,* when the mitral valve closes. The initial decrease in left ventricular pressure (*A* to *B*), despite the rapid inflow of blood from the atrium, is attributed to progressive ventricular relaxation and distensibility. During the remainder of diastole (*B* to *C*), the increase in ventricular pressure reflects ventricular filling and the passive elastic characteristics of the ventricle. Note that only a small increase in pressure occurs with the increase in ventricular volume during diastole (*B* to *C*). The small increase in pressure just to the left of *C* is caused by the contribution of atrial contraction to ventricular filling. With isovolumic contraction (*C* to *D*), pressure rises steeply, but no change occurs in ventricular volume. At *D,* the aortic valve opens, and during the first phase of ejection (rapid ejection, *D* to *E*), the large reduction in volume is associated with a steady increase in ventricular pressure that is less steep than the pressure increase that occurred during isovolumic contraction. This volume reduction is followed by reduced ejection (*E* to *F*) and a small decrease in ventricular pressure. The aortic valve closes at *F,* and this event is followed by isovolumic relaxation (*F* to *A*), which is characterized by a sharp drop in pressure and no change in volume. The mitral valve opens at A to complete one cardiac cycle.

In certain disease states, the AV valves may be markedly narrowed **(stenotic).** Under such conditions, atrial contraction plays a much more important role in ventricular filling than it does in the normal heart.

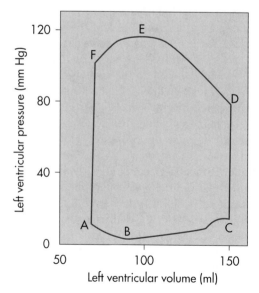

■ **Fig. 23-16**   Pressure-volume loop of the left ventricle for a single cardiac cycle *(ABCDEF).*

■ *Measurement of Cardiac Output*

■ *Fick Principle*

In 1870 the German physiologist Adoph Fick contrived the first method for measuring cardiac output in intact animals and people. The basis for this method, called the **Fick principle,** is simply an application of the law of conservation of mass. It is derived from the fact that the quantity of oxygen (O_2) delivered to the pulmonary capillaries via the pulmonary artery, plus the quantity of O_2 that enters the pulmonary capillaries from the alveoli, must equal the quantity of O_2 that is carried away by the pulmonary veins.

The Fick principle is depicted schematically in Fig. 23-17. The rate, q_1, of O_2 delivery to the lungs equals the O_2 concentration in the pulmonary arterial blood, $[O_2]_{pa}$, times the pulmonary arterial blood flow, Q, which equals the cardiac output; that is

$$q_1 = Q[O_2]_{pa} \qquad (23\text{-}1)$$

Let q_2 be the net rate of O_2 uptake by the pulmonary capillaries from the alveoli. At equilibrium, q_2 equals the **O_2 consumption** of the body. The rate, q_3, at which O_2 is carried away by the pulmonary veins equals the O_2 concentration in the pulmonary venous blood, $[O_2]_{pv}$, times the total pulmonary venous flow, which is virtually equal to the pulmonary arterial blood flow, Q; that is,

$$q_3 = Q[O_2]_{pv} \qquad (23\text{-}2)$$

From conservation of mass,

$$q_1 + q_2 = q_3 \qquad (23\text{-}3)$$

Therefore,

$$Q[O_2]_{pa} + q_2 = Q[O_2]_{pv} \qquad (23\text{-}4)$$

Solving for cardiac output,

$$Q = q_2/([O_2]_{pv} - [O_2]_{pa}) \qquad (23\text{-}5)$$

Equation 23-5 is the statement of the Fick principle.

The clinical determination of cardiac output requires three values: (1) O_2 consumption of the body, (2) the O_2 concentration in the pulmonary venous blood ($[O_2]_{pv}$, and (3) the O_2 concentration in the pulmonary arterial blood ($[O_2]_{pa}$). O_2 consumption is computed from measurements of the volume and O_2 content of expired air over a given interval of time. Because the O_2 concentration of peripheral arterial blood is essentially identical to that in the pulmonary veins, $[O_2]_{pv}$ is determined on a sample of peripheral arterial blood withdrawn by needle puncture. Pulmonary arterial blood, $[O_2]_{pa}$, actually represents mixed systemic venous blood. Samples for O_2 analysis are obtained from the pulmonary artery or right ventricle through a catheter. In the past, a relatively stiff catheter was used and it had to be introduced into the pul-

monary artery under fluoroscopic guidance. Today, a very flexible catheter with a small balloon near the tip can be inserted into a peripheral vein. As the tube is advanced, it is carried by the flowing blood toward the heart. By following the pressure changes, the physician is able to advance the catheter tip into the pulmonary artery without the aid of fluoroscopy.

An example of the calculation of cardiac output in a normal, resting adult is illustrated in Fig. 23-17. With an O_2 consumption of 250 ml/min, an arterial (pulmonary venous) O_2 content of 0.20 ml O_2/ml blood, and a mixed venous (pulmonary arterial) O_2 content of 0.15 ml O_2/ml blood, the cardiac output equals $250/(0.20 - 0.15)$ = 5000 ml/min.

The Fick principle is also used for estimating the O_2 consumption of organs when blood flow and the O_2 contents of the arterial and venous blood can be determined. Algebraic rearrangement reveals that O_2 consumption equals the blood flow times the arteriovenous O_2 concentration difference. For example, if the blood flow through one kidney is 700 ml/min, arterial O_2 content is 0.20 ml O_2/ml blood, and renal venous O_2 content is 0.18 ml O_2/ml blood, the rate of O_2 consumption by that kidney must be $700 (0.2 \times 0.18)$ = 14 ml O_2/min.

■ *Indicator Dilution Techniques*

The indicator dilution technique for measuring cardiac output is also based on the law of conservation of mass and is illustrated by the model in Fig. 23-18. In this model, a liquid flows through a tube at a rate of Q ml/sec, and q mg of dye is injected as a slug into the stream at point *A*. Mixing occurs at some point downstream. If a small sample of liquid is continually withdrawn from point *B* farther downstream and passed through a densitometer, a curve of the dye concentration, *c*, may be recorded as a function of time, *t*, as shown in the lower half of Fig. 23-18.

If no dye is lost between points *A* and *B*, the amount of dye, *q*, passing point *B* between times t_1 and t_2 will be

$$q = \bar{c}Q(t_1 - t_2) \qquad (23\text{-}6)$$

where $\bar{c}$ is the mean concentration of dye. The value of $\bar{c}$ may be computed by dividing the area of the dye concentration by the duration ($t_2 - t_1$) of the curve; that is

$$\bar{c} = \int_{t_1}^{t_2} cdt/(t_2 - t_1) \qquad (23\text{-}7)$$

Substituting this value of $\bar{c}$ into equation 23-6 and solving for Q yields

$$Q = \frac{q}{\int_{t_1}^{t_2} cdt} \qquad (23\text{-}8)$$

Thus, flow may be measured by dividing the amount of indicator (the dye) injected upstream by the area under the downstream concentration curve.

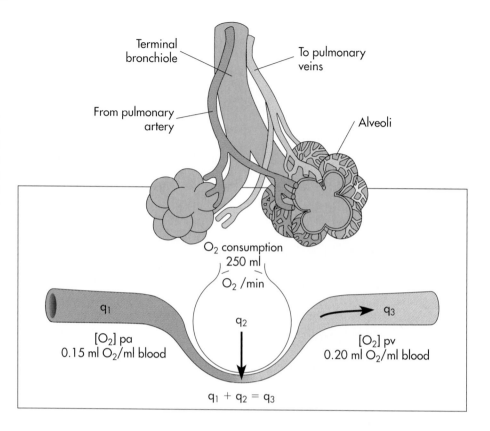

■ **Fig. 23-17** Schema illustrating the Fick principle for measuring cardiac output. The change in color from pulmonary artery to pulmonary vein represents the change in color of the blood as venous blood becomes fully oxygenated.

■ **Fig. 23-18** Indicator dilution technique for measuring cardiac output. In this model, in which there is no recirculation, q mg of dye are injected instantaneously at point *A* into a stream flowing at Q ml/min. A mixed sample of the fluid flowing past point *B* is withdrawn at a constant rate through a densitometer; *C* is concentration of dye in the fluid. The resultant dye concentration curve at point *B* has the configuration shown in the lower section of the figure.

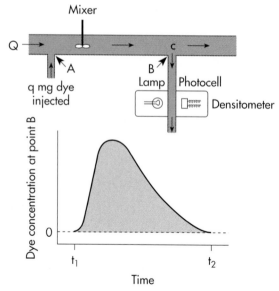

This technique has been widely used to estimate cardiac output in humans. A measured quantity of some indicator (a dye or isotope that remains within the circulation) is injected rapidly into a large central vein or into the right side of the heart through a catheter. Arterial blood is continuously drawn through a detector (densitometer or isotope rate counter), and a curve of indicator concentration is recorded as a function of time.

Currently, the most popular indicator dilution technique is **thermodilution.** The indicator used in this method is cold saline. The temperature and volume of the saline are measured accurately before injection. A flexible catheter is introduced into a peripheral vein and advanced so that the tip lies in the pulmonary artery. A small thermistor at the catheter tip records the changes in temperature. The opening in the catheter lies a few inches proximal to the tip. When the tip is in the pulmonary artery, the opening lies in or near the right atrium. The

cold saline is injected rapidly into the right atrium through the catheter and flows out through the opening in the catheter. The change in temperature downstream is recorded by the thermistor in the pulmonary artery.

The thermodilution technique has the following advantages: (1) an arterial puncture is not necessary; (2) the small volumes of saline used in each determination are innocuous, and thus repeated determinations can be made; and (3) recirculation is negligible. Temperature equilibration takes place as the cooled blood flows through the pulmonary and systemic capillary beds, before it flows by the thermistor in the pulmonary artery the second time.

■ *Summary*

1. An increase in myocardial fiber length, as occurs with augmented ventricular filling (preload) during diastole, produces a more forceful ventricular contraction. This relation between fiber length and strength of contraction is known as the Frank-Starling relationship or Starling's law of the heart.

2. Although the myocardium is made up of individual cells with discrete membrane boundaries, the cardiac myocytes that make up the ventricles contract almost in unison, as do those of the atria. The myocardium functions as a syncytium with an all-or-none response to excitation. Cell-to-cell conduction occurs through gap junctions that connect the cytosol of adjacent cells.

3. On excitation, voltage-gated calcium channels open to admit extracellular Ca^{++} into the cell. The influx of Ca^{++} triggers the release of Ca^{++} from the sarcoplasmic reticulum. The elevated intracellular $[Ca^{++}]$ produces contraction of the myofilaments. Relaxation is accomplished via restoration of the resting cytosolic Ca^{++} level by pumping it back into the sarcoplasmic reticulum and exchanging it for extracellular Na^+ across the sarcolemma.

4. Velocity and force of contraction are functions of the intracellular concentration of free calcium ions. Force and velocity are inversely related, so that with no load, velocity is maximal. In an isovolumic contraction, where no external shortening occurs, total load is maximal and velocity is zero.

5. In ventricular contraction, the preload is the stretch of the fibers by the blood during ventricular filling. The afterload is the aortic pressure against which the left ventricle ejects the blood.

6. Contractility is an expression of cardiac performance at a given preload and afterload.

7. Simultaneous recording of left atrial, left ventricular, and aortic pressures; ventricular volume; heart sounds; and the electrocardiogram graphically portray the sequential and related electrical and cardiodynamic events throughout a cardiac cycle.

8. The first heart sound is caused mainly by abrupt closure of the AV valve; the second heart sound is caused by abrupt closure of the semilunar valves.

9. Cardiac output can be determined, according to the Fick principle, by measuring the oxygen consumption of the body (q_2) and the oxygen content of arterial $[O_2]_a$ and mixed venous $[O_2]_v$ blood. Cardiac output $= q_2 /([O_2]_a - [O_2]_v)$. It can also be measured by dye dilution or thermodilution techniques. The greater the cardiac output, the greater is the dilution of the injected dye or cold saline by the arterial blood.

■ *Self-Study Problems*

1. Increase of force in skeletal muscle is accomplished by recruitment of muscle fibers via motor nerve activity. How does the heart increase its contractile force?

2. What are cardiac preload and afterload, and how do they affect developed pressure and velocity of contraction?

3. How is myocardial contractility evaluated?

4. What is the function of the pericardium, and how can it affect cardiac filling and performance?

5. In a patient with severe mitral stenosis, where precisely in the cardiac cycle does the murmur occur?

6. If the arterial blood oxygen content is 19 ml/dl, the mixed venous oxygen content 12 ml/dl, and the oxygen consumption 280 ml/min, what is the cardiac output? In the same person, if the coronary sinus blood oxygen content is 5 ml/dl and the coronary sinus blood flow 150 ml/min, what is the oxygen consumption of the myocardium drained via the coronary sinus?

■ *Bibliography*

Journal articles

Bers DM, Lederer WJ, Berlin JR: Intracellular Ca transients in rat cardiac myocytes: role of Na-Ca exchange in excitation-contraction coupling, *Am J Physiol* 258:C944, 1990.

Brutsaert DL, Sys SU: Relaxation and diastole of the heart, *Physiol Rev* 69:1228, 1989.

Cannell MB, Cheng H, Lederer WJ: The control of calcium release in heart muscle, *Science* 268:1045, 1995.

Carafoli E: Calcium pump of the plasma membrane, *Physiol Rev* 71:129, 1991.

Chapman RA: Control of cardiac contractility at the cellular level, *Am J Physiol* 245:H535, 1983.

Elzinga G, Westerhof N: Matching between ventricle and arterial load, *Circ Res* 68:1495, 1991.

Fabiato A, Fabiato F: Calcium and cardiac excitation-contraction coupling, *Annu Rev Physiol* 41:473, 1979.

Fleischer S, Inui M: Biochemistry and biophysics of excitation-contraction coupling, *Annu Rev Biophys Chem* 18:333, 1989.

Ford LE: Mechanical manifestations of activation in cardiac muscle, *Circ Res* 68:621, 1991.

Gilbert JC, Glantz SA: Determinants of left ventricular filling and of the diastolic pressure-volume relation, *Circ Res* 64:827, 1989.

Katz AM: Cyclic adenosine monophosphate effects on the myocardium: a man who blows hot and cold with one breath, *J Am Coll Cardiol* 2:143, 1983.

Katz AM: Interplay between inotropic and lusitropic effects of cyclic adenosine monophosphate on the myocardial cell, *Circulation* 82:1-7, 1990.

Landesberg A, Sideman S: Mechanical regulation of cardiac muscle by coupling calcium kinetics with crossbridge cycling: a dynamic model, *Am J Physiol* 267:H779, 1994.

Luo W et al: Targeted ablation of the phospholamban gene is associated with markedly enhanced myocardial contractility and loss of β-agonist stimulation, *Circ Res* 75:401, 1994.

Sagawa K: The ventricular pressure-volume diagram revisited, *Circ Res* 43:677, 1978.

Schwinger RHG et al: The failing human heart is unable to use the Frank-Starling mechanism, *Circ Res* 74:959, 1994.

Smith JS, Rousseau E, Meissner G: Single sarcoplasmic reticulum Ca^{2+}-release channels from calmodulin modulation of cardiac and skeletal muscle, *Circ Res* 64:352, 1989.

Stern MD, Lakatta EG: Excitation-contraction coupling in the heart: the state of the question, *FASEB J* 6:3092, 1992.

Streeter DD Jr et al: Fiber orientation in the canine left ventricle during diastole and systole, *Circ Res* 24:339, 1969.

Zhang R, Zhao J, Mandveno A, Potter JD: Cardiac troponin I phosphorylation increases the rate of cardiac muscle relaxation, *Circ Res* 76:1028, 1995.

Books and monographs

Brady AJ: *Mechanical properties of cardiac fibers.* In *Handbook of physiology,* sect 2: *The cardiovascular system—the heart,* vol I, Bethesda, Md, 1979, American Physiological Society.

Frank GB, Bianchi CP, ten Keurs HEDJ, editors: *Excitation-contraction coupling in skeletal cardiac and smooth muscle,* New York, 1992, Plenum Press.

Gibbons WR, Zygmunt AC: *Excitation-contraction coupling in the heart.* In Fozzard HA et al, editors: *The heart and cardiovascular system,* ed 2, New York, 1991, Raven Press.

Lakatta EG: *Length modulation of muscle performance: Frank-Starling law of the heart.* In Fozzard HA et al, editors: *The heart and cardiovascular system,* ed 2, New York, 1991, Raven Press.

Lytton J, MacLennan DH: *Sarcoplasmic reticulum.* In Fozzard HA et al, editors: *The heart and cardiovascular system,* ed 2, New York, 1991, Raven Press.

Parmley WW, Talbot L: *Heart as a pump.* In *Handbook of physiology,* sect 2: *The cardiovascular system—the heart,* vol I, Bethesda, Md, 1979, American Physiological Society.

Ruegg JC: *Calcium in muscle activation,* Heidelberg, 1988, Springer-Verlag.

Sheu SS, Blaustein MP: *Sodium/calcium exchange and control of cell calcium and contractility in cardiac muscle and vascular smooth muscle.* In Fozzard HA et al, editors: *The heart and cardiovascular system,* ed 2, New York, 1991, Raven Press.

Sommer JR, Johnson EA: *Ultrastructure of cardiac muscle.* In *Handbook of physiology,* sect 2: *The cardiovascular system—the heart,* vol I, Bethesda, Md, 1979, American Physiological Society.

Regulation of the Heartbeat

The **cardiac output** (CO) is defined as the quantity of blood pumped by the heart each minute. Cardiac output may be varied by changing the frequency of the heartbeat (i.e., the **heart rate** [HR]) or the volume of blood ejected from one ventricle with each heartbeat; this volume is called the **stroke volume** (SV). In mathematical terms, cardiac output can be expressed as the product of heart rate and stroke volume:

$$CO = HR \times SV$$

As this equation demonstrates, an understanding of how cardiac activity is controlled can be gained by considering how heart rate and stroke volume are regulated. Heart rate is regulated through the activity of the pacemaker, and stroke volume is directly related to myocardial performance. These two determinants cannot be considered independently, however. A change in one of these determinants of cardiac output almost invariably alters the other determinant.

■ *Nervous Control of Heart Rate*

Although certain local factors, such as temperature changes and tissue stretch, can affect the heart rate, the autonomic nervous system is the principal means by which heart rate is controlled.

The average resting heart rate is approximately 70 beats per minute in normal adults, and it is significantly greater in children. During sleep, the heart rate diminishes by 10 to 20 beats per minute, and during emotional excitement or muscular activity it may accelerate to rates considerably above 100. In well-trained, resting athletes, the rate is usually only about 50 beats per minute.

Both divisions of the autonomic nervous system tonically influence the cardiac pacemaker, or SA node. The sympathetic system enhances automaticity, whereas the parasympathetic system inhibits it. Changes in heart rate usually involve a reciprocal action of these two divisions of the autonomic nervous system. Thus, the heart rate increases with a decrease in parasympathetic activity and an increase in sympathetic activity; it decreases with the opposite activity.

Parasympathetic tone usually predominates in healthy, resting individuals. When a healthy individual is given **atropine,** a muscarinic receptor antagonist that blocks parasympathetic effects, heart rate usually increases substantially. If a healthy individual is given **propranolol,** a β-adrenergic receptor antagonist that blocks sympathetic effects, heart rate decreases only slightly (Fig. 24-1). When both divisions of the autonomic nervous system are blocked, the heart rate of young adults averages about 100 beats per minute. The rate that prevails after complete autonomic blockade is called the **intrinsic heart rate.**

■ *Parasympathetic Pathways*

The cardiac parasympathetic fibers originate in the medulla oblongata, in cells that lie in the **dorsal motor nucleus of the vagus** or in the **nucleus ambiguus** (see Chapter 15). The precise location of the parasympathetic fibers varies from species to species. In humans, centrifugal vagal fibers (Fig. 24-2) pass inferiorly through the neck close to the common carotid arteries and then through the mediastinum to synapse with postganglionic cells. These cells are located either on the epicardial surface or within the walls of the heart. Most of the cardiac ganglion cells are located near the SA node and the atrioventricular (AV) conduction tissue.

The right and left vagi are distributed to different cardiac structures. The right vagus nerve affects the SA node predominantly. Stimulation of this nerve slows SA nodal firing and can even stop it for several seconds. The left vagus nerve mainly inhibits AV conduction tissue to produce various degrees of AV block (see Chapter 22). However, the distribution of the efferent vagal fibers is overlapping. As a result of this overlap, left vagal stimulation also depresses the SA node, and right vagal stimulation impedes AV conduction.

The SA and AV nodes are rich in **cholinesterase,** an enzyme that breaks down the neurotransmitter acetylcholine. Acetylcholine released at the nerve terminals is thus rapidly hydrolyzed. Owing to this rapid breakdown of acetylcholine, the effects of any given vagal stimula-

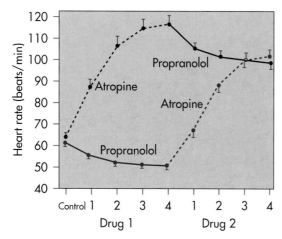

■ **Fig. 24-1** Effects of four equal doses of atropine (0.04 mg/kg total) and of propranolol (0.2 mg/kg total) on the heart rate of 10 healthy young men (mean age, 21.9 years). In half of the trials, atropine was given first *(top curve)*; in the other half, propranolol was given first *(bottom curve)*. (Redrawn from Katona PG, McLean M, Dighton DH, Guz A: *J Appl Physiol* 52:1652, 1982.)

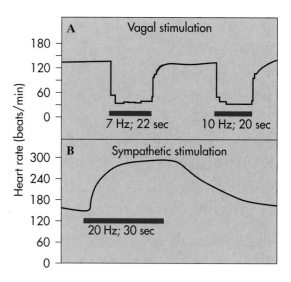

■ **Fig. 24-3** Changes in heart rate evoked by stimulation *(horizontal bars)* of the vagus **(A)** and sympathetic nerves **(B)** in an anesthetized dog. (Modified from Warner HR, Cox A: *J Appl Physiol* 17:349, 1962.)

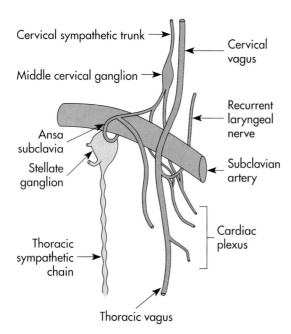

■ **Fig. 24-2** Sympathetic and parasympathetic (vagal) innervation of the heart on the right side of the body in humans.

such as the adenylyl cyclase system. The combination of these two features of the vagus nerves—brief latency and the rapid decay of the response—permits these nerves to exert a beat-by-beat control of SA and AV nodal function.

Parasympathetic influences usually preponderate over sympathetic effects at the SA node. The experiment shown in Fig. 24-4 shows that as the frequency of sympathetic stimulation increases from 0 to 4 Hz in an anesthetized dog, the heart rate increases by about 80 beats per minute in the absence of vagal stimulation (*Vag =* 0 Hz). However, when the vagi are stimulated at 8 Hz, increasing the sympathetic stimulation frequency from 0 to 4 Hz has only a negligible influence on heart rate.

■ *Sympathetic Pathways*

The cardiac sympathetic fibers originate in the **intermediolateral columns** of the upper five or six thoracic and lower one or two cervical segments of the spinal cord (see Chapter 15). These fibers emerge from the spinal column through the white communicating branches and enter the paravertebral chains of ganglia (Fig. 24-2). The preganglionic and postganglionic neurons synapse mainly in the stellate or middle cervical ganglia, depending on the species. In the mediastinum, the postganglionic sympathetic fibers and preganglionic parasympathetic fibers join to form a complex plexus of mixed efferent nerves to the heart.

The postganglionic cardiac sympathetic fibers in this plexus approach the base of the heart along the adventitial surface of the great vessels. On reaching the base of the heart, these fibers are distributed to the various cham-

tion decay very quickly (Fig. 24-3, *A*) when vagal stimulation is discontinued. Furthermore, the effects of vagal activity on SA and AV nodal function have a very short latency (about 50 to 100 msec), because the released acetylcholine activates special acetylcholine-regulated K+ channels in the cardiac cells. The reason these channels open so quickly is that the acetylcholine obviates the need for an intermediate second messenger system,

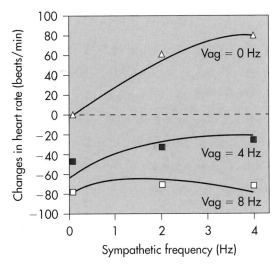

■ **Fig. 24-4** Changes in heart rate in an anesthetized dog when the vagus and cardiac sympathetic nerves were stimulated simultaneously. The sympathetic nerves were stimulated at 0, 2, and 4 Hz; the vagus nerves at 0, 4, and 8 Hz. The symbols represent the observed changes in heart rate; the curves were derived from the computed regression equation. (Modified from Levy MN, Zieske H: *J Appl Physiol* 27:465, 1969.)

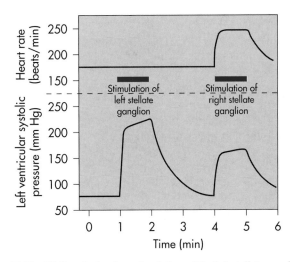

■ **Fig. 24-5** In the dog, stimulation of the left stellate ganglion has a greater effect on ventricular contractility than does right-sided stimulation, but it has a lesser effect on heart rate. In this example, traced from an original record, left stellate ganglion stimulation had no detectable effect at all on heart rate but had a considerable effect on ventricular performance in an isovolumic left ventricle preparation. (From Levy MN: Unpublished tracing.)

bers as an extensive epicardial plexus. They then penetrate the myocardium, usually accompanying the coronary vessels.

As with the vagus nerves, the left and right sympathetic fibers are distributed to different areas of the heart. In the dog, for example, the fibers on the left side have more pronounced effects on myocardial contractility than do fibers on the right side, whereas the fibers on the left side exert much less effect on heart rate than do the fibers on the right side (Fig. 24-5). In some dogs, left cardiac sympathetic nerve stimulation may not affect heart rate at all. This bilateral asymmetry probably also exists in humans.

In contrast to the abrupt termination of the response after vagal activity, the effects of sympathetic stimulation decay only gradually after stimulation is stopped (Fig. 24-3, *B*). Nerve terminals take up most of the norepinephrine released during sympathetic stimulation, and much of the remainder is carried away by the bloodstream. These processes are relatively slow. Furthermore, at the beginning of sympathetic stimulation, the stimulatory effects on the heart attain steady-state values much more slowly than do the inhibitory effects of vagal stimulation. The onset of the cardiac response to sympathetic stimulation is slow for two main reasons. First, norepinephrine appears to be released from the cardiac sympathetic nerve terminals at a relatively slow rate. Second, the effects of the neurally released norepinephrine on the heart are mediated mainly via a relatively slow second messenger system, principally the adenylyl cyclase system (see Chapter 5). Hence, sympathetic activity alters

heart rate and AV conduction much more slowly than does vagal activity. Consequently, although vagal activity can exert beat-by-beat control of cardiac function, sympathetic activity cannot.

■ ***Control by Higher Centers***

Stimulation of various regions of the brain can have significant effects on cardiac rate, rhythm, and contractility (see Chapter 15). In the cerebral cortex, the centers that regulate cardiac function are located mostly in the anterior half of the brain, principally in the frontal lobe, the orbital cortex, the motor and premotor cortex, the anterior part of the temporal lobe, the insula, and the cingulate gyrus. Stimulation of the midline, ventral, and medial nuclei of the thalamus causes tachycardia. Stimulation of the posterior and posterolateral regions of the hypothalamus can also change the heart rate. Stimuli applied to the H2 fields of Forel in the diencephalon cause a variety of cardiovascular responses, including tachycardia; these changes are very similar to those observed during muscular exercise. Undoubtedly the cortical and diencephalic centers are responsible for initiating the cardiac reactions that occur during excitement, anxiety, and other emotional states. The hypothalamic centers are also involved in the cardiac response to alterations in environmental temperature. Experimentally induced temperature changes in the preoptic anterior hypothalamus alter heart rate and peripheral resistance.

Stimulation of the parahypoglossal area of the medulla reciprocally activates cardiac sympathetic pathways and inhibits cardiac parasympathetic pathways. In certain dorsal regions of the medulla, distinct cardiac accelerator and augmentor sites have been detected in animals with transected vagi. Stimulation of accelerator sites increases heart rate, whereas stimulation of augmentor sites increases cardiac contractility. The accelerator regions are more abundant on the right side, whereas the augmentor sites are more prevalent on the left side. A similar distribution also exists in the hypothalamus. Therefore, the sympathetic fibers mainly descend ipsilaterally through the brainstem.

■ Baroreceptor Reflex

Sudden changes in arterial blood pressure initiate a reflex that leads to an inverse change in heart rate (Fig. 24-6). Baroreceptors located in the aortic arch and carotid sinuses (see Chapter 28) are responsible for this reflex. The inverse relationship between heart rate and arterial blood pressure is usually most pronounced over an intermediate range of arterial blood pressures. In experiments conducted on conscious, chronically instrumented monkeys (Fig. 24-6), this range varied between about 70 and 160 mm Hg. Below this intermediate range of pressures, the heart rate maintains a constant, high value; above this pressure range, the heart rate maintains a constant, low value.

The effects of these changes in carotid sinus pressure on the activity in the cardiac autonomic nerves of an anesthetized dog are shown in Fig. 24-7. This experiment shows that over an intermediate range of arterial pressures (100 to 180 mm Hg), the heart rate changes with

reciprocal changes in vagal and sympathetic neural activity. Below this range of arterial blood pressures, the heart rate increases when sympathetic activity is intense and vagal activity is virtually absent. Conversely, above the intermediate range of arterial blood pressures, the heart rate decreases when vagal activity is intense and sympathetic activity is low.

■ Bainbridge Reflex, Atrial Receptors, and Atrial Natriuretic Peptide

In 1915, Bainbridge reported that infusing dogs with blood or saline accelerated their heart rate. This increase did not seem to be tied to arterial blood pressure—the heart rate rose regardless of whether arterial blood pressure did or did not rise. However, Bainbridge also noted that the heart rate increased whenever central venous pressure rose sufficiently to distend the right side of the heart. Bilateral transection of the vagi abolished this response.

Numerous investigators have confirmed Bainbridge's observations and have made the additional discovery that the magnitude and direction of the response depend on the prevailing heart rate. When the heart rate is slow, intravenous infusions usually accelerate the heart. At more rapid heart rates, however, infusions ordinarily slow the heart. What accounts for these different responses?

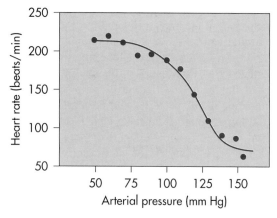

■ **Fig. 24-6**   Heart rate as a function of mean arterial pressure in a group of five conscious, chronically instrumented monkeys. The mean control arterial pressure was 114 mm Hg. Pressure was increased above the control value by infusing phenylephrine and was decreased below the control value by infusing nitroprusside. (Adapted from Cornish KG, Barazanji MW, Yong T, Gilmore JP: *Am J Physiol* 257:R595, 1989.)

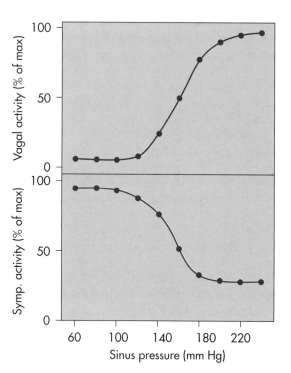

■ **Fig. 24-7**   Effects of changes in pressure in the isolated carotid sinuses on the neural activity in cardiac vagal and sympathetic nerve fibers in an anesthetized dog. (Adapted from Kollai M, Koizumi K: *Pflugers Arch Ges Physiol* 413:365, 1989.)

Increases in blood volume not only evoke the so-called **Bainbridge reflex** but also activate other reflexes (notably the baroreceptor reflex). These other reflexes tend to cause opposite changes in the heart rate. Therefore, changes in heart rate evoked by an alteration of blood volume are the result of these antagonistic reflex effects (Fig. 24-8).

The antagonistic effects of the Bainbridge and baroreceptor reflexes can be seen in the experiment shown in Fig. 24-9. In a group of unanesthetized dogs, volume loading with blood increases heart rate and cardiac output proportionately. Consequently, stroke volume remains virtually constant. Conversely, reductions in blood volume diminish the cardiac output but increase heart rate. Undoubtedly, the Bainbridge reflex predominates over the baroreceptor reflex when the blood volume rises, but the baroreceptor reflex prevails over the Bainbridge reflex when the blood volume diminishes.

Both atria have receptors that are affected by changes in blood volume and that influence heart rate. These receptors are located principally in the venoatrial junctions: in the right atrium at its junctions with the venae cavae and in the left atrium at its junctions with the pulmonary veins. Distention of these atrial receptors sends impulses centripetally in the vagi. The efferent impulses are carried by fibers from both autonomic divisions to the SA node. The cardiac response to these changes in autonomic neural activity is highly selective. Even when the reflex increase in heart rate is large, changes in ventricular contractility have been negligible. Furthermore, the neurally induced increase in heart rate is not accompanied by an increase of sympathetic activity to the peripheral arterioles.

Not only does stimulation of the atrial receptors increase heart rate, but it also increases urine volume. Reduced activity in the renal sympathetic nerve fibers may be partially responsible for this diuresis. However, the principal mechanism appears to be a neurally mediated reduction in the secretion of **vasopressin** (antidiuretic hormone) by the posterior pituitary gland (see Chapter 49).

Stretch of the atrial walls also releases **atrial natriuretic peptide (ANP)** from the atrial tissues. ANP exerts potent diuretic and natriuretic effects on the kidneys (see also Chapter 42) and vasodilator effects on the resistance and capacitance blood vessels. Thus, ANP plays an important role in the regulation of blood volume and blood pressure.

In **congestive heart failure,** NaCl and water are retained, mainly because of the increased release of aldosterone from the adrenal cortex that results from stimulation by the renin-angiotensin system. The plasma level of ANP is also increased in congestive heart failure. By enhancing the renal excretion of NaCl and water, this peptide gradually reduces the fluid retention and consequent elevations of central venous pressure and cardiac preload.

■ *Respiratory Sinus Arrhythmia*

Rhythmic variations in heart rate, occurring at the frequency of respiration, are detectable in most individuals and tend to be more pronounced in children. The heart rate typically accelerates during inspiration and decelerates during expiration (Fig. 24-10).

Recordings from the autonomic nerves to the heart reveal that neural activity increases in the sympathetic fibers during inspiration, whereas neural activity in the vagal fibers increases during expiration (Fig. 24-11). As previously noted, the heart rate response to cessation of vagal stimulation is very quick because the acetylcholine released from the vagus nerves is rapidly broken down by cholinesterase. It is this short latency period that permits the heart rate to vary rhythmically at the respiratory frequency. Conversely, the norepinephrine released periodically at the sympathetic endings is removed very slowly. Therefore, the rhythmic variations in sympathetic activity do not induce any appreciable oscillatory changes in heart rate. Hence, this **respiratory sinus arrhythmia** is

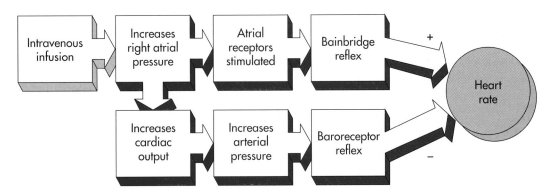

■ **Fig. 24-8**   Intravenous infusions of blood or electrolyte solutions tend to increase heart rate via the Bainbridge reflex and to decrease heart rate via the baroreceptor reflex. The actual change in heart rate induced by such infusions is the result of these two opposing effects.

almost entirely accomplished by changes in vagal activity. In fact, respiratory sinus arrhythmia is exaggerated when vagal tone is enhanced.

Both reflex and central factors help initiate respiratory cardiac arrhythmia (Fig. 24-12). Stretch receptors in the lungs are stimulated during inspiration, and this action may lead to a reflex increase in heart rate. The afferent and efferent limbs of this reflex are located in the vagus nerves. Intrathoracic pressure also decreases during inspiration, and thereby increases venous return to the right side of the heart (see Chapter 29). The consequent stretch of the right atrium elicits the Bainbridge reflex (Fig. 24-12). After the time delay required for the increased venous return to reach the left side of the heart, left ventricular output increases and raises arterial blood pressure. This rise in blood pressure in turn reduces heart rate through the baroreceptor reflex (Fig. 24-12).

Central factors are also responsible for respiratory cardiac arrhythmia. The respiratory center in the medulla directly influences the cardiac autonomic centers (Fig. 24-12). In heart-lung bypass experiments conducted in animals, the chest is open, the lungs are collapsed, venous return is diverted to a pump-oxygenator, and arterial blood pressure is maintained at a constant level. In such experiments, rhythmic movements of the rib cage attest to the activity of the medullary respiratory centers.

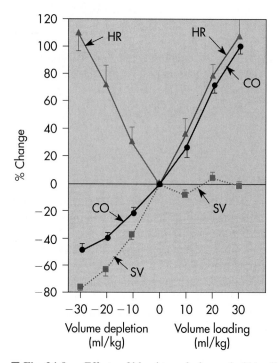

■ **Fig. 24-9** Effects of blood transfusion and of bleeding on cardiac output *(CO)*, heart rate *(HR)*, and stroke volume *(SV)* in unanesthetized dogs. (From Vatner SF, Boettcher DH: *Circ Res* 42:557, 1978, with permission of the American Heart Association.)

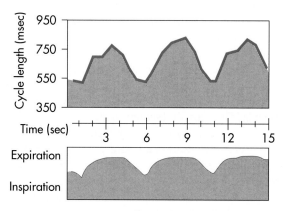

■ **Fig. 24-10** Respiratory sinus arrhythmia in a resting, unanesthetized dog. Note that the cardiac cycle length increases during expiration and decreases during inspiration. (Modified from Warner MR, de Tarnowsky JM, Whitson CC, Loeb JM: *Am J Physiol* 251:H1134, 1986.)

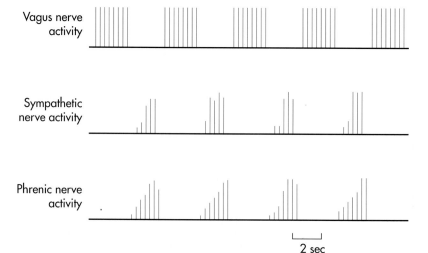

■ **Fig. 24-11** The respiratory fluctuations in efferent activity in the cardiac nerves of an anesthetized dog. Note that the sympathetic nerve activity occurs synchronously with the phrenic nerve discharges (which initiate diaphragmatic contraction), whereas the vagus nerve activity occurs between the phrenic nerve discharges. (From Kollai M, Koizumi K: *J Auton Nerv Syst* 1:33, 1979.)

These movements of the rib cage are often accompanied by rhythmic changes in heart rate at the respiratory frequency. This respiratory cardiac arrhythmia is almost certainly induced by a direct interaction between the respiratory and cardiac centers in the medulla.

■ *Chemoreceptor Reflex*

The cardiac response to peripheral chemoreceptor stimulation merits special consideration, because it illustrates the complex interactions that may ensue when one stimulus excites two organ systems simultaneously. In intact animals, stimulation of the carotid chemoreceptors consistently increases ventilatory rate and depth (see Chapter 36), but ordinarily it changes heart rate only slightly. The magnitude of the ventilatory response determines whether the heart rate increases or decreases as a result of carotid chemoreceptor stimulation, as shown in Fig. 24-13. Mild respiratory stimulation decreases heart rate moderately; more pronounced stimulation increases heart rate only slightly. If the pulmonary response to chemoreceptor stimulation is blocked, the heart rate response may be greatly exaggerated, as described below.

The cardiac response to peripheral chemoreceptor stimulation is the result of primary and secondary reflex mechanisms (Fig. 24-14). The principal effect of this primary stimulation is to excite the medullary vagal center and thereby to decrease heart rate. Secondary reflex effects are mediated by the respiratory system. The respiratory stimulation by the arterial chemoreceptors tends to inhibit the medullary vagal center. This inhibitory effect varies with the level of concomitant stimulation of respiration; small increases in respiration inhibit the vagal center slightly, whereas greater increases in ventilation inhibit the vagal center more profoundly.

An example of this primary inhibitory influence is shown in Fig. 24-15. In this experiment on an anesthetized dog, the lungs were completely collapsed and blood oxygenation was accomplished by an artificial oxygenator. When the carotid chemoreceptors were stimulated, an intense bradycardia and some degree of AV block ensued. Such effects are mediated primarily by efferent vagal fibers.

The identical primary inhibitory effect also operates in humans. The electrocardiogram in Fig. 24-16 was recorded from a **quadriplegic patient** who could not breathe spontaneously but required tracheal intubation and artificial respiration. When the tracheal catheter was briefly disconnected (near the beginning of the top strip in the figure) to permit nursing care, the patient quickly developed a profound bradycardia. His heart rate was 65 beats per minute just before the tracheal catheter was disconnected. In less than 10 seconds after cessation of artificial respiration, his heart rate dropped to about 20 beats per minute. This bradycardia could be prevented by blocking the effects of efferent vagal activity with atropine, and its onset could be delayed considerably by hyperventilating the patient before disconnecting the tracheal catheter.

The pulmonary hyperventilation that is ordinarily evoked by carotid chemoreceptor stimulation influences heart rate secondarily, both by initiating more pronounced pulmonary inflation reflexes and by producing hypocapnia (Fig. 24-14). Both influences tend to depress the primary cardiac response to chemoreceptor stimula-

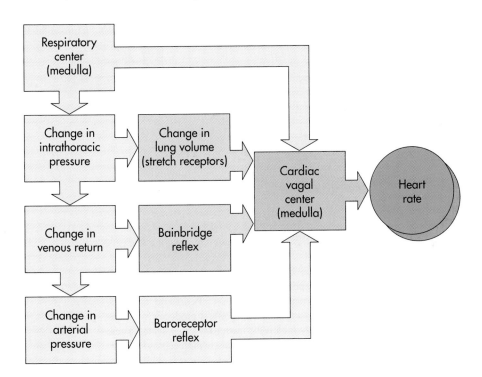

■ Fig. 24-12 Respiratory sinus arrhythmia is generated by a direct interaction between the respiratory and cardiac centers in the medulla, as well as by reflexes that originate from stretch receptors in the lungs, stretch receptors in the right atrium (Bainbridge reflex), and baroreceptors in the carotid sinuses and aortic arch.

tion and thereby accelerate the heart. Hence, when pulmonary hyperventilation is not prevented, the primary and secondary effects neutralize each other, and carotid chemoreceptor stimulation affects heart rate only moderately (Fig. 24-13).

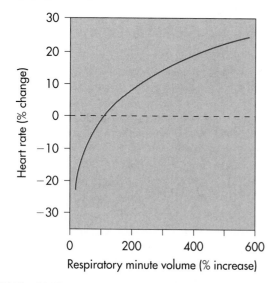

■ **Fig. 24-13** Relationship between the change in heart rate and the change in respiratory minute volume during carotid chemoreceptor stimulation in spontaneously breathing cats and dogs. When respiratory stimulation was relatively slight, heart rate usually diminished; when respiratory stimulation was more pronounced, heart rate usually increased. (Modified from Daly MdeB, Scott MJ: *J Physiol* 144:148, 1958.)

■ *Ventricular Receptor Reflexes*

Sensory receptors located near the endocardial surfaces of the ventricular walls initiate reflex effects similar to those elicited by the arterial baroreceptors. Excitation of these endocardial receptors diminishes the heart rate and peripheral resistance. Other sensory receptors have been identified in the epicardial regions of the ventricles. Although it is known that all these ventricular receptors are excited by various mechanical and chemical stimuli, their exact physiological functions remain unclear.

Ventricular receptors have been implicated in the initiation of **vasovagal syncope,** which is a feeling of lightheadedness or brief loss of consciousness that may be triggered by psychological or orthostatic stress. The ventricular receptors are believed to be stimulated by a reduced ventricular filling volume combined with a vigorous ventricular contraction. In a person standing quietly, ventricular filling is diminished because blood tends to pool in the veins in the abdomen and legs, as explained in Chapter 29. Consequently, the reduction in cardiac output and arterial blood pressure leads to a generalized increase in sympathetic neural activity via the baroreceptor reflex (Fig. 24-7). The enhanced sympathetic activity to the heart evokes a vigorous ventricular contraction, which thereby stimulates the

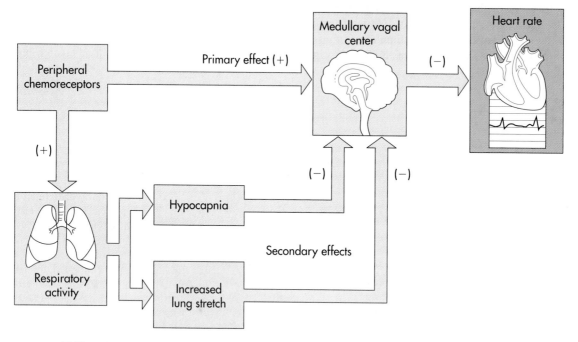

■ **Fig. 24-14** The primary effect of stimulation of the peripheral chemoreceptors on heart rate is to excite the cardiac vagal center in the medulla and thus to decrease heart rate. Peripheral chemoreceptor stimulation also excites the respiratory center in the medulla. This effect produces hypocapnia and increases lung inflation, both of which secondarily inhibit the medullary vagal center. Thus, these secondary influences attenuate the primary reflex effect of peripheral chemoreceptor stimulation on heart rate.

ventricular receptors. Excitation of the ventricular receptors is widely believed to initiate the autonomic neural changes that evoke the vasovagal syncope, namely, a combination of a profound, vagally mediated bradycardia and a generalized arteriolar vasodilation mediated by a reduction in sympathetic neural activity.

■ *Regulation of Myocardial Performance*

■ *Intrinsic Regulation of Myocardial Performance*

Just as the heart can initiate its own beat in the absence of any nervous or hormonal control, so also can the myocardium adapt to changing hemodynamic conditions by means of mechanisms that are intrinsic to cardiac muscle itself. Experiments on denervated hearts reveal that this organ adjusts remarkably well to stress. For example, racing greyhounds with denervated hearts perform almost as well as those with intact innervation. Their maximal running speed was found to decrease only 5% after complete cardiac denervation. In these dogs, the threefold to fourfold increase in cardiac output during a race was achieved principally by an increase in stroke volume. In normal dogs, the increase of cardiac output with exercise is accompanied by a proportionate increase of heart rate; stroke volume does not change much (see Chapter 31). It is unlikely that the cardiac adaptation in the denervated animals is achieved entirely by intrinsic mechanisms; circulating catecholamines undoubtedly contribute. If β-adrenergic receptor antagonists are given to greyhounds with denervated hearts, their racing performance is severely impaired.

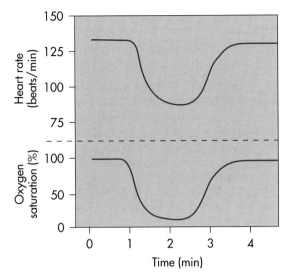

■ **Fig. 24-15** Changes in heart rate during carotid chemoreceptor stimulation in an anesthetized dog on total heart bypass. The lungs remain deflated and respiratory gas exchange is accomplished by an artificial oxygenator. The lower tracing represents the oxygen saturation of the blood perfusing the carotid chemoreceptors. The blood perfusing the remainder of the animal, including the myocardium, was fully saturated with oxygen throughout the experiment. (Modified from Levy MN, DeGeest H, Zieske H: *Circ Res* 18:67, 1966, with permission of the American Heart Association.)

The heart is partially or completely denervated in various clinical situations: (1) the surgically transplanted heart is totally decentralized, although the intrinsic, postganglionic parasympathetic fibers persist; (2) atropine blocks vagal effects on the heart, and propranolol blocks sympathetic β-adrenergic influences; (3) certain drugs, such as reserpine, deplete cardiac norepinephrine stores and thereby restrict or abolish sympa-

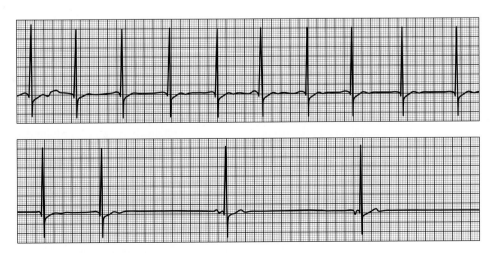

■ **Fig. 24-16**   Electrocardiogram of a 30-year-old quadriplegic man who could not breathe spontaneously and required tracheal intubation and artificial respiration. The two strips are continuous. (Modified from Berk JL, Levy MN: *Eur Surg Res* 9:75, 1977.)

thetic control; and (4) in chronic congestive heart failure, cardiac norepinephrine stores are often severely diminished, thereby attenuating any sympathetic influences.

Two principal intrinsic mechanisms, namely the **Frank-Starling mechanism** and **rate-induced regulation,** enable the myocardium to adapt to changes in hemodynamic conditions. The Frank-Starling mechanism (also referred to as **Starling's law of the heart**), is invoked in response to changes in the resting length of the myocardial fibers. The physiological basis of this mechanism is explained in Chapter 23. Rate-induced regulation is invoked in response to changes in the frequency of the heartbeat. The physiological basis of this mechanism is explained in Chapter 22. How these two mechanisms allow the heart to adapt to alterations in hemodynamic conditions is explained below.

Frank-Starling mechanism. About one century ago, the German physiologist Otto Frank and the English physiologist Ernest Starling independently studied the responses of isolated hearts to changes in preload and afterload (see Chapter 23). When the ventricular filling pressure (the preload) was increased (e.g., by raising a blood reservoir connected to the right atrium), the ventricular volume initially increased progressively. After several beats, however, the ventricles attained a constant, larger volume. At equilibrium, the volume of blood ejected by the ventricles (the stroke volume) with each heartbeat had increased to equal the greater quantity of venous return to the right atrium with each heartbeat.

The increased ventricular volume had somehow facilitated ventricular contraction and had enabled the ventricles to pump a greater stroke volume, resulting in an exact match between the cardiac output and the increased venous return at equilibrium. Other researchers noted subsequently that the increased ventricular volume was associated with an increase in the length of the individual myocardial fibers that make up the ventricular chambers. On the basis of this observation, they concluded that the increase in fiber length altered cardiac performance mainly by altering the number of myofilament cross-bridges that could interact. However, more recent evidence indicates that the principal mechanism involves a stretch-induced change in the sensitivity of the cardiac myofilaments to calcium (see Chapter 23). An optimal fiber length exists, however. Excessively high filling pressures that overstretch the myocardial fibers may depress rather than enhance the pumping capacity of the ventricles.

Starling also showed that isolated heart preparations were able to adapt to changes in the counterforce to the ventricular ejection of blood during systole. As the left ventricle contracts, it does not eject blood into the aorta until the ventricle has developed a pressure that just exceeds the prevailing aortic pressure (see Chapter 23). The aortic pressure during ventricular ejection essentially constitutes the left ventricular afterload. In Starling's experiments, the arterial pressure was controlled by a hydraulic device in the tubing that led from the ascending aorta to the right atrial blood reservoir, and venous return to the right atrium was held constant by maintaining the hydrostatic level of the blood reservoir. As Starling raised the arterial pressure to a new, constant level, the left ventricle responded at first to the increased afterload by pumping a diminished stroke volume. Because venous return was held constant, the diminution of stroke volume was attended by a rise in ventricular diastolic volume as well as an increase in the length of the myocardial fibers. This change in end-diastolic fiber length finally enabled the ventricle to pump a normal stroke volume against the greater peripheral resistance. Although again a change in the number of cross-bridges between the thick and thin filaments probably contributes to this adaptation, the major factor appears to be a stretch-induced change in the sensitivity of the contractile proteins to calcium.

Changes in ventricular volume are also involved in the cardiac adaptation to alterations in heart rate. During bradycardia, for example, the increased duration of diastole permits greater ventricular filling. The consequent increase in myocardial fiber length increases stroke volume. Therefore, the reduction in heart rate may be fully compensated by the increase in stroke volume, and the cardiac output therefore remains constant (see Fig. 29-16).

When cardiac compensation involves ventricular dilation, it is necessary to consider how the increased size of the ventricle affects the generation of the intraventricular pressure. If the ventricle enlarges, the force required by each myocardial fiber to generate a given intraventricular systolic pressure must be appreciably greater than that developed by the fibers in a ventricle of normal size. The Laplace relationship between wall tension and cavity pressure for the cardiac ventricles resembles that for cylindrical tubes (see Chapter 27), in that for a constant internal pressure, wall tension varies directly with the radius. As a consequence, more energy is required for the dilated heart to perform a given amount of external work than for the normal-sized heart. Hence, in the computation of the afterload on the contracting myocardial fibers in the walls of the ventricles, the dimensions of the ventricles must be considered along with the intraventricular (and aortic) pressure.

The relatively rigid pericardium that encloses the heart determines the pressure-volume relationship at high levels of pressure and volume. The pericardium exerts this limitation of volume even under normal conditions, when an individual is at rest and the heart rate is slow. In patients with chronic **congestive heart failure,** the cardiac dilation and hypertrophy may stretch the pericardium considerably. In such patients, the pericardial limitation of cardiac filling is exerted at pressures and volumes entirely different from those in normal individuals (Fig. 24-17).

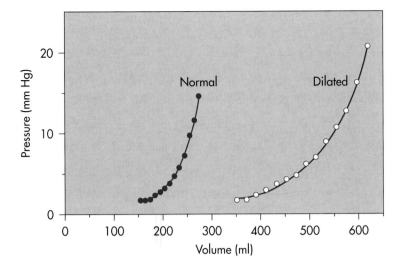

■ **Fig. 24-17**   Pericardial pressure-volume relations in a normal dog and in a dog with experimentally induced chronic cardiac hypertrophy. (Modified from Freeman GL, Le Winter MM: *Circ Res* 54:294, 1984, with permission of the American Heart Association.)

The major problem in assessing the role of the Frank-Starling mechanism in intact animals and humans is the difficulty of measuring end-diastolic volume or end-diastolic myocardial fiber length. In intact subjects, the Frank-Starling mechanism has been represented graphically by plotting some index of ventricular performance along the ordinate and some index of end-diastolic ventricular volume or fiber length along the abscissa. The most commonly used indices of ventricular performance have been cardiac output, stroke volume, and stroke work; stroke work is the product of stroke volume and mean arterial pressure. The indices of end-diastolic ventricular volume and fiber length have been end-diastolic ventricular pressure and mean atrial pressure.

In plotting these indices, the Frank-Starling mechanism is better represented by a family of so-called **ventricular function curves,** rather than by a single curve. To construct a given ventricular function curve, blood volume is altered over a range of values, and stroke work and end-diastolic ventricular pressure are measured at each step. Similar observations are then made during the desired experimental intervention. For example, the ventricular function curve obtained during a norepinephrine infusion in an anesthetized dog lies above and to the left of a control ventricular function curve (Fig. 24-18). It is evident that, for a given level of left ventricular end-diastolic pressure (an index of the preload), the left ventricle performs more work during a norepinephrine infusion than during control conditions. In this experiment, the change in arterial blood pressure (an index of the afterload) was relatively small. Hence, a shift of the ventricular function curve to the left usually signifies an improvement of ventricular **contractility,** which denotes a change in ventricular performance that is independent of a change in either preload or afterload (see Chapter 23). A shift to the left in a ventricular function curve usually signifies an enhancement of contractility, whereas a shift to the right usually indicates an impairment of contractility, and a consequent tendency toward **cardiac failure.**

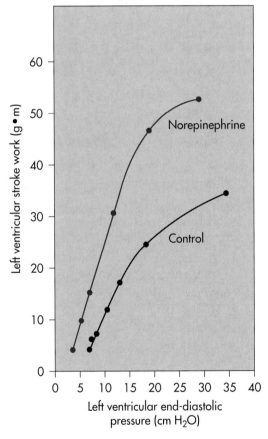

■ **Fig. 24-18**   A constant infusion of norepinephrine in a dog shifts the ventricular function curve to the left. This shift signifies an enhancement of ventricular contractility. (Redrawn from Sarnoff SJ et al: *Circ Res* 8:1108, 1960, with permission of the American Heart Association.)

The Frank-Starling mechanism is ideally suited to matching the cardiac output to the venous return. Any sudden, excessive output by one ventricle soon causes an increase in the venous return to the other ventricle. The consequent increase in diastolic fiber length augments the output of the second ventricle to correspond with that of its mate. In this way, the Frank-Starling mechanism maintains a precise balance between the outputs of the right and left ventricles. Because the two ventricles are arranged in series in a closed circuit, any small, but maintained, imbalance in the outputs of the two ventricles would otherwise be catastrophic.

The curves that relate cardiac output to mean atrial pressure for the two ventricles do not coincide; the curve for the left ventricle usually lies below that for the right ventricle (Fig. 24-19). At equal right and left atrial pressures (points *A* and *B*), right ventricular output would exceed left ventricular output. Hence, venous return to the left ventricle (a function of right ventricular output) would exceed left ventricular output, and left ventricular diastolic volume and pressure would rise. By the Frank-Starling mechanism, left ventricular output would therefore increase (from *B* toward *C*). Only when the outputs of both ventricles are identical (points *A* and *C*) would equilibrium be reached. Under such conditions, however, left atrial pressure *(C)* would exceed right atrial pressure *(A)*, and this is precisely the relationship that ordinarily prevails.

This greater left than right atrial pressure accounts for the observation that in individuals with **congenital atrial septal defects,** in which the two atria communicate with each other via a **patent foramen ovale,** the direction of the shunt flow is usually from left to right.

Rate-induced regulation. Myocardial performance is also regulated by changes in the frequency at which the myocardial fibers contract. The effects of changes in the frequency of contraction on the force developed in an isometrically contracting cat papillary muscle are shown in Fig. 24-20. Initially the strip of cardiac muscle was stimulated to contract only once every 20 seconds (Fig. 24-20, *A*). When the muscle was suddenly made to contract once every 0.63 second, the developed force increased progressively over the next several beats. At the new steady state, the developed force was more than five times as great as it was at the larger contraction interval. A return to the larger interval (20 seconds) had the opposite influence on developed force.

The effects of a wide range of intervals between contractions on the steady-state levels of developed force are shown in Fig. 24-20, *B*. As the interval was diminished from 300 seconds down to about 20 seconds, little change occurred in developed force. As the interval was reduced further, to a value of about 0.5 second, force increased sharply. Further reduction of the interval to 0.2 second had little additional effect on developed force.

The initial progressive rise in developed force when the interval between beats was suddenly decreased (e.g., from 20 seconds to 0.63 second in Fig. 24-20, *B*) is caused by a gradual increase in intracellular Ca^{++} concentration. Two mechanisms contribute to the rise in

Ca^{++} concentration: (1) an increase in the number of depolarizations per minute and (2) an increase in the inward Ca^{++} current per depolarization.

In the first mechanism, Ca^{++} enters the myocardial cell during each action potential plateau (see Fig. 22-8). As the interval between beats is diminished, the number of plateaus per minute increases. Although the duration of each action potential (and of each plateau) decreases as the interval between beats is reduced (see Fig. 22-17), the overriding effect of the increased number of plateaus per minute on the influx of Ca^{++} prevails, and the intracellular concentration of Ca^{++} increases.

In the second mechanism, as the interval between beats is suddenly diminished, the inward Ca^{++} current (i_{Ca}) progressively increases with each successive beat until a new steady state is attained at the new basic cycle length. Fig. 24-21 shows that in an isolated ventricular myocyte subjected to repetitive depolarizations, the influx of Ca^{++} into the myocyte increased on successive beats. For example, the maximal i_{Ca} was considerably greater during the seventh depolarization than it was during the first depolarization. Furthermore, the decay of that current (i.e., its rate of inactivation) was substantially slower during the seventh depolarization than during the first depolarization. Both of these characteristics of the i_{Ca} would result in a greater influx of Ca^{++} into the myocyte during the seventh depolarization than during the first depolarization. The greater influx of Ca^{++} would, of course, strengthen the contraction.

Transient changes in the intervals between beats also profoundly affect the strength of contraction. When the left ventricle contracts prematurely (Fig. 24-22, beat *A*),

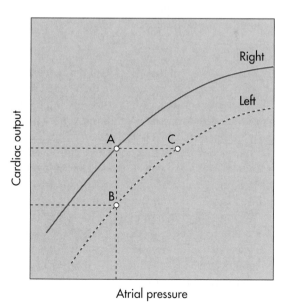

■ **Fig. 24-19** Relationships between the outputs of the right and left ventricles and the mean pressures in the right and left atria, respectively. At any given level of cardiac output, mean left atrial pressure (e.g., point *C*) exceeds mean right atrial pressure (point *A*).

the premature contraction (extrasystole) itself is feeble, whereas beat *B* (postextrasystolic contraction) after the compensatory pause is very strong. In the intact circulatory system, this response depends partly on the Frank-Starling mechanism. Inadequate ventricular filling just before the premature beat accounts partly for the weak premature contraction. Subsequently, the exaggerated degree of filling associated with the compensatory pause (see p 356) explains in part the vigorous postextrasystolic contraction.

Although the Frank-Starling mechanism is certainly involved in the usual ventricular adaptation to a premature beat, it is not the exclusive mechanism. Fig. 24-22 shows the ventricular pressure curves recorded from an isovolumic left ventricle preparation, in which neither filling nor ejection takes place during the cardiac cycle. Although the left ventricular volume remained constant throughout the entire tracing, the premature beat *(A)* was feeble and the postextrasystolic contraction *(B)* was supernormal. Such enhanced contractility in the postextrasystolic contraction is an example of **postextrasys-**

tolic potentiation, and it may persist for one or more additional beats (e.g., contraction *C*).

The weakness of the premature beat is directly related to its degree of prematurity. In other words, the earlier the premature beat occurs, the weaker is its force of contraction. Conversely, as the time (**coupling interval**) between the premature beat and the preceding beat increases, the strength of contraction of the premature beat moves toward normal. The curve that relates the strength of contraction of a premature beat to the coupling interval is called a **mechanical restitution curve.** Fig. 24-23 shows the restitution curve obtained by varying the coupling intervals of test beats in an isolated ventricular muscle preparation from a guinea pig.

The restitution of the force of contraction probably depends on the time course of the intracellular circulation of Ca^{++} in the cardiac myocytes during the contraction and relaxation process. During relaxation, the Ca^{++} that dissociates from the contractile proteins is taken up by the sarcoplasmic reticulum for subsequent release. However, there is a lag of about 500 to 800

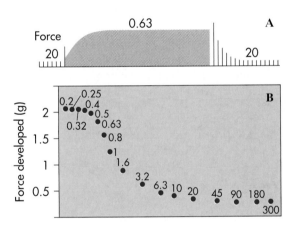

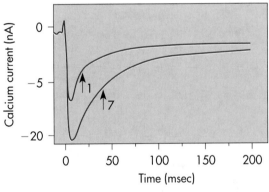

■ **Fig. 24-20** Changes in force development in an isolated papillary muscle from a cat as the interval between contractions is varied from 20 seconds to 0.63 second, and then back to 20 seconds **(A)**. In **B,** the points represent the steady-state forces developed by the same papillary muscle at each of the indicated intervals (in seconds). (Redrawn from Koch-Weser J, Blinks JR: *Pharmacol Rev* 15:601, 1963.)

■ **Fig. 24-21** Calcium currents induced in a guinea pig myocyte during the first and seventh depolarizations in a consecutive sequence of depolarizations. The arrows indicate the half-times of inactivation. Note that during the seventh depolarization, the maximal inward Ca^{++} current and the half-time of inactivation were greater than the respective values for the first depolarization. (Modified from Lee KS: *Proc Natl Acad Sci* 84:3941, 1987.)

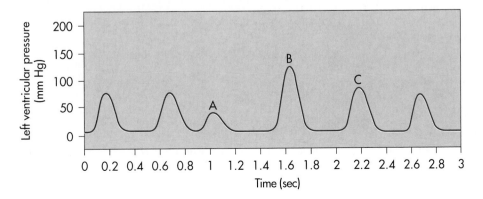

■ **Fig. 24-22** In an isovolumic canine left ventricle preparation, a premature ventricular systole (beat *A*) is typically feeble, whereas the postextrasystolic contraction (beat *B*) is characteristically strong, and the enhanced contractility may diminish over a few beats (e.g., contraction *C*). (From Levy MN: Unpublished tracing.)

msec before this Ca⁺⁺ becomes available for release from the sarcoplasmic reticulum in response to the next depolarization.

If we look once again at the experiment depicted in Fig. 24-22 (beat *A*), the premature beat itself was feeble, probably because there is insufficient time during the preceding relaxation to allow much of the Ca⁺⁺ taken up by the sarcoplasmic reticulum to become available for release during the premature beat. The postextrasystolic beat (*B*), conversely, was considerably stronger than normal. A plausible explanation for the increase in contraction force developed in beat *B* is that a relatively large

quantity of Ca⁺⁺ was taken up by the sarcoplasmic reticulum during the time that had elapsed from the end of the last regular beat until the beginning of the postextrasystolic beat, and this quantity of Ca⁺⁺ would have been available for release during beat *B*.

■ *Extrinsic Regulation of Myocardial Performance*

Although the completely isolated heart can adapt well to changes in preload and afterload, various extrinsic factors also influence the heart in the intact animal. Under many natural conditions, these extrinsic regulatory mechanisms may even overwhelm the intrinsic mechanisms. The extrinsic regulatory factors may be subdivided into nervous and chemical components.

Nervous control

Sympathetic influences. Sympathetic nervous activity enhances atrial and ventricular contractility. Effects of increased cardiac sympathetic activity on the ventricular myocardium are asymmetric. As shown in Fig. 24-5, the cardiac sympathetic nerves on the left side of the body usually have a much greater effect on ventricular contraction than do those on the right side.

The alterations in ventricular contraction evoked by electrical stimulation of the left stellate ganglion in a canine isovolumic left ventricle preparation are shown in Fig. 24-24. The peak pressure and the maximal rate of pressure rise (dP/dt) during systole are markedly increased. Also, the duration of systole is reduced and the rate of ventricular relaxation is increased during the early phases of diastole; both of these responses assist ventricular filling. For any given cycle length, the abbreviation

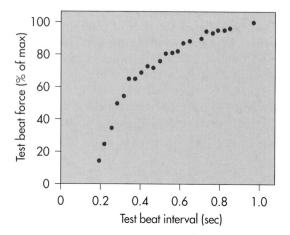

■ **Fig. 24-23**   Force generated during premature contractions in an isolated ventricular muscle preparation from a guinea pig. The muscle was stimulated to contract once per second. Periodically the muscle was stimulated prematurely. The scale along the X axis denotes the time between the driven and the premature beat. The Y axis denotes the ratio of the contractile force of the premature beat to that of the driven beat. (Modified from Seed WA, Walker JM: *Cardiovasc Res* 22:303, 1988.)

■ **Fig. 24-24**   In an isovolumic left ventricle preparation, stimulation of cardiac sympathetic nerves evokes a substantial rise in peak left ventricular pressure and in the maximal rates of intraventricular pressure rise and fall *(dP/dt)*. (From Levy MN: Unpublished tracing.)

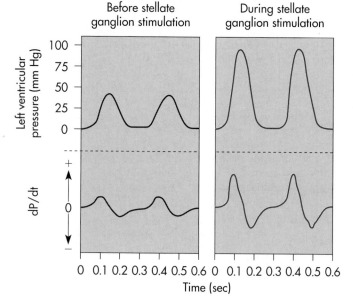

of systole allows more time for diastole and hence for ventricular filling. In the experiment shown in Fig. 24-25, for example, the animal's heart was paced at a constant rapid rate. Sympathetic stimulation *(right panel)* shortened systole, which allowed substantially more time for ventricular filling.

Sympathetic nervous activity also enhances myocardial performance by activating calcium channels in myocardial cell membranes. Neurally released norepinephrine or circulating catecholamines interact with β-adrenergic receptors on the cardiac cell membranes (Fig. 24-26). This interaction activates adenylyl cyclase, which raises the intracellular levels of cyclic AMP (see Chapter 5). Consequently, protein kinases are activated that promote the phosphorylation of various proteins within the myocardial cells. Phosphorylation of specific sarcolemmal proteins activates the calcium channels in the membranes of myocardial cells.

Activation of the calcium channels increases the influx of Ca^{++} during the action potential plateau, and more Ca^{++} is released from the sarcoplasmic reticulum in response to each cardiac excitation. The contractile strength of the heart is thereby increased. Fig. 24-27 shows the correlation between the contractile force in a

thin strip of ventricular muscle and the Ca^{++} concentration (as reflected by the aequorin light signal) in the myocytes as the concentration of isoproterenol (a β-adrenergic agonist) was increased in the tissue bath.

The overall effect of increased cardiac sympathetic activity in intact animals can best be appreciated in terms of families of ventricular function curves. When stepwise increases in the frequency of electrical stimulation are applied to the left stellate ganglion, the ventricular function curves shift progressively to the left. The changes parallel those produced by norepinephrine infusions (Fig. 24-18). Hence, for any given left ventricular end-diastolic pressure, the ventricle is capable of performing more work as the level of sympathetic nervous activity is increased.

During cardiac sympathetic stimulation, the increase in work is usually accompanied by a reduction in left ventricular end-diastolic pressure. An example of the response to stellate ganglion stimulation in a heart paced at a constant frequency is shown in Fig. 24-25. In this experiment, stroke work increased by about 50%, despite a reduction in left ventricular end-diastolic pressure. The reason for the reduction in ventricular end-diastolic pressure is explained on p 466.

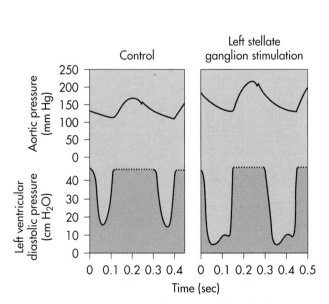

■ **Fig. 24-25** Stimulation of the left stellate ganglion of a dog increases arterial pressure, stroke volume, and stroke work but decreases the ventricular end-diastolic pressure. Note also the abridgement of systole, which allows more time for ventricular filling; the heart was paced at a constant rate. In the ventricular pressure tracings the pen excursion is limited at 45 mm Hg; actual ventricular pressures during systole can be estimated from the aortic pressure tracings. (Redrawn from Mitchell JH, Linden RJ, Sarnoff SJ: *Circ Res* 8:1100, 1960, with permission of the American Heart Association.)

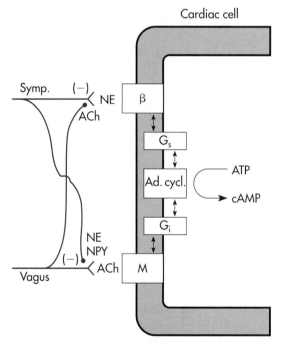

■ **Fig. 24-26** The interneuronal and intracellular mechanisms responsible for the interactions between the sympathetic and parasympathetic systems in the neural control of cardiac function. *NE*, Norepinephrine; *ACh*, acetylcholine; *NPY*, neuropeptide Y; β, β-adrenergic receptor; *M*, muscarinic receptor; G_s and G_i, stimulatory and inhibitory G proteins; *Ad. cycl.*, adenylyl cyclase; *ATP*, adenosine triphosphate; *cAMP*, cyclic adenosine monophosphate. (From Levy MN. In Kulbertus HE, Franck G, editors: *Neurocardiology*, Mt. Kisco, NY, 1988, Futura.)

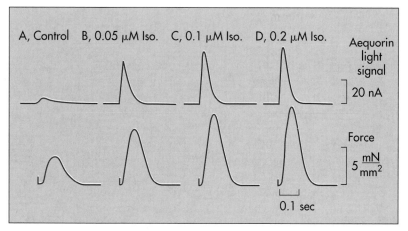

■ **Fig. 24-27**   Effects of various concentrations of isoproterenol *(Iso)* on aequorin light signal (in *nA*) and contractile force (in *mN/mm²*) in a rat ventricular muscle injected with aequorin. The aequorin light signal reflects the instantaneous changes in intracellular Ca⁺⁺ concentration. (Modified from Kurihara S, Konishi M: *Pflugers Arch* 409:427, 1987.)

Parasympathetic influences. The vagus nerves inhibit the cardiac pacemaker, atrial myocardium, and AV conduction tissue (see Chapter 22). The vagus nerves also depress the ventricular myocardium, but the effects are less pronounced in the ventricles than in the atria. In the isovolumic left ventricle preparation encountered on p 391, vagal stimulation decreases the peak left ventricular pressure, maximal rate of pressure development (dP/dt), and maximal rate of pressure decline during diastole (Fig. 24-28). In pumping heart preparations, the ventricular function curve shifts to the right during vagal stimulation.

At least two mechanisms are responsible for the vagal effects on the ventricular myocardium. In one mechanism, acetylcholine *(ACh)* released from the vagal endings can interact with muscarinic *(M)* receptors in the cardiac cell membrane (Fig. 24-26). This interaction leads to the inhibition of adenylyl cyclase. The consequent diminution in the intracellular concentration of cyclic AMP leads to a reduction in Ca⁺⁺ conductance of the cell membrane, and hence to a decrease in myocardial contractility.

In another mechanism, ACh released from the vagal endings can also inhibit the release of norepinephrine from neighboring sympathetic nerve endings (Fig. 24-26). The experiment illustrated in Fig. 24-29 demonstrates that stimulation of the cardiac sympathetic nerves *(S)* causes a substantial overflow of norepinephrine into the coronary sinus blood. Concomitant vagal stimulation *(S + V)* reduces the overflow of norepinephrine by about 30%. The amount of norepinephrine that enters the coronary sinus blood probably parallels the amount released at the sympathetic terminals. Thus, vagal activity can decrease ventricular contractility partly by antagonizing any stimulatory effects that concomitant sympathetic activity may be exerting on ventricular contractility. Similarly, sympathetic nerves release norepinephrine and certain neuropeptides, including neuropeptide Y (NPY). Norepinephrine and NPY both inhibit the release of acetylcholine from neighboring vagal fibers (Fig. 24-26).

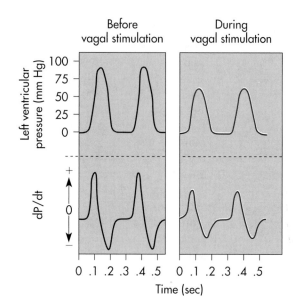

■ **Fig. 24-28**   In an isovolumic left ventricle preparation, when the ventricle is paced at a constant frequency, vagal stimulation decreases the peak left ventricular pressure and diminishes the maximal rates of pressure rise and fall *(dP/dt)*. (From Levy MN: Unpublished tracing.)

Chemical control

Hormones

ADRENOMEDULLARY HORMONES. The adrenal medulla is essentially a component of the autonomic nervous system (see Chapters 15 and 51). The principal hormone secreted by the adrenal medulla is epinephrine, although some norepinephrine is also released. The rate of secretion of these catecholamines by the adrenal medulla is largely regulated by the same mechanisms that control the activity of the sympathetic nervous system. The concentrations of catecholamines in the blood rise under the same conditions that activate the sympathoadrenal system. However, the cardiovascular effects of circulating catecholamines are probably minimal under normal conditions.

The changes in myocardial contractility induced by norepinephrine infusions have been tested in resting, unanesthetized dogs. The maximal rate of rise of left ventricular pressure (dP/dt), an index of myocardial contractility, was found to be proportional to the norepinephrine concentration in the blood (Fig. 24-30). In these same animals, moderate exercise increased the maximum dP/dt by almost 100%, but it raised the circulating catecholamines by only 0.5 ng/ml. By itself, such a rise in blood norepinephrine concentration would have had only a negligible effect on left ventricular dP/dt (Fig. 24-30). Therefore, the pronounced change in dP/dt observed during exercise must have been mediated mainly by the norepinephrine released from the cardiac sympathetic nerve fibers rather than by the catecholamines released from the adrenal medulla.

ADRENOCORTICAL HORMONES. Information about the influence of adrenocortical steroids on myocardial contractility is sketchy and controversial. Cardiac muscle removed from adrenalectomized animals and placed in a tissue bath is more likely to fatigue than that obtained from normal animals. In some species, however, the adrenocortical hormones enhance contractility. Furthermore, hydrocortisone potentiates the cardiotonic effects of catecholamines. This potentiation may be mediated in part by the ability of the adrenocortical steroids to inhibit the catecholamine uptake mechanisms.

> Cardiovascular problems are common in adrenocortical insufficiency (**Addison's disease**). The blood volume tends to fall, which may lead to severe hypotension and cardiovascular collapse, the so-called **addisonian crisis** (see Chapter 51).

THYROID HORMONES. Numerous studies in intact animals and humans have demonstrated that thyroid hormones enhance myocardial contractility. The rates of adenosine triphosphate (ATP) hydrolysis and of Ca^{++} uptake by the sarcoplasmic reticulum are increased in experimental hyperthyroidism, and the opposite effects occur in hypothyroidism. Thyroid hormones increase protein synthesis in the heart, which leads to cardiac hypertrophy. These hormones also affect the composition of myosin isoenzymes in cardiac muscle. By principally increasing those isoenzymes with the greatest ATPase activity, thyroid hormones enhance myocardial contractility.

The cardiovascular changes in thyroid dysfunction also depend on indirect mechanisms. Thyroid hyperactivity increases the body's metabolic rate, which in turn results in arteriolar vasodilation. The consequent reduction in the total peripheral resistance increases cardiac output, as explained in Chapter 29.

> Cardiac activity is sluggish in patients with inadequate thyroid function (**hypothyroidism**). The converse is true in patients with overactive thyroid glands (**hyperthyroidism**). Characteristically, hyperthyroid patients

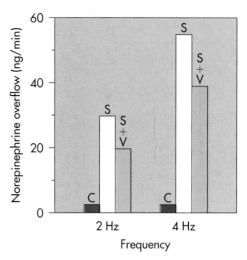

■ **Fig. 24-29** Mean rates of overflow of norepinephrine into the coronary sinus blood in a group of seven dogs under control conditions *(C)*, during cardiac sympathetic stimulation *(S)* at 2 or 4 Hz, and during combined sympathetic and vagal stimulation *(S + V)*. The combined stimulus consisted of sympathetic stimulation at 2 or 4 Hz and vagal stimulation at 15 Hz. (Redrawn from Levy MN, Blattberg B: *Circ Res* 38:81, 1976, with permission of the American Heart Association.)

> exhibit tachycardia, high cardiac output, palpitations, and arrhythmias, such as atrial fibrillation (see Chapter 50). In hyperthyroid subjects, either sympathetic neural activity is increased, or the sensitivity of the heart to such activity is enhanced. Studies have shown that thyroid hormone increases the density of β-adrenergic receptors in cardiac tissue (see also Chapter 50). In experimental animals, the cardiovascular manifestations of hyperthyroidism may be simulated by the administration of thyroxine.

INSULIN. Insulin has a prominent, direct, positive inotropic effect on the heart (see Chapter 47). The effect of insulin is evident even when hypoglycemia is prevented by glucose infusions and when the β-adrenergic receptors are blocked. In fact, the positive inotropic effect of insulin is potentiated by β-adrenergic receptor antagonists. The enhancement of contractility cannot be explained satisfactorily by the concomitant augmentation of glucose transport into the myocardial cells.

GLUCAGON. Glucagon has potent positive inotropic and chronotropic effects on the heart (see Chapter 47). This endogenous hormone is probably not important in the normal regulation of the cardiovascular system, but it has been used clinically to enhance cardiac performance. The effects of glucagon on the heart closely resemble those of the catecholamines, and certain metabolic effects are similar. Both glucagon and catecholamines activate adenylyl cyclase to increase the myocardial tissue levels of cyclic AMP. The catecholamines activate adenylyl cyclase by interacting with β-adrenergic recep-

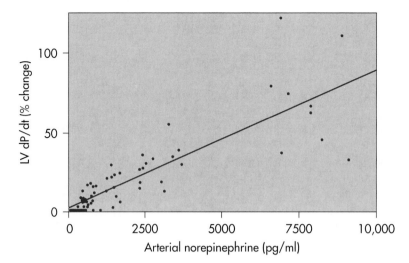

■ Fig. 24-30   Effect of norepinephrine infusions on ventricular contractility in a group of resting, unanesthetized dogs. The plasma concentrations of norepinephrine *(pg/ml)* plotted along the abscissa are the increments above the control values. The maximal rate of rise of left ventricular pressure *(LV dP/dt)*, an index of contractility, is plotted along the ordinate as percentage change from the control value. (Redrawn from Young MA, Hintze TH, Vatner SF: *Am J Physiol* 248:H82, 1985.)

tors, but glucagon activates this enzyme through a different mechanism. Nevertheless, the consequent rise in cyclic AMP increases Ca^{++} influx through the Ca^{++} channels in the sarcolemma, and facilitates Ca^{++} release and reuptake by the sarcoplasmic reticulum, just as do the catecholamines.

ANTERIOR PITUITARY HORMONES. The cardiovascular derangements in hypopituitarism are related principally to the associated deficiencies in adrenocortical and thyroid function (see Chapter 49). Growth hormone does affect the myocardium, at least in combination with thyroxine. In hypophysectomized animals, growth hormone alone has little effect on the depressed heart, whereas thyroxine by itself restores adequate cardiac performance under basal conditions. However, when blood volume or peripheral resistance is increased, thyroxine alone does not restore adequate cardiac function, but the combination of growth hormone and thyroxine does reestablish normal cardiac performance. In certain animal models of heart failure, administration of growth hormone alone has been reported to increase cardiac output and myocardial contractility.

Blood gases

Oxygen. Changes in oxygen tension (Pao_2) of the blood perfusing the brain and the peripheral chemoreceptors affect the heart through nervous mechanisms, as described earlier in this chapter. These indirect effects of hypoxia are usually prepotent. When a subject is exposed to moderate degrees of hypoxia, heart rate, cardiac output, and myocardial contractility are usually enhanced. These changes are largely abolished by β-adrenergic receptor antagonists.

The Po_2 of the arterial blood perfusing the myocardium also influences myocardial performance directly. The effect of hypoxia is biphasic: mild hypoxia is stimulatory, but more severe hypoxia is depressant, because oxidative metabolism is limited.

Carbon dioxide and acidosis. Changes in $Paco_2$ may also affect the myocardium directly and indirectly. The direct effects on the heart elicited by changes of Pco_2 in the coronary arterial blood are illustrated in Fig. 24-31. In this experiment on an isolated left ventricle preparation, the control $Paco_2$ was 45 mm Hg (arrow *A*). Decreasing the Pco_2 to 34 mm Hg (arrow *B*) was stimulatory, whereas increasing Pco_2 to 86 mm (arrow *C*) was depressant.

The indirect, neurally mediated effects produced by an increased Pco_2 in the systemic arterial blood are similar to those evoked by a decrease in Pao_2. An increase in systemic arterial Pco_2 stimulates the central and peripheral chemoreceptors, which then leads to a generalized increase in sympathetic neural activity. The effect of moderate increases in systemic arterial Pco_2 on the cardiovascular system is to increase heart rate, cardiac output, and arterial blood pressure. Thus, in intact animals, the activation of the sympathoadrenal system by moderate increases in systemic arterial Pco_2 tends to prevail over the direct depressant effect on the heart imposed by the increased arterial Pco_2 in the coronary arterial blood.

Neither the arterial Pco_2 nor the blood pH is a primary determinant of myocardial behavior; the associated change in intracellular pH is the critical factor. The reduced intracellular pH diminishes the amount of Ca^{++} released from the sarcoplasmic reticulum in response to excitation. The diminished pH also decreases the sensitivity of the myofilaments to Ca^{++}. The effect of this aci-

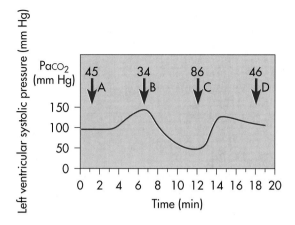

Fig. 24-31 Decrease in Paco$_2$ increases left ventricular systolic pressure (arrow *B*) in an isovolumic left ventricle preparation; a rise in Paco$_2$ (arrow *C*) has the reverse effect. When the Paco$_2$ is returned to the control level (arrow *D*), left ventricular systolic pressure returns to its original value (arrow *A*). (Levy MN: Unpublished tracing.)

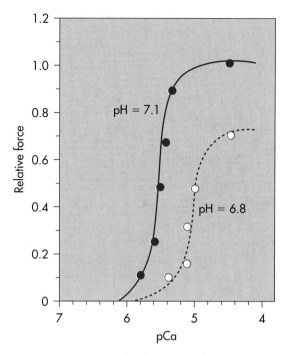

Fig. 24-32 Effect of pH on the relationship between relative force and pCa (negative logarithm of the Ca concentration) in a "skinned" ventricular fiber from a rat. Relative force is the force developed by the preparation at various combinations of pH and pCa, expressed as a percentage of the maximal force developed by the preparation when the intracellular pH was 7.1 and the pCa was less than 4.6. The "skinned" fiber was prepared by treating the preparation with a detergent to solubilize the cell membranes, and thereby to expose the contractile proteins in the fiber to the concentrations of H$^+$ and of Ca^{++} that prevailed in the bathing solution. (Modified from Mayoux E et al: *Am J Physiol* 266:H2051, 1994.)

dosis on the sensitivity to Ca^{++} is reflected by a shift in the relationship between developed force and pCa (the negative logarithm of the intracellular Ca^{++} concentration). Increases in intracellular pH have the opposite effect; that is, they enhance the sensitivity to Ca^{++}.

Fig. 24-32 illustrates such a shift in sensitivity to Ca^{++} in an experiment on isolated ventricular fibers immersed in a tissue bath. When the pH of the bath was changed from 7.1 to 6.8, the curve of contractile force as a function of pCa was shifted substantially to the right (the normal intracellular pH is about 7.1). Furthermore, in this same preparation, at high intracellular Ca^{++} concentrations (i.e., at values of pCa below about 4.6), a reduction in pH diminished the maximal developed force. This reduction in maximal force suggests that the low pH depresses the actomyosin interactions.

■ *Summary*

1. Cardiac function is regulated by a number of intrinsic and extrinsic mechanisms.

2. Heart rate is regulated mainly by the autonomic nervous system. Sympathetic nervous activity increases heart rate, whereas parasympathetic (vagal) activity decreases heart rate. When both systems are active, the vagal effects usually dominate.

3. The following reflexes regulate heart rate: baroreceptor, chemoreceptor, pulmonary inflation, atrial receptor (Bainbridge), and ventricular receptor reflexes.

4. The principal intrinsic mechanisms that regulate myocardial contraction are the Frank-Starling mechanism and rate-induced regulation.

a. Frank-Starling mechanism: a change in the resting length of the muscle influences subsequent contraction by altering the affinity of the myofilaments for calcium and by altering the number of interacting cross-bridges between the thick and thin filaments.

b. Rate-induced regulation: a sustained change in contraction frequency affects the strength of contraction by altering the rate of influx of Ca^{++} into the cell per minute, whereas a transient change in contraction frequency alters contractile strength because an appreciable delay exists between the time that Ca^{++} is taken up by the sarcoplasmic reticulum and the time that it becomes available again for release.

5. The autonomic nervous system regulates myocardial performance mainly by varying the Ca^{++} conductance of the cell membrane via the adenylyl cyclase system.

6. Certain hormones, such as epinephrine, adrenocortical steroids, thyroid hormones, insulin, glucagon, and anterior pituitary hormones, regulate myocardial performance by various mechanisms.

7. Changes in the arterial blood concentrations of O_2, CO_2, and H^+ alter cardiac function directly and via the chemoreceptors reflexly.

■ *Self-Study Problems*

1. What are the temporal characteristics of the changes in heart rate induced by (a) a 1-minute period of vagus nerve stimulation and (b) a 1-minute period of cardiac sympathetic nerve stimulation, and what are the main factors responsible for those characteristics?

2. What changes in heart rate occur when the cardiac sympathetic and vagus nerves are both stimulated strongly and simultaneously, and what factors operate to induce the changes evoked by simultaneous stimulation?

3. What changes in heart rate would occur if a vasoconstrictor drug were given to raise a subject's arterial blood pressure by about 25 mm Hg? What changes in efferent vagal and sympathetic neural activity would be elicited?

4. If 200 ml of blood were rapidly infused intravenously, what would be the temporal sequence of the changes in stroke volume of the right and left ventricles?

5. What changes would take place in the stroke volumes of the right and left ventricles if a substantial opening was made in the interatrial septum in the course of a cardiac catheterization?

6. During a cardiac catheterization, manipulation of the catheter in the right ventricle induced a premature ventricular beat, which was followed by a relatively long pause that was terminated by a postextrasystolic ventricular beat. Compare the magnitudes of the stroke volumes ejected during a normal beat, during the premature beat, and during the postextrasystolic beat.

■ *Bibliography*

Journal articles

Bouchard RA, Bose D: Analysis of the interval-force relationship in rat and canine ventricular myocardium, *Am J Physiol* 257:H2036, 1989.

Dampney RAL: Functional organization of central pathways regulating the cardiovascular system, *Physiol Rev* 74:323, 1994.

Endoh M, Blinks JR: Actions of sympathomimetic amines on the Ca^{2+} transients and contractions of rabbit myocardium: reciprocal changes in myofibrillar responsiveness to Ca^{2+} mediated through α- and β-adrenoceptors, *Circ Res* 62:247, 1988.

Fuchs F: Mechanical modulation of the Ca^{2+} regulatory protein complex in cardiac muscle, *News Physiol Sci* 10:6, 1995.

Gwathmey JK, Hajjar RJ: Relation between steady-state force and intracellular [Ca^{2+}] in intact human myocardium: index of myofibrillar responsiveness to Ca^{2+}, *Circulation* 82:1266, 1990.

Hainsworth R: Reflexes from the heart, *Physiol Rev* 71:617, 1991.

Hakumäki MOK: Seventy years of the Bainbridge reflex, *Acta Physiol Scand* 130:177, 1987.

Josephson RA, Spurgeon HA, Lakatta EG: The hyperthyroid heart. An analysis of systolic and diastolic properties in single rat ventricular myocytes, *Circ Res* 66:773, 1990.

Kohmoto O, Spitzer KW, Movsesian MA, Barry WH: Effects of intracellular acidosis on $(Ca^{2+})_i$ transients, transsarcolemmal Ca^{2+} fluxes, and contraction in ventricular myocytes, *Circ Res* 66:622, 1990.

Koizumi K, Kollai M: Multiple modes of operation of cardiac autonomic control: development of the ideas from Cannon and Brooks to the present, *J Auton Nerv Syst* 41:19, 1992.

Kowallik P, Meesman M: Independent autonomic modulation of the human sinus and AV nodes: evidence from beat-to-beat measurements of PR and PP intervals during sleep, *J Cardiovasc Electrophysiol* 6:993, 1995.

Kuhn HJ, Bletz C, Rüegg JC: Stretch-induced increase in the Ca^{2+} sensitivity of myofibrillar ATPase activity in skinned fibres from pig ventricles, *Pflügers Arch* 415:741, 1990.

Lakatta EG: Starling's law of the heart is explained by an intimate interaction of muscle length and myofilament calcium activation, *J Am Coll Cardiol* 10:1157, 1987.

Levy MN: Autonomic interactions in cardiac control, *Ann N Y Acad Sci* 601:209, 1990.

Marshall JM: Peripheral chemoreceptors and cardiovascular regulation, *Physiol Rev* 74:543, 1994.

Mayoux E et al: Effects of acidosis and alkalosis on mechanical properties of hypertrophied rat heart fiber bundles, *Am J Physiol* 266:H2051, 1994.

Mohabir R, Lee H-C, Kurz RW, Clusin WT: Effects of ischemia and hypercarbic acidosis on myocyte calcium transient, contraction, and pH_i in perfused rabbit hearts, *Circ Res* 69:1525, 1991.

Morgan JP: Abnormal intracellular modulation of calcium as a major cause of cardiac contractile dysfunction, *N Engl J Med* 325:625, 1991.

Onishi K et al: Decrease in oxygen cost of contractility during hypocapnic alkalosis in canine hearts, *Am J Physiol* 270:H1905, 1996.

Polikar R et al: The thyroid and the heart, *Circulation* 87:1435, 1993.

Rea RF, Thames MD: Neural control mechanisms and vasovagal syncope, *J Cardiovasc Electrophysiol* 4:587, 1993.

Reiter M: Calcium mobilization and cardiac inotropic mechanisms, *Pharmacol Rev* 40:189, 1988.

Sauvadet A, Rohn T, Pecker F, Pavoine C: Synergistic actions of glucagon and miniglucagon on Ca^{2+} mobilization in cardiac cells, *Circ Res* 78:102, 1996.

Seals DR et al: Respiratory modulation of muscle sympathetic nerve activity in intact and lung denervated humans, *Circ Res* 72:440, 1993.

Spyer KM: Central nervous mechanisms contributing to cardiovascular control, *J Physiol (Lond)* 474:1, 1994.

Taha BH et al: Respiratory sinus arrhythmia in humans: an obligatory role for vagal feedback from the lungs, *J Appl Physiol* 78:638, 1995.

Walley KR, Ford LE, Wood LDH: Effects of hypoxia and hypercapnia on the force-velocity relation of rabbit myocardium, *Circ Res* 69:1616, 1991.

Books and monographs

Armour JA, Ardell JL, editors: *Neurocardiology,* New York, 1994, Oxford University Press.

Bishop VS, Malliani A, Thorén P: *Cardiac mechanoreceptors.* In *Handbook of physiology: sect 2: The cardiovascular system—peripheral circulation and organ blood flow,* vol 3, Bethesda, Md, 1983, American Physiological Society.

Fozzard HA et al, editors: *Heart and cardiovascular system: Scientific foundations,* ed 2 (2 vols), New York, 1991, Raven Press.

Garfein OB, editor: *Current concepts in cardiovascular physiology,* San Diego, 1990, Academic Press.

Katz AM: *Physiology of the heart,* ed 2, New York, 1991, Raven Press.

Levy MN, Schwartz PJ, editors: *Vagal control of the heart: experimental basis and clinical implications,* Armonk, NY, 1994, Futura Publishing.

Opie LH: *Heart: physiology and metabolism,* ed 2, New York, 1991, Raven Press.

Persson PB, Kirchheim HR, editors: *Baroreceptor reflexes: integrative functions and clinical aspects,* Berlin, 1991, Springer-Verlag.

Rowell LB: *Human cardiovascular control,* New York, 1993, Oxford University Press.

Shepherd JT, Vatner SF, editors: *Nervous control of the heart,* Amsterdam, 1996, Harwood Academic.

Sperelakis N, editor: *Physiology and pathophysiology of the heart,* ed 3, Boston, 1995, Kluwer Academic.

Zucker IH, Gilmore JP: *Reflex control of the circulation,* Boca Raton, Fla, 1990, CRC Press.

CHAPTER

25

Hemodynamics

The definition of precise mathematical terms for the pulsatile flow of blood through the cardiovascular system is fraught with problems. The heart is a complicated pump, and many physical and chemical factors affect its behavior. The blood vessels are multibranched, and their elasticity allows continuous variation in their dimensions. The blood itself is not a simple, homogeneous solution but instead a complex suspension of red and white corpuscles, platelets, and lipid globules dispersed in a colloidal solution of proteins.

Despite this complexity, it is possible to gain insight into the dynamics of the cardiovascular system by applying the elementary principles of fluid mechanics as they pertain to simple hydraulic systems. These principles are explored in this chapter to explain the interrelationships among velocity of blood flow, blood pressure, and the dimensions of the various components of the systemic circulation.

■ *Velocity of the Bloodstream*

Before describing the variations in blood flow in different vessels, it is first necessary to distinguish between the terms **velocity** and **flow.** Velocity, which is sometimes called **linear velocity,** refers to the rate of displacement of fluid with respect to time, and it is expressed in units of distance per unit time (e.g., cm/sec). Flow, which is frequently called **volume flow,** is expressed in units of volume per unit time (e.g., cm³/sec). In a tube with varying cross-sectional dimensions, velocity (v), flow (Q), and cross-sectional area (A) are related by the equation:

$$v = Q/A \qquad (25\text{-}1)$$

The interrelationships among velocity, flow, and area are shown in Fig. 25-1. The principle of conservation of mass requires that the flow of an incompressible fluid past successive cross-sections of a rigid tube must be constant. For a given flow, the velocity of the fluid varies inversely with the cross-sectional area. Thus, as fluid flows from section *a* into section *b,* where the cross-sectional area is five times greater, the velocity diminishes to

one fifth of its previous value, because the area of section *b* is five times greater than that of section *a* (Fig. 25-1). Conversely, when the fluid flows from section *b* to section *c,* where the cross-sectional area is one tenth as great as that of section *b,* the velocity of each particle of fluid increases tenfold.

The velocity of the fluid at any point in the system depends not only on the area, but also on the flow, Q. Flow, in turn, depends on the pressure gradient, properties of the fluid, and dimensions of the entire hydraulic system, as discussed in the following section. For any given flow, however, the ratio of the velocity past one cross-section relative to that past a second cross-section depends only on the inverse ratio of the respective areas, that is,

$$v_1/v_2 = A_2/A_1 \qquad (25\text{-}2)$$

This rule applies whether the system is composed of a single large tube or several smaller tubes in parallel.

As shown in Fig. 21-3, velocity decreases progressively as the blood traverses the aorta, its larger primary branches, the smaller secondary branches, and the arterioles. Finally, at the capillaries, the velocity decreases to a minimal value. As the blood then passes through the venules and continues centrally toward the venae cavae, the velocity progressively increases again. The relative velocities in the various components of the circulatory system are related only to the respective cross-sectional areas. Thus, each point on the cross-sectional area curve is inversely proportional to the corresponding point on the velocity curve (see Fig. 21-3).

■ *Relationship between Velocity and Pressure*

In the specific portion of a hydraulic system in which the total energy remains virtually constant, changes in velocity may be accompanied by appreciable changes in measured pressure. Consider three sections (*A, B,* and *C*) of the hydraulic system depicted in Fig. 25-2. Six pressure probes, or **Pitot tubes,** have been inserted at various

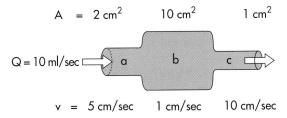

$A = 2\ cm^2 \qquad 10\ cm^2 \qquad 1\ cm^2$

$Q = 10\ ml/sec$

$v = 5\ cm/sec \qquad 1\ cm/sec \qquad 10\ cm/sec$

■ **Fig. 25-1** As fluid flows through a tube of variable cross-sectional area, *A*, the linear velocity, *v*, varies inversely as the cross-sectional area.

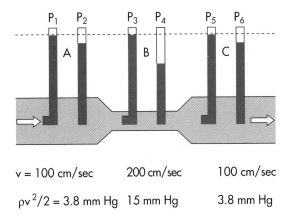

$v = 100\ cm/sec \qquad 200\ cm/sec \qquad 100\ cm/sec$

$\rho v^2/2 = 3.8\ mm\ Hg \quad 15\ mm\ Hg \qquad 3.8\ mm\ Hg$

■ **Fig. 25-2** In a narrow section, *B*, of a tube, the linear velocity, *v*, and hence the dynamic component of pressure, $\rho v^2/2$, are greater than in the wide sections, *A* and *C*, of the same tube. If the total energy is virtually constant throughout the tube (i.e., if the energy loss because of viscosity is negligible), the total pressures $(P_1, P_3, and P_5)$ will not be detectably different from each other, but the lateral pressure, P_4, in the narrow section will be less than the lateral pressures $(P_2 and P_6)$ in the wide sections of the tube.

points in the system. The openings of three of these tubes (2, 4, and 6) are tangential to the direction of flow, and hence they measure the **lateral,** or **static,** pressure within the tube. The openings of the remaining three Pitot tubes (1, 3, and 5) face upstream. These Pitot tubes detect the **total pressure,** which is the lateral pressure plus a dynamic pressure component that is affected by the kinetic energy of the flowing fluid. This dynamic component, P_d, of the total pressure may be calculated from the following equation:

$$P_d = \rho v^2/2 \qquad (25\text{-}3)$$

where ρ is the density of the fluid and v is the velocity. If the midpoints of segments *A, B,* and *C* are at the same hydrostatic level, then the corresponding total pressures, P_1, P_3, and P_5, will be equal, provided that the energy loss from viscosity in these segments is negligible (in other words, the fluid we are studying here is an "ideal fluid"). However, because of the differences in cross-sectional area along the system, the concomitant velocity changes alter the dynamic component, as defined by equation 25-3.

In tube sections *A* and *C,* let ρ equal 1 g/cm^3 and let v equal 100 cm/sec; note also that 1 mm Hg equals 1330 $dynes/cm^2$. From equation 25-3

$$P_d = 5000\ dynes/cm^2,\ = 3.8\ mm\ Hg$$

In the narrow section, *B,* of the tube, let the velocity be twice as great as in sections *A* and *C.* In the narrow section, therefore,

$$P_d = 20{,}000\ dynes/cm^2 = 15\ mm\ Hg$$

Hence, in the wide sections of the tube (*A* and *C*), the lateral pressures (P_2 and P_6) will be only 3.8 mm Hg less than the respective total pressures (P_1 and P_5), whereas in the narrow section (*B*), the lateral pressure (P_4) is 15 mm Hg less than the total pressure (P_3).

We can make two generalizations from these calculations. First, as velocity decreases, the dynamic component (which, you will recall, is affected by the kinetic energy of the flowing fluid) becomes a less significant component of the total pressure. Second, in narrowed sections of a tube, the dynamic component increases significantly, because the flow velocity is associated with a

large kinetic energy. For example, the peak velocity of flow in the ascending aorta of normal dogs is about 150 cm/sec. Because the dynamic component is a significant fraction of the total pressure, the measured pressure may vary significantly, depending on the orientation of the pressure probe. In the descending thoracic aorta, the peak velocity is substantially less than that in the ascending aorta (Fig. 25-3), and lesser velocities have been recorded in still more distal arterial sites. In most arterial locations, the dynamic component will be a negligible fraction of the total pressure, and the orientation of the pressure probe will not materially influence the pressure recorded. At the site of a constriction, however, the high flow velocity is associated with a large kinetic energy, and therefore the dynamic pressure component may increase significantly. Hence, the lateral pressure would be reduced correspondingly.

The pressure tracings shown in Fig. 25-4 were obtained from two pressure transducers inserted into the left ventricle of a patient with **aortic stenosis,** a condition in which the aortic orifice narrows. The transducers were located on the same catheter and were 5 cm apart. When both transducers were well within the left ventricular cavity (Fig. 25-4, *A*), they both recorded the same pressures. However, when the proximal transducer was positioned in the aortic valve orifice (Fig. 25-4, *B*), the lateral pressure recorded during ejection was much less than that recorded by the transducer in the ventricular cavity. This pressure difference was associated almost entirely with the much greater velocity of flow in the narrowed valve orifice than in the ventricular cavity. The pressure difference reflects mainly the conversion of some potential energy to kinetic energy. When the catheter was withdrawn still farther, so that the proximal transducer was in the aorta (Fig. 25-4, *C*), the pressure difference was even more pronounced, because substantial energy was lost through friction (viscosity) as blood flowed rapidly through the narrow orifice.

The reduction of lateral pressure in the region of the narrowed aortic valve orifice may influence the coronary blood flow in patients with aortic stenosis. The orifices of the right and left coronary arteries are located in the sinuses of Valsalva, just behind the valve leaflets. The initial segments of these vessels are thus oriented at right angles to the direction of blood flow through the aortic valves. Therefore, the lateral pressure is that component of the total pressure that propels the blood through the two major coronary arteries. During the ejection phase of the cardiac cycle, the lateral pressure is diminished by the conversion of potential energy to kinetic energy.

Angiographic studies in patients with aortic stenosis have revealed that the direction of flow often reverses in the large coronary arteries toward the end of the ejection phase of systole (i.e., blood flows toward the aorta rather than toward the myocardial capillaries). The decreased lateral pressure in the aorta in aortic stenosis is undoubtedly an important factor in causing this reversal of coronary blood flow. An important feature that aggravates this condition is that the demands of the heart muscle for oxygen are greatly increased. Therefore, the pronounced drop in lateral pressure during cardiac ejection may contribute to the tendency for patients with severe aortic stenosis to experience **angina pectoris** (anterior chest pain associated with inadequate blood supply to the heart muscle), which can lead to sudden death.

■ *Relationship between Pressure and Flow*

The most fundamental law that governs the flow of fluids through cylindrical tubes was derived empirically by Poiseuille. He was primarily interested in the physical determinants of blood flow, but he substituted simpler liquids for blood in his measurements of flow through glass capillary tubes. His work was so precise and important that his observations have been designated **Poiseuille's law.** Subsequently, this same law has been derived theoretically.

■ *Application of Poiseuille's Law*

Poiseuille's law applies only to the steady, laminar flow of newtonian fluids through cylindrical tubes. (The term *newtonian fluid* is described in more detail below.) The term **steady flow** signifies the absence of variations of flow in time (i.e., a nonpulsatile flow). **Laminar flow** is

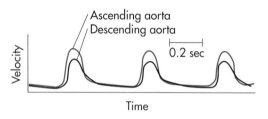

■ **Fig. 25-3** Velocity of blood in the ascending and descending aorta of a dog. (Redrawn from Falsetti HL, Kiser KM, Francis GP, Belmore ER: *Circ Res* 31:328, 1972, with permission of the American Heart Association.)

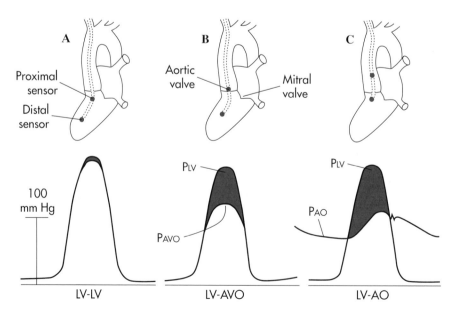

■ **Fig. 25-4** Pressures (*P*) recorded by two transducers in a patient with aortic stenosis. **A,** Both transducers were in the left ventricle *(LV-LV).* **B,** One transducer was in the left ventricle and the other was in the aortic valve orifice *(LV-AVO).* **C,** One transducer was in the left ventricle and the other in the ascending aorta *(LV-AO).* (Redrawn from Pasipoularides A, Murgo JP, Bird JJ, Craig WE: *Am J Physiol* 246:H542, 1984.)

the type of motion in which the fluid moves as a series of individual layers, with each layer moving at a different velocity from its neighboring layers (Fig. 25-5). In the case of laminar flow through a tube, the fluid consists of a series of infinitesimally thin concentric tubes sliding

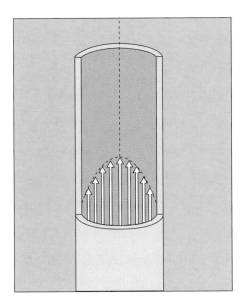

■ **Fig. 25-5** When flow is laminar, all elements of the fluid move in streamlines that are parallel to the axis of the tube; the fluid does not move in a radial or circumferential direction. The layer of fluid in contact with the wall is motionless; the fluid that moves along the axis of the tube has the maximal velocity.

past one another. Laminar flow is described in greater detail below, where it is distinguished from turbulent flow. For the present discussion, laminar flow is considered a homogeneous fluid, such as water, in contrast to a suspension, such as blood.

At the most basic level, Poiseuille's law describes the flow of fluids through cylindrical tubes in terms of flow, pressure, the dimensions of the tube, and the viscosity of liquid in the tube. In the following pages, these terms are explained in detail and are then related to each other to yield Poiseuille's law.

Pressure is one of the principal determinants of the rate of flow. The pressure, P, in dynes/cm², at a distance h centimeters below the surface of a liquid is

$$P = h\rho g \qquad (25\text{-}4)$$

where ρ is the density of the liquid, in g/cm³, and g is the acceleration of gravity, in cm/sec². For convenience, however, pressure is frequently expressed simply in terms of the height (h) of the column of liquid above some arbitrary reference point.

Consider the tube that connects reservoirs R_1 and R_2 in Fig. 25-6, *A*. Reservoir R_1 is filled with liquid to height h_1, and reservoir R_2 is empty. The outflow pressure, P_o, is therefore equal to the atmospheric pressure, which shall be designated as the zero, or reference, level. The inflow pressure, P_i, is then equal to the same reference level plus the height, h_1, of the column of liquid in reservoir R_1. Under these conditions, let the flow (Q) through the tube be 5 ml/sec.

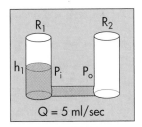

A, When R_2 is empty, fluid flows from R_1 to R_2 at a rate proportional to the pressure in R_1.

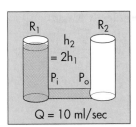

B, When the fluid level in R_1 is increased twofold, the flow increases proportionately.

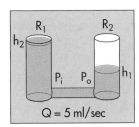

C, Flow from R_1 to R_2 is proportional to the difference between the pressures in R_1 and R_2.

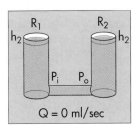

D, When pressure in R_2 rises to equal the pressure in R_1, flow ceases in the connecting tube.

■ **Fig. 25-6** **A** to **D,** The flow, *Q*, of fluid through a tube connecting two reservoirs, R_1 and R_2, is proportional to the difference between the pressure, P_i, at the inflow end and the pressure, P_o, at the outflow end of the tube.

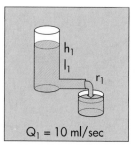

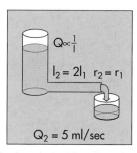

■ **Fig. 25-7   A** to **D,** The flow, Q, of fluid through a tube is inversely proportional to the length, l, and the viscosity, η, and is directly proportional to the fourth power of the radius, r.

A, Reference condition: for a given pressure, length, radius, and viscosity, let the flow (V₁) equal 10 ml/sec.

B, If tube length doubles, flow decreases by 50%.

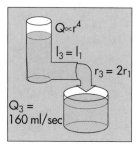

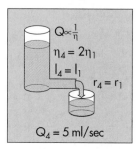

C, If tube radius doubles, flow increases 16-fold.

D, If viscosity doubles, flow decreases by 50%.

In Fig. 25-6, *B,* reservoir R₁ is filled to height h₂, which is twice h₁, and reservoir R₂ is again empty. The flow in *B* is twice as great (i.e., 10 ml/sec) as that in panel *A.* Thus, when the outflow pressure (P₀) in reservoir R₂ equals zero, the flow is directly proportional to the inflow pressure, Pᵢ. If reservoir R₂ is now allowed to fill to height h₁, and the fluid level in R₁ is maintained at h₂ (as in Fig. 25-6, *C*), the flow will again become 5 ml/sec. Thus, *flow is directly proportional to the difference between the inflow and outflow pressures:*

$$Q \propto P_i - P_o \qquad (25\text{-}5)$$

If the fluid level in R₂ attains the same height as in R₁, flow will cease (Fig. 25-6, *D*).

Now, consider how the dimensions of a tube affect flow. For any given pressure difference between the two ends of a tube, the flow depends on the dimensions of the tube. Consider the tube connected to the reservoir in Fig. 25-7, *A.* With length l₁ and radius r₁, the flow Q₁ is 10 ml/sec. The tube connected to the reservoir in Fig. 25-7, *B* has the same radius but is twice as long as the tube in *A.* Under these conditions, the flow Q₂ is 5 ml/sec, or only half as great as Q₁. Conversely, for a tube half as long as l₁, the flow would be twice as great as Q₁. In other words, *flow is inversely proportional to the length of the tube:*

$$Q \propto 1/l \qquad (25\text{-}6)$$

The tube connected to the reservoir in Fig. 25-7, *C* is

the same length as l₁, but the radius, r₃, is twice as great as r₁. Under these conditions the flow Q₃ is found to increase to 160 ml/sec, which is 16 times greater than Q₁. The precise measurements of Poiseuille revealed that *flow varies directly as the fourth power of the radius:*

$$Q \propto r^4 \qquad (25\text{-}7)$$

Thus, in the example above, because r₃ = 2r₁, Q₃ will be proportional to (2r₁)⁴, or 16r₁⁴; therefore, Q₃ will equal 16Q₁.

Finally, for a given pressure difference and for a cylindrical tube of given dimensions, the flow varies as a function of the nature of the fluid itself. This flow-determining property of fluids is termed **viscosity,** η, which has been defined by Newton as the ratio of **shear stress** to the **shear rate** of the fluid.

These terms can be understood most clearly by considering the flow of a homogeneous fluid between parallel plates. In Fig. 25-8, the bottom plate (the bottom of a large basin) is stationary, and the upper plate moves along the upper surface of the fluid. The **shear stress,** τ, is defined as the ratio of F:A, where F is the force applied to the upper plate in the direction of its motion along the upper surface of the fluid, and A is the area of the upper plate that is in contact with the fluid. The **shear rate** is du/dy, where u is the velocity of a minute fluid element in the direction parallel to the motion of the upper plate, and y is the distance of that fluid element above the bottom, stationary plate.

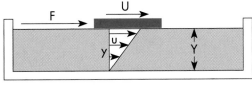

$$\eta = \frac{\tau}{du/dy} = \frac{F/A}{U/Y}$$

■ **Fig. 25-8** For a newtonian fluid, the viscosity, η, is defined as the ratio of shear stress, τ, to shear rate, du/dy. For a plate of contact area, A, moving across the surface of a liquid, τ equals the ratio of the force, F, applied in the direction of motion to the contact area, A, and du/dy equals the ratio of the velocity of the plate, U, to the depth of the liquid, Y.

For a plate that travels with constant velocity, U, across the surface of a homogeneous fluid, the velocity profile of the fluid will be linear. The fluid layer in contact with the upper plate will adhere to it and therefore will move at the same velocity, U, as the plate. Each minute element of fluid between the plates will move at a velocity, u, that is proportional to its distance, y, from the lower plate. Therefore, the shear rate will be U/Y where Y is the distance between the two plates. Because viscosity, η, is defined as the ratio of shear stress, τ, to the shear rate, du/dy, in the example illustrated in Fig. 25-8,

$$\eta = (F/A)/(U/Y) \qquad (25\text{-}8)$$

Thus, the dimensions of viscosity are dynes/cm^2 divided by (cm/sec)/cm, or dyne·sec/cm^2. In honor of Poiseuille, 1 dyne·sec/cm^2 has been termed a **poise**. The viscosity of water at 20° C is approximately 0.01 poise, or 1 centipoise. In the case of certain nonhomogeneous fluids, notably suspensions such as blood, the ratio of the shear stress to the shear rate is not constant; that is, the fluid does not possess a characteristic viscosity. Such fluids are said to be **non-newtonian**. *With regard to the flow of newtonian fluids through cylindrical tubes, the flow varies inversely with the viscosity.*

$$Q \propto 1/\eta \qquad (25\text{-}9)$$

Looking back at the example of flow from the reservoir in Fig. 25-6, *D*, if the viscosity of the fluid in the reservoir were doubled, the flow would be halved (5 ml/sec instead of 10 ml/sec).

In summary, *for the steady, laminar flow of a newtonian fluid through a cylindrical tube, the flow, Q, varies directly as the pressure difference, $P_i - P_o$, and the fourth power of the radius, r, of the tube, and it varies inversely as the length, l, of the tube and the viscosity, η, of the fluid.* The full statement of Poiseuille's law is

$$Q = \frac{\pi (P_i - P_o) r^4}{8\eta l} \qquad (25\text{-}10)$$

where $\pi/8$ is the constant of proportionality.

■ *Resistance to Flow*

In electrical theory, **Ohm's law** states that the resistance, R, equals the ratio of voltage drop, E, to current flow, I. Similarly, in fluid mechanics, *the hydraulic resistance, R, may be defined as the ratio of pressure drop, $P_i - P_o$, to flow, Q*. P_i and P_o are the pressures at the inflow and outflow ends, respectively, of the hydraulic system. For the steady, laminar flow of a newtonian fluid through a cylindrical tube, the physical components of hydraulic resistance may be appreciated by rearranging Poiseuille's law to give the **hydraulic resistance equation:**

$$R = (P_i - P_o)/Q = 8 \eta l/\pi r^4 \qquad (25\text{-}11)$$

Thus, when Poiseuille's law applies, the resistance to flow depends only on the dimensions of the tube and on the characteristics of the fluid.

Because resistance varies inversely as the fourth power of the radius of the tube, the principal determinant of the resistance to blood flow through any individual vessel within the circulatory system is the caliber of the vessel. In Fig. 25-9, the resistance to flow through small blood vessels in cat mesentery was measured and the resistance per unit length of vessel (R/l) plotted against the vessel diameter. The resistance is highest in the capillaries (diameter 7 μm), and it diminishes as the vessels increase in diameter on the arterial and venous sides of the capillaries. The values of R/l are virtually proportional to the fourth power of the diameter (or radius) of the larger vessels on both sides of the capillaries.

Changes in vascular resistance induced by natural stimuli occur when the caliber of vessels changes. The most important factor that leads to a change in vessel caliber is the contraction of the circular smooth muscle cells in the vessel wall. However, changes in internal pressure also alter the caliber of the blood vessels, and therefore alter the resistance to blood flow through those vessels. The blood vessels are elastic tubes. Hence, the greater the **transmural pressure** (i.e., the difference between internal and external pressures) across the wall of a vessel, the greater is the caliber of the vessel and the less is its hydraulic resistance.

It is apparent from Fig. 21-2 that the greatest upstream-to-downstream drop in internal pressure occurs in the very small arteries and arterioles. Because the total flow is the same through each of the various series components of the circulatory system, it follows that the greatest resistance to flow resides in the small arteries and arterioles. For example, if R_a represents the resistance of all these small arterial vessels and R_x represents the resistance of any other group of vessels that are in series with these high-resistance vessels, then by the definition of hydraulic resistance (equation 25-11), the resistance of all the small arterial vessels is:

$$R_a = (P_i - P_o)/Q_a \qquad (25\text{-}12)$$

Similarly, the resistance of any other group of vessels in

series with the group of high resistance small arterial vessels is:

$$R_x = (P_i - P_o)/Q_x \qquad (25\text{-}13)$$

However, at equilibrium, the flow, Q_a, through all the small arterial vessels must equal the flow, Q_x, through each of the other groups of vessels in series with these small arterial vessels. Because Q_a equals Q_x, division of equation 25-11 by equation 25-12 yields the following relationship between relative resistances and relative pressure drops:

$$R_a/R_x = (P_i - P_o)_a/(P_i - P_o)_x \qquad (25\text{-}14)$$

That is, *the ratio of the pressure drop across the length of the small arterial vessels to the pressure drop across the length of any other vascular component in series equals the ratio of the hydraulic resistances of these two vascular components.*

With regard to individual vessels, capillaries that have a mean diameter of about 7 μm (Fig. 25-9) have the greatest resistance to blood flow. Nevertheless, it is the arterioles, not the capillaries, that have the greatest resistance of all the different varieties of blood vessels that lie in series with one another (as in Fig. 21-2). This seeming paradox is related to the relative numbers of parallel capillaries and parallel arterioles, as explained on p 407. For

now, a simple explanation is that there are far more capillaries than arterioles in the systemic circulation, and total resistance across the many capillaries is much less than the total resistance across the fewer arterioles. Furthermore, arterioles have a thick coat of circularly arranged smooth muscle fibers, which can vary the lumen radius. Even small changes in radius alter resistance greatly, as we can see from the hydraulic resistance equation (equation 25-11), wherein R varies inversely with r^4.

■ *Resistances in Series and in Parallel*

In the cardiovascular system, the various types of vessels listed along the horizontal axis in Fig. 21-3 lie in series with one another. Furthermore, the individual members of each category of vessels are ordinarily arranged in parallel with one another (see Fig. 21-4). For example, the capillaries throughout the body are in most instances parallel elements, except for the renal vasculature (in which the peritubular capillaries are in series with the glomerular capillaries) and the splanchnic vasculature (in which the intestinal and hepatic capillaries are aligned in series with each other). Formulas for the total hydraulic resistance of components arranged in series or in parallel have been derived in the same manner as those for similar combinations of electrical resistances.

Resistance of vessels in series. Three hydraulic resistances, R_1, R_2, and R_3, are arranged in series in the system depicted in Fig. 25-10. The pressure drop across the entire system—that is, the difference between inflow pressure, P_i, and outflow pressure, P_o—consists of the sum of the pressure drops across each of the individual resistances (equation *a*). Under steady-state conditions, the flow, Q, through any given cross-section must equal the flow through any other cross-section. By dividing each component in equation *a* by Q (equation *b*), it becomes evident from the definition of resistance (equation 25-11, above) that *for resistances in series, the total resistance, R_t, of the entire system equals the sum of the individual resistances,* that is,

$$R_t = R_1 + R_2 + R_3 \qquad (25\text{-}15)$$

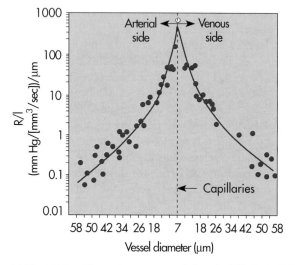

■ Fig. 25-9 The resistance per unit length *(R/l)* for individual small blood vessels in the cat mesentery. The capillaries, diameter 7 μm, are denoted by the vertical dashed line. Resistances of the arterioles are plotted to the left and resistances of the venules to the right of the vertical dashed line. The solid circles represent the actual data. The two curves through the data represent the following regression equations for the arteriole and venule data, respectively: (a) arterioles, $R/l = 1.02 \times 10^6 D^{-4.04}$, and (b) venules, $R/l = 1.07 \times 10^6 D^{-3.94}$. Note that for both types of vessels, the resistance per unit length is inversely proportional to the fourth power (within 1%) of the vessel diameter *(D)*. (Redrawn from Lipowsky HH, Kovalcheck S, Zweifach BW: *Circ Res* 43:738, 1978, with permission of the American Heart Association.)

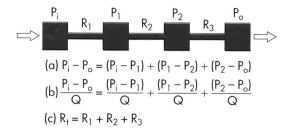

■ Fig. 25-10 For resistances $(R_1, R_2,$ and $R_3)$ arranged in series, the total resistance, R_t, equals the sum of the individual resistances. *P,* Pressure; *Q,* flow.

Resistance of vessels in parallel. For resistances in parallel, as illustrated in Fig. 25-11, the inflow and outflow pressures are the same for all tubes. Under steady-state conditions, the total flow, Q_t, through the system equals the sum of the flows through the individual parallel elements (equation *a*). Because the pressure gradient $(P_i - P_o)$ is identical for all parallel elements, each term in equation *a* may be divided by that pressure gradient to yield equation *b*. From the definition of resistance, equation *c* may be derived. This equation states that *for resistances in parallel, the reciprocal of the total resistance, R_t, equals the sum of the reciprocals of the individual resistances,* that is,

$$1/R_t = 1/R_1 + 1/R_2 + 1/R_3 \qquad (25\text{-}16)$$

A simpler way of stating this relation is to use the term hydraulic **conductance,** which can be defined as the reciprocal of resistance. It then becomes evident that, *for tubes in parallel, the total conductance is the sum of the individual conductances.*

By considering a few simple illustrations, some of the fundamental properties of parallel hydraulic systems become apparent. For example, if the resistances of the three parallel elements in Fig. 25-11 were all equal, then

$$R_1 = R_2 = R_3 \qquad (25\text{-}17)$$

Therefore, from equation 25-16:

$$1/R_t = 3/R_1 \qquad (25\text{-}18)$$

By equating the reciprocals of these terms:

$$R_t = R_1/3 \qquad (25\text{-}19)$$

Thus, the total resistance is less than the individual resistances. In other words, *for any parallel arrangement, the total resistance must be less than that of any*

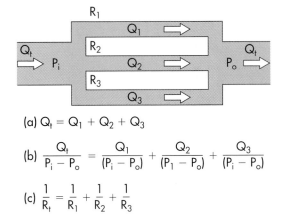

$$(a) \quad Q_t = Q_1 + Q_2 + Q_3$$

$$(b) \quad \frac{Q_t}{P_i - P_o} = \frac{Q_1}{(P_i - P_o)} + \frac{Q_2}{(P_1 - P_o)} + \frac{Q_3}{(P_i - P_o)}$$

$$(c) \quad \frac{1}{R_t} = \frac{1}{R_1} + \frac{1}{R_2} + \frac{1}{R_3}$$

■ **Fig. 25-11** For resistances (R_1, R_2, and R_3) arranged in parallel, the reciprocal of the total resistance, R_t, equals the sum of the reciprocals of the individual resistances. *P,* Pressure; *Q,* flow.

individual component. For example, consider a system in which a very-high-resistance tube is added in parallel to a low-resistance tube. The total resistance of the system must be less than that of the low-resistance component by itself, because the high-resistance component affords an additional pathway, or conductance, for fluid flow.

As a physiological illustration of these principles, consider the relationship between the **total peripheral resistance** (TPR) of the entire systemic vascular bed and the resistance of one of its components, such as the renal vasculature. TPR is the ratio of the arteriovenous pressure difference $(P_a - P_v)$ to the flow through the entire systemic vascular bed (i.e., the cardiac output, Q_t). The renal vascular resistance (R_r) would be the ratio of the same arteriovenous pressure difference $(P_a - P_v)$ to the renal blood flow (Q_r).

In an individual with an arterial pressure of 100 mm Hg, a peripheral venous pressure of about 0 mm Hg, and a cardiac output of 5000 ml/min, TPR will be 0.02 mm Hg/ml/min, or 0.02 PRU (peripheral resistance units). Normally, blood flow through one kidney would be approximately 600 ml/min. Renal resistance would therefore be 100 mm Hg ÷ 100 ml/min, or 0.17 PRU, which is 8.5 times greater than the TPR. One might be surprised initially that an organ such as the kidney, which weighs only about 1% as much as the whole body, has a vascular resistance much greater than that of the entire systemic circulation. But consider that the entire systemic circulation possesses many more alternate pathways for blood to flow than just one kidney. Hence, it is not surprising that the resistance to flow would be greater for a component organ, such as the kidney, than for the entire systemic circulation.

In looking at Fig. 21-2, it may seem paradoxical that the resistance to flow through the small arteries and arterioles (as manifested by the pressure drop from the arterial to the capillary ends of these vessels) is considerably greater than that through certain other vascular components, such as the large arteries, despite the fact that the total cross-sectional area of the small arterial vessels exceeds that for the large arteries.

Consideration of simple models of tubes in parallel will help resolve this apparent paradox. In Fig. 25-12 the resistance to flow through one wide tube of cross-sectional area A_w is compared with that through four narrower tubes in parallel, each of area A_n. The total cross-sectional area of the parallel system of four narrow tubes equals the area of the wide tube; that is,

$$A_w = 4A_n \qquad (25\text{-}20)$$

For a cylindrical tube,

$$A = \pi r^2 \qquad (25\text{-}21)$$

From equation (25-11), resistance, R, is inversely proportional to the fourth power of the radius, r. It follows from equation 25-21, therefore, that

$$R = k/A^2 \qquad (25\text{-}22)$$

The proportionality constant, k, is related to tube length and fluid viscosity, both of which will be held constant in this example. From equation 25-22, the resistances of the wide tube, R_w, and a single narrow tube, R_n, are

$$R_w = k/A_w^2 \qquad (25\text{-}23)$$

$$R_n = k/A_n^2 \qquad (25\text{-}24)$$

From equation 25-16,

$$1/R_t = 1/R_n + 1/R_n + 1/R_n + 1/R_n = 4/R_n \qquad (25\text{-}25)$$

Substituting the value of R_n in equation 25-24 into equation 25-25, and rearranging,

$$R_t = k/4A_n^2 \qquad (25\text{-}26)$$

From equations 25-20 and 25-23,

$$R_t = 4k/A_w^2 = 4 R_w \qquad (25\text{-}27)$$

Hence, the total resistance, R_t, of four such narrow tubes in parallel is four times as great as the resistance, R_w, of a single wide tube of equal total cross-sectional area.

If a similar calculation is made for eight such tubes in parallel, with each tube having one fourth the cross-sectional area of the single wide tube, it will be found that the total resistance equals $2R_w$. In this circumstance, the resistance to flow through eight such narrow tubes in parallel will still be twice as great as that through the single tube, despite the fact that the total cross-sectional area for the eight narrow tubes is twice as great as for the single wide tube. This relationship is analogous to the relationship that exists between resistance and area in the circulatory system when the small arteries and arterioles are compared with the large arteries. Although the total cross-sectional area of all the small arterial vessels greatly exceeds that of all the large arteries (see Fig. 21-3), the resistance to flow through the small arterial vessels is considerably greater than that through the large arteries (see Fig. 21-2).

If we expand this example still further, it will be found that 16 such narrow tubes in parallel, now with four times the total cross-sectional area of the single wide tube, will exert a resistance to flow just equal to the resistance through the wide tube. Any number of these narrow tubes in excess of 16, then, will have a lower resistance than that of the single wide tube. This situation is analogous to the comparison of the arterioles and capillaries that we encountered in Fig. 21-2. The resistance to flow through a single capillary is much greater than that through a single arteriole (Fig. 25-9), yet the number of capillaries so greatly exceeds the number of arterioles, as reflected by the relative difference in total cross-sectional areas (see Fig. 21-3), that the pressure drop across the arterioles is considerably greater than the pressure drop across the capillaries (see Fig. 21-2).

◼ Laminar and Turbulent Flow

Under certain conditions, the flow of a fluid in a cylindrical tube will be **laminar** (sometimes called **streamlined**), as illustrated in Fig. 25-5. As the fluid moves through the tube, a thin layer of fluid in contact with the tube wall adheres to the wall and hence is motionless. The layer of fluid just central to this external lamina must shear against this motionless layer, and therefore the layer moves slowly, but with a finite velocity. Similarly, the next more central layer moves still more rapidly; the longitudinal velocity profile is that of a paraboloid (Fig. 25-5). The fluid elements in any given lamina remain in that lamina as the fluid progresses longitudinally along the tube. The velocity at the center of the stream is maximal and equal to twice the mean velocity of flow across the entire cross-section of the tube.

◼ **Fig. 25-12**   When four narrow tubes, each of area A_n, are connected in parallel, the total cross-sectional area equals the area, A_w, of a wide tube of area such that $A_w = 4A_n$. Although the total areas are equal, the total resistance, R_t, to flow through the parallel narrow tubes is four times as great as the resistance, R_w, through the single wide tube. R_n is the resistance of one narrow tube; k is a constant of proportionality.

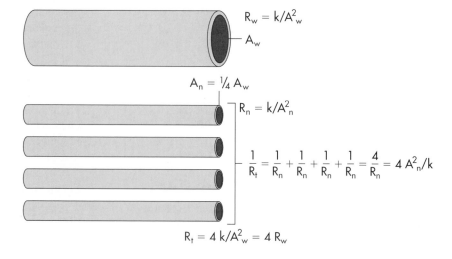

$$R_w = k/A_w^2$$
$$A_w$$
$$A_n = \tfrac{1}{4} A_w$$
$$R_n = k/A_n^2$$
$$\frac{1}{R_t} = \frac{1}{R_n} + \frac{1}{R_n} + \frac{1}{R_n} + \frac{1}{R_n} = \frac{4}{R_n} = 4 A_n^2/k$$
$$R_t = 4 k/A_w^2 = 4 R_w$$

Irregular motions of the fluid elements may develop in the flow of fluid through a tube; such flow is called **turbulent.** Under such conditions, fluid elements do not remain confined to definite laminae, but rapid, radial mixing occurs (Fig. 25-13). A considerably greater pressure is required to force a given flow of fluid through the same tube when the flow is turbulent than when it is laminar. In turbulent flow, the pressure drop is approximately proportional to the square of the flow rate, whereas in laminar flow the pressure drop is proportional to the first power of the flow rate. Hence, to produce a given flow, a pump such as the heart must do considerably more work if turbulence develops.

Whether turbulent or laminar flow will exist in a tube under given conditions may be predicted on the basis of a dimensionless number, called **Reynold's number, N_R.** This number represents the ratio of inertial to viscous forces. For a fluid flowing through a cylindrical tube,

$$N_R = \rho D v / \eta \qquad (25\text{-}28)$$

where ρ is the fluid density, D is the tube diameter, v is the mean velocity, and η is the viscosity. For N_R less than 2000, the flow will usually be laminar; for N_R greater than 3000, the flow will be turbulent; and for N_R between 2000 and 3000, the flow will be transitional between laminar and turbulent. Equation 25-28 indicates that high fluid densities, large tube diameters, high flow velocities, and low fluid viscosities predispose to turbulence. In addition to these factors, abrupt variations in tube dimensions or irregularities in the tube walls may produce turbulence.

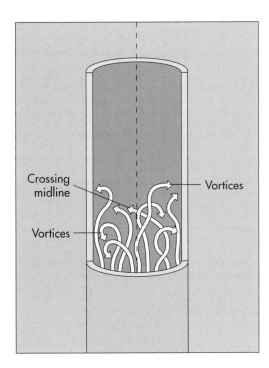

■ **Fig. 25-13** In turbulent flow the elements of the fluid move irregularly in axial, radial, and circumferential directions. Vortices frequently develop.

Crossing midline

Vortices

Vortices

Turbulence is usually accompanied by audible vibrations. When turbulent flow exists within the cardiovascular system, it may be detected during a physical examination as a **murmur.** The factors listed above that predispose to turbulence may account for murmurs heard clinically. In severe anemia, **functional cardiac murmurs** (murmurs not caused by structural abnormalities) are frequently detectable. The physical basis for such murmurs resides in (1) the reduced viscosity of blood in anemia and (2) the high flow velocities associated with the high cardiac output that usually prevails in anemic patients.

Blood clots, or **thrombi,** are much more likely to develop in turbulent than in laminar flow. One of the problems with the use of artificial valves in the surgical treatment of **valvular heart disease** is that thrombi may occur in association with the prosthetic valve. The thrombi may be dislodged and occlude a crucial blood vessel. It is thus important to design such valves to avert turbulence.

■ *Shear Stress on the Vessel Wall*

In Fig. 25-8, an external force was applied to a plate floating on the surface of a liquid in a large basin. This force, directed parallel to the surface, exerted a shearing stress on the liquid below, and thus it produced a differential motion of each layer of liquid relative to the adjacent layers. At the bottom of the basin, the flowing liquid exerted a shearing stress on the surface of the basin in contact with the liquid. Rearranging the equation for viscosity shown in Fig. 25-8 discloses that the shear stress, τ, equals η (du/dy) (i.e., the shear stress equals the product of the viscosity and the shear rate). Hence, the greater the rate of flow, the greater is the shear stress (i.e., the **viscous drag**) that the liquid exerts on the walls of the container in which it flows.

For precisely the same reasons, the rapidly flowing blood in a large artery tends to pull the endothelial lining of the artery along with it. This force, the viscous drag, is proportional to the shear rate (du/dy) of the layers of blood near the wall. For a flow regimen that obeys Poiseuille's law,

$$\tau = 4\eta Q / \rho r^3 \qquad (25\text{-}29)$$

The greater the rate of blood flow (Q) in the artery, the greater is the shear rate (du/dy) near the arterial wall, and therefore the greater the viscous drag (τ).

In certain types of arterial disease, particularly in patients with hypertension, the subendothelial layers of vessels tend to degenerate locally, and small regions of the endothelium may lose their normal support. The viscous drag on the arterial wall may cause a tear between a normally supported and an unsupported region of the endothelial lining. Blood may then flow from the vessel lumen through the rift in the lining and dissect between the various layers of the artery. Such a lesion is called a **dissecting aneurysm.** It occurs most often in the proximal portions of the aorta and is extremely serious. One reason for its predilection for this site is the high velocity of blood flow, with the associated large values of du/dy at the endothelial wall. The shear stress at the vessel wall also influences many other vascular functions, such as the permeability of the vascular walls to large molecules, the biosynthetic activity of the endothelial cells, the integrity of the formed elements in the blood, and the coagulation of the blood. An increase in shear stress on the endothelial wall is also an effective stimulus for the release of nitric oxide (NO) from the vascular endothelial cells; NO is a potent vasodilator.

Rheologic Properties of Blood

The viscosity of a newtonian fluid, such as water, may be determined by measuring the steady, laminar flow of the fluid at a given pressure gradient through a cylindrical tube of known length and radius. The viscosity is then computed by substituting these values into Poiseuille's equation. The viscosity of a given newtonian fluid at a specified temperature will be constant over a wide range of tube dimensions and flows. However, for a non-newtonian fluid, the viscosity calculated by substituting into Poiseuille's equation may vary considerably as a function of tube dimensions and flows. Therefore, in considering the rheologic properties of a suspension such as blood, the term **viscosity** does not have a unique meaning. The terms **anomalous viscosity** and **apparent viscosity** are frequently applied to the value of viscosity obtained for blood under the particular conditions of measurement.

Rheologically, blood is a suspension of formed elements, principally erythrocytes, in a relatively homogeneous liquid, the blood plasma. Because blood is a suspension, the apparent viscosity of blood varies as a function of the **hematocrit ratio** (ratio of volume of red blood cells to volume of whole blood). In Fig. 25-14, the upper curve represents the ratio of the apparent viscosity of whole blood to that of plasma over a range of hematocrit ratios from 0% to 80%; the measurements were made in a tube 1 mm in diameter. The viscosity of plasma is 1.2 to 1.3 times that of water. Fig. 25-14 *(upper curve)* shows that blood, with a normal hematocrit ratio of 45%, has an apparent viscosity 2.4 times that of plasma. In severe anemia (in which the concentration of erythrocytes is low), blood viscosity is low. With greater hematocrit ratios, the slope of the curve increases progressively; it is especially steep at the upper range of erythrocyte concentrations.

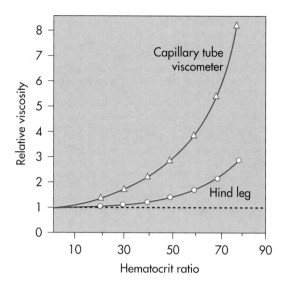

■ **Fig. 25-14**   The viscosity of whole blood, relative to that of plasma, increases at a progressively greater rate as the hematocrit ratio increases. For any given hematocrit ratio, the apparent viscosity of blood is less when measured in a biological viscometer (such as the hind leg of a dog) than in a conventional capillary tube viscometer. (Redrawn from Levy MN, Share L: *Circ Res* 1:247, 1953, with permission of the American Heart Association.)

A rise in hematocrit ratio from 45% to 70% (such as occurs in the blood disease **polycythemia vera**) increases the apparent viscosity more than twofold. This change in viscosity tends to exert a proportionate effect on the resistance to blood flow. The change in peripheral resistance that occurs with an increase in blood viscosity may be appreciated when it is recognized that even in the most severe cases of **essential hypertension,** which is the most common type of arterial hypertension, the total peripheral resistance rarely increases by more than a factor of two. In this type of hypertension, the increase in peripheral resistance is achieved by arteriolar vasoconstriction.

For any given hematocrit ratio, the apparent viscosity of blood depends on the dimensions of the tube employed in estimating the viscosity. Fig. 25-15 demonstrates that the apparent viscosity of blood diminishes progressively as tube diameter decreases below a value of about 0.3 mm. The diameters of the highest-resistance blood vessels, the arterioles, are considerably less than this critical value. This phenomenon therefore reduces the resistance to flow in the blood vessels that possess the greatest resistance.

The apparent viscosity of blood, when measured in living tissues, is considerably less than when measured in a conventional capillary tube viscometer with a diameter greater than 0.3 mm. In the lower curve of Fig. 25-14, the apparent relative viscosity of blood was assessed by using the hind leg of an anesthetized dog as a bio-

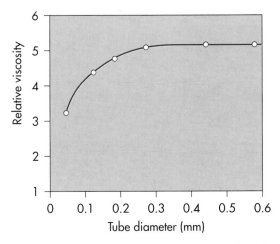

■ **Fig. 25-15** Viscosity of blood, relative to that of water, increases as a function of tube diameter up to a diameter of about 0.3 mm. (Redrawn from Fåhraeus R, Lindqvist T: *Am J Physiol* 96:562, 1931.)

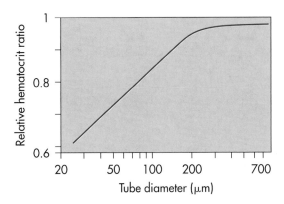

■ **Fig. 25-16** The relative hematocrit ratio of blood flowing from a feed reservoir through capillary tubes of various calibers as a function of the tube diameter. The relative hematocrit ratio equals the hematocrit ratio of the blood in the tubes divided by that of the blood in the feed reservoir. (Redrawn from Barbee JH, Cokelet GR: *Microvasc Res* 3:6, 1971.)

logical viscometer. Over the entire range of hematocrit ratios, the apparent viscosity was less as measured in the living tissue than in the capillary tube viscometer *(upper curve),* and the disparity was greater the higher the hematocrit ratio.

The influence of tube diameter on apparent viscosity is explained in part by the actual change in composition of the blood as it flows through small tubes. The composition changes because the red blood cells tend to accumulate in the faster axial stream, whereas plasma tends to flow in the slower marginal layers. To illustrate this phenomenon, a reservoir such as R_1 in Fig. 25-6, *C* has been filled with blood with a given hematocrit ratio. The blood in R_1 was constantly agitated to prevent settling and the blood was permitted to flow through a narrow capillary tube into reservoir R_2. As long as the tube diameter was substantially greater than the diameter of the red blood cells, the hematocrit ratio of the blood in R_2 was not detectably different from that in R_1. Surprisingly, however, the hematocrit ratio of the blood contained within the tube was found to be considerably lower than the hematocrit ratio of the blood in either reservoir.

In Fig. 25-16, the relative hematocrit is the ratio of the hematocrit in the tube to that in the reservoir at either end of the tube. For tubes 300 μm in diameter or greater, the relative hematocrit ratio was close to 1. However, as the tube diameter was diminished below 300 μm, the relative hematocrit ratio progressively diminished; for a tube diameter of 30 μm, the relative hematocrit ratio was only 0.6; that is, *the erythrocyte content of a given volume of blood in the capillary tube was 40% less than that in the blood reservoirs at either end of the tube.*

That this situation results from a disparity in the relative velocities of the red cells and plasma can be appreciated in the following analogy. Consider the flow of automobile traffic across a bridge that is 3 miles long. Let the cars move in one lane at a speed of 60 mph and the trucks in another lane at 20 mph, as illustrated in Fig. 25-17. If one car and one truck start out across the bridge each minute, then except for the initial few minutes of traffic flow across the bridge, one car and one truck will arrive at the other end each minute. Yet if one counts the actual number of cars and trucks on the bridge at any moment, three times as many slower-moving trucks will be on the bridge than rapidly traveling cars.

Because the axial portions of the bloodstream contain a greater proportion of red cells and move with a greater velocity, the red cells tend to traverse the tube in less time than does the plasma. Therefore, the red cells correspond to the rapidly moving cars in the analogy, and the plasma corresponds to the slowly moving trucks. Measurement of transit times through various organs has shown that red cells do travel faster than the plasma. Furthermore, the hematocrit ratios of the blood contained in various tissues are lower than those in blood samples withdrawn from large arteries or veins in the same animal (Fig. 25-18).

The physical forces responsible for the drift of the erythrocytes toward the axial stream and away from the vessel walls are not fully understood. One factor is the great flexibility of the red blood cells. At low flow rates, comparable with those in the microcirculation, rigid particles do not migrate toward the axis of a tube, whereas flexible particles do migrate. The concentration of flexible particles near the tube axis is enhanced by increasing the shear rate.

The apparent viscosity of blood diminishes as the flow rate is increased (Fig. 25-19), a phenomenon called **shear thinning** (the greater the flow, the greater the rate that one lamina of fluid shears against an adjacent lamina). The greater tendency for the erythrocytes to accumulate in the axial laminae at higher flow rates is partly responsible for this non-newtonian behavior. However, a

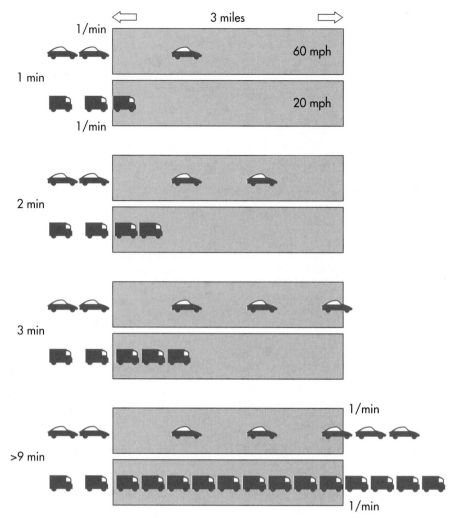

■ **Fig. 25-17** When the car velocity is three times as great as the truck velocity, the ratio of the number of cars to trucks on the bridge will be 1:3 after 9 minutes, even though one of each type of vehicle enters and leaves the bridge each minute.

■ **Fig. 25-18** The hematocrit ratio (H_{micro}) of the blood in various-sized arterial and venous microvessels in the cat mesentery, relative to the hematocrit ratio (H_{sys}) in the large systemic vessels. The hematocrit ratio is least in the capillaries and tiny venules. (Modified from Lipowsky HH, Usami S, Chien S: *Microvasc Res* 19:297, 1980.)

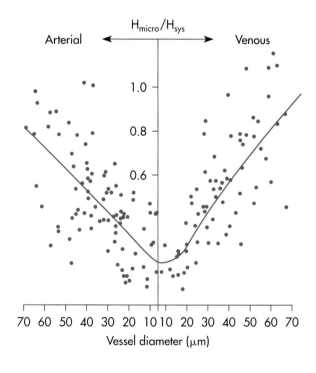

more important factor is that at very slow flow rates, the suspended cells tend to form aggregates, which would increase viscosity. As the flow is increased, this aggregation decreases and so also does the apparent viscosity (Fig. 25-19).

The tendency for the erythrocytes to aggregate at low flows depends on the concentration in the plasma of the larger protein molecules, especially fibrinogen. For this reason, the changes in blood viscosity with flow rate are much more pronounced when the concentration of fibrinogen is high. Also, at low flow rates, leukocytes tend to adhere to the endothelial cells of the microvessels and thereby increase the apparent viscosity.

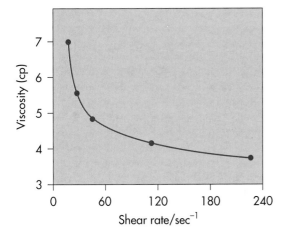

■ **Fig. 25-19** Decrease in the viscosity of blood (centipoise) at increasing rates of shear (s^{-1}). The shear rate refers to the velocity of one layer of fluid relative to that of the adjacent layers and is directionally related to the rate of flow. (Redrawn from Amin TM, Sirs JA: *Q J Exp Physiol* 70:37, 1985.)

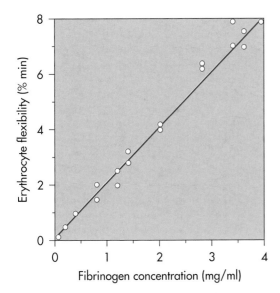

■ **Fig. 25-20** Effect of the plasma fibrinogen concentration on the flexibility of human erythrocytes. (Redrawn from Amin TM, Sirs JA: *Q J Exp Physiol* 70:37, 1985.)

The deformability of the erythrocytes is also a factor in shear thinning, especially when hematocrit ratios are high. The mean diameter of human red blood cells is about 7 μm, yet they are able to pass through openings with a diameter of only 3 μm. As blood with densely packed erythrocytes flows at progressively greater rates, the erythrocytes become more and more deformed, which diminishes the apparent viscosity of the blood. The flexibility of human erythrocytes is enhanced as the concentration of fibrinogen in the plasma increases (Fig. 25-20). If the red blood cells become hardened, as they are in certain **spherocytic anemias,** shear thinning may become much less prominent.

■ *Summary*

1. The vascular system is composed of two major subdivisions in series with one another: the systemic circulation and the pulmonary circulation.

2. Each subdivision comprises a number of types of vessels (e.g., arteries, arterioles, capillaries) that are aligned in series with one another. In general, the vessels of a given type are arranged in parallel with each other.

3. The mean velocity (v) of blood flow in a given type of vessel is directly proportional to the total blood flow (Q_t) being pumped by the heart, and it is inversely proportional to the cross-sectional area (A) of all the parallel vessels of that type (i.e., $v = Q_t/A$).

4. The laterally directed pressure in the bloodstream decreases as the flow velocity increases; the decrement in lateral pressure is proportional to the square of the velocity. The changes are insignificant, however, except when flow is very great.

5. When blood flow is steady and laminar in vessels larger than arterioles, the flow (Q) is proportional to the pressure drop down the vessel ($P_i - P_o$) and to the fourth power of the radius (r), and it is inversely proportional to the length (l) of the vessel and to the viscosity (η) of the fluid; that is, $Q = \rho(P_i - P_o)r^4/8\eta l$ (Poiseuille's law).

6. For resistances aligned in series, the total resistance equals the sum of the individual resistances.

7. For resistances aligned in parallel, the reciprocal of the total resistance equals the sum of the reciprocals of the individual resistances.

8. Flow tends to become turbulent when (1) flow velocity is high, (2) fluid viscosity is low, (3) fluid density is great, (4) tube diameter is large, or (5) the wall of the vessel is irregular.

9. Blood flow is non-newtonian in very small blood vessels (i.e., Poiseuille's law is not applicable).

10. The apparent viscosity of the blood diminishes as shear rate (flow) increases and as the tube dimensions decrease.

■ *Self-Study Problems*

1. A renal physiologist found that the mean arterial pressure in an anesthetized animal was 100 mm Hg, and the blood flow to each kidney 200 ml/min. What was the resistance to blood flow through one kidney, and what was the resistance to blood flow through both kidneys? Explain the reason for the disparity in the resistances for one and two kidneys.

2. A patient is found to have a loud cardiac murmur, but his cardiac valves appear to function normally. Laboratory examinations revealed that he was severely anemic and that his cardiac output was abnormally high. What factors operated in this patient to produce the "functional" murmur?

3. In a patient who has a small dissecting aneurysm of the thoracic aorta, what is the rationale for giving a drug that will reduce cardiac output?

4. Why is the hematocrit ratio of the blood in small blood vessels, such as the arterioles, consistently less than the hematocrit ratio in the large blood vessels?

■ *Bibliography*

Journal articles

Alonso C et al: Transient rheological behavior of blood in low-shear tube flow: velocity profiles and effective viscosity, *Am J Physiol* 268:H25, 1995.

Amin TM, Sirs JA: The blood rheology of man and various animal species, *Q J Exp Physiol* 70:37, 1985.

Chien S: Role of blood cells in microcirculatory regulation, *Microvasc Res* 29:129, 1985.

Cokelet GR, Goldsmith HL: Decreased hydrodynamic resistance in the two-phase flow of blood through small vertical tubes at low flow rates, *Circ Res* 68:1, 1991.

Goldsmith HL: The microrheology of human blood, *Microvasc Res* 31:121, 1986.

Hoeks APG et al: Noninvasive determination of shear-rate distribution across the arterial wall, *Hypertension* 26:26, 1995.

Klanchar M, Tarbell JM, Wang DM: In vitro study of the influence of radial wall motion on wall shear stress in an elastic tube model of the aorta, *Circ Res* 66:1624, 1990.

Lee RT, Kamm RD: Vascular mechanics for the cardiologist, *J Am Coll Cardiol* 23:1289, 1994.

Lipowsky HH, Usami S, Chien S: In vivo measurements of "apparent viscosity" and microvessel hematocrit in the mesentery of the cat, *Microvasc Res* 19:297, 1980.

Maeda N, Shiga T: Velocity of oxygen transfer and erythrocyte rheology, *News Physiol Sci* 9:22, 1994.

McKay CB, Meiselman HJ: Osmolality-mediated Fåhraeus and Fåhraeus-Lindqvist effects for human RBC suspensions, *Am J Physiol* 254:H238, 1988.

Melkumyants AM, Balashov SA, Khayutin VM: Control of arterial lumen by shear stress on endothelium, *News Physiol Sci* 10:204, 1995.

Morita T et al: Role of Ca^{2+} and protein kinase C in shear stress–induced actin depolymerization and endothelin 1 gene expression, *Circ Res* 75:630, 1994.

Pries AR, Secomb TW, Gaetgens P: Design principles of vascular beds, *Circ Res* 77:1017, 1995.

Pries AR et al: Resistance to blood flow in microvessels in vivo, *Circ Res* 75:904, 1994.

Reinhart WH et al: Influence of endothelial surface on flow velocity in vitro, *Am J Physiol* 265:H523, 1993.

Sarelius IH, Duling BR: Direct measurement of microvessel hematocrit, red cell flux, velocity, and transit time, *Am J Physiol* 243:H1018, 1982.

Secomb TW: Flow-dependent rheological properties of blood in capillaries, *Microvasc Res* 34:46, 1987.

Tangelder GJ et al: Wall shear rate in arterioles in vivo: least estimates from platelet velocity profiles, *Am J Physiol* 254:H1059, 1988.

Thompson TN, La Celle PL, Cokelet GR: Perturbation of red blood cell flow in small tubes by white blood cells, *Pflugers Arch* 413:372, 1989.

White KC et al: Hemodynamics and wall shear rate in the abdominal aorta of dogs: effects of vasoactive agents, *Circ Res* 75:637, 1994.

Books and monographs

Chien S, Usami S, Skalak R: *Blood flow in small tubes.* In Renkin EM, Michel CC, editors: *Handbook of physiology:* sect 2: *The cardiovascular system—microcirculation,* vol 4, Bethesda, Md, 1984, American Physiological Society.

Fung YC: *Biodynamics: circulation,* New York, 1984, Springer-Verlag.

Lowe GDO: *Clinical blood rheology,* vol 1, Boca Raton, Fla, 1988, CRC Press.

Milnor WR: *Hemodynamics,* Baltimore, 1982, Williams & Wilkins.

Taylor DEM, Stevens AI, editors: *Blood flow: theory and practice,* New York, 1983, Academic Press.

The Arterial System

The principal function of the systemic and pulmonary arterial systems is to distribute blood to the capillary beds throughout the body. The arterioles, the terminal components of this system, are high-resistance vessels that regulate the distribution of flow to the various capillary beds. Because of their elasticity, the aorta, the pulmonary artery, and their major branches form a system of channels capable of handling considerable volume. These two features of the arterial system—its elastic conduits and high-resistance terminals—are also shared by fluid systems called **hydraulic filters,** which tend to dampen fluctuations in flow. Thus, the body's arterial system constitutes a hydraulic filter; these filters are analogous to the resistance-capacitance filters of electrical circuits.

The main advantage of hydraulic filtering in the arterial system is that it *converts the intermittent output of the heart to a steady flow through the capillaries.* This important function of the large elastic arteries has been likened to the Windkessels of antique fire engines. The Windkessel contained a large volume of trapped air. The compressibility of the air that remained trapped above the water in the Windkessel converted the intermittent inflow of water from the water source to a steady outflow of water at the nozzle of the fire hose. Without the Windkessel, water would flow only in spurts, making firefighting inefficient at best and dangerous at worst.

■ *Overview of the Hydraulic Filter*

The role that the large elastic arteries play in the hydraulic filtering function is illustrated in Fig. 26-1. Because the heart pumps intermittently, the entire stroke volume is discharged into the arterial system during systole. Systole usually occupies only about one third of the cardiac cycle. In fact, however, as described in Chapter 23, most of the stroke volume is actually pumped during the rapid ejection phase, which constitutes about half of systole. A small part of the energy of cardiac contraction is dissipated as forward capillary flow during systole; the remainder is stored as potential energy, as much of the

stroke volume is retained by the distensible arteries (Fig. 26-1, *A,* and *B*). During diastole, the elastic recoil of the arterial walls converts this potential energy into capillary blood flow. If the arterial walls were rigid, capillary flow would not occur during diastole (Fig. 26-1, *C* and *D*).

Hydraulic filtering minimizes the workload of the heart. More work is required to pump a given flow intermittently than steadily. The more effective the hydraulic filtering, the less work is required. A simple example illustrates this point.

Consider first the steady flow of a fluid at a rate of 100 ml/sec through a hydraulic system with a resistance of 1 mm Hg/ml/sec. This combination of flow and resistance would result in a constant pressure of 100 mm Hg, as shown in Fig. 26-2, *A*. If we neglect any inertial effect, the hydraulic work, W, may be defined as

$$W = \int_{t_1}^{t_2} P dV \qquad (26\text{-}1)$$

That is, each small increment of volume that is pumped, dV, is multiplied by the associated pressure, P, and the products (PdV) are integrated over the time interval of interest, $t_2 - t_1$, to give the total work, W. For steady flow,

$$W = PV \qquad (26\text{-}2)$$

In the example in Fig. 26-2, *A*, the work done in pumping the fluid for 1 second would be 10,000 mm Hg · ml (or 1.33×10^7 dyne · cm).

Next, consider an intermittent pump that puts out the same volume per second but pumps the entire volume at a steady rate over 0.5 second and then pumps nothing during the next 0.5 second. Hence, it pumps at the rate of 200 ml/sec for 0.5 second, as shown in Fig. 26-2, *B* and *C*. In *B*, the conduit is rigid and the fluid is incompressible, but the hydraulic system has the same resistance as in *A*. During the pumping phase of the cycle (systole), the flow of 200 ml/sec through a resistance of 1 mm Hg/ml/sec would produce a pressure of 200 mm Hg. During the filling phase of the pump (diastole), the pressure would be 0 mm Hg in this rigid system. The work done during systole would be 20,000 mm Hg · ml, which is twice that required in the example shown in Fig. 26-2, *A*.

The more distensible the system, the more efficient is the hydraulic filtering. The reason for this increased efficiency is that in a very distensible system, the pressure remains virtually constant throughout the entire cycle (Fig. 26-2, *C*). Of the 100 ml of fluid pumped during the 0.5 second of systole, only 50 ml would be emitted through the high-resistance outflow end of the

system during systole. The remaining 50 ml would be stored by the distensible conduit during systole and would flow out during diastole. Hence, the pressure would be virtually constant at 100 mm Hg throughout the cycle. The fluid pumped during systole would be ejected at only half the pressure that prevailed in Fig. 26-2, *B*, and therefore the work would be only half as great. With nearly perfect filtering, as in Fig. 26-2, *C*, the work would be identical to that for steady flow (Fig. 26-2, *A*).

Compliant arteries

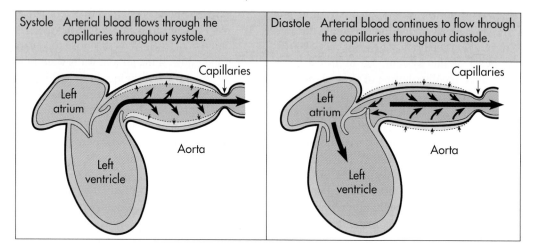

A, When the arteries are normally compliant, a substantial fraction of the stroke volume is stored in the arteries during ventricular systole. The arterial walls are stretched.

B, During ventricular diastole the previously stretched arteries recoil. The volume of blood that is displaced by the recoil furnishes continuous capillary flow throughout diastole.

Rigid arteries

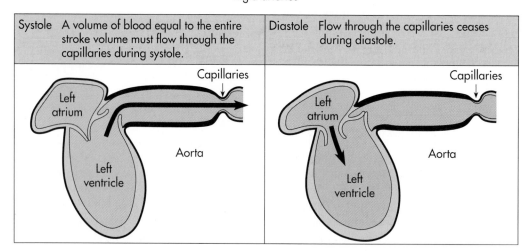

C, When the arteries are rigid, virtually none of the stroke volume can be stored in the arteries.

D, Rigid arteries cannot recoil appreciably during diastole.

■ **Fig. 26-1** **A** to **D,** When the arteries are normally compliant, blood flows through the capillaries throughout the cardiac cycle. When the arteries are rigid, blood flows through the capillaries during systole, but flow ceases during diastole.

The filtering accomplished by the systemic and pulmonic arterial systems is intermediate between the system with rigid conduits shown in Fig. 26-2, *B* and the system with infinitely distensible conduits in Fig. 26-2, *C*. Ordinarily, the additional work imposed by intermittency of pumping, in excess of that for steady flow, is about 35% for the right ventricle and about 10% for the left ventricle. These fractions change, however, with variations in heart rate, peripheral resistance, and arterial distensibility.

Rigid conduits in a hydraulic system create the need for more energy to pump fluid through the system. The increased cardiac energy requirements imposed by a rigid arterial system are illustrated by the experimental results shown in Fig. 26-3. In a group of anesthetized dogs, the cardiac output pumped by the left ventricle could be allowed to flow through the natural route (the aorta), or it could be diverted into a stiff plastic tube attached to the peripheral arteries. The total peripheral resistances were found to be virtually identical, regardless of which pathway was selected. The data (Fig. 26-3) from a representative animal show that for any given stroke volume, the myocardial oxygen consumption was substantially greater when the blood was diverted through the plastic tubing than when it flowed through the aorta. This increase in oxygen consumption indicates that the left ventricle had to expend more energy to pump blood through a less compliant conduit than through a more compliant conduit.

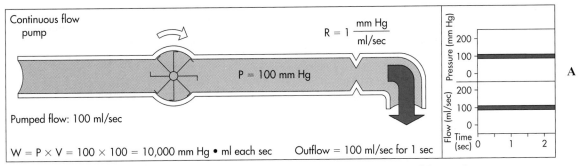

The flow is steady, and pressure will remain constant regardless of the distensibility of the conduit.

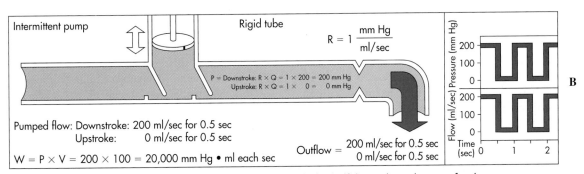

The flow (Q) produced by the pump is intermittent; it is steady for half the cycle and ceases for the remainder of the cycle. The conduit is rigid, and therefore the flow produced by the pump during its downstroke must exit through the resistance during the same 0.5 second that elapses during the downstroke. The pump must do twice as much work as the pump in **A**.

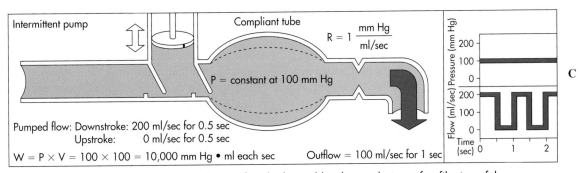

The pump operates as in **B,** but the conduit is infinitely distensible. This results in perfect filtering of the pressure; that is, the pressure is steady, and the flow through the resistance is also steady. The work equals that in **A.**

■ **Fig. 26-2** **A** to **C,** Relationships between pressure and flow for three hydraulic systems. In each the overall flow is 100 ml/sec, and the resistance is 1 mm Hg/(ml/sec).

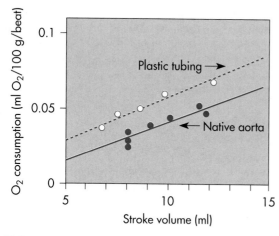

■ Fig. 26-3 Relationship between myocardial oxygen consumption *(ml/100 g/beat)* and stroke volume *(ml)* in an anesthetized dog whose cardiac output could be pumped by the left ventricle either through the aorta or through a stiff plastic tube to the peripheral arteries. (Modified from Kelly RP, Tunin R, Kass DA: *Circ Res* 71:490, 1992, with permission of the American Heart Association.)

■ *Arterial Elasticity*

A good way to appreciate the elastic properties of the arterial wall is to consider the **static pressure-volume relationship** for the aorta. To obtain the curves shown in Fig. 26-4, aortas were obtained at autopsy from individuals in different age groups. All branches of the aorta were tied off, and successive volumes of liquid were injected into this closed elastic system, just as successive amounts of water might be introduced into a balloon. After each increment of volume had been introduced, the internal pressure was measured. In Fig. 26-4, the curve that relates pressure to volume for the youngest age group (curve *a*) is sigmoidal. Although the curve is nearly linear over most of its extent, the slope decreases at the upper and lower ends. The aortic **compliance** at any point on the curve is represented by the slope, dV/dP, at that point. Thus, in young individuals, the aortic compliance is least at both very high and very low pressures and greatest over the pressure range (75 to 140 mm Hg) that prevails in healthy people. This sequence of compliance changes induced by increasing fluid volumes resembles the familiar compliance changes encountered when one inflates a balloon. The greatest difficulty in introducing air into the balloon is encountered at the beginning of inflation and again when the volume is near maximum, just before rupture of the balloon. At intermediate fluid volumes the balloon is relatively easy to inflate; that is, it is very compliant.

As people age, the pressure-volume curves of their arterial systems shift downward, and the slopes of these curves diminish (Fig. 26-4). Thus, for any pressure above about 80 mm Hg, the compliance decreases with age. This change in compliance is a

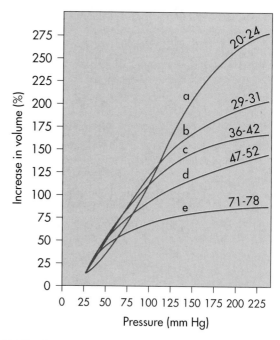

■ Fig. 26-4 Pressure-volume relationships for aortas obtained at autopsy from humans in different age groups (denoted by the numbers at the right end of each of the curves). (Redrawn from Hallock P, Benson IC: *J Clin Invest* 16:595, 1937.)

manifestation of the increased rigidity (**atherosclerosis**) of the system caused by progressive changes in the collagen and elastin contents of the arterial walls.

The effects of the subject's age on the elastic characteristics of the arterial system, as shown in Fig. 26-4, were derived from aortas removed at autopsy. Age-related changes have also been confirmed in living subjects by ultrasound imaging techniques. These studies show that the increase in the diameter of the aorta produced by each cardiac contraction is much less in elderly persons than in young persons (Fig. 26-5). The effects of aging on the **elastic modulus** of the aorta in healthy subjects are shown in Fig. 26-6. The elastic modulus, E_p, is defined as

$$E_p = \Delta P/(\Delta D/D) \qquad (26\text{-}3)$$

where ΔP is the aortic pulse pressure (i.e., the change in aortic pressure during a cardiac cycle; Fig. 26-7), D is the mean aortic diameter during the cardiac cycle, and ΔD is the maximal change in aortic diameter during the cardiac cycle.

The fractional change in diameter ($\Delta D/D$) of the aorta during the cardiac cycle reflects the change in aortic volume as the left ventricle ejects its stroke volume into the aorta with each systole. Thus, E_p is **inversely** related to compliance, which is the ratio of ΔV to ΔP. Consequently, the **increase** in elastic modulus with aging (Fig. 26-6) and the **decrease** in compliance with aging (Fig. 26-4) both reflect the stiffening of the arterial walls as individuals age.

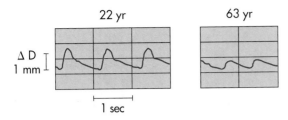

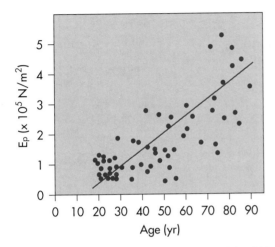

■ **Fig. 26-5** Pulsatile changes in diameter, measured ultrasonically, in a 22-year-old and a 63-year-old man. (Modified from Imura T et al: *Cardiovasc Res* 20:208, 1986.)

■ **Fig. 26-6** Effects of age on the elastic modulus (E_p) of the abdominal aorta in a group of 61 human subjects. (Modified from Imura T et al: *Cardiovasc Res* 20:208, 1986.)

■ *Determinants of Arterial Blood Pressure*

The determinants of arterial blood pressure cannot be evaluated precisely. However, arterial blood pressure is routinely measured in patients, and it provides a useful clue to their cardiovascular status. We therefore present a simplified explanation of the principal determinants of arterial blood pressure. First, we will analyze the determinants of **mean arterial pressure,** which is the pressure averaged over time (Fig. 26-7). The **systolic** (maximal) and **diastolic** (minimal) **arterial pressures** within the cardiac cycle (Fig. 26-7) will then be considered as the upper and lower limits of periodic oscillations about this mean pressure. Finally, the changes in arterial pressure as the pulse wave progresses from the origin of the aorta toward the capillaries will be discussed.

In our discussion, we arbitrarily divide the determinants of the arterial blood pressure into "physical" and "physiological" factors (Fig. 26-8). The physical factors relate to the fluid mechanical characteristics, whereas the physiological factors relate to certain features of the cardiovascular system of living subjects. Because we will assume that the arterial system is a static, elastic system, the only two physical factors that we will consider are **fluid volume** (i.e., blood volume) within the arterial system and the **elastic characteristics** (compliance) of the system. Certain physiological factors will be considered, namely, **cardiac output** (which equals **heart rate × stroke volume**) and **peripheral resistance.** Such physiological factors will be shown to operate through one or both of the physical factors.

■ *Mean Arterial Pressure*

The mean arterial pressure, $\bar{P}_a$, may be estimated from an arterial blood pressure tracing by measuring the area under the curve and dividing this area by the time interval involved, as shown in Fig. 26-7. Alternatively, $\bar{P}_a$ can usually be approximated satisfactorily from the measured values of the systolic (P_s) and diastolic (P_d) pressures by means of the following formula:

$$\bar{P}_a = P_d + (P_s - P_d)/3 \qquad (26\text{-}4)$$

As noted previously, in this discussion we consider that the mean arterial pressure depends on only two physical factors: the mean blood volume in the arterial system and the arterial compliance (Fig. 26-8). The arterial volume, V_a, in turn depends on the rate of inflow, Q_h, into the arteries from the heart (**cardiac output**) and on the rate of outflow, Q_r, from the arteries through the resistance vessels (**peripheral runoff**). These relationships can be expressed mathematically as

$$dV_a/dt = Q_h - Q_r \qquad (26\text{-}5)$$

This equation is actually an expression of the law of conservation of mass. It states that the change in arterial blood volume per unit time (dV_a/dt) represents the difference between the rate at which blood is pumped into the arterial system by the heart (Q_h) and the rate at which it leaves the arterial system through the resistance vessels (Q_r). If arterial inflow exceeds outflow, arterial volume increases, the arterial walls are stretched further, and pressure rises. The converse happens when arterial outflow exceeds inflow. When inflow equals outflow, arterial pressure remains constant.

The change in pressure in response to an alteration of cardiac output can be better appreciated by considering the simple example in the box below.

Under control conditions, let cardiac output be 5 L/min and mean arterial pressure ($\bar{P}_a$) be 100 mm Hg (Fig. 26-9, *A*). From the definition of total peripheral resistance

$$R \equiv (\bar{P}_a - P_{ra})/Q_r \qquad (26\text{-}6)$$

If $\bar{P}_{ra}$ (mean right atrial pressure) is negligible in comparison with $\bar{P}_a$, then

$$R \equiv \bar{P}_a/Q_r \qquad (26\text{-}7)$$

In this example, therefore, R is 100/5, or 20 mm Hg/L/min.

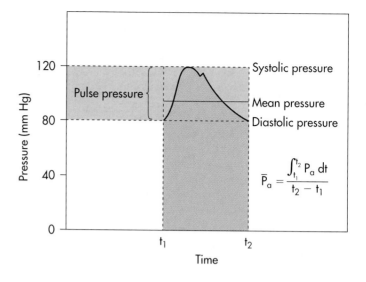

■ **Fig. 26-7**   Arterial systolic, diastolic, pulse, and mean pressures. The mean arterial pressure $(\bar{P}_a)$ represents the area under the arterial pressure curve *(shaded area)* divided by the cardiac cycle duration $(t_2 - t_1)$.

$$\bar{P}_a = \frac{\int_{t_1}^{t_2} P_a \, dt}{t_2 - t_1}$$

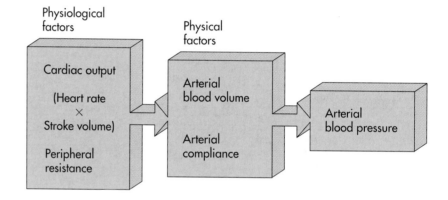

■ **Fig. 26-8**   The arterial blood pressure is determined directly by two major physical factors, the arterial blood volume and the arterial compliance. These physical factors are affected in turn by certain physiological factors, namely, heart rate, stroke volume, cardiac output (heart rate × stroke volume), and peripheral resistance.

Now let cardiac output, Q_h, suddenly increase to 10 L/min (Fig. 26-9, *B*). Instantaneously, $\bar{P}_a$ will be unchanged. Because the outflow, Q_r, from the arteries depends on P_a and R, Q_r will also remain unchanged at first. Therefore, Q_h, now 10 L/min, will exceed Q_r, still only 5 L/min. This will increase the mean arterial blood volume $(\bar{V}_a)$. From equation 26-5, when $Q_h > Q_r$, then $d\bar{V}_a/dt > 0$; that is, volume is increasing.

Because $\bar{P}_a$ depends on the mean arterial blood volume, $\bar{V}_a$, and the arterial compliance, C_a, an increase in $\bar{V}_a$ will increase $\bar{P}_a$. By definition,

$$C_a \equiv dV_a/d\bar{P}_a \qquad (26\text{-}8)$$

After rearranging this equation, and dividing both sides by dt,

$$dV_a/dt = C_a \, dP_a/dt \qquad (26\text{-}9)$$

From equation 26-5, we can substitute $Q_h - Q_r$ for $d\bar{V}_a/dt$ in equation 26-9. Therefore,

$$d\bar{P}_a/dt = (Q_h - Q_r)/C_a \qquad (26\text{-}10)$$

Hence, $\bar{P}_a$ will rise when $Q_h > Q_r$, will fall when $Q_h < Q_r$, and will remain constant when $Q_h = Q_r$.

In this example, in which cardiac output (Q_h) is suddenly increased to 10 L/min, mean arterial pressure $(\bar{P}_a)$ continues to rise as long as cardiac output exceeds arterial outflow (Q_r). Equation 26-7 indicates that arterial outflow will not reach 10 L/min until the mean arterial pressure reaches a level of 200 mm Hg and as long as peripheral resistance (R) remains constant at 20 mm Hg/L/min. Hence, as the mean arterial pressure approaches 200, arterial outflow will almost equal cardiac output, and mean arterial pressure will rise very slowly. When cardiac output is first raised, however, it greatly exceeds arterial outflow, and therefore mean arterial pressure rises sharply. The pressure-time tracing in Fig. 26-10 indicates that, regardless of the value of arterial compliance (C_a), the slope gradually diminishes as pressure rises and approaches its final asymptotic value (equilibrium).

Furthermore, the *height* that mean arterial pressure will attain at equilibrium is independent of the elastic characteristics of the arterial walls (Fig. 26-10). We have seen that, at equilibrium, mean arterial pressure must rise to a level such that arterial outflow equals cardiac output. Equation 26-6 indicates that cardiac output depends only on pressure gradient and resistance to flow. Hence, com-

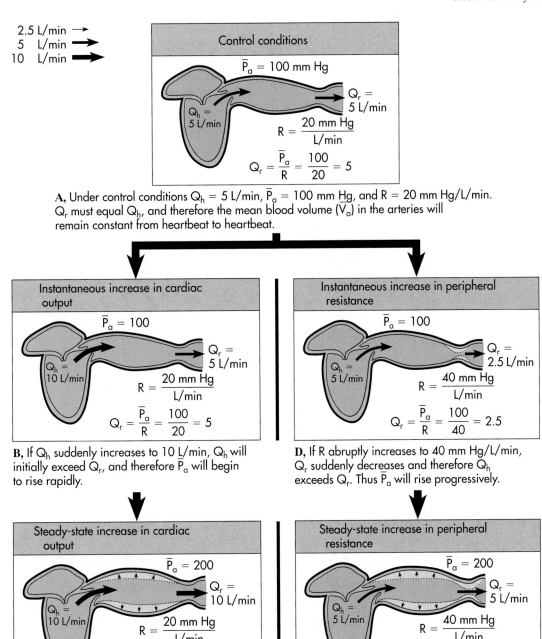

A, Under control conditions Q_h = 5 L/min, $\bar{P}_a$ = 100 mm Hg, and R = 20 mm Hg/L/min. Q_r must equal Q_h, and therefore the mean blood volume (V_a) in the arteries will remain constant from heartbeat to heartbeat.

B, If Q_h suddenly increases to 10 L/min, Q_h will initially exceed Q_r, and therefore $\bar{P}_a$ will begin to rise rapidly.

D, If R abruptly increases to 40 mm Hg/L/min, Q_r suddenly decreases and therefore Q_h exceeds Q_r. Thus $\bar{P}_a$ will rise progressively.

C, The disparity between Q_h and Q_r progressively increases arterial blood volume. The volume continues to increase until $\bar{P}_a$ reaches a level of 200 mm Hg.

E, The excess of Q_h over Q_r accumulates blood in the arteries. Blood continues to accumulate until $\bar{P}_a$ rises to a level of 200 mm Hg.

■ **Fig. 26-9**   Relationship of mean arterial blood pressure $(\bar{P}_a)$ to cardiac output (Q_h), peripheral runoff (Q_r), and peripheral resistance *(R)* under control conditions **(A),** in response to an increase in cardiac output **(B** and **C),** and in response to an increase in peripheral resistance **(D** and **E).**

pliance determines only the *rate* at which the new equilibrium value of mean arterial pressure will be approached, as illustrated in Fig. 26-10. When compliance is small (rigid vessels), a relatively slight increment in mean arterial blood volume (caused by a transient excess of cardiac output over arterial outflow) greatly increases mean arterial pressure. Hence, mean arterial pressure attains its new equilibrium level quickly. Conversely, when compliance is large, considerable volumes can be accommodated with relatively small pressure changes. Therefore, the new equilibrium value of mean arterial pressure is reached at a slower rate.

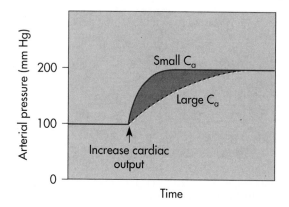

■ Fig. 26-10 When cardiac output is suddenly increased, the arterial compliance *(C$_a$)* determines the rate at which the mean arterial pressure will attain its new, elevated value, but it does not determine the *magnitude* of the new pressure.

■ Peripheral Resistance

Similar reasoning may now be used to explain the changes in mean arterial pressure that accompany alterations in peripheral resistance. Let the control conditions be identical with those of the preceding example; that is, let $Q_h = 5$, $\overline{P}_a = 100$, and $R = 20$ (Fig. 26 9, *A*). Then, let R suddenly be increased to 40 (Fig. 26-9, *D*). Instantaneously, $\overline{P}_a$ will be unchanged. With $\overline{P}_a = 100$ and $R = 40$, $Q_r = \overline{P}_a/R = 2.5$ L/min. If Q_h remained constant at 5 L/min, $Q_h > Q_r$, and therefore $\overline{V}_a$ would increase. Hence, $\overline{P}_a$ would rise, and it would continue to rise until it reached 200 mm Hg (Fig. 26-9, *E*). At this level $Q_r = 200/40 = 5$ L/min, which equals Q_h. $\overline{P}_a$ would then remain at this new elevated equilibrium level as long as Q_h and R did not change again.

These examples indicate, therefore, that *the level of the mean arterial pressure depends on two physiological factors: cardiac output and peripheral resistance* (Fig. 26-11). It does not matter whether changes in cardiac output are accomplished by an alteration of heart rate, stroke volume, or both. Any change in heart rate that is balanced by an opposite change in stroke volume would not alter cardiac output. Hence, mean arterial pressure would not be affected.

■ Arterial Pulse Pressure

Arterial pulse pressure is defined as the difference between systolic and diastolic pressures. The following discussion will show that *the arterial pulse pressure is principally a function of just one physiological factor, namely, stroke volume*, which would determine the change in arterial blood volume (a physical factor) during ventricular systole. This physical factor, plus the second physical factor (arterial compliance), would determine the arterial pulse pressure (Fig. 26-11).

Stroke volume. The effect of a change in stroke volume on pulse pressure may be analyzed under conditions in which arterial compliance (C_a) remains virtually constant over a substantial range of pressures. In the example described below and illustrated in Fig. 26-12, we assume that C_a remains constant over the range of pressures and volumes that prevail in the example.

Under steady-state conditions, the arterial blood pressure of a subject oscillates about some mean value (e.g., $\overline{P}_A$ in Fig. 26-12) that, as previously explained, depends entirely on cardiac output and peripheral resistance. This mean arterial pressure corresponds to some mean arterial blood volume, $\overline{V}_A$. The coordinates, $\overline{P}_A$, $\overline{V}_A$ (point *A* on the graph), represent the mean arterial pressure and volume that prevail for the existing cardiac output and peripheral resistance. During the period of ventricular diastole, peripheral runoff from the arterial system occurs. At the same time, no blood is ejected from the ventricles into the arterial system. As a result, P_A and V_A diminish to minimal values, P_1 and V_1, just before the next ventricular ejection. P_1 is then, by definition, the **diastolic pressure.**

During the rapid ejection phase of systole, the volume of blood introduced into the arterial system exceeds the volume that exits the system through the arterioles (see Chapter 23). Arterial pressure and volume therefore rise from point A_1 toward point A_2 in Fig. 26-12. The maximal arterial volume, V_2, is reached at the end of the rapid ejection phase (see Fig. 23-10), and this volume corresponds to a peak pressure, P_2, which is the **systolic pressure.**

The **pulse pressure** is the difference between systolic and diastolic pressures ($P_2 - P_1$ in Fig. 26-12). Pulse pressure can also be understood in terms of a concept called the **arterial volume increment,** $V_2 - V_1$. *This increment equals the volume of blood discharged into the aorta by the left ventricle during the rapid ejection phase minus the volume that has run off from the arteries and through the microcirculation during this same phase of the cardiac cycle.* Pulse pressure corresponds to this volume increment. For instance, when a normal heart beats at a normal frequency, the volume increment during the rapid ejection phase constitutes a large part of the stroke volume (about 80%). It is this increment that raises arterial volume rapidly from V_1 to V_2, and hence that causes the arterial pressure to rise from the diastolic to the systolic level (P_1 to P_2 in Fig. 26-12). During the remainder of the cardiac cycle, peripheral runoff greatly exceeds cardiac ejection. During ventricular diastole, of course, cardiac ejection equals zero. The resultant arterial blood volume decrement thus causes volumes and pressures to fall from point A_2 back to point A_1.

If stroke volume is now doubled while heart rate and peripheral resistance remain constant, the mean arterial

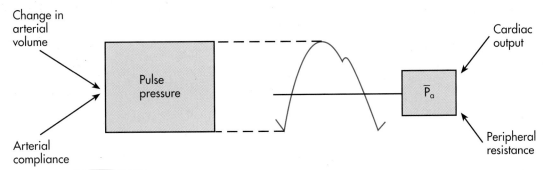

■ **Fig. 26-11**   The two physiological determinants of the mean arterial pressure $(\overline{P_a})$ are the cardiac output and the total peripheral resistance. The two physical determinants of the pulse pressure are the arterial compliance (C_a) and the change in arterial volume.

pressure doubles, to $\overline{P}_B$ in Fig. 26-12. The arterial pressure will now oscillate each heartbeat about this new value of the mean arterial pressure. A normal, vigorous heart ejects this greater stroke volume mainly during the rapid ejection phase of the cardiac cycle; the duration of this phase is approximately equal to the duration of this phase that prevailed at the lower stroke volume. Therefore, the arterial volume increment, $V_4 - V_3$, will be a large fraction of the new stroke volume, and hence the volume increment will be approximately twice as great as the previous volume increment $(V_2 - V_1)$. If compliance remains constant, the greater volume increment will be reflected by a pulse pressure $(P_4 - P_3)$ approximately twice as great as the original pulse pressure $(P_2 - P_1)$. Inspection of Fig. 26-12 reveals that when both mean pressure and pulse pressure increase, the rise in systolic pressure (from P_2 to P_4) exceeds the rise in diastolic pressure (from P_1 to P_3).

The arterial pulse pressure gives valuable clues about a person's stroke volume, provided that the arterial compliance is essentially normal. Patients who have severe **congestive heart failure** or who have had a severe hemorrhage are likely to have very small arterial pulse pressures, because their stroke volumes are abnormally small. Conversely, individuals with large stroke volumes, as in **aortic regurgitation,** are likely to have increased arterial pulse pressures. Similarly, well-trained athletes at rest tend to have large stroke volumes because their heart rates are usually low. The prolonged ventricular filling times in these individuals induce the ventricles to pump a large stroke volume, and hence their pulse pressures are large.

Arterial compliance. Arterial compliance also affects pulse pressure. To see how, compare the relative effects of a given volume increment $(V_2 - V_1$ in Fig. 26-13) in a young person (curve *A*) with that in an

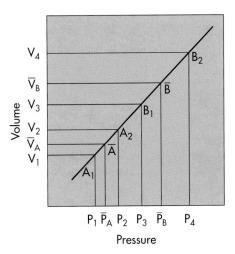

■ **Fig. 26-12**   Effect of a change in stroke volume on pulse pressure in a system in which arterial compliance remains constant over the prevailing range of pressures and volumes. A larger volume increment $[(V_4 - V_3) > (V_2 - V_1)]$ results in a greater mean pressure $(\overline{P}_B > \overline{P}_A)$ and a greater pulse pressure $[(P_4 - P_3) > (P_2 - P_1)]$.

elderly person (curve *B*). Let cardiac output and total peripheral resistance be the same in both people; therefore, $\overline{P}_a$ will be the same. Fig. 26-13 shows that the same volume increment $(V_2 - V_1)$ will generate a greater pulse pressure $(P_4 - P_1)$ in the less compliant arteries of the elderly individual than in the more compliant arteries of the young person $(P_3 - P_2)$. The reason for this discrepancy is shown in Fig. 26-2. Diminished arterial compliance imposes a greater workload on the left ventricle of the elderly person than on that of the young person, even if the stroke volumes, total peripheral resistances (TPRs), and mean arterial pressures are equal in the two individuals.

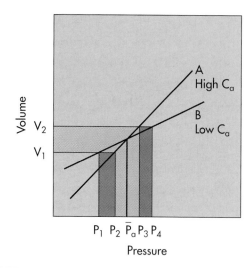

■ Fig. 26-13   For a given volume increment ($V_2 - V_1$), a reduced arterial compliance (compliance *B* < compliance *A*) results in an increased pulse pressure [($P_4 - P_1$) > ($P_3 - P_2$)].

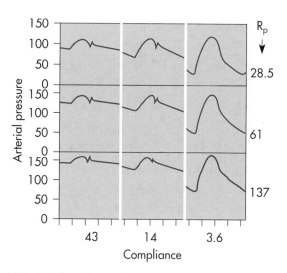

■ Fig. 26-14   Changes in aortic pressure induced by changes in arterial compliance and peripheral resistance (R_p) in an isolated cat heart preparation. (Modified from Elizinga G, Westerhof N: *Circ Res* 32:178, 1973, with permission of the American Heart Association.)

We can also see this same effect on pulse pressure in Fig. 26-14, which shows how changes in arterial compliance and peripheral resistance, R_p, affect the arterial pressure in an isolated cat heart preparation. As the compliance was reduced from 43 to 14 to 3.6 units, the pulse pressure increased significantly. However, in contrast to our human example, in which stroke volume was held at a constant value, the stroke volume decreased in the cat heart preparation as the compliance was diminished (not shown). This change in stroke volume accounts for the failure of the mean arterial pressure to remain constant in the cat heart preparation at different levels of arterial compliance. The effects of changes in peripheral resistance on the arterial pulse pressure are described in the next section.

Total peripheral resistance and arterial diastolic pressure. Clinicians have often proclaimed that TPR mainly affects the level of the diastolic arterial pressure, but is this true? To investigate this assertion, first let TPR be increased in an individual whose arterial system has a P_a:V_a curve that is virtually linear over a wide range of pressures and volumes, as depicted in Fig. 26-15, *A*. If heart rate and stroke volume remain constant, then an increase in TPR will increase mean arterial pressure ($\overline{P}_a$) proportionately (from $\overline{P}_2$ to $\overline{P}_5$). If the arterial volume increments ($V_2 - V_1$ and $V_4 - V_3$) are equal at both levels of TPR, the pulse pressures ($P_3 - P_1$ and $P_6 - P_4$) will also be equal. Hence, systolic (P_6) and diastolic (P_4) pressures will have been elevated by exactly the same amounts from their respective control levels (P_3 and P_1). Therefore, we can safely say that the above assertion is not true, because in the absence of a pressure-induced change in arterial compliance, an increase in peripheral

resistance will not have a differential effect on the levels of systolic and diastolic arterial pressures.

In chronic **hypertension,** a condition characterized by a persistent elevation of TPR, the P_a:V_a curve resembles that shown in Fig. 26-15, *B*. The changing slope of the curve in Fig. 26-15, *B*, reveals that the arteries are less compliant at higher than at lower arterial pressures. Any given arterial volume increment will produce a greater pressure increment (i.e., a greater pulse pressure) when the arteries are more rigid than when they are more compliant. Hence, the rise in arterial systolic pressure ($P_6 - P_3$) will exceed the increase in arterial diastolic pressure ($P_4 - P_1$). Thus, if the arteries become substantially less compliant when arterial pressure rises, an increase in peripheral resistance will elevate systolic pressure more than it will elevate diastolic pressure.

These hypothetical changes in arterial pressure closely resemble those actually seen in patients with hypertension. Diastolic pressure is indeed elevated in such individuals, but ordinarily not more than 10 to 40 mm Hg above the average normal level of 80 mm Hg. Not uncommonly, however, systolic pressures are elevated by 50 to 100 mm Hg above the average normal level of 120 mm Hg. The combination of increased resistance and diminished arterial compliance would be represented in Fig. 26-14 by a shift in direction from the top left panel to the bottom right panel; that is, both the mean pressure and the pulse pressure would be increased significantly. These results also coincide with the systolic and diastolic arterial pressure changes predicted by Fig. 26-15, *B*.

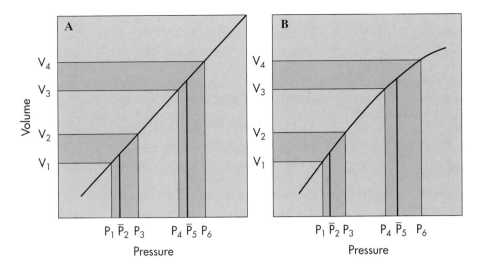

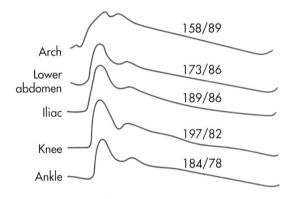

■ **Fig. 26-15** Comparison of the effects of a given change in peripheral resistance on pulse pressure when the pressure-volume curve for the arterial system is either rectilinear (**A**) or curvilinear (**B**). The arterial volume increment is the same for both conditions: $[(V_4 - V_3) = (V_2 - V_1)]$.

■ *Peripheral Arterial Pressure Curves*

The radial stretch of the ascending aorta brought about by left ventricular ejection initiates a pressure wave that is propagated down the aorta and its branches. The pressure wave travels much faster than does the blood itself. This pressure wave is the "pulse" that can be detected by palpating a peripheral artery.

The velocity of the pressure wave varies inversely with the arterial compliance. Accurate measurement of the transmission velocity has provided valuable information about the elastic characteristics of the arterial tree. In general, transmission velocity increases with age, confirming the observation that the arteries become less compliant with advancing age (Figs. 26-4 and 26-6). Velocity also increases progressively as the pulse wave travels from the ascending aorta toward the periphery. This increase in velocity reflects the decrease in vascular compliance in the more distal than in the more proximal portions of the arterial system. This spatial change in compliance has been confirmed by direct measurement.

The arterial pressure contour becomes distorted as the wave is transmitted down the arterial system. This distortion in the pressure wave contour is demonstrated by changes in configuration of the pulse at distant sites; these changes are shown in Fig. 26-16. Aside from the increasing delay in the onset of the initial pressure rise, three major changes occur in the arterial pulse contour as the pressure wave travels distally. First, the systolic portions of the pressure wave become narrowed and elevated. In the curves shown in Fig. 26-16, the systolic pressure at the level of the knee was 39 mm Hg greater than that recorded in the aortic arch. Second, the high-frequency components of the pulse, such as the incisura (i.e., the notch that appears at the end of ventricular ejection), are damped out and soon disappear. Third, a hump may appear on the diastolic portion of the pressure wave, in a point in the pressure wave near which the incisura initially appeared. These changes in contour are pro-

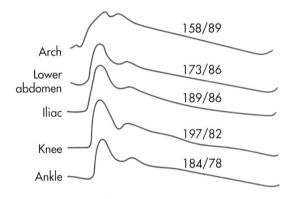

■ **Fig. 26-16** Arterial pressure curves recorded from various sites in an anesthetized dog. (From Remington JW, O'Brien LJ: *Am J Physiol* 218:437, 1970.)

nounced in young individuals, but they diminish with age. In elderly patients, the pulse wave may be transmitted virtually unchanged from the ascending aorta to the periphery.

The damping of the high-frequency components of the arterial pulse is largely caused by the viscoelastic properties of the arterial walls. Several factors, including wave reflection and resonance, vascular tapering, and pressure-induced changes in transmission velocity, contribute to the peaking of the arterial pressure wave.

■ *Blood Pressure Measurement in Humans*

In hospital intensive care units, needles or catheters may be introduced into peripheral arteries of patients, and arterial blood pressure can then be measured **directly** by means of strain gauges. Ordinarily, however, blood pressure is estimated **indirectly** by means of a **sphygmomanometer.** This instrument consists of a noncompliant cuff that contains an inflatable bag. The cuff is wrapped around an extremity (usually an arm); the inflatable bag lies between the cuff and the skin, directly over the artery to be compressed. The artery is occluded by inflating the bag, by means of a rubber squeeze bulb, to a pressure in excess of the arterial systolic pressure. The pressure in the bag is measured by means of a mercury or an aneroid manometer. Pressure is released from the bag at a rate of 2 or 3 mm Hg per second by means of a needle valve in the inflating bulb (Fig. 26-17).

When blood pressure readings are taken from the arm, the systolic pressure may be estimated by palpating the radial artery at the wrist (**palpatory method**). While pressure in the bag exceeds the systolic level, no pulse is perceived. As the pressure falls just below the systolic level (Fig. 26-17, *A*), a spurt of blood passes through the brachial artery under the cuff during the peak of systole, and a slight pulse will be felt at the wrist.

The **auscultatory method** is a more sensitive and therefore more precise method for measuring systolic pressure, and it also permits the diastolic pressure level to be estimated. The practitioner listens with a stethoscope applied to the skin of the antecubital space over the brachial artery. While the pressure in the bag exceeds the

systolic pressure, the brachial artery is occluded and no sounds are heard (Fig. 26-17, *B*). When the inflation pressure falls just below the systolic level (120 mm Hg in Fig. 26-17, *A*), a small spurt of blood escapes the pressure of the cuff, and slight tapping sounds (called **Korotkoff sounds**) are heard with each heartbeat. The pressure at which the first sound is detected represents the **systolic pressure.** It usually corresponds closely with the directly measured systolic pressure.

As the inflation pressure of the cuff continues to fall, more blood escapes under the cuff per beat and the sounds become louder. When the inflation pressure approaches the diastolic level, the Korotkoff sounds become muffled. When the inflation pressure falls just below the diastolic level (80 mm Hg in Fig. 26-17, *A*), the sounds disappear; the pressure reading at this point indicates the **diastolic pressure.** The origin of the Korotkoff sounds is related to the discontinuous spurts of blood that pass under the cuff and meet a static column of blood beyond the cuff; the impact and turbulence generate audible vibrations. Once the inflation pressure is less than the diastolic pressure, flow is continuous in the brachial artery, and sounds are no longer heard (Fig. 26-17, *C*).

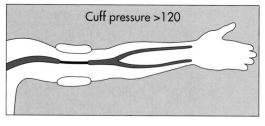

B, When the cuff pressure exceeds the systolic arterial pressure (120 mm Hg), no blood progresses through the arterial segment under the cuff, and no sounds can be detected by a stethoscope bell placed on the arm distal to the cuff.

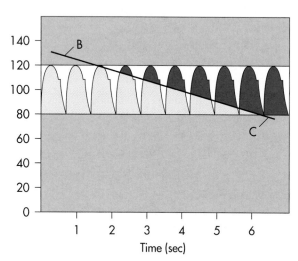

A, Consider that the arterial blood pressure is being measured in a patient whose blood pressure is 120/80 mm Hg. The pressure (represented by the *oblique line*) in a cuff around the patient's arm is allowed to fall from greater than 120 mm Hg (point *B*) to below 80 mm Hg (point *C*) in about 6 seconds.

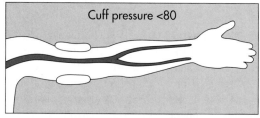

C, When the cuff pressure falls below the diastolic arterial pressure, arterial flow past the region of the cuff is continuous, and no sounds are audible. When the cuff pressure is between 120 and 80 mm Hg, spurts of blood traverse the artery segment under the cuff with each heartbeat, and the Korotkoff sounds are heard through the stethoscope.

■ **Fig. 26-17**   **A to C,** Measurement of arterial blood pressure with a sphygmomanometer.

■ *Summary*

1. The arteries not only conduct blood from the heart to the capillaries but also store some of the ejected blood during each cardiac systole. Hence, blood flow continues through the capillaries during cardiac diastole.

2. The aging process diminishes the compliance of the arteries.

3. The less compliant the arteries, the more work the heart must do to pump a given cardiac output.

4. The mean arterial pressure varies directly with the cardiac output and total peripheral resistance.

5. The arterial pulse pressure varies directly with the stroke volume but inversely with the arterial compliance.

6. The contour of the systemic arterial pressure wave is distorted as it travels from the ascending aorta to the periphery. The high-frequency components of the pulse wave are damped, the pressure components of the wave during ventricular systole are elevated, and a hump appears in the early diastolic component of the wave.

7. When blood pressure is measured by a sphygmomanometer, (a) the systolic pressure is manifested by a tapping sound that is produced by the spurts of blood that pass through the compressed artery as the cuff pressure falls below the peak arterial pressure and (b) the diastolic pressure is manifested by the disappearance of the sound as the flow through the artery becomes continuous when the cuff pressure falls below the minimal arterial pressure.

■ *Self-Study Problems*

1. Why would a patient with a normal cardiac output and a normal total peripheral resistance (TPR), but with generalized atherosclerosis, require a greater coronary blood flow than would a patient with a normal arterial system?

2. How would the systolic, diastolic, and mean arterial pressures in a well-trained, resting athlete, with a heart rate of 45 beats/min, differ from the systolic, diastolic, and mean arterial pressures in a resting, nonathletic person of the same age and with the same cardiac output and total peripheral resistance, but with a heart rate of 75 beats/min?

3. A 20-year-old and a 70-year-old person each had the same cardiac output, heart rate, and TPR under basal conditions. Assume that a vasoconstrictor drug was given to each person, and that it increased their TPR identically by 50%, but did not affect their cardiac output or heart rate. What changes in systolic, diastolic, and mean arterial pressures would you expect in each of these subjects?

4. The left ventricle of a patient with aortic valve insufficiency ejects 100 ml of blood during systole, but 30 ml leaks back into the ventricle during diastole. Hence, the patient's net stroke volume (i.e., the quantity of blood pumped through the peripheral vasculature at each heartbeat) is 70 ml. If the patient's heart rate were 70 beats/min, cardiac output would be 4.9 L/min. How would the systolic, diastolic, and mean arterial pressures in this patient compare with those pressures in a normal person without aortic valve disease but with the same cardiac output, heart rate, and TPR as the patient with aortic valve insufficiency?

■ *Bibliography*

Journal articles

Alexander J Jr, Burkhoff D, Schipke J, Sagawa K: Influence of mean pressure on aortic impedance and reflections in the systemic arterial system, *Am J Physiol* 257:H969, 1989.

Armentano RL et al: Arterial wall mechanics in conscious dogs: assessment of viscous, inertial, and elastic moduli to characterize aortic wall behavior, *Circ Res* 76:468, 1995.

Burattini R, Campbell KB: Effective distributed compliance of the canine descending aorta estimated by modified T-tube model, *Am J Physiol* 264:H1977, 1993.

Farrar DJ et al: Anatomic correlates of aortic pulse wave velocity and carotid artery elasticity during atherosclerosis progression and regression in monkeys, *Circulation* 83:1754, 1991.

Folkow B, Svanborg A: Physiology of cardiovascular aging, *Physiol Rev* 73:725, 1993.

Frasch HF, Kresh JY, Noordergraaf A: Two-port analysis of microcirculation: an extension of Windkessel, *Am J Physiol* 270:H376, 1996.

Imura T et al: Non-invasive ultrasonic measurement of the elastic properties of the human abdominal aorta, *Cardiovasc Res* 20:208, 1986.

Kelly RP et al: Effective arterial elastance as index of arterial vascular load in humans, *Circulation* 86:513, 1992.

Kingwell BA et al: Arterial compliance may influence baroreflex function in athletes and hypertensives, *Am J Physiol* 268:H411, 1995.

Lee RT, Kamm RD: Vascular mechanics for the cardiologist, *J Am Coll Cardiol* 23:1289, 1994.

Mulvany MJ, Aalkjaer C: Structure and function of small arteries, *Physiol Rev* 70:921, 1990.

O'Rourke M: Mechanical principles in arterial disease, *Hypertension* 26:2, 1995.

Perloff D et al: Human blood pressure determination by sphygmomanometry, *Circulation* 88:2460, 1993.

Rose WC, Schwaber JS: Analysis of heart rate–based control of arterial blood pressure, *Am J Physiol* 271:H812, 1996.

Stergiopulos N, Meister J-J, Westerhof N: Evaluation of methods for estimation of total arterial compliance, *Am J Physiol* 268:H1540, 1995.

Stergiopulos N, Meister J-J, Westerhof N: Determinants of stroke volume and systolic and diastolic aortic pressure, *Am J Physiol* 270:H2050, 1996.

Van Gorp A et al: Technique to assess aortic distensibility and compliance in anesthetized and awake rats, *Am J Physiol* 270:H780, 1996.

Books and monographs

Fung YC: *Biodynamics: circulation,* Heidelberg, 1984, Springer-Verlag.

Li J K-J: *Arterial system dynamics: hemodynamics of arteries,* New York, 1987, New York University Press.

Milnor WR: *Hemodynamics,* Baltimore, 1982, Williams & Wilkins.

O'Rourke M, Kelly R, Avolio A: *Arterial pulse,* Baltimore, 1992, Williams & Wilkins.

Taylor DEM, Stevens AL, editors: *Blood flow: theory and practice,* New York, 1983, Academic Press.

Westerhof N, Gross DR, editors: *Vascular dynamics: physiological perspectives,* New York, 1989, Plenum Press.

The Microcirculation and Lymphatics

The circulatory system is geared to supply the body tissues with blood in amounts that meet their requirements for oxygen and nutrients. The capillaries, whose walls consist of a single layer of endothelial cells, permit rapid exchange of gases, water, and solutes with interstitial fluid. The muscular arterioles, which are the major **resistance vessels,** regulate regional blood flow to the capillary beds. The venules and veins serve primarily as collecting channels and storage, or **capacitance, vessels.**

The lymphatic system is composed of lymphatic vessels, nodes, and lymphoid tissue. This system transports fluid and proteins that have escaped from the blood to the veins for recirculation in the blood. In this chapter, the network of the smallest vessels of the body, as well as the lymphatic vessels, is explored in detail.

■ *The Microcirculation*

The microcirculation is defined as the circulation of blood through the smallest vessels of the body—the arterioles, capillaries, and venules. Arterioles, which range in diameter from about 5 to 100 μm, have a thick smooth muscle layer, a thin adventitial layer, and an endothelial lining (see Fig. 21-1). The arterioles give rise directly to the capillaries (5 to 10 μm in diameter) or in some tissues to **metarterioles** (10 to 20 μm in diameter), which then give rise to capillaries (Fig. 27-1). The metarterioles can either bypass the capillary bed and thus serve as thoroughfare channels to the venules, or serve as direct conduits to supply the capillary bed. Cross-connections are often made between arterioles and between venules, as well as in the capillary network. Arterioles that give rise directly to capillaries regulate flow through these capillaries by constriction or dilation. The capillaries form an interconnecting network of tubes of different lengths, with an average length of 0.5 to 1 mm.

■ *Functional Properties of Capillaries*

Capillary distribution varies from tissue to tissue. In metabolically active tissues, such as cardiac and skeletal muscle and glandular structures, capillary density is high. In less active tissues, such as subcutaneous tissue or cartilage, capillary density is low.

Capillary diameter also varies. Some capillaries have diameters less than those of erythrocytes. Passage through these tiny capillaries requires the erythrocytes to become temporarily deformed. Fortunately, normal erythrocytes are quite flexible and readily change their shape to conform with that of the small capillaries.

Blood flow in the capillaries is not uniform and depends chiefly on the contractile state of the arterioles. The average velocity of blood flow in the capillaries is approximately 1 mm/sec; however, it can vary from zero to several millimeters per second in the same vessel within a brief period. These changes in capillary blood flow may be random or rhythmical. The rhythmical oscillatory behavior of capillaries is caused by contraction and relaxation (**vasomotion**) of the precapillary vessels (i.e., the arterioles and small arteries).

Vasomotion is to some extent an intrinsic contractile behavior of the vascular smooth muscle and is independent of external input. In addition, changes in **transmural pressure** (intravascular minus extravascular pressure) influence the contractile state of the precapillary vessels. An increase in transmural pressure, whether produced by an increase in venous pressure or by dilation of arterioles, results in contraction of the terminal arterioles at the points of origin of the capillaries. A decrease in transmural pressure causes precapillary vessel relaxation (see "Myogenic Response," p 445). Humoral and possibly neural factors also affect vasomotion. For example, when the precapillary vessels contract in response to increased transmural pressure, the contractile response can be overridden and vasomotion abolished. This effect is accomplished by metabolic (humoral) factors (see p 446) when the oxygen supply becomes too low to meet the requirements of the parenchymal tissue, as occurs in muscle during exercise.

Although reduction of transmural pressure induces relaxation of the terminal arterioles, blood flow through the capillaries obviously cannot increase if the reduction in intravascular pressure is caused by severe constriction of the parent arterioles, metarterioles, or small arteries. Large arterioles and metarterioles also exhibit vasomotion. However, in the contraction phase they usually do not completely occlude the lumen of the vessel and arrest blood flow, whereas contraction of the terminal arterioles may arrest blood flow (Fig. 27-2). Thus, *flow rate in the*

capillaries may be altered by contraction and relaxation of small arteries, arterioles, and metarterioles.

Because blood flow through the capillaries provides for exchange of gases and solutes between blood and tissue, it has been called **nutritional flow,** whereas blood flow that bypasses the capillaries in traveling from the arterial to the venous side of the circulation has been termed **non-nutritional,** or **shunt, flow** (Fig. 27-1). In some areas of the body (e.g., fingertips, ears), true **arteriovenous shunts** exist (see p 487). However, in many tissues, such as muscle, evidence of anatomic shunts is lacking. Even in the absence of these shunts, non-nutritional flow can occur; this flow has been called **physiological shunting** of blood flow. Physiological shunting results from a greater flow of blood through previously open capillaries, with either no change or an increase in the number of closed capillaries. In tissues that have metarterioles, non-nutritional flow may be continuous from arteriole to venule during low metabolic activity when many precapillary vessels are closed. When metabolic activity increases in these tissues, more precapillary vessels open. Blood passing through the metarterioles is then readily available for capillary perfusion.

True capillaries are devoid of smooth muscle and are therefore incapable of active constriction. Nevertheless, the endothelial cells that form the capillary wall contain actin and myosin and can alter their shape in response to certain chemical stimuli. No evidence exists, however, that changes in endothelial cell shape regulate blood flow

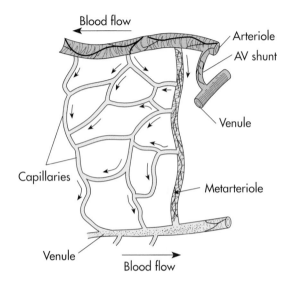

■ **Fig. 27-1**   Composite schematic drawing of the microcirculation. The circular structures on the arteriole and venule represent smooth muscle fibers, and the branching solid lines represent sympathetic nerve fibers. The arrows indicate the direction of blood flow.

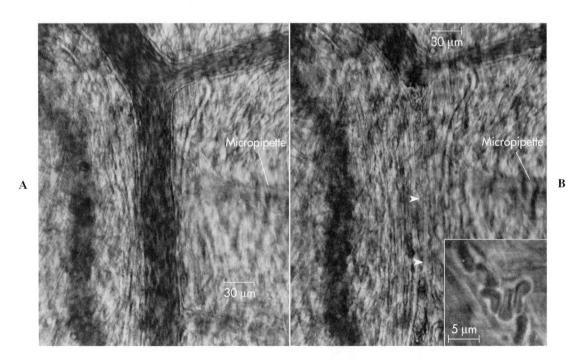

■ **Fig. 27-2**   **A,** Arterioles of a hamster cheek pouch before microinjection of norepinephrine. **B,** After injection of norepinephrine. Note the complete closure of the arteriole between the arrows, and the narrowing of a branch arteriole at the upper right. *Inset:* Capillary with red cells during a period of complete closure of the feeding arteriole. Scale in **A** and **B,** 30 μm; in inset, 5 μm. (Courtesy of David N. Damon.)

through the capillaries. Hence, *changes in capillary diameter are passive and are caused by alterations in precapillary and postcapillary resistance.*

Because of their narrow lumen, the thin-walled capillaries can withstand high internal pressures without bursting. This property can be explained in terms of the **law of Laplace,** which is illustrated in the following comparison of wall tension of a capillary with that of the aorta (Table 27-1). The Laplace equation is

$$T = Pr \qquad (27\text{-}1)$$

where

T = tension in the vessel wall
P = transmural pressure
r = radius of the vessel

Wall tension (T) is the force per unit length of the vessel wall. Wall tension opposes the distending force (Pr) that tends to pull apart a theoretical longitudinal slit in the vessel (Fig. 27-3). Transmural pressure of a blood vessel in vivo is essentially equal to intraluminal pressure, because extravascular pressure is usually negligible. The Laplace equation applies to very thin-walled vessels, such as capillaries.

Wall thickness must be taken into consideration when the equation is applied to thick-walled vessels, such as the aorta. To account for wall thickness of the aorta, Pr (pressure × radius) is divided by wall thickness (w).

The equation now becomes

$$\sigma \text{ (wall stress)} = Pr/w \qquad (27\text{-}2)$$

Pressure in mm Hg is converted to dynes per square centimeter according to the equation $P = h\rho g$, where h = the height of a Hg column in centimeters, ρ = the density of Hg in g/cm^3, g = gravitational acceleration in cm/s^2, and wall stress (σ) = force per unit area within the vascular wall.

Thus, at normal aortic and capillary pressures, the wall tension of the aorta is about 12,000 times greater than that of the capillary (Table 27-1). In a person standing quietly, capillary pressure in the feet may reach 100 mm Hg. Under such conditions, capillary wall tension increases to 66.5 dyne/cm, a value that is still only one three-thousandth of the wall tension in the aorta at the same internal pressure. However, σ (wall stress),

which takes wall thickness into account, is only about tenfold greater in the aorta than in the capillary.

In addition to providing an explanation for the ability of capillaries to withstand large internal pressures, the above calculations also point out that as vessels dilate, wall stress increases if internal pressure remains constant.

Syphilitic aortic aneurysm, which is now rare, and **abdominal aneurysm** (caused by atherosclerotic degeneration of the aortic wall) are associated with murmurs that result from turbulence in the dilated segment of the aorta. The diseased part of the aorta is also under severe stress because of its increased radius and thinner wall. Unless treated, the aneurysm can rupture and cause immediate death. Treatment consists of resection of the aneurysm and replacement with a Dacron graft.

The diameter of the resistance vessels (arterioles) is determined by the balance between the contractile force of the vascular smooth muscle and the distending force produced by the intraluminal pressure. The greater the contractile activity of the vascular smooth muscle of an arteriole, the smaller is its diameter. In small arterioles, contraction can continue to the point where the vessel is completely occluded. Occlusion is caused by infolding of the endothelium and by trapping of the cells in the vessel.

With progressive reduction in the intravascular pressure, vessel diameter decreases (as does tension in the vessel wall—law of Laplace) and blood flow eventually ceases although pressure within the arteriole or small artery is still greater than tissue pressure. This phenomenon has been referred to as the **critical closing pressure,**

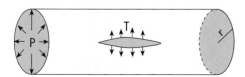

■ **Fig. 27-3**   Diagram of a small blood vessel to illustrate the law of Laplace—T = Pr, where *P* = intraluminal pressure, *r* = radius of the vessel, and *T* = wall tension as the force per unit length tangential to the vessel wall, tending to pull apart a theoretical longitudinal slit in the vessel.

■ **Table 27-1**   Vessel wall tension in the aorta and a capillary

	Aorta	*Capillary*
Radius (r)	1.5 cm	5×10^{-4} cm
Height of Hg column (h)	10 cm Hg	2.5 cm Hg
ρ	$13.6\ g/cm^3$	$13.6\ g/cm^3$
g	$980\ cm/sec^2$	$980\ cm/sec^2$
P	$10 \times 13.6 \times 980$ $= 1.33 \times 10^5$ $dyne/cm^2$	$2.5 \times 13.6 \times 980$ $= 3.33 \times 10^4$ $dyne/cm^2$
w	0.2 cm	1×10^{-4} cm
T = Pr	$(1.33 \times 10^5)(1.5)$ $= 2 \times 10^5$ dyne/cm	(3.33×10^4) (5×10^{-4}) $= 16.7$ dyne/cm
$\sigma = \dfrac{Pr}{w}$	$\dfrac{2 \times 10^5}{0.2} =$ 1×10^6 $dyne/cm^2$	$\dfrac{16.7}{1 \times 10^{-4}} =$ 1.67×10^5 $dyne/cm^2$

and its mechanism is still controversial. This critical closing pressure is low when vasomotor activity is reduced by inhibition of sympathetic nerve activity to the vessel, and is increased when vasomotor tone is enhanced by activation of the vascular sympathetic nerve fibers.

If the heart becomes greatly dilated, as may occur in heart failure caused by **idiopathic cardiomyopathy,** the combination of a weakened myocardium and increased left ventricular wall stress (predicted by the Laplace equation) may result in a dangerously low cardiac output. Recently, a small number of patients with severely dilated hearts have been treated successfully by resection of the myocardium (a remodeling procedure called **ventriculotomy**) to reduce the diastolic volume of the left ventricle and thereby enhance its efficiency.

■ *Vasoactive Role of the Capillary Endothelium*

For many years, the endothelium of capillaries was thought to be an inert single layer of cells that served solely as a passive filter to permit passage of water and small molecules across the blood vessel wall, and to retain blood cells and large molecules (proteins) within the vascular compartment. However, it is now recognized that the endothelium is an important source of substances that cause contraction or relaxation of the vascular smooth muscle.

One of these substances is **prostacyclin.** As shown in Fig. 27-4, prostacyclin can relax vascular smooth muscle via an increase in the cyclic adenosine monophosphate (cAMP) concentration. Prostacyclin is formed in the endothelium from arachidonic acid, and the process is catalyzed by prostacyclin synthase. The mechanism by which prostacyclin synthesis is triggered is not known. However, prostacyclin may be released by shear stress caused by the pulsatile blood flow. The primary function of prostacyclin is to inhibit platelet adherence to the endothelium and platelet aggregation, and thus prevent intravascular clot formation.

Of far greater importance in endothelium-mediated vascular dilation is the formation and release of **endothelium-derived relaxing factor (EDRF)** (Fig. 27-4), which has been identified as **nitric oxide (NO).** When endothelial cells are stimulated by acetylcholine or several other agents (adenosine triphosphate [ATP], bradykinin, serotonin, substance P, histamine), NO is produced and released. In blood vessels from which the endothelium has been mechanically removed, these agents do not cause vasodilation. NO (synthesized from L-arginine) activates guanylyl cyclase in the vascular smooth muscle to increase the cyclic guanosine monophosphate (cGMP) concentration, which produces relaxation by decreasing cytosolic free Ca^{++}. NO release can be stimulated by the shear stress of blood flow on the

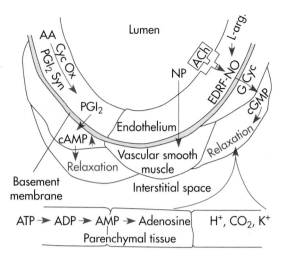

■ **Fig. 27-4** Endothelium- and nonendothelium-mediated vasodilation. Prostacyclin (PGI_2) is formed from arachidonic acid *(AA)* by the action of cyclooxygenase *(Cyc Ox)* and prostacyclin synthase *(PGi₂ Syn)* in the endothelium, and elicits relaxation of the adjacent vascular smooth muscle via increases in cyclic adenosine monophosphate *(cAMP)*. Stimulation of the endothelial cells with acetylcholine *(ACh)* or other agents (see text) results in the formation and release of an endothelium-derived relaxing factor *(EDRF)*, identified as nitric oxide *(NO)*. The NO stimulates guanylyl cyclase *(G Cyc)* to increase cyclic guanosine monophosphate *(cGMP)* in the vascular smooth muscle to produce relaxation. The vasodilator agent nitroprusside *(NP)* acts directly on the vascular smooth muscle. Substances such as adenosine, hydrogen ions *(H^+)*, CO_2, and potassium ions *(K^+)* can arise in the parenchymal tissue and elicit vasodilation by direct action on the vascular smooth muscle (see p 447).

endothelium, but the physiological role of NO in the local regulation of blood flow remains to be determined. The drug nitroprusside also increases cGMP, which produces vasodilation, but it acts directly on the vascular smooth muscle and is not endothelium-mediated (Fig. 27-4). Vasodilator agents such as adenosine, hydrogen ions, CO_2, and potassium may be released from parenchymal tissue and act locally on the resistance vessels (Fig. 27-4).

The endothelium can also synthesize **endothelin,** a potent vasoconstrictor peptide. Endothelin can affect vascular tone and blood pressure in humans and may be involved in pathological states such as atherosclerosis, pulmonary hypertension, congestive heart failure, and renal failure.

■ *Passive Role of the Capillary Endothelium*

Transcapillary exchange. Solvent and solute move across the capillary endothelial wall by three processes: diffusion, filtration, and pinocytosis. Diffusion is the most important process for transcapillary exchange and pinocytosis is the least important.

Diffusion. Under normal conditions, only about 0.06 ml of water per minute moves back and forth across the capillary wall per 100 g of tissue as a result of filtration and absorption. In contrast, 300 ml of water per minute per 100 g of tissue moves across the capillary wall by diffusion, a 5000-fold difference.

When filtration and diffusion are related to blood flow, about 2% of the plasma passing through the capillaries is filtered. In contrast, the diffusion of water is 40 times greater than the rate by which it is brought to the capillaries by blood flow. The transcapillary exchange of solutes is also primarily governed by diffusion. Thus, *diffusion is the key factor in providing exchange of gases, substrates, and waste products between the capillaries and the tissue cells.*

The process of diffusion is described by Fick's law:

$$J = -DA \frac{dc}{dx} \qquad (27\text{-}3)$$

where

> J = quantity of a substance moved per unit time (t)
> D = free diffusion coefficient for a particular molecule (the value is inversely related to the square root of the molecular weight)
> A = cross-sectional area of the diffusion pathway
> dc/dx = concentration gradient of the solute

Fick's law is also expressed as

$$J = -PS(C_o - C_i) \qquad (27\text{-}4)$$

where

> P = capillary permeability to the substance
> S = capillary surface area
> C_i = concentration of the substance inside the capillary
> C_o = concentration of the substance outside the capillary

Hence, the PS product provides a convenient expression of available capillary surface, because permeability is rarely substantially altered under physiological conditions.

In the capillaries, diffusion of lipid-insoluble molecules is not free but is restricted to the pores. The mean size of the pores can be calculated by measurement of the diffusion rate of an uncharged molecule whose free diffusion coefficient is known. Movement of solutes across the capillary endothelium is complex and involves corrections for attractions between solute and solvent molecules, interactions between solute molecules, pore configuration, and charge on the molecules relative to charge on the endothelial cells. It is not simply a matter of random thermal movements of molecules down a concentration gradient.

For small molecules, such as water, NaCl, urea, and glucose, the capillary pores offer little restriction to diffusion (in other words, they have a low **reflection coefficient,** see p 436). Diffusion of these substances is so rapid that the mean concentration gradient across the capillary endothelium is extremely small. With lipid-insoluble molecules of increasing size, diffusion through muscle capillaries becomes progressively more restricted. Diffusion eventually becomes minimal with molecules of a molecular weight above about 60,000. With small molecules, the only limitation to net movement across the capillary wall is the rate at which blood flow transports the molecules to the capillary. The transport of these molecules is said to be **flow limited.**

With flow-limited small molecules, the concentration of the molecule in the blood reaches equilibrium with its concentration in the interstitial fluid near the origin of the capillary from its parent arteriole. Its concentration falls to negligible levels near the arterial end of the capillary (Fig. 27-5, *A*). If the flow is large, the small molecule can still be present farther downstream in the capillary. A somewhat larger molecule moves farther along the capillary before it reaches an insignificant concentration in the blood, and the number of still larger molecules that enter the arterial end of the capillary and cannot pass through the capillary pores is the same as the number leaving the venous end of the capillary (Fig. 27-5, *A*).

With large molecules, diffusion across the capillaries becomes the limiting factor (**diffusion limited**). In other words, capillary permeability to a large molecule solute limits its transport across the capillary wall (Fig. 27-5, *A*). The diffusion of small lipid-insoluble molecules is so rapid that diffusion becomes limiting in blood-tissue exchange only when the distances between capillaries and parenchymal cells are large (e.g., tissue edema or very low capillary density) (Fig. 27-5, *B*).

Movement of lipid-soluble molecules across the capillary wall is not limited to capillary pores (only about 0.02% of the capillary surface), because these molecules can pass directly through the lipid membranes of the entire capillary endothelium. Consequently, *lipid-soluble molecules move rapidly between blood and tissue. The degree of lipid solubility (oil-to-water partition coefficient) provides a good index of the ease of transfer of lipid molecules through the capillary endothelium.*

Oxygen and carbon dioxide are both lipid soluble and readily pass through the endothelial cells. Calculations based on (1) the diffusion coefficient for O_2, (2) capillary density and diffusion distances, (3) blood flow, and (4) tissue O_2 consumption indicate that the O_2 supply of normal tissue at rest and during activity is not limited by diffusion or the number of open capillaries.

Measurements of Po_2 and saturation of blood in the microvessels indicate that, in many tissues, O_2 saturation at the entrance of the capillaries has already decreased to a saturation of about 80% as a result of diffusion of O_2 from arterioles and small arteries. Also, CO_2 loading and the resultant intravascular shifts in the oxyhemoglobin dissociation curve occur in the precapillary vessels. Hence, in addition to gas exchange at the level of the capillaries, direct flux of O_2 and CO_2 occurs between adjacent arterioles and venules, and possibly between arteries

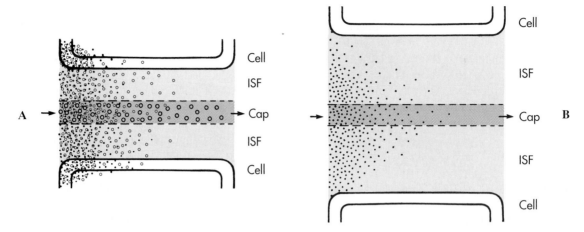

■ **Fig. 27-5**   Flow- and diffusion-limited transport from capillaries *(Cap)* to tissue. **A,** Flow-limited transport. The smallest water-soluble inert tracer particles *(black dots)* reach negligible concentrations after passing only a short distance down the capillary. Larger particles *(colored circles)* with similar properties travel farther along the capillary before reaching insignificant intracapillary concentration. Both substances cross the interstitial fluid *(ISF)* and reach the parenchymal tissue *(Cell)*. Because of their size, more of the smaller particles are taken up by the tissue cells. The largest particles *(black circles)* cannot penetrate the capillary pores and hence do not escape from the capillary lumen except by pinocytotic vesicle transport. An increase in the volume of blood flow or an increase in capillary density increases tissue supply for the diffusible solutes. Note that capillary permeability is greater at the venous end of the capillary (also in the venule, not shown) because of the larger number of pores in this region. **B,** Diffusion-limited transport. When the distance between the capillaries and the parenchymal tissue is large, as a result of edema or low capillary density, diffusion becomes a limiting factor in the transport of solutes from capillary to tissue even at high rates of capillary blood flow.

and veins (**countercurrent exchange**). This countercurrent exchange of gas represents a diffusional shunt of gas away from the capillaries, and, at low blood flow rates, it may limit the supply of O_2 to the tissue.

Capillary filtration. The permeability of the capillary endothelial membrane is not uniform throughout all body tissues. For example, the liver capillaries are quite permeable, and albumin escapes from them at a rate several times greater than that from the less permeable muscle capillaries. Also, permeability is not uniform along the length of the capillary. The venous ends are more permeable than the arterial ends, and permeability is greatest in the venules. The greater permeability at the venous end of the capillaries and in the venules is attributed to the greater number of pores (see below) in these regions of the microvessels.

The sites where filtration occurs have been a controversial subject for a number of years. Some water flows through the capillary endothelial cell membranes, but most flows through apertures (**pores**) in the endothelial wall of the capillaries (Figs. 27-6 and 27-7). It is estimated that pores in skeletal and cardiac muscle have diameters of about 4 nm. In agreement with this estimate, electron microscopy has revealed clefts between adjacent endothelial cells in mouse cardiac muscle with a gap at the narrowest point of about 4 nm (Figs. 27-6 and 27-7). The clefts (pores) are sparse and represent only about

0.02% of the capillary surface area. In cerebral capillaries, where the blood-brain barrier blocks the entrance of many small molecules, pores are absent.

In addition to clefts, some of the more porous capillaries (e.g., in kidney, intestine) contain **fenestrations** (Fig. 27-7) 20 to 100 nm wide, whereas others (e.g., in the liver) have a **discontinuous endothelium** (Fig. 27-7). Fenestrations and discontinuous endothelium permit passage of molecules that are too large to pass through the intercellular clefts of the endothelium. *The direction and magnitude of the movement of water across the capillary wall can be determined by the algebraic sum of the hydrostatic and osmotic pressures that exist across the membrane.* An increase in intracapillary hydrostatic pressure favors movement of fluid from the vessel to the interstitial space, whereas an increase in the concentration of osmotically active particles within the vessels favors movement of fluid into the vessels from the interstitial space.

Hydrostatic forces. The hydrostatic pressure (blood pressure) within the capillaries is not constant. Instead, it depends on arterial pressure, venous pressure, and precapillary (arterioles) and postcapillary (venules and small veins) resistances. An increase in arterial or venous pressure elevates capillary hydrostatic pressure, whereas a reduction in either has the opposite effect. An increase in arteriolar resistance or closure of arteries reduces capil-

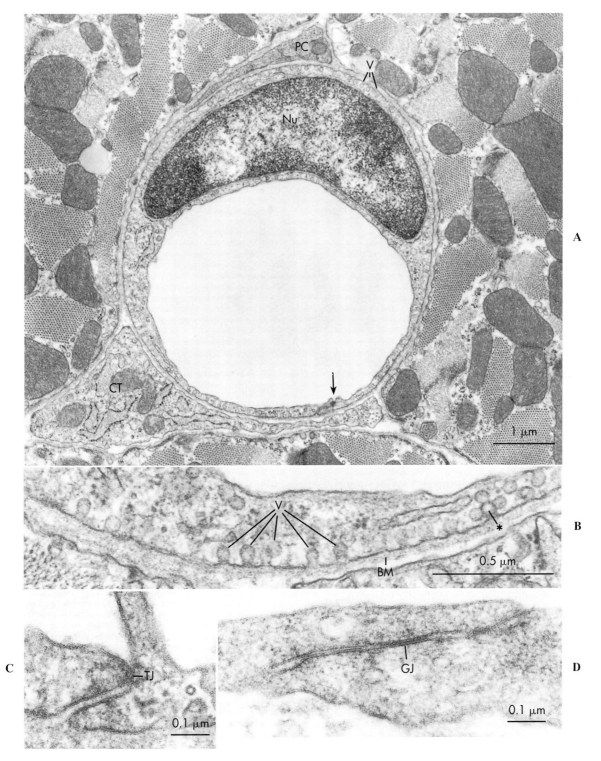

■ **Fig. 27-6** **A,** Cross-sectioned capillary in a mouse ventricular wall. The luminal diameter is approximately 4 μm. In this thin section, the capillary wall is formed by a single endothelial cell *(Nu,* endothelial nucleus), which forms a functional complex *(arrow)* with itself. The thin pericapillary space is occupied by a pericyte *(PC)* and a connective tissue *(CT)* cell ("fibroblast"). Note the numerous endothelial vesicles *(V).* **B,** Detail of the endothelial cell in **A,** showing plasmalemmal vesicles *(V),* attached to the endothelial cell surface. These vesicles are especially prominent in vascular endothelium and are involved in transport of substances across the blood vessel wall. Note the complex alveolar vesicle (∗). *BM,* Basement membrane. **C,** Junctional complex in a capillary of mouse heart. "Tight" junctions *(TJ)* typically form in these small blood vessels and appear to consist of fusions between apposed endothelial cell surface membranes. **D,** Interendothelial junction in a muscular artery of monkey papillary muscle. Although tight junctions similar to those of capillaries are found in these large blood vessels, extensive junctions that resemble gap junctions in the intercalated disks between myocardial cells often appear in arterial endothelium (example shown at *GJ*).

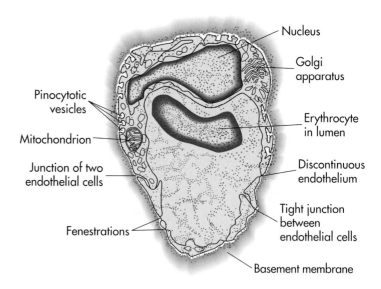

■ **Fig. 27-7**   Diagrammatic sketch of an electron micrograph of a composite capillary in cross-section.

lary pressure, whereas greater resistance in the venules and veins increases capillary pressure.

Hydrostatic pressure is the principal force in capillary filtration. However, changes in the venous resistance affect capillary hydrostatic pressure more than changes in arteriolar resistance. A given change in venous pressure produces a greater effect on capillary hydrostatic pressure than the same change in arterial pressure. About 80% of an increase in venous pressure is transmitted back to the capillaries.

Capillary hydrostatic pressure (P_c) varies from tissue to tissue. Average values, obtained from direct measurements in human skin, are about 32 mm Hg at the arterial end of the capillaries and 15 mm Hg at the venous end of the capillaries at the level of the heart (Fig. 27-8). When a person stands, the hydrostatic pressure increases in the legs and decreases in the head.

Tissue pressure, or more specifically interstitial fluid pressure (P_i) outside the capillaries, opposes capillary filtration. $P_c - P_i$ constitutes the driving force for filtration. In the normal (nonedematous) state, P_i is close to zero, so that P_c essentially represents the hydrostatic driving force.

Osmotic forces. The key factor that restrains fluid loss from the capillaries is the osmotic pressure of the plasma proteins (such as albumin). This osmotic pressure is called the **colloid osmotic** or **oncotic pressure** (π_p). The total osmotic pressure of plasma is about 6000 mm Hg, whereas the oncotic pressure is only about 25 mm Hg (see Chapter 1). Nevertheless, this small oncotic pressure plays an important role in fluid exchange across the capillary wall. The reason oncotic pressure is important in fluid exchange is that the plasma proteins are essentially confined to the intravascular space, whereas the electrolytes, that are in large part responsible for the plasma osmotic pressure, are practically of equal concentration on both sides of the

capillary endothelium. The relative permeability of solute to water influences the actual magnitude of the osmotic pressure. The **reflection coefficient** (σ) is the relative impediment to the passage of a substance through the capillary membrane. The reflection coefficient of water is zero and that of albumin (to which the endothelium is essentially impermeable) is 1. Filterable solutes have reflection coefficients between 0 and 1. Also, different tissues have different reflection coefficients for the same molecule, and therefore movement of a given solute across the endothelial wall varies with the tissue. The true oncotic pressure (π) is defined by the equation

$$\pi = \sigma RT (C_i - C_o) \qquad (27-5)$$

where

σ = reflection coefficient
R = gas constant
T = absolute temperature
C_i and C_o = solute (albumin) concentration, respectively, inside and outside the capillary

Of the plasma proteins, albumin is the most important in determining oncotic pressure. The average albumin molecule (molecular weight 69,000) is approximately half the size of the average globulin molecule (molecular weight 150,000) and is present in almost twice the concentration as the globulins (4.5 vs. 2.5 g/dl of plasma). Albumin also exerts a greater osmotic force than can be accounted for solely on the basis of the number of molecules dissolved in a unit volume of plasma. Therefore, it cannot be completely replaced by inert substances of appropriate molecular size, such as dextran. This additional osmotic force becomes disproportionately great at high concentrations of albumin (as in plasma) and is weak to absent in dilute solutions of albumin (as in interstitial fluid).

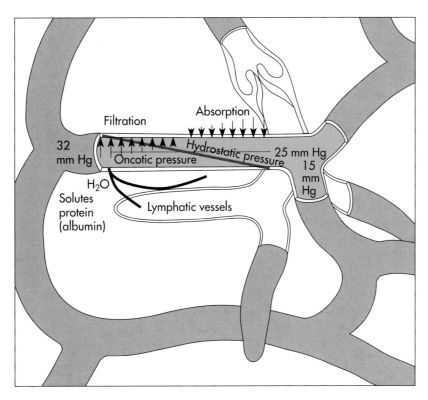

■ **Fig. 27-8** Schematic representation of the factors responsible for filtration and absorption across the capillary wall and the formation of lymph.

The reason for this behavior of albumin is its negative charge when the blood pH is normal. Albumin binds a small number of chloride ions, which increases its negative charge, and hence its ability to retain more sodium ions inside the capillaries (see Chapter 2). This small increase in electrolyte concentration of the plasma over that of the interstitial fluid produced by the negatively charged albumin enhances its osmotic force to that of an ideal solution containing a solute of molecular weight 37,000. If albumin did indeed have a molecular weight of 37,000, it would not be retained by the capillary endothelium because of its small size. Hence, albumin could not function as a counterforce to capillary hydrostatic pressure. If, however, albumin did not exert this enhanced osmotic force, a concentration of about 12 g of albumin/per deciliter of plasma would be required to achieve a plasma oncotic pressure of 25 mm Hg. Such a high albumin concentration would greatly increase blood viscosity and hence the resistance to blood flow through the vascular system.

Small amounts of albumin escape from the capillaries and enter the interstitial fluid, where they exert a very small osmotic force (0.1 to 5 mm Hg). This force, π_i, is small because of the low concentration of albumin in the interstitial fluid, and because at low concentrations albumin cannot enhance the osmotic force as much as it does at high concentrations.

With prolonged standing, particularly when associated with some elevation of venous pressure in the legs (such as that caused by pregnancy) or with sustained increases in venous pressure (as seen in congestive heart failure), filtration is greatly enhanced and exceeds the capacity of the lymphatic system to remove the capillary filtrate from the interstitial space.

The concentration of the plasma proteins may also change in different pathological states and thus alter the osmotic force and movement of fluid across the capillary membrane. The plasma protein concentration is increased in **dehydration** (e.g., water deprivation, prolonged sweating, severe vomiting, diarrhea). In this condition, water moves by osmotic forces from the tissues to the vascular compartment. In contrast, the plasma protein concentration is reduced in **nephrosis** (a renal disease characterized by protein loss, which appears in the urine), and edema may occur.

When capillary injury is extensive, as in burns, intravascular fluid and plasma protein leak into the interstitial space. The protein that escapes from the vessel lumen increases the oncotic pressure of the interstitial fluid. This greater osmotic force outside the capillaries leads to additional fluid loss and possibly to severe dehydration of the patient.

Balance of hydrostatic and osmotic forces. The relationship between hydrostatic pressure and oncotic pressure, and the role of these forces in regulating fluid passage across the capillary endothelium, were expounded by Starling in 1896 and constitute the **Starling hypothesis.** It can be expressed by the equation

$$Q_f = k[(P_c + \pi_i) - (P_i + \pi_p)] \qquad (27\text{-}6)$$

where

> Q_f = fluid movement
> P_c = capillary hydrostatic pressure
> P_i = interstitial fluid hydrostatic pressure
> π_p = plasma oncotic pressure
> π_i = interstitial fluid oncotic pressure
> k = filtration constant for capillary membrane

Filtration occurs when the algebraic sum is positive; absorption occurs when it is negative.

Traditionally, it has been thought that filtration occurs at the arterial end of the capillary and absorption at its venous end because of the gradient of hydrostatic pressure along the capillary. This scheme is true for the idealized capillary, as depicted in Fig. 27-8. However, direct observations have revealed that many capillaries only filter whereas others only absorb. In some vascular beds (e.g., the renal glomerulus), hydrostatic pressure in the capillary is high enough to result in filtration along the entire length of the capillary. In other vascular beds (e.g., the intestinal mucosa), the hydrostatic and oncotic forces are such that absorption occurs along the whole capillary.

As discussed earlier in this chapter, capillary pressure is variable and depends on several factors, the principal one being the contractile state of the precapillary vessel. In the normal steady state, arterial pressure, venous pressure, postcapillary resistance, interstitial fluid hydrostatic and oncotic pressures, and plasma oncotic pressure are relatively constant. A change in precapillary resistance is the determining factor that influences fluid movement across the wall for any given capillary. Because water moves so quickly across the capillary endothelium, the hydrostatic and osmotic forces are nearly in equilibrium along the entire capillary. Hence, in the normal state, filtration and absorption occur only with slight degrees of imbalance of pressure across the capillary wall. Only a small percentage (2%) of the plasma that flows through the vascular system is filtered. Of this, about 85% is absorbed in the capillaries and venules. The remainder returns to the vascular system as lymph fluid along with the albumin that escapes from the capillaries.

In the lungs, the mean capillary hydrostatic pressure is only about 8 mm Hg (see Chapter 34). Because the plasma oncotic pressure is 25 mm Hg and the lung interstitial fluid pressure approximately 15 mm Hg, the net force slightly favors reabsorption. Despite the favoring of reabsorption, pulmonary lymph is formed. This lymph consists of fluid that is drawn out of the capillaries osmotically by the small amount of plasma protein that escapes through the capillary endothelium.

In pathological conditions, such as left ventricular failure or stenosis of the mitral valve, pulmonary capillary hydrostatic pressure may exceed plasma oncotic pressure. When this occurs, it may cause **pulmonary edema,** a condition that seriously interferes with gas exchange in the lungs.

Capillary filtration coefficient. The rate of movement of fluid across the capillary membrane (Q_f) depends not only on the algebraic sum of the hydrostatic and osmotic forces across the endothelium (ΔP), but also on the area of the capillary wall available for filtration (A_m), the distance across the capillary wall (Δx), the viscosity of the filtrate (η), and the filtration constant of the membrane (k). These factors may be expressed by the equation

$$Q_r = \frac{kA_m \Delta P}{\eta \Delta x} \qquad (27\text{-}7)$$

The dimensions are units of flow per unit of pressure gradient across the capillary wall per unit of capillary surface area. This expression, which describes the flow of fluid through a membrane (pores), is essentially Poiseuille's law for flow through tubes (see Chapter 25).

Because the thickness of the capillary wall and the viscosity of the filtrate are relatively constant, they can be included in the filtration constant, k. If the area of the capillary membrane is not known, the rate of filtration can be expressed per unit weight of tissue. Hence, the equation can be simplified to

$$Q_f = k_t \Delta P \qquad (27\text{-}8)$$

where k_t is the capillary filtration coefficient for a given tissue, and the units for Q_f are milliliters per minute per 100 g of tissue per mm Hg pressure.

In any given tissue, the filtration coefficient per unit area of capillary surface, and hence capillary permeability, is not changed by different physiological conditions, such as arteriolar dilation and capillary distention, or by such adverse conditions as hypoxia, hypercapnia, or reduced pH. When capillaries are injured (as by toxins or severe burns) significant amounts of fluid and protein leak out of them into the interstitial space. This increase in capillary permeability is reflected by an increase in the filtration coefficient.

Because capillary permeability is constant under normal conditions, the filtration coefficient can be used to determine the relative number of open capillaries (total capillary surface area available for filtration in tissue). For example, increased metabolic activity of contracting skeletal muscle induces relaxation of precapillary resistance vessels with opening of more capillaries. This process, called **capillary recruitment,** increases the filtering surface area.

Disturbances in hydrostatic-osmotic balance. Relatively small changes in arterial pressure may have little effect on filtration. The change in pressure may be countered by adjustments of the precapillary resistance vessels (autoregulation, see p 445), so that hydrostatic pressure in the open capillaries remains the same. However, a severe reduction in arterial pressure usually evokes constriction of the arterioles that is mediated by the sympathetic nervous system. This may occur in hemorrhage and is often accompanied by a fall in venous pressure caused by the blood loss. These changes lead to a decrease in capillary hydrostatic pressure. However, the low blood pressure in hemorrhage causes a decrease in blood flow (and hence O_2 supply) to the tissue, with the result that vasodilator metabolites accumulate and induce relaxation of the arterioles. Precapillary vessel relaxation also occurs because of the reduced transmural pressure (autoregulation, see p 445). As a consequence of these several factors, absorption predominates over filtration, and it occurs at a larger capillary surface area. These responses to hemorrhage constitute one of the compensatory mechanisms employed by the body to restore blood volume (see Chapter 31).

An increase in venous pressure alone, as occurs in the feet when a person stands up from a lying position, would elevate capillary pressure and enhance filtration. However, the increase in transmural pressure causes precapillary vessel closure (myogenic mechanism, see p 445), so that the capillary filtration coefficient actually decreases. This reduction in capillary surface available for filtration prevents large amounts of fluid from leaving the capillaries and entering interstitial space (edema).

A large amount of fluid can move rapidly across the capillary wall. In a normal individual, the filtration coefficient (k_t) for the whole body is about 0.0061 ml/min/100 g of tissue/mm Hg. For a 70-kg man, elevation of venous pressure of 10 mm Hg for 10 minutes would increase filtration from capillaries by 342 ml. Edema does not usually occur because the fluid is returned to the vascular compartment by the lymphatic vessels. When edema does develop, it usually appears in the dependent parts of the body, where the hydrostatic pressure is greatest, but its location and magnitude are also determined by the type of tissue. Loose tissues, such as the subcutaneous tissue around the eyes or in the scrotum, are more prone to collect larger quantities of interstitial fluid than are firm tissues, such as muscle, or encapsulated structures, such as the kidney.

Pinocytosis. Some transfer of substances across the capillary wall can occur in tiny pinocytotic vesicles (pinocytosis). These vesicles (Fig. 27-6 and 27-7), formed by a pinching off of the endothelial cell membrane, can take up substances on one side of the capillary wall, move them by thermal kinetic energy across the cell, and deposit their contents at the other side. The amount of material that can be transported in this way is very small relative to that moved by diffusion. However, pinocytosis may be responsible for the movement of large lipid-insoluble molecules (30 nm) between the blood and interstitial fluid. The number of pinocytotic vesicles in endothelium varies with the tissue (muscle > lung > brain) and increases from the arterial to the venous end of the capillary.

■ *Lymphatics*

The terminal vessels of the lymphatic system consist of a widely distributed, closed-end network of highly permeable lymph capillaries. These lymph capillaries resemble blood capillaries, with two important differences: tight junctions are not present between endothelial cells, and fine filaments anchor lymph vessels to the surrounding connective tissue. With muscular contraction, these fine strands pull on the lymphatic vessels to open spaces between the endothelial cells, and permit the entrance of protein and large particles and cells present in the interstitial fluid. The lymph capillaries drain into larger vessels that finally enter the right and left subclavian veins, where they connect with the respective internal jugular veins.

Only cartilage, bone, epithelium, and tissues of the central nervous system are devoid of lymphatic vessels. The function of lymphatic vessels is to return the plasma capillary filtrate to the circulation. This task is accomplished by virtue of tissue pressure, facilitated by intermittent skeletal muscle activity, contractions of the lymphatic vessels, and an extensive system of one-way valves. In this respect, lymphatic vessels resemble the veins, although even the larger lymphatic vessels have thinner walls than the corresponding veins, and they contain only a small amount of elastic tissue and smooth muscle.

The volume of fluid transported through the lymphatics in 24 hours is about equal to an animal's total plasma volume. The protein returned by the lymphatics to the blood in a day is about one fourth to one half of the circulating plasma proteins. The lymphatic vessels are the only means whereby protein (albumin) that leaves the vascular compartment can be returned to the blood. Net back diffusion of albumin into the capillaries cannot occur against the large albumin concentration gradient. If the protein were not removed by the lymph vessels, it would accumulate in the interstitial fluid and act as an oncotic force to draw fluid from the blood capillaries to produce edema.

In addition to returning fluid and protein to the vascular bed, the lymphatic system filters the lymph at the **lymph nodes** and removes foreign particles, such as bacteria. The largest lymphatic vessel, the **thoracic duct,** in addition to draining the lower extremities, returns protein lost through the permeable liver capillaries. It also carries substances absorbed from the gastrointestinal tract, principally fat in the form of chylomicrons, to the circulating blood.

Lymph flow varies considerably. It is almost nil from resting skeletal muscle and increases during exercise in proportion to the degree of muscular activity. It is increased by any mechanism that enhances the rate of blood capillary filtration: for example, increased capillary pressure or permeability, or decreased plasma oncotic pressure. When either the volume of interstitial fluid exceeds the drainage capacity of the lymphatics or the lymphatic vessels become blocked, as may occur in certain disease states, interstitial fluid accumulates, chiefly in the more compliant tissues (e.g., subcutaneous tissue), and gives rise to clinical edema.

■ *Summary*

1. Blood flow through the capillaries is chiefly regulated by contraction and relaxation of the arterioles (resistance vessels).

2. The capillaries, which consist of a single layer of endothelial cells, can withstand high transmural pressure by virtue of their small diameter. According to the law of Laplace, T (wall tension) = P (transmural pressure) × r (radius of the capillary).

3. The endothelium is the source of an endothelium-derived relaxing factor (EDRF—identified as nitric oxide) and prostacyclin, which relax vascular smooth muscles.

4. Movement of water and small solutes between the vascular and interstitial fluid compartments occurs through capillary pores mainly by diffusion but also by filtration and absorption.

5. Because the rate of transcapillary diffusion is about 40 times greater than the blood flow in the tissue, exchange of small lipid-insoluble molecules is flow limited. The larger the molecules, the slower is their diffusion. Large lipid-insoluble molecules are diffusion limited. Molecules larger than about 60,000 kD are essentially confined to the vascular compartment.

6. Lipid-soluble substances, such as CO_2 and O_2, pass directly through the lipid membranes of the capillary, and the ease of transfer is directly proportional to the degree of lipid solubility of the substance.

7. Capillary filtration and absorption are described by the Starling equation: Fluid movement = $k[(P_c + \pi_i) - (P_i + \pi_p)]$, where P_c = capillary hydrostatic pressure, P_i = interstitial fluid hydrostatic pressure, π_i = interstitial fluid oncotic pressure, and π_p = plasma oncotic pressure. Filtration occurs when the algebraic sum is positive; absorption occurs when it is negative.

8. Large molecules can move across the capillary wall in vesicles by a process called pinocytosis. The vesicles are formed from the lipid membrane of the capillaries.

9. Fluid and protein that have escaped from the blood capillaries enter the lymphatic capillaries and are transported via the lymphatic system back to the blood vascular compartment.

■ *Self-Study Problems*

1. What physiological factors influence capillary blood flow?

2. When a person is standing quietly, the pressure in the capillaries of the feet can reach as high as 100 nm Hg. Why do the thin-walled capillaries not rupture when subjected to such a high pressure?

3. If mean capillary hydrostatic pressure is 20 mm Hg, tissue pressure 4 mm Hg, plasma oncotic pressure 25 mm Hg, and tissue oncotic pressure 2 mm Hg, is there absorption or filtration in this capillary? Why? In the passage of solute across the capillary wall, how do filtration and absorption compare with diffusion?

4. In the movement of lipid-insoluble solutes from the capillary lumen to the interstitial fluid, what is meant by flow limited and diffusion limited?

5. By what mechanisms do lipid-soluble and lipid-insoluble solutes pass from the capillary lumen to the interstitial space?

6. How is albumin that has escaped from the capillaries returned to the systemic circulation?

■ *Bibliography*

Journal articles

Aukland K: Why don't our feet swell in the upright position?, *News Physiol Sci* 9:214, 1994.

Aukland K, Reed RK: Interstitial-lymphatic mechanisms in the control of extracellular fluid volume, *Physiol Rev* 73:1, 1993.

Curry FRE: Regulation of water and solute exchange in microvessel endothelium: studies in single perfused capillaries, *Microcirculation* 1:11, 1994.

Davies PF: Flow-mediated endothelial mechanotransduction, *Physiol Rev* 75:519, 1995.

Duling BR, Klitzman B: Local control of microvascular function: role in tissue oxygen supply, *Annu Rev Physiol* 42:373, 1980.

Feng Q, Hedner T: Endothelium-derived relaxing factor (EDRF) and nitric oxide. II. Physiology, pharmacology, and pathophysiological implications, *Clin Physiol* 10:503, 1990.

Furchgott RF, Vanhoutte PM: Endothelium-derived relaxing and contracting factors, *FASEB J* 3:2007, 1989.

Krogh A: The number and distribution of capillaries in muscles with calculation of the oxygen pressure head necessary for supplying the tissue, *J Physiol* 52:409, 1919.

Lewis DH, editor: Symposium on lymph circulation, *Acta Phyiol Scand Suppl* 463:9, 1979.

Michel CC: One hundred years of Starling's hypothesis, *News Physiol Sci* 11:229, 1996.

Pries AR et al: Resistance to blood flow in microvessels in vivo, *Circ Res* 75:904, 1994.

Rippe B, Haraldsson B: Transport of macromolecules across microvascular walls: the two-pore theory, *Physiol Rev* 74:163, 1994.

Rosell S: Neuronal control of microvessels, *Annu Rev Physiol* 42:359, 1980.

Starling EH: On the absorption of fluids from the connective tissue spaces, *J Physiol* 19:312, 1896.

Books and monographs

Bert JL, Pearce RH: *The interstitium and microvascular exchange.* In *Handbook of physiology,* sect 2: *The cardiovascular system—microcirculation,* vol IV, Bethesda, Md, 1984, American Physiological Society.

Crone C, Levitt DG: *Capillary permeability to small solutes.* In *Handbook of physiology,* sect 2: *The cardiovascular system—microcirculation,* vol IV, Bethesda, Md, 1984, American Physiological Society.

Hudlicka O: *Development of microcirculation: capillary growth and adaptation.* In *Handbook of physiology,* sect 2: *The cardiovascular system—microcirculation,* vol IV, Bethesda, Md, 1984, American Physiological Society.

Krogh A: *The anatomy and physiology of capillaries,* New York, 1959, Hafner.

Luscher TF, Vanhoutte PM: *The endothelium: modulator of cardiovascular function,* Boca Raton, Fla, 1990, CRC Press.

Michel CC: *Fluid movements through capillary walls.* In *Handbook of physiology,* sect 2: *The cardiovascular system—microcirculation,* vol IV, Bethesda, Md, 1984, American Physiological Society.

Mortillaro NA: *Physiology and pharmacology of the microcirculation,* vol 1, New York, 1983, Academic Press.

Renkin EM: *Control microcirculation and blood-tissue exchange.* In *Handbook of physiology,* sect 2: *The cardiovascular system—microcirculation,* vol IV, Bethesda, Md, 1984, American Physiological Society.

Shepro D, D'Amore PA: *Physiology and biochemistry of the vascular wall endothelium.* In *Handbook of physiology,* sect 2: *The cardiovascular system—microcirculation,* vol IV, Bethesda, Md, 1984, American Physiological Society.

Simionescu M, Simionescu N: *Ultrastructure of the microvascular wall: functional correlations.* In *Handbook of physiology,* sect 2: *The cardiovascular system—microcirculation,* vol IV, Bethesda, Md, 1984, American Physiological Society.

Taylor AE, Granger DN: *Exchange of macromolecules across the microcirculation.* In *Handbook of physiology,* Sect 2: *The cardiovascular system—microcirculation,* vol IV, Bethesda, Md, 1984, American Physiological Society.

Wiedeman MP: *Architecture.* In *Handbook of physiology,* sect 2: *The cardiovascular system—microcirculation,* vol IV, Bethesda, Md, 1984, American Physiological Society.

Zweifach BW, Lipowsky HH: *Pressure-flow relations in blood and lymph microcirculation.* In *Handbook of physiology,* sect 2: *The cardiovascular system—microcirculation,* vol IV, Bethesda, Md, 1984, American Physiological Society.

The Peripheral Circulation and Its Control

The peripheral circulation is essentially under dual control: centrally through the nervous system, and locally by the conditions in the immediate vicinity of the blood vessels. The relative importance of these two control mechanisms is not the same in all tissues. In some areas of the body, such as the skin and splanchnic regions, neural regulation of blood flow predominates, whereas in others, such as the heart and brain, this mechanism plays only a minor role.

The vessels chiefly involved in regulating the rate of blood flow throughout the body are called the **resistance vessels** (arterioles). As their name implies, these vessels offer the greatest resistance to the flow of blood pumped to the tissues by the heart, and thus they are important in the maintenance of arterial blood pressure. The walls of these resistance vessels are composed in large part of smooth muscle fibers (see Fig. 21-1). The presence of smooth muscle in these vessels allows the vessel lumen diameter to vary. When this smooth muscle contracts strongly, the endothelial lining folds inward and completely obliterates the vessel lumen. When the smooth muscle is completely relaxed, the vessel lumen is maximally dilated. Some resistance vessels are closed at any given time. In addition, the smooth muscle in these vessels is partially contracted (which accounts for the tone of these vessels). Were all the resistance vessels in the body to dilate simultaneously, blood pressure would fall precipitously.

■ Vascular Smooth Muscle

Vascular smooth muscle is responsible for the control of total peripheral resistance, arterial and venous tone, and the distribution of blood flow throughout the body. The smooth muscle cells are small, mononucleate, and spindle shaped. They are generally arranged in helical or circular layers around the larger blood vessels and in a single circular layer around arterioles (Fig. 28-l, A and B).

Parts of endothelial cells project into the vascular smooth muscle layer (**myoendothelial junctions**) at various points along the arterioles (Fig. 28-1, C). These projections suggest a functional interaction between endothelium and adjacent vascular smooth muscle. In general, the close association between action potentials and contraction observed in skeletal and cardiac muscle cells cannot be demonstrated in vascular smooth muscle. Vascular smooth muscle also lacks transverse tubules.

Graded changes in the membrane potential of smooth muscle cells are often associated with increases or decreases in force. Contractile activity of these cells is generally elicited by neural or humoral stimuli. However, the behavior of smooth muscle varies in different vessels. For example, some vessels, particularly in the portal or mesenteric circulation, contain longitudinally oriented smooth muscle that is spontaneously active. The smooth muscle cells of these vessels show action potentials that correlate with the contractions and the electrical coupling between cells.

The vascular smooth muscle cells contain large numbers of thin (actin) filaments and comparatively small numbers of thick (myosin) filaments. These filaments are aligned in the long axis of the cell, but they do not form visible sarcomeres with striations. Nevertheless, the sliding filament mechanism is believed to operate in this tissue, and phosphorylation of cross-bridges regulates their rate of cycling. Compared with skeletal muscle, smooth muscle contracts more slowly; develops high forces, which can be maintained for long periods with low adenosine triphosphate (ATP) utilization; and operates over a considerable range of lengths under physiological conditions (see Chapter 19). Cell-to-cell conduction is via gap junctions, just as in cardiac muscle (see p 361).

The interaction between myosin and actin leads to contraction in smooth muscle cells, as in skeletal muscle cells. This interaction, again as in skeletal muscle, is controlled by the myoplasmic Ca^{++} concentration. However, the molecular mechanism whereby Ca^{++} regulates con-

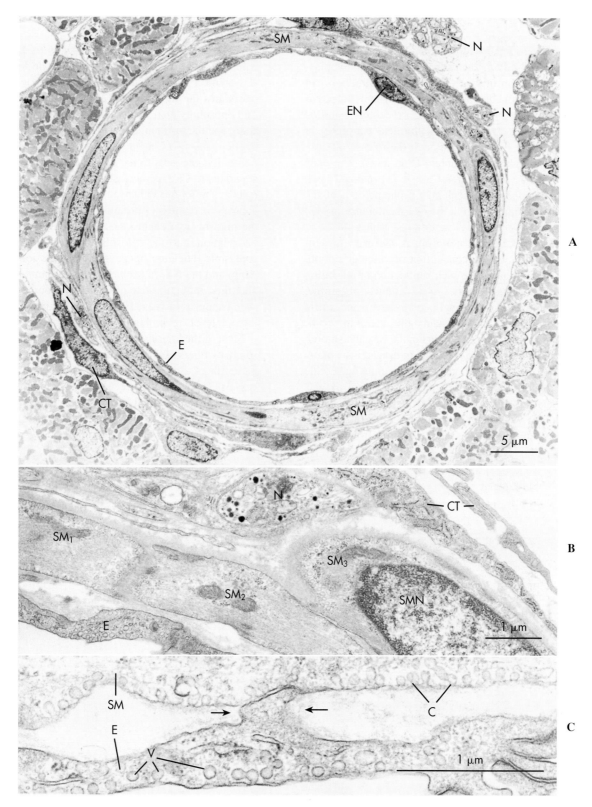

■ **Fig. 28-1** **A,** Low-magnification electron micrograph of an arteriole in cross-section (inner diameter of approximately 40 μm) in cat ventricle. The wall of the blood vessel is composed largely of vascular smooth muscle cells *(SM)* whose long axes are directed approximately circularly around the vessel. A single layer of endothelial cells *(E)* forms the innermost portion of the blood vessel. Connective tissue elements *(CT)* such as fibroblasts and collagen make up the adventitial layer at the periphery of the vessel; nerve bundles also appear in this layer *(N)*. *EN,* Endothelial cell nucleus. **B,** Detail of the wall of the blood vessel in **A.** This field contains a single endothelial layer *(E),* the medial smooth muscle layer (three smooth muscle cell profiles: SM_1, SM_2, SM_3), and the adventitial layer (containing nerves *[N]* and connective tissue *[CT]*). *SMN,* Smooth muscle nucleus. **C,** Another region of the arteriole, showing the area in which the endothelial *(E)* and smooth muscle *(SM)* layers are apposed. A projection of an endothelial cell *(between arrows)* is closely applied to the surface of the overlying smooth muscle, forming a "myoendothelial junction." Plasmalemmal vesicles are prominent in both the endothelium *(V)* and the smooth muscle cell (where such vesicles are known as "caveolae," *C*).

traction differs. For example, smooth muscle lacks troponin and fast sodium channels. The increased myoplasmic concentration of Ca⁺⁺ that elicits contraction can come through voltage-gated calcium channels **(electromechanical coupling)** and through receptor-mediated calcium channels **(pharmacomechanical coupling)** in the sarcolemma, as well as through the release of Ca⁺⁺ from the sarcoplasmic reticulum (Fig. 28-2). The cells relax when intracellular free Ca⁺⁺ is (1) pumped back into the sarcoplasmic reticulum, (2) pumped out of the cell by the calcium pump in the cell membrane, and (3) removed by the Na-Ca exchanger (see Chapter 19).

Pharmacomechanical coupling is the predominant mechanism for eliciting contraction of vascular smooth muscle. Stimuli that cause such contraction or relaxation include substances such as catecholamines, histamine, acetylcholine, serotonin, angiotensin, adenosine, nitric oxide, CO_2, K^+, H^+, and prostaglandins (see Fig. 27-4). Such substances activate receptors in the vascular smooth muscle membrane. These receptors in turn activate phospholipase C in a reaction coupled to guanine nucleotide binding proteins (G proteins). The phospholipase C hydrolyzes phosphatidyl inositol bisphosphate in the membrane to yield diacylglycerol and inositol trisphosphate; the latter causes the release of Ca⁺⁺ from the sar-

coplasmic reticulum. The Ca⁺⁺ binds to calmodulin, which in turn binds to myosin light chain kinase. This activated Ca⁺⁺-calmodulin-myosin kinase complex phosphorylates the light chains (20,000 daltons) of myosin. The phosphorylated myosin ATPase is then activated by actin, and the resultant cross-bridge cycling initiates contraction (see also Chapter 17).

Finally, the sensitivity of the contractile regulatory apparatus to Ca⁺⁺ is increased by agonists. Although the mechanism for this enhanced sensitivity is still unclear, it appears to involve G proteins. Relaxation occurs when the myosin light chain kinase is inactivated by dephosphorylation, and the cytosolic Ca⁺⁺ is lowered by sarcoplasmic reticulum uptake and by extrusion by the Ca pump and the Na-Ca exchanger. Local humoral changes alter the contractile state of vascular smooth muscle, and such factors as increased temperature or increased carbon dioxide levels relax this tissue.

Most of the arteries and veins of the body are supplied solely by fibers of the sympathetic nervous system. These nerve fibers exert a tonic contractile effect on the blood vessels. This effect has been demonstrated by cutting or freezing the sympathetic nerves to a vascular bed (such as muscle), which results in an increase in blood flow (the blood vessels relax). Activation of the sympathetic

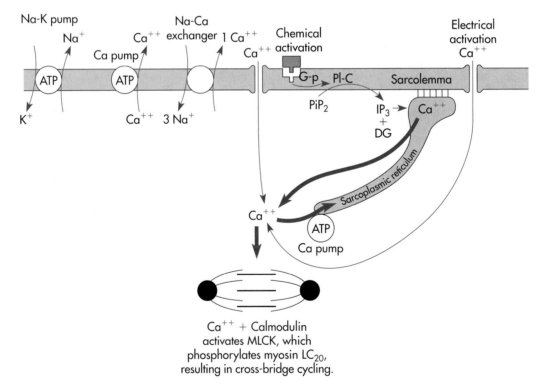

■ **Fig. 28-2**   Excitation-contraction coupling in vascular smooth muscle. Calcium can enter the cell via electrically activated channels (electromechanical coupling) or via receptor-operated channels (chemical activation, termed *pharmacomechanical coupling*) in the sarcolemma. Calcium is also released from the sarcoplasmic reticulum in response to inositol trisphosphate *(IP₃)* stimulation and is taken back into the sarcoplasmic reticulum by a calcium pump. Calcium is extruded from the cell by a calcium pump and by the Na-Ca exchanger. *G-p,* Guanine nucleotide binding protein; *Pl-C,* phospholipase C; *PiP₂,* phosphatidyl inositol bisphosphate; *DG,* diacyglycerol; *MLCK,* myosin light chain kinase; *LC,* light chain kinase, molecular weight 20,000.

nerves either directly or through a reflex (see pp 448 and 450) enhances vascular resistance. In contrast to the sympathetic nerves, the parasympathetic nerves tend to decrease vascular resistance, but they innervate only a small fraction of the blood vessels in the body, mainly in certain viscera and pelvic organs.

■ Intrinsic or Local Control of Peripheral Blood Flow

■ Autoregulation and Myogenic Regulation

In certain tissues, the blood flow is adjusted to the existing metabolic activity of the tissue. Furthermore, changes that occur in perfusion pressure (arterial blood pressure) at constant levels of tissue metabolism are met with vascular resistance changes that tend to maintain a constant blood flow. This mechanism is commonly referred to as **autoregulation** of blood flow and is illustrated graphically in Fig. 28-3.

In the skeletal muscle preparation from which these data were gathered, the muscle was completely isolated from the rest of the animal and was in a resting state. From a control pressure of 100 mm Hg, the pressure was abruptly increased or decreased. The blood flows observed immediately after changing the perfusion pressure are represented by the closed circles. Maintenance of the altered pressure at each new level was followed within 30 to 60 seconds by a return of flow to or toward the control levels; the open circles represent these steady-state flows. Over the pressure range of 20 to 120 mm Hg, the steady-state flow is relatively constant. Calculation of resistance (pressure/flow) across the vascular bed during steady-state conditions shows that the resistance vessels

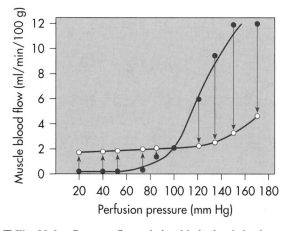

■ **Fig. 28-3** Pressure-flow relationship in the skeletal muscle vascular bed of the dog. Closed circles represent the flows obtained immediately after abrupt changes in perfusion pressure from the control level (*point where lines cross*). Open circles represent the steady-state flows obtained at the new perfusion pressure. (Redrawn from Jones RD, Berne RM: *Circ Res* 14:126, 1964.)

constrict with elevation of the perfusion pressure but dilate with reduction of perfusion pressure.

Why blood flow remains constant in the presence of an altered perfusion pressure is not known, but it appears to be explained best by the **myogenic mechanism.** *According to the myogenic mechanism, the vascular smooth muscle contracts in response to an increase in pressure difference across the wall of a blood vessel (the transmural pressure) and it relaxes in response to a decrease in transmural pressure.* Therefore, the initial increase in blood flow produced by an abrupt increase in perfusion pressure that passively distends the blood vessels would be followed by a return of flow to the previous control level by contraction of the smooth muscles of the resistance vessels.

An example of a myogenic response is shown in Fig. 28-4. Arterioles isolated from the hearts of young pigs were cannulated at each end, and the transmural pressure (intravascular pressure minus extravascular pressure) and flow through the arteriole could be adjusted to desired levels. With no flow through the arteriole, successive increase of transmural pressure elicited progressive decreases in the vessel diameter (Fig. 28-4, *A*). This response was independent of the endothelium because it was identical in intact vessels and in vessels that had been stripped of endothelium (Fig. 28-4, *B*). Arterioles that were relaxed by direct action of nitroprusside on the vascular smooth muscle showed only a passive increase in diameter when transmural pressure was increased. The mechanism that allows vessel distention to elicit contraction is still unknown. However, because stretch of vascular smooth muscle elevates the intracellular concentration of Ca^{++}, it has been proposed that an increase in transmural pressure activates membrane calcium channels.

In normal subjects, blood pressure is maintained at a fairly constant level via the baroreceptor reflex, and it might be expected that a myogenic mechanism would be ineffectual under normal conditions. However, when one changes from a lying to a standing position, a large change in transmural pressure occurs in the lower extremities, and the precapillary vessels constrict in response to this imposed stretch. This constriction, coupled with the hydrostatic pressure imposed by the vertical column of blood from the heart to the feet, results in cessation of flow in most capillaries. After flow stops, capillary filtration diminishes until the increase in plasma oncotic pressure and the increase in interstitial fluid pressure balance the elevated capillary hydrostatic pressure produced by the change from a horizontal to a vertical position.

■ Endothelium-Mediated Regulation

As discussed on p 432, stimulation of the endothelium can elicit a vasoactive response of the vascular smooth muscle. To demonstrate this response experimentally, transmural pressure is kept constant in an isolated arteriole. The flow is then increased progressively by raising

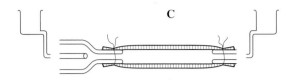

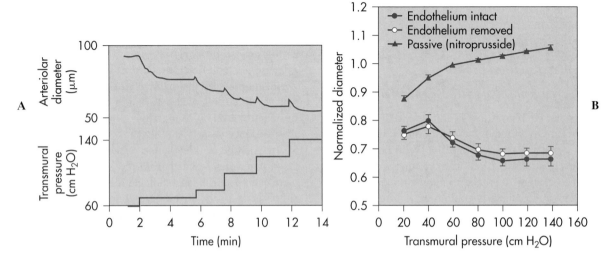

■ **Fig. 28-4** **A,** Constriction of an isolated cardiac arteriole in response to increases in transmural pressure without flow through the blood vessel. **B,** Constrictor response of the arteriole to an increase in transmural pressure is unaffected by removal of its endothelium. **C,** Diagram of cannulated arteriole. When the smooth muscle is relaxed by nitroprusside, the arteriole is passively distended by the increase in transmural pressure. (Redrawn from Kuo L, Davis MJ, Chilian WM: *Am J Physiol* 259:H1063, 1990.)

the perfusion fluid reservoir connected to one end of the arteriole, while the reservoir connected to the other end of the arteriole is simultaneously lowered by an equal distance. This maneuver increases the longitudinal pressure gradient along the vessel, and vasodilation occurs (Fig. 28-5, *A*) The vasodilation is presumably caused by the endothelium-derived relaxing factor (nitric oxide) (see p 432), which is released from the endothelium in response to the shear stress caused by the increase in velocity of flow. If the arteriole is stripped of endothelium, the dilation of the vessel in response to increased flow does not occur (Fig. 28-5, *B*).

> If arteriolar resistance did not increase when a subject stands, the hydrostatic pressure in the lower parts of the legs would reach such high levels that large volumes of fluid would pass from the capillaries into the interstitial fluid compartment and produce edema.

■ *Metabolic Regulation*

According to the metabolic mechanism, blood flow is governed by the metabolic activity of the tissue. Any intervention that results in an O_2 supply that is inade- *quate for the requirements of the tissue prompts the formation of vasodilator metabolites.* These metabolites are released from the tissue and act locally to dilate the resistance vessels. When the metabolic rate of the tissue increases or the O_2 delivery to the tissue decreases, more vasodilator substance is released and the metabolite concentration in the tissue increases.

Candidate vasodilator substances. Many substances have been proposed as mediators of metabolic vasodilation. Some of the earliest ones suggested were lactic acid, CO_2, and hydrogen ions. However, the decrease in vascular resistance induced by supernormal concentrations of these dilator agents falls considerably short of the dilation observed when metabolic activity is increased physiologically.

Changes in O_2 tension can change the contractile state of vascular smooth muscle. An increase in Po_2 elicits contraction; a decrease elicits relaxation. However, measurements of Po_2 at the resistance vessels indicate that over a wide range of Po_2 (11 to 343 mm Hg), no correlation between O_2 tension and arteriolar diameter exists. Furthermore, if Po_2 were directly responsible for vascular smooth muscle tension, one would not expect a correlation between the duration of arterial occlusion and the duration of reactive hyperemia (flow above control level upon release of an arterial occlusion) (Fig. 28-6). With

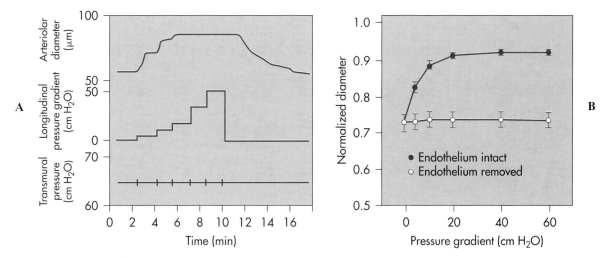

■ **Fig. 28-5**   **A,** Flow-induced vasodilation in an isolated cardiac arteriole at constant transmural pressure. Flow was increased progressively by increasing the pressure gradient in the long axis of the arteriole (longitudinal pressure gradient). **B,** Flow-induced vasodilation is abolished by removal of the endothelium of the arteriole. (Redrawn from Kuo L, Davis MJ, Chilian WM: *Am J Physiol* 259:H1063, 1990.)

either short (5 to 10 seconds) or long (1 to 3 minutes) occlusions, the venous blood becomes bright red (well oxygenated) within 1 or 2 seconds after release of the arterial occlusion. Hence, the smooth muscle of the resistance vessels must be exposed to a high Po_2 in each instance. Nevertheless, the longer occlusions result in longer periods of reactive hyperemia. These observations are more compatible with the release of a vasodilator metabolite from the tissue than with a direct effect of Po_2 on the vascular smooth muscle.

Potassium ions, inorganic phosphate, and interstitial fluid osmolarity can also induce vasodilation. Both K^+ and phosphate are released and osmolarity is increased during skeletal muscle contraction. Therefore, these factors may contribute to **active hyperemia** (increased blood flow caused by enhanced tissue activity). However, significant increases of phosphate concentration and osmolarity are not consistently observed during muscle contraction, and they may increase blood flow only transiently. Therefore, they probably do not mediate the vasodilation observed with muscular activity. Potassium is released with the onset of skeletal muscle contraction or with an increase in cardiac activity, and could be responsible for the initial decrease in vascular resistance observed with exercise or increased cardiac work. However, K^+ release is not sustained, despite continued arteriolar dilation throughout the period of enhanced muscle activity. Furthermore, reoxygenated venous blood obtained from active cardiac and skeletal muscles under steady-state conditions of exercise does not elicit vasodilation when infused into a test vascular bed. It is difficult to see how oxygenation of the venous blood could alter its K^+ or phosphate content or its osmolarity and thereby destroy its vasodilator effect. Therefore, some agent other

than potassium must mediate the vasodilation associated with the metabolic activity of the tissue.

Adenosine, which is involved in the regulation of coronary blood flow, may also participate in the control of the resistance vessels in skeletal muscle. Also, some of the prostaglandins may be important vasodilator mediators in certain vascular beds. Thus, a number of candidates have been proposed as mediators of metabolic vasodilation, and the relative contribution of each of the various factors remains a subject for future investigation.

Basal vessel tone. Metabolic control of vascular resistance by the release of a vasodilator substance is predicated on the existence of basal vessel tone. This tonic activity, or **basal tone,** in vascular smooth muscle is readily demonstrable, but, in contrast to tone in skeletal muscle, it is independent of the nervous system. Thus, some metabolic factor must be responsible for maintaining this tone. The factor responsible for basal tone in blood vessels is not known, but the following factors may be involved: (1) an expression of myogenic activity in response to the stretch imposed by the blood pressure, (2) the high O_2 tension of arterial blood, or (3) the presence of calcium ions.

Reactive hyperemia. Experiments that test the duration of reactive hyperemia after a vessel is occluded provide evidence for the existence of a metabolic factor that locally regulates tissue blood flow. If arterial inflow to a vascular bed is stopped for a few seconds to several minutes, the blood flow, on release of the occlusion, immediately exceeds the flow before occlusion and only gradually returns to the control level. This increase in blood flow is called **reactive hyperemia.** In Fig. 28-6, blood flow to the leg was stopped by clamping the femoral artery for 15, 30, and 60 seconds. Release of the 60-sec-

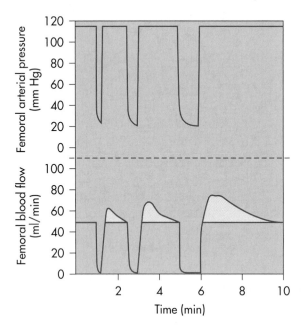

■ **Fig. 28-6**   Reactive hyperemia in the hind limb of the dog after 15-, 30-, and 60-second occlusions of the femoral artery. (Berne RM: Unpublished observations.)

ond occlusion resulted in a peak blood flow that was 70% greater than the control flow, with a return to control flow within about 110 seconds.

When this same experiment is performed in humans by inflating a blood pressure cuff on the upper arm, dilation of the resistance vessels of the hand and forearm, immediately after release of the cuff, is evident from the bright red color of the skin and the fullness of the veins. Within limits the peak flow, and particularly the duration of the reactive hyperemia, are proportional to the duration of the occlusion (Fig. 28-6). If the extremity is exercised during the occlusion period, reactive hyperemia is increased. These observations, and the close relationship that exists between metabolic activity and blood flow in the unoccluded limb, are consonant with a metabolic mechanism in the local regulation of tissue blood flow.

Coordination of arterial and arteriolar dilation. When the vascular smooth muscle of the arterioles relaxes in response to vasodilator metabolites whose release is caused by a decrease in the ratio of the oxygen supply to the oxygen demand of the tissue, resistance may diminish in the arteries that feed these arterioles. The result is a greater blood flow than that produced by arteriolar dilation alone. Two possible mechanisms can account for this coordination of arterial and arteriolar dilation. First, vasodilation in the microvessels is propagated, and when dilation is initiated in the arterioles, it can propagate along the vessels from arterioles back to arteries. Second, the metabolite-mediated dilation of the arterioles accelerates blood

flow in the feeder arteries. This greater velocity of blood flow increases the shear stress on the arterial endothelium, which can in turn induce vasodilation by release of nitric oxide (Fig. 28-5).

Disease of the arterial walls can lead to obstruction of the arteries and symptoms, called **intermittent claudication,** when it occurs in the legs. The symptoms consist of leg pain when the subject walks or climbs stairs, and the pain is relieved by rest. The disease is called **thromboangiitis obliterans** and is seen most frequently in men who are smokers. With minimal walking, the resistance vessels become maximally dilated by local metabolite release; when the oxygen demand of the muscles increases with further walking, blood flow cannot increase sufficiently to meet the muscle needs for oxygen, and pain caused by muscle ischemia results.

■ *Extrinsic Control of Peripheral Blood Flow*

■ *Sympathetic Neural Vasoconstriction*

A number of regions in the medulla influence cardiovascular activity. Stimulation of the dorsal lateral medulla (**pressor** region) evokes vasoconstriction, cardiac acceleration, and enhanced myocardial contractility. Stimulation caudal and ventromedial to the pressor region produces a decrease in blood pressure. This **depressor** area exerts its effect by direct spinal inhibition and by inhibition of the medullary pressor region. These areas are not true anatomic centers, in which a discrete group of cells is discernible, but constitute a "physiological" center.

From the vasoconstrictor regions, fibers descend in the spinal cord and synapse at different levels of the thoracolumbar region (T1 to L2 or L3). Fibers from the intermediolateral gray matter of the cord emerge with the ventral roots, but they leave the motor fibers to join the paravertebral sympathetic chains through the white communicating branches (see Chapter 15). These preganglionic white (myelinated) fibers may pass up or down the sympathetic chains to synapse in the various ganglia within the chains or in certain outlying ganglia. Postganglionic gray branches (unmyelinated) then join the corresponding segmental spinal nerves and accompany them to the periphery to innervate the arteries and veins. Postganglionic sympathetic fibers from the various ganglia join the larger arteries and accompany them as an investing network of fibers to the resistance and capacitance vessels.

The vasoconstrictor regions are tonically active. Reflexes or humoral stimuli that enhance this activity result in an increase in the frequency of impulses that reach the terminal branches to the vessels. A constrictor neurohumor (**norepinephrine**) is then released at the terminals and elicits constriction (α-adrenergic effect) of the resistance vessels. Inhibition of the vasoconstrictor areas reduces their tonic activity and hence diminishes the frequency of impulses in the efferent nerve fibers, with resultant vasodilation. In this way, neural regulation of the peripheral circulation is accomplished primarily by alteration of the number of impulses passing down the vasoconstrictor fibers of the sympathetic nerves to the blood vessels.

> Surgical section of the sympathetic nerves to an extremity abolishes sympathetic vascular tone and thereby increases limb blood flow. With time, vascular tone is regained by an increase in basal (intrinsic) tone.

Both the pressor and depressor regions may undergo rhythmic changes in tonic activity, manifested as oscillations of arterial pressure. Some rhythmic changes (**Traube-Hering waves**) occur at the frequency of respiration and are caused by a cyclic increase in sympathetic impulses to the resistance vessels. Other fluctuations in sympathetic activity (**Mayer waves**) occur at a frequency lower than that of respiration.

■ *Sympathetic Constrictor Influence on Resistance and Capacitance Vessels*

The vasoconstrictor fibers of the sympathetic nervous system supply the arteries, arterioles, and veins, but neural influence on the larger vessels is of far less functional importance than it is on the arterioles and small arteries. Capacitance vessels (veins) are more responsive to sympathetic nerve stimulation than are resistance vessels; they reach maximal constriction at a lower frequency of stimulation than do the resistance vessels. However, capacitance vessels lack β-adrenergic receptors and do not respond to vasodilator metabolites. Norepinephrine is the neurotransmitter released at the sympathetic nerve terminals in the blood vessel. Many factors, such as circulating hormones and particularly locally released substances, modify the release of norepinephrine from the vesicles of the nerve terminals.

The response of the resistance and capacitance vessels of the cat to stimulation of the sympathetic fibers is illustrated in Fig. 28-7. At constant arterial pressure, sympathetic fiber stimulation reduces blood flow (constriction of the resistance vessels) and decreases blood volume of the tissue (constriction of the capacitance vessels). The abrupt decrease in tissue volume is caused by movement of blood out of the capacitance vessels and out of the hindquarters of the cat, whereas the late, slow progressive decline in volume (*to the right of the arrow*) is caused by movement of extravascular fluid

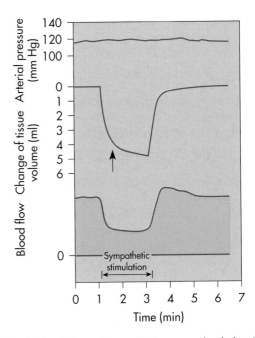

■ **Fig. 28-7**   Effect of sympathetic nerve stimulation (2 Hz) on blood flow and tissue volume in the hindquarters of the cat. The arrow denotes the change in slope of the tissue volume curve where the volume decrease caused by emptying of capacitance vessels ceases and loss of extravascular fluid becomes evident. (Redrawn from Mellander S: *Acta Physiol Scand* 50 (suppl 176):1, 1960.)

into the capillaries and hence away from the tissue. The loss of tissue fluid is a consequence of the lowered capillary hydrostatic pressure brought about by constriction of the resistance vessels. With constriction of the resistance vessels, a new equilibrium of the forces responsible for filtration and absorption across the capillary wall (see p 437) is established.

In addition to active changes (contraction and relaxation of the vascular smooth muscle) in vessel caliber, passive changes are also caused solely by alteration in intraluminal pressure. An increase in intraluminal pressure distends the vessels, and a decrease reduces the caliber of the vessels caused by recoil of the elastic components of the vessel walls.

At the level of basal vascular tone, approximately one third of the blood volume of a tissue can be mobilized when the sympathetic nerves are stimulated at physiological frequencies. The basal tone is very low in capacitance vessels; if these vessels are denervated experimentally, the increases in volume evoked by maximal doses of acetylcholine are small. Therefore, the blood volume at basal vascular tone is close to the maximal blood volume of the tissue. More blood can be mobilized from the skin than from the muscle capacitance vessels. This disparity depends in part on the greater sensitivity of the skin vessels to sympathetic stimulation, but also in part because basal tone is lower in skin vessels than in muscle vessels. Therefore, in the absence of neural influence, the skin capacitance vessels contain more blood than do the muscle capacitance vessels.

Blood is mobilized from capacitance vessels in response to physiological stimuli. For example, during exercise, activation of the sympathetic nerve fibers constricts the veins and hence augments the cardiac filling pressure. In arterial hypotension (as in hemorrhage), the capacitance vessels constrict to help correct the decreased central venous pressure associated with blood loss.

In hemorrhagic shock, the resistance vessels constrict and thereby assist in the maintenance or restoration of arterial pressure. With arterial hypotension, the enhanced arteriolar constriction also leads to a small mobilization of blood from the tissue by virtue of recoil of the postarteriolar vessels when intraluminal pressure is reduced. Furthermore, extravascular fluid is mobilized because of greater absorption into the capillaries in response to the lowered capillary hydrostatic pressure (see also Chapter 31).

Parasympathetic Neural Influence

The efferent fibers of the cranial division of the parasympathetic nervous system supply the blood vessels of the head and viscera, whereas fibers of the sacral division supply blood vessels of the genitalia, bladder, and large bowel. Skeletal muscle and skin do not receive parasympathetic innervation. Because only a small proportion of the resistance vessels of the body receive parasympathetic fibers, the effect of these cholinergic fibers on total vascular resistance is small.

Stimulation of the parasympathetic fibers to the salivary glands induces marked vasodilation. A vasodilator polypeptide, **bradykinin,** formed locally from the action of an enzyme on a plasma protein substrate present in the glandular lymphatics mediates the vasodilation produced by this stimulation. Bradykinin is formed in other exocrine glands, such as the lacrimal and sweat glands. Its presence in sweat may be partly responsible for the dilation of cutaneous blood vessels that occurs with sweating.

Humoral Factors

Epinephrine and norepinephrine exert a powerful effect on the peripheral blood vessels. In skeletal muscle, epinephrine in low concentrations dilates resistance vessels (**β-adrenergic effect**) and in high concentrations produces constriction (**α-adrenergic effect).** In skin, epinephrine causes only vasoconstriction, whereas in *all* vascular beds the primary effect of norepinephrine is vasoconstriction. When stimulated, the adrenal gland can release epinephrine and norepinephrine into the systemic circulation.

However, under physiological conditions, the effect of catecholamine release from the adrenal medulla is of lesser importance than norepinephrine release produced by sympathetic nerve activation (see also Chapter 24).

Vascular Reflexes

Areas of the medulla that mediate sympathetic and vagal effects are under the influence of neural impulses that arise in the baroreceptors, chemoreceptors, hypothalamus, cerebral cortex, and skin. These areas of the medulla are also affected by changes in the blood concentrations of CO_2 and O_2.

Arterial baroreceptors. The **baroreceptors** (or **pressoreceptors**) are stretch receptors located in the carotid sinuses. The carotid sinuses are the slightly widened areas of the internal carotid arteries. Baroreceptors are also located in the aortic arch (Figs. 28-8 and 28-9). Impulses that arise in the carotid sinus travel up the sinus nerve (nerve of Hering) to the glossopharyngeal nerve and, via the latter, to the **nucleus of the tractus solitarius** (**NTS**) in the medulla. The NTS is the site of central projection of the chemoreceptors and baroreceptors. Stimulation of the NTS inhibits sympathetic nerve impulses to the peripheral blood vessels (depressor), whereas lesions of the NTS produce vasoconstriction (pressor). Impulses that arise in the baroreceptors of the aortic arch reach the NTS via afferent fibers in the vagus nerves. The baroreceptor nerve terminals in the walls of the carotid sinus and aortic arch respond to the stretch and deformation of the vessel induced by changes in the arterial blood pressure. The frequency of firing of these nerve terminals is enhanced by an increase in blood pressure and diminished by a reduction in blood pressure. An increase in impulse frequency, as occurs with a rise in arterial pressure, inhibits the vasoconstrictor regions and results in peripheral vasodilation and a lowering of blood pressure. Contributing to this lowering of the blood pressure is a bradycardia brought about by activation of the cardiac branches of the vagus nerves.

The carotid sinus and aortic baroreceptors do not cause equally powerful effects on peripheral resistance in response to nonpulsatile alterations in blood pressure. The carotid sinus baroreceptors are more sensitive than those in the aortic arch. Changes in pressure in the carotid sinus evoke greater alterations in systemic arterial pressure than do equivalent changes in aortic arch pressure. However, the two sets of baroreceptors respond similarly to pulsatile changes in blood pressure.

The carotid sinus with its sinus nerve can be isolated from the rest of the circulation and perfused by either a donor animal or an artificial perfusion system. Under these conditions, changes in the pressure within the carotid sinus are associated with reciprocal changes in the blood pressure of the donor animal. The receptors in

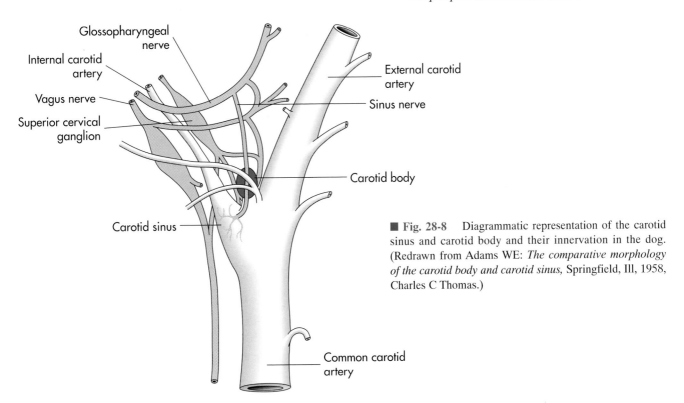

Glossopharyngeal
nerve

Internal carotid
artery

Vagus nerve

Superior cervical
ganglion

Carotid sinus

External carotid
artery

Sinus nerve

Carotid body

Common carotid
artery

■ **Fig. 28-8**   Diagrammatic representation of the carotid sinus and carotid body and their innervation in the dog. (Redrawn from Adams WE: *The comparative morphology of the carotid body and carotid sinus,* Springfield, Ill, 1958, Charles C Thomas.)

the walls of the carotid sinus are more responsive to constantly changing pressures than to sustained constant pressures. This is illustrated in Fig. 28-10, which shows that at normal levels of mean blood pressure (about 100 mm Hg) a barrage of impulses from a single fiber of the sinus nerve is initiated in early systole by the pressure rise, and only a few spikes are observed during late systole and early diastole. At lower pressures, these phasic changes are even more evident, but the overall frequency of discharge is reduced. The blood pressure threshold for eliciting sinus nerve impulses is about 50 mm Hg, and a maximal sustained firing is reached at around 200 mm Hg. Because the baroreceptors show some degree of adaptation, their response at any level of mean arterial pressure is greater to a large than to a small pulse pressure. This response is illustrated in Fig. 28-11, which shows the effects of damping pulsations in the carotid sinus on the firing frequency in a fiber of the sinus nerve and on the systemic arterial pressure. When the pulse pressure in the carotid sinuses is reduced with an air chamber, but mean pressure remains constant, the rate of electrical impulses recorded from a sinus nerve fiber decreases and the systemic arterial pressure increases. Restoration of the pulse pressure in the carotid sinus restores the frequency of sinus nerve discharge and systemic arterial pressure to control levels (Fig. 28-11).

The resistance increases that occur in response to reduced pressure in the carotid sinus vary from one peripheral vascular bed to another. These variations allow blood flow to be redistributed. In the dog, for example, the resistance changes elicited by altering carotid sinus

pressure around the normal operating sinus pressure are greatest in the femoral vessels, less in the renal vessels, and least in the mesenteric and celiac vessels.

Furthermore, the sensitivity of the carotid sinus reflex can be altered. Local application of norepinephrine or stimulation of sympathetic nerve fibers to the carotid sinuses enhances the sensitivity of the receptors in the sinus, so that a given increase in intrasinus pressure produces a greater depressor response. Baroreceptor sensitivity decreases in hypertension because the carotid sinuses become stiffer and less deformable as a result of the high intra-arterial pressure. Under these conditions, a given increase in carotid sinus pressure elicits a smaller decrease in systemic arterial pressure than it does at normal levels of blood pressure. In other words, the set point of the baroreceptors is raised in hypertension so that the threshold is increased and the pressure receptors are less sensitive to changes in transmural pressure.

As would be expected, denervation of the carotid sinus can produce temporary, and in some instances prolonged, hypertension.

The arterial baroreceptors play a key role in short-term adjustments of blood pressure in response to relatively abrupt changes in blood volume, cardiac output, or peripheral resistance (as in exercise). However, long-term control of blood pressure—that is, over days, weeks, and longer—is determined by the fluid balance of the individual, namely, the balance between fluid intake and fluid output. By far the single most important organ in the control of body fluid volume, and hence of blood pressure, is the kidney (see also Chapter 42). In overhydra-

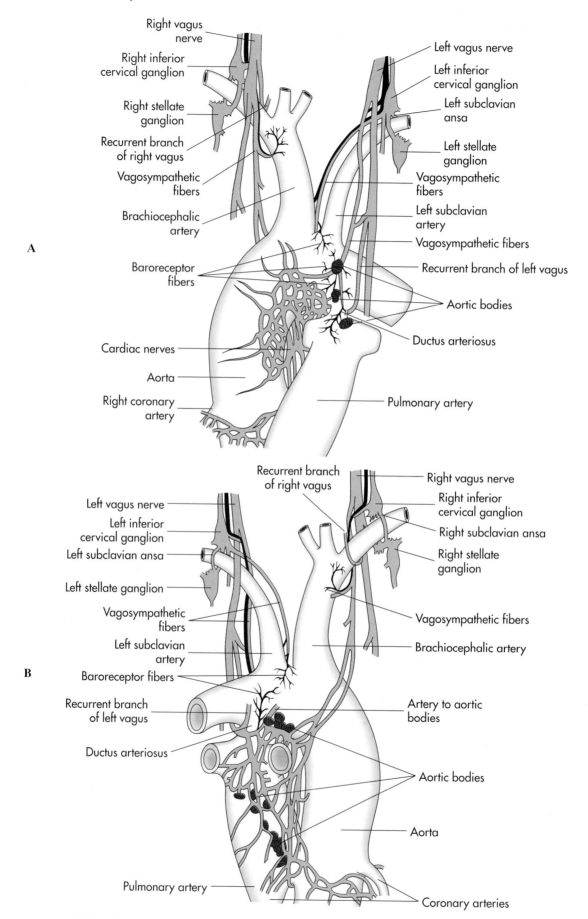

■ **Fig. 28-9**   **A,** Anterior view and **B,** posterior view of the aortic arch showing the innervation of the aortic bodies and pressoreceptors in the dog. (Modified from Nonidez JF: *Anat Rec* 69:299, 1937.)

tion, excessive fluid is excreted, whereas in dehydration, urine output is markedly reduced.

In some individuals, the carotid sinus is abnormally sensitive to external pressure. Hence, tight collars or other forms of external pressure over the region of the carotid sinus may elicit marked hypotension and fainting.

Cardiopulmonary baroreceptors. Cardiopulmonary receptors are located in the atria, ventricles, and pulmonary vessels. These baroreceptors are innervated by

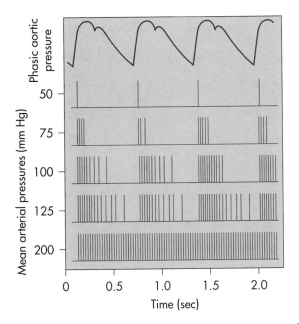

■ **Fig. 28-10**   Relationship of phasic aortic blood pressure in the firing of a single afferent nerve fiber from the carotid sinus at different levels of mean arterial pressure.

vagal and sympathetic afferent nerves. Cardiopulmonary reflexes are tonically active and can alter peripheral resistance in response to changes in intracardiac, venous, or pulmonary vascular pressure.

The atria contain two types of cardiopulmonary baroreceptors: those activated by the tension developed during atrial contraction (**A receptors**) and those activated by the stretch of the atria during atrial filling (**B receptors**) (see also Chapter 24). Stimulation of these atrial receptors sends impulses up vagal fibers to the vagal center in the medulla. Consequently, the sympathetic activity is decreased to the kidney and increased to the sinus node. These changes in sympathetic activity increase renal blood flow, urine flow, and heart rate.

Activation of the cardiopulmonary receptors can also initiate a reflex that lowers blood pressure by inhibiting the vasoconstrictor center in the medulla. Stimulation of the receptors inhibits angiotensin, aldosterone, and vasopressin (antidiuretic hormone) release; interruption of the reflex pathway has the opposite effects.

An example of the role that activation of these baroreceptors plays in the regulation of blood volume can be seen in the body's responses to hemorrhage. In hemorrhage, blood volume decreases (hypovolemia). Hypovolemia enhances sympathetic vasoconstriction in the kidney and increases secretion of renin, angiotensin, aldosterone, and antidiuretic hormone (see also Chapters 31 and 42). The renal vasoconstriction (primarily afferent arterioles) reduces glomerular filtration and increases renin release from the kidney. Renin acts on a plasma substrate to form angiotensin, which increases aldosterone release from the adrenal cortex. The enhanced release of antidiuretic hormone increases water reabsorption and the greater release of aldosterone increases sodium reabsorption, and with it water.

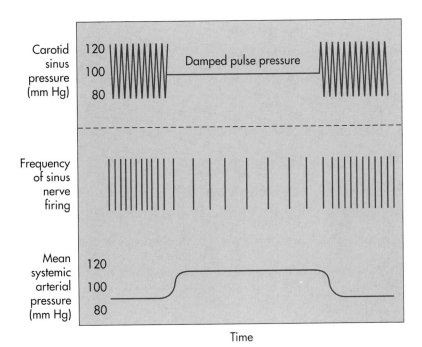

■ **Fig. 28-11**   Effect of reducing pulse pressure in the vascularly isolated perfused carotid sinuses *(top record)* on impulses recorded from a fiber of a sinus nerve *(middle record)* and on mean systemic arterial pressure *(bottom record)*. Mean pressure in the carotid sinuses *(horizontal line, top record)* is held constant when pulse pressure is damped.

The net results are retention of salt and water by the kidney, which increases the blood volume and evokes a sensation of thirst. Angiotensin II (formed from antiotensin I by converting enzyme) also raises systemic arteriolar tone.

Peripheral chemoreceptors. These chemoreceptors consist of small, highly vascular bodies in the region of the aortic arch (**aortic bodies,** Fig. 28-9) and just medial to the carotid sinuses (**carotid bodies,** Fig. 28-8). They are sensitive to changes in the Po_2, Pco_2, and pH of the blood. Although they are primarily involved in the regulation of respiration, they influence the vasomotor regions through reflexes to a minor degree. A reduction in arterial blood O_2 tension (Pao_2) stimulates the chemoreceptors, and the increase in the number of impulses in the afferent nerve fibers from the carotid and aortic bodies stimulates the vasoconstrictor regions, and results in increased tone of the resistance and capacitance vessels.

The chemoreceptors are also stimulated by increased arterial blood CO_2 tension ($Paco_2$) and reduced pH, but the reflex effect induced is quite small compared with the direct effect of hypercapnia (high $Paco_2$) and hydrogen ions on the vasomotor regions in the medulla. When hypoxia and hypercapnia occur at the same time, the stimulation of the chemoreceptors is greater than the sum of the two stimuli when they each act alone. The effects of hypoxia plus hypercapnia on blood pressure, heart rate, and respiration are shown in Fig. 28-12 (see also Chapters 24 and 36).

When the chemoreceptors are stimulated simultaneously by a reduction in pressure in the baroreceptors, the chemoreceptors elicit the vasoconstriction observed in the peripheral vessels. However, when the baroreceptors and chemoreceptors are both stimulated (e.g, with high carotid sinus pressure and low Pao_2), the effects of the baroreceptors predominate.

Chemoreceptors with sympathetic afferent fibers are also located in the heart. These cardiac chemoreceptors are activated by ischemia and transmit the precordial pain (**angina pectoris**) associated with an inadequate blood supply to the myocardium.

Hypothalamus. Optimal function of the cardiovascular reflexes requires the integrity of the pontine and hypothalamic structures. Furthermore, these structures are responsible for behavioral and emotional control of the cardiovascular system (see also Chapter 15). Stimulation of the anterior hypothalamus produces a drop in blood pressure and bradycardia, whereas stimulation of the posterolateral region of the hypothalamus produces a rise in blood pressure and tachycardia. The hypothalamus also contains a temperature-regulating center that affects the skin vessels. Stimulation by cold applications to the skin or by cooling of the blood perfusing the hypothalamus results in constriction of the skin vessels and heat conservation, whereas warm stimuli result in cutaneous vasodilation and enhanced heat loss (see p 488).

When subjects are exposed to high altitudes, the low Pao_2 stimulates the peripheral chemoreceptors to increase the rate and depth of respiration. This is the main mechanism involved in an attempt to restore the oxygen supply to the body (see also Chapter 36).

Cerebrum. The cerebral cortex can also exert a significant effect on blood flow distribution in the body. Stimulation of the motor and premotor areas can affect blood pressure; usually a pressor response is obtained. However, vasodilation and depressor responses may be evoked, as in blushing or fainting, in response to an emotional stimulus.

Skin and viscera. Painful stimuli can elicit either pressor or depressor responses, depending on the magnitude and location of the stimulus. Distention of the viscera often evokes a depressor response, whereas painful stimuli on the body surface usually evoke a pressor response.

Pulmonary reflexes. Inflation of the lungs initiates a reflex that induces systemic vasodilation and a decrease in arterial blood pressure. Conversely, collapse of the lungs evokes systemic vasoconstriction. Afferent fibers that mediate this reflex run in the vagus nerves and possibly also in the sympathetic nerves. Their stimulation by stretch of the lungs inhibits the vasomotor areas. The magnitude of the depressor response to lung inflation is directly related to the degree of inflation and to the existing level of vasoconstrictor tone (see also Chapter 24).

Central chemoreceptors. Increases in $Paco_2$ stimulate chemosensitive regions of the medulla (or central chemoreceptors) and elicit vasoconstriction and increased peripheral resistance. Reduction in $Paco_2$ below normal levels (as with hyperventilation) decreases the degree of tonic activity of these areas in the medulla and thereby releases peripheral resistance. The chemosensitive regions are also affected by changes in pH. A lowering of blood pH stimulates, and a rise in blood pH inhibits, these areas. These effects of changes in $Paco_2$ and blood pH possibly operate through changes in cerebrospinal fluid pH, as does also the respiratory center.

Oxygen tension has relatively little direct effect on the medullary vasomotor region. The primary effect of hypoxia is mediated by reflexes via the carotid and aortic chemoreceptors. Moderate reduction of Pao_2 stimulates the vasomotor region, but severe reduction depresses vasomotor activity in the same manner in which other areas of the brain are depressed by very low O_2 tensions.

Cerebral ischemia, which may occur because of excessive pressure exerted by an expanding intracranial tumor, results in a marked increase in peripheral vasoconstriction. The stimulation is probably caused by a local accumulation of CO_2 and reduction of O_2, and possibly by excitation of intracranial baroreceptors. With prolonged, severe ischemia, central depression eventually supervenes and blood pressure falls.

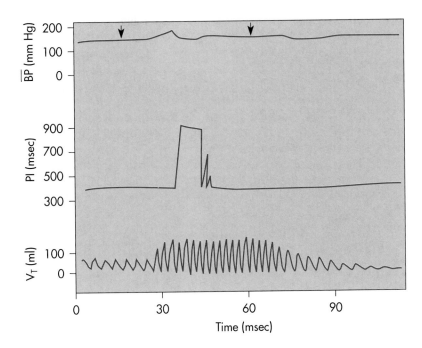

■ **Fig. 28-12**   Effects of stimulation of the isolated perfused carotid body chemoreceptors at constant carotid sinus perfusion pressure, by substituting hypoxic blood (Po_2, 31.1 mm Hg; Pco_2, 84.9 mm Hg; pH, 7.242) for arterial blood (Po_2, 140.4 mm Hg; Pco_2, 42.1 mm Hg; pH, 7.33) between arrows. Note that the bradycardia was transient. The enhanced respiratory response abolishes bradycardia and can produce tachycardia, especially with sustained stimulation of the carotid body receptors (see Figs. 24-14 and 24-15). The increase in pulse interval *(PI)* indicates a decrease in heart rate. $\overline{BP}$, Mean arterial blood pressure; V_T, tidal volume. (Redrawn from Daly MdeB, Kouner PI, Angell-James JE, Oliver JA: *Clin Exp Pharmacol Physiol* 5:511, 1978.)

■ *Balance between Extrinsic and Intrinsic Factors in Regulation of Peripheral Blood Flow*

Dual control of the peripheral vessels by intrinsic and extrinsic mechanisms evokes a number of vascular adjustments that enable the body to direct blood flow to areas where it is most needed and away from areas that have fewer requirements. In some tissues, the effect of extrinsic and intrinsic mechanisms is fixed; in other tissues, the ratio is changeable, depending on the state of activity of that tissue.

In the brain and heart, which are vital structures with a limited tolerance for a reduced blood supply, intrinsic flow-regulating mechanisms are dominant. For instance, massive discharge of the vasoconstrictor region over the sympathetic nerves, which might occur in severe, acute hemorrhage, has negligible effects on the cerebral and cardiac resistance vessels, whereas skin, renal, and splanchnic blood vessels become greatly constricted (see also Chapter 31).

In the skin, the extrinsic vascular control is dominant. Not only do the cutaneous vessels participate strongly in a general vasoconstrictor discharge, but they also respond selectively through hypothalamic pathways to subserve the heat loss and heat conservation function required in body temperature regulation. However, intrinsic control can be demonstrated by local temperature changes that can modify or override the central influence on resistance and capacitance vessels (see also Chapter 30).

In skeletal muscle, extrinsic and intrinsic mechanisms interact. In resting skeletal muscle, neural control (vasoconstrictor tone) is dominant, as can be demonstrated by the large increase in blood flow that occurs immediately after section of the sympathetic nerves to the tissue. In anticipation of and at the start of exercise, such as running, blood flow increases in the leg muscles. After the onset of exercise, the intrinsic flow-regulating mechanism assumes control, and vasodilation occurs in the active muscles because of the local increase in metabolites. Vasoconstriction occurs in the inactive tissues as a manifestation of the general sympathetic discharge. However, constrictor impulses that reach the resistance vessels of the active muscles are overridden by the local metabolic effect. Operation of this dual control mechanism thus provides increased blood flow where it is required and shunts it away from relatively inactive areas (see also Chapter 30). Similar effects may be achieved with an increase in $Paco_2$. Normally, the hyperventilation associated with exercise keeps $Paco_2$ at normal levels. However, were $Paco_2$ to increase, a generalized vasoconstriction would occur because of stimulation of the medullary vasoconstrictor region by CO_2. In the active muscles, where the CO_2 concentration is highest, the smooth muscle of the arterioles relaxes in response to the local Pco_2. Factors that affect and are affected by the vasomotor region are summarized in Fig. 28-13.

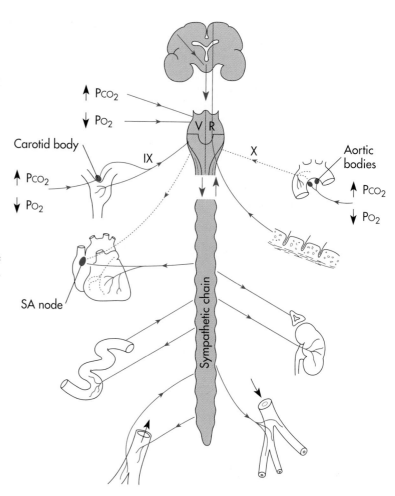

■ **Fig. 28-13**   Schematic diagram illustrating the neural input and output of the vasomotor region *(SR)*. *IX*, Glossopharyngeal nerve; *X*, vagus nerve.

■ *Summary*

1. The arterioles (resistance vessels) mainly regulate blood flow through their capillaries. The smooth muscle, which makes up a major fraction of the walls of the arterioles, contracts and relaxes in response to neural and humoral stimuli.

2. Autoregulation of blood flow occurs in most tissues. Autoregulation is characterized by a constant blood flow in the face of a change in perfusion pressure. A logical explanation of autoregulation is the myogenic mechanism, whereby an increase in transmural pressure elicits a contractile response of the vascular smooth muscle, whereas a decrease in transmural pressure elicits relaxation.

3. The striking parallelism between tissue blood flow and tissue oxygen consumption indicates that blood flow is largely regulated by a metabolic mechanism. A decrease in the oxygen supply:oxygen demand ratio of a tissue releases a vasodilator metabolite that dilates arterioles to enhance the oxygen supply.

4. Neural regulation of blood flow is almost completely accomplished by the sympathetic nervous system. Sympathetic nerves to blood vessels are tonically active;

inhibition of the vasoconstrictor center in the medulla reduces peripheral vascular resistance. Stimulation of the sympathetic nerves constricts resistance and capacitance (veins) vessels.

5. Parasympathetic fibers innervate the head, viscera, and genitalia; they do not innervate skin and muscle.

6. The baroreceptors (pressoreceptors) in the internal carotid arteries and aorta are tonically active and regulate blood pressure on a moment-to-moment basis. Stretch of these receptors by an increase in arterial pressure initiates a reflex that inhibits the vasoconstrictor center in the medulla and induces vasodilation, whereas a decrease in arterial pressure disinhibits the vasoconstrictor center and induces vasoconstriction.

7. The carotid baroreceptors predominate over those in the aorta and respond more vigorously to changes in pressure (stretch) than they do to elevated or reduced nonpulsatile pressures. In other words, they adapt to an imposed constant pressure.

8. Baroreceptors are also present in the cardiac chambers and large pulmonary vessels (cardiopulmonary baroreceptors); they have less influence on blood pressure but participate in blood volume regulation.

9. Peripheral chemoreceptors (carotid and aortic bodies) and central chemoreceptors in the medulla oblongata are stimulated by a decrease in blood oxygen tension (PaO_2) and an increase in blood carbon dioxide tension ($PaCO_2$). Stimulation of these chemoreceptors primarily increases the rate and depth of respiration but also produces peripheral vasoconstriction.

10. Peripheral resistance, and hence blood pressure, are affected by stimuli arising in the skin, viscera, lungs, and brain.

11. The combined effect of neural and local metabolic factors distributes blood to active tissues and diverts it from inactive tissues. In vital structures such as the heart and brain and in contracting skeletal muscle, the metabolic factors predominate.

■ *Self-Study Problems*

1. What is meant by autoregulation of blood flow and what is the mechanism involved?

2. How can the endothelium affect the contractile state of vascular smooth muscle?

3. What is vascular tone?

4. Briefly describe the local and neural effects on vascular resistance in resting and contracting skeletal muscle.

5. How is blood pressure regulated by the carotid baroreceptors?

■ *Bibliography*

Journal articles

Berne RM, Knabb RM, Ely SW, Rubio R: Adenosine in the local regulation of blood flow: a brief overview, *Fed Proc* 42:3136, 1983.

Brown AM: Receptors under pressure—an update on baroreceptors, *Circ Res* 46:1, 1980.

Cowley AW Jr: Long-term control of blood pressure, *Physiol Rev* 72:231, 1992.

Donald DE, Shepherd JT: Autonomic regulation of the peripheral circulation, *Annu Rev Physiol* 42:429, 1980.

Ellsworth ML, Forrester T, Ellis CG, Dietrich HH: The erythrocyte as a regulator of vascular tone, *Am J Physiol* 269:H2155, 1995.

Hainsworth R: Reflexes from the heart, *Physiol Rev* 71:617, 1991.

Hilton SM, Spyer KM: Central nervous regulation of vascular resistance, *Annu Rev Physiol* 42:399, 1980.

Hirst GDS, Edwards FR: Sympathetic neuroeffector transmission in arteries and arterioles, *Physiol Rev* 69:546, 1989.

Kuo L, Davis JJ, Chilian WM: Endothelium-dependent flow-induced dilation of isolated coronary arterioles, *Am J Physiol* 259:H1063, 1990.

Marshall JM: Peripheral chemoreceptors and cardiovascular regulation, *Physiol Rev* 74:543, 1994.

Monos E, Berczi V, Nadasy G: Local control of veins: biomechanical, metabolic, and humoral aspects, *Physiol Rev* 75:611, 1995.

Shen Y-T, Knight DR, Thomas JX Jr, Vatner SF: Relative roles of cardiac receptors and arterial baroreceptors during hemorrhage in conscious dogs, *Circ Res* 66:397, 1990.

Shepherd JT: Reflex control of arterial blood pressure, *Cardiovasc Res* 16:357, 1982.

Books and monographs

Abboud FM, Thames MD: *Interaction of cardiovascular reflexes in circulatory control.* In *Handbook of physiology,* sect 2: *The cardiovascular system—peripheral circulation and organ blood flow,* vol III, Bethesda, Md, 1983, American Physiological Society.

Bishop VS, Malliani A, Thoren P: *Cardiac mechanoreceptors.* In *Handbook of physiology,* sect 2: *The cardiovascular system—peripheral circulation and organ blood flow,* vol III, Bethesda, Md, 1983, American Physiological Society.

Eyzaguirre C, Fitzgerald RS, Lahiri S, Zapata P: *Arterial chemoreceptors.* In *Handbook of physiology,* sect 2: *The cardiovascular system—peripheral circulation and organ blood flow,* vol III, Bethesda, Md, 1980, American Physiological Society.

Kovach AGB, Sandos P, Kollii M, editors: *Cardiovascular physiology: neural control mechanisms,* New York, 1981, Academic Press.

Mancia G, Mark AL: *Arterial baroreflexes in humans,* In *Handbook of physiology,* sect 2: *The cardiovascular system—peripheral circulation and organ blood flow,* vol III, Bethesda, Md, 1983, American Physiological Society.

Mark AL, Mancia G: *Cardiopulmonary baroreflexes in humans.* In *Handbook of physiology,* sect 2: *The cardiovascular system—peripheral circulation and organ blood flow,* vol III, Bethesda, Md, 1983, American Physiological Society.

Mulvany MJ, Strandgaard S, Hammersen F, editors: *Resistance vessels: physiology, pharmacology and hypertensive pathology,* Basel, Switzerland, 1985, S Karger.

Persson PB, Kirchheim HR, editors: *Baroreceptor reflexes,* Berlin, 1991, Springer-Verlag.

Rothe CF: *Venous system: physiology of the capacitance vessels.* In *Handbook of physiology,* sect 2: *The cardiovascular system—peripheral circulation and organ blood flow,* vol III, Bethesda, Md, 1983, American Physiological Society.

Sagawa K: *Baroreflex control of systemic arterial pressure and vascular bed.* In *Handbook of physiology,* sect 2: *The cardiovascular system—peripheral circulation and organ blood flow,* vol III, Bethesda, Md, 1983, American Physiological Society.

Shepherd JT: *Cardiac mechanoreceptors.* In Fozzard HA et al, editors: *The heart and cardiovascular system, scientific foundations,* ed 2, New York, 1991, Raven Press.

Somlyo AP, Somlyo AV: *Smooth muscle structure and function.* In Fozzard HA et al, editors: *The heart and cardiovascular system, scientific foundations,* ed 2, New York, 1991, Raven Press.

Sparks HR Jr: *Effect of local metabolic factors on vascular smooth muscle.* In *Handbook of physiology,* sect 2: *The cardiovascular system—vascular smooth muscle,* vol II, Bethesda, Md, 1980, American Physiological Society.

Zucker IH, Gilmore JP, editors: *Reflex control of the circulation,* Boca Raton, Fla, 1991, CRC Press.

CHAPTER
29

Control of Cardiac Output: Coupling of Heart and Blood Vessels

Four factors control cardiac output: heart rate, myocardial contractility, preload, and afterload (Fig. 29-1). Heart rate and myocardial contractility are strictly **cardiac factors;** that is, these factors originate in the cardiac tissues, although they are controlled by various neural and humoral mechanisms. Preload and afterload, however, are factors that are mutually dependent on the behavior of the heart and the vasculature. On the one hand, preload and afterload are important *determinants of* cardiac output. On the other hand, preload and afterload are themselves *determined by* the cardiac output and by certain vascular characteristics. Because these factors constitute a functional coupling between the heart and blood vessels, preload and afterload will be called **coupling factors.**

To understand the regulation of cardiac output, therefore, the nature of the coupling between the heart and the vascular system must be appreciated. In this chapter, we use two kinds of graphs to analyze the interactions between the cardiac and vascular components of the circulatory system. These graphs represent two important functional relationships between **cardiac output** and **central venous pressure** (i.e., the pressure in the right atrium and thoracic venae cavae).

The curve that defines one of these relationships is called the **cardiac function curve.** It is an expression of the well-known Frank-Starling relationship and it illustrates the dependence of cardiac output on preload (i.e., the central venous, or right atrial, pressure). The cardiac function curve is a characteristic of the heart itself; in fact, it is usually studied in hearts completely isolated from the rest of the circulatory system. This curve has already been discussed in detail in Chapters 23 and 24. We use it later in this chapter in association with the other characteristic curve to analyze the interactions between the heart and the vasculature.

The second curve, called the **vascular function curve,** defines the dependence of central venous pressure on cardiac output. This relationship depends only on certain vascular system characteristics, namely, the peripheral resistance, the arterial and venous compliances, and the blood volume. The vascular function curve is entirely independent of the characteristics of the heart. Because of this independence, it can be derived experimentally even if the heart is replaced by a mechanical pump.

■ *Vascular Function Curve*

The vascular function curve defines the changes in central venous pressure that are caused by changes in cardiac output. In this curve, the central venous pressure is the **dependent variable** (or **response**), and cardiac output is the **independent variable** (or **stimulus**). These variables are opposite to those of the cardiac function curve, in which the central venous pressure (or preload) is the **independent variable** and the cardiac output is the **dependent variable.**

The simplified model of the circulation illustrated in Fig. 29-2 helps explain how the cardiac output determines the level of central venous pressure. In this simplified model, all the essential components of the cardiovascular system have been lumped into four basic elements. The right and left sides of the heart, as well as the pulmonary vascular bed, constitute a **pump-oxygenator,** much like the artificial heart-lung machine that is used to perfuse the body during open heart surgery. The high-resistance microcirculation is designated the **peripheral resistance.** Finally, the compliance of the system is subdivided into two components, the **arterial compliance,** C_a, and the **venous compliance,** C_v. As defined in Chapter 26, the compliance (C) of a blood vessel is the increase in volume (ΔV) that is accommodated in that vessel per unit change of transmural pressure (ΔP); that is,

$$C \equiv \Delta V/\Delta P \qquad (29\text{-}1)$$

The venous compliance is about 20 times greater than the arterial compliance. In the example that follows, the

458

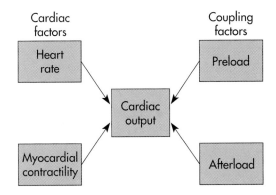

■ **Fig. 29-1** The four factors that determine cardiac output.

ratio of C_v to C_a is set at 19:1 to simplify the calculations. Thus, if it were necessary to add x ml of blood to the arterial system to produce a 1 mm Hg increase in arterial pressure, 19x ml of blood would need to be added to the venous system to raise venous pressure by the same amount.

To show why a change in cardiac output causes an inverse change in central venous pressure, let us first endow our hypothetical model with certain characteristics that mimic those of an average adult person (Fig. 29-2, *A*). Therefore, the flow (Q_h) generated by the heart (i.e., the cardiac output) will be 5 L/min; the mean arterial pressure, P_a, 102 mm Hg; and the central venous pressure, P_v, 2 mm Hg. The peripheral resistance, R, is the ratio of arteriovenous pressure difference ($P_a - P_v$) to flow (Q_r) through the resistance vessels; this ratio equals 20 mm Hg/L/min. An arteriovenous pressure difference of 100 mm Hg is sufficient to force a flow (Q_r) of 5 L/min through a peripheral resistance of 20 mm Hg/L/min. Under equilibrium conditions, this flow (Q_r) is precisely equal to the flow (Q_h) pumped by the heart. From heartbeat to heartbeat the volume (V_a) of blood in the arteries and the volume (V_v) of blood in the veins remain constant, because the volume of blood transferred from the veins to the arteries by the heart equals the volume of blood that flows from the arteries through the resistance vessels and into the veins.

■ *Effects of Cardiac Arrest on Arterial and Venous Pressures*

Fig. 29-2, *B*, illustrates the status of the circulation at the very beginning of an episode of cardiac arrest; that is, $Q_h = 0$. In the instant immediately after the arrest of the heart, the volumes of blood in the arteries (V_a) and veins (V_v) have not had time to change appreciably. Because the arterial and venous pressures depend on V_a and V_v, respectively, these pressures are identical to the respective pressures in panel *A* (i.e., $P_a = 102$ and $P_v = 2$). This arteriovenous pressure gradient of 100 mm Hg forces a flow (Q_r) of 5 L/min through the peripheral resistance of

20 mm Hg/L/min. Thus, although cardiac output (Q_h) now equals 0 L/min, the flow through the microcirculation equals 5 L/min. In other words, the potential energy stored in the arteries by the pumping action of the heart that occurred immediately before the cardiac arrest causes blood to be transferred from arteries to veins, initially at the control rate, even though the heart can no longer transfer blood from the veins into the arteries.

As time passes and the heart continues in arrest, the blood flow through the resistance vessels causes the blood volume in the arteries to decrease progressively and the blood volume in the veins to increase progressively. Because the arteries and veins are elastic structures, the arterial pressure falls gradually and the venous pressure rises gradually. This process continues until the arterial and venous pressures become equal (Fig. 29-2, *C*). Once this condition is reached, the flow (Q_r) from the arteries to the veins through the resistance vessels is zero, as is the cardiac output (Q_h).

When the effects of cardiac arrest reach this equilibrium (Fig. 29-2, *C*), the pressure attained in the arteries and veins depends on the relative compliances of these vessels. If the arterial (C_a) and venous (C_v) compliances are equal, the decline in P_a would equal the rise in P_v, because the decrease in arterial volume would equal the increase in venous volume (principle of conservation of mass). Both P_a and P_v would attain the average of their combined values in panel *A*; that is, $P_a = P_v = (102 + 2)/2 = 52$ mm Hg.

However, C_a and C_v compliances in a living subject are *not* equal. The veins are much more compliant than the arteries; the compliance ratio (C_v:C_a) is approximately 19, which is the ratio that we have assumed for the model. Consequently, when the effects of cardiac arrest reach equilibrium in an intact subject, the pressure in the arteries and veins is much less than the average value of 52 mm Hg that occurs when C_a and C_v compliances are equal. Hence, the transfer of blood from arteries to veins at equilibrium induces a fall in arterial pressure 19 times as great as the concomitant rise in venous pressure. As Fig. 29-2, *C* shows, P_v would increase by 5 mm Hg (to 7 mm Hg), whereas P_a would fall by $19 \times 5 = 95$ mm Hg (to 7 mm Hg). This equilibrium pressure, which prevails in the circulatory system in the absence of flow, is referred to as either the **mean circulatory pressure** or the **static pressure.** The pressure in the static system reflects the total volume of blood in the system and the overall compliance of the system.

We have used the example of cardiac arrest because it facilitates understanding of the vascular function curve. Using this example, we can now begin to assemble a vascular function curve (Fig. 29-3.) As stated previously, the independent variable (plotted along the abscissa) is the cardiac output, and the dependent variable (plotted along the ordinate) is the central venous pressure. Two important points on this curve can be derived from Fig. 29-2. One point (*A* in Fig. 29-3) represents the control state;

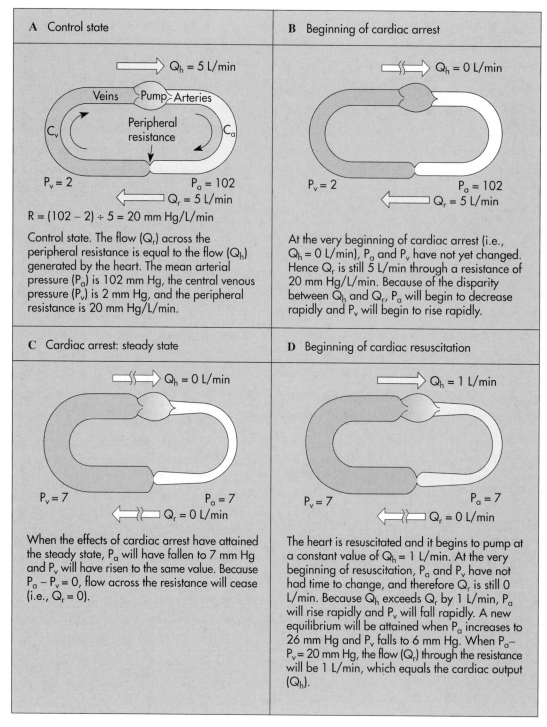

A   Control state

Veins   Pump   Arteries

C_v C_a

Peripheral resistance

$Q_h = 5$ L/min

$P_v = 2$ $P_a = 102$

$Q_r = 5$ L/min

$R = (102 - 2) \div 5 = 20$ mm Hg/L/min

Control state. The flow (Q_r) across the peripheral resistance is equal to the flow (Q_h) generated by the heart. The mean arterial pressure (P_a) is 102 mm Hg, the central venous pressure (P_v) is 2 mm Hg, and the peripheral resistance is 20 mm Hg/L/min.

B   Beginning of cardiac arrest

$Q_h = 0$ L/min

$P_v = 2$ $P_a = 102$

$Q_r = 5$ L/min

At the very beginning of cardiac arrest (i.e., $Q_h = 0$ L/min), P_a and P_v have not yet changed. Hence Q_r is still 5 L/min through a resistance of 20 mm Hg/L/min. Because of the disparity between Q_h and Q_r, P_a will begin to decrease rapidly and P_v will begin to rise rapidly.

C   Cardiac arrest: steady state

$Q_h = 0$ L/min

$P_v = 7$ $P_a = 7$

$Q_r = 0$ L/min

When the effects of cardiac arrest have attained the steady state, P_a will have fallen to 7 mm Hg and P_v will have risen to the same value. Because $P_a - P_v = 0$, flow across the resistance will cease (i.e., $Q_r = 0$).

D   Beginning of cardiac resuscitation

$Q_h = 1$ L/min

$P_v = 7$ $P_a = 7$

$Q_r = 0$ L/min

The heart is resuscitated and it begins to pump at a constant value of $Q_h = 1$ L/min. At the very beginning of resuscitation, P_a and P_v have not had time to change, and therefore Q_r is still 0 L/min. Because Q_h exceeds Q_r by 1 L/min, P_a will rise rapidly and P_v will fall rapidly. A new equilibrium will be attained when P_a increases to 26 mm Hg and P_v falls to 6 mm Hg. When $P_a - P_v = 20$ mm Hg, the flow (Q_r) through the resistance will be 1 L/min, which equals the cardiac output (Q_h).

■ **Fig. 29-2**   **A** to **D,** Simplified model of the cardiovascular system, consisting of a pump, arterial compliance (C_a), peripheral resistance, and venous compliance (C_v).

that is, when cardiac output is 5 L/min, P_v is 2 mm Hg (as depicted in Fig. 29-2, *A*). Then, when the heart is arrested (cardiac output = 0), P_v becomes 7 mm Hg at equilibrium (Fig. 29-2, *C*); this pressure is the mean circulatory pressure (P_{mc} in Fig. 29-3).

The inverse relation between P_v and cardiac output simply denotes that when cardiac output is suddenly decreased, the rate at which blood flows from arteries to

veins through the capillaries is temporarily greater than the rate at which the heart pumps it from the veins back into the arteries. During that transient period, a net volume of blood is transferred from arteries to veins; hence, P_a falls and P_v rises.

Now, let us see what happens when cardiac output is suddenly increased. This example will illustrate how a third point (*B* in Fig. 29-3) on the vascular function curve

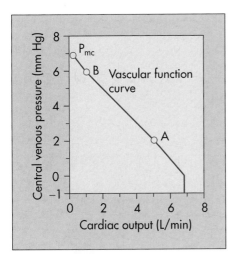

■ **Fig. 29-3** Changes in central venous pressure produced by changes in cardiac output. The mean circulatory pressure (or static pressure), P_{mc}, is the equilibrium pressure throughout the cardiovascular system when cardiac output is 0. Points *B* and *A* represent the values of venous pressure at cardiac outputs of 1 and 5 L/min, respectively.

is derived. Consider that the arrested heart is suddenly restarted and immediately begins pumping blood from the veins into the arteries at a rate of 1 L/min (Fig. 29-2, *D*). When the heart first begins to beat, the arteriovenous pressure gradient is zero, and hence no blood is transferred from the arteries through the capillaries and into the veins. Thus, when beating at first resumes, blood is depleted from the veins at the rate of 1 L/min, and the arterial blood volume is repleted from the venous blood volume at that same rate. Hence, P_v begins to fall and P_a begins to rise. Because of the difference in arterial and venous compliances, P_a will rise at a rate 19 times greater than the rate at which P_v will fall.

The resultant pressure gradient causes blood to flow through the resistance. If the heart maintains a constant output of 1 L/min, P_a will continue to rise and P_v will continue to fall until the pressure gradient becomes 20 mm Hg. This gradient will force a flow of 1 L/min through a resistance of 20 mm Hg/L/min. This gradient will be achieved by a 19 mm Hg rise (to 26 mm Hg) in P_a and a 1 mm Hg fall (to 6 mm Hg) in P_v. This equilibrium value of $P_v = 6$ mm Hg for a cardiac output of 1 L/min also appears on the vascular function curve of Fig. 29-3 (point *B*). The 1 mm Hg reduction in P_v reflects a net transfer of blood from the venous to the arterial side of the circuit.

The reduction of P_v that can be evoked by a sudden increase in cardiac output is limited. At some critical maximal value of cardiac output, sufficient fluid will be transferred from the venous to the arterial side of the circuit for P_v to fall below the ambient pressure. In a system of very distensible vessels, such as the venous system, the vessels will be collapsed by the greater external pressure. This venous collapse acts as an impediment to venous return to the heart. Hence, it limits the maximal

value of cardiac output to 7 L/min in this example (Fig. 29-3), regardless of the capabilities of the pump. For readers interested in the mathematical derivation of these results, the basic equations are presented here.

Mathematical analysis of the vascular function curve

The definition of peripheral resistance (equation 26-6 on p 419) is:

$$R \equiv (P_a - P_v)/Q_r, \qquad (29\text{-}2)$$

where R is peripheral resistance, P_a is arterial pressure, P_v is venous pressure, and Q_r is blood flow through the resistance vessels. At equilibrium, Q_r equals cardiac output, Q_h. Assume that R = 20, and that Q_r had been 0, but that it had then been increased to a constant value of 1 L/min (Fig. 29-4, arrow *1*). If we solve equation 29-2 for the value of P_a when the system has reached equilibrium (i.e., $Q_r = Q_h$):

$$P_a = P_v + Q_r R = P_v + (1 \times 20) \qquad (29\text{-}3)$$

Thus, P_a will increase to a value 20 mm Hg greater than Pv. It will continue to be 20 mm Hg above P_v as long as the pump output is maintained at 1 L/min and the peripheral resistance remains at 20 mm Hg/L/min.

We can calculate what the actual changes in P_a and P_v will be when Q_h attains a constant value of 1 L/min. The arterial volume increase needed to achieve the required level of P_a depends entirely on the arterial compliance C_a. For a rigid arterial system (low compliance), this volume will be small; for a very distensible system (like the human vascular system), the volume will be large. Whatever the magnitude, however, the change in volume represents the transfer of some quantity of blood from the venous to the arterial side of the circuit.

For a given total blood volume, any increase in arterial volume (ΔV_a) must equal the decrease in venous volume (ΔV_v); that is,

$$\Delta V_a = -\Delta V_v \qquad (29\text{-}4)$$

From the general definition of compliance,

$$C_a = \Delta V_a /\Delta P_a , \text{ and } C_v = \Delta V_v /\Delta P_v \qquad (29\text{-}5)$$

By solving equation 29-5 for ΔV_a and ΔV_v , and substituting the results into equation 29-4:

$$\Delta P_v /\Delta P_a = -C_a /C_v \qquad (29\text{-}6)$$

Given that C_v is 19 times greater than C_a, then the increment in P_a will be 19 times greater than the decrement in P_v; that is,

$$\Delta P_a = -19 \, \Delta P_v \qquad (29\text{-}7)$$

To calculate the absolute values of P_a and P_v, let ΔP_a represent the difference between the prevailing P_a and the mean circulatory pressure (P_{mc}); that is, let

$$\Delta P_a = P_a - P_{mc} \qquad (29\text{-}8)$$

and let ΔP_v represent the difference between the prevailing P_v and the mean circulatory pressure:

$$\Delta P_v = P_v - P_{mc} \qquad (29\text{-}9)$$

Substituting these values for ΔP_a and ΔP_v into equation 29-7,

$$P_a - P_{mc} = -19(P_v - P_{mc}) \qquad (29\text{-}10)$$

By solving equations 29-3 and 29-10 simultaneously:

$$P_a = P_{mc} + 19, \text{ and } P_v = P_{mc} - 1 \qquad (29\text{-}11)$$

Hence, if the mean circulatory pressure equals 7 mm Hg, P_a increases to 26 mm Hg and P_v decreases to 6 mm Hg when Q_h increases from 0 to 1 L/min (Fig. 29-4). These pressure changes provide the required arteriovenous pressure gradient of 20 mm Hg.

If the pump output is abruptly increased to a constant level of 5 L/min (Fig. 29-4, arrow 2) and peripheral resistance remains constant at 20 mm Hg/L/min, an additional volume of blood again will be transferred from the venous to the arterial side of the circuit. It will progressively accumulate in the arteries until P_a reaches a level of 100 mm Hg above P_v, as shown by substitution into equation 29-3:

$$P_a = P_v + Q_r R = P_v + (5 \times 20) \qquad (29\text{-}12)$$

By solving equations 29-10 and 29-12 simultaneously, we find that when the pump output is increased to 5 L/min, P_a rises to a value of 95 mm Hg above P_{mc}, and P_v falls to a value 5 mm Hg below P_{mc}. In Fig. 29-4, therefore, P_v declines to 2 mm Hg and P_a rises to 102 mm Hg. The resultant pressure gradient of 100 mm Hg will force a cardiac output of 5 L/min through a constant peripheral resistance of 20 mm Hg/L/min.

The following equation for the vascular function curve (P_v as a function of Q_r) in the model is derived from equations 29-2, 29-6, 29-8, and 29-9:

$$P_v = -[RC_a/(C_a + C_v)] Q_r + P_{mc} \qquad (29\text{-}13)$$

Note that the slope of the vascular function curve depends only on R, C_a, and C_v. Note also that when $Q_r = 0$, $P_v = P_{mc}$; that is, when flow is zero, P_v (and P_a) equal the mean circulatory pressure.

■ *Factors That Influence the Vascular Function Curve*

Venous pressure dependence on cardiac output. Experimental and clinical observations have shown that changes in cardiac output do indeed evoke the alterations in P_a and P_v that have been predicted by our simplified model. In an experiment on an anesthetized dog, a mechanical pump was substituted for the right ventricle (Fig. 29-5). As the pump output, Q, was decreased grad-

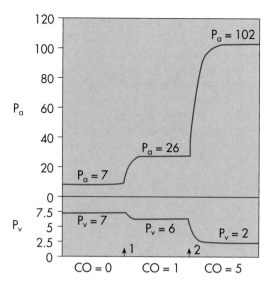

■ **Fig. 29-4** The changes in arterial *(Pₐ)* and venous *(Pᵥ)* pressures in the circulatory model shown in Fig. 29-3. The total peripheral resistance is 20 mm Hg/L/min, and the ratio of C_v to C_a is 19:1. The cardiac output *(CO)* is 0 to the left of arrow *1*. It is increased to 1 L/min at arrow *1* and to 5 L/min at arrow *2*.

ually in a series of small steps, P_a fell and P_v rose progressively. The changes in P_a and P_v evoked by the alterations in blood flow in this experiment resemble those derived from our simplified model (Fig. 29-4).

Similarly, cardiac output may decrease abruptly when a major coronary artery suddenly becomes occluded in a human patient. The **acute heart failure** that occurs as a result of **myocardial infarction** (death of myocardial tissue) is usually accompanied by a fall in arterial blood pressure and a rise in central venous pressure.

Blood volume. The vascular function curve is affected by variations in total blood volume. During circulatory standstill (zero cardiac output, such as occurs during cardiac arrest), the mean circulatory pressure depends only on total vascular compliance and blood volume, as stated previously. Thus, for a given vascular compliance, the mean circulatory pressure is increased when blood volume is expanded (**hypervolemia**) and is decreased when blood volume is diminished (**hypovolemia**). This relationship is illustrated by the Y-axis intercepts in Fig. 29-6, where the mean circulatory pressure is 5 mm Hg after hemorrhage and 9 mm Hg after transfusion, as compared with the value of 7 mm Hg at normal blood volume (**normovolemia**).

Furthermore, the differences in P_v during hypervolemia, normovolemia, and hypovolemia in the static system are preserved at each level of cardiac output. As a result, the vascular function curves parallel each other (Fig. 29-6). To illustrate, consider the example

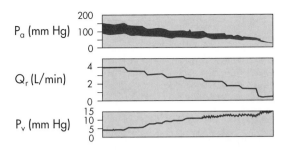

P_a (mm Hg)
Q_r (L/min)
P_v (mm Hg)

■ **Fig. 29-5**   The changes in arterial *(P_a)* and central venous *(P_v)* pressures produced by changes in systemic blood flow *(Q_r)* in a canine right-heart bypass preparation. Stepwise changes in Q_r were produced by altering the rate of a mechanical pump. (From Levy MN: *Circ Res* 44:739, 1979, with permission of the American Heart Association.)

of hypervolemia, in which the mean circulatory pressure is 9 mm Hg. In Fig. 29-6, both P_a and P_v would be 9 mm Hg, instead of 7 mm Hg, when the cardiac output is zero. If the peripheral resistance is 20 mm Hg/L/min, and if cardiac output is suddenly increased to 1 L/min (e.g., at arrow *1* in Fig. 29-4), an arteriovenous pressure gradient of 20 mm Hg is still necessary for 1 L/min to flow through the resistance vessels. This condition does not differ from the example for normovolemia. If we assume the same ratio of C_v to C_a (19:1), the pressure gradient would be achieved by a 1 mm Hg decline in P_v and a 19 mm Hg rise in P_a. Hence, a change in cardiac output from 0 to 1 L/min would evoke the same 1 mm Hg reduction in P_v irrespective of the blood volume, as long as C_a, C_v, and peripheral resistance were independent of blood volume. Equation 19-13 also shows that the slope of the vascular function curve remains constant as long as C_a, C_v, and R do not change.

From Fig. 29-6, it is also apparent that the cardiac output at which P_v = 0 varies directly with the blood volume. Therefore, the maximal value of cardiac output becomes progressively more limited as the total blood volume is reduced. However, the central venous pressure at which the veins collapse (illustrated by the sharp change in slope of the vascular function curve) is not significantly altered by changes in blood volume. This pressure depends only on the ambient pressure surrounding the central veins.

Venomotor tone. The effects of changes in venomotor tone on the vascular function curve closely resemble those for changes in blood volume. In Fig. 29-6, for example, the transfusion curve could just as well represent increased venomotor tone, whereas the hemorrhage curve could represent decreased tone. During circulatory standstill, for a given blood volume, the pressure within the vascular system will rise as the tension exerted by the smooth muscle within the vascular walls increases (these contractile

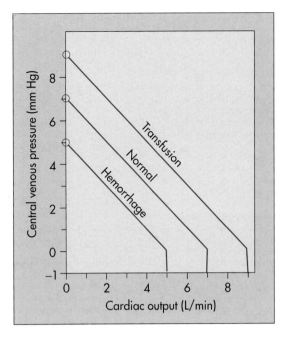

■ **Fig. 29-6**   Effects of increased blood volume *(transfusion curve)* and of decreased blood volume *(hemorrhage curve)* on the vascular function curve. Similar shifts in the vascular function curve can be produced by increases and decreases, respectively, in venomotor tone.

changes in the arteriolar and venous smooth muscle are under nervous and humoral control). The fraction of the blood volume located within the arterioles is very small, whereas the blood volume in the veins is large (see Fig. 21-2). Therefore, changes in peripheral resistance (arteriolar tone) will have no significant effect on the mean circulatory pressure, but changes in venous tone can alter the mean circulatory pressure appreciably. Hence, mean circulatory pressure rises with increased venomotor tone and falls with diminished venomotor tone.

Experimentally, the mean circulatory pressure attained about 1 minute after abrupt circulatory standstill is usually substantially above 7 mm Hg, even when blood volume is normal. This high pressure level is attributable to the generalized venoconstriction that is caused by cerebral ischemia, activation of the chemoreceptors, and reduced excitation of the baroreceptors. If resuscitation is not successful, this reflex response subsides as central nervous activity ceases, and the mean circulatory pressure usually falls to a value close to 7 mm Hg.

Blood reservoirs. Venoconstriction is considerably greater in certain regions of the body than in others. In effect, vascular beds that undergo significant venoconstriction constitute blood reservoirs. The vascular bed of the skin is one of the major blood reservoirs in humans. Blood loss evokes profound subcutaneous venoconstriction, which gives rise to the pale appearance of the skin characteristic of hemorrhage. The resultant diversion of blood away from the skin frees up several hundred milliliters of blood that can be perfused through more vital regions of the body. The vascular beds of the liver, lungs, and spleen are also important blood reservoirs. In the dog, the spleen is packed with red blood cells, and it can constrict to a small fraction of its normal size. During hemorrhage, this mechanism autotransfuses blood of high erythrocyte content into the general circulation. In humans, however, the volume changes of the spleen are considerably less extensive (see also Chapter 31).

Peripheral resistance. The changes in the vascular function curve induced by changes in arteriolar tone are shown in Fig. 29-7. As noted, the amount of blood in the arterioles is small—they contain only about 3% of total blood volume (see p 327). Hence, changes in the contractile state of these vessels do not significantly alter the mean circulatory pressure. Thus, a collection of vascular function curves that represent different peripheral resistances converges at a common point on the abscissa.

Equation 29-13 above indicates that P_v varies inversely with the total peripheral resistance (TPR) when all other factors remain constant. Physiologically, the relationship between P_v and TPR can be explained as follows: if cardiac output is held constant, a sudden increase in TPR causes a progressively greater volume of blood to be retained in the arterial system. Blood volume in the arterial system continues to increase until P_a rises sufficiently to force a flow of blood equal to the cardiac output through the resistance vessels. In the absence of any change in total blood volume, this increase in arterial blood volume is accompanied by an equivalent decrease in venous blood volume. Hence, an increase in TPR induces a reduction in P_v. Furthermore, the magnitude of the reduction in P_v will be proportionate to the increment in TPR. This relationship between TPR and the decrease in P_v, together with the inability of peripheral resistance to affect the mean circulatory pressure, accounts for the clockwise rotation of the vascular function curves with increased arteriolar constriction (Fig. 29-7). Similarly, arteriolar dilation produces a counterclockwise rotation from the same vertical axis intercept. A higher maximal level of cardiac output is attainable when the arterioles are dilated than when they are constricted (Fig. 29-7).

Interrelationships between cardiac output and venous return. Cardiac output and venous return are tightly linked. Except for small, transient disparities, the heart is unable to pump any more blood than is delivered to it through the venous system. Similarly, because the circulatory system is a closed circuit, the venous return to the heart must equal the cardiac output over any appreciable time interval. The flow around the entire closed circuit depends on the capability of the pump, the characteristics of the circuit, and the total volume of fluid in the system.

Thus, we can say that cardiac output and venous return are simply two terms for the flow around this closed circuit. Cardiac output is the volume of blood being pumped by the heart per unit time. Venous return is the volume of

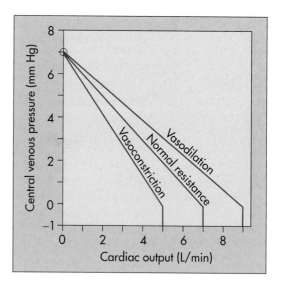

■ **Fig. 29-7** Effects of arteriolar dilation and constriction on the vascular function curve.

blood returning to the heart per unit time. At equilibrium, these two flows are equal. In the following section, we apply certain techniques of circuit analysis to gain some insight into the control of flow around the circuit.

■ *Relating the Cardiac Function Curve to the Vascular Function Curve*

■ *Coupling between the Heart and the Vasculature*

In accordance with Starling's law of the heart, cardiac output depends closely on right atrial or central venous pressure. Furthermore, right atrial pressure is approximately equal to right ventricular end-diastolic pressure, because the normal tricuspid valve acts as a low-resistance junction between the right atrium and ventricle. In the discussion that follows, graphs of cardiac output as a function of central venous pressure (P_v) are called **cardiac function curves.** Extrinsic regulatory influences may be expressed as shifts in such curves, as indicated in Chapter 24.

A typical cardiac function curve is plotted on the same coordinates as a normal vascular function curve in Fig. 29-8. The cardiac function curve is plotted according to the usual convention; that is, the independent variable (P_v) is plotted along the abscissa, and the dependent variable (cardiac output) is plotted along the ordinate. However, here is where the similarities between these two curves end. In accordance with the Frank-Starling mechanism, the cardiac function curve reveals that a rise in P_v increases cardiac output. Conversely, the vascular function curve describes an inverse relationship between cardiac output and P_v; that is, a rise in cardiac output

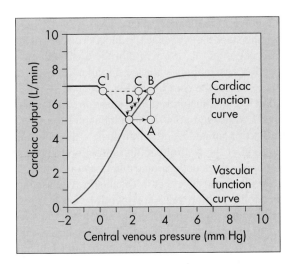

■ Fig. 29-8 Typical vascular and cardiac function curves plotted on the same coordinate axes. Note that to plot both curves on the same graph, the X and Y axes for the vascular function curves had to be reversed; compare the assignment of axes with that in Figs. 29-3, 29-6, and 29-7. The coordinates of the equilibrium point, at the intersection of the cardiac and vascular function curves, represent the stable values of cardiac output and central venous pressure at which the system tends to operate. Any perturbation (e.g., a sudden increase in venous pressure to point *A*) institutes a sequence of changes in cardiac output and venous pressure that restore these variables to their equilibrium values.

diminishes P_v. P_v is the dependent variable (or response) and cardiac output is the independent variable (or stimulus) for the vascular function curve. Therefore, to plot a vascular function curve in the conventional manner, P_v should be scaled along the Y axis and cardiac output should be scaled along the X axis. Note that this convention is honored for the vascular function curves displayed in Figs. 29-3, 29-6, and 29-7.

To plot the two curves on the same axes requires a drastic modification. *To include the cardiac and vascular function curves on the same set of coordinate axes, as in Fig. 29-8, it is necessary to violate the plotting convention for one of these curves. We have arbitrarily chosen to violate the convention for the vascular function curve.* Note that the vascular function curve in Fig. 29-8 is intended to reflect how P_v (scaled along the X axis) varies in response to a change of cardiac output (scaled along the Y axis).

When a cardiovascular system is represented by a given pair of cardiac and vascular function curves, the intersection of these two curves defines the **equilibrium point** of that system. The coordinates of this equilibrium point represent the values of cardiac output and P_v at which the system tends to operate. Only transient deviations from such values for cardiac output and P_v are possible, as long as the given cardiac and vascular function curves accurately describe the system.

The tendency of the cardiovascular system to operate about this equilibrium point may best be illustrated by examining its response to a sudden perturbation in the system. Consider the changes caused by a sudden rise in P_v from the equilibrium point to point *A* in Fig. 29-8. Such a change in P_v might be induced by rapid injection, during ventricular diastole, of a given volume of blood on the venous side of the circuit, and simultaneous withdrawal of an equal volume from the arterial side of the circuit. Thus, although P_v rises, the total blood volume remains constant.

As defined by the cardiac function curve, this elevated P_v would increase cardiac output (from *A* to *B*) during the next ventricular systole. The increased cardiac output in turn would transfer a net quantity of blood from the venous to the arterial side of the circuit, with a consequent reduction in P_v. In one heartbeat the reduction in P_v would be small (from *B* to *C*) because the heart would transfer only a tiny fraction of the total venous blood volume over to the arterial side. Because of this reduction in P_v, the cardiac output during the very next beat diminishes (from *C* to *D*) by an amount dictated by the cardiac function curve. Because *D* is still above the intersection point, the heart will pump blood from the veins to the arteries at a rate greater than that at which the blood will flow across the peripheral resistance from arteries to veins. Hence, P_v will continue to fall. This process will continue in diminishing steps until the point of intersection is reached. Only one specific combination of cardiac output and venous pressure—the equilibrium point, denoted by the coordinates of the point of the curves' intersection—will satisfy simultaneously the requirements of the cardiac and vascular function curves.

■ Myocardial Contractility

Combinations of cardiac and vascular function curves may also help explain the effects of alterations in ventricular contractility on cardiac output and P_v. In Fig. 29-9, the lower cardiac function curve represents the control state, whereas the upper curve reflects improved myocardial contractility. This pair of curves is analogous to the "family" of ventricular function curves shown in Fig. 24-19. The enhancement of ventricular contractility represented by the upper curve in Fig. 29-9 might be achieved experimentally by electrical stimulation of the cardiac sympathetic nerves. When the effects of such stimulation are restricted to the heart, the vascular function curve is unaffected. Therefore, only one vascular function curve is needed for this hypothetical intervention, as shown in Fig. 29-9.

During the control state of our hypothetical model, the equilibrium values for cardiac output and P_v are designated by point *A* in Fig. 29-9. Cardiac sympathetic nerve stimulation abruptly raises cardiac output to point *B*, because of the enhanced myocardial contractility.

However, this high cardiac output increases the net transfer of blood from the venous to the arterial side of the circuit, and consequently P_v then begins to fall (to point *C*). The reduction in P_v then leads to a small decrease in cardiac output. However, the cardiac output is still sufficiently high to effect the net transfer of blood from the venous to the arterial side of the circuit. Thus, P_v and cardiac output both continue to fall gradually until a new equilibrium point *(D)* is reached. This equilibrium point is located at the intersection of the vascular function curve with the new cardiac function curve. Point *D* lies above and to the left of the control equilibrium point *(A)*, and indicates that sympathetic stimulation can evoke a greater cardiac output at a lower level of P_v.

The actual biological response of an experimental animal to an enhancement of myocardial contractility is mimicked by the hypothetical change predicted by our model. In the experiment depicted in Fig. 29-10, the left stellate ganglion of an anesthetized dog was stimulated between the two arrows. During neural stimulation, the cardiac output (aortic flow) rose quickly to a peak value and then fell gradually to a steady-state value significantly greater than the control level. The increased aortic flow was accompanied by reductions in right and left atrial pressures (P_{RA} and P_{LA}).

Blood Volume

Changes in blood volume do not directly affect myocardial contractility, but they do influence the vascular func-

tion curve in the manner shown in Fig. 29-6. Therefore, to understand how changes in blood volume affect cardiac output and P_v, we will plot the appropriate cardiac function curve along with the vascular function curves that represent the control and experimental states.

Fig. 29-11 illustrates the response to a blood transfusion. Equilibrium point *B*, which denotes the values for cardiac output and P_v after transfusion, lies above and to the right of the control equilibrium point *A*. Thus, transfusion increases both cardiac output and P_v. Hemorrhage causes the opposite effect. Mechanistically, the change in ventricular filling pressure (central venous pressure) evoked by a given change in blood volume alters cardiac output by changing the sensitivity of the contractile proteins to the prevailing concentration of intracellular Ca^{++}, as explained in Chapters 23 and 24. For reasons explained earlier in this chapter, pure increases or decreases in venomotor tone elicit responses analogous to those evoked by increases or decreases, respectively, of total blood volume.

Heart failure is a general term that applies to conditions in which the pumping capability of the heart is impaired to the point that the tissues of the body are not adequately perfused. In heart failure, myocardial contractility is impaired. Heart failure may be acute or

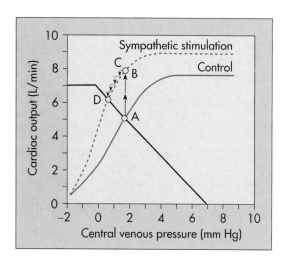

■ **Fig. 29-9**   An enhancement of myocardial contractility, as by cardiac sympathetic nerve stimulation, causes the equilibrium values of cardiac output and central venous pressure (P_v) to shift from the intersection (point *A*) of the control vascular and cardiac function curves *(continuous curve)* to the intersection (point *D*) of the same vascular function curve with the cardiac function curve *(dashed curve)* that represents the response to sympathetic stimulation.

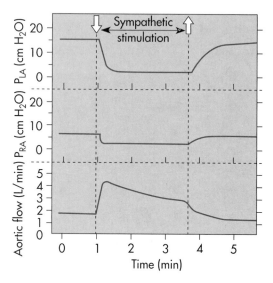

■ **Fig. 29-10**   During electrical stimulation of the left stellate ganglion (which contains cardiac sympathetic nerve fibers), the aortic blood flow (cardiac output) increased while pressures in the left atrium *(P_{LA})* and right atrium *(P_{RA})* diminished. These data conform with the conclusions derived from Fig. 29-9, in which the equilibrium values of cardiac output and venous pressure are observed to shift from point *A* to point *D* (i.e., cardiac output increased, but central venous pressure decreased) during cardiac sympathetic nerve stimulation. (Redrawn from Sarnoff SJ et al: *Circ Res* 8:1108, 1960, with permission of the American Heart Association.)

chronic. Consequently, in a graph of cardiac and vascular function curves, the cardiac function curve is shifted downward and to the right, as depicted in Fig. 29-12.

Acute heart failure may be caused by **toxic quantities of drugs or anesthetics** or by certain pathological conditions, such as sudden **coronary artery occlusion.** In acute heart failure, blood volume does not change immediately. In Fig. 29-12, therefore, the equilibrium point shifts from the intersection *(A)* of the normal curves to the intersection *(B* or *C)* of the normal vascular function curve with one of the curves that depict depressed cardiac function.

Chronic heart failure may occur in such conditions as **essential hypertension** or **ischemic heart disease.** In chronic heart failure, both the cardiac function and the vascular function curves shift. The vascular function curve shifts because of an increase in blood volume caused in part by fluid retention by the kidneys. The fluid retention is related to the concomitant reduction in glomerular filtration rate and to the increased secretion of aldosterone by the adrenal cortex (see also Chapters 42 and 51). The resultant hypervolemia is reflected by a rightward shift of the vascular function curve, as shown in Fig. 29-12. Hence, with moderate degrees of heart failure, P_v is elevated, but cardiac output may be normal *(D)*. With more severe degrees of heart failure, P_v is still greater, but cardiac output is subnormal *(E)*.

the cardiac and vascular function curves shift. When peripheral resistance increases (Fig. 29-13), the vascular function curve is rotated counterclockwise, but it converges on the same P_v axis intercept as the control curve (Fig. 29-7). Note that vasoconstriction causes a counterclockwise rotation of the vascular function curve in Fig. 29-13, but a clockwise rotation in Fig. 29-7. The direction of rotation differs, because the axes for the vascular function curves were reversed in these two figures, for reasons explained earlier in this chapter. The cardiac function curve in Fig. 29-13 is also shifted downward, because at any given P_v the heart is able to pump less blood against the greater cardiac afterload imposed by the increased peripheral resistance. Because both curves in Fig. 29-13 are displaced downward, the new equilibrium point, *B*, falls below the control point, *A*; that is, an increase in peripheral resistance diminishes the cardiac output.

Whether point *B* falls directly below point *A* or lies to the right or left of it depends on the magnitude of the shift in each curve. For example, if a given increase in peripheral resistance shifts the vascular function curve more than it does the cardiac function curve, equilibrium point *B* falls below and to the left of *A*; that is, both cardiac output and P_v diminish. Conversely, if the cardiac function curve is displaced more than the vascular function curve, point *B* falls below and to the right of point *A;* that is, cardiac output decreases, but P_v rises.

■ *Peripheral Resistance*

Analysis of the effects of changes in peripheral resistance on cardiac output and P_v is also complex, because both

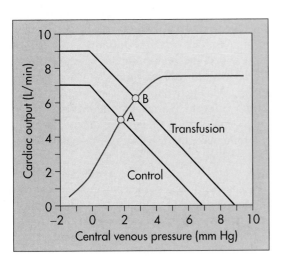

■ **Fig. 29-11** After a blood transfusion, the vascular function curve is shifted to the right. Therefore, cardiac output and venous pressure are both increased, as denoted by the translocation of the equilibrium point from *A* to *B*.

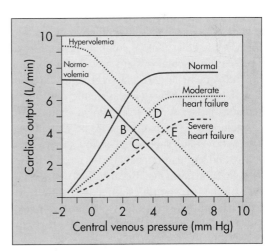

■ **Fig. 29-12** Moderate or severe heart failure shifts the cardiac function curves downward and to the right. Before blood volume changes, the cardiac output decreases and central venous pressure rises (from control equilibrium point *A* to point *B* or point *C*). After the increase in blood volume that usually occurs in heart failure, the vascular function curve is shifted to the right. Hence, central venous pressure may be elevated with no reduction in cardiac output (point *D*) or (in severe heart failure) with some reduction in cardiac output (point *E*).

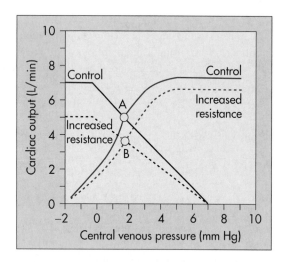

■ **Fig. 29-13** An increase in peripheral resistance shifts the cardiac and the vascular function curves downward. At equilibrium, the cardiac output is less *(B)* when the peripheral resistance is high than when it is normal *(A)*.

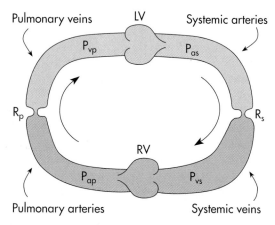

■ **Fig. 29-14** A simplified cardiovascular system model that consists of left *(LV)* and right *(RV)* ventricles, systemic *(R_s)* and pulmonary *(R_p)* vascular resistances, systemic arterial and venous compliances, and pulmonary arterial and venous compliances. P_{as} and P_{vs} are the pressures in the systemic arteries and veins, respectively; P_{ap} and P_{vp} are the pressures in the pulmonary arteries and veins, respectively.

■ *A More Complete Theoretical Model: The Two Pump System*

The preceding discussion shows that the interrelations between cardiac output and central venous pressure are complicated and perplexing even in an oversimplified circulation model that includes only one pump and only the systemic circulation. However, in reality, the cardiovascular system includes the systemic and pulmonary circulations and two pumps: the left and right ventricles. The interrelations are therefore much more complex.

Fig. 29-14 shows a more complete, but still oversimplified, cardiovascular system model that contains two pumps in series (the left and right ventricles) and two vascular beds in series (the systemic and pulmonary vasculature). The series arrangement requires that the flows pumped by the two ventricles be virtually equal to each other over any substantial period; otherwise, all the blood would ultimately accumulate in one or the other of the vascular systems. Because the cardiac function curves for the two ventricles differ substantially, the filling (atrial) pressures for the two ventricles must differ appropriately in order to ensure equal stroke volumes (see Fig. 24-18).

Any contractility change that affects the two ventricles differently alters the distribution of blood volume in the two vascular systems. For example, if a coronary artery to the left ventricle becomes suddenly occluded, left ventricular contractility will be impaired, and **acute left ventricular failure** will ensue. In the instant after occlusion, left atrial pressure will not change and the left ventricle will begin to pump a diminished flow. If the right ventricle is not

affected by the acute coronary artery occlusion, the right ventricle will initially continue to pump the normal flow. The disparate right and left ventricular outputs will result in a progressive increase in left atrial pressure and a progressive decrease in right atrial pressure. Therefore, left ventricular output will increase toward the normal value and right ventricular output will fall below the normal value. This process will continue until the outputs of the two ventricles again become equal. At this new equilibrium, the outputs of the two ventricles will be subnormal. The elevated left atrial pressure will be accompanied by an equally elevated pulmonary venous pressure, which can have serious clinical consequences. The high pulmonary venous pressure can increase lung stiffness and lead to respiratory distress by increasing the mechanical work of pulmonary ventilation. Furthermore, the high pulmonary venous pressure will elevate the hydrostatic pressure in the pulmonary capillaries and may therefore lead to the transudation of fluid from the pulmonary capillaries to the pulmonary interstitium or into the alveoli themselves **(pulmonary edema).** The last of these consequences may be lethal.

Two basic principles to keep in mind about ventricular function are that (1) the left ventricle pumps blood through the systemic vasculature and (2) the right ventricle pumps blood through the pulmonary vasculature. However, these principles do not necessarily imply that both ventricles are essential for the systemic and pulmonary vascular beds to be perfused adequately. To understand better the relationships between the two ventricles and the two vascular beds, let us examine right ventricular function in more detail.

In the circulatory system model shown in Fig. 29-14, consider the hemodynamic consequences that would prevail if the right ventricle suddenly ceased to function as a pump but instead served merely as a passive, low-resistance conduit between the systemic veins and the pulmonary arteries. Under these conditions, the only remaining functional pump would be the left ventricle. The left ventricle would then be required to pump blood through both the systemic and pulmonary resistances (for our purposes, consider the resistance to the flow of blood through the inactive right ventricle to be negligible).

Normally, the pulmonary resistance is about 10% as great as the systemic resistance. Because the two resistances are in series with one another, the total resistance would be 10% greater than the systemic resistance alone (see Chapter 25). In a normal cardiovascular system, a 10% increase in systemic vascular resistance would increase mean arterial pressure (and hence left ventricular afterload) by approximately 10%. This increase would not drastically affect left ventricular function. However, if certain conditions are in place, this increase in mean arterial pressure can significantly alter the function of the cardiovascular system. *If the 10% increase in total resistance is achieved by adding a small resistance (i.e., the pulmonary vascular resistance) to that of the much larger systemic resistance, and if the pulmonary vascular resistance is separated from the systemic resistance by a large compliance (the combined systemic venous and pulmonary arterial compliance), the 10% increase in total resistance will drastically impair the operation of the cardiovascular system.*

The simulated effects of inactivating the pumping action of the right ventricle in a hydraulic analog of the circulatory system are shown in Fig. 29-15. In the model, the right and left ventricles generate cardiac outputs that vary directly with their respective filling pressures. Under control conditions (when the right ventricle is functioning normally), the outputs of the left and right ventricles are equal (5 L/min). The right ventricular pumping action causes the pressure in the pulmonary artery (not shown) to exceed the pressure in the pulmonary veins (P_{vp}) by an amount that will force fluid through the pulmonary vascular resistance at a rate of 5 L/min.

When the right ventricle ceases pumping (arrow *1*), the systemic venous and pulmonary arterial systems, along with the right ventricle itself, become a common passive conduit with a large compliance (Fig. 29-14). When the right ventricle ceases to transfer blood actively from the pulmonary veins to the pulmonary arteries, the pulmonary arterial pressure (P_{ap}) decreases rapidly (not shown), and systemic venous pressure (P_{vs}) rises rapidly to a common value (about 5 mm Hg in Fig. 29-15). At this low pressure, however, fluid flows from the pulmonary arteries to the pulmonary veins at a greatly reduced rate. At the start of right ventricular arrest, the left ventricle is pumping fluid from the pulmonary veins

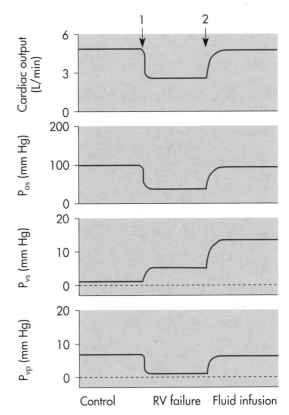

■ **Fig. 29-15** The changes in cardiac output, systemic arterial pressure (P_{as}), systemic venous pressure (P_{vs}), and pulmonary venous pressure (P_{vp}) evoked by simulated right ventricular failure and by simulated fluid infusion in the circulatory model shown in Fig. 29-14. At arrow *1*, the pumping action of the right ventricle was discontinued (simulated right ventricular failure), and the right ventricle served only as a low-resistance conduit. At arrow *2*, the fluid volume in the system was expanded, and the right ventricle continued to serve only as a conduit. (Modified from Furey SA, Zieske HA, Levy MN: *Am Heart J* 107:404, 1984.)

to the systemic arteries at the control rate of 5 L/min, which greatly exceeds the rate at which blood returns to the pulmonary veins once the right ventricle ceases to operate. Hence, the pulmonary venous pressure (P_{vp}) drops sharply. Because the pulmonary venous pressure is the preload for the left ventricle, the left ventricular (cardiac) output drops abruptly as well, to attain a steady-state value of about 2.5 L/min. This effect in turn leads to a rapid reduction in systemic arterial pressure (P_{as}). In short, *stoppage of right ventricular pumping markedly curtails cardiac output, systemic arterial pressure, and pulmonary venous pressure and raises systemic venous pressure moderately* (Fig. 29-15).

Most of the hemodynamic problems induced by inactivation of the right ventricle can be reversed by increasing the fluid (blood) volume of the system (arrow *2*, Fig. 29-15). If fluid is added until the pulmonary venous pressure (left ventricular preload) is raised to its control value, the cardiac output and systemic arterial pressure are restored almost to normal, but systemic venous pressure is abnormally elevated. If left ventricular function is normal, adding a normal left ventricular preload will evoke a normal left ventricular output; the 10% increase in peripheral resistance caused by adding the pulmonary vascular resistance to that of the systemic vascular resistance does not impose a serious burden on the left ventricular pumping capacity. When the right ventricle is inoperative, however, the pulmonary blood flow will not be normal unless the usual pulmonary arteriovenous pressure gradient (about 10 to 15 mm Hg) prevails. Hence, the systemic venous pressure (P_{vs}) must exceed the pulmonary venous pressure (P_{vp}) by this amount. Maintenance of high systemic venous pressures may lead to the accumulation of fluid (**edema**) in the dependent regions of the body. Such edema is a characteristic finding in patients with **right ventricular heart failure.**

With these findings in mind, we may state the principal function of the right ventricle as follows. From the viewpoint of providing sufficient flow of blood to all the tissues in the body, the left ventricle alone is adequate to carry out this function. The operation of two ventricles in series is not essential to provide adequate blood flow to the tissues. *The crucial function of the right ventricle is to prevent the rise in systemic venous (and pulmonary arterial) pressure that would be required to force the normal cardiac output through the pulmonary vascular resistance.* A normal right ventricle, by preventing an abnormal rise in systemic venous pressure, prevents the occurrence of extensive dependent edema.

Clinically, **right ventricular heart failure** may be caused by occlusive disease predominantly of the coronary vessels to the right ventricle. These vessels are affected much less commonly than are the vessels to the left ventricle. The major hemodynamic effects of acute right heart failure are pronounced reductions in cardiac output and in arterial blood pressure, and the principal treatment is the infusion of blood or plasma. Bypass of the right ventricle (by anastomosing the right atrium to the pulmonary artery) may be performed surgically for patients with certain **congenital cardiac defects,** such as severe narrowing of the tricuspid valve or maldevelopment of the right ventricle. The effects of acute right heart failure or of right ventricular bypass are directionally similar to those predicted above by the model analysis (Fig. 29-15).

■ *Role of Heart Rate in Control of Cardiac Output*

Cardiac output is the product of stroke volume and heart rate. The above analysis of the control of cardiac output has been restricted to the control of stroke volume, and the role of the heart rate has been ignored. We now consider the effects of changes in heart rate on cardiac output. The analysis is complex, because a change in heart rate alters the other three factors (preload, afterload, and contractility) that determine stroke volume (Fig. 29-1). An increase in heart rate, for example, shortens the duration of diastole. Hence, ventricular filling is diminished; that is, preload is reduced. If an increase in heart rate did alter cardiac output, the arterial pressure would change; that is, afterload would be altered. Finally, a rise in heart rate would increase the net influx of Ca^{++} per minute into the myocardial cells (see also Chapter 24), and this influx would enhance myocardial contractility.

The effects of changes in heart rate on cardiac output have been studied extensively in human subjects and in experimental animals, and the results are similar to those shown in Fig. 29-16. This experiment was performed on an anesthetized dog. As the atrial pacing frequency was gradually increased, the stroke volume (SV) progressively diminished (Fig. 29-16, *A*). Presumably, the decrease in SV was caused by the reduced time for ventricular filling. The changes in SV were evidently not inversely proportional to the changes in heart rate (HR), because the direction of the change in cardiac output (Q_h) was influenced markedly by the actual level of HR (Fig. 29-16, *B*). For example, as the pacing frequency was increased over the range of 50 to 100 beats/min, an increase in HR augmented Q_h. Because $Q_h = SV \times HR$, it is evident that over this frequency range, the decrease in SV must have been proportionately less than the increase in HR.

Over the frequency range from about 100 to 200 beats/min, however, Q_h was not affected significantly by changes in pacing frequency (Fig. 29-16, *B*). Hence, as

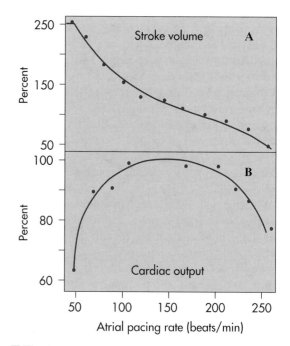

■ **Fig. 29-16**   The changes in stroke volume (**A**) and cardiac output (**B**) induced by changing the rate of atrial pacing in an anesthetized dog. (Redrawn from Kumada M, Azuma T, Matsuda K: *Jpn J Physiol* 17:538, 1967.)

the pacing frequency was increased, the decrease in SV must have been approximately equal to the increase in HR. Also, generalized vascular autoregulation tends to keep tissue blood flow constant (see also Chapter 28). This adaptation leads to changes in preload and afterload that keep Q_h nearly constant.

Finally, at excessively high pacing frequencies (above 200 beats/min in Fig. 29-16), further increases in HR decreased Q_h. Therefore, the induced decrease in SV must have exceeded the increase in HR over this high range of pacing frequencies. Evidently, at such high pacing frequencies, the ventricular filling time was so severely restricted that compensation was inadequate and cardiac output decreased sharply. Although the relationship of Q_h to HR is characteristically that of an inverted U in the general population, the relationship varies quantitatively among subjects and among physiological states in any given subject.

The characteristic relationship between cardiac output and heart rate explains the urgent need for treatment of patients who have excessively slow or excessively fast heart rates. Profound **bradycardias** (slow rates) may occur as a result of a very slow sinus rhythm in patients with **sick sinus syndrome** or as a result of a slow idioventricular rhythm in patients with **complete atrioventricular block.** In either rhythm disturbance, the capacity of the ventricles to fill during a prolonged diastole is limited (often by the noncompliant pericardium). Hence, cardiac output usually decreases substantially, because the very slow heart rate cannot be counterbalanced by a sufficiently large stroke volume. Consequently, these rhythm disturbances often require the installation of an artificial pacemaker.

Excessively high heart rates in patients with **supraventricular** or **ventricular tachycardias** often require emergency treatment, because these patients have cardiac outputs that may be critically low. In such patients, the filling time is so restricted at very high heart rates that even small additional reductions in filling time cause disproportionately severe reductions in filling volume. Slowing the tachycardia to a more normal rhythm can usually be accomplished pharmacologically, but **cardioversion,** by delivering a strong electric current across the thorax or directly to the heart through an implanted device, may be required in emergencies.

Strong correlations between heart rate and cardiac output must be interpreted cautiously, as must all correlations between important factors. Interpretation of the correlation between the changes in heart rate and cardiac output that prevail in physical exercise provides an excellent example of why this caution is needed. In exercising subjects, cardiac output and heart rate usually increase proportionately, and the stroke volume may remain constant or increase slightly (see also Chapter 31). The temptation is great to conclude that the increase in cardiac output must be caused by the observed increase in heart rate, because of the striking correlation between cardiac output and heart rate. However, Fig. 29-16 emphasizes that, over a wide range of heart rates, a change in heart rate per se has little influence on cardiac output. Several studies on exercising subjects have confirmed that even during exercise, changes in pacing frequency do not alter cardiac output very much.

The principal increase in cardiac output during exercise must therefore be attributed to other factors, notably the pronounced reduction in peripheral vascular resistance because of the vasodilation in the active skeletal muscles, and the increased contractility of the cardiac muscle associated with the generalized increase in sympathetic neural activity. Nevertheless, the increase in heart rate is still an important factor, even if it cannot be assigned a key causative role for the increase in cardiac output. Abundant data show that if the heart rate cannot increase normally during exercise, the augmentation of cardiac output and the capacity for exercise are severely limited. Stroke volume changes only slightly during exercise. Therefore, *the increase in heart rate plays an important permissive role in augmenting cardiac output during physical exercise.*

■ Ancillary Factors That Affect the Venous System and Cardiac Output

In earlier sections of this chapter, we oversimplified the interrelationships between central venous pressure and cardiac output by restricting our discussion to the effects evoked by individual variables. However, because the cardiovascular system is regulated by so many feedback control loops, its responses are rarely simple. A change in blood volume, for example, not only affects cardiac output directly by the Frank-Starling mechanism, but also triggers reflexes that alter other aspects of cardiac function (such as heart rate, atrioventricular conduction, and myocardial contractility) and other characteristics of the vascular system (such as peripheral resistance and venomotor tone). Several ancillary factors, especially gravity and respiration, also regulate cardiac output. These ancillary factors may be considered to operate by means of some of the more basic mechanisms that have already been considered.

■ Gravity

Gravitational forces may profoundly affect cardiac output. For example, soldiers standing at attention for a long time may faint because gravity causes blood to pool in the dependent blood vessels, thereby reducing cardiac output. Warm ambient temperatures interfere with the compensatory vasomotor reactions, and the absence of muscular activity exaggerates these effects. Gravitational effects are amplified in airplane pilots during pullouts from dives. The centrifugal force in the footward direction may be several times greater than the force of gravity. Pilots characteristically black out momentarily during the maneuver, as blood is drained from the cephalic regions and pooled in the lower parts of the body.

Some of the explanations for the reduction in cardiac output under such conditions are not accurate. It is argued that when an individual is standing, the forces of gravity impede venous return to the heart from the dependent regions of the body. This statement is incomplete, however, because it ignores the gravitational counterforce on the arterial side of the same vascular circuit, and this counterforce facilitates venous return.

In this sense, the vascular system resembles a U tube. To understand the effects of gravity on flow through this U-shaped hydraulic system, look at the models depicted in Figs. 29-17 and 29-18. In Fig. 29-17, all the U tubes represent rigid cylinders of constant diameter. With both limbs of the U tube oriented horizontally *(A)*, the flow depends only on the pressures at the inflow and outflow ends of the tube (P_i and P_o, respectively), the viscosity of the fluid, and the length and radius of the tube, in accordance with Poiseuille's equation (see Chapter 25). When the cross-sectional area of the tube limbs is constant, the pressure gradient is uniform; hence, the pressure midway down the tube (P_m) equals the average of the inflow and outflow pressures.

However, when the U tube is oriented vertically *(B* to *D)*, hydrostatic forces must now be considered. In tube *B*, both limbs are open to atmospheric pressure and both ends are located at the same hydrostatic level; hence, there is no flow. The pressure, P_m, at the midpoint of the tube equals ρhg, where ρ is the density of the fluid; h is the height of the U tube; and g is the acceleration of gravity. In this example, the midpoint pressure of tube *B* is 80 mm Hg.

Now consider tube *C*. This tube is oriented in the same way as tube *B*, but a 100 mm Hg pressure difference is applied across the two ends. The flow precisely equals that in *A*, because the pressure gradient, tube dimensions, and fluid viscosity are all the same. Gravitational forces are precisely equal in magnitude but opposite in direction in the two limbs of the U tube. Because the flow will be the same as that in *A*, the pressure drop will be 50 mm Hg at the midpoint, because of the viscous losses that result from flow. Furthermore, gravity will tend to increase pressure by 80 mm Hg at the midpoint, just as in tube *B*. The actual pressure at the midpoint of tube *C* will be the algebraic sum of the viscous loss and hydrostatic gain, or 130 mm Hg in this example.

In tube *D*, a pressure gradient of 100 mm Hg is applied to the same U tube (i.e., *C*), but the tube is oriented in the opposite direction ("upside down"). Gravitational forces will be so directed that the pressure at the midpoint will

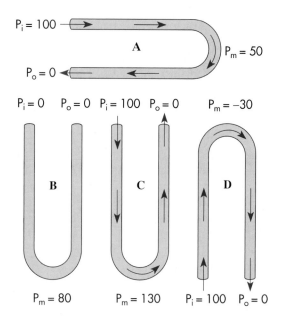

■ **Fig. 29-17**   Pressure distributions in rigid U tubes, all with the same dimensions. For a given inflow pressure ($P_i = 100$) and outflow pressure ($P_o = 0$), the pressure at the midpoint (P_m) depends on the orientation of the U tube, but the flow through the tube is independent of the orientation.

tend to be 80 mm Hg less than that at the end of the U tube. However, viscous losses will still produce a 50 mm Hg pressure drop at the midpoint relative to P_i. Hence, when the tube is oriented as in tube *D*, pressure at the midpoint of the U tube will be -30 mm Hg (i.e., 30 mm Hg below the ambient pressure). Flow will of course be the same as in tubes *A* and *C*, for the reasons stated for tube *C*.

As we can see from Fig. 29-17, in a system of rigid U tubes, gravitational effects do not alter the rate of fluid flow. However, experience does show that gravity affects the cardiovascular system, sometimes dramatically. The reason is that the vessels are *distensible*, not rigid. These gravitational effects can be explained by analyzing the pressures in a set of U tubes with distensible components (at the bends in the tubes of Fig. 29-18). In tubes *A* and *B*, the pressure distributions will resemble those in tubes *A* and *C*, respectively, of Fig. 29-17. Because the pressure is higher at the bend of tube *B* than at the bend of tube *A* in Fig. 29-18 and because the segments are distensible in this region, the distention at the bend in tube *B* will exceed that at the bend in tube *A*. The extent of the distention will depend on the compliance of these tube segments. Because flow varies directly with the tube diameter, the flow through tube *B* in Fig. 29-18 will exceed the flow through tube *A* for a given pressure difference applied at the ends.

Because orienting a U tube with its bend downward actually increases rather than diminishes flow, how then is the observed impairment of cardiovascular function explained when the orientation of the body is similarly changed? The reason is that the cardiovascular system is

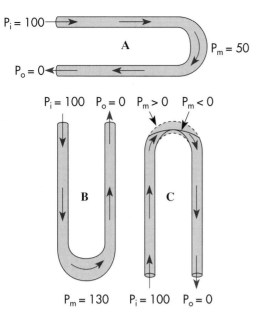

■ **Fig. 29-18** In U tubes with a *distensible section* at the bend, even when inflow pressures *(P_i)* are the same for each tube and the outflow pressures *(P_o)* are the same for each tube, the resistance to flow and the fluid volume contained within each tube vary with the orientation of the tube. *P_m* is the pressure at the midpoint of each tube.

a closed circuit of constant fluid (blood) volume, whereas the U tube is an open conduit supplied by a fluid source of unlimited volume. In the dependent regions of the cardiovascular system, the distention occurs more on the venous than on the arterial side of the circuit, because the venous compliance is so much greater than the arterial compliance. Such venous distention is readily observed on the back of the hands when the arms are allowed to hang down below the level of the right atrium.

The hemodynamic effects of such venous distention **(venous pooling)** resemble those caused by the hemorrhage of an equivalent volume of blood from the body. When an adult person shifts from a supine position to a relaxed standing position, 300 to 800 ml of blood pools in the legs. This pooling may reduce cardiac output by about 2 L/min. The compensatory adjustments to assumption of a standing position are similar to the adjustments to blood loss. For example, the diminished baroreceptor excitation triggers a reflex that speeds the heart rate, strengthens the cardiac contraction, and constricts the arterioles and veins. The baroreceptor reflex has a greater effect on the resistance than on the capacitance vessels.

Many of the drugs used to treat chronic **hypertension** interfere with the reflex adaptation to standing. Similarly, astronauts exposed to weightlessness lose their adaptations after a few days in space, and they experience pronounced difficulties when they first return to earth. When astronauts and other individuals with impaired reflex adaptations stand, their blood pressures may drop substantially. This response is called **orthostatic hypotension,** which may cause lightheadedness or fainting.

When the U tube is rotated so that the bend is directed upward (Fig. 29-18, tube *C*), the effects are opposite to those that take place in tube *B*. The pressure at the bend of tube *C* would tend to be −30 mm Hg, just as in tube *D* of Fig. 29-17. However, because the ambient pressure exceeds the internal pressure, the distensible segment of tube *C* will collapse. Flow will then cease, and therefore the decline of pressure associated with viscous flow will disappear. When flow stops in U tube C, the pressure at the top of each limb will be 80 mm Hg less than at the bottom (the hydrostatic pressure difference). Hence, in the left (or inflow) limb, the pressure will approach 20 mm Hg. As soon as this pressure exceeds ambient pressure (0 mm Hg), the collapsed tubing will be forced open and flow will begin. With the initiation of flow, however, pressure at the bend will again drop below the ambient pressure. Thus, the tubing at the bend will flutter; that is, it will fluctuate between the open and closed states.

When a subject raises an arm, the cutaneous veins in the hand and forearm collapse, for the reasons already described. Fluttering does not occur here, because the deeper veins are protected from collapse by being tethered to surrounding structures. This protection allows the deep veins to accommodate the flow that is ordinarily carried by the collapsed superficial veins. In our hydraulic model, this protection can be simulated by adding a rigid tube (representing the deeper veins) in parallel with the collapsible tube (representing the superficial veins) at the bend of tube *C* in Fig. 29-18. The collapsible tube would no longer flutter but would remain closed. All flow would occur through the rigid tube, just as in tube *D* in Fig. 29-17.

The superficial veins in the neck are ordinarily partially collapsed when a normal individual is upright. Venous return from the head is conducted largely through the deeper cervical veins. However, when central venous pressure is abnormally elevated, the superficial neck veins are distended and they do not collapse even when the subject sits or stands. Such cervical venous distention is an important clinical sign of **congestive heart failure.**

■ *Muscular Activity and Venous Valves*

When a recumbent person stands but remains at rest, the pressure rises in the veins in the dependent regions of the body. The venous pressure in the legs increases gradually and does not reach an equilibrium value until almost 1 minute after standing. The slowness of this rise in P_v is attributable to the venous valves, which permit flow only toward the heart. When a person stands, the valves prevent blood in the veins from falling toward the feet. Hence, the column of venous blood is supported at numerous levels by these valves. Because of these valves, the venous column can be thought of as consisting of many discontinuous segments. However, blood continues to enter the column from many venules and small tributary veins, and the pressure continues to rise. As soon as the pressure in one segment exceeds that in the segment just above it, the intervening valve is forced open. Ultimately all the valves are open and the column is continuous, similar to the status in the outflow limbs of the U tubes shown in Figs. 29-17 and 29-18.

Precise measurement reveals that the final level of P_v in the feet during quiet standing is only slightly greater than that in a static column of blood extending from the right atrium to the feet. This finding indicates that the pressure drop caused by blood flow from the foot veins to the right atrium is very small. This very low resistance justifies considering all the veins as a common venous compliance in the circulatory system model illustrated in Fig. 29-2.

When an individual who has been standing quietly begins to walk, the venous pressure in the legs decreases appreciably (Fig. 29-19). Because of the intermittent venous compression exerted by the contracting leg muscles and because of the operation of the venous valves, blood is forced from the veins toward the heart (see Fig. 30-11). Hence, muscular contraction lowers the mean venous pressure in the legs and serves as an **auxiliary pump.** Furthermore, muscular contraction prevents venous pooling and lowers capillary hydrostatic pressure. In this way, muscular contraction reduces the tendency for edema fluid to collect in the feet during standing.

This auxiliary pumping mechanism generated by skeletal muscle contractions is not effective in people with **varicose veins** in their legs. The valves in these defective veins do not function properly, and therefore when the leg muscles contract, the blood in the leg veins is forced in the retrograde as well as in the antegrade direction. Thus, when an individual with varicose veins stands or walks, the venous pressure in the ankles and feet is excessively high. The consequent high capillary pressure leads to the accumulation of edema fluid in the ankles and feet.

■ *Circulatory Effects of Respiratory Activity*

The normal, periodic activity of the respiratory muscles causes rhythmic variations in vena caval flow (Fig. 29-20). During respiration, the reduction in intrathoracic pressure is transmitted to the lumina of the thoracic blood vessels. The reduction in central venous pressure during inspiration increases the pressure gradient between extrathoracic and intrathoracic veins. The consequent acceleration of venous return to the right atrium is shown in Fig. 29-20 as an increase in superior vena caval blood flow from 5.2 ml/sec during expiration to 11 ml/sec during inspiration.

The exaggerated reduction in intrathoracic pressure achieved by a strong inspiratory effort against a closed glottis (called **Müller's maneuver**) does not increase venous return proportionately. The extrathoracic veins collapse near their entry into the chest when their internal pressures fall below the ambient level. As the veins collapse, flow into the chest momentarily stops. The cessation of flow raises pressure upstream, forcing the col-

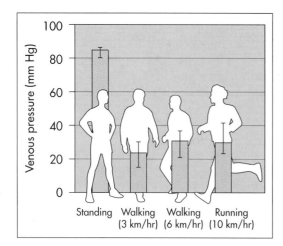

■ **Fig. 29-19**   Mean pressures ($\pm$ 95% confidence intervals) in the foot veins of 18 human subjects during quiet standing, walking, and running. (From Stick C, Jaeger H, Wizleb E: *J Appl Physiol* 72:2063, 1992.)

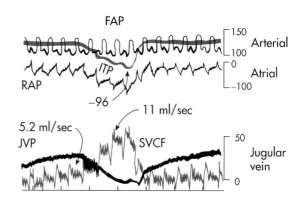

■ **Fig. 29-20**   During a normal inspiration intrathoracic *(ITP)*, right atrial *(RAP)*, and jugular venous *(JVP)* pressures decrease, and flow in the superior vena cava *(SVCF)* increases (from 5.2 to 11 ml/sec). All pressures are in mm H_2O, except for femoral arterial pressure *(FAP)*, which is in mm Hg. (Modified from Brecher GA: *Venous return,* New York, 1956, Grune & Stratton.)

lapsed segment to open again. The process is repetitive; the venous segments adjacent to the chest alternately open and close.

During normal expiration, flow into the central veins decelerates. However, the mean rate of venous return during normal respiration exceeds the flow during a brief period of **apnea** (cessation of respiration). Hence, normal inspiration apparently facilitates venous return more than normal expiration impedes it. In part, this facilitation of venous return is implemented by the valves in the veins of the extremities and neck. These valves prevent any reversal of flow during expiration. Thus, the respiratory muscles and venous valves constitute an **auxiliary pump** for venous return.

Sustained expiratory efforts increase intrathoracic pressure and thereby impede venous return. Straining against a closed glottis (termed **Valsalva's maneuver**) regularly occurs during coughing, defecation, and heavy lifting. Intrathoracic pressures in excess of 100 mm Hg have been recorded in trumpet players, and pressures over 400 mm Hg have been observed during paroxysms of coughing. Such pressure increases are transmitted directly to the lumina of the intrathoracic arteries. After coughing stops, the arterial blood pressure may fall precipitously because of the preceding impediment to venous return.

> The dramatic increase in intrathoracic pressure induced by coughing constitutes an **auxiliary pumping mechanism** for the blood, despite its concurrent tendency to impede venous return. Patients undergoing certain diagnostic procedures, such as coronary angiography or electrophysiological testing, are at increased risk for ventricular fibrillation. Such patients are trained to cough rhythmically on command. If ventricular fibrillation does occur, each cough can generate substantial arterial blood pressure increases, and enough cerebral blood flow may be promoted to sustain consciousness. The cough raises the intravascular pressure equally in intrathoracic arteries and veins. Blood is propelled through the extrathoracic tissues, however, because the increased pressure is transmitted to the extrathoracic arteries, but not to the extrathoracic veins, because the venous valves prevent backflow from the intrathoracic to the extrathoracic veins.

■ *Artificial Respiration*

In most forms of artificial respiration (mouth-to-mouth resuscitation, mechanical respiration), lung inflation is achieved by applying endotracheal pressures above atmospheric pressure, and expiration occurs by passive recoil of the thoracic cage. Thus, lung inflation is accompanied by an appreciable rise in intrathoracic pressure. Vena caval flow decreases sharply during the phase of positive-pressure lung inflation (indicated by the progressive rise in endotracheal pressure in the central portion of Fig. 29-21). When negative endotracheal pressure (indicated by the abrupt decrease in endotracheal pressure in the right half of Fig. 29-21) is used to facilitate deflation, vena caval flow accelerates more than when the lungs are allowed to deflate passively (near the left border of Fig. 29-21).

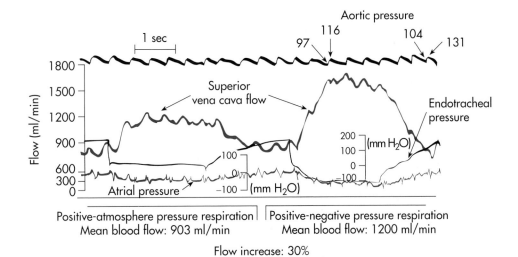

■ **Fig. 29-21** During intermittent positive-pressure respiration, the flow in the superior vena cava is approximately 30% greater when the lungs are deflated actively by applying negative endotracheal pressure *(right side)* than when they are allowed to deflate passively against atmospheric pressure *(left side)*. (Modified from Brecher GA: *Venous return,* New York, 1956, Grune & Stratton.)

■ *Summary*

1. Two important relationships between cardiac output (Q_h) and central venous pressure (P_v) prevail in the cardiovascular system: one applies to the heart and the other to the vascular system.

2. With respect to the heart, Q_h varies directly with P_v (or preload) over a very wide range of P_v. This relationship is represented by the cardiac function curve, and it expresses the Frank-Starling mechanism.

3. With respect to the vascular system, P_v varies inversely with Q_h. This relationship is represented by the vascular function curve, and it reflects the fact that as Q_h increases, a greater fraction of the total blood volume resides in the arteries and a smaller volume resides in the veins.

4. The principal mechanisms that govern the cardiac function curve are the changes in numbers of crossbridges that interact and in the affinity of the contractile proteins for calcium. These mechanisms are evoked by changes in the cardiac filling pressure (preload).

5. The principal factors that govern the vascular function curve are the arterial and venous compliances, the peripheral vascular resistance, and the total blood volume.

6. The equilibrium values of Q_h and P_v that prevail under a given set of conditions are determined by the intersection of the cardiac and vascular function curves.

7. At very low and very high heart rates, the heart is unable to pump adequate Q_h. At very low heart rates, the increase in filling during diastole cannot compensate for the small number of cardiac contractions per minute. At very high heart rates, the large number of contractions per minute cannot compensate for the inadequate filling time.

8. Gravity influences Q_h because the veins are so compliant, and substantial quantities of blood tend to pool in the veins of the dependent portions of the body.

9. Respiration changes the pressure gradient between the intrathoracic and extrathoracic veins. Hence, respiration serves as an auxiliary pump, which may affect the mean level of Q_h and may induce rhythmic changes in stroke volume during the various phases of the respiratory cycle.

■ *Self-Study Problems*

1. Is the ventricular preload a determinant of cardiac performance, or does cardiac performance determine the preload?

2. What effect does the arterial blood pressure have on cardiac performance?

3. If isoproterenol were infused into the left coronary artery at such a rate that it would influence myocardial contractility exclusively, what effects would that infusion have on cardiac output and central venous pressure?

4. If 2 L of blood were infused into a normal human subject, what influence would that transfusion have on cardiac output and central venous pressure?

5. If a person with a healthy myocardium suddenly develops complete atrioventricular block, and the ventricular rate becomes 35 beats/min, what will happen to cardiac output and central venous pressure?

6. If a person is strapped to a tilt table in such a manner that he will not have to use his skeletal muscles when he is tilted to the upright position, what will happen to his cardiac output, mean arterial pressure, central venous pressure, and pressure in a foot vein when he is tilted to that position?

■ *Bibliography*

Journal articles

Aukland K: Why don't our feet swell in the upright position?, *News Physiol Soc* 9:214, 1994.

Bedford TG, Dormer KJ: Arterial hemodynamics during head-up tilt in conscious dogs, *J Appl Physiol* 65:1556, 1988.

Bromberger-Barnea B: Mechanical effects of inspiration on heart functions: a review, *Fed Proc* 40:2172, 1981.

Ferlinz J: Right ventricular function in adult cardiovascular disease, *Prog Cardiovasc Dis* 25:225, 1982.

Furey SA, Zieske HA, Levy MN: The essential function of the right ventricle, *Am Heart J* 107:404, 1984.

Geddes LA, Wessale JL: Cardiac output, stroke volume, and pacing rate, *J Cardiovasc Electrophysiol* 2:408, 1991.

Lacolley PJ et al: Microgravity and orthostatic intolerance: carotid hemodynamics and peripheral responses, *Am J Physiol* 264:H588, 1993.

Levy MN: The cardiac and vascular factors that determine systemic blood flow, *Circ Res* 44:739, 1979.

Monos E, Bérczi V, Nadasy G: Local control of veins: biomechanical, metabolic, and humoral aspects, *Physiol Rev* 75:611, 1995.

Risøe C, Tan W, Smiseth OA: Effect of carotid sinus baroreceptor reflex on hepatic and splenic vascular capacitance in vagotomized dogs, *Am J Physiol* 266:H1528, 1994.

Rothe CF: Mean circulatory filling pressure: its meaning and measurement, *J Appl Physiol* 74:499, 1993.

Rothe CF, Gaddis ML: Autoregulation of cardiac output by passive elastic characteristics of the vascular capacitance system, *Circulation* 81:360, 1990.

Seymour RS, Hargens AR, Pedley TJ: The heart works against gravity, *Am J Physiol* 265:R715, 1993.

Sheriff DD, Zhou XP, Scher AM, Rowell LB: Dependence of cardiac filling pressure on cardiac output during rest and dynamic exercise in dogs, *Am J Physiol* 265:H316, 1993.

Shoukas AA: Overall systems analysis of the carotid sinus baroreceptor reflex control of the circulation, *Anesthesiology,* 79:1402, 1993.

Shoukas AA, Bohlen HG: Rat venular pressure-diameter relationships are regulated by sympathetic activity, *Am J Physiol* 259:H674, 1990.

Stick C, Jaeger H, Witzleb E: Measurement of volume changes and venous pressure in the human lower leg during walking and running, *J Appl Physiol* 72:2063, 1992.

Tyberg JV: Venous modulation of ventricular preload, *Am Heart J* 123:1098, 1992.

Ursino M, Antonucci M, Belardinelli E: Role of active changes in venous capacity by the carotid baroreflex: analysis with a mathematical model, *Am J Physiol* 267:H2531, 1994.

Books and monographs

Guyton AC, Jones CE, Coleman TG: *Circulatory physiology: cardiac output and its regulation,* ed 2, Philadelphia, 1973, WB Saunders.

Rothe CF: Venous system: physiology of the capacitance vessels. In *Handbook of physiology,* sect 2, *The cardiovascular system—peripheral circulation and organ blood flow,* vol III, Bethesda, Md, 1983, American Physiological Society.

Smith JJ, editor: *Circulatory response to the upright posture,* Boca Raton, Fla, 1990, CRC Press.

Yin FCP, editor: *Ventricular/vascular coupling,* New York, 1987, Springer-Verlag.

Special Circulations

■ *Coronary Circulation*
■ *Functional Anatomy of Coronary Vessels*

The right and left coronary arteries arise at the root of the aorta behind the right and left cusps of the aortic valve, respectively. These arteries provide the entire blood supply to the myocardium. The right coronary artery principally supplies the right ventricle and atrium; the left coronary artery, which divides near its origin into the anterior descending and the circumflex branches, principally supplies the left ventricle and atrium. However, some overlap exists between the left and right arteries. In humans, the right coronary artery is dominant (supplying most of the myocardium) in 50% of individuals. The left coronary artery is dominant in another 20%, and the flow delivered by each main artery is about equal in the remaining 30%. The epicardial distribution of the coronary arteries and veins is illustrated in Fig. 30-1.

After the coronary venous blood passes through the capillary beds, most of it returns to the right atrium through the coronary sinus, but some reaches the right atrium by way of the anterior coronary veins. In addition, vascular communications directly link the vessels of the myocardium and the cardiac chambers; these communications are the **arteriosinusoidal, arterioluminal,** and **thebesian vessels.** The arteriosinusoidal channels consist of small arteries or arterioles that lose their arterial structure as they penetrate the chamber walls, where they divide into irregular, endothelium-lined sinuses. These sinuses anastomose with other sinuses and with capillaries and communicate with the cardiac chambers. The arterioluminal vessels are small arteries or arterioles that open directly into the atria and ventricles. The thebesian vessels are small veins that connect capillary beds directly with the cardiac chambers and also communicate with cardiac veins. On the basis of anatomic studies, all the minute vessels of the myocardium communicate in the form of an extensive plexus of subendocardial vessels. However, the myocardium does not receive significant nutritional blood flow directly from the cardiac chambers.

■ *Measurement of Coronary Blood Flow*

Coronary blood flow is most commonly measured in humans by a technique called *thermodilution.* Thermodilution is the same procedure used to measure cardiac output (see p 375) except that the indicator (cold saline) is ejected at the tip of a catheter inserted into the coronary sinus via a peripheral vein. The thermal sensor (thermistor) is located on the catheter a few centimeters from the catheter tip. The greater the coronary sinus outflow, the less is the temperature decrease produced by the cold saline injection. This method does not measure total coronary blood flow because only about two thirds of coronary arterial inflow returns to the venous circulation through the coronary sinus. However, almost all the blood flow that does empty into the coronary sinus comes from the left ventricle. Hence, the thermodilution method provides a good estimate of left ventricular coronary blood flow.

Right and left coronary artery flow, as well as flow in the major branches of the left coronary artery, can be measured with reasonable accuracy by injection of a radioactive tracer (e.g., ^{133}Xe) through a catheter threaded into one of the coronary arteries via a peripheral artery. Myocardial clearance of the isotope is monitored with a detector appropriately placed over the precordium.

In the major coronary arteries, blood flow can also be measured by the **pulsed Doppler technique.** An ultrasound signal is emitted from a crystal at the tip of a cardiac catheter inserted, via a peripheral (e.g., femoral) artery, into the origin of the coronary artery to be studied. The sound is reflected by the flowing blood, and the frequency shift of the reflected sound is proportional to the velocity of the blood flow. The blood flow can be calculated from the measured flow velocity and the estimated cross-sectional area of the coronary artery.

Coronary blood flow can also be estimated by video densitometry, in which the movement of a bolus of a radiopaque substance injected into the coronary artery is monitored by rapid sequential radiographs. Similarly, intracoronary injection of microbubbles and tracking of their movement by echocardiography is used to measure

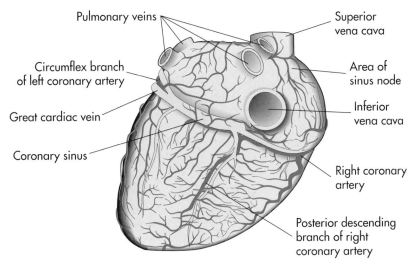

Pulmonary veins

Circumflex branch
of left coronary artery

Great cardiac vein

Coronary sinus

Superior
vena cava

Area of
sinus node

Inferior
vena cava

Right coronary
artery

Posterior descending
branch of right
coronary artery

POSTERIOR VIEW

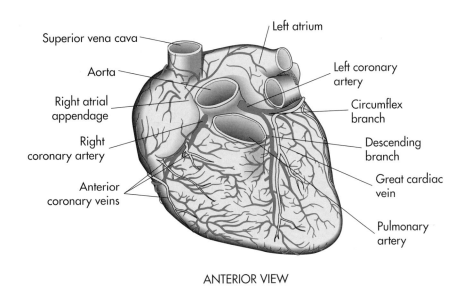

Superior vena cava

Aorta

Right atrial
appendage

Right
coronary artery

Anterior
coronary veins

Left atrium

Left coronary
artery

Circumflex
branch

Descending
branch

Great cardiac
vein

Pulmonary
artery

ANTERIOR VIEW

■ **Fig. 30-1**   Anterior and posterior surfaces of the heart, illustrating the location and distribution of the principal coronary vessels.

coronary blood flow. Cine computed tomography and magnetic resonance imaging are also used to determine total and regional myocardial blood flow.

■ *Factors That Influence Coronary Blood Flow*

Physical Factors. *The primary factor responsible for perfusion of the myocardium is the aortic pressure, which is, of course, generated by the heart itself.* Changes in aortic pressure generally evoke parallel directional changes in coronary blood flow. This is in part caused by changes in coronary perfusion pressure. However, the major factor in the regulation of coronary blood flow is a change in arteriolar resistance engendered by changes in myocardial metabolic activity. When the metabolic activ-

ity of the heart increases, coronary resistance decreases; when cardiac metabolism decreases, coronary resistance increases (see p 446).

If a cannulated coronary artery is perfused by blood from a pressure-controlled reservoir, perfusion pressure can be altered without changing aortic pressure and cardiac work. Under these conditions, abrupt variations in perfusion pressure produce equally abrupt changes in coronary blood flow in the same direction. However, maintenance of the perfusion pressure at the new level is associated with a return of blood flow toward the level observed before the induced changes in perfusion pressure (Fig. 30-2). This phenomenon is an example of autoregulation of blood flow and is discussed in Chapter 28. Under normal conditions, blood pressure is kept within relatively narrow limits by the baroreceptor reflex mechanisms, so that changes in coronary blood flow are mainly caused by changes in the diameter of the coronary resistance vessels in response to metabolic demands of the heart.

In addition to providing the head of pressure to drive blood through the coronary vessels, the heart also influences its blood supply by the squeezing effect of the contracting myocardium on the blood vessels that course through it (**extravascular compression** or **extracoronary resistance**). This force is so great during early ventricular systole that blood flow, as measured in a large coronary artery that supplies the left ventricle, is briefly reversed. Maximal left coronary inflow occurs in early diastole, when the ventricles have relaxed and extravascular compression of the coronary vessels is virtually absent. This flow pattern is seen in the phasic coronary flow curve for the left coronary artery (Fig. 30-3). After an initial reversal in early systole, left coronary blood flow follows the aortic pressure until early diastole, when it rises abruptly and then declines slowly as aortic pressure falls during the remainder of diastole.

The minimal extravascular resistance and absence of left ventricular work during diastole can be used to improve myocardial perfusion in patients with damaged myocardium and low blood pressure. In a method called **counterpulsation,** an inflatable balloon is inserted into the thoracic aorta through a femoral artery. The balloon is inflated during ventricular diastole and deflated during systole. This procedure enhances coronary blood flow during diastole by raising diastolic pressure at a time when coronary extravascular resistance is lowest. Furthermore, it reduces cardiac energy requirements by lowering aortic pressure (afterload) during ventricular ejection.

Left ventricular myocardial pressure (pressure within the wall of the left ventricle) is greatest near the endocardium and lowest near the epicardium. However, under normal conditions, this pressure gradient does not impair endocardial blood flow, because a greater blood flow to the endocardium during diastole compensates for the greater blood flow to the epicardium during systole. In fact, when radioactive spheres 10 μm in diameter are injected into the coronary arteries, their distribution indicates that the blood flow to the epicardial and endocardial halves of the left ventricle is approximately equal under normal conditions. Because extravascular compression is greatest at the endocardial surface of the ventricle, an explanation for the equality of epicardial and endocardial blood flow is that the tone of the endocardial resistance vessels is less than the tone of the epicardial vessels.

The flow pattern in the right coronary artery is similar to that in the left coronary artery (Fig. 30-3). However, because of the lower pressure developed during systole by the thin right ventricle, reversal of blood flow does not

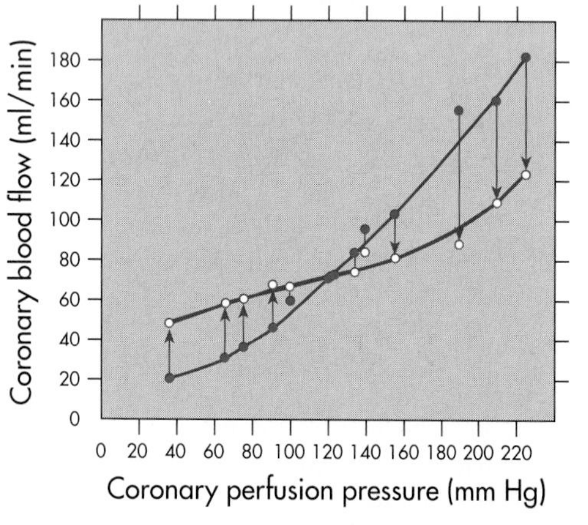

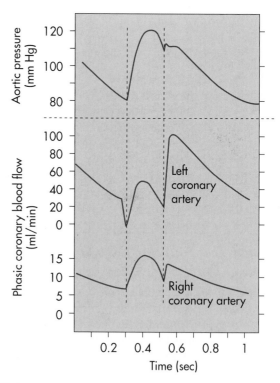

■ **Fig. 30-2**   Pressure-flow relationships in the coronary vascular bed. At constant aortic pressure, cardiac output, and heart rate, coronary artery perfusion pressure was abruptly increased or decreased from the control level indicated by the point where the two lines cross. The closed circles represent the flows that were obtained immediately after the change in perfusion pressure; the open circles represent the steady-state flows at the new pressures. There is a tendency for flow to return toward the control level (autoregulation of blood flow), and this is most prominent over the intermediate pressure range (about 60 to 180 mm Hg). (From Berne RM, Rubio R: *Coronary circulation.* In *Handbook of physiology,* sect 2, *The cardiovascular system—the heart,* vol I, Bethesda, Md, 1979, American Physiological Society.)

■ **Fig. 30-3**   Comparison of phasic coronary blood flow in the left and right coronary arteries.

occur in early systole. Hence, systolic blood flow constitutes a much greater proportion of total coronary inflow than it does in the left coronary artery.

The extent to which extravascular compression restricts coronary inflow can be readily seen when the heart is suddenly arrested in diastole, or with the induction of ventricular fibrillation. Fig. 30-4 depicts mean left coronary flow when the vessel was perfused with blood at a constant pressure from a reservoir. At the arrow in Fig. 30-4, *A*, ventricular fibrillation was electrically induced and an immediate and substantial increase in blood flow occurred. Subsequent increase in coronary resistance over a period of many minutes reduced myocardial blood flow to below the level existing before induction of ventricular fibrillation (Fig. 30-4, *B*, before stellate ganglion stimulation).

Under abnormal conditions, when diastolic pressure in the coronary arteries is low (such as in severe hypotension, partial **coronary artery occlusion,** or severe **aortic stenosis**), the ratio of endocardial to epicardial blood flow falls below a value of l. This ratio indicates that the blood flow to the endocardial regions is more severely impaired than that to the epicardial regions of the ventricle. The redistribution of coronary blood flow is also reflected in an increase in the gradient of myocardial lactic acid and adenosine concentrations from epicardium to endocardium. For this reason, the myocardial damage observed in **arteriosclerotic heart disease** (e.g., after coronary occlusion) is greatest in the inner wall of the left ventricle.

Tachycardia and bradycardia have dual effects on coronary blood flow. A change in heart rate is accomplished chiefly by shortening or lengthening of diastole. In tachycardia the proportion of time spent in systole, and consequently the period of restricted inflow, increases. However, this mechanical reduction in mean coronary flow is overridden by the dilation of the coronary resistance vessels associated with the increased metabolic activity of the more rapidly beating heart. With bradycardia the opposite is true; restriction of coronary inflow is less (more time in diastole), but so are the metabolic (O_2) requirements of the myocardium.

Neural and neurohumoral factors. *Stimulation of the sympathetic nerves to the heart elicits a marked increase in coronary blood flow.* However, the increase in flow is associated with cardiac acceleration and a more forceful systole. The stronger myocardial contraction and the tachycardia (with the consequence that a greater proportion of time is spent in systole) tend to restrict coronary flow. The increase in myocardial metabolic activity, however, as evidenced by the rate and contractility changes, tends to evoke dilation of the coronary resistance vessels. The increase in coronary blood flow elicited by cardiac sympathetic nerve stimulation is the sum of these factors. In perfused hearts in which the mechanical effect of extravascular compression is eliminated by cardiac arrest or ventricular fibrillation, an initial coronary vasoconstriction is often observed. After this initial vasoconstriction, vasodilation attributable to the metabolic effect comes into play (Fig. 30-4, *B*).

Furthermore, if the β-adrenergic receptors are blocked to eliminate the chronotropic effects (those that affect the heart rate) and inotropic effects (those that affect contractility), direct reflex activation of the sympathetic nerves to the heart increases coronary resistance. These observations indicate that the *primary action of the sympathetic nerve fibers on the coronary resistance vessels is vasoconstriction.*

α- and β-Adrenergic agonists, as well as α- and β-adrenergic blocking agents, reveal the presence of α-

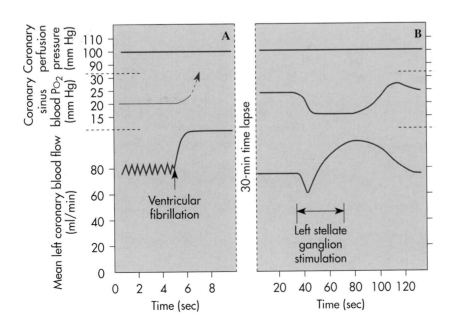

■ **Fig. 30-4** **A,** Unmasking of the restricting effect of ventricular systole on mean coronary blood flow by induction of ventricular fibrillation during constant pressure perfusion of the left coronary artery. **B,** Effect of cardiac sympathetic nerve stimulation on coronary blood flow and coronary sinus blood O_2 tension in the fibrillating heart during constant pressure perfusion of the left coronary artery. (Berne RM: Unpublished observations.)

adrenergic receptors (constrictors) and β-adrenergic receptors (dilators) on the coronary vessels. Coronary resistance vessels also participate in the baroreceptor and chemoreceptor reflexes, and the sympathetic constrictor tone of the coronary arterioles can be modulated by such reflexes. Nevertheless, coronary resistance is predominantly under local non-neural control.

Vagus nerve stimulation slightly dilates the coronary resistance vessels, and activation of the carotid and aortic chemoreceptors can elicit a small decrease in coronary resistance via the vagus nerves to the heart. The failure of strong vagal stimulation to evoke a large increase in coronary blood flow is not due to insensitivity of the coronary resistance vessels to acetylcholine; intracoronary demonstration of this agent elicits marked vasodilation.

Reflexes that originate in the myocardium and alter vascular resistance in peripheral systemic vessels, including the coronary vessels, have been conclusively demonstrated. However, the existence of extracardiac reflexes, with the coronary resistance vessels as the effector sites, has not been established.

Metabolic factors. One of the most striking characteristics of the coronary circulation is the close parallel relationship between the level of myocardial metabolic activity and the magnitude of the coronary blood flow (Fig. 30-5). This relationship is also found in the denervated heart or the completely isolated heart, whether in the beating or in the fibrillating state. The ventricles continue to fibrillate for many hours when the coronary arteries are perfused with arterial blood from some external source. With the onset of ventricular fibrillation, an abrupt increase in coronary blood flow occurs because of the removal of extravascular compression (Fig. 30-4). Flow then gradually returns toward, and often falls below, the prefibrillation level. The increase in coronary resistance that occurs despite the elimination of extravascular compression demonstrates the heart's ability to adjust its blood flow to meet its energy requirements. The fibrillating heart uses less O_2 than the pumping heart, and blood flow to the myocardium is reduced accordingly.

The mechanism that links cardiac metabolic rate and coronary blood flow remains unsettled. However, it appears that a *decrease in the ratio of oxygen supply to oxygen demand (whether produced by a decrease in oxygen supply or by an increase in oxygen demand) releases a vasodilator substance from the myocardium into the interstitial fluid, where it relaxes the coronary resistance vessels.* As diagrammed in Fig. 30-6, a decrease in arterial blood oxygen content, coronary blood flow, or both, or an increase in metabolic rate, decreases the oxygen supply/demand ratio. In response to the decrease in oxygen supply/demand ratio, a vasodilator substance, such as adenosine, is released. This substance dilates the arterioles and thereby adjusts oxygen supply to demand. A decrease in oxygen demand would reduce the vasodilator release and permit greater expression of basal tone.

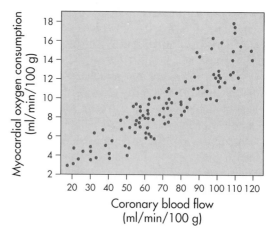

■ **Fig. 30-5**   Relationship between myocardial oxygen consumption and coronary blood flow during a variety of interventions that increased or decreased myocardial metabolic rate. (Redrawn from Berne RM, Rubio R: *Coronary circulation.* In *Handbook of physiology,* sect 2, *The cardiovascular system—the heart,* vol I, Bethesda, Md, 1979, American Physiological Society.)

■ **Fig. 30-6**   Imbalance in the oxygen supply/oxygen demand ratio alters coronary blood flow by the rate of release of a vasodilator metabolite from the cardiomyocytes. A decrease in the ratio elicits an increase in vasodilator release, whereas an increase in the ratio has the opposite effect.

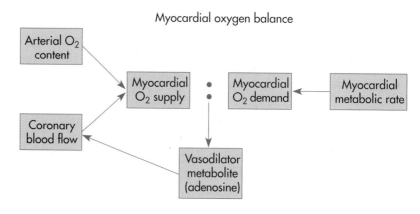

Numerous agents, generally referred to as metabolites, have been suggested as mediators of the vasodilation observed with increased cardiac work. Accumulation of vasoactive metabolites may also be responsible for reactive hyperemia (see p 447), because the duration of the enhanced coronary flow after release of the briefly occluded vessel is, within certain limits, proportional to the duration of the period of occlusion. Among the substances implicated are CO_2, O_2 (reduced O_2 tension), hydrogen ions (lactic acid), potassium ions, and adenosine.

Of these agents, adenosine comes closest to satisfying the criteria for the physiological mediator. According to the adenosine hypothesis, a reduction in myocardial O_2 tension produced by low coronary blood flow, hypoxemia, or increased metabolic activity of the heart, leads to the myocardial formation of adenosine. This nucleoside crosses the interstitial fluid space to reach the coronary resistance vessels, and induces vasodilation by activating an adenosine receptor.

Potassium release from the myocardium can account for about half of the initial decrease in coronary resistance. However, it cannot be responsible for the increased coronary flow observed with prolonged enhancement of cardiac metabolic activity, because its release from the cardiac muscle is transitory. Little evidence exists that CO_2 hydrogen ions or O_2 play a significant *direct* role in the regulation of coronary blood flow. Factors that alter coronary vascular resistance are schematized in Fig. 30-7.

■ *Effects of Diminished Coronary Blood Flow*

Most of the oxygen in the coronary arterial blood is extracted during one passage through the myocardial capillaries. Thus, the supply of oxygen to the myocardial cells is **flow limited:** any substantial reduction in coronary blood flow will curtail the delivery of oxygen to the myocardium, because the extraction of oxygen from each unit volume of blood is nearly maximal even when blood flow is normal.

A reduction of coronary flow that is neither too prolonged nor too severe to cause myocardial necrosis can still cause substantial (but temporary) dysfunction of the heart. For example, a relatively brief period of severe ischemia followed by reperfusion can cause a pronounced mechanical dysfunction (called **myocardial stunning**). The heart eventually fully recovers from the dysfunction.

The pathophysiological basis for myocardial stunning appears to be a combination of calcium overload, initiated during the period of ischemia, combined with the generation of hydroxyl and superoxide free radicals early in the period of reperfusion. These changes in turn are believed to impair the responsiveness of the myofilaments to calcium.

> Myocardial stunning may be evident in patients who have had an **acute coronary artery occlusion** (a so-called heart attack). If the patient is treated sufficiently early by **coronary bypass surgery** or **balloon angioplasty** and if adequate blood flow is restored to the ischemic region, the myocardial cells in this region may eventually recover fully. However, for many days or even weeks, the contractility of the myocardium in the affected region may be grossly subnormal.

> Reductions in coronary blood flow (**myocardial ischemia**) may critically impair the mechanical and electrical behavior of the heart. Diminished coronary blood flow as a consequence of coronary artery disease (usually **coronary atherosclerosis**) is one of the most common causes of serious cardiac disease. The ischemia may be global (it affects an entire ventricle) or regional (it affects some fraction of the ventricle). The impairment of the mechanical contraction of the affected myocardium is produced not only by the diminished delivery of oxygen and metabolic substrates, but also by the accumulation of potentially harmful substances (e.g., K^+, lactic acid, H^+) in the cardiac tissues. If the reduction of coronary flow to

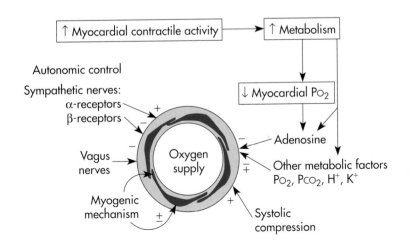

■ **Fig. 30-7** Schematic representation of factors that increase ($+$) or decrease ($-$) coronary vascular resistance. The intravascular pressure (arterial blood pressure) stretches the vessel wall.

any region of the heart is sufficiently severe and prolonged, **necrosis** (death) of the affected cardiac cells will result.

The relationships between coronary perfusion pressure, cardiac behavior, and myocardial metabolic activity in an experimental model of **myocardial hibernation** are shown in Fig. 30-8. When the perfusion pressure in isolated hearts was diminished over the range from 160 to about 70 mm Hg, the intraventricular pressure developed by those hearts progressively diminished. However, the intracellular pH and inorganic phosphate concentrations and the efflux of lactic acid remained essentially unaffected. Only when the perfusion pressure was reduced below 60 mm Hg did these metabolic variables change substantially. The changes in developed force and in cardiac metabolism were readily reversible when perfusion pressure was restored. The changes in developed pressure correlated directly with the transient intracellular Ca^{++} currents measured during each ventricular contraction. However, the reasons why the current Ca^{++} current transient diminished when perfusion pressure was reduced remain to be established.

Myocardial hibernation occurs mainly in patients with coronary artery disease just as does myocardial stunning. The coronary blood flow in these patients is diminished persistently and significantly, and the mechanical function of the heart is impaired concomitantly. However, the metabolic activity of the heart does not reflect the extent of the ischemia; the process is called hibernation because the down-regulation of metabolism tends to preserve the viability of the cardiac tissues. If coronary blood flow is restored to normal by bypass surgery or angioplasty, mechanical function returns to normal.

■ *Coronary Collateral Circulation and Vasodilators*

In the normal human heart, there are virtually no functional intercoronary channels, whereas in the dog, a few small vessels link branches of the major coronary arteries. Abrupt occlusion of a coronary artery or one of its branches in a human or dog leads to ischemic necrosis and eventual fibrosis of the areas of myocardium supplied by the occluded vessel. However, if a coronary artery narrows slowly and progressively over a period of days, weeks, or longer, collateral vessels develop and may furnish sufficient blood to the ischemic myocardium to prevent or reduce the extent of necrosis. The development of collateral coronary vessels has been extensively studied in dogs. The clinical picture of human coronary atherosclerosis can be simulated by gradual narrowing of

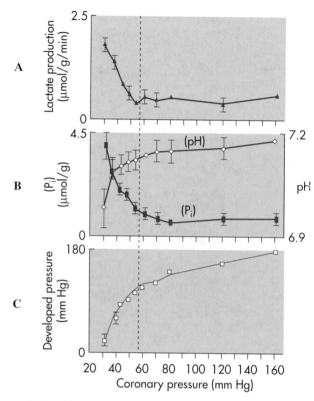

■ **Fig. 30-8**   Effects of changes in coronary perfusion pressure on myocardial lactate production **(A),** on inorganic phosphate levels *(p$_i$)* and intracellular pH **(B),** and on the pressure developed during left ventricular contraction **(C),** in a group of five ferret hearts. (Modified from Kitikaze M, Marban E: *J Physiol (Lond)* 414:455, 1989.)

the normal dog's coronary arteries. Collateral vessels develop between branches of occluded and nonoccluded arteries. They originate from preexisting small vessels that undergo proliferative changes of the endothelium and smooth muscle. These changes are possibly in response to wall stress and chemical agents released by the ischemic tissue.

Numerous surgical attempts have been made to enhance the development of coronary collateral vessels. However, the techniques used do not increase the collateral circulation over and above that produced by coronary artery narrowing alone. When discrete occlusions or severe narrowing occur in coronary arteries, as in **coronary atherosclerosis,** the lesions can be bypassed with an artery (internal mammary) or a vein graft. In many cases the narrow segment can be dilated by inserting a balloon-tipped catheter into the diseased vessel via a peripheral artery and inflating the balloon. Distention of the vessel by balloon inflation (**angioplasty**) can produce a lasting dilation of a narrowed coronary artery (Fig. 30-9).

A variety of drugs that induce coronary vasodilation are available and are used in patients with coronary

Cusps of aortic valve   Cardiac catheter

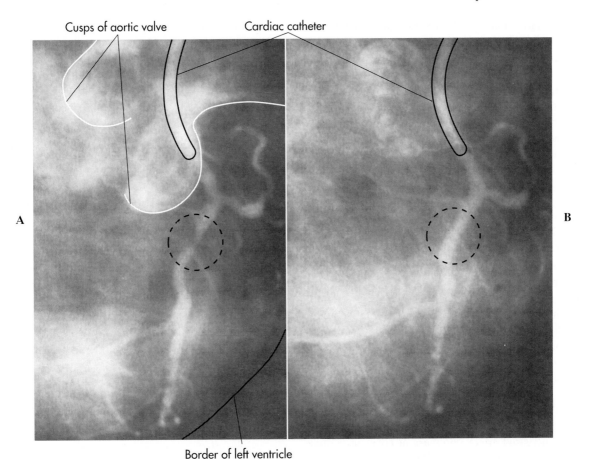

A   B

Border of left ventricle

■ **Fig. 30-9**   **A,** Angiogram (intracoronary radiopaque dye) of a person with marked narrowing of the circumflex branch of the left coronary artery *(encircled)*. Reflux of dye into the root of the aorta outlines two of the aortic valve cusps. **B,** The same segment of the coronary artery after angioplasty. (Courtesy of Dr. Eric R. Powers.)

artery disease to relieve **angina pectoris,** the chest pain associated with myocardial ischemia. Many of these compounds are organic nitrates and nitrites. They do not selectively dilate the coronary vessels, and the mechanism whereby they accomplish their beneficial effects has not been established. The arterioles that would dilate in response to the drugs are undoubtedly already maximally dilated by the ischemia responsible for the symptoms.

In fact, in a patient with marked narrowing of a coronary artery, administration of a vasodilator can fully dilate normal vessel branches that are parallel to the narrowed segment, and thereby reduce the head of pressure to the partially occluded vessel. The reduced pressure to the narrowed vessel will further compromise blood flow to the ischemic myocardium and elicit pain and electrocardiographic changes indicative of tissue injury. This phenomenon is known as **coronary steal,** and it can occur in response to vasodilator drugs such as dipyridamole, which acts by blocking cellular uptake and metabolism of endogenous adenosine. Nitrites and nitrates alleviate angina pectoris, at

least partly, by reducing cardiac work and myocardial oxygen requirements. This is accomplished by relaxing the great veins, which reduces preload, and by decreasing blood pressure, which reduces afterload. In short, to prevent coronary steal, the reduction in pressure work and O_2 requirement must be greater than the reduction in coronary blood flow and O_2 supply consequent to the lowered coronary perfusion pressure. Also, nitrites and nitrates dilate large coronary arteries and coronary collateral vessels, and thereby increase blood flow to ischemic myocardium and alleviate precordial pain.

■ *Cardiac Oxygen Consumption and Work*

The volume of O_2 consumed by the heart depends on the amount and type of activity the heart performs. Under basal conditions, myocardial O_2 consumption is about 8 to 10 ml/min/100 g of heart. It can increase several-fold during exercise and decrease moderately under conditions such as hypotension and hypothermia. The O_2 content of cardiac venous blood is normally quite low (about 5 ml/dl), and the myocardium can receive little additional O_2 by further O_2 extraction from the coronary blood. Therefore, increased O_2 demands of the heart must be met mainly by an increase in coronary blood flow. In experiments in which the heartbeat is arrested, as with administration of potassium, but coronary perfusion is maintained, O_2 consumption falls to 2 ml/min/100 g or less, which is still six to seven times greater than that for resting skeletal muscle.

Left ventricular work per beat (**stroke work,** see Chapter 26) is approximately equal to the product of the stroke volume and the mean aortic pressure against which the blood is ejected by the left ventricle. At resting levels of cardiac output, the kinetic energy component is negligible (see p 401). However, at high cardiac outputs, as in strenuous exercise, the kinetic component can account for up to 50% of total cardiac work. Simultaneously halving the aortic pressure and doubling the cardiac output, or vice versa, will result in the same value for cardiac work. However, *the O_2 requirements are greater for any given amount of cardiac work when a major proportion of the work is pressure work as opposed to volume work.* An increase in cardiac output at a constant aortic pressure (volume work) is accomplished with a small increase in left ventricular O_2 consumption, whereas increased arterial pressure at constant cardiac output (pressure work) is accompanied by a large increase in myocardial O_2 consumption. Thus, myocardial O_2 consumption may not correlate well with overall cardiac work. The magnitude and duration of left ventricular pressure do correlate with left ventricular O_2 consumption.

The work of the right ventricle is one seventh that of the left ventricle, because pulmonary vascular resistance is much less than systemic vascular resistance.

The greater energy demand of pressure work than of volume work is clinically important, especially in **aortic stenosis.** In this condition, left ventricular O_2 consumption is increased mainly because of the high intraventricular pressures developed during systole. However, coronary perfusion pressure, and hence oxygen supply, is either normal or reduced because of the pressure drop across the narrowed orifice of the diseased aortic valve (see also Chapter 25).

■ *Cardiac Efficiency*

As with an engine, the efficiency of the heart can be calculated as the ratio of the work accomplished to the total energy utilized. Assuming an average O_2 consumption of 9 ml/min/100 g for the two ventricles, a 300-g heart consumes 27 ml O_2/min, which is equivalent to 130 small

calories when the respiratory quotient is 0.82. Together, the two ventricles do about 8 kg-m of work per minute, which is equivalent to 18.7 small calories. Therefore, the gross efficiency of the heart is 14%.

$$\frac{18.7}{130} \times 100 = 14\% \qquad (30\text{-}1)$$

The net efficiency of the heart is slightly higher (18%) and is determined by subtracting the O_2 consumption of the nonbeating (asystolic) heart (about 2 ml/min/100 g) from the total cardiac O_2 consumption in the calculation of efficiency. It is thus evident that the efficiency of the heart as a pump is relatively low and is comparable with the efficiency of many common mechanical devices. With exercise, efficiency improves, because mean blood pressure shows little change, whereas cardiac output and work increase considerably without a proportional increase in myocardial O_2 consumption. The energy expended in cardiac metabolism that does not contribute to the propulsion of blood through the body is dissipated in the form of heat. The energy of the flowing blood is also dissipated as heat, chiefly in passage through the arterioles.

■ *Substrate Utilization*

The heart is versatile in its use of substrates, and within certain limits the uptake of a particular substrate is directly proportional to its arterial concentration. The use of one substrate by the heart is also influenced by the presence or absence of other substrates. For example, the addition of lactate to the blood that perfuses a heart metabolizing glucose leads to a reduction in glucose uptake, and vice versa. At normal blood concentrations, glucose and lactate are consumed at about equal rates. In contrast, pyruvate uptake is very low, as is its arterial concentration. For glucose, the threshold concentration is about 4 mM. Below this blood level, no glucose is taken up by the myocardium. Insulin reduces the glucose threshold and increases the rate of glucose uptake by the heart. A very low threshold exists for cardiac utilization of lactate; insulin does not affect its uptake by the myocardium. Under hypoxic conditions, glucose utilization is facilitated by an increase in the rate of transport across the myocardial cell wall. However, lactate cannot be metabolized by the hypoxic heart and is in fact produced by the heart under anaerobic conditions. Associated with lactate production by the hypoxic heart is the breakdown of cardiac glycogen.

Of the total cardiac O_2 consumption, only 35% to 40% can be accounted for by the oxidation of carbohydrate. Thus, the heart derives the major part of its energy from oxidation of noncarbohydrate sources. The chief noncarbohydrate fuel used by the heart is esterified and nonesterified fatty acid, which accounts for about 60% of myocardial O_2 consumption in subjects in the postabsorptive state. The various fatty acids show different thresholds for myocardial uptake, but they are generally used in direct proportion to their arterial concentration. Ketone bodies, especially acetoacetate, are readily oxidized by the heart and contribute a major source of energy in diabetic acidosis. As is true of carbohydrate substrates, utilization of a specific noncarbohydrate is influenced by the presence of other substrates, whether noncarbohydrate or carbohydrate. Therefore, within certain limits, the heart preferentially uses the substrate available in the largest concentration. The contribution to myocardial energy expenditure provided by the oxidation of amino acids is small.

Normally the heart derives its energy by oxidative phosphorylation, in which each mole of glucose yields 36 moles of adenosine triphosphate (ATP). However, during hypoxia, glycolysis takes over, and 2 moles of ATP are provided by each mole of glucose; beta oxidation of fatty acids is also curtailed. If hypoxia is prolonged, cellular creatine phosphate and eventually ATP are depleted.

In ischemia, lactic acid accumulates (lack of washout) and causes a decrease in intracellular pH. This condition inhibits glycolysis, fatty acid use, and protein synthesis, which results in cellular damage and eventually in necrosis of myocardial cells.

■ *Cutaneous Circulation*

The oxygen and nutrient requirements of the skin are relatively small. In contrast to most other body tissues, the supply of oxygen and nutrients is not the chief factor in the regulation of cutaneous blood flow. The primary function of the cutaneous circulation is maintenance of a constant body temperature. Consequently, the skin shows wide fluctuation in blood flow, depending on whether the body needs to lose or conserve heat. Mechanisms responsible for alterations in skin blood flow are mainly activated by changes in ambient and internal body temperatures.

■ *Regulation of Skin Blood Flow*

Neural factors. The skin contains essentially two types of resistance vessels: arterioles and **arteriovenous (AV) anastomoses.** The arterioles are similar to those found elsewhere in the body. AV anastomoses shunt blood from the arterioles to venules and venous plexuses; hence, they bypass the capillary bed. The anastomoses are found in the fingertips, palms of the hands, toes, soles of the feet, ears, nose, and lips. AV anastomoses differ morphologically from the arterioles: they are either short, straight, or long coiled vessels about 20 to 40 μm in luminal diameter, with thick muscular walls richly supplied with nerve fibers (Fig. 30-10). These vessels are almost exclusively under sympathetic neural control and dilate maximally when their nerve supply is interrupted. Conversely, reflex stimulation of the sympathetic fibers to these vessels may produce constriction to the point of complete obliteration of the vascular lumen. Although AV anastomoses do not exhibit **basal tone** (tonic activity of the vascular smooth muscle independent of innervation), they are highly sensitive to vasoconstrictor agents such as epinephrine and norepinephrine. Furthermore, AV anastomoses are *not* under metabolic control, and they do *not* show reactive hyperemia or autoregulation of blood flow. *Thus, the regulation of blood flow through these anastomotic channels is governed principally by the nervous system in response to reflex activation by temperature receptors or from higher centers of the central nervous system.*

Most of the skin resistance vessels exhibit some basal tone and are under dual control of the sympathetic nervous system and local regulatory factors, in much the same manner as are resistance vessels in other vascular beds. However, neural control is more important than local control in the skin vessels. Stimulation of sympathetic nerve fibers to skin blood vessels (arteries and veins, as well as arterioles) induces vasoconstriction, and cutting the sympathetic nerves induces vasodilation. After chronic denervation of the cutaneous blood vessels, the degree of tone that existed before denervation is gradually regained over a period of several weeks. This restoration of tone is accomplished by an enhancement of basal tone that compensates for the degree of tone previously contributed by sympathetic nerve fiber activity. As noted, epinephrine and norepinephrine elicit only vasoconstriction in cutaneous vessels. Denervation of the skin vessels results in enhanced sensitivity to circulation catecholamines (**denervation hypersensitivity**).

Parasympathetic vasodilator nerve fibers do not supply the cutaneous blood vessels. However, stimulation of the sweat glands, which are innervated by cholinergic fibers of the sympathetic nervous system, causes the skin resistance vessels to dilate. Sweat contains an enzyme that acts on a protein moiety in the tissue fluid to produce **bradykinin,** a polypeptide with potent vasodilator properties. Bradykinin formed in the tissue acts locally to dilate the arterioles and increase blood flow to the skin.

The skin vessels of certain regions, particularly the head, neck, shoulders, and upper chest, are regulated by the higher centers in the brain. Blushing, in response to embarrassment or anger, and blanching, in response to fear or anxiety, are examples of cerebral inhibition and stimulation, respectively, of the sympathetic nerve fibers to the affected regions.

In contrast to AV anastomoses in the skin, the cutaneous resistance vessels show autoregulation of blood flow and reactive hyperemia. If the arterial inflow to a

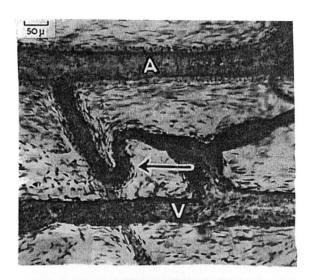

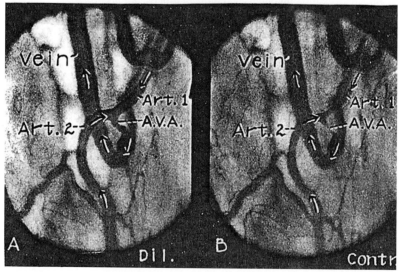

■ **Fig. 30-10** *Top,* Arteriovenous anastomosis in the human ear injected with Berlin blue. *A,* Artery; *V,* vein; arrow points to AV anastomosis. The walls of the AV anastomosis in the fingertips are thicker and more cellular. (From Pritchard MML, Daniel PM: *J Anat* 90:309, 1956.) *Bottom,* Two frames from a motion picture record of the same relatively large artiovenous anastomosis *(A.V.A.)* in a stable rabbit ear chamber installed 3¹/₂ months previously. *Frame A,* A.V.A. dilated; *Frame B,* contracted. On this day the lumen of the A.V.A. measured 51 μm dilated and 5 μm contracted at its narrowest point. (From Clark ER, Clark EL: *Am J Anat* 54:229, 1934.)

limb is stopped with an inflated blood pressure cuff for a brief period, the skin becomes bright red below the point of vascular occlusion when the cuff is deflated. This increased cutaneous blood flow (reactive hyperemia) is also manifested by distention of the superficial veins in the erythematous extremity. Autoregulation of blood flow in the skin is best explained by a myogenic mechanism (see p 445).

The fingers (and sometimes the toes) of some individuals are very sensitive to cold. Upon exposure to cold, the arteries and arterioles to the hands constrict, producing ischemia of the fingers characterized by blanching of the skin associated with tingling, numbness, and pain. The blanching is followed by cyanosis and later by redness as the arterial spasm subsides. This condition, called **Raynaud's disease,** is of unknown cause and occurs most frequently in young women.

Ambient and body temperature in regulation of skin blood flow. *The primary function of the skin is to maintain a constant internal environment and protect the body from adverse changes. Ambient (outside) temperature is one of the most important external variables with which the body must contend. Thus, it is not surprising that the vasculature of the skin is chiefly influenced by environmental temperature.* Exposure to cold elicits a generalized cutaneous vasoconstriction that is most pronounced in the hands and feet. This response is chiefly mediated by the nervous system. Arrest of the circulation to a hand with a pressure cuff, and immersion of that hand in cold water, result in vasoconstriction in the skin of the other extremities that are exposed to room temperature. When the circulation to the chilled hand is not occluded, the reflex vasoconstriction is caused in part by the cooled blood that returns to the general circulation. This returned blood then stimulates the temperature-regulating center in the anterior hypothalamus. Direct application of cold to this region of the brain produces cutaneous vasoconstriction.

The skin vessels of the cooled hand also respond directly to cold. Moderate cooling or exposure for brief periods to severe cold (0° to 15° C) results in constriction of the resistance and capacitance vessels, including AV anastomoses. However, prolonged exposure to severe cold evokes a secondary vasodilator response. Prompt vasoconstriction and severe pain are elicited by immersion of the hand in water near 0° C but are soon followed by dilation of the skin vessels, with reddening of the immersed part and alleviation of the pain. With continued immersion of the hand, alternating periods of constriction and dilation occur, but the skin temperature rarely drops as much as it did with the initial vasoconstriction. Prolonged severe cold, of course, damages tissue. The rosy faces of people working or playing in a cold environment are examples of cold vasodilation. However, the blood flow through the skin of the face may be greatly reduced despite the flushed appearance. The red color of the slowly flowing blood is in large measure caused by reduced oxygen uptake by the cold skin and the cold-induced shift to the left of the oxyhemoglobin dissociation curve.

Direct application of heat to the skin produces not only local vasodilation of resistance and capacitance vessels and AV anastomoses but also reflex dilation in other parts of the body. The local effect is independent of the vascular nerve supply, whereas the reflex vasodilation is a combination of anterior hypothalamic stimulation by the returning warmed blood and of stimulation of receptors in the heated part.

The close proximity of the major arteries and veins permits considerable heat exchange (**countercurrent**) *between them.* Cold blood that flows in veins from a cooled hand toward the heart takes up heat from adjacent arteries; this warms the venous blood and cools the arterial blood. Heat exchange is, of course, in the opposite direction when the extremity is exposed to heat. Thus, heat conservation is enhanced and heat gain is minimized during exposure of extremities to cold and warm environments, respectively.

■ *Skin Color: Relationship to Skin Blood Volume, Oxyhemoglobin, and Blood Flow*

The color of the skin is caused in large part by pigment. However, in all but very dark skin, the degree of pallor or ruddiness is mainly a function of the amount of blood in the skin. With little blood in the venous plexus, the skin appears pale, whereas with moderate to large quantities of blood in the venous plexus, the skin shows color. This color may be red, blue, or some shade between, depending on the degree of oxygenation of the blood in the subcutaneous vessels. For example, a combination of vasoconstriction and reduced hemoglobin can produce an ashen gray color of the skin. A combination of venous engorgement and reduced hemoglobin can result in a dark purple hue.

Skin color provides little information about the rate of cutaneous blood flow. Rapid blood flow may be accom-panied by pale skin when the AV anastomoses are open and slow blood flow may be associated with red skin when the extremity is exposed to cold.

■ *Skeletal Muscle Circulation*

The rate of blood flow in skeletal muscle varies directly with the contractile activity of the tissue and the type of muscle. Blood flow and capillary density in red (slow-twitch, high-oxidative) muscle are greater than in white (fast-twitch, low-oxidative) muscle. In resting muscle, the precapillary arterioles exhibit asynchronous intermittent contractions and relaxations. Thus, at any given moment a very large percentage of the capillary bed is not perfused. Consequently, total blood flow through quiescent skeletal muscle is low (1.4 to 4.5 ml/min/100 g). During exercise, the resistance vessels relax and the muscle blood flow may increase to up to 15 to 20 times the resting level. The magnitude of this increase depends largely on the strenuousness of the exercise.

■ *Regulation of Skeletal Muscle Blood Flow*

Muscle circulation is regulated by neural and local factors. As with all tissues, physical factors such as arterial pressure, tissue pressure, and blood viscosity influence muscle blood flow. However, another physical factor comes into play during exercise—the squeezing effect of the active skeletal muscle on the vessels. With intermittent contractions, inflow is restricted and venous outflow is enhanced during each brief contraction (Fig. 30-11). The venous valves prevent backflow of blood in the veins between contractions, and the valves thereby aid in the forward propulsion of the blood (see also p 474). With strong sustained contractions such as those that occur during exercise, the vascular bed can be compressed to the point at which blood flow actually ceases temporarily.

When the valves of the superficial leg veins are incompetent, as may occur with pregnancy, thrombophlebitis, or obesity, the veins become dilated and tortuous. Such **varicose veins** can be treated by surgical removal, injection of sclerosing solutions, or the use of elastic stockings.

Neural factors. Although the resistance vessels of muscle possess a high degree of basal tone, they also display tone attributable to continuous low-frequency activity in the sympathetic vasoconstrictor nerve fibers. The basal frequency of firing in the sympathetic vasoconstrictor fibers is quite low (about 1 to 2 per second), and maximal vasoconstriction is observed at frequencies as low as 8 to 10 per second.

The vasoconstriction evoked by sympathetic nerve

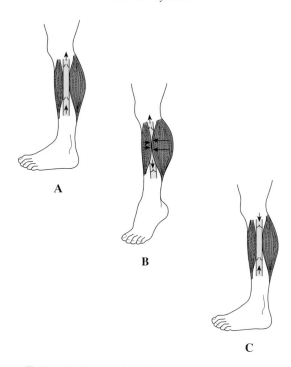

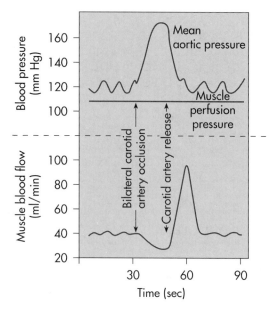

■ Fig. 30-11   Action of the muscle pump in venous return from the legs. **A,** Standing at rest, the venous valves are open and blood flows upward toward the heart by virtue of the pressure generated by the heart and transmitted through the capillaries to the veins from the arterial side of the vascular system (vis a tergo). **B,** Contraction of the muscle compresses the vein so that the increased pressure in the vein drives blood toward the thorax through the upper valve and closes the lower valve in the uncompressed segment of the vein just below the point of muscular compression. **C,** Immediately after muscle relaxation, the pressure in the previously compressed venous segment falls and the reversed pressure gradient causes the upper valve to close. The valve below the previously compressed segment opens because pressure below it exceeds that above it. The segment then fills with blood from the foot. As blood flow continues from the foot, the pressure in the previously compressed segment rises. When it exceeds the pressure above the upper valve, this valve opens and continuous flow occurs as in **A.**

■ Fig. 30-12   Evidence for participation of the muscle vascular bed in vasoconstriction and vasodilation mediated by the carotid sinus baroreceptors after common carotid artery occlusion and release. In this preparation, the sciatic and femoral nerves constituted the only direct connection between the hind leg muscle mass and the rest of the dog. The muscle was perfused by blood at a constant pressure that was completely independent of the animal's arterial pressure. (Redrawn from Jones RD, Berne RM: *Am J Physiol* 204:461, 1963.)

stimulation is caused by the release of norepinephrine from nerve fiber endings. Intra-arterial injection of norepinephrine in skeletal muscle elicits only vasoconstriction, whereas low doses of epinephrine produce vasodilation and large doses cause vasoconstriction.

The tonic activity of the sympathetic nerves is greatly influenced by reflexes from the baroreceptors. An increase in carotid sinus pressure results in dilation of the vascular bed of muscle, and a decrease in carotid sinus pressure elicits vasoconstriction (Fig. 30-12). When the existing sympathetic constrictor tone is high, as in the experiment illustrated in Fig. 30-12, the decrease in blood flow associated with common carotid artery occlusion is small, but the increase after the release of occlusion is large. The vasodilation produced by baroreceptor stimulation is caused by inhibition of sympathetic vasoconstrictor activity.

The muscle resistance vessels contribute significantly to maintenance of blood pressure, because skeletal muscle constitutes a large fraction of the body's mass, and hence the muscle vasculature represents the largest vascular bed. Therefore, participation of its resistance vessels in vascular reflexes is important in maintaining a constant arterial blood pressure.

A comparison of the vasoconstrictor and vasodilator effects of the sympathetic nerves to blood vessels of muscle and skin is summarized in Fig. 30-13. Note the lower basal tone of the skin vessels, their greater constrictor response, and the absence of active cutaneous vasodilation.

Local factors. In active muscle, blood flow is regulated by metabolic factors (see Chapter 28). In resting muscle, neural factors predominate and superimpose neurogenic tone on the non-neural basal tone (Fig. 30-13). Cutting the sympathetic nerves to muscle abolishes the neural component of vascular tone and unmasks the intrinsic basal tone of the blood vessels. *Neural and local blood flow regulating mechanisms oppose each other, and during muscle contraction the local vasodilator mechanism supervenes.* However, during exercise, strong sympathetic nerve stimulation slightly reduces the vasodilation induced by locally released metabolites.

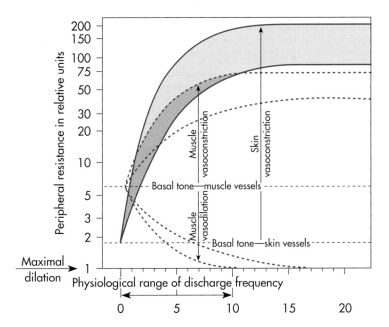

■ **Fig. 30-13**   Basal tone and the range of response of the resistance vessels in muscle *(dashed lines)* and skin *(shaded area)* to stimulation and section of the sympathetic nerves. Peripheral resistance plotted on a logarithmic scale. (Redrawn from Celander O, Folkow B: *Acta Physiol Scand* 29:241, 1953.)

■ *Cerebral Circulation*

Blood reaches the brain through the internal carotid and vertebral arteries. The vertebral arteries join to form the basilar artery, which, in conjunction with branches of the internal carotid arteries, forms the **circle of Willis.**

A unique feature of the cerebral circulation is that it lies within a rigid structure, the cranium. Because intracranial contents are incompressible, any increase in arterial inflow, as with arteriolar dilation, must be associated with a comparable increase in venous outflow. The volume of blood and of extravascular fluid can vary considerably in most tissues. In the brain, however, the volume of blood and extravascular fluid is relatively constant; a change in either of these fluid volumes must be accompanied by a reciprocal change in the other. In contrast to most other organs, the rate of total cerebral blood flow is maintained within a relatively narrow range; in humans, it averages 55 ml/min/100 g of brain.

■ *Estimation of Cerebral Blood Flow*

Total cerebral blood flow can be measured in humans by the nitrous oxide (N_2O) method, which is based on the Fick principle (see p 375). The subject breathes a gas mixture of 15% N_2O, 21% O_2, and 64% N_2 for 10 minutes, which is sufficient time to permit equilibration of the N_2O between the brain tissue and the blood leaving the brain. Simultaneous samples of arterial blood (which can be taken from any artery) and mixed cerebral venous blood (taken from the internal jugular vein) are taken at the start of N_2O administration. From these samples, the cerebral blood flow can be calculated by the Fick equation (see p 375):

$$CBF = \frac{(q_{N_2O})\,t_2 - (q_{N_2O})t_1}{\int_{t_1}^{t_2}([N_2O]_a - [N_2O]_v)dt}$$

where

CBF = cerebral blood flow
$(q_{N_2O})t_1$ = brain content of N_2O at time t_1
$(q_{N_2O})t_2$ = brain content of N_2O at time t_2
$[N_2O]_a$ = N_2O concentration in cerebral arterial blood
$[N_2O]_v$ = N_2O concentration in cerebral venous blood

The development of multiple collimated scintillation detectors built into a helmet that fits over the cranium has made possible the measurement of regional blood flow (cortical blood flow) in animals and humans. To measure regional blood flow in the brain using this technology, an inert radioactive gas (e.g.,[133]Xe) is injected into an internal carotid artery. From its rate of washout from the brain, regional cerebral blood flow can be determined. The radioactive gas may also be given by inhalation, but inhalation of the gas requires more sophisticated analytical techniques in order to identify and disregard noncerebral blood flow and to distinguish between blood flow to cortical (gray matter) and deep cerebral (white matter) tissue.

■ *Regulation of Cerebral Blood Flow*

Of all the body tissues, the brain is the least tolerant of ischemia. Interruption of cerebral blood flow for as little as 5 seconds results in loss of consciousness, and ischemia lasting just a few minutes results in irreversible tissue damage. Fortunately, regulation of the cerebral circulation is primarily under direction of the brain itself. Local regulatory mechanisms and reflexes originating in the brain maintain cerebral circulation at a relatively constant level in the presence of possible adverse extrinsic effects such as sympathetic vasomotor nerve activity, circulating humoral vasoactive agents, and changes in arterial blood pressure. Under certain conditions, the brain also regulates its blood flow by initiating changes in systemic blood pressure.

Neural factors. The cerebral vessels receive innervation from the cervical sympathetic nerve fibers that accompany the internal carotid and vertebral arteries into the cranial cavity. The importance of neural regulation of the cerebral circulation is controversial. Currently, it is thought that sympathetic control of the cerebral vessels is weaker than in other vascular beds, and that the contractile state of the cerebrovascular smooth muscle depends mainly on local metabolic factors. There are no known sympathetic vasodilator nerves to the cerebral vessels, although the vessels do receive parasympathetic fibers from the facial nerve. Stimulation of these fibers produces only a slight vasodilation.

Elevation of intracranial pressure, as by a brain tumor, results in an increase in systemic blood pressure. This response, called **Cushing's phenomenon,** is apparently caused by ischemic stimulation of vasomotor regions in the medulla. Cushing's phenomenon helps maintain cerebral blood flow in such conditions as expanding intracranial tumors.

Local factors. *Generally, total cerebral blood flow is constant. However, regional cortical blood flow is associated with regional neural activity.* For example, movement of one hand results in increased blood flow only in the hand area of the contralateral sensorimotor and premotor cortex. Also, talking, reading, and other stimuli to the cerebral cortex are associated with increased blood flow in the appropriate regions of the contralateral cortex (Fig. 30-14). Glucose uptake also corresponds with regional cortical neuronal activity. For example when the retina is stimulated by light, uptake of ^{14}C-2-deoxyglucose is enhanced in the visual cortex.

The cerebral vessels are very sensitive to carbon dioxide tension. Increases in arterial blood CO_2 tension (Pa_{CO_2}) elicit marked cerebral vasodilation; inhalation of 7% CO_2 increases cerebral blood flow twofold. Conversely, decreases in Pa_{CO_2}, which can be caused by hyperventilation, decrease cerebral blood flow. CO_2 causes these changes by altering perivascular (and probably intracellular vascular smooth muscle) pH, which in turn alters arterial resistance. By independently changing P_{CO_2} and bicarbonate concentration, pial vessel diameter (and presumably blood flow) and pH have been shown to be inversely related, regardless of the level of the P_{CO_2}.

Carbon dioxide can diffuse to the vascular smooth muscle from the brain tissue or from the lumen of the vessels, whereas hydrogen ions in the blood are prevented from reaching the arteriolar smooth muscle by the **blood-brain barrier.** Hence, the cerebral vessels dilate when the hydrogen ion concentration of the cerebrospinal fluid is increased, but they dilate only minimally in response to an increase in the hydrogen ion concentration of the arterial blood.

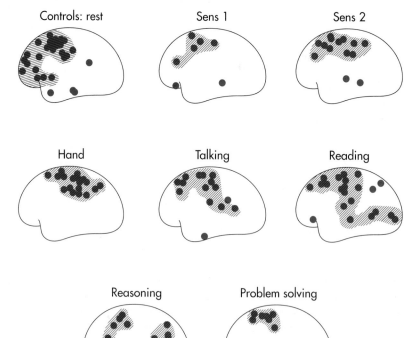

■ **Fig. 30-14** Effects of different stimuli on regional blood flow in the contralateral human cerebral cortex. *Sens 1,* Low-intensity electrical stimulation of the hand; *Sens 2,* high-intensity electrical stimulation of the hand (pain). (Redrawn from Ingvar DH: *Brain Res* 107:181, 1976.)

The K+ concentration also affects cerebral blood flow. Stimuli such as hypoxia, electrical stimulation of the brain, and seizures elicit rapid increases in cerebral blood flow that are associated with increases in perivascular K+ concentration. The increases in K+ concentration are similar to those that produce pial arteriolar dilation when K+ is applied topically to these vessels. However, the increase in K+ is not sustained throughout the period of stimulation. Hence, only the initial increase in cerebral blood flow can be attributed to the release of K+.

Adenosine is another factor that affects cerebral blood flow. Adenosine levels of the brain increase in response to ischemia, hypoxemia, hypotension, hypocapnia, electrical stimulation of the brain, and induced seizures. When applied topically, adenosine is a potent dilator of the pial arterioles. In fact, any intervention that either reduces the O₂ supply to the brain or increases the O₂ need of the brain results in rapid (within 5 seconds) formation of adenosine in the cerebral tissue. Unlike pH or K+, the adenosine concentration of the brain increases with initiation of the stimulus and remains elevated throughout the period of O₂ imbalance. The adenosine released into the cerebrospinal fluid during conditions associated with an inadequate brain O₂ supply becomes incorporated into cerebral tissue adenine nucleotides.

These local factors—pH, K+, and adenosine—may all act in concert to adjust the cerebral blood flow to the metabolic activity of the brain.

The cerebral circulation shows reactive hyperemia and excellent autoregulation between pressures of about 60 and 160 mm Hg. Mean arterial pressures below 60 mm Hg result in reduced cerebral blood flow and syncope, whereas mean pressures above 160 may lead to increased permeability of the blood-brain barrier and cerebral edema. Autoregulation of cerebral blood flow is abolished by hypercapnia or any other potent vasodilator. None of the candidates for metabolic regulation of cerebral blood flow accounts for this phenomenon. Hence, autoregulation of cerebral blood flow is probably attributable to a myogenic mechanism, although experimental proof is still lacking.

■ *Intestinal Circulation*
■ *Anatomy*

The gastrointestinal tract is supplied by the celiac, superior mesenteric, and inferior mesenteric arteries. The superior mesenteric artery is the largest of all the aortic branches and carries over 10% of the cardiac output. Small mesenteric arteries form an extensive vascular network in the submucosa of the gastrointestinal tract (Fig. 30-15). Their branches penetrate the longitudinal and circular muscle layers of the tract and give rise to third- and fourth-order arterioles. Some third-order arterioles in the submucosa become the main arterioles that supply the tips of the villi.

The direction of the blood flow in the capillaries and venules in a villus is opposite to that in the main arteriole (Fig. 30-16). This arrangement is a **countercurrent exchange system** (see Chapter 42). An effective countercurrent exchange also permits diffusion of O₂ from arterioles to venules. At low flow rates, a substantial portion of the O₂ of the blood may be shunted from arterioles to venules near the base of the villus. Thus, the supply of O₂ to the mucosal cells at the tip of the villus is reduced. When intestinal blood flow is very low, the shunting of O₂ is exaggerated, which may cause extensive necrosis of the intestinal villi.

■ *Neural Regulation*

The neural control of the mesenteric circulation is almost exclusively sympathetic. Increased sympathetic activity constricts the mesenteric arterioles and capacitance vessels. These responses are mediated by α-adrenergic receptors, which are prepotent in the mesenteric circulation; however, β-adrenergic receptors are also present. Infusion of a β-receptor agonist, such as isoproterenol, causes vasodilation.

During aggressive behavior or in response to artificial stimulation of the hypothalamic "defense" area, pro-

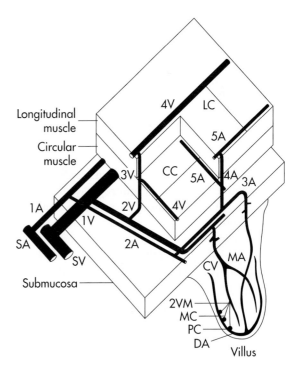

■ **Fig. 30-15** Distribution of small blood vessels to the rat intestinal wall. *Sa,* Small artery; *SV,* small vein: *1A* to *5A,* first- to fifth-order arterioles; *IV* to *4V,* first- to fourth-order venules; *CC* and *LC,* capillaries in circular and longitudinal muscle layers; *MA* and *CV,* main arteriole and collecting venule of a villus; *DA,* distribution arteriole; *2VM,* second-order mucosal venule; *PC,* precapillary sphincter; *MC,* mucosal capillary. (From Gore RW, Bohlen HG: *Am J Physiol* 233:H685, 1977.)

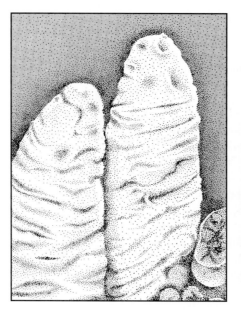 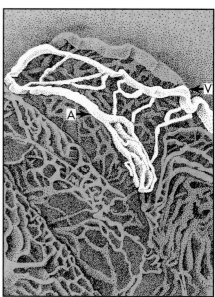

■ **Fig. 30-16** Scanning electron micrographs of rabbit intestinal villi *(left panel)* and corrosion cast of the microcirculation in the villus *(right panel)*. *A,* Arteriole; *V,* venule. (From Gannon BJ, Gore RW, Rogers PAW: *Biomed Res 2(suppl):*235, 1981.)

nounced vasoconstriction occurs in the mesenteric vascular bed. This vasoconstriction shifts blood flow from the temporarily less important intestinal circulation to the more crucial skeletal muscles, heart, and brain.

■ *Autoregulation*

Autoregulation of blood flow in the intestinal circulation is not as well developed as in certain other vascular beds, such as those in the brain and kidney. The principal mechanism responsible for autoregulation is metabolic, although a myogenic mechanism probably also participates (see Chapter 28). The adenosine concentration in the mesenteric venous blood rises fourfold after brief arterial occlusion. It also rises during enhanced metabolic activity of the intestinal mucosa, such as during absorption of food substances. Adenosine is a potent vasodilator in the mesenteric vascular bed and may be the principal metabolic mediator of autoregulation. However, potassium and altered osmolality may also contribute to autoregulation.

The O_2 consumption of the small intestine is more rigorously controlled than is the blood flow. In one series of experiments, the O_2 uptake of the small intestine remained constant when arterial perfusion pressure was varied between 30 and 125 mm Hg.

■ *Functional Hyperemia*

Food ingestion increases intestinal blood flow. The secretion of certain gastrointestinal hormones contributes to this hyperemia. Gastrin and cholecystokinin augment intestinal blood flow, and they are secreted when food is ingested. The absorption of food also affects intestinal blood flow. Undigested food has no vasoactive influence,

whereas several products of digestion are potent vasodilators. Among the various constituents of chyme, the principal mediators of mesenteric hyperemia are glucose and fatty acids.

■ *Hepatic Circulation*
■ *Anatomy*

The blood flow to the liver is normally about 25% of cardiac output. The *hepatic blood flow is derived from two sources: the portal vein and the hepatic artery.* Ordinarily, the portal vein provides about three fourths of the blood flow. Because the portal venous blood has already passed through the gastrointestinal capillary bed, much of the O_2 of the portal vein blood flow has been already extracted. The hepatic artery delivers the remaining one fourth of the blood, which is fully saturated with O_2. Hence, *about three fourths of the O_2 used by the liver is derived from the hepatic arterial blood.*

The small branches of the portal vein and hepatic artery give rise to terminal portal venules and hepatic arterioles (Fig. 30-17). These terminal vessels enter the hepatic acinus (the functional unit of the liver) at its center. Blood flows from these terminal vessels into the sinusoids, which constitute the capillary network of the liver. The sinusoids radiate toward the periphery of the acinus, where they connect with the terminal hepatic venules. Blood from these terminal venules drains into progressively larger branches of the hepatic veins, which are tributaries of the inferior vena cava.

■ *Hemodynamics*

The mean blood pressure in the portal vein is about 10 mm Hg, and the mean blood pressure in the hepatic

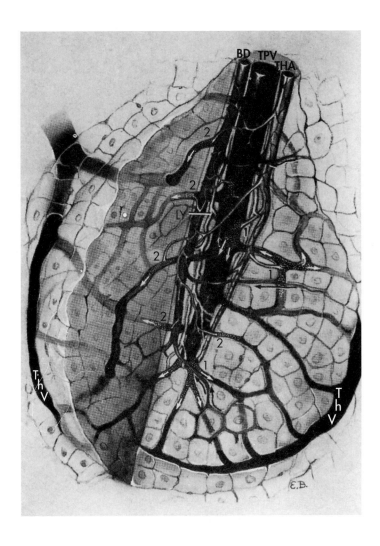

■ **Fig. 30-17** Microcirculation to a hepatic acinus. *THA,* Terminal hepatic arteriole; *TPV,* terminal portal venule; *BD,* bile ductule; *ThV,* terminal hepatic venule; *LY,* lymphatic. The hepatic arterioles empty either directly *(1)* or through the peribiliary plexus *(2)* into the sinusoids that run from the terminal portal venule to the terminal hepatic venules. (From Rappaport SM: *Microvasc Res* 6:212, 1973.)

artery about 90 mm Hg. The resistance of the vessels upstream to the hepatic sinusoids is considerably greater than that of the downstream vessels. Consequently, the pressure in the sinusoids is only 2 or 3 mm Hg greater than that in the hepatic veins and inferior vena cava. The ratio of presinusoidal to postsinusoidal resistance in the liver is much greater than is the ratio of precapillary to postcapillary resistance in almost any other vascular bed. Hence, drugs and other interventions that alter the presinusoidal resistance usually affect the pressure in the sinusoids only slightly. Such changes in presinusoidal resistance have little effect on the fluid exchange across the sinusoidal wall. However, *changes in hepatic venous (and in central venous) pressure are transmitted almost quantitatively to the hepatic sinusoids and profoundly affect the transsinusoidal exchange of fluids.*

■ *Regulation of Flow*

Blood flows in the portal venous and hepatic arterial systems vary reciprocally. When blood flow is curtailed in one system, the flow increases in the other system. However, the ensuing increase in flow in one system usu-

ally does not fully compensate for the reduction in flow in the other system.

The portal venous system does not autoregulate. As portal venous pressure and flow are raised, resistance either remains constant or decreases. The hepatic arterial system does autoregulate, however, and adenosine may be involved in this adjustment of blood flow.

When central venous pressure is elevated, as in **congestive heart failure,** large quantities of plasma water transude from the liver into the peritoneal cavity; such a fluid accumulation in the abdomen is known as **ascites.** Extensive fibrosis of the liver, as in the various types of **hepatic cirrhosis,** leads to a pronounced increase in hepatic vascular resistance, which raises the pressure substantially in the portal venous system. The consequent increase in capillary hydrostatic pressure through the splanchnic circulation also leads to extensive fluid transudation into the abdominal cavity. Furthermore, the pressure may rise substantially in other veins that anastomose with the portal vein. For example, the esophageal veins may enlarge considerably to form **esophageal varices.** These varices may rupture and lead to severe, frequently fatal, internal bleeding. To prevent these grave problems associated with elevated portal venous pressure in cirrhosis of the liver, an anastomosis **(portacaval shunt)** is often created surgically between the portal vein and inferior vena cava to lower portal venous pressure.

The liver tends to maintain a constant O_2 consumption, because the extraction of O_2 from the hepatic blood is very efficient.

The rate of O_2 delivery to the liver is varied; the liver compensates by an appropriate change in the fraction of O_2 extracted from the blood. This extraction is facilitated by the distance between the presinusoidal vessels at the acinar center and the postsinusoidal vessels at the periphery of the acinus (Fig. 30-17). The substantial distance between these types of vessels prevents a countercurrent exchange of O_2, contrary to the countercurrent exchange that occurs in an intestinal villus (Fig. 30-16).

The sympathetic nerves constrict the presinusoidal resistance vessels in the portal venous and hepatic arterial systems. Neural effects on the capacitance vessels are more important, however. The liver contains about 15% of the total blood volume of the body. Under appropriate conditions, such as in response to hemorrhage, about half of the hepatic blood volume can be rapidly expelled with constriction of the capacitance vessels (see also Chapter 31). Hence, *the liver constitutes an important blood reservoir in humans.* In certain other species, such as the dog, the spleen is a more important blood reservoir.

■ *Fetal Circulation*

■ *In Utero*

Before birth, the circulation of the fetus differs from that of the postnatal infant. The most important difference is that the fetal lungs are functionally inactive, and the fetus depends completely on the placenta for O_2 and nutrient supply. Oxygenated fetal blood from the placenta passes through the umbilical vein to the liver. Approximately half of the flow from the placenta passes though the liver, and the remainder bypasses the liver and reaches the inferior vena cava through the **ductus venosus** (Fig. 30-18). In the inferior vena cava, blood from the ductus venosus joins blood returning from the lower trunk and extremities, and this combined stream is in turn joined by blood from the liver through the hepatic veins.

The streams of blood tend to maintain their identities in the inferior vena cava and are divided into two streams of unequal size by the edge of the interatrial septum **(crista dividens).** The larger stream, which contains mainly blood from the umbilical vein, is shunted from the inferior vena cava to the left atrium through the **foramen ovale** (Fig. 30-18). The other stream passes into the right atrium, where it is joined by blood returning from the upper parts of the body through the superior vena cava and by blood from the myocardium.

In contrast to the adult, in whom the right and left ventricles pump in series, the ventricles in the fetus operate essentially in parallel. Because the pulmonary vascular resistance of the fetus is large, only one tenth of right ventricular output passes through the lungs. The remainder passes from the pulmonary artery through the ductus arteriosus to the aorta at a point distal to the origins of the arteries to the head and upper extremities. Blood flows from the pulmonary artery to the aorta, because the pulmonary vascular resistance is high and the diameter of the ductus arteriosus is as large as that of the descending aorta.

The large volume of blood that passes through the foramen ovale into the left atrium is joined by blood returning from the lungs, and it is pumped out by the left ventricle into the aorta. Most of the blood in the ascending aorta goes to the head, upper thorax, and arms; the remainder joins blood from the ductus arteriosus and supplies the rest of the body. The amount of blood pumped by the left ventricle is about half that pumped by the right ventricle. The major fraction of the blood that passes down the descending aorta comes from the ductus arteriosus and right ventricle and flows by way of the two umbilical arteries to the placenta.

Fig. 30-18 indicates the O_2 saturations of the blood at various points of the fetal circulation. Fetal blood that leaves the placenta is 80% saturated, but the saturation of the blood that passes through the foramen ovale is reduced to 67%. This reduction in O_2 saturation is caused by mixing with desaturated blood returning from the lower part of the body and the liver. Addition of the desaturated blood from the lungs reduces the O_2 saturation of left ventricular blood to 62%, which is the level of saturation of the blood reaching the head and upper extremities.

The blood in the right ventricle, which is a mixture of desaturated superior vena caval blood, coronary venous blood, and inferior vena caval blood, is only 52% saturated with O_2. When the major portion of this blood traverses the ductus arteriosus and joins that pumped out by the left ventricle, the resultant O_2 saturation of blood traveling to the lower part of the body and back to the placenta is 58%. Thus, the tissues that receive blood of the highest O_2 saturation are the liver, heart, and upper parts of the body, including the head.

At the placenta, the chorionic villi dip into the maternal sinuses, and O_2, CO_2, nutrients, and metabolic waste products are exchanged across the membranes. The barrier to exchange prevents equilibration of Po_2 between the two circulations at normal rates of blood flow. Therefore, the O_2 tension of the fetal blood that leaves the placenta is very low. Were it not for the fact that fetal hemoglobin has a greater affinity for O_2 than does adult hemoglobin, the fetus would not receive an adequate O_2 supply. The fetal oxyhemoglobin dissociation curve is shifted to the left so that, at equal pressures of O_2, fetal blood carries significantly more O_2 than does maternal blood.

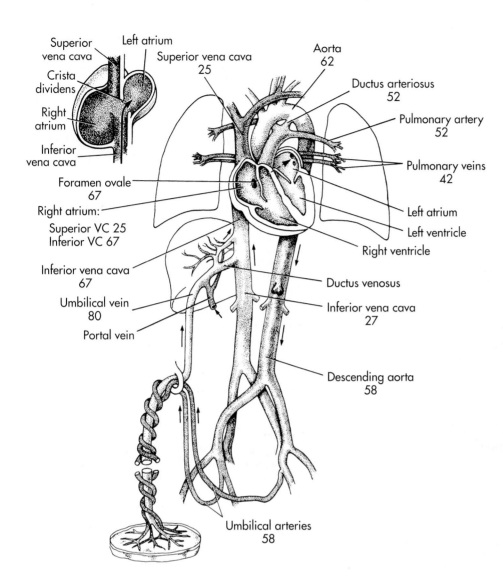

Superior vena cava
Left atrium
Superior vena cava 25
Aorta 62
Ductus arteriosus 52
Crista dividens
Right atrium
Pulmonary artery 52
Inferior vena cava
Pulmonary veins 42
Foramen ovale 67
Right atrium:
Superior VC 25
Inferior VC 67
Left atrium
Left ventricle
Right ventricle
Inferior vena cava 67
Umbilical vein 80
Ductus venosus
Inferior vena cava 27
Portal vein
Descending aorta 58
Umbilical arteries 58

■ **Fig. 30-18** Schematic diagram of the fetal circulation. The numbers represent the percentage of O_2 saturation of the blood flowing in the indicated blood vessel. The inset at upper left illustrates the direction of flow of a major portion of the inferior vena caval blood through the foramen ovale to the left atrium. (Values for O_2 saturations are from Dawes GS, Mott JC, Widdicombe JG: *J Physiol* 126:563, 1954.)

In early fetal life, the high cardiac glycogen levels that prevail may protect the heart from acute periods of hypoxia. The glycogen levels decrease in late fetal life and reach adult levels by term.

> If the mother is subjected to hypoxia, the reduced blood O_2 tension is reflected in the fetus by tachycardia and an increase in blood flow through the umbilical vessels. If the hypoxia persists or if flow through the umbilical vessels is impaired, **fetal distress** occurs and is first manifested as bradycardia.

■ *Circulatory Changes That Occur at Birth*

The umbilical vessels have thick muscular walls that react to trauma, tension, sympathomimetic amines, bradykinin, angiotensin, and changes in Po_2. In animals in which the umbilical cord is not tied, hemorrhage of the newborn is prevented by constriction of these large vessels in response to one or more of these stimuli.

Closure of the umbilical vessels produces an increase in total peripheral resistance and of blood pressure. When blood flow through the umbilical vein ceases, the ductus venosus, a thick-walled vessel with a muscular sphincter, closes. The factor that initiates closure of the ductus venosus is still unknown.

Immediately after birth, the asphyxia caused by constriction or clamping of the umbilical vessels, together with the cooling of the body, activates the respiratory center of the newborn infant. As the lungs fill with air, pulmonary vascular resistance decreases to about one tenth of the value that existed before lung expansion. This resistance change is not caused by the presence of O_2 in the lungs, because the change is just as great if the lungs are filled with nitrogen. However, filling the lungs with liquid does not reduce pulmonary vascular resistance.

After birth, the left atrial pressure is raised above that in the inferior vena cava and right atrium by (1) the decrease in pulmonary resistance, with the resultant large flow of blood through the lungs to the left atrium; (2) the reduction of flow to the right atrium caused by occlusion of the umbilical vein; and (3) the increased resistance to left ventricular output produced by occlusion of the umbilical arteries. This reversal of the pressure gradient across the atria abruptly closes the valve over the foramen ovale, and the septal leaflets fuse over several days.

The decrease in pulmonary vascular resistance causes the pressure in the pulmonary artery to fall to about one half its previous level (to about 35 mm Hg). This change in pressure, coupled with a slight increase in aortic pressure, reverses the flow of blood through the ductus arteriosus. However, within several minutes, the large ductus arteriosus begins to constrict. This constriction produces turbulent flow, which is manifested as a murmur in the newborn. Constriction of the ductus arteriosus is progressive and is usually complete within 1 to 2 days after birth. Closure of the ductus arteriosus appears to be initiated by the high O_2 tension of the arterial blood passing through it; pulmonary ventilation with O_2 closes the ductus, whereas ventilation with air low in O_2 opens this shunt vessel. Whether O_2 acts directly on the ductus or through the release of a vasoconstrictor substance is not known.

The ductus arteriosus occasionally fails to close after birth. This congenital cardiovascular abnormality, called **patent ductus arteriosus,** can be corrected surgically.

At the time of birth, the walls of the two ventricles are about equal in thickness. In addition, the muscle layer of the pulmonary arterioles is thick; this thickness is partly responsible for the high pulmonary vascular resistance of the fetus. After birth, the thickness of the walls of the right ventricle diminishes, as does the muscle layer of the pulmonary arterioles. The left ventricular walls also become thicker. These changes are progressive over a period of weeks after birth.

■ *Summary*

■ *Coronary Circulation*

1. The physical factors that influence coronary blood flow are the viscosity of the blood, the frictional resistance of the vessel walls, the aortic pressure, and the extravascular compression of the vessels within the walls of the left ventricle. Left coronary blood flow is restricted during ventricular systole by extravascular compression, and it is greatest during diastole when the intramyocardial vessels are not compressed.

2. Neural regulation of coronary blood flow is much less important than metabolic regulation. Activation of the cardiac sympathetic nerves constricts the coronary resistance vessels. However, the enhanced myocardial metabolism caused by the associated increase in heart rate and contractile force produces vasodilation, which overrides the direct constrictor effect of sympathetic nerve stimulation. Stimulation of the cardiac branches of the vagus nerves slightly dilates the coronary arterioles.

3. A striking parallelism exists between metabolic activity of the heart and coronary blood flow. A decrease in oxygen supply or an increase in oxygen demand apparently releases a vasodilator substance that decreases coronary resistance. Of the known factors (CO_2, O_2, H^+, K^+, adenosine) that can mediate this response, adenosine appears to be the most likely candidate.

4. Prolonged, severe reduction in coronary blood flow leads to myocardial cell necrosis and thereby impairs cardiac contraction. Moderate, sustained reductions in coronary blood flow may evoke myocardial hibernation, which is a reversible impairment of mechanical performance associated with a down-regulation of cardiac metabolism. Transient periods of severe ischemia followed by reperfusion may induce myocardial stunning, a temporary stage of impaired mechanical performance by the heart.

5. In response to gradual occlusion of a coronary artery, collateral vessels from adjacent unoccluded arteries develop and supply blood to the compromised myocardium distal to the point of occlusion.

6. The myocardium functions only aerobically and in general uses substrates in proportion to their arterial concentration.

■ *Skin Circulation*

1. Most of the resistance vessels in the skin are under dual control of the sympathetic nervous system and local vasodilator metabolites. The arteriovenous anastomoses found in the hands, feet, and face, however, are solely under neural control.

2. The main function of skin blood vessels is to aid in the regulation of body temperature by constricting to conserve heat and dilating to lose heat.

3. Skin blood vessels dilate directly and reflexly in response to heat and constrict directly and reflexly in response to cold.

■ *Skeletal Muscle Circulation*

1. Skeletal muscle blood flow is regulated centrally by the sympathetic nerves and locally by the release of vasodilator metabolites.

2. In subjects at rest, neural regulation of blood flow is paramount, but it yields to metabolic regulation during muscle contractions (such as during exercise).

■ Cerebral Circulation

1. Cerebral blood flow is predominantly regulated by metabolic factors, especially CO_2, K^+, and adenosine.

2. Increased regional cerebral activity produced by stimuli such as touch, pain, hand motion, talking, reading, reasoning, and problem solving are associated with enhanced blood flow in the activated area of the contralateral cerebral cortex.

■ Intestinal Circulation

1. The microcirculation in the intestinal villi constitutes a countercurrent exchange system for O_2. The presence of this countercurrent exchange system places the villi in jeopardy in states of low blood flow.

2. The splanchnic resistance and capacitance vessels are very responsive to changes in sympathetic neural activity.

■ Hepatic Circulation

1. The liver receives about 25% of cardiac output; about three fourths of this output is from the portal vein and about one fourth from the hepatic artery. When flow is diminished in either the portal or hepatic system, flow in the other system usually increases, but not proportionately.

2. The liver tends to maintain a constant O_2 consumption, in part because its mechanism for extracting O_2 from the blood is so efficient.

3. The liver normally contains about 15% of total blood volume. It serves as an important blood reservoir for the body.

■ Fetal Circulation

1. In the fetus, a large percentage of right atrial blood passes through the foramen ovale to the left atrium, and a large percentage of pulmonary arterial blood passes through the ductus arteriosus to the aorta.

2. At birth, the umbilical vessels, ductus venosus, and ductus arteriosus close by contraction of their muscle layers. The reduction in pulmonary vascular resistance caused by lung inflation is the main factor that reverses the pressure gradient between the atria, thereby closing the foramen ovale.

■ Self-Study Problems

1. What is the effect of cardiac sympathetic nerve stimulation on coronary blood flow?

2. What is meant by metabolic regulation of coronary blood flow?

3. How do tachycardia and bradycardia affect coronary blood flow?

4. With regard to the various disturbances in cardiac function induced by diminished coronary blood flow, distinguish among myocardial infarction, stunning, and hibernation.

5. Compare and contrast the chief factors in the regulation of skin and skeletal muscle blood flow.

6. How is cerebral blood flow regulated?

7. What problem in transcapillary fluid exchange in the abdominal viscera occurs as a consequence of chronic inflammatory processes in the liver (hepatic cirrhosis)?

8. What happens to the distribution of right ventricular output when the newborn infant takes his or her first few breaths?

■ Bibliography

Journal articles

Abboud FM, editor: Regulation of the cerebral circulation (symposium), *Fed Proc* 40:2296, 1981.

Baron JF, Vicaut E, Hou X, Duvelleroy M: Independent role of arterial O_2 tension in local control of coronary blood flow, *Am J Physiol* 258:H1388, 1990.

Belardinelli L, Linden J, Berne RM: The cardiac effects of adenosine, *Prog Cardiovasc Dis* 32:73, 1989.

Berne RM: Role of adenosine in the regulation of coronary artery blood flow, *Circ Res* 47:807, 1980.

Berne RM, Winn HR, Rubio R: The local regulation of cerebral blood flow, *Prog Cardiovasc Dis* 24:243, 1981.

Bolli R: Myocardial "stunning" in man, *Circulation* 86:1671, 1992

Brunner JJ, Greene AS, Frankle AE, Shoukas AA: Carotid sinus baroreceptor control of splanchnic resistance and capacity, *Am J Physiol* 255:H1305, 1988.

Clyman RI, Saugstad OD, Mauray F: Reactive oxygen metabolites relax the lamb ductus arteriosus by stimulating prostaglandin production, *Circ Res* 64:1, 1989.

Escourrou P et al: Cardiopulmonary and carotid baroflex control of splanchnic and forearm circulation, *Am J Physiol* 264:H777, 1993.

Feigl EO: Coronary physiology, *Physiol Rev* 63:1, 1983.

Greenway CV, Lautt WW: Distensibility of hepatic venous resistance sites and consequences on portal pressure, *Am J Physiol* 254:H452, 1988.

Heymann MA, Iwamoto HS, Rudolf AM: Factors affecting changes in the neonatal systemic circulation, *Annu Rev Physiol* 43:371, 1981.

Hoffman JIE, Spaan JAE: Pressure-flow relations in coronary circulation, *Physiol Rev* 70:331, 1990.

Iwata F et al: Role of EDRF in splanchnic blood flow of normal and chronic portal hypertensive rats, *Am J Physiol* 263:G149, 1992.

Klocke FJ, Ellis AK: Control of coronary blood flow, *Annu Rev Med* 31:489, 1980.

Klocke FJ, Mates RE, Canty JM Jr, Ellis AK: Coronary pressure-flow relationships—controversial issues and probable implications, *Circ Res* 56:310, 1985.

Kusuoka H, Marban E: Cellular mechanisms of myocardial stunning, *Annu Rev Physiol* 54:243, 1992.

Laughlin MH: Skeletal muscle blood flow capacity: role of muscle pump in exercise hyperemia, *Am J Physiol* 253:H993, 1987.

Lautt WW, Legare DJ: Passive autoregulation of portal venous pressure: distensible hepatic resistance, *Am J Physiol* 263: G702, 1992.

Lautt WW, Schafer J, Legare DJ: Hepatic blood flow distribution: consideration of gravity, liver surface, and norepinephrine on regional heterogeneity, *Can J Physiol* 71:128, 1993.

Maass-Moreno R, Rothe CF: Contribution of large hepatic veins to postsinusoidal vascular resistance, *Am J Physiol* 262:G14, 1992.

Manor D et al: Modulation of coronary flow by left ventricular volume in the presence and absence of vasomotor tone, *Am J Physiol* 269:H2010, 1995.

Marban E: Myocardial stunning and hibernation: the physiology behind the colloquialisms, *Circulation* 83:681, 1991.

Marshall JM: Skeletal muscle vasculature and systemic hypoxia, *News Physiol Sci* 10:274, 1995.

Mohabir R et al: Effects of ischemia and hypercarbic acidosis on myocyte calcium transient, contraction and pHi in perfused rabbit hearts, *Circ Res* 69:1525, 1991.

Mohri M et al: Duration of ischemia is vital for collateral development: repeated brief coronary artery occlusions in conscious dogs, *Circ Res* 64:287, 1989.

Morgan JP: Abnormal intracellular modulation of calcium as a major cause of cardiac contractile dysfunction, *N Engl J Med* 325:625, 1991.

Olsson RA: Local factors regulating cardiac and skeletal muscle blood flow, *Annu Rev Physiol* 43:385, 1981.

Olsson RA, Bunger R: Metabolic control of coronary blood flow, *Prog Cardiovasc Dis* 29:369, 1987.

Olsson RA, Pearson JD: Cardiovascular purinoceptors, *Physiol Rev* 70:761, 1990.

Reller MD et al: Nitric oxide is an important determinant of coronary flow at rest and during hypoxemic stress in fetal lambs, *Am J Physiol* 269:H2074, 1995.

Schaper W: Molecular mechanisms of coronary collateral vessel growth, *Circ Res* 79:911, 1996.

Schwartz LM, McKenzie JE: Adenosine and active hyperemia in soleus and gracilis muscle of cats, *Am J Physiol* 259:H1295, 1990.

Symons JD, Firoozmand E, Longhurst JC: Repeated dipyridamole administration enhances collateral-dependent flow and regional function during exercise: a role for adenosine, *Circ Res* 73:503, 1993.

Tysebnko VA, Yanchuk PI: Central nervous control of hepatic circulation, *J Auton Nerv Syst* 33:255, 1991.

Wearn JT, Mettier SR, Klumpp TG, Zschiesche LJ: The nature of the vascular communications between the coronary arteries and the chambers of the heart, *Am Heart J* 9:143, 1933.

White CW, Wilson RF, Marcus ML: Methods of measuring myocardial blood flow in humans, *Prog Cardiovasc Dis* 31:79, 1988.

Zellers TM, McCormick J, Wu Y: Interaction among ET-1, endothelium-derived nitric oxide, and prostacyclin in pulmonary arteries and veins, *Am J Physiol* 267:H139, 1994.

Books and monographs

Berne RM, Rubio R: *Coronary circulation.* In *Handbook of physiology,* sect 2, *The cardiovascular system—the heart,* vol I, Bethesda, Md, 1979, American Physiological Society.

Berne RM, Winn HR, Rubio R: *Metabolic regulation of cerebral blood flow.* In *Mechanisms of vasodilation—second symposium,* New York, 1981, Raven Press.

Donald DE: *Splanchnic circulation.* In *Handbook of physiology,* sect 2, *The cardiovascular system—peripheral circulation and organ blood flow,* vol III, Bethesda, Md, 1983, American Physiological Society.

Faber JJ, Thornburg K: *Placental physiology,* New York, 1983, Raven Press.

Granger DN, Kvietys PR, Korthuis RJ, Premen AJ: *Microcirculation of the intestinal mucosa.* In *Handbook of physiology,* sect 6, *The gastrointestinal system—motility and circulation,* vol I, Bethesda, Md, 1989, American Physiological Society.

Greenway CV, Lautt WW: *Hepatic circulation.* In *Handbook of physiology,* sect 6, *The gastrointestinal system—motility and circulation,* vol I, Bethesda, Md, 1989, American Physiological Society.

Gregg DE: *Coronary circulation in health and disease,* Philadelphia, 1950, Lea & Febiger.

Guth PH, Leung FW, Kauffman GL Jr: *Physiology of gastric circulation.* In *Handbook of physiology,* sect 6, *The gastrointestinal system—motility and circulation,* vol I, Bethesda, Md, 1989, American Physiological Society.

Heistad DD, Kontos HA: *Cerebral circulation.* In *Handbook of physiology,* sect 2, *The cardiovascular system—peripheral circulation and organ blood flow,* vol III, Bethesda, Md, 1983, American Physiological Society.

Hellon R: *Thermoreceptors.* In *Handbook of physiology,* sect 2, *The cardiovascular system—peripheral circulation and organ blood flow,* vol III, Bethesda, Md, 1983, American Physiological Society.

Lewis T: *Blood vessels of the human skin and their responses,* London, 1927, Shaw & Son.

Marcus ML: *The coronary circulation in health and disease,* New York, 1983, McGraw-Hill.

Mott JC, Walker DW: *Neural and endocrine regulation of circulation in the fetus and newborn.* In *Handbook of physiology,* sect 2, *The cardiovascular system—peripheral circulation and organ blood flow,* vol III, Bethesda, Md, 1983, American Physiological Society.

Olsson RA, Bunger R, Spaan JAE: *The coronary circulation.* In Fozzard HA et al, editors: *The heart and cardiovascular system,* ed 2, New York, 1991, Raven Press.

Owman C, Hardebo JE, editors: *Neural regulation of brain circulation,* Amsterdam, 1985, Elsevier.

Phillis JW, editor: *The regulation of cerebral blood flow,* Boca Raton, Fla, 1993, CRC Press.

Roddie EC: *Circulation to skin and adipose tissue.* In *Handbook of physiology,* sect 2, *The cardiovascular system—peripheral circulation and organ blood flow,* vol III, Bethesda, Md, 1983, American Physiological Society.

Schaper W, Bernotat-Danielowski S, Niennaber C, Schaper J: *Collateral circulation.* In Fozzard HA et al, editors: *The heart and cardiovascular system,* ed 2, New York, 1991, Raven Press.

Shepherd JT: *Circulation to skeletal muscle.* In *Handbook of physiology,* sect 2, *The cardiovascular system—peripheral circulation and organ blood flow,* vol III, Bethesda, Md, 1983, American Physiological Society.

Sparks HV Jr, Wangler RD, Groman MW: *Control of the coronary circulation.* In Sperelakis N, editor: *Physiology and pathophysiology of the heart,* ed 2, Boston, 1989, Wolters-Kluwer.

CHAPTER

31

Interplay of Central and Peripheral Factors in the Control of the Circulation

The primary function of the circulatory system is to deliver the supplies needed for tissue metabolism and growth and to remove the products of metabolism. In previous chapters, to explain how the heart and blood vessels serve this function, we have analyzed the system morphologically and functionally. Specifically, we have discussed the contributions of the component parts of the cardiovascular system to maintain adequate tissue perfusion under different physiological conditions.

With this understanding of the functions of the various components in mind, it is now essential to explore their interrelationships in the overall role of the circulatory system. Tissue perfusion depends on arterial pressure and local vascular resistance. Arterial pressure in turn depends on cardiac output and total peripheral resistance (TPR). Arterial pressure is maintained within a relatively narrow range in the normal individual, a feat accomplished by reciprocal changes in cardiac output and TPR. However, cardiac output and peripheral resistance are each influenced by a number of factors, and it is the interplay among these factors that determines the level of these two variables.

The autonomic nervous system and the baroreceptors play key roles in regulating blood pressure. However, from the long-range point of view, the control of fluid balance by the kidney, adrenal cortex, and central nervous system, with maintenance of a constant blood volume, is of the greatest importance.

In any well-regulated system, one way to study the extent and sensitivity of its regulatory mechanisms is to disturb the system and observe how it restores the preexisting steady state. Disturbances in the form of physical exercise and hemorrhage are used in the following sections to illustrate the effects of the various regulatory factors.

■ Exercise

The cardiovascular adjustments that take place during exercise consist of a combination and integration of neural and local (chemical) factors. The neural factors include (1) **central command,** (2) reflexes that originate in the contracting muscle, and (3) the baroreceptor reflex.

Central command is the cerebrocortical activation of the sympathetic nervous system that produces cardiac acceleration, increased myocardial contractile force, and peripheral vasoconstriction. Reflexes are activated intramuscularly by stimulation of mechanoreceptors (by stretch, tension) and chemoreceptors (by products of metabolism) in response to muscle contraction. Impulses from these receptors travel centrally via small myelinated (group III) and unmyelinated (group IV) afferent nerve fibers. The group IV unmyelinated fibers may represent the muscle chemoreceptors, as no morphologic chemoreceptor has been identified. The central connections of this reflex are unknown, but the efferent limb consists of sympathetic nerve fibers to the heart and peripheral blood vessels. The baroreceptor reflex is described on p 450, and the local factors that influence skeletal muscle blood flow (metabolic vasodilators) are described on pp 446 and 490. Vascular chemoreceptors are important in the regulation of the cardiovascular system during exercise. Evidence for this assertion comes from the observations that the pH, Pco_2, and Po_2 of arterial blood remain normal during exercise, and that the vascular chemoreceptors are located on the arterial side of the circulatory system.

■ Mild to Moderate Exercise

In humans or trained animals, anticipation of physical activity inhibits the vagal nerve impulses to the heart and increases sympathetic discharge. The simultaneous inhibition of parasympathetic areas and activation of sympathetic areas of the medulla increase heart rate and myocardial contractility. The tachycardia and enhanced contractility increase cardiac output.

Peripheral resistance. At the same time that cardiac stimulation occurs, the sympathetic nervous system also changes vascular resistance in the periphery. In skin, kidneys, splanchnic regions, and inactive muscle, sympathetic-mediated vasoconstriction increases vascular resistance, and thereby diverts blood away from these areas (Fig. 31-1). This increased vascular resistance persists throughout the period of exercise.

As cardiac output and blood flow to active muscles increase with progressive increases in the intensity of exercise, visceral blood flow (i.e., to the splanchnic and renal vasculatures) decreases. Blood flow to the myocardium increases, whereas flow to the brain is unchanged. Skin blood flow initially decreases during exercise and then increases as body temperature rises with increments in the duration and intensity of exercise. Skin blood flow finally decreases when the skin vessels constrict as total body O_2 consumption nears its maximal value (Fig. 31-1).

The major circulatory adjustment to prolonged exercise occurs in the vasculature of the active muscles. Local formation of vasoactive metabolites dilates the resistance vessels markedly. This dilation progresses with increases in the intensity level of exercise. Potassium is one of the vasodilator substances released by the contracting muscle, and it may be partly responsible for the initial decrease in vascular resistance in the active muscles. Other contributing factors may be the release of adenosine and a decrease in pH during sustained exercise. The local accumulation of metabolites relaxes the terminal arterioles. As a result, blood flow through the muscle may increase fifteenfold to twentyfold above the resting level. This metabolic vasodilation of the precapillary vessels in active muscles occurs very soon after the onset of exercise. The decrease in total peripheral resistance (TPR) enables the heart to pump more blood at a lesser load and more efficiently (less pressure work, see p 486) than if TPR were unchanged (see Chapters 29 and 30).

Marked changes in the capillary circulation also occur during exercise. Only a small percentage of the capillaries are perfused at rest, whereas in actively contracting muscle, all or nearly all of the capillaries contain flowing blood **(capillary recruitment).** The surface area available for exchange of gases, water, and solutes is increased many times. Furthermore, the hydrostatic pressure in the capillaries is increased because of the relaxation of the resistance vessels. Hence, water and solutes move into the muscle tissue. Tissue pressure rises and remains elevated during exercise as fluid continues to move out of the capillaries; this fluid is carried away by the lymphatics. Lymph flow is increased as a result of the increase in capillary hydrostatic pressure and the mas-

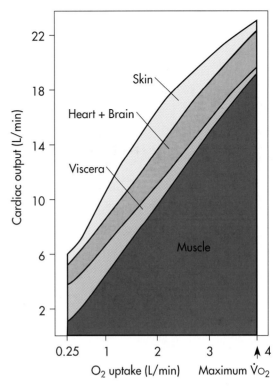

■ **Fig. 31-1** Approximate distribution of cardiac output at rest and at different levels of exercise up to the maximal O_2 consumption (Vo_{2max}) in a normal young man. (Redrawn from Ruch HP, Patton TC: *Physiology and biophysics,* ed 12, Philadelphia, 1974, WB Saunders.)

saging effect of the contracting muscles on the valve-containing lymphatic vessels (see p 489).

Contracting muscle avidly extracts O_2 from the perfusing blood and thereby increases arteriovenous O_2 difference, Fig. 31-2). This release of O_2 from the blood is facilitated by the shift in the oxyhemoglobin dissociation curve during exercise. During exercise, the high concentration of CO_2 and the formation of lactic acid reduce the pH. This decrease in pH plus the increase in temperature in the contracting muscle shifts the oxyhemoglobin dissociation curve to the right (see Chapter 35). Therefore, at any given partial pressure of O_2, less O_2 is held by the hemoglobin in the red cells, and consequently more O_2 is available for the tissues. Oxygen consumption may increase as much as sixtyfold with only a fifteenfold increase in muscle blood flow. Muscle myoglobin may serve as a limited O_2 store during exercise, and it can release attached O_2 at very low partial pressures. However, the myoglobin can also facilitate O_2 transport from capillaries to mitochondria by serving as an O_2 carrier.

Cardiac output. Because the enhanced sympathetic drive and the reduced parasympathetic inhibition of the sinoatrial node continue during exercise, tachycardia persists. If the workload is moderate and constant, the heart rate will reach a certain level and remain there through-

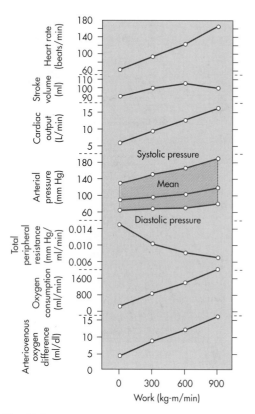

■ **Fig. 31-2** Effect of different levels of exercise on several cardiovascular variables. (Data from Carlsten A, Grimby G: *The circulatory response to muscular exercise in man,* Springfield, Ill, 1966, Charles C Thomas.)

out the period of exercise. However, if the workload increases, the heart rate increases concomitantly until a plateau is reached in strenuous exercise at about 180 beats/min. In contrast to the large increase in heart rate, the increase in stroke volume is only about 10% to 35%, the larger values occurring in trained individuals (Fig. 31-2). In very-well-trained distance runners, whose cardiac outputs can reach six to seven times the resting level, stroke volume reaches about twice the resting value.

Thus, the increase in cardiac output observed during exercise is correlated principally with an increase in heart rate. If the baroreceptors are denervated, the cardiac output and heart rate responses to exercise are sluggish compared with the changes in animals with normally innervated baroreceptors. However, in dogs with total cardiac denervation, exercise still increases cardiac output as much as it does in normal animals. This increase in cardiac output is achieved chiefly by means of an elevated stroke volume. However, if a β-adrenergic receptor blocking agent is given to the dogs with denervated hearts, exercise performance is impaired. The β-adrenergic receptor blocker apparently prevents the cardiac acceleration and enhanced contractility caused by increased amounts of circulating catecholamines, and hence limits the increase in cardiac output necessary for maximal exercise performance.

Venous return. In addition to the contribution made by sympathetically mediated constriction of the capacitance vessels in both exercising and nonexercising parts of the body, venous return is aided by the auxillary pumping action of the working skeletal muscles and the muscles of respiration (see also Chapter 29). The intermittently contracting muscles compress the veins that course through them. Because the venous valves are oriented toward the heart, the contracting muscle pumps blood back toward the right atrium (see Chapter 30). In exercise, the flow of venous blood to the heart is also aided by the deeper and more frequent respirations that increase the pressure gradient where the veins enter the thorax (intrathoracic pressure becomes more negative during exercise).

In humans, blood reservoirs do not contribute much to the circulating blood volume. In fact, blood volume is usually reduced slightly during exercise, as evidenced by a rise in the hematocrit ratio. This decrease in blood volume is caused by water loss externally through sweating and enhanced ventilation, and fluid movement into the contracting muscle.

However, fluid loss is counteracted in several ways. The fluid loss from vascular compartment into contracting muscles eventually reaches a plateau as interstitial fluid pressure rises and opposes the increased hydrostatic pressure in the capillaries of the active muscle. Fluid loss is partially offset by movement of fluid from the splanchnic regions and inactive muscle into the bloodstream. This influx of fluid occurs as a result of a decrease of hydrostatic pressure in the capillaries of these tissues, and of an increase in the plasma osmolarity because of movement of osmotically active molecules into the blood from the contracting muscle. In addition, reduced urine formation by the kidneys helps to conserve body water.

The large volume of blood returning to the heart is so effectively pumped through the lungs and out into the aorta that central venous pressure remains essentially constant. Thus, the Frank-Starling mechanism of a greater initial fiber length does not account for the greater stroke volume in moderate exercise. Chest x-ray films of individuals at rest and during exercise reveal a decrease in heart size during exercise. This observation is in harmony with the observation of a constant ventricular filling pressure. However, during maximal or near-maximal exercise, right atrial pressure and end-diastolic ventricular volume do increase. Thus, the Frank-Starling mechanism contributes to the enhanced stroke volume in very vigorous exercise.

Arterial pressure. If the exercise involves a large proportion of the body musculature, such as in running or swimming, the reduction in total vascular resistance can be considerable. Nevertheless, arterial pressure starts to rise with the onset of exercise, and the increase in blood pressure roughly parallels the severity of the exercise performed (Fig. 31-2). Therefore, the increase in cardiac output is proportionally greater than the decrease in TPR.

The vasoconstriction produced in the inactive tissues by the sympathetic nervous system (and to some extent by the release of catecholamines from the adrenal medulla) is important for maintenance of normal or increased blood pressure. Sympathectomy- or drug-induced block of the adrenergic sympathetic nerve fibers results in a decrease in arterial pressure (hypotension) during exercise.

Sympathetic neural activity also elicits vasoconstriction in active skeletal muscle when additional muscles are recruited. In experiments in which one leg is working at maximal levels and then the other leg starts to work, blood flow decreases in the first working leg. Furthermore, blood levels of norepinephrine rise significantly during exercise, and most of it is released from the sympathetic nerves in the active muscles.

As body temperature rises during exercise, the skin vessels dilate in response to thermal stimulation of the heat-regulating center in the hypothalamus, and TPR decreases further. This reduction in TPR would reduce blood pressure were it not for the increased cardiac output and the constriction of arterioles in the renal, splanchnic, and other tissues.

In general, then, mean arterial pressure rises during exercise as a result of the increase in cardiac output. However, the effect of enhanced cardiac output is offset by the overall decrease in TPR, so that the mean blood pressure increases only slightly. Vasoconstriction in the inactive vascular beds helps maintain a normal arterial blood pressure for adequate perfusion of the active tissues. The actual mean arterial pressure attained during exercise thus represents a balance between cardiac output and TPR (see p 422). Systolic pressure usually increases more than diastolic pressure, which results in an increase in pulse pressure (Fig. 31-2). The larger pulse pressure is primarily attributable to a greater stroke volume, and to a lesser degree to a more rapid ejection of blood by the left ventricle with less peripheral runoff during the brief ventricular ejection period (see also Chapters 23 and 26).

■ *Severe Exercise*

In severe exercise taken to the point of exhaustion, the compensatory mechanisms begin to fail. Heart rate attains a maximal level of about 180 beats/min, and stroke volume reaches a plateau and often decreases, resulting in a fall in blood pressure. The subject also becomes dehydrated. Sympathetic vasoconstrictor activity supersedes the vasodilator influence on the vessels of the skin, resulting in the hemodynamic effect of a slight increase in effective blood volume. However, vasoconstriction of skin vessels also decreases the rate of heat loss. Body temperature is normally elevated in exercise, and reduction in heat loss through cutaneous vasoconstriction can lead to very high body temperatures with associated feelings of acute distress during severe exer-

cise. The tissue and blood pH decrease as a result of increased lactic acid and CO_2 production. The reduced pH is probably the key factor that determines the maximal amount of exercise a given individual can tolerate because of muscle pain, a subjective feeling of exhaustion, and an inability or loss of will to continue. A summary of the neural and local effects of exercise on the cardiovascular system is diagrammed in Fig. 31-3.

■ *Postexercise Recovery*

When exercise stops, heart rate and cardiac output abruptly decrease—the sympathetic drive to the heart is essentially removed. In contrast, TPR remains low for some time after the exercise is stopped, presumably because of the accumulation of vasodilator metabolites in the muscles during the exercise period. As a result of the reduced cardiac output and persistence of vasodilation in the muscles, arterial pressure falls, often below pre-exercise levels, for brief periods. Blood pressure is then stabilized at normal levels by the baroreceptor reflexes.

■ *Limits of Exercise Performance*

The two main factors that could limit skeletal muscle performance in the human body are the rate of O_2 utilization by the muscles and the O_2 supply to the muscles. O_2 usage by muscle is probably not a critical factor. During exercise, maximal O_2 consumption ($\dot{V}o_{2max}$) by a large percentage of the body muscle mass is unchanged or increases only slightly when additional muscles are activated. In fact, during exercise of a large muscle mass, as in vigorous bicycling, the addition of bilateral arm exercise without change in the cycling efforts produces only a small increase in cardiac output and $\dot{V}o_{2max}$. However, it decreases blood flow to the legs. This centrally mediated (baroreceptor reflex) vasoconstriction during maximal cardiac output prevents the fall in blood pressure that would otherwise be caused by metabolically induced vasodilation in the active muscle. If muscle O_2 usage were a significant limiting factor, recruitment of more contracting muscles would use much more O_2 to meet the enhanced O_2 requirements (about the amount equal to the sum of oxygen consumption of the arms and legs exercised alone).

Limitation of O_2 supply could be caused by inadequate oxygenation of blood in the lungs or limitation of the supply of O_2-laden blood to the muscles. Failure to fully oxygenate blood by the lungs can be excluded, because even with the most strenuous exercise at sea level, arterial blood is fully saturated with O_2. Therefore, O_2 delivery (or blood flow, because arterial blood O_2 content is normal) to the active muscles appears to be the limiting factor in muscle performance. This limitation could be caused by the inability to increase cardiac output beyond

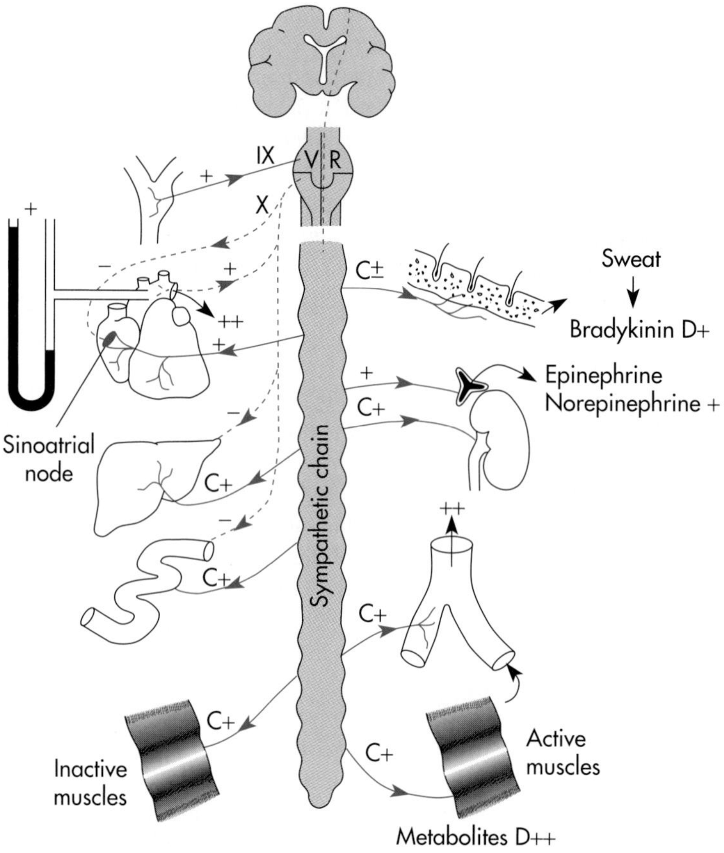

■ **Fig. 31-3** Cardiovascular adjustments in exercise. *VR,* Vasomotor region; *C,* vasoconstrictor activity; *D,* vasodilator activity; *IX,* glossopharyngeal nerve; *X,* vagus nerve, + , increased activity; − , decreased activity.

a certain level. In turn, this inability is caused by a limitation of stroke volume, because heart rate reaches maximal levels before $\dot{V}o_{2max}$ is reached. *Hence, the major factor that limits muscle performance is the pumping capacity of the heart.*

During exercise of a small group of muscles, such as those found in the hand, the limiting factor is unknown but appears to lie within the muscle.

■ *Physical Training and Conditioning*

The response of the cardiovascular system to regular exercise is to increase its capacity to deliver O_2 to the active muscles and to improve the ability of the muscle to utilize O_2. The $\dot{V}o_{2max}$ varies with the level of physical conditioning. Training progressively increases the $\dot{V}o_{2max}$, which reaches a plateau at the highest level of conditioning. Highly trained athletes have a lower resting heart rate, a greater stroke volume, and lower peripheral resistance than they had before training or after deconditioning (becoming sedentary). The low resting heart rate is caused by a higher vagal tone and a lower sympathetic tone. During exercise, the maximal heart rate of the trained individual is the same as that in the untrained, but it is attained at a higher level of exercise.

The trained person also exhibits a low vascular resistance that is inherent in the muscle. For example, if an individual exercises one leg regularly over an extended period and does not exercise the other leg, the vascular resistance is lower and the $\dot{V}o_{2max}$ is higher in the "trained" leg than in the "untrained" leg. Physical conditioning is also associated with greater extraction of O_2 from the blood (greater arteriovenous O_2 difference) by the muscles. With long-term training, capillary density in skeletal muscle increases. Also, an increase in the number of arterioles may account for the decrease in muscle vascular resistance. The numbers of mitochondria increase, as do the oxidative enzymes in the mitochondria. In addition, the levels of ATPase activity, myoglobin, and enzymes involved in lipid metabolism increase with physical conditioning.

Endurance training, such as running or swimming, increases left ventricular volume without increasing left ventricular wall thickness. In contrast, strength exercises, such as weight lifting, increase left ventricular wall thickness (hypertrophy) with little effect on ventricular volume. However, this increase in wall thickness is small relative to that observed in chronic hypertension, in which afterload is persistently elevated because of high peripheral resistance.

■ *Hemorrhage*

In an individual who has lost a large quantity of blood, the principal system affected is the cardiovascular system. The arterial systolic, diastolic, and pulse pressures decrease and the arterial pulse is rapid and feeble. The cutaneous veins collapse and fill slowly when compressed centrally. The skin is pale, moist, and slightly cyanotic. Respiration is rapid, but the depth of respiration may be shallow or deep.

■ *Course of Arterial Blood Pressure Changes*

Cardiac output decreases as a result of blood loss (see Chapter 29). The changes in mean arterial pressure evoked by an acute hemorrhage in experimental animals are illustrated in Fig. 31-4. If sufficient blood is rapidly withdrawn to decrease the mean arterial pressure to 50 mm Hg, the pressure tends to rise spontaneously toward a control level over the next 20 or 30 minutes. In some animals (curve *A,* Fig. 31-4), this trend continues and normal pressures are regained within a few hours. In other animals (curve *B*), after an initial pressure rise, the pressure begins to decline and continues to fall at an accelerating rate until death ensues. This progressive deterioration of cardiovascular function is termed **hemorrhagic shock.** *At some point, the deterioration of the cardiovascular system becomes irreversible. A lethal outcome can be prevented only temporarily by any known therapy, including massive transfusions of donor blood.*

■ *Compensatory Mechanisms*

The changes in arterial pressure immediately after an acute blood loss (Fig. 31-4) indicate that certain compensatory mechanisms must operate. Any mechanism that senses the level of blood pressure and raises the pressure toward normal in response to the reduction in pressure may be designated a **negative feedback mechanism.** This mechanism is termed *negative* because the secondary change in pressure is opposite to the initiating change after acute blood loss. The following negative feedback responses are evoked: (1) the baroreceptor reflexes, (2) the chemoreceptor reflexes, (3) cerebral ischemia responses, (4) reabsorption of tissue fluids, (5) release of endogenous vasoconstrictor substances, and (6) renal conservation of salt and water.

Baroreceptor reflexes. The reduction in mean arterial pressure and in pulse pressure during hemorrhage decreases the stimulation of the baroreceptors in the carotid sinuses and aortic arch (see Chapter 28). Several cardiovascular responses are thus evoked, all of which tend to restore the normal level of arterial pressure. Reduction of vagal tone and enhancement of sympathetic tone increase heart rate and enhance myocardial contractility.

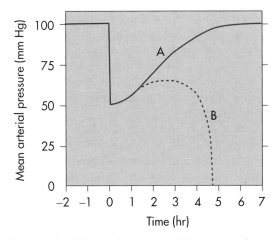

■ **Fig. 31-4** Changes in mean arterial pressure after a rapid hemorrhage. At time zero, the animal is bled rapidly to a mean arterial pressure of 50 mm Hg. After a period in which the pressure returns toward the control level, some animals continue to improve until the control pressure is attained (curve *A*). However, in other animals, the pressure will begin to decline until death ensues (curve *B*).

The increased sympathetic tone also produces generalized venoconstriction, which has the same hemodynamic consequences as a transfusion of blood (see Chapters 28 and 29). Sympathetic activation constricts certain blood reservoirs. In effect, this vasoconstriction acts as an autotransfusion of blood into the circulating bloodstream. In the dog, considerable quantities of blood are mobilized by the contraction of the spleen. In humans, the cutaneous, pulmonary, and hepatic vasculatures constitute the principal blood reservoirs.

Generalized arteriolar constriction is a prominent response to the diminished baroreceptor stimulation during hemorrhage. The reflex increase in peripheral resistance minimizes the fall in arterial pressure caused by the reduction of cardiac output. Fig. 31-5 shows the effect of an 8% blood loss on mean aortic pressure in a group of dogs. If both vagi are cut to eliminate the influence of the aortic arch baroreceptors, and only the carotid sinus baroreceptors are operative (Fig. 31-5, *A*), this hemorrhage decreases mean aortic pressure by 14%. This pressure change does not differ significantly from the pressure decline (12%) evoked by the same hemorrhage before vagotomy (not shown). When the carotid sinuses are denervated and the aortic baroreceptor reflexes are intact, the 8% blood loss decreases mean aortic pressure by 38% (Fig. 31-5, *B*). Hence, the carotid sinus baroreceptors are more effective than the aortic baroreceptors in attenuating the fall in pressure. The aortic baroreceptor must also be operative, however, because when both sets of afferent baroreceptor pathways are interrupted (Fig. 31-5, *C*), an 8% blood loss reduces arterial pressure by 48%.

Although the arteriolar constriction is widespread during hemorrhage, it is by no means uniform. Vasoconstriction is most pronounced in the cutaneous, skeletal muscle, and splanchnic vascular beds and is slight or absent in the cerebral and coronary circulations. In many instances, the cerebral and coronary vascular resistances are diminished. *Thus, the reduced cardiac output is redistributed to favor flow through the brain and the heart.*

In early stages of mild to moderate hemorrhage, the changes in renal resistance are usually slight. The tendency for increased sympathetic activity to constrict the renal vessels is counteracted by autoregulatory mechanisms (see Chapters 28 and 40). With more prolonged and severe hemorrhages, however, renal vasoconstriction becomes intense. The reductions in renal circulation are most severe in the outer layers of the renal cortex. The inner zones of the cortex and outer zones of the medulla are spared.

The severe renal and splanchnic vasoconstriction during hemorrhage favors the heart and brain. However, if such constriction persists too long, it may be detrimental. Frequently, patients survive the acute hypotensive period of a prolonged, severe hemorrhage, only to die several days later from kidney failure that results from renal ischemia. Intestinal ischemia may also have dire effects. In the dog, for example, intestinal bleeding and extensive sloughing of the mucosa occur after only a few hours of hemorrhagic hypotension. Furthermore, the diminished splanchnic flow swells the centrilobular cells in the liver. The resultant obstruction of the hepatic sinusoids raises portal venous pressure, which intensifies intestinal blood loss. Fortunately, the pathological changes in the liver and intestine are usually much less severe in humans than in dogs.

Chemoreceptor reflexes. Reductions in arterial pressure below about 60 mm Hg do not evoke any additional responses through the baroreceptor reflexes, because this pressure level constitutes the threshold for stimulation (see Chapter 28). However, low arterial pressure may stimulate peripheral chemoreceptors because of hypoxia in the chemoreceptor tissue that results from inadequate local blood flow. Chemoreceptor excitation enhances the already existent peripheral vasoconstriction evoked by the baroreceptor reflexes. Also, respiratory stimulation assists venous return by the auxiliary pumping mechanism described in Chapter 29.

Cerebral ischemia. When the arterial pressure falls below about 40 mm Hg, the resultant cerebral ischemia activates the sympathoadrenal system. The sympathetic nervous discharge is several times greater than the maximal neural activity that occurs when the baroreceptors cease to be stimulated. Therefore, the vasoconstriction and facilitation of myocardial contractility may be pronounced. With more severe degrees of cerebral ischemia, however, the vagal centers also become activated. The resultant bradycardia may aggravate the hypotension that initiated the cerebral ischemia

Reabsorption of tissue fluids. The arterial hypotension, arteriolar constriction, and reduced venous pressure during hemorrhagic hypotension lower the hydrostatic pressure in the capillaries. The balance of these forces promotes the net reabsorption of interstitial fluid into the vascular compartment (see Chapter 27). The rapidity of this response is displayed in Fig. 31-6. In a group of cats, 45% of the estimated blood volume was removed over a 30-minute period. The mean arterial blood pressure

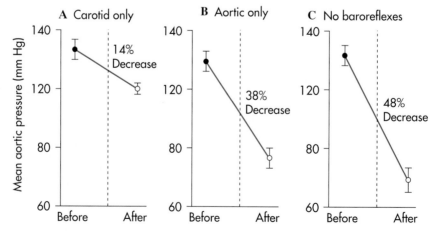

■ **Fig. 31-5** Changes in mean aortic pressure in response to an 8% blood loss in 3 groups of dogs. **A,** The carotid sinus baroreceptors were intact and the aortic reflexes were interrupted. **B,** The aortic reflexes were intact and the carotid sinus reflexes were interrupted. **C,** All sinoaortic reflexes were abrogated. (From Shepherd JT: *Circulation* 50:418, 1974, with permission of the American Heart Association; derived from the data of Edis AJ: *Am J Physiol* 221:1352, 1971.)

declined rapidly to about 45 mm Hg. The pressure then returned rapidly, but only temporarily, to near the control level. The plasma colloid osmotic pressure declined markedly during the bleeding and continued to decrease more gradually for several hours. The reduction in colloid osmotic pressure reflects the dilution of the blood by tissue fluids that contain little protein.

Considerable quantities of fluid may thus be drawn into the circulation during hemorrhage. About 0.25 ml of fluid per minute per kilogram of body weight may be reabsorbed. Approximately 1 L of fluid per hour might be autoinfused from the interstitial spaces into the circulatory system of the average individual after an acute blood loss.

Substantial quantities of fluid may also be slowly shifted from intracellular to extracellular spaces. This fluid exchange is probably mediated by secretion of cortisol from the adrenal cortex in response to hemorrhage. Cortisol appears to be essential for the full restoration of plasma volume after hemorrhage.

Endogenous vasoconstrictors. The **catecholamines** epinephrine and norepinephrine are released from the adrenal medulla in response to the same stimuli that evoke widespread sympathetic nervous discharge (see Chapter 51). Blood levels of catecholamines are high during and after hemorrhage. When animals are bled to an arterial pressure level of 40 mm Hg, the level of catecholamines increases as much as 50 times.

Epinephrine comes almost exclusively from the adrenal medulla, whereas norepinephrine is derived from both the adrenal medulla and the peripheral sympathetic nerve endings. These humoral substances reinforce the effects of sympathetic nervous activity listed previously.

Vasopressin (antidiuretic hormone), a potent vasoconstrictor, is actively secreted by the posterior pituitary gland in response to hemorrhage (see Chapter 49). The plasma concentration of vasopressin rises progressively as the arterial blood pressure diminishes (Fig. 31-7). The receptors responsible for the augmented release of vasopressin are the sinoaortic baroreceptors and stretch receptors in the left atrium.

The diminished renal perfusion during hemorrhagic hypotension leads to the secretion of **renin** from the juxtaglomerular apparatus (see Chapter 42). This enzyme acts on a plasma protein, **angiotensinogen,** to form the decapeptide **angiotensin I,** which in turn is cleaved to the active octapeptide, **angiotensin II**, by the angiotensin converting enzyme; angiotensin II is a very powerful vasoconstrictor

Renal conservation of salt and water. Fluid and electrolytes are conserved by the kidneys during hemorrhage in response to various stimuli, including the increased secretion of vasopressin noted previously (Fig. 31-7). The lower arterial pressure decreases the glomerular filtration rate and thus curtails the excretion of water and electrolytes. Also, the diminished renal blood flow raises the blood levels of angiotensin II, as described above. This polypeptide accelerates the release of **aldosterone** from the adrenal cortex. Aldosterone in turn stimulates sodium reabsorption by the renal tubules. Sodium is actively reabsorbed, and water accompanies the sodium passively (see also Chapter 42).

■ *Decompensatory Mechanisms*

In contrast to the negative feedback mechanisms just described, latent **positive feedback mechanisms** are also evoked by hemorrhage. These mechanisms exaggerate any primary change initiated by the blood loss. Specifically, positive feedback mechanisms aggravate the hypotension induced by blood loss and tend to initiate "vicious" cycles, which may lead to death.

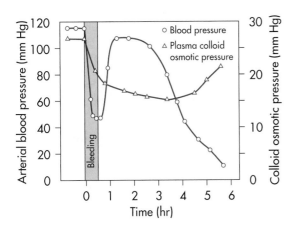

■ **Fig. 31-6** Changes in arterial blood pressure and plasma colloid osmotic pressure in response to withdrawal of 45% of the estimated blood volume over a 30-minute period, beginning at time zero. The data are the average values for 23 cats. (Redrawn from Zweifach BW: *Anesthesiology* 41:157, 1974.)

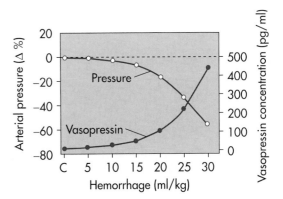

■ **Fig. 31-7** Mean percentage changes in arterial blood pressure and in plasma vasopressin concentration in response to blood loss (0.5 mg/kg/min) in a group of 12 dogs; the maximal volume of blood withdrawn was 30 ml/kg. (Redrawn from Shen YT, Cowley AW Jr, Vatner SF: *Circ Res* 68:1422, 1991, with permission of the American Heart Association.)

Whether a positive feedback mechanism will lead to a vicious cycle depends on the gain of that mechanism. Gain is defined as the ratio of the secondary change evoked by a given mechanism to the initiating change itself. A gain greater than 1 induces a vicious cycle; a gain less than 1 does not. For example, consider a positive feedback mechanism with a gain of 2. If mean arterial pressure were to decrease by 10 mm Hg, a positive feedback mechanism with a gain of 2 would then evoke a secondary pressure reduction of 20 mm Hg, which in turn would cause a further decrease of 40 mm Hg. In other words, each change would induce a subsequent change that is twice as great. Hence, mean arterial pressure would decline at an ever-increasing rate until death occurred. This process is depicted in curve *B* in Fig. 31-4.

Conversely, a positive feedback mechanism with a gain of 0.5 would also exaggerate any change in mean arterial pressure, but the change would not necessarily lead to death. For example, if arterial pressure suddenly decreased by 10 mm Hg, the positive feedback mechanism would initiate a secondary, additional fall of 5 mm Hg. This decrease in turn would provoke a further decrease of 2.5 mm Hg. The process would continue in ever-diminishing steps until the arterial pressure approached an equilibrium value.

Some of the more important positive feedback mechanisms that are evident during hemorrhage include (1) cardiac failure, (2) acidosis, (3) central nervous system depression, (4) aberrations of blood clotting, and (5) depression of the reticuloendothelial system.

Cardiac failure. The role of cardiac failure in the progression of shock during hemorrhage is controversial. All investigators agree that the heart fails terminally, but opinions differ about the importance of cardiac failure during earlier stages of hemorrhagic hypotension. Shifts to the right in ventricular function curves (Fig. 31-8) constitute experimental evidence of a progressive depression of myocardial contractility during hemorrhage.

The hypotension induced by hemorrhage reduces the coronary blood flow and therefore depresses ventricular function. The consequent reduction in cardiac output leads to a further decline in arterial pressure, a classic example of a positive feedback mechanism. Furthermore, the reduced blood flow to the peripheral tissues leads to an accumulation of vasodilator metabolites. The accumulation of these substances decreases peripheral resistance and therefore aggravates the fall in arterial pressure.

Acidosis. The inadequate blood flow during hemorrhage affects the metabolism of all cells in the body. The decreased oxygen delivery to the cells accelerates the production of lactic acid and other acid metabolites by the tissues. Furthermore, impaired kidney function prevents adequate excretion of the excess H^+, and generalized metabolic acidosis ensues (Fig. 31-9). The resultant depressant effect of acidosis on the heart (see Chapter 24) further reduces tissue perfusion and thus aggravates the metabolic acidosis. Acidosis also diminishes the reactivity of the heart and resistance vessels to neurally released and circulating catecholamines, and thereby intensifies the hypotension.

Central nervous system depression. The hypotension in shock reduces cerebral blood flow. Moderate degrees of cerebral ischemia induce a pronounced sympathetic nervous stimulation of the heart, arterioles, and veins, as noted above. In severe hypotension, however, the cardiovascular centers in the brainstem eventually become depressed because of inadequate cerebral blood flow. The resultant loss of sympathetic tone then reduces cardiac output and peripheral resistance. The consequent reduction in mean arterial pressure intensifies the inadequate cerebral perfusion.

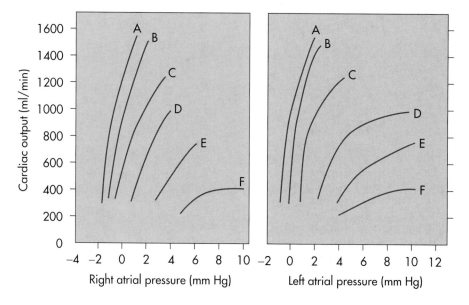

■ **Fig. 31-8** Ventricular function curves for the right and left ventricles during the course of hemorrhagic shock. Curves *A* represent the control function curve; curves *B,* 117 min; curves *C,* 247 min; curves *D,* 280 min; curves *E,* 295 min; and curves *F,* 310 min after the initial hemorrhage. (Redrawn from Crowell JW, Guyton AC: *Am J Physiol* 203:248, 1962.)

Various endogenous **opioids,** such as **enkephalins** and **β-endorphin,** may be released into the brain substance or into the circulation in response to the same stresses that provoke circulatory shock. Opioids are contained, along with catecholamines, in secretory granules in the adrenal medulla and sympathetic nerve terminals, and they are released together in response to stress. Similar stimuli release β-endorphin and adrenocorticotropic hormone (ACTH) from the anterior pituitary gland. Opioids depress the brainstem centers that mediate some of the compensatory autonomic adaptations to blood loss, endotoxemia, and other shock-provoking stresses. Conversely, the opioid antagonist **naloxone** improves cardiovascular function and survival in various forms of shock.

Aberrations of blood clotting. *The alterations of blood clotting after hemorrhage are typically biphasic. An initial phase of hypercoagulability is followed by a secondary phase of hypocoagulability and fibrinolysis.* In the initial phase, platelets and leukocytes adhere to the vascular endothelium, and intravascular clots, or **thrombi,** develop within a few minutes of the onset of severe hemorrhage. Coagulation may be extensive throughout the small blood vessels.

The initial phase is further enhanced by the release of thromboxane A_2 from various ischemic tissues. Thromboxane A_2 aggregates platelets. As more platelets aggregate, more thromboxane A_2 is released and more platelets are trapped. This form of positive feedback intensifies and prolongs the clotting tendency. The mortality from certain standard shock-provoking procedures has been reduced considerably by the administration of anticoagulants such as heparin (see Chapter 20).

Reticuloendothelial system. During the course of hemorrhagic hypotension, reticuloendothelial system (RES) function becomes depressed. The phagocytic activity of the RES is modulated by an **opsonic protein.** The opsonic activity in plasma diminishes during shock, which may account in part for the depression of RES function. As a result, the antibacterial and antitoxin defense mechanisms are impaired. Endotoxins from the normal bacterial flora of the intestine constantly enter the circulation. Ordinarily, they are inactivated by the RES, principally in the liver. When the RES is depressed, these endotoxins invade the general circulation. *Endotoxins produce profound, generalized vasodilation, mainly by inducing the abundant synthesis of an isoform of nitric oxide synthase in the smooth muscle of blood vessels throughout the body.* The profound vasodilation aggravates the hemodynamic changes caused by blood loss.

In addition to their role in inactivating endotoxin, the macrophages release many of the mediators associated with shock. These mediators include acid hydrolases, neutral proteases, oxygen free radicals, certain coagulation factors, and arachidonic acid derivatives: prostaglandins, thromboxanes, and leukotrienes. Macrophages also release certain **monokines** that modulate temperature regulation, intermediary metabolism, hormone secretion, and the immune system.

■ *Interactions of Positive and Negative Feedback Mechanisms*

Hemorrhage provokes a multitude of circulatory and metabolic derangements. As we have seen, some of these changes are compensatory, others are decompensatory. Some of these feedback mechanisms possess a high gain, others a low gain. Furthermore, the gain of any specific mechanism varies with the severity of the hemorrhage. For example, with only a slight loss of blood, mean arterial pressure is within the normal range and the gain of the baroreceptor reflexes is high. With greater losses of blood, when mean arterial pressure is below 60 mm Hg (i.e., below the threshold for the baroreceptors), further reductions of pressure have no additional influence through the baroreceptor reflexes. Hence, below this critical pressure, the baroreceptor reflex gain is zero or near zero.

As a general rule, with minor degrees of blood loss, the gains of the negative feedback mechanisms are high, whereas those of the positive feedback mechanisms are low. The opposite is true with more severe hemorrhages. The gains of the various mechanisms are additive algebraically. Therefore, whether a vicious cycle develops depends on whether the sum of the positive and negative gains exceeds 1. Total gains in excess of 1 are of course more likely with severe losses of blood. Therefore, to avert a vicious cycle, serious hemorrhages must be treated quickly and intensively, preferably by whole blood transfusions, before the process becomes irreversible.

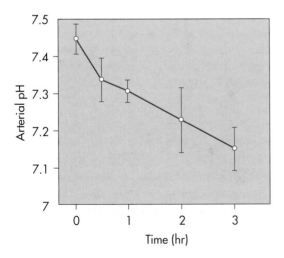

■ **Fig. 31-9** Reduction in arterial blood pH (mean ± SD) in a group of 11 dogs whose blood pressure had been held at a level of 35 mm Hg by bleeding into a reservoir, beginning at time zero. (Modified from Markov AK, Oglethorpe N, Young DB, Hellems HK: *Circ Shock* 8:9, 1981.)

■ *Summary*

■ *Exercise*

1. In anticipation of exercise, the vagus nerve impulses to the heart are inhibited and the sympathetic nervous system is activated by central command. The result is an increase in heart rate, myocardial contractile force, and regional vascular resistance.

2. With exercise, vascular resistance increases in the skin, kidneys, splanchnic regions, and inactive muscles and decreases markedly in the active muscles. The overall effect is a pronounced reduction in total peripheral resistance. This change in resistance, along with the auxiliary pumping action of the contracting skeletal muscles, leads to a large increase in venous return.

3. The increase in heart rate and the enhanced myocardial contractility, both induced by activation of the cardiac sympathetic nerves, enable the heart to transfer the blood to the pulmonary and systemic circulations, thereby increasing cardiac output. Stroke volume increases only slightly. Oxygen consumption and blood oxygen extraction increase, and systolic and mean blood pressure increase slightly.

4. As body temperature rises during exercise, the skin blood vessels dilate. However, when heart rate becomes maximal during severe exercise, the skin vessels constrict. This increases the effective blood volume but causes greater increases in body temperature and a feeling of exhaustion.

5. The limiting factor in exercise performance is the delivery of blood to the active muscles.

■ *Hemorrhage*

1. Acute blood loss induces the following hemodynamic changes: tachycardia, hypotension, generalized arteriolar constriction, and generalized venoconstriction.

2. Acute blood loss invokes a number of negative feedback (compensatory) mechanisms, such as baroreceptor and chemoreceptor reflexes, responses to moderate cerebral ischemia, reabsorption of tissue fluids, release of endogenous vasoconstrictors, and renal conservation of water and electrolytes.

3. Acute blood loss also induces a number of positive feedback (decompensatory) mechanisms, such as cardiac failure, acidosis, central nervous system depression, aberrations of blood coagulation, and depression of the reticuloendothelial system.

4. The outcome of acute blood loss depends on the sum of gains of the positive and negative feedback mechanisms and on the interactions between these mechanisms.

■ *Self-Study Problems*

1. What are the major cardiovascular changes that occur with exercise?

2. What is the limiting factor in the performance of strenuous exercise such as distance running and swimming? Why?

3. What are the major compensatory responses to blood loss?

4. What factors tend to aggravate the hemodynamic effects of blood loss?

■ *Bibliography*

Journal articles

Abboud FM et al: Role of vasopressin in cardiovascular and blood pressure regulation, *Blood Vessels* 27:106, 1990.

Astiz ME, Rackow EC, Weil MH: Pathophysiology and treatment of circulatory shock, *Crit Care Clin* 9:183, 1993.

Baker CH, Sutton ET: Arteriolar endothelium-dependent vasodilation occurs during endotoxin shock, *Am J Physiol* 264:H1118, 1993.

Blomqvist CG, Saltin B: Cardiovascular adaptations to physical training, *Annu Rev Physiol* 45:169, 1983.

Booth FW, Thomason DB: Molecular and cellular adaptation of muscle in response to exercise: perspectives of various models, *Physiol Rev* 71:541, 1991.

Brengelmann GL: Circulatory adjustments to exercise and heat stress, *Annu Rev Physiol* 45:191, 1983.

Cameron JD, Dart AM: Exercise training increases total systemic arterial compliance in humans, *Am J Physiol* 266:H693, 1994.

Cheng K-P, Igarashi Y, Little WC: Mechanism of augmented rate of left ventricular filling during exercise, *Circ Res* 70:9, 1992.

Christensen NJ, Galbo H: Sympathetic nervous activity during exercise, *Annu Rev Physiol* 45:139, 1983.

Clausen JP: Effect of physical training on cardiovascular adjustments to exercise in man, *Physiol Rev* 57:779, 1977.

Courneya C-A, Korner PI, Oliver JR, Woods RL: Afferent vascular resistance control during hemorrhage in normal and autonomically blocked rabbits, *Am J Physiol* 261:H380, 1991.

Eldridge FL, Millhorn DE, Kiley JP, Waldrop TG: Stimulation by central command of locomotion, respiration and circulation during exercise, *Respir Physiol* 59:313, 1985.

Fitts RH: Cellular mechanisms of muscle fatigue, Physiol Rev 74:49, 1994.

Geerdes BP, Frederick KL, Brunner MJ: Carotid baroreflex control during hemorrhage in conscious and anesthetized dogs, *Am J Physiol* 265:R195, 1993.

Herbertson MJ, Werner HA, Walley KR: Nitric oxide synthase inhibition partially prevents decreased LV contractility during endotoxemia, *Am J Physiol* 270:H1979, 1996.

Herd JA: Cardiovascular response to stress, *Physiol Rev* 71:305, 1991.

Kovach AGB, Lefler AM: Endothelial dysfunction in shock states, *News Physiol Sci* 8:145, 1993.

Laughlin MH, Armstrong RB: Muscle and blood flow during locomotory exercise, *Exerc Sport Sci Rev* 13:95, 1985.

Lefer AM, Lefer DJ: Pharmacology of the endothelium in ischemia-reperfusion and circulatory shock, *Annu Rev Pharmacol Toxicol* 33:71, 1993.

Ludbrook J: Reflex control of blood pressure during exercise, *Annu Rev Physiol* 45:155, 1983.

Mitchell JH, Kaufman MP, Iwamoto GA: The exercise pressor reflex: its cardiovascular effects, afferent mechanisms, and central pathways, *Annu Rev Physiol* 45:229, 1983.

Rea RG, Eckberg DL, Fritsch JM, Goldstein DS: Relation of plasma norepinephrine and sympathetic traffic during hypotension in humans, *Am J Physiol* 258:R982, 1990.

Redl H, Gasser H, Schlag G, Marzi I: Involvement of oxygen radical in shock related cell injury, *Br Med Bull* 49:556, 1993.

Schadt JC, Gaddis RR: Renin-angiotensin system and opioids during acute hemorrhage in conscious rabbits, *Am J Physiol* 258:R543, 1990.

Share L: Control of vasopressin release: an old but continuing story, *News Physiol Sci* 11:7, 1996.

Sheriff DD, Zhou XP, Scher Am, Rowell LB: Dependence of cardiac filling pressure on cardiac output during rest and dynamic exercise in dogs, *Am J Physiol* 265:H316, 1993.

Stoclet J-C et al: Nitric oxide and endotoxemia, *Circulation* 87:V-77, 1993.

Szabo C: Alterations in nitric oxide production in various forms of circulatory shock, *New Horizons* 3:2, 1995.

Thiemermann C: Role of L-arginine: nitric oxide pathway in circulatory shock, *Adv Pharmacol* 28:45, 1994.

Vissing SF, Scherrer U, Victor RG: Stimulation of skin sympathetic nerve discharge by central command: differential control of sympathetic outflow to skin and skeletal muscle during exercise, *Circ Res* 69:229, 1991.

Westerblad H, Lee JA, Lannergren J, Allen DG: Cellular mechanisms of fatigue in skeletal muscle, *Am J Physiol* 261:C195, 1991.

Yao Y-M et al: Significance of NO in hemorrhage-induced hemodynamic alterations, organ injury, and mortality in rats, *Am J Physiol* 270:J1615, 1996.

Books and monographs

Bond RF, Adams HR, Chaudry IH, editors: *Perspectives in shock research,* New York, 1988, Alan R Liss.

Brooks GA, Fahey TD: *Exercise physiology—human bioenergetics and its applications,* New York, 1984, John Wiley.

Janssen HF, Barnes CD, editors: *Circulatory shock: basic and clinical implications,* New York, 1985, Academic Press.

Lind AR: *Cardiovascular adjustments to isometric contractions: static effort. In Handbook of physiology,* sect 2, *The cardiovascular system—peripheral circulation and organ blood flow,* vol III, Bethesda, Md, 1983, American Physiological Society.

Mitchell JH, Schmidt RF: Cardiovascular reflex control by afferent fibers from skeletal muscle receptors. In *Handbook of physiology,* sect 2, *The cardiovascular system—peripheral circulation and organ blood flow,* vol III, Bethesda, Md, 1983, American Physiological Society.

Roth BL, Nielsen TB, McKee AE, editors: *Molecular and cellular mechanisms of septic shock. In Progress in clinical and biological research,* vol 286, New York, 1988, Alan R Liss.

Rowell LB: *Integration of body system in exercise.* In Berne RM, Levy MN, editors: *Principles of physiology,* St Louis, 1990, Mosby–Year Book.

Rowell LB: *Human circulation: regulation during physical stress,* New York, 1986, Oxford University Press.

THE RESPIRATORY SYSTEM

Norman C. Staub, Sr.

Structure and Function of the Respiratory System

Although pulmonary disease does not receive the publicity that cancer and heart disease do, **chronic obstructive pulmonary disease (COPD)** ranks fifth and **influenza** and **pneumonia** rank seventh as leading causes of death in the United States. Combined, these diseases account for 8% of deaths, ahead of accidents and strokes. A large portion of modern medical practice, critical care medicine, and nursing care involves treating people with lung diseases. Thus, an understanding of pulmonary physiology and pathophysiology is important and relevant.

Breathing is an automatic, rhythmic, and centrally regulated mechanical process. In breathing, the contraction and relaxation of the skeletal muscles of the diaphragm, abdomen, and rib cage cause gas to move into and out of the **terminal respiratory units** (functional alveoli) of the lung. **Respiration** is the overall process of controlled oxidation of metabolites for the production of useful energy by living organisms; it includes breathing.

Respiring cells require a supply of oxygen (O_2) and other nutrients; in addition, carbon dioxide (CO_2) and other waste products must be removed. Large animals, including humans, make use of two systems for this process: a circulatory system, which carries substances to and from the tissue cells, and a breathing system (a gas exchanger), which carries O_2 and CO_2 between the environment (ambient atmosphere) and the alveoli of the lung.

Cardiopulmonary resuscitation includes both breathing and blood circulation. Contrary to media presentations, resuscitation by well-meaning citizens infrequently succeeds. Chest compression alone may move some blood by altering pleural pressure, but it does not adequately ventilate the lungs. Modern emergency resuscitation demands mouth-to-mouth breathing after every five or six chest compressions. Hospital emergency teams and paramedics are trained and equipped to resuscitate people properly.

■ Functions and Definitions

■ Principal Function of the Lung

The lungs (Fig. 32-1) are designed to provide an adequate distribution of inspired air and pulmonary blood flow. This design allows the exchange of O_2 and CO_2 between the alveolar gas and the pulmonary capillary blood to be accomplished with a minimal expenditure of energy (work of breathing and of the right ventricle).

Ventilation and perfusion. The process of breathing is measured by **ventilation** (frequency × depth of breathing). The exchange of O_2 and CO_2 in the lung is measured by their respective concentration differences between inspired air and expired gas.

Lung **perfusion** is the cardiac output (heart rate × stroke volume of the right ventricle). The exchanges of O_2 and of CO_2 in pulmonary capillary blood are measured by their concentration differences between blood in the pulmonary artery (mixed venous blood) and in the pulmonary veins, left atrium, or any systemic artery.

The differences between O_2 and CO_2 **partial pressures** (fraction of total gas pressure caused by a particular molecular species) in alveolar gas and systemic arterial blood are useful in determining the overall efficiency of lung function. Lung efficiency depends on how closely the alveolar ventilation (volume flow rate of fresh air to each part of the lung) matches perfusion (volume flow rate of blood to each part of the lung). Ideally, **ventilation/perfusion ratios** (which illustrate the distribution of fresh air and pulmonary capillary blood flow) of every lung unit are identical.

Blood gas transport. Oxygenated blood leaves the lungs via the pulmonary veins and is pumped by the left ventricle through the systemic arteries. These arteries conduct the oxygenated blood to the systemic capillaries, which are associated with all the respiring cells of the body. Likewise, the principal waste product of metabolism, CO_2, is transported away from the respiring cells via the systemic veins to the lung for elimination. The

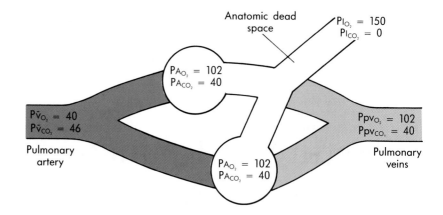

■ **Fig. 32-1**   Simplified lung model showing two normal parallel lung units. Both units receive equal quantities of fresh air and blood flow for their size. The blood and alveolar gas partial pressures, P, are normal values in a resting person.

transport of O_2 and CO_2 in the blood is an important part of respiration.

For the convective transport of O_2 in the blood, the *concentration* of O_2 is the important variable. Because oxygen is only slightly soluble in water, one must know how the special protein **hemoglobin** carries oxygen within erythrocytes. The remarkable property of hemoglobin is its ability to combine *rapidly* and *reversibly* with oxygen, and thus effectively increases the solubility of oxygen in blood many times. The **hemoglobin-oxygen equilibrium curve** (Fig. 32-2) depicts the empiric (experimental) relationship between the partial pressure of oxygen in blood and the relative amount (percentage saturation) bound to normal hemoglobin. The normal blood hemoglobin concentration is 150 g/L. Thus, when the blood is well oxygenated, the hemoglobin increases arterial blood oxygen concentration by twentyfold. In normal humans, arterial blood contains nearly 200 ml O_2/L in the arterial oxygen partial pressure range (Pa_{O_2} = 85 to 100 mm Hg) that prevails at sea level. See Table 32-1 and Box 32-1 for summaries of respiratory abbreviations and normal values.

The cardiac output in a resting human adult is about 5 L/min. On average, only 25% of the oxygen bound to hemoglobin dissociates during passage through the systemic capillaries (arterial − venous O_2 difference = 50 ml/L). This rather small difference has two beneficial effects. First, it maintains a reasonably high oxygen partial pressure difference between systemic capillary blood (Pc_{O_2} = 50 mm Hg) and tissue cells (Pt_{O_2} ≈ 10 mm Hg). This pressure difference drives the diffusion of oxygen from the blood into the cells. Second, it provides a reserve of oxygen bound to hemoglobin for use by cells in an emergency, as when capillary flow is stopped briefly by muscle contraction.

Even during the most strenuous exercise sustainable by average normal humans, cardiac output is unlikely to increase to more than three times the resting level (about 15 L/min). Because oxygen usage by the body (oxygen consumption) in steady-state exercise may increase sixfold from the resting value (from 250 to 1500 ml O_2/min), an additional 25% of the O_2 bound to hemoglo-

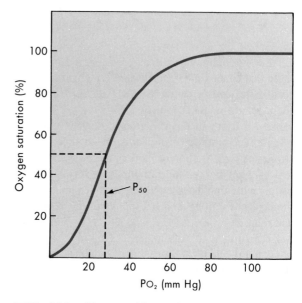

■ **Fig. 32-2**   The normal human hemoglobin-oxygen equilibrium curve (HbO_2). It is used to convert between oxygen partial pressure (abscissa) and fractional saturation of the hemoglobin, So_2, in erythrocytes (ordinate). The P_{50} is used to compare different chemical species of hemoglobins.

bin in systemic arterial blood must be unloaded in the capillaries. The threefold increase in blood flow multiplied by the doubling of O_2 removal from blood accounts for the sixfold increase in O_2 consumption.

Some highly trained athletes (e.g., cross-country Olympic skiers) can briefly increase their exercise cardiac output, ventilation, or oxygen consumption to more than twice the values stated above, but such people are not "average normal." An enlarged heart in a healthy person is especially common in people who begin strenuous training in childhood. Such growth and development do not regress when the exercise ceases.

Gas transport from the environment to cells takes place primarily by the two bulk (convective) processes, venti-

■ **Table 32-1** Some values of cardiopulmonary physiological variables for a normal adult, 70-kg body weight, at rest and during steady-state exercise

	Units	*Rest*	*Exercise*
Constants			
Hemoglobin concentration	g/L	150	
O_2 capacity of hemoglobin	O_2/g Hb	1.34	
Atmospheric pressure (sea level)	mm Hg	760	
Water vapor pressure (37° C)	mm Hg	47	
Standard conditions (STPS)	°K, mm Hg, mm Hg	273, 760, 0	
Body conditions (BTPS)	°K, mm Hg, mm Hg	310, 760, 47	
Cardiovascular			
Cardiac output	L/min	5	15
Heart rate	per min	60	180
Systemic arterial pressure, mean	mm Hg	90	100
Right atrial pressure, mean	cm H_2O	2	4
Pulmonary vascular pressures (left atrial level)			
Pulmonary arterial, mean	cm H_2O	19	30
Left atrial, mean	cm H_2O	11	15
Lung variables, BTPS			
Functional residual capacity (FRC)	L	2.4	2.4
Total lung capacity (TLC)	L	6	6
Tidal volume (V_T)	L	0.5	2
Breathing frequency (f)	per min	12	15
Metabolism, STPD			
Carbon dioxide production ($\dot{V}_{CO_2}$)	ml/min	200	1200
Oxygen consumption ($\dot{V}_{CO_2}$)	ml/min	250	1500
Respiratory exchange ratio (R)	—	.80	.80
Mechanics			
Pleural pressure, mean (Ppl)	cm H_2O	−5	−3.5
Chest wall compliance at FRC (Cw)	L/cm H_2O	0.2	0.2
Lung compliance at FRC (C$_L$)	L/cm H_2O	0.2	0.2
Airway resistance (Raw)	cm H_2O × L/sec	2.0	1.5

STPS, Standard temperature, pressure, saturated with water vapor; *BTPS,* body temperature, pressure, saturated with water vapor; *STPD,* standard temperature, pressure, dry; *ATPS,* ambient temperature, pressure, saturated with water vapor; *V,* volume; *V̇,* rate of change of volume.

lation and blood flow, as mentioned previously. However, at two key interfaces of gas transport (i.e., between the air spaces of the lung and the blood flowing through the pulmonary capillaries, and between the blood flowing through the systemic capillaries and the mitochondria of the respiring cells), the only process available is **diffusion.** Diffusion is the passive flow of molecules between regions in which the specified molecules have different chemical activities (see Chapters 1 and 27).

The control system. *The overall efficiency of breathing depends on the regulation of ventilation, blood flow, and ventilation/perfusion matching. Various external mechanisms (nervous system, humoral substances) and internal mechanisms (terminal respiratory unit distensibility, resistance to airflow, resistance to blood flow)* (Fig. 32-3) *are responsible for this regulation.* The cellular demand for oxygen is not ordinarily regulated. Thus, steady-state oxygen consumption is not affected by changes in breathing, inspired gas composition, cardiac output, or blood composition. In a larger sense, however,

respiration of cells is regulated on demand through complex local and central events (Fig. 32-4).

■ *Structural Basis of Breathing*

In the normal human adult, the lungs weigh 800 to 1200 g. Blood accounts for 40% of the weight of the lung. At end-expiration (**functional residual capacity [FRC]**) the gas volume of the lungs is 2 to 3 L, whereas at maximal inspiration (**total lung capacity, [TLC]**) it may be 5 to 6 L.

Inspiration is the active phase of breathing. Breathing is initiated by the coordinated neural activity in the respiratory control centers in the brainstem (pons and medulla). Motor impulses from these centers pass down the phrenic nerves and spinal cord to stimulate the diaphragm and external intercostal muscles to contract. The muscle contraction causes the thoracic cavity to expand, which lowers the pressure in the pleural space

---

Box 32-1 *Glossary of standard symbols and abbreviations used in respiratory physiology and medicine*

Pressures (P)

P_B, barometric (ambient)

H_2O, water vapor

Respiratory gases

P_{GAS}, gas in general

PA_{GAS}, gas in alveolar air

Pa_{GAS}, gas in arterial blood

Pv_{GAS}, gas in mixed venous blood (pulmonary artery)

Pt_{GAS}, gas in tissue

Volumes (V)

FRC (functional residual capacity) is the volume of gas in the lungs at the end of expiration.

TLC (total lung capacity) is the maximal volume of gas that the lung can hold under given circumstances.

RV (residual volume) is the gas volume left in the lungs after a maximal expiration, always less than FRC.

V_T (tidal volume) is the normal breath volume.

VC (vital capacity) is the maximal tidal volume. It equals TLC − RV.

V_I and V_E are the inspired and expired volumes, respectively. The former is slightly larger than the latter. Normally, more oxygen is taken up than carbon dioxide is removed, because the expiratory exchange ratio is < 1.0.

V_D (anatomic dead space volume) is mainly the air in the cartilaginous airways at end-inspiration.

Blood flow (Q)

Pulmonary blood flow and cardiac output are normally synonymous but need not be, as in some types of congenital heart disease. Bronchial blood flow is usually neglected as insignificant.

Ventilation (V̇)

$\dot{V}_{O_2}$ is oxygen consumption.

$\dot{V}_{CO_2}$ is carbon dioxide production.

$\dot{V}_A$ is alveolar ventilation/min.

$\dot{V}/Q$ is the ventilation/perfusion ratio.

Concentration (C)

Generally refers to dissolved gas concentrations; for example, Ca_{O_2}—arterial oxygen concentration.

Fraction (F)

Refers to decimal fraction of dry gas of a particular species in a gas mixture; for example, FA_{CO_2} is the alveolar CO_2 fraction, normally 0.056.

Blood oxygen transport

Hb, hemoglobin concentration in circulating blood—normally, 150 g/L.

HbO_2, oxyhemoglobin, the amount of oxygen (ml/L) bound to hemoglobin under a given condition.

So_2, the percentage of Hb bound with oxygen.

Gas conditions

STPD (standard temperature, pressure, dry)—273° K, 760 mm Hg.

BTPS (body temperature, pressure, saturated)—37° C, ambient pressure, P_{H_2O} = 47 mm Hg.

ATPS (ambient temperature and pressures).

---

that surrounds the lungs. As the pressure falls in the pleural space, the distensible lungs expand passively, which causes the pressure in the terminal air spaces (alveolar ducts and alveoli) to decrease. As the pressure decreases, fresh air flows down the branching airways into the terminal air spaces until the pressures are equalized, which marks the end of inspiration. During **expi-**ration (the mostly passive phase of breathing), the process is reversed. As the chest wall muscles relax, pleural and alveolar pressures rise, and gas flows out of the lung.

During growth and development, the lung conforms to the shape of the pleural cavities in a manner that minimizes structural stress. During breathing, the lung

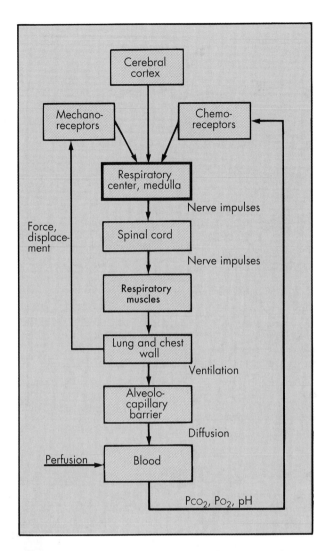

■ Fig. 32-3 Block diagram of the respiratory control system. Ventilation and perfusion come together near the bottom, and their output sets arterial and alveolar carbon dioxide and oxygen partial pressures, and in part arterial hydrogen ion concentration, pH. These outputs feed back to the controllers via chemoreceptors located in strategic places.

expands in all directions as the chest cavity expands caudally and enlarges owing to the movement of the diaphragm and rib cage.

Fig. 32-5 is a light microscopic picture of a thin slice of an expanded normal lung. The alveolar tissue occupies only a tiny fraction of the total area. Fig. 32-6 is an electron micrograph of several alveolar walls.

Oxygen transport from ambient (surrounding) air via the lungs to all systemic tissue cells is accomplished by two efficient convective processes: alveolar ventilation and pulmonary blood flow. The efficiency of these processes depends on ventilation/perfusion matching. At two key points—namely, between the alveoli and the blood in the pulmonary capillaries, and between the blood in the systemic capillaries and the mitochondria of the respiring cells—**diffusion** is the only gas transport process available. The diffusion of O_2 is rate limiting at the two key points mentioned, because it has a low solubility in tissue water and blood plasma. However, various strategies have developed in the course of evolution to reduce the resistance to O_2 diffusion. The prime example is that the average distance between the alveolar gas and the hemoglobin in the red blood cells is only 1.5 μm. Diffusion requires little time over such short distances. In the systemic tissues, the limitation of oxygen diffusion is much more important, because the diffusion distance cannot be easily reduced.

The many alveoli give the human lung at FRC a total internal surface area of approximately 1 m^2/kg body weight. This vast area (70 m^2 total) is not necessary for the distribution of gas within the lung. Rather, it fulfills the need for distributing the pulmonary blood flow (cardiac output) into a very thin film (about one red blood cell thick), so that even under stressful circumstances, such as exercise, the time each erythrocyte spends flowing along the capillaries is sufficiently long to permit equilibration of O_2 and CO_2 between blood and gas. The tissue phase of gaseous diffusion from air to blood is minimized; the resistance to blood flow is low because of the large number of parallel pathways.

■ *The Airways*

The two main types of conduction airways are cartilaginous **bronchi** and **bronchioles** (Fig. 32-7). Because these conducting airways do not generally participate in gas exchange, the air in them at end-inspiration is wasted **(anatomic dead space)**. Dead space accounts for about 30% of each normal breath.

In addition to their supporting cartilage, the bronchi are lined by a pseudostratified columnar epithelium, which rests on spiral bands of smooth muscle. The bronchi can dilate or constrict independently of lung volume. Among the numerous cell types in the epithelium that lines the bronchi are cells with cilia. The rhythmic beating of the ciliated cells effectively transports the surface film of mucus and particles out of the lung by way of the trachea.

Although the diameter and length of the bronchi decrease with each successive branching, the sum of the cross-sectional areas of each pair of daughter bronchi is actually greater than that of the parent bronchus. The cartilage support also gradually decreases, and it disappears completely in airways about 1 mm in diameter. By convention, all distal airways are called bronchioles. In addition to being small and lacking cartilage, the bronchioles have a simple cuboidal epithelium. An important functional difference between bronchioles and bronchi is that bronchioles are embedded directly into the connective tissue framework of the lung. Thus, in contrast to bronchi, their diameter depends on lung volume.

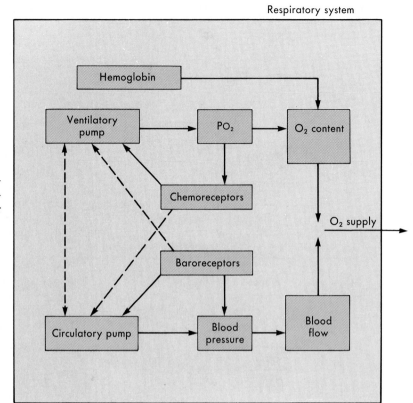

■ **Fig. 32-4** Because the main purpose of breathing is to supply O_2 to all cells of the body, the interactions between the respiratory and cardiovascular system require tight control.

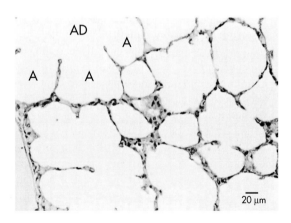

■ **Fig. 32-5** A low-power microscopic view from a normal inflated human lung. The space occupied by gas is very large and the alveolar to capillary tissue pathway for diffusion is minimized. *A,* Alveoli; *AD,* alveolar duct. (Courtesy of K.H. Albertine, Thomas Jefferson University, Philadelphia.)

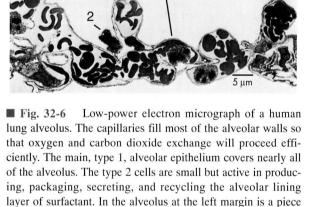

■ **Fig. 32-6** Low-power electron micrograph of a human lung alveolus. The capillaries fill most of the alveolar walls so that oxygen and carbon dioxide exchange will proceed efficiently. The main, type 1, alveolar epithelium covers nearly all of the alveolus. The type 2 cells are small but active in producing, packaging, secreting, and recycling the alveolar lining layer of surfactant. In the alveolus at the left margin is a piece of an alveolar macrophage *(AM).* (Courtesy of K.H. Albertine, Thomas Jefferson University, Philadelphia.)

The blood supply of the airways, from the trachea to the terminal bronchioles, is via the **bronchial arteries,** a systemic source. Bronchial blood flow is normally about 1% of cardiac output. *The functions of the bronchial circulation are to provide nutrition to the airways and larger pulmonary blood vessels, to warm and add water vapor in order to condition inspired air, and to provide substrate for airway cellular metabolism and secretions.*

The motor and sensory nerves of the airways participate in the reflex regulation of breathing, airway caliber,

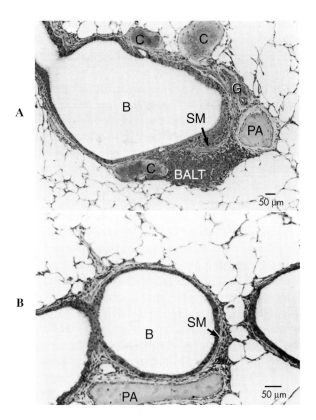

Fig. 32-7 Two human airways. **A,** A 2-mm diameter cartilaginous bronchus *(B)*. Bits of cartilage *(C)* and submucosal glands *(G)* are indicated. *BALT* refers to bronchus-associated lymphoid tissue. **B,** A membranous bronchiole about 0.2 mm in diameter. There is no cartilage and the lining epithelium is simple cuboidal. Both sections show the accompanying pulmonary artery *(PA)* and the submucosal smooth muscle *(SM)*. (Courtesy of K.H. Albertine, Thomas Jefferson University, Philadelphia.)

glandular secretion, and bronchial vasomotor control. The subepithelial smooth muscle bands receive their motor innervation from the parasympathetic branch of the autonomic nervous system (vagus nerves). When the airway muscle contracts, the lumen is narrowed.

Sensory fibers are located beneath and within the intercellular junctions of the epithelial cells. The best understood sensory receptors are located in the bronchi (chiefly, the trachea and mainstem bronchi), and are sensitive to physical distortion (stretch) and chemical substances (irritants). All along the airways, particularly in the bronchioles and in the alveolar walls, are many small, nonmyelinated, slowly conducting C fibers. Although these fibers are nonspecific, they can be stimulated by various chemical mediators. Various pulmonary-cardiac reflex responses are elicited by such stimulation. The role of the C fibers in the regulation of the lungs and heart, however, is not well understood.

The distal bronchioles have outpouchings that are the primitive alveoli. During development, the first bronchioles with alveoli that appear are called **respiratory bron-**

chioles, because these bronchioles actually participate in gas exchange. With successive branching (generations) of the respiratory bronchioles, the number and size of the anatomic alveoli increase until the walls of the bronchioles are almost completely replaced by the "mouths" of the alveoli. These final airway branches are called **alveolar ducts.**

The airways are involved in several major pulmonary diseases. One such disease is **asthma,** in which the airway smooth muscle is very sensitive (hyperactive) to certain external stimuli. During an asthma attack, the airways constrict tightly and their glands secrete excessive amounts of mucus. Both effects greatly narrow the bronchi and bronchioles, so that the person with asthma has to work much harder than normal to breathe adequately. The wheezing noises made by asthmatics are caused by turbulent airflow in the narrowed airways. Asthma can cause serious dysfunction and engender great expense. Another lung disease that often seriously damages the airways is **chronic obstructive pulmonary disease.** Actually, this disease constitutes a group of lung diseases that is a major cause of illness and death.

Pulmonary Circulation

The pulmonary artery accompanies and branches in close relationship with the airways. Thus, the physiological theme we stress throughout this section—that *ventilation/perfusion matching is necessary for efficient lung function*—is reflected in the anatomic relationships within the lungs. The pulmonary veins, on the other hand, lie within the interlobular and interlobar connective tissue septa, where they receive blood from many terminal respiratory units. At rest, about 10% of the total circulating blood volume is stored in the lungs.

Pulmonary arteries and veins with diameters larger than about 50 μm in the normal adult human contain smooth muscle. These vessels can actively regulate their diameter and thus alter resistance to blood flow. Normally, the pulmonary vessels are relaxed, so that resistance to blood flow is low.

In the fetus, the pulmonary vessels are constricted, and therefore only a small fraction of right ventricular output flows through the lungs. Pulmonary vascular resistance is high. At the onset of air breathing, the vessels dilate, and vascular resistance normally falls precipitously. However, in a tiny percentage of babies, a congenital opening in the septum between the right and left ventricles persists (**interventricular septal defect),** so that left ventricular blood flows at high pressure into the right ventricle. This defect causes an abnormally high pressure and flow in the pulmonary arteries, which respond by constricting and increasing their smooth muscle coat. These responses eventually result in a permanent increase in pulmonary vascular resistance. If the congenital septal defect can be corrected early (even before birth, if the defect is severe), the long-term effects on the pulmonary vessels can be prevented or reversed.

The pulmonary vasculature is richly innervated. The motor nerve to the smooth muscle comes from the sympathetic branch of the autonomic nervous system. In contrast to the systemic circulation, however, the normal pulmonary circulation shows little evidence of active external regulation. The extensive sensory innervation, located in the adventitia surrounding the blood vessels, can be stimulated by vascular pressure changes (stretch) and by various chemical substances, but its role in regulation of pulmonary and cardiac events is unclear. Most active regulation is mediated by local metabolic influences.

The bronchial circulation supplies nutrients to all lung support structures (airways, vessels, connective tissue, septa, and pleura). The pulmonary circulation supplies nutrients to the alveolar walls.

The pulmonary capillaries form an extensive interdigitating network within the alveolar walls. About 70% to 80% of the surface area of the alveolar wall overlies red blood cells when the capillaries are well filled with blood. The total capillary surface area is nearly as great as the alveolar surface area. Anatomically, the functional capillary volume in resting humans is about 70 ml (1 ml/kg body weight), but during exercise the functional volume increases and approaches the maximal anatomic volume of about 200 ml. The capillary volume can be increased by opening of closed or compressed segments. This process, called **recruitment,** occurs as increased cardiac output raises pulmonary vascular pressures. Capillary volume can also be increased by enlarging open capillaries as their internal pressure rises. This process is called **distention,** and it occurs when the lungs become congested by rising left atrial pressure, as in left heart failure.

Another feature of the alveolocapillary network is that the capillaries are continuous over several alveoli. The average path traveled by red blood cells in the capillaries is 600 to 800 μm before they enter the venous drainage system. The pulmonary capillary blood volume at any instant is about equal to the stroke volume of the right ventricle. Therefore, at an average heart rate of 75 beats/min, red blood cells will remain within the capillaries for one cardiac cycle (about 0.8 second). This time is more than adequate for the diffusion of O_2 and CO_2. Less than 0.25 second is required to reach equilibration through the very thin alveolocapillary barrier mentioned above.

From the top to the bottom of the lung (Fig. 32-8), the hydrostatic pressure in the pulmonary circulation changes by approximately 1 cm H_2O/cm height (higher at the bottom). Thus, when the lung is at FRC, the pressure in the pulmonary artery near the bottom of the lung is about 25 cm H_2O greater than that near the top of the lung.

The pressures in the pulmonary veins vary in the same manner. Left atrial pressure is less than pulmonary arterial pressure, so that the pressure in the veins near the top of the lung may fall below atmospheric pressure (alveolar pressure) at end-expiration or end-inspiration. The anatomic effect of this compressive transmural pressure is that the pulmonary capillaries and venules will collapse and limit blood flow through that region.

The physiological importance of the distribution of pulmonary arterial and venous pressures over the height of the lung is that the lung can be divided into functional zones of blood flow. Blood flow depends on the pressures in the pulmonary vessels relative to alveolar pressure.

Finally, the pulmonary vessels can be divided into alveolar and extra-alveolar vessels; the former are directly affected by alveolar pressure, while the latter are not. The alveolar vessels include most of the capillaries. If the lung is expanded by high positive alveolar gas pressure, most of the alveolar capillaries can be squeezed so that they contain no blood. However, the blood cannot be squeezed out of the arteries and veins, because the surrounding lung tissue elements are effectively pulling them open as lung volume increases.

■ *Terminal Respiratory Unit*

The functional unit of the lung, in terms of O_2 and CO_2 exchange, is called the **terminal respiratory unit.** The

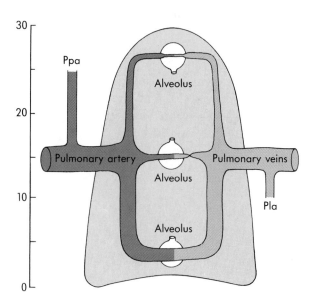

■ **Fig. 32-8** The distribution of pulmonary blood flow in the lung is sensitive to both the pulmonary arterial *(Ppa)* and left atrial *(Pla)* pressures because pulmonary vascular pressures are typically low compared with systemic ones. The three main blood flow zones are shown.

human adult lung has about 60,000 terminal respiratory units. Each unit contains approximately 5000 anatomic alveoli and 250 alveolar ducts. Fig. 32-9 is a model that shows the relationship among the various structural elements of the lung.

■ *Chest Wall*

The functional chest wall includes not only the rib cage and diaphragm but also the abdominal cavity and anterior abdominal muscles. The lungs are passive during breathing. Thus, the muscles of the chest wall, principally the diaphragm, must lower pleural pressure in order to expand the thoracic cavity and implement inspiration. The thoracic cavity enlarges in all dimensions as the rib cage rises and the diaphragm moves caudally, displacing the abdominal contents (Fig. 32-10).

The shape of the lungs must conform to the shape of the thoracic cavity. Membranes called pleuras allow for this conformation. The **visceral** and **parietal** pleuras cover the surfaces of the lungs and thoracic cavity, respectively. The lung and the chest wall pleuras are coupled together by a thin layer of liquid (about 20 μm thick). The liquid coupling acts as a lubricant and allows the lung to move relative to the chest wall during breathing. It also allows the lung to accommodate to changes in thoracic configuration with minimal stress.

The diaphragm is the main muscle of the chest wall. In a chest radiograph, the diaphragm appears as a dome-shaped structure that separates the thoracic and abdominal cavities. Blood is supplied to the diaphragm from branches of the intercostal arteries. The veins drain centrally into the inferior vena cava. The diaphragm is innervated by the right and left phrenic nerves. These nerves have their origins at the third to fifth cervical segments of the spinal cord and descend laterally in the mediastinum to the right and left leaves of the diaphragm.

In humans, the 12 ribs on each side articulate with the thoracic vertebrae. The only motion permitted for the ribs is rotation upward like a pail handle, toward the horizontal plane. This motion increases the cross-sectional area of the thorax when the thorax is viewed along its cephalocaudal axis. Even this motion is limited mainly to the lower ribs; the first and second ribs do not usually move appreciably.

The principal inspiratory muscles of the rib cage are the **external intercostals,** which act to rotate the ribs in the cephalic direction. The first and second ribs and the apex of the sternum are anchored by the neck fascia and neck muscles. The **internal intercostals** are expiratory muscles, which act to rotate the ribs caudally. The ventral neck muscles (**sternocleidomastoids** and **scalenes**) are called the **accessory muscles of breathing.** Normally, they do not contract, but act passively to anchor the sternum and upper ribs. In forced ventilation, however, they contract and actively pull up on the rib cage. This motion assists chest expansion. Individuals in respiratory distress often use the accessory muscles to assist breathing. All the rib cage muscles are voluntary muscles, supplied by intercostal arteries and veins and innervated by motor and sensory intercostal nerves.

An important characteristic of the rib cage is its stiffness. In normal, quiet breathing, the rib cage may contribute up to half of the active inspiratory volume change. Diaphragmatic contraction causes the remainder. The rib cage also contributes passively, because it prevents inward movement of the thoracic wall, as pleural pressure becomes more subatmospheric during inspiration.

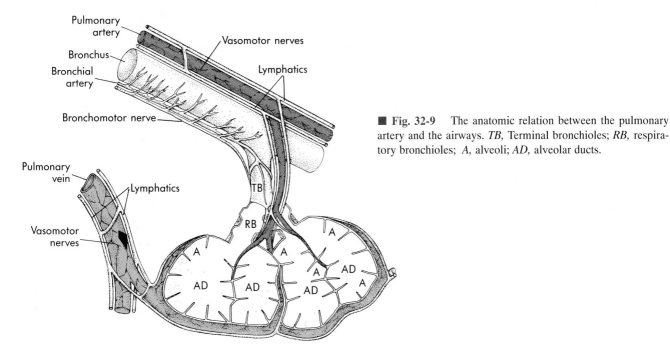

■ **Fig. 32-9**   The anatomic relation between the pulmonary artery and the airways. *TB,* Terminal bronchioles; *RB,* respiratory bronchioles; *A,* alveoli; *AD,* alveolar ducts.

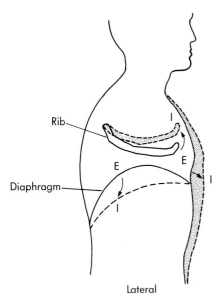

■ **Fig. 32-10**   Chest and rib movements both contribute to the expansion of the chest cavity during breathing. Note that the anterior abdominal wall is included in the functional chest wall because it influences functional residual capacity and also diaphragm movement.

When lung volume is low (**residual volume [RV]**) a large negative intrathoracic pressure (-80 mm Hg) can be generated if an individual inspires against a closed glottis **(Müller's maneuver).** When lung volume is near **TLC** (the maximal lung volume that one can achieve voluntarily), the ability of chest wall muscles to generate a more negative pleural pressure decreases rapidly to zero. This effect limits maximal inspiratory volume.

Inspiratory muscles do the work of breathing. This work is low under normal conditions, and therefore the respiratory muscles have a large reserve capacity. In certain diseases, the chest wall muscles, especially the diaphragm, may fatigue and cause respiratory failure.

> In many diseases, the end-expiratory lung volume (FRC) is increased. Such disorders include **asthma,** which is characterized by episodes of markedly increased airway resistance, and **emphysema,** which is characterized by destruction of lung elastic tissue and degeneration of airway support and structural elements. In these diseases, the muscles of inspiration operate at a disadvantage. Their ability to generate lower pleural pressures and expand the lungs is reduced.

■ *Review of Some Basic Physical Gas Laws*

Table 32-1 lists many of the commonly used respiratory variables, together with their units, for a normal adult in resting and steady-state exercise conditions.

■ *Universal Gas Law*

The equation of state for ideal gases relates three variables—pressure (P), temperature (T), and volume (V)—to the number (n) of moles of gas by a proportionality factor, R, the gas constant. Thus,

$$nR = PV/T \qquad (32\text{-}1)$$

This law is mainly used by respiratory physiologists to convert the **volumes** between different conditions by setting two PV/T conditions (denoted by subscripts 1 and 2) equal to each other. This is allowed, as long as the term *nR* is constant:

$$V_2 = V_1 \times \frac{P_1}{P_2} \times \frac{T_2}{T_1} \qquad (32\text{-}2)$$

■ *Partial Pressure*

In any volume, the total gas pressure of all molecular species in the volume is the sum of the individual pressures that would exist if each species were alone in the same volume. The law of partial pressures is based on the assumption that the gas molecules do not interact. This assumption is nearly valid for the respiratory gases (O_2, CO_2, N_2, H_2O). The law of partial pressures is a direct consequence of the universal gas law, which can be readily seen by keeping volume and temperature constant and relating n (moles of gas) to pressure (P), as shown above.

Dry room air at sea level contains 21% O_2, 79% N_2, and 0% CO_2, and the pressure, PB, is 760 mm Hg. If we remove all of the nitrogen and let the oxygen fill the room at constant temperature, the universal gas law requires that the partial pressure of oxygen (PO_2) equals the fractional content of oxygen (0.21) times the barometric pressure (PB), which equals 0.21 × 760 mm Hg = 160 mm Hg. By a similar calculation, the partial pressure of nitrogen (PN_2) at sea level is 600 mm Hg.

The partial pressure of any gas dissolved in water (blood plasma, interstitial or intracellular liquids) is equal to the partial pressure of that gas in a gas mixture that is in equilibrium with the liquid. In the normal resting human, blood that leaves the pulmonary capillaries has come into equilibrium with all of the alveolar gases. However, small quantities of venous blood from the bronchial venules and the thebesian vessels (heart) contaminate the pulmonary venous outflow. Because of this contamination, the partial pressure of O_2 (Pa_{O_2}) in systemic arterial blood (a) is normally 5 to 15 mm Hg less than that in alveolar gas. Thus, Pa_{O_2} = 85 to 95 mm Hg. Table 32-2 lists the normal partial pressures of the respiratory gases at various physiologically important locations in the body.

■ *Water Vapor Pressure*

When air is inspired, it is warmed to 37° C in the nose, throat, and trachea and becomes saturated with water

■ **Table 32-2**   Total and partial pressures of respiratory gases in ideal alveolar gas and blood at sea level barometric pressure (760 mm Hg)

	Ambient air (dry)	Moist tracheal air	Alveolar gas (R = 0.80)	Systemic arterial blood	Mixed venous blood
P_{O_2}	160	150	102	90	40
P_{CO_2}	0	0	40	40	46
P_{H_2O}, 37°C	0	47	47	47	47
P_{N_2}	600	563	571*	571	571
P_{TOTAL}	760	760	760	760	704†

*P_{N_2} is increased in alveolar gas by 1% because R is < 1 normally.

†P_{TOTAL} is less in venous than in arterial blood because P_{O_2} has decreased more than P_{CO_2} has increased.

vapor at 37° C. This event is obligatory and occurs rapidly. The water vapor exerts a mandatory partial pressure, $P_{H_2O} = 47$ mm Hg at 37° C.

Air inhaled through the nose is almost completely equilibrated to body temperature and water vapor partial pressure before it passes into the trachea. However, air inhaled through the mouth may reach the distal cartilaginous bronchi before complete equilibrium is attained, and hence the inhaled air may draw heat from the surrounding lungs. It is impossible to breathe rapidly enough or deeply enough for air to reach the alveolar surfaces unequilibrated.

■ *Conditions*

The universal gas law is used to correct respiratory gas volumes among three conditions. These are ambient temperature and pressure saturated (with H_2O) (ATPS), body temperature and pressure saturated (BTPS), and standard temperature and pressure dry (STPD).

In clinical pulmonary function reports, the various lung volumes, such as **tidal volume (V_T)** and **vital capacity (VC),** are reported as BTPS, which is the condition that prevails in life. However, in the laboratory, if a spirometer is used (Fig. 32-11), the volumes are obtained under ambient conditions (ATPS) and must be corrected.

Standard conditions (273° K, 760 mm Hg, dry; STPD) must be used when referring to O_2 and CO_2 consumptions. The reason is that the physician and physiologist want to know the number of molecules that are exchanging. Standard conditions are independent of location (sea level, under the sea, or on top of a mountain) and ambient or body temperature.

■ *Blood Oxygen Concentration*

The hemoglobin-oxygen (HbO_2) equilibrium curve (Fig 32-2) is a plot of HbO_2 saturation (S_{O_2}, the percentage of hemoglobin that is bound to oxygen) as a function of the partial pressure of O_2 (P_{O_2}). This graph is used mainly to determine one of the variables when other variables are known.

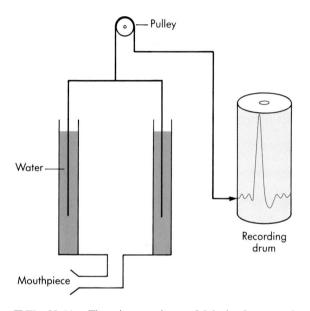

■ **Fig. 32-11**   The spirometer is a useful device for measuring all lung volumes (except residual volume). The subject breathes in and out of the water-sealed chamber, which moves the delicately balanced float that moves a pen on a rotating drum.

What the curve does not show is that, even at equilibrium, rapid association and dissociation chemical reactions are occurring. In other words, any point on the equilibrium curve corresponds to the condition that the rate of formation of oxyhemoglobin, $O_2 + Hb \rightarrow HbO_2$, exactly equals the rate of its dissociation, $HbO_2 \rightarrow Hb + O_2$. It is necessary to know the speed (kinetics) of these two simultaneous reactions in order to understand fully the physiological value of the HbO_2 equilibrium curve in life.

From the equilibrium curve (Fig. 32-2), one can read that at $P_{O_2} = 100$ mm Hg, $S_{O_2} = 97.4\%$. However, some oxygen is also dissolved (in physical solution), although oxygen is not very soluble in water. The dissolved oxygen concentration is determined by the solubility coefficient, $\alpha = 22.8$ ml/L × 760 mm Hg. Thus, 1 L of blood holds 3.0 ml O_2 in solution at $P_{O_2} = 100$ mm Hg.

Because hemoglobin can chemically bind 1.34 ml O_2/g and the normal hemoglobin concentration (Hb) in blood is 150 g/L, the **O_2 capacity of hemoglobin** = 1.34 ml O_2/g Hb × 150 g Hb/L = 200 ml O_2/L.

In normal systemic arterial blood, $S_{O_2} = 97\%$ because $Pa_{O_2} \approx 90$ mm Hg. This means that the bound oxygen concentration is 97% of capacity. To obtain the total oxygen concentration in blood, add the chemically bound O_2 to that dissolved at the appropriate P_{O_2}. For systemic arterial blood, the total concentration of oxygen $Ca_{O_2} = [(0.97 \times 200) + (0.03 \times 100)]$ ml O_2/L = 197 ml O_2/L. The correction for dissolved O_2 is usually small, but when a person breathes 100% O_2 it may be substantial—18 to 20 ml/L of blood.

■ Conservation of Mass

A physical principle widely used in physiology is the **conservation of mass law.** This law states that in a closed system (such as the body), the total number of atoms remains constant, as long as the body is in a steady state. Because oxygen enters the body at a rate of 250 ml/min, the same quantity of oxygen must leave the body. If it does not, the body will accumulate oxygen; that is, the conservation of mass law will be violated. The oxygen that enters the human body leaves either as carbon dioxide (CO_2) or water vapor (H_2O).

The ratio of carbon dioxide production ($\dot{V}_{CO_2}$) to oxygen consumption ($\dot{V}_{O_2}$) is the **respiratory exchange ratio (R),** also called the **respiratory quotient** $= \dot{V}_{CO_2} / \dot{V}_{O_2}$. R in the steady state ranges between 0.7 and 1.0. The value of the respiratory exchange ratio is determined by the metabolic fuel being burned by the body; the fuel mixture determines the number of CO_2 molecules produced for a given number of O_2 molecules consumed. In Table 32-1, the average respiratory quotient is 0.80, which is reasonable for a person on a mixed diet of carbohydrates, protein, and fat. Thus, for a resting person $\dot{V}_{O_2} = 250$ ml/min, $\dot{V}_{CO_2} = 0.80 \times 250$ ml/min = 200 ml/min.

■ Lung Volumes and Ventilation

Because tissues engaged in aerobic metabolism use O_2 and produce CO_2, they remove O_2 from systemic capillary blood and add CO_2 to it. This exchange lowers the partial pressure of oxygen in mixed venous blood ($P\bar{v}_{O_2}$) to below that of alveolar gas and raises the partial pressure of CO_2 in mixed venous blood ($P\bar{v}_{CO_2}$) to above that of alveolar gas. The normal partial pressures of the common respiratory gases in systemic arterial and mixed venous (pulmonary arterial) blood are listed in Table 32-2.

Half of the process of ventilation/perfusion matching involves ventilation of the alveoli in such a way that it increases PA_{O_2} well above that of mixed venous blood. Increasing PA_{O_2} causes oxygen to diffuse along its partial pressure gradient and loads oxygen into the pulmonary capillary blood. Ventilation also lowers the PA_{CO_2} below

that in mixed venous blood. Decreasing PA_{O_2} causes CO_2 to diffuse along its partial pressure gradient and reduces the CO_2 content of the pulmonary capillary blood.

When body metabolism increases, as in exercise, $P\bar{v}_{O_2}$ will decrease and $P\bar{v}_{O_2}$ will increase as the body consumes more oxygen and produces more CO_2. To maintain the arterial O_2 and CO_2 partial pressures close to resting steady-state levels, **alveolar ventilation** (the amount of fresh air in each breath that reaches the gas exchange units) increases. The increase in alveolar ventilation supplies the alveoli with an amount of O_2 equal to the amount that diffuses out of systemic capillary blood in the metabolizing tissues. Furthermore, alveolar ventilation removes the increased quantity of CO_2 from the alveoli that was added to the venous blood in the systemic capillaries.

The main purpose of ventilation is to maintain an optimal composition of alveolar gas. Think of alveolar gas as a buffer (stabilizing) compartment of gas that lies between the environment (ambient air) and pulmonary capillary blood. Oxygen is continuously removed from alveolar gas, and CO_2 is continuously added to it by blood that flows through the pulmonary capillary network. Oxygen is supplied to the alveolar gas, and CO_2 is removed from it by the cyclic process of ventilation—the inspiration of fresh air followed by the expiration of alveolar gas. The cyclic nature of ventilation suggests the importance of the buffering effect of a large alveolar gas volume.

■ Total Ventilation and Alveolar Ventilation

Total ventilation is the volume of air that enters or leaves the nose or mouth during each breath or each minute. It can be measured breath to breath by volume recorders, such as the spirometer in Fig. 32-11.

The volume of each breath is called the **tidal volume (V_T)** which varies with age, sex, body position, and metabolic activity. The average normal value of V_T in a resting adult is 0.5 L (500 ml). The largest possible tidal volume of anyone is the **vital capacity (VC).**

Alveolar ventilation (V_A) is the volume of fresh air that enters the alveoli each minute (or each breath). Alveolar ventilation is always less than total ventilation; how much less depends on the anatomic dead space and tidal volume.

■ Anatomic Dead Space and Tidal Volume

Fresh air does not go directly to the terminal respiratory units. It first flows through the conducting airways (nose, mouth, pharynx, larynx, trachea, bronchi, and bronchioles). In the conducting airways, little, if any, O_2 and CO_2 exchange occurs between gas and blood. Therefore, the portion of the fresh inspired air that fills the airways is called the **anatomic dead space (VD).** Although the anatomic dead space can be measured, it is generally assumed to be approximately 2 ml/kg ideal body weight.

At the end of a normal expiration (just before the next inspiration begins), the conducting airways are filled with alveolar gas, which has a PA_{O_2} of 100 mm Hg and a PA_{CO_2} of 40 mm Hg. Thus, as inspiration begins, the alveoli must first receive the gas that was in the anatomic dead space from the last exhalation. This gas does not raise alveolar PO_2 or lower alveolar PCO_2, because it has the same composition as the alveolar gas. After the dead space gas is inspired, the alveoli receive fresh air until the tidal volume is reached. The last portion of the fresh air, of course, remains in the conducting airways. The volume of the dead space, VD, and the volume of the breath, VT, are important factors in determining the amount of alveolar ventilation per breath (Fig. 32-12).

■ *Lung Volumes and Capacities*

The lungs do not collapse to the airless state with each expiration, partly because the chest wall (ribs, intercostal muscles, diaphragm) becomes stiffer at the end of expiration. Indeed, the lungs cannot be completely emptied of gas, even by the most forceful expiration. Some gas still remains—the **residual volume (RV)**—as shown in Fig. 32-13.

The **functional residual capacity (FRC)** is the volume of air that remains at the end of a normal expiration. The FRC is not actively regulated; it is determined by the passive mechanical relationship between the chest wall and the lungs, although airflow dynamics may contribute in some conditions.

The FRC acts as a buffer against large changes in alveolar PO_2 with each breath. If FRC were very small, PA_{O_2} would fluctuate markedly with each breath; it would decrease toward that of mixed venous blood in the pulmonary capillaries at end-expiration ($P\bar{v}_{O_2}$ = 40 mm Hg), and it would rise toward that of moist tracheal air (PO_2 = 150 mm Hg) during inspiration. The advantage of cyclic ventilation of a relatively large space (e.g., FRC = 2.4 L; 40% of TLC in normal young adult males) by a small volume of alveolar ventilation per breath (VT − VD) is that fluctuations of PA_{O_2} and PA_{CO_2} are minimal: about 4 mm Hg for the former and 3 mm Hg for the latter.

The various static lung **volumes** and **capacities** are shown in Fig. 32-13, which also includes a tracing of a normal spirogram. There are four non-overlapping volumes together with several capacities, each of which includes two or more volumes. Of the four volumes named above, all, except residual volume, can be measured directly by volume recorders, such as the spirometer in Fig. 32-11.

Diseases of the lungs or chest wall affect lung volumes and capacities in various ways. The most frequent change is in the vital capacity (VC), which may be greatly reduced. The reduction may be caused by limited expansion (**restrictive disease**) or by an abnormally large residual volume (**chronic obstructive pulmonary disease**). In strenuous exercise, tidal volume may have to increase to one half the vital

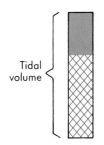

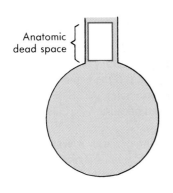

End-expiration

■ **Fig. 32-12** Tidal volume and alveolar ventilation are equal, but the air entering the alveoli contains the dead space gas from the previous breath plus some of the new air. The fresh air in the anatomic dead space is wasted (i.e., it does not contribute to gas exchange).

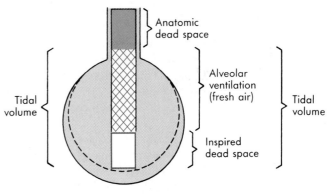

End-inspiration

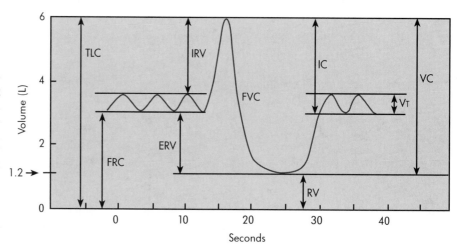

■ **Fig. 32-13** The various volumes and capacities. *TLC,* Total lung capacity; *FRC,* functional residual capacity; *IRV,* inspiratory reserve volume; *ERV,* expiratory reserve volume; *RV,* residual volume; *IC,* inspiratory capacity; *VT,* tidal volume; *VC,* vital capacity; *FVC,* forced vital capacity.

capacity to ensure adequate alveolar ventilation. Thus, limitation of exercise capacity is often an early sign of lung disease that limits VC.

Changes in RV are important in the assessment of lung function; hence it is frequently measured in the pulmonary function laboratory. The single breath volume of dilution, used to measure RV, is another application of the widely used law of conservation of mass. In this method, the subject inspires a known volume of gas of markedly different composition from normal alveolar gas. The dilution of the expired gas is measured and the conservation of mass law is then used to calculate the residual volume. Insoluble inert gases, such as helium or neon, are most commonly used in this test. For example, a normal subject inspires 4.4 L, V_I, of a mixture that contains 10% helium from a spirometer at 21° C. On expiration, a sample of alveolar gas contains 8% helium. The inspired volume is diluted by the gas already in the lungs. To compute RV, we use the conservation of mass law to set up the mixing equation:

$$(C_1 \times V_1) + (C_2 \times V_2) = (C_3 \times V_3) \qquad (32\text{-}3)$$

If V_1 = RV, then C_1 is zero, because helium is not present in air. Hence, the first term drops out (which is convenient and explains why foreign inert gases are used). Let V_3 be the total volume of gas (RV + V_2). Substitute the necessary helium concentrations to obtain residual volume. One small problem must be overcome: the inspired gas in the spirometer is ATPS. Therefore, the inspired volume has to be corrected to 37° C, as described earlier, to obtain the correct RV to BTPS conditions.

Because alveolar O_2 tension is the main determinant of the rate of diffusion of O_2 from alveolar gas into pulmonary capillary blood, the amount of alveolar ventilation is more important in determining $P_{A_{O_2}}$ than is the size of the FRC.

■ *Alveolar Ventilation*

The alveolar ventilation/breath, when multiplied by the frequency of breathing, f, gives the alveolar ventilation per minute, $\dot{V}_A$, just as tidal volume × frequency gives the total expired ventilation per minute, $\dot{V}_E$. If V_T = 500 ml and the normal breathing rate is 12/min, then $\dot{V}_E$ = V_T × f = 500 ml × 12/min = 6000 ml/min. To obtain alveolar ventilation, the anatomic dead space is simply subtracted from the tidal volume and multiplied by the frequency of breathing: $\dot{V}_A$ = f × (V_T − V_D).

In the lung function laboratory, the anatomic dead space is not often measured. Alveolar ventilation is calculated using the same volume of dilution principle employed to calculate residual volume. In this application, however, it is more convenient to use CO_2 than helium, a foreign gas. CO_2 is used because, as mentioned earlier, it is not exchanged in the anatomic dead space. Therefore, ventilation of the dead space contributes nothing to the expired CO_2, although it does contribute to expired volume. Usually, all gas concentrations are expressed as fractions, F, of total dry gas pressure. In terms of F_{CO_2}, the volume of dilution equation is as follows:

$$(\dot{V}_A \times F_{A_{CO_2}}) + (V_D \times F_{D_{CO_2}}) = \dot{V}_E \times F_{E_{CO_2}} \quad (32\text{-}4)$$

where the second term on the left represents dead space CO_2 production, which is normally zero. Normal alveolar gas contains 5.6% CO_2 [$F_{A_{CO_2}}$ = 40 mm Hg/(760 − 47 mm Hg) = 0.056]. If the expired ventilation had been collected in a spirometer, ATPS, a correction to BTPS would be required because $\dot{V}_A$ is always reported under body conditions.

Because the main purpose of ventilation is to maintain an optimal concentration of alveolar gases, alveolar ventilation is in balance (steady state) for oxygen when it matches O_2 use with O_2 supply. For example, if we use the normal values of tidal volume of 500 ml and dead

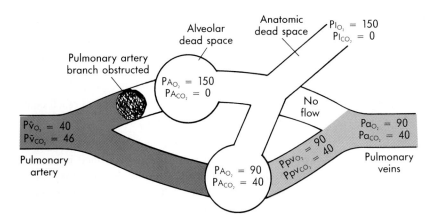

■ **Fig. 32-14** Wasted ventilation includes the anatomic dead space plus any portion of the alveolar ventilation that does not exchange O_2 or CO_2 with the pulmonary blood flow. This simple sketch shows one pulmonary artery completely obstructed by a blood clot, but in most patients an anatomic definition of the wasted ventilation is not easily made.

space volume of 150 ml, the alveolar ventilation per breath is 350 ml. If a normal person breathes 12 times/min, the alveoli are supplied with an alveolar ventilation, $\dot{V}A$, of 4200 ml/min.

As discussed later, it is not the oxygen supply to the alveoli but the partial pressure of CO_2 in arterial blood, PA_{CO_2}, that is closely regulated. If PA_{CO_2} is held at 40 mm Hg, which can be equated with the average $Pa_{CO_2} = 40$ mm Hg, then while the subject breathes air at sea level, the PA_{O_2} is maintained at 100 mm Hg.

The adequacy of ventilation is described in terms of PA_{CO_2} because sometimes the inspired oxygen concentration is decreased (e.g., when one goes to higher altitude) or increased (e.g., when one breathes enriched oxygen mixtures). Normal alveolar ventilation means that $PA_{CO_2} = 40$ mm Hg. **Hyperventilation** (overventilation) for a particular metabolic state means that PA_{CO_2} is < 40 mm Hg. **Hypoventilation** (underventilation), which is the more common condition encountered in patients with severe lung diseases, means that PA_{CO_2} is > 40 mm Hg.

■ *Wasted Ventilation (Physiological Dead Space)*

In a perfect lung, all alveoli would receive ventilation ($\dot{V}$) and blood flow (Q) in the same proportion. In other words, the perfect lung would have a uniform ventilation/perfusion ratio ($\dot{V}/Q$). However, these ideal conditions do not exist even in the healthiest individuals and may be markedly abnormal in diseased lungs. The concept of **wasted ventilation** or **physiological dead space** is used clinically to describe the deviation from ideal ventilation relative to blood flow (Fig. 32-14).

Clearly, ventilation of the anatomic dead space is necessary, but it is wasted because no useful gas exchange occurs there. In addition, some terminal lung units may not receive their normal allotment of blood flow. For example, imagine that one of the pulmonary artery branches is blocked by a blood clot (embolus). The alveolar ventilation to that lung is wasted because it does not participate in any useful gas exchange. Thus, the physiological dead space is the sum of anatomic dead space and

a portion of the ventilation that goes to units that receive low blood flow. Because the expired alveolar volume contains gas from unperfused and normally perfused alveoli, the true PA_{CO_2} is underestimated. *The systemic arterial carbon dioxide partial pressure is generally accepted as being equal to the carbon dioxide partial pressure for the properly ventilated and perfused lung.*

■ *Alveolar Ventilation Equation*

The **alveolar ventilation** equation describes the reciprocal (hyperbolic) relationship between alveolar ventilation and PA_{CO_2}. It is the most important relationship in pulmonary physiology. All discussions of the adequacy of ventilation and of alveolar oxygen or carbon dioxide partial pressures come directly from this equation:

$$\dot{V}A = \frac{\dot{V}_{CO_2} \times K}{PA_{CO_2}} \tag{32-5}$$

If the barometric pressure is 760 mm Hg and body temperature 33° C, then the correction factor, K, is 0.863 mm Hg × L/ml, when $\dot{V}A$ is given in L/min, BTPS, and the CO_2 production, $\dot{V}_{CO_2}$, is in ml/min, STPD (Fig. 32-15).

The alveolar ventilation equation is correct for any CO_2 production, even during heavy exercise, when $\dot{V}_{CO_2}$ may be six times the resting value. Fig. 32-15 shows two plots of the alveolar ventilation equation for different metabolic states. The equation implies that P_{CO_2} is the controlled variable for the regulation of alveolar ventilation, which is correct.

The alveolar ventilation equation can be used to compute the wasted ventilation to obtain an index of the efficiency of ventilation. Normally, wasted ventilation is less than 35% of $\dot{V}E$.

■ *Alveolar Gas Equation*

If PA_{CO_2} is known, one can calculate PA_{O_2} by the alveolar gas equation. This calculation is used clinically to determine the alveolar-arterial oxygen tension difference

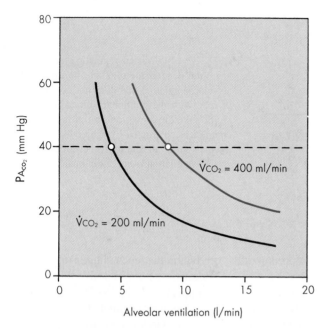

■ **Fig. 32-15** The relationship between alveolar ventilation and alveolar P_{CO_2} is a hyperbola. The other variable required is the CO_2 production. In the examples shown, the dashed line shows that for the same P_{CO_2} the alveolar ventilation must be doubled when CO_2 production is doubled.

and for assessing the underlying pathophysiology.

$$P_{A_{O_2}} = [F_{I_{O_2}} \times (P_B - P_{H_2O})] -$$

$$P_{a_{CO_2}} \times \left[F_{I_{O_2}} + \frac{1 - F_{I_{O_2}}}{R} \right] \qquad (32\text{-}6)$$

$P_B - P_{H_2O}$ is the total dry gas pressure as previously defined. If R (the respiratory exchange ratio) = 1 or if one breathes 100% oxygen ($F_{I_{O_2}} = 1.0$), the complex term in the square brackets equals one. Normally, the term in the right brackets evaluates to 1.2 ($F_I = 0.21$; R = 0.80).

As we generally use $P_{a_{CO_2}}$ (arterial blood), not $P_{A_{CO_2}}$ (alveolar gas), in the alveolar gas equation, the $P_{a_{O_2}}$ we obtain is for the effectively ventilated lung.

■ *Summary*

1. The main function of the lung is to bring fresh air (ventilation) into close contact with blood flowing in the pulmonary capillaries (perfusion), so that the exchange of oxygen and carbon dioxide will take place efficiently.

2. The lung effectively matches ventilation to perfusion, as reflected by the coordinated branching pattern of the airways and the pulmonary arteries.

3. The airways are of two types: cartilaginous bronchi and membranous bronchioles. One pulmonary artery branch accompanies each airway and branches with it. The lung has the most extensive capillary network surface area of any organ. The erythrocytes remain in the capillaries long enough for gas exchange to reach equilibrium, even in heavy exercise.

4. Groups of alveolar ducts and their alveoli, together with their supplying arteries, are combined into small functional elements called terminal respiratory units. Their parallel arrangement helps to ensure the efficient distribution of inspired air and mixed venous blood.

5. Functionally, the chest wall includes not only the diaphragm and rib cage but also the abdomen. Coordinated muscle contraction in the chest wall enlarges the thoracic cavity during inspiration, while the lungs expand passively in all directions to fill the cavity.

6. The universal gas law is used to convert gas volumes between differing pressures and temperatures. In both the gas and liquid phases, each kind of gas in a mixture, including water vapor, exerts a partial pressure that is proportional to its fractional concentration in the gas phase.

7. The red protein, hemoglobin, in erythrocytes binds O_2 rapidly and reversibly. The oxygen capacity (100% saturation) of normal blood is 200 ml O_2/L.

8. The conservation of mass law is used to measure cardiac output and various components of breathing, such as alveolar ventilation, oxygen consumption, and CO_2 production. Alveolar ventilation is the useful portion of fresh air that reaches the gas exchange units each minute. The portion of each breath that fills the airway is called the anatomic dead space.

9. Total lung capacity is composed of several separate volumes and overlapping capacities, of which the most important are the residual volume, functional residual capacity, and vital capacity. Except for residual volume, all volumes and capacities can be directly measured with a spirometer or equivalent device in the pulmonary function laboratory.

10. Alveolar P_{CO_2} or its equivalent arterial P_{CO_2} reflects the adequacy of alveolar ventilation. The alveolar ventilation equation describes the relationship among alveolar ventilation, arterial P_{CO_2}, and CO_2 production (metabolism).

11. The alveolar gas equation permits the calculation of mean alveolar P_{O_2}, if P_{CO_2} is known. The $O_2 - CO_2$ diagram shows all possible alveolar O_2 and CO_2 partial pressures under given physiological conditions.

■ Self-Study Problems

1. Compare the main anatomic differences between the pathways of ventilation and perfusion in the lung. Compare the physiological aspects of ventilation and perfusion.

2. When a pulmonary artery branch is completely obstructed by a blood clot (pulmonary embolus), the lung tissue served by that artery is metabolically depressed for days or weeks, but the involved lung tissue does not usually die. What pathways for nutritional blood supply sustain life in the obstructed segment?

3. If one inspires from FRC to TLC, then expires back to FRC, all the terminal respiratory units expand and contract. How do the units at the cephalic end of the lung under the first and second ribs expand, if those ribs do not move?

4. In some of the classic science fiction stories about space exploration, death by loss of pressure (explosive decompression) was imaginatively described in gory detail. What occurs physiologically when part or all of the body is exposed quickly to an atmospheric pressure $P_B = 0$ mm Hg. What happens when normal people are exposed to ambient pressures less than 100 mm Hg?

■ Bibliography

Journal articles

Staub NC: The interdependence of pulmonary structure and function, *Anesthesiology* 24:831, 1963.

Books and monographs

Hayek HV: *The human lung,* New York, 1960, Hafner.
Macklem PT: *Symbols and abbreviations.* In *Handbook of physiology,* sect 3, *Respiration,* Bethesda, Md, 1985, American Physiological Society, pp ix and endpapers.
Staub NC: *Basic respiratory physiology.* New York, 1991, Churchill Livingstone.
Staub NC, Albertine KN: *Anatomy of the lungs.* In Murray JF, Nadel JA, editors: *Textbook of respiratory medicine,* ed 2, vol 1, Philadelphia, 1994, WB Saunders, p 3.
Tyler WS, Julian MD: *Gross and subgross anatomy of lungs, pleura, connective tissue septa, distal airways and structural units.* In Parent RA, editor: *Comparative biology of the normal lung,* Boca Raton, Fla, 1991, CRC Press, p 37.
Weibel ER: *Morphometry of the human lung,* New York, 1963, Academic Press.

CHAPTER
33

Mechanical Properties in Breathing

■ *Statics*

The *static* mechanical properties of the lung and chest wall encompass a major part of modern respiratory physiology, and have important manifestations in such diverse diseases as emphysema, pulmonary fibrosis, and respiratory distress syndromes. In this section, we treat the lungs and chest wall as *passive;* that is, the muscles of the chest wall (diaphragm and intercostal muscles) are relaxed. In normal breathing, this condition occurs only when the lungs are at functional residual capacity (FRC) (end-expiration). However, this passive condition can also be achieved when the lungs and chest wall are moved by a mechanical ventilator in a relaxed subject or in a patient who is paralyzed.

■ *Lung Distensibility*

Compliance, *C,* is the usual term used to describe lung distensibility. Compliance reflects the ease with which an object can be deformed, whereas **elastance, E,** reflects the opposition of an object to deformation by an external force. Elastance is thus expressed as the inverse of compliance: E = 1/C.

■ *Elastic Recoil of the Lung*

The compliance of the lung is determined from the pressure-volume curve or loop; a normal loop for the human lung is shown in Fig. 33-1. Clearly, the lung does not behave as a perfectly elastic body, owing to the lung's complex anatomic structure and the alveolar air-liquid surface tension. Two main points concerning the pressure-volume loop are emphasized here: (1) inflation and deflation follow different paths and (2) the end points exhibit sharp discontinuities.

The structures of the lung are not uniformly elastic; they consist of collagen and elastic fibers, giant glycoprotein molecules in the interstitial matrix, and various cells, such as the alveolar epithelium and capillary endothelium. Many lung tissues, such as cells, interstitial

ground substance molecules, and elastic fibers, are extensible. The collagen fibers, however, are not very stretchable. As lung volume increases above 75% of total lung capacity (TLC), the collagen restricts lung expansion more and more. The lung becomes stiffer and the slope of the pressure-volume curve decreases.

■ *The Measure of Lung Distensibility*

Lung compliance, C_L, is the measure of its distensibility. Lung compliance is the slope of the line between any two points on the deflation limb of the pressure-volume loop; the deflation limb is shown in Fig. 33-2:

$$C_L = \Delta V_L / \Delta P_L \qquad (33\text{-}1)$$

where ΔV_L is the change in lung volume, and ΔP_L is the change in translung pressure. The units of lung compliance are liters per centimeter of H_2O (L/cm H_2O). Lung elastance, E_L, is the measure of the lung's opposition to distention:

$$E_L = \Delta P_L / \Delta V_L \qquad (33\text{-}2)$$

With reference to trans-organ pressures, the pressure difference across the wall must be measured from the inside to the outside. For the lung, trans-organ pressure, P_L, is defined as: $P_L = P_A - P_{pl}$, where P_A is total alveolar gas pressure and P_{pl} is the pressure in the pleural space.

■ *The Deflation Pressure-Volume Curve*

The static deflation limb of the pressure-volume curve of a normal, air-filled human lung is shown in Fig. 33-2. Zero applied translung pressure is indicated by the vertical line. Pressures to the right of this line are positive and act to distend the lung; pressures to the left of the line are negative and act to compress it.

The ordinate shows relative lung volume from zero to **total lung capacity (TLC).** Also marked are **residual volume (RV), functional residual capacity (FRC),** and **minimal volume (MV).** MV represents the *unstressed*

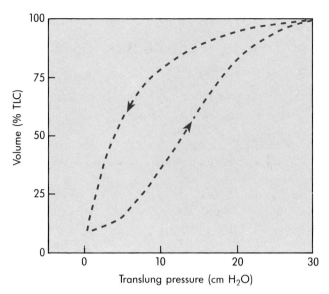

■ **Fig. 33-1**　The air pressure-volume curve is rich in information about the static mechanical properties of the lung. The curve must be traced in the counterclockwise direction *(arrows)*. Inflation and deflation limbs are different chiefly because of differences in the alveolar air-liquid interfacial surface tension.

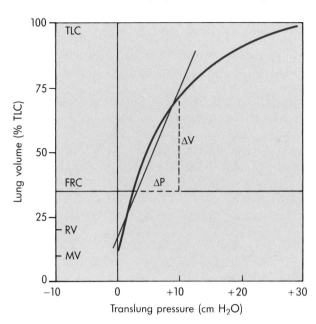

■ **Fig. 33-2**　Deflation pressure-volume curve of a normal human lung demonstrates how compliance can be measured as the slope of the line between two different volumes. *TLC,* Total lung capacity; *FRC,* functional residual capacity; *RV,* residual volume; *MV,* minimal volume; *ΔV,* change in lung volume; *ΔP,* change in translung pressure that corresponds to the change in lung volume, ΔV.

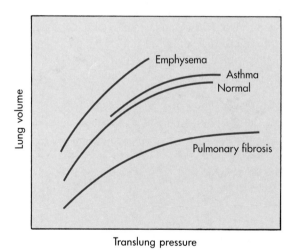

■ **Fig. 33-3**　Deflation pressure-volume curves. Normal and asthma are the same, except that the latter has a higher FRC. Emphysema has a high TLC as well as FRC but at lower translung distending pressures because the lung is easily inflated. Fibrosis stiffens the lung and reduces TLC and FRC.

volume (i.e., the volume that exists when PL = 0). When the chest is opened, as during thoracic surgery, and the lungs are allowed to recoil until the translung pressure equals zero, they do not collapse to the airless condition; rather, they retain approximately 10% of their total gas capacity. In Figs. 33-1 and 33-2, notice that volume is not zero when PL is zero.

Minimal volume for the lung as a whole does not actually occur in life, because the chest wall becomes rigid and does not permit the lung volume to decrease below residual volume. However, some regions may reach minimal volume during quiet breathing, especially in older people, whose lungs tend to be more compliant.

> In **chronic obstructive pulmonary disease (COPD, emphysema)** the alveolar walls progressively degenerate, which *increases* lung compliance. Small changes in transpulmonary pressure evoke larger than normal changes in lung volume (Fig. 33-3). In **chronic restrictive lung disease (pulmonary fibrosis),** which is characterized by decreased compliance of the lung, changes in transpulmonary pressure evoke smaller than normal changes in lung volume. In **asthma** (hyperactive airway smooth muscle), lung compliance is normal. However, FRC may be much increased because the airways narrow excessively during expiration.

The deflation pressure-volume curve shown in Fig. 33-2 is for a normal adult human lung that has been inflated with air to total lung capacity and then allowed to deflate very slowly. This standard procedure is performed to ensure reproducible initial conditions.

Notice that the deflation limb is curvilinear. Over its upper third, the slope of the line is not very steep, which indicates a low compliance. Over the lower portion of the curve, however, the slope is steep, which denotes a high compliance. To calculate the compliance of the lung between any two points on the pressure-volume curve, the change in volume, ΔVL, is divided by the change in translung pressure, ΔPL.

The lung can easily be distended when transpulmonary pressure is low. This property is beneficial, because normally, even in exercise, we breathe at pressures and volumes that represent the lower 70% of the curve. Tidal volume in exercise seldom exceeds half of vital capacity. Thus, in normal subjects, the work of breathing, $\int PdV$, is less than the work that would be expended if one breathed at high lung volumes. Such a condition may occur in a person during an asthma attack, during which the narrowed airways markedly increase airflow resistance (see p 543). This condition would lead to an increased FRC, even though lung elastic recoil is normal (Fig. 33-3).

The end-expiratory point of the pressure-volume curve is the FRC, which is represented by the horizontal line in Fig. 33-2. The translung pressure (elastic recoil pressure) when the lung volume is at FRC averages 3.5 cm H_2O; the FRC is about 35% of the TLC.

■ *Surface Forces and Lung Recoil*

The adult human lung contains about 300 million alveoli. This large number provides a vast surface area for O_2 and CO_2 exchange. However, each anatomic alveolus has a very small radius (about 110 μm in the adult human at FRC). This geometric condition, together with the interface between air in the alveoli and the watery alveolar tissue, introduces the complication of surface tension.

The significance of the air-liquid surface tension in the alveoli is best demonstrated by determining the complete lung pressure-volume curve when the lung is filled with

saline, and comparing it with that obtained when the lung is filled with air. The comparison is shown in Fig. 33-4, in which the air pressure-volume loop is the same as in Fig. 33-1.

The pressure-volume loop of the liquid-filled lung is displaced to the left of the loop of the air-filled lung at any given volume. This displacement is especially pronounced on the inflation limb. *The significance of the shift is that it requires much less pressure to maintain lung volume when the lung is filled with liquid (saline) than when it is filled with gas.*

The difference between the air and liquid pressure-volume loops is not caused by tissue elastic recoil forces (e.g., collagen, elastin). These elements are not affected differently by filling the lung with saline or air. What has changed is that the alveolar air-liquid interface has disappeared. Therefore, the pressure necessary to maintain a given lung volume is the sum of the pressures necessary to overcome the elastic recoil of the tissue elements and of the elastic air-liquid interface at the alveolar surface.

What is surface tension? On a clean glass plate that has not been washed with dishwashing compound a drop of water will form a raised bead. If some liquid dishwashing soap is added to the droplet, the droplet will spread over the surface of the plate. The large surface tension difference between the water and the plate caused the bead to form; the decrease of surface tension caused by the liquid soap allows the drop to spread. Surface tension has its largest effects on sharply curved surfaces, such as those that prevail in the alveoli.

Within the bulk phase of a polar liquid, such as water (Fig. 33-5, *A*), forces of attraction exist among the water

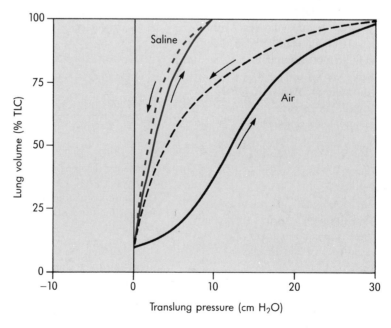

■ **Fig. 33-4** Note the marked difference between the air pressure-volume curve and the saline-filled lung. The latter is much easier to inflate, suggesting that lung distensibility is increased by the absence of the alveolar air-liquid interface.

molecules. Throughout most of the liquid, these forces are equal in all directions, but not at the surface (Fig. 33-5, *B*). The attraction of the molecules under the surface is not balanced by molecules in the vapor phase. Thus, the surface molecules are pulled inward and compressed together, and they exert a force within the plane of the surface. This force acts as an elastic tension.

Surface tension is expressed as the units of force (millinewtons, [mN]) per unit length (centimeters). In a hemisphere, which in this discussion is analogous to an alveolus, the surface tension acts as if it were concentrated along a circumferential curvature in the surface. In a soap bubble, it is the surface tension alone that holds the sphere together in opposition to the transmural distending pressure, as shown schematically in Fig. 33-6. In the alveoli, the situation is similar: the distending air pressure, P_L, is opposed by the air-liquid surface tension. For this reason, the air pressure-volume loop requires more distending pressure at any given volume (Fig. 33-4).

The relationship between the tension, T, in the surface and the transmural distending pressure, Ptm, is described by the law of Laplace (see also Chapter 27). For hemispherical alveoli, the law is:

$$Ptm = 2 \times T/r \tag{33-3}$$

Ptm is the portion of the translung pressure, P_L, caused by surface tension.

In addition, the surface active material in the alveoli has a special property not found in commercial detergents. Not only can the alveolar surface tension be low, but it also *varies* as a function of lung volume (as alveolar surface area changes). In Fig. 33-4, the inflation limb of the air pressure-volume curve requires a higher translung pressure at any volume than does the deflation limb. This requirement can be explained only if the surface tension is different between inflation and deflation—higher as the lung surface expands and lower as the lung surface contracts. The variable surface tension accounts for most of the hysteresis (disparity between responses to inflation and deflation) seen in the air pressure-volume curve. The saline-filled lung displays very little hysteresis.

An amazing feature of the lung's surface is the presence of special phospholipid molecules. These molecules allow the surface tension to vary in a cyclic manner as alveolar surface area changes during breathing. In the usual range of breathing, the variation in surface tension is small because alveolar surface area does not change much; surface tension cycles around its equilibrium value of 28 mN/cm at 37° C. With a large breath, however, as the surface expands, the surface tension rises to 50 mN/cm (about the same value as for plasma or interstitial liquid). This rising tension opposes expansion of the lung; increased transpulmonary pressure is required during inspiration. However, the expansion has the beneficial effect of allowing more molecules of the surface tension–lowering material to enter the air-liquid interface.

As the lung begins to deflate, the alveolar surface active molecules are squeezed together. Their physical structure causes them to resist compression. This resistance acts to lower surface tension to less than 10 mN/cm. Consequently, transpulmonary pressure decreases substantially before lung volume changes much, as the deflation limb of the air pressure-volume curve in Fig. 33-4 illustrates. The decreasing surface tension during deflation also stabilizes the smallest alveoli, so that they do not shrink faster than the largest alveoli as the lung deflates.

In Fig. 33-4, the pressure difference between the air and liquid deflation curves at 50% TLC is 2 cm H_2O, whereas the pressure difference between air and liquid inflation curves is about 8 cm H_2O (1 cm H_2O = 980 mN/cm). If the average radius of the anatomic alveoli in the human lung is 120 μm (120 × 10^{-4} cm) at 50% TLC, then the surface tension on deflation must be: P = 2 × T/r; 1960 = 2T/(120 × 10^{-4}); T = 12 mN/cm. On inflation, T = 47 mN/cm at the same volume.

Many substances, called **surfactants** (wetting agents or detergents), lower the surface tension of water. Even the proteins in plasma reduce the air-liquid surface tension from 70 mN/cm (pure water) to 50 mN/cm.

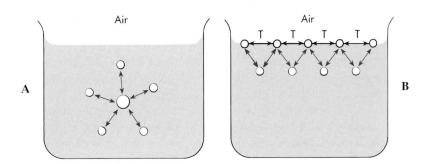

■ **Fig. 33-5** Intermolecular forces generate surface tension. **A,** Force is relatively uniform on molecules in the interior. **B,** At the surface the molecules are pulled toward the interior and generate a compressive tension (**T**) in the plane of the surface.

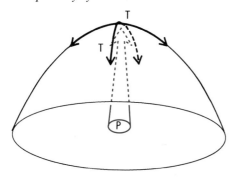

■ Fig. 33-6   As translung pressure *(P)* inflates an alveolus, it is opposed by air-liquid surface tension, which can be summarized by considering the tension *(T)* along a circumferential curvature on the surface of the alveolus. The pressure is also opposed by the tensile strength of the alveolar wall structures. However, their tensile strength is low until the lung is inflated to near TLC.

The alveolar surfactant molecules are less attracted by the water molecules in the bulk phase, because the lipid portion of the molecule is hydrophobic. When the surface area of the alveoli changes, the surfactant molecules at the air-liquid interface are compacted (during deflation) or spread apart (during inflation). It is this effect that causes the alveolar surface tension to vary with lung volume.

The physiological advantages of lung surfactant are that: (1) it reduces the muscular effort needed to expand the lungs (the work of breathing); (2) it lowers the elastic recoil at low lung volume (FRC), and thus helps to prevent the alveoli from collapsing at the end of each expiration; and (3) it stabilizes alveoli that tend to deflate at different rates. The alveoli that deflate more rapidly generate a lower surface tension. This slows the rate of volume decrease and allows a more slowly deflating unit with a higher surface tension to catch up.

In **respiratory distress syndrome,** which is a leading cause of morbidity and mortality in babies with immature lungs, the key defect is failure of the type 2 alveolar epithelial cells to secrete adequate quantities of surfactant. The lungs are somewhat more difficult to inflate, but the main problem is that during deflation the alveoli readily collapse, because surface tension does not fall. Thus, the *deflation* limb of the pressure-volume curve is similar to the *inflation* curve. Therefore, each lung inflation is like the first breath of air after birth, when the liquid-filled lungs have to be inflated with air. The increased work required to inflate the lungs fatigues the diaphragm (see p 545).

Origin, composition, turnover, and regulation of the surface-active material. Lung surfactant consists of a complex phospholipid-protein material, which is produced and secreted onto the alveolar surface by the type 2 alveolar epithelial cells. The main surface tension–low-ering substance in lung surfactant is **dipalmitoyl phosphatidylcholine (DPPC),** which contains two 16-carbon, saturated, fatty acid chains. The lipid chains are nonpolar (hydrophobic), but the phosphatidylcholine is polar (hydrophilic). Therefore, the molecules orient themselves at the air-liquid interface with the fatty acid residues arranged vertically, and they project out from the bulk phase. This arrangement is mechanically stable. Thus, the surface film resists compression during lung deflation, and this leads to lower surface tension.

Beginning in late fetal development (third trimester), the production of surface-active material is "turned on" as the lung matures and becomes ready for air breathing. Immediately after birth, babies have to fill their liquid-filled lungs with air. The first cry of the newborn signifies that its lungs have been successfully inflated. Although surfactant does not make the initial air inflation easier, it does keep the alveoli inflated during successive expirations, which markedly reduces the work of breathing.

As people breathe, some surfactant molecules leave the surface film and some new ones enter it. The stability of the alveolar air-liquid interfacial film depends on the sustained metabolism of the type 2 alveolar epithelial cells, which not only produce and secrete surfactant but also recycle it.

■ *Chest Wall Distensibility*

The functional chest wall includes the rib cage, diaphragm, and abdomen. The importance of the abdomen in breathing may not be immediately obvious. The chest wall components must work together, under central nervous control, to implement the cyclic process of breathing. Diseases that affect the chest wall can be serious and may be the immediate cause of death. For example, multiple broken ribs can cause a collapsible rib cage; inspiratory neuron degeneration may lead to chest wall muscle paralysis in poliomyelitis; and liquid accumulation in the abdomen **(ascites)** can interfere with motion of the diaphragm.

■ *Elastic Recoil of the Chest Wall*

Consider the condition of the chest wall relative to that of the lungs at end-expiration (FRC). In this relaxed position of the lungs it is the chest wall that opposes lung collapse. In Fig. 33-2, the translung static recoil pressure when the lungs are at FRC is 3.5 cm H_2O. At that point, alveolar pressure, P_A, is zero (equal to atmospheric pressure). Thus, pleural pressure, P_{pl}, must be -3.5 cm H_2O. Therefore, the static recoil pressure across the chest wall, P_w, must be equal to pleural pressure, P_{pl}, minus body surface pressure, P_{bs} (normally atmospheric pressure).

Recall that transorgan pressure is always read from inside to outside the organ. Thus, $Pw = Ppl - Pbs$. Therefore, at FRC, the trans–chest wall pressure is: $Pw = -3.5 - 0 = -3.5$ cm H_2O. The transorgan pressure is subatmospheric (negative), which indicates that the chest wall is being compressed; that is, it is being squeezed below its relaxed or unstressed configuration.

At FRC, the lungs are above their unstressed volume and the chest wall is below its unstressed volume. *It is these equal but opposite elastic recoil forces that determine the configuration of the respiratory system (lungs + chest wall) at end-expiration.* If air is injected between the parietal and visceral pleurae (creating a pneumothorax) to break the liquid seal that couples the lungs to the chest wall, the lungs will get smaller and the thoracic cavity will get larger.

When the chest wall is opened during thoracic surgery, air enters the pleural space because the pleural pressure is less than atmospheric pressure; this condition is called a **pneumothorax.** The lungs tend to collapse as they approach their minimal volume, whereas the chest cavity gets larger as the chest wall springs outward toward its relaxed position. A traumatic or spontaneous pneumothorax may be life threatening. If the lungs become completely uncoupled from the chest wall pump, they will not move when the diaphragm contracts. This condition occurs when the air leak is large and continuous.

In Fig. 33-7, the passive pressure-volume curve of the chest wall is added to that of the lung. If the pressure-volume curve of the chest wall is compared with that of the lungs, the former is always to the left of the latter. When the lung volume is below FRC, the chest wall becomes progressively stiffer, until at residual volume, Pw may be -20 cm H_2O or lower. When the lung volume is above FRC, the pressure-volume curve of the chest wall is steep (high compliance) and nearly linear. When the lung volume is at TLC, trans–chest wall pressure is about $+7$ cm H_2O.

When the lung volume is near TLC, the stiffness of the lung limits thoracic expansion. This phenomenon explains why the TLC of a person with degenerative lung disease **(emphysema)** may be above normal, as shown in Fig. 33-3. As a person expires to residual volume, the stiff chest wall becomes the factor that limits collapse of the lungs to minimal volume.

Although the chest wall is normally under compression, the compliance of the chest wall, Cw, is a positive number, because the slope of the pressure-volume curve is positive. *Over the range of normal breathing, the chest wall and lung compliances are similar,* as can be seen in Fig. 33-7 and Table 32-1.

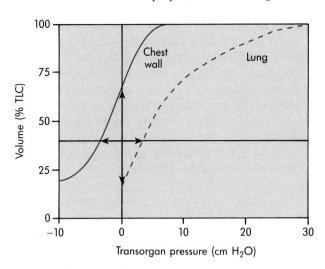

■ **Fig. 33-7** The pressure-volume curve of the chest wall. The trans–chest wall pressure difference is pleural pressure minus body surface pressure. At FRC, the chest wall and lung are recoiling equally but in opposite directions *(horizontal arrows).* At zero transorgan pressure, the chest is expanded, while the lung collapses to minimal volume *(vertical arrows).*

■ *Transdiaphragmatic Pressure*

One of the least intuitive aspects of chest wall mechanics is that the diaphragm and abdomen are important components of the chest wall. When the lungs are at FRC, and trans–chest wall pressure is equal everywhere, the pressure across the diaphragm, Pdi, must also equal Pw. In supine humans with the diaphragm and abdominal muscles relaxed, the abdominal pressure is equal to atmospheric pressure (Fig. 33-8, *A*). The unbalanced pressure difference pushes the diaphragm cephalad into the thoracic cavity until the passive stretch develops sufficient force to oppose the inwardly acting (compressive) pressure difference.

FRC is smaller and pleural pressure is less subatmospheric when a person lies in the dorsally recumbent (supine) position. In intensive care units, this position can cause serious problems in patients with lungs that tend to collapse because of increased alveolar surface tension. These patients often require mechanical ventilation. Sometimes, high pressures are required to inflate the lungs adequately for gas exchange. The high inflation pressure imposes the attendant danger of **barotrauma** (rupture of the lung caused by the high pressure). If the patient is turned to the prone (face-down) position, abdominal pressure on the diaphragm is reduced and it becomes easier to ventilate the lungs.

When a person is standing, abdominal pressure decreases because the weight of the abdominal contents pushes down and out against the anterior abdominal wall

(Fig. 33-8, *B*). At end-expiration, the pressure beneath the diaphragm equals the pleural pressure; that is, transdiaphragm pressure is zero, and thus there is no tension on the diaphragm. The diaphragm moves caudally into the abdominal cavity until the anterior abdominal wall is sufficiently stretched to oppose the elevated abdominal pressure. The transfer of Pw from across the diaphragm when the subject is supine to across the anterior abdominal wall when the subject is standing explains why FRC increases when one assumes the upright position.

In the third trimester of pregnancy, especially with multiple fetuses, the enlarged uterus pushes upward and outward. The high abdominal wall tension raises the intra-abdominal pressure, even when the woman is upright. The diaphragm does not descend appreciably, and therefore the FRC remains reduced.

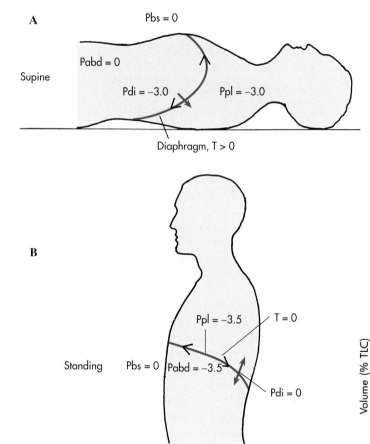

■ **Fig. 33-8** The role of the diaphragm and abdominal wall as part of the functional chest wall. **A,** In the supine position, the weight of abdominal contents pushes against the diaphragm until appropriate passive tension develops. **B,** In the upright position, the liver and other abdominal contents tend to fall, and the abdominal wall protrudes until adequate tension is created in it. The transdiaphragmatic pressure is zero; there is no passive tension in the diaphragm. *Pbs,* Pressure at body surface; *Ppl,* pleural pressure; *Pabd,* intraabdominal pressure; *Pdi,* transdiaphragmatic pressure.

■ *Elastic Recoil of the Total Respiratory System*

Normally, the lungs and chest wall move together because the lungs are coupled to the chest wall by the cohesion of a thin pleural layer of interstitial liquid. The total pressure across the respiratory system (Prs) is the sum of translung (PL) and trans–chest wall (Pw) pressures:

$$Prs = P_L + Pw = P_L - Pbs \qquad (33\text{-}4)$$

When the lungs are at FRC, Prs = 0 because PA = Pbs. All muscles of breathing, including the abdominal muscles, are relaxed, and the alveolar pressure (PA) is equal to the pressure at the body surface (Pbs). Regardless of volume, the passive pressure across the respiratory system must be the sum of the trans–chest wall pressure and the translung pressure. Fig. 33-9 shows the pressure-volume curves for the respiratory system, lung, and chest wall. For any transorgan pressure, the slope of the pressure-volume curve for the respiratory system is less positive than that for either the lung or the chest wall. Hence, the compliance of the respiratory system (Crs) must be less than that of either the lung or the chest wall.

Calculation of compliance for the respiratory system is complicated by the fact that compliances in series must be added as reciprocals: 1/Crs = 1/CL + 1/Cw. Thus, it is preferable to use elastance for these relationships, because elastance is the reciprocal of compliance. The elastance of the respiratory system (Ers) is readily calculated by adding the elastances of the lung (EL) and chest wall (Ew):

$$Ers = E_L + Ew \qquad (33\text{-}5)$$

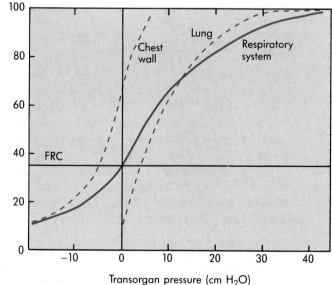

■ **Fig. 33-9** Pressure-volume curve of the entire respiratory system during passive deflation. At FRC, there is no pressure difference between the alveoli and the body surface *(junction of black lines and heavy colored line).*

When the lungs are at FRC in a standing subject, if Ppl = −3.5 cm H_2O and if EL = Ew, then Ers = 7.0 cm H_2O/L. Similarly, compliance, Crs, = 1/Ers = 0.17 L/cm H_2O, which is half of either lung or chest wall compliance.

In disease, the distensibility of the various components of the respiratory system, individually or together, may change profoundly. For example, in pulmonary fibrosis, the lungs may become stiff because of increased deposition of collagen. In emphysema, the lungs may become flaccid because of destruction of their elastic fibers (Fig. 33-3). The chest wall may be distorted by congenital malformations or by disorders that produce stiffening (**kyphoscoliosis, extreme obesity**).

■ *Dynamics*

The normal resting breathing rate of 12/min allows only 2 seconds for inspiration and 3 seconds for expiration: scarcely a static condition. Indeed, breathing adds a set of dynamic mechanical properties that affect the pressures within the lung-thorax system.

Dynamic lung compliance. A dynamic pressure-volume loop can be derived when a subject breathes over the normal range of lung volumes from FRC to FRC + VT, as shown in Fig. 33-10. The figure also includes the static curve from Fig. 33-1 as reference. The tidal loop is located approximately in the center of the static pressure-volume loop.

The mean dynamic compliance of the lung (dynCL) during breathing can be calculated as the slope of the line that joins the end-inspiratory and end-expiratory points of no flow. Thus,

$$\text{dynCL} = \Delta V_L / \Delta P_L = 0.5/2.5 = 0.2 \text{ L/cm } H_2O \quad (33\text{-}6)$$

The dynamic compliance can never exceed the static compliance; that is, it must always be somewhere within the dashed loop in Fig. 33-10.

The dynamic compliance is 0.2 L/cm H_2O in subjects at rest, but it is 0.3 L/cm H_2O in subjects during exercise. The dynamic compliance is greater during exercise, because the tidal volume is larger (up to half of vital capacity). Because the tidal volume is larger, the surface area changes more, and more surfactant material is incorporated into the air-liquid interface.

Dynamic compliance is less than static compliance, because the minimal change in alveolar surface area associated with tidal breathing is inadequate to bring new surfactant molecules into the air-liquid interface. The elastance of the lung increases with time as surface tension rises. The slowly decreasing FRC is detected by lung deflation receptors, which drive the central (brain) breathing controller to occasionally increase tidal volume. Sighing is a single large breath that occurs every few minutes. It restores the normal surfactant layer and the FRC. Yawning accomplishes the same beneficial result.

■ *Dynamic Chest Wall Compliance*

The dynamic compliance of the chest wall is not different from its static compliance. However, the trans–chest wall pressure at FRC during tidal breathing is −5 cm H_2O, because it must balance the translung pressure. To appreciate the slowly changing lung dynamics, imagine inspiring to TLC, slowly expiring to FRC, and then breathing quietly. Immediately after the large breath, dynCL is high, but over the next several minutes, the lungs become stiffer. FRC decreases with each breath as pleural pressure becomes more subatmospheric. This process continues until the trans–chest wall pressure, Pw, equals −5 cm H_2O, which is sufficient to balance the rising translung pressure. *Note that when the lung volume is at FRC, the lungs and chest wall are recoiling equally but in opposite directions. The pressure across the respiratory system (Prs) must equal zero at the beginning or end of an inspiration.*

■ *Resistance to Airflow*

The loop of the tidal breathing pressure-volume curve indicates that some of the work (P × ΔV) of breathing done by the contracting chest wall muscles during inspiration is not recovered during expiration, chiefly because of frictional losses (resistance) during airflow.

During breathing, the total pressure difference across the lung is the sum of the pressure required to overcome

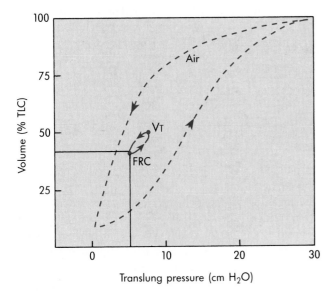

■ **Fig. 33-10** Dynamic pressure-volume loop during tidal breathing. All possible air pressure-volume curves lie within the boundaries of the larger pressure-volume curve.

elastic recoil (PA − Ppl) and the pressure caused by airflow resistance (Pao − PA):

$$P_L = (P_A - P_{pl}) + (P_{ao} - P_A) = P_{ao} - P_{pl} \qquad (33\text{-}7)$$

where Pao represents pressure at the airway opening (nose or mouth). At end-inspiration and end-expiration, when airflow stops momentarily, Pao = PL. Dynamic compliance can be calculated at the points of no airflow, if one assumes that the alveolar pressure equilibrates rapidly with ambient pressure at the airway opening. During airflow, however, Pao ≠ PA. The difference may be positive (inspiration) or negative (expiration).

Physical factors that determine resistance to air flow in rigid tubes. Resistance in the airways (Raw) is calculated as driving pressure divided by flow ($\dot{V}$):

$$R_{aw} = \frac{P_{ao} - P_A}{\dot{V}} \qquad (33\text{-}8)$$

The factors that affect laminar airflow resistance are described by Poiseuille's equation (see also Chapter 25):

$$P_{aw} = \frac{8}{\pi} \times \eta \times \frac{1}{r^4} \qquad (33\text{-}9)$$

which consists of a constant ($8/\pi$), viscosity (η), and geometry ($1/r^4$). *Resistance is inversely proportional to the fourth power of the airway radius, r, which is the main factor that affects airway resistance.* Small changes may greatly affect airway resistance. For example, if mean airway diameter decreases by half, resistance increases sixteenfold.

Airflow resistance is also affected by the fact that, even in quiet breathing, flow is turbulent in the upper airways (nose, mouth, glottis, bronchi), which is why breath sounds within the chest can be heard through a stethoscope. Laminar flow is silent. Because of turbulence, an additional term must be added to the driving pressure:

$$P = 2.4 \times \dot{V} + 0.03 \times \dot{V}^2 \qquad (33\text{-}10)$$

where the first term describes the pressure drop caused by laminar flow and the second term (airflow velocity squared) describes the pressure drop caused by turbulence. Turbulence has little effect until V^2 becomes large, as in exercise.

Airflow resistance is sometimes divided between the upper airways (>2 mm diameter; bronchi) and the lower airways (<2 mm diameter; bronchioles):

$$R_{aw} = R_{large} + R_{small} \qquad (33\text{-}11)$$

Normally, most of the total airway resistance is in the large airways. Small airway resistance is low because airflow velocity is very low as the effective cross-sectional area of the many bronchioles in parallel increases. This condition stands in marked contrast to the pulmonary blood vessels, in which most of the resistance is in the smaller vessels. Resistances of tubes in parallel are added reciprocally (see also Chapter 25).

In disease, the longitudinal distribution of airway resistance may vary markedly. In infants, a life-threatening viral disease known as **bronchiolitis** (inflamed bronchioles) causes edema (swelling) of the mucosa that lines the bronchioles. The edema may drastically reduce the radii of the bronchioles. A reduction by half increases their contribution to resistance sixteenfold because of the fourth power factor (equation 33-8).

Measurement of airway resistance. To measure total airway resistance, alveolar pressure, PA, and airflow velocity, V, must be measured. An easy way to measure airflow velocity is with a device known as a pneumotachograph. This instrument detects the very small pressure decrease caused by flow across a low fixed resistance. A more difficult problem is measuring the alveolar pressure. As our brief discussion of dynamic compliance has shown, alveolar pressure is not the same as ambient pressure during airflow. Thus, PA can be measured by briefly occluding the airway opening during breathing. At the instant after airflow stops, Pao = PA.

During normal tidal breathing, airflow reaches a peak velocity of about +0.5 L/sec during inspiration and about −0.5 L/sec during expiration; the minus sign signifies flow out of the lung. Alveolar pressure decreases below the pressure at the airway opening by 0.8 cm H$_2$O at peak airflow during inspiration, and it exceeds the pressure at the airway opening by 1.2 cm H$_2$O during expiration. The difference between these measurements is explained by the fact that the airways are narrower during expiration, and therefore resistance is increased. Thus, at peak velocity during inspiration Raw = $\Delta P/\dot{V}$ = (Pao − PA)/$\dot{V}$ = 1.6 cm H$_2$O × sec/L. Likewise, during expiration Raw = 2.4 cm H$_2$O × sec/L.

The normal range for airway resistance in adult humans is 1.5 to 2.0 cm H$_2$O × sec/L (Table 32-2). Because the signs of the airflow and the alveolar pressure differences are always the same, resistance is always a positive number.

Total translung pressure during breathing. The total pressure difference from ambient to pleural space during airflow is the pressure difference caused by lung distensibility (dynamic compliance) plus the pressure difference caused by airflow resistance. The sum of these pressures equals PL (see equation 33-7).

Physical factors that influence airway resistance. In rigid cylindrical tubes, resistance during laminar flow is fixed, because the physical dimensions of the tube never change, regardless of the transmural pressure across the tube walls. However, if the tube is distensible and collapsible (similar to conditions that prevail in the lung), the transmural pressure may have important nonlinear effects. Fig. 33-11 is a model of flow in a nonrigid tube. In *A*, the pressure in the tube always exceeds the external pressure. Therefore, the transmural pressure is positive. The tube expands and flow resistance decreases. In *B*, the external pressure is raised above the outflow or down-

A

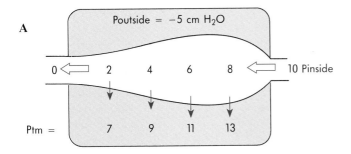

B

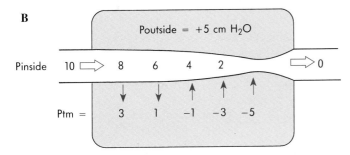

■ **Fig. 33-11** Flow in a distensible and collapsible tube is affected by the lateral transmural distending pressure as well as the longitudinal driving pressure. **A,** An analogy to lung inflation, where the pressure outside the airways is subatmospheric, which distends the tubes as air flows into the lungs. **B,** An analogy to lung deflation, where the pressure outside the airways may become positive and compresses them near the outlet. This leads to dynamic airway compression and limits airflow. *Pinside* and *Poutside*, Pressures inside and outside a collapsible tube; *Ptm,* transmural pressure (Pinside − Poutside).

stream pressure. Thus, as flow resistance dissipates the driving pressure, the pressure inside the tube falls. When it falls below the external pressure, the tube begins to narrow. As transmural pressure becomes more negative, the tube is compressed more and more until a new stable condition is reached in which the collapsed zone (always at the outflow end of the tube) limits the flow rate.

Regulation of airflow in this manner is called **dynamic airway compression.** Under such conditions, airflow is independent of the total driving pressure. During expiration, pleural pressure rises and increases alveolar pressure above the pressure at the airway opening. The cartilaginous airways narrow during expiration, which explains why airway resistance is higher during expiration. The bronchioles, however, are much less sensitive to the phases of breathing because they depend on lung volume, which in normal tidal breathing does not change much (<20%).

When a healthy person takes a very large inspiration from FRC to TLC, and then breathes out as hard and fast as possible (**forced vital capacity,** Fig. 33-12), pleural pressure rises to a high level and generates a large driving pressure. When pleural pressure rises above the pressure at the airway opening, as shown in Fig. 33-12, the large airways are compressed near the thoracic outlet (main-

stem bronchi or trachea). As the airways are compressed, flow velocity is increased, which reduces the lateral pressure, according to the **Bernoulli principle** (see Chapter 25) and leads to further compression. This process limits expiratory airflow. The dynamic compression quickly becomes stable; no matter how great the respiratory effort, the expiratory flow cannot be increased. The reason for this cut-off point is that any further rise in pleural pressure causes more airway compression, which prevents any increase in flow. A maximal expiratory flow rate is generated that is *independent of effort* (Fig. 33-12).

Coughing is an example of dynamic airway compression. In the degenerative lung disease emphysema, cartilaginous airway support is lost. As the transpulmonary pressure at any lung volume is reduced, pleural pressure at the end of a normal inspiration is less negative than it is in a normal individual. In addition, the airways are often weakened by degeneration of their cartilage and elastic fibers. During expiration, to generate sufficient airflow in a reasonable period to provide adequate minute alveolar ventilation, the individual unconsciously tries to increase expiratory airflow by increasing pleural pressure. However, the elevated pleural pressure needed to increase flow further compresses the large airways, and thus increases expiratory resistance further. See the pressure-volume curve of emphysema in Fig. 33-3.

Emphysema belongs to a large group of serious pulmonary diseases called **chronic obstructive pulmonary disease (COPD).** Emphysematous patients learn to inspire quickly and breathe out slowly to avoid airway collapse. As COPD becomes more severe, the patient generates less and less maximal expiratory flow. When ventilation falls, alveolar CO_2 tension rises, according to the alveolar gas equation.

A person with hyperirritable airway disease **(asthma)** has a different problem. The airways are narrowed by smooth muscle contraction, mucosal edema, or excessive secretions. Thus, both inspiratory *and* expiratory flow resistances are increased. However, patients with asthma usually have a normal lung elastance. They breathe at an increased FRC (see the pressure-volume curve for asthma in Fig. 33-3), which acts to distend the airways during inspiration and limits compression during expiration.

Flow-volume relationship. A flow-volume curve can be generated by plotting airflow velocity as a function of lung volume throughout a respiratory cycle. Fig. 33-13 shows two stylized flow-volume curves. The small loop is the flow-volume curve of a normal tidal breath. The large loop is a maximal flow-volume curve. Inspiratory flow is limited only by effort, but the expiratory flow curve is the maximal flow that can be achieved no matter how much effort is expended. The maximal flow-volume curve makes it possible to assess dynamic airway compression.

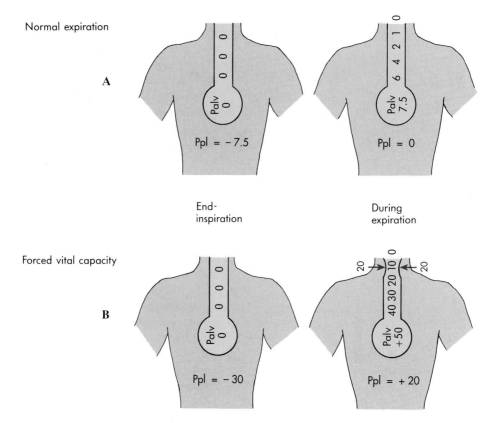

■ **Fig. 33-12**   **A** and **B**, Generation of dynamic airway compression during a forced vital capacity maneuver. *Palv*, Alveolar pressure.

During inspiration, normal humans cannot produce a flow velocity as high as during expiration. The reason for this inability is that inspiratory effort decreases as the thorax enlarges. The strongest inspiratory effort occurs before the diaphragm and the chest wall muscles have expanded the thoracic cavity. Although the force available decreases, inspiratory flow tends to remain constant until lung volume nears total lung capacity, at which point flow falls rapidly to zero.

During expiration, the flow-volume curve is different. Contracting the powerful anterior abdominal muscles and the intercostal muscles generates a high pleural pressure and high flow velocity when thoracic volume is near TLC. Velocity decreases rapidly (approximately linearly) as volume decreases, but not because of decreasing muscular effort. Once the linear portion of the expiratory flow-volume curve is reached, it is effort independent. No matter how hard the subject tries, he or she cannot exceed the maximal flow at the given volume. Dynamic compression of the airways limits expiratory flow, and this limitation increases as lung volume decreases.

Neurohumoral regulation of airway resistance. The vagus nerves innervate the smooth muscle of all the cartilaginous airways and probably of the membranous bronchioles and alveolar ducts also. Stimulation of the efferent vagal fibers, either via a reflex or directly, leads to airway constriction, a decrease in anatomic dead space volume (V_D), and an increase in airway resistance (Raw).

Stimulation of the sympathetic nerves has the opposite effect. In humans, sympathetic nerves to the lungs innervate vascular smooth muscle, submucosal glands, and parasympathetic ganglia, but probably not airway smooth muscle. However, the airway smooth muscle has adrenergic receptors, so that local diffusion of the sympathetic postganglionic neurotransmitter norepinephrine inhibits airway constriction.

A number of agents act through a reflex via the vagus nerves to constrict the airways or to induce cough. Inhalation of smoke, dust, cold air, and irritant substances has this effect. For example, exercise-induced asthma is common among people with hyperirritable airways.

Some substances affect airway smooth muscle directly. Agents that constrict airways in this manner include histamine, acetylcholine, adrenergic-receptor antagonists, thromboxane A_2, prostaglandin F_2, and leukotrienes C_4 and D_4. Histamine-like compounds, such as methylcholine, are sometimes used as provocative agents in tests in patients who may have hypersensitive airways (asthma).

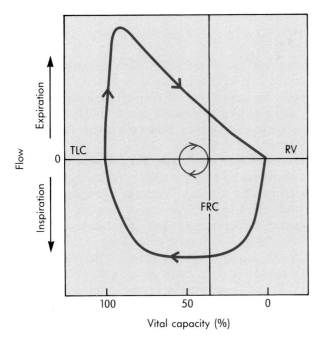

■ **Fig. 33-13** Normal flow-volume loops for tidal breathing *(small)* and forced vital capacity. Expiration exhibits dynamic compression, which becomes more flow limiting as lung volume decreases.

Agents that tend to dilate airways include increased PA_{CO_2} (hypoventilation or inspired CO_2), adrenergic α- and β-receptor agonists, atropine (which blocks postganglionic parasympathetic impulses), and prostaglandin E_2.

In the normal lung, airway smooth muscle tone is continuously modulated, presumably to provide a balance between airway resistance (Raw) and anatomic dead space (VD), and thereby to diminish the work of breathing.

■ *The Work of Breathing*

The work (W) involved in taking a single breath is defined as $W = P \times \Delta V$. Work is measured in joules (1 joule = 1 L $\times$ 10 cm H_2O), and the rate of doing work (power) is measured in watts (1 watt = 1 joule/sec). Clearly, if a person increases tidal volume, he or she does more work to inflate the lung; if a person increases minute ventilation (increased volume flow/time), he or she increases power utilization.

The work of breathing is commonly divided into two kinds of work: the work of moving the lungs and the work of moving the chest wall. Many diseases affect the work of breathing.

In **respiratory distress syndrome** of the newborn, the deflation limb of the air pressure-volume curve is displaced to the right (closer to the inflation limb), and

thus the alveoli tend to collapse at end-expiration. Therefore, higher pressures are necessary to reinflate the lungs at each breath. The enormous increase in the work of breathing required under these conditions is the principal cause of respiratory failure and death, if the baby is untreated. The use of positive-pressure ventilation for the affected babies markedly reduces mortality. Inhalation of artificially produced surfactant is also beneficial.

■ *Assessing the Work of Breathing*

The work of moving the chest wall cannot be assessed during active breathing, because there is no simple way to measure the mechanical work done by the muscles of breathing alone. However, if a person is paralyzed either by disease or through a neuromuscular blocking drug, ventilation can be maintained by a mechanical device. Under these conditions, the lungs and thorax are moved passively by the ventilator, and therefore the total work of breathing can be determined. From such measurements, the total work of a single breath at normal tidal volume is about 0.25 joule, of which half is expended in moving the lung and half is stored in the expanded lung's elastic recoil. The power requirement of normal breathing is 50 milliwatts (0.25 joule/breath $\times$ 1 breath/5 sec = 0.05 watts). These quantities of work are very small; for example, an ordinary nightlight uses 7.5 watts. Thus, normal breathing does not require much work.

In Fig. 33-14, *A,* the work done to inflate the lung is represented by the shaded area bounded by FRC (point *E*) and FRC + VT (point *I*) and the pressure axis. During expiration (Fig. 33-14, *B*), work is done by the potential energy stored in the stretched lung to restore FRC. The difference between inspiratory and expiratory work represents the energy (heat) generated to overcome frictional (resistive) losses. Normally, more potential energy is available to do work in expiration (because of the change in surface tension) than is necessary to overcome airway resistance. In the steady state, no energy can be left over, so the extra energy is used to compress the chest wall back to its resting configuration. Some of the excess energy is used to impart velocity to the air leaving the airway opening.

During exercise, the work of each breath increases proportionally more than does tidal volume, because airflow velocity is greater during exercise, and this increased airflow velocity increases turbulence. A tenfold increase in airflow rate increases the turbulence factor by 100.

During the maximal voluntary ventilation test, an average person may move 160 L/min. Reasonable values are 4 L/breath $\times$ 40 breaths/min. The resistive driving pressure across the respiratory system may reach 20 cm H_2O. The power requirement is 5 watts (100 times normal), even though ventilation is increased only thirtyfold.

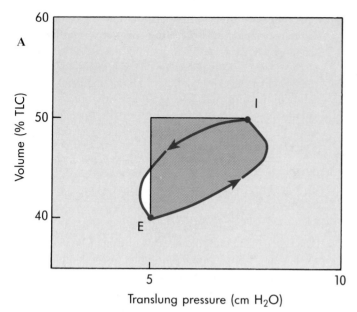

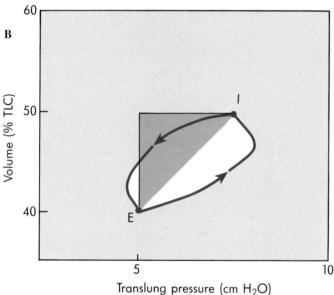

■ **Fig. 33-14**   Work done on the lung during a normal inspiration (**A**) includes frictional losses not recoverable during expiration (**B**).

■ *Oxygen Cost and Efficiency of Breathing*

During tidal breathing in a resting subject, the oxygen cost of quiet breathing ($\dot{V}O_2$ of the respiratory muscles) cannot be measured reliably. The increase in oxygen consumption associated with forced ventilation, however, can be measured; it amounts to an O_2 cost of breathing of 1% to 2% (3 to 5 ml O_2/min) of the resting oxygen consumption of the whole body (250 ml/min). The mechanical efficiency of breathing is defined as the work required to inflate the lungs divided by the energy consumed by the muscles of breathing:

$$\text{Efficiency} = \frac{P \times \Delta V}{O_2 \text{ cost of breathing}} \qquad (33\text{-}12)$$

The efficiency of the breathing apparatus is less than 10%, whereas that of skeletal muscle in general is about 20%.

In patients with pulmonary diseases that reduce lung compliance or increase airway resistance, the work of breathing may be markedly increased. Ordinarily, a large safety factor prevails for the muscles of breathing: they are adequately supplied with oxygen and metabolic substrates to do their work indefinitely (aerobic metabolism). However, muscle fatigue occurs when the elastic or resistive load is too great for the available blood supply. Under such conditions, **respiratory fatigue** occurs. In respiratory fatigue, the muscles of breathing cannot generate enough pressure to ventilate the lungs adequately to supply the body's oxygen requirements and to dispose of the CO_2 formed. Thus, PA_{CO_2} rises. Respiratory muscle fatigue can be corrected by reducing the workload (e.g., by dilating the airways in a patient with asthma) or by mechanically assisting ventilation (e.g., in a patient with emphysema complicated by bronchitis).

Although the normal oxygen cost of breathing is less than 2% of resting oxygen consumption, up to 30% of total oxygen consumption may be used to move the lungs and chest wall during voluntary hyperventilation. Obviously, in patients who are already using more O_2 than normal to move air at rest, the oxygen cost of breathing may limit their exercise capability.

Sufficient potential energy is stored in the lungs and thorax during inspiration to restore the breathing apparatus to its FRC position. If the work of inspiration is increased because of increased resistance to airflow, as in asthma, the potential energy stored in the lungs and chest wall is not increased, because the extra work is dissipated as frictional heat loss during inspiration. Because expiratory resistance is also increased, sufficient elastic potential energy may not be available to move air fast enough for the lungs to reach their original FRC position within the time available during expiration. If expiratory airflow is not completed at the beginning of the next inspiration, alveolar pressure will be greater than the pressure at the airway opening at the end of expiration. This condition is referred to as "intrinsic PEEP," a form of **positive end-expiratory pressure** not caused by an external device. Consequently, FRC will increase until sufficient elastic energy is stored by the lungs to achieve a new steady state. The need to store elastic energy explains why patients have hyperinflated lungs during attacks of asthma (Fig. 33-3).

One of the difficulties associated with an increased work of breathing in pulmonary disease is that, as breathing becomes more labored, the low efficiency of the breathing apparatus greatly increases the oxygen cost of breathing. If all the increase in oxygen consumption is required just to meet the demands of the breathing apparatus, additional oxygen is not available for other metabolic requirements. The lack of oxygen for metabolism can severely limit patients with advanced lung disease, such as elderly people with pronounced emphysema or infants with marked airway narrowing (severe asthma).

Whether a control mechanism exists to sense the work of breathing is not clear. In disease, the tendency is to breathe rapidly and shallowly when lung compliance is increased, and to breathe slowly and deeply when airflow resistance is increased. These two factors, resistance and compliance (R and C), affect breathing in opposite ways. Their product, R × C (the time constant tau, τ) is another important variable.

■ *Summary*

1. The normal lungs are compliant at low volume, but they become much less compliant when lung volume is near total lung capacity. Lung compliance is determined from the slope of the pressure-volume curve during deflation.

2. Lung distensibility during inflation is low compared with its distensibility during deflation. The main reason is the variable air-liquid surface tension in the alveoli, which have a very small radius. The reason for the variable surface tension is surfactant, a special surface active material (secreted by type 2 alveolar epithelial cells) whose main component is dipalmitoyl phosphatidylcholine.

3. At end-expiration, the lungs recoil toward a smaller volume, but the chest wall recoils in the opposite direction, toward a larger volume. Thus, the chest wall is normally under compression in the range of tidal breathing.

4. The pressure difference across the diaphragm–abdominal wall is the same as across the rib cage.

5. Because the lungs and chest wall move together, the total compliance of the respiratory system is less than that of either part alone.

6. The dynamic compliance of the lung is less than its static compliance, which is due mainly to a rise in air-liquid surface tension toward its equilibrium value during tidal breathing. An occasional large sighing breath restores the surfactant and increases compliance. Chest wall dynamic compliance is the same as its static compliance.

7. Because of resistance to flow in the airways, alveolar pressure equals ambient pressure only when air does not flow. During breathing, the pressure difference across the lung is the sum of the elastic and resistive components. Breath sounds are caused by turbulence in the upper airways.

8. An important physical factor that affects airway resistance is the transmural pressure across the bronchi, whose walls are distensible and collapsible. During a forced expiratory maneuver, pleural pressure may rise above large airway pressure, dynamically compressing the airways and limiting peak expiratory flow velocity.

9. The vagus nerves regulate airway resistance via a reflex. Many substances can cause constriction and increased airflow resistance (histamine, thromboxane, leukotrienes), whereas high CO_2, catecholamines, and atropine lead to dilation.

10. The work of breathing is small in a normal, resting subject. In pulmonary disease, work may be increased to such an extent that respiratory failure occurs.

■ *Self-Study Problems*

1. At an ocean depth of 100 m (328 ft), the pressure at the airway opening necessary to maintain normal FRC of a skin diver is roughly 10 atmospheres. Suppose the pressure at the airway opening suddenly dropped to zero. What would happen immediately in the lungs and chest wall?

2. If Ppl = + 5 cm H_2O when the lung volume is at normal FRC, what are two likely explanations? Consider both static and dynamic events.

3. A normal adult woman's peak inspiratory airflow is 5.0 L/sec when she is running. How would you estimate the driving pressure for air flow?

4. Compare the possible consequences of breathing too rapidly with the possible consequences of breathing too slowly.

■ *Bibliography*

Journal articles

Clements JA: Surface phenomena in relation to pulmonary function, *Physiologist* 5:11, 1962.

Cookson WOCM, Moffatt MF: Asthma: an epidemic in the absence of infection?, *Science* 275:41, 1997.

Derenne JPH, Macklem PT, Roussos CS: The respiratory muscles: mechanics, control and pathophysiology, Parts I, II, III, *Am Rev Respir Dis* 48:119, 373, 581, 1978.

Fry DL, Hyatt RE: Pulmonary mechanics: a unified analysis of the relationship between pressure, volume and gas flow in the lungs of normal and diseased human subjects, *Am J Med* 29:672, 1960.

Mead J: Mechanical properties of lungs, *Physiol Rev* 41:281, 1961.

Shirakawa T, Enomoto T, Shimazu S, Hopkin JM: The inverse association between tuberculin responses and atopic disorder, *Science* 275:77, 1997.

Books and monographs

Bates DV, Macklem PT, Christie RV: *Respiratory function in disease*, ed 2, Philadelphia, 1971, WB Saunders.

Forgars P: *Lung sounds.* London, 1978, Bailliere Tindall.

Murray JF: *The normal lung*, ed 2, Philadelphia, 1986, WB Saunders.

Nunn JF: *Applied respiratory physiology.* ed 3, London, 1987, Butterworths.

Pulmonary and Bronchial Circulations: Ventilation/Perfusion Ratios

■ *Overview*

Pulmonary blood flow is the denominator of the ventilation/perfusion ratio ($\dot{V}/\dot{Q}$). It is as important as ventilation in determining the overall efficiency of gas exchange. The pulmonary circulation begins in the right ventricle, which pumps the mixed venous blood through the pulmonary arterial distribution system. The pulmonary arterial blood flows through the alveolar wall capillaries (where O_2 is added and CO_2 is removed), and then through the veins to the left atrium.

The cardiac output flows through the lung at a much lower arterial pressure than it does through the systemic circulation. The difference in arterial pressures between the two circulations is due to the enormous number of small, muscular pulmonary arteries; the enormous pulmonary capillary bed; and the normally dilated state (low vascular tone) of the pulmonary resistance vessels. The low vascular tone of the pulmonary resistance vessels does not mean that the pulmonary vascular bed has no active vasomotor control. The pulmonary circulation has potent mechanisms to balance perfusion with ventilation and thereby to maintain arterial P_{O_2} and P_{CO_2} near their ideal values. However, the smaller muscular arteries and arterioles of the pulmonary circulation have much less smooth muscle than do comparable vessels of the systemic circulation. The importance of having low resistance is that the entire cardiac output can flow through the lungs without expending a large amount of metabolic energy (right ventricular work).

One of the most serious pulmonary vascular diseases is **essential pulmonary hypertension**—an unrelenting narrowing and occlusion of the small muscular pulmonary arteries. As the vessels narrow, pulmonary arterial pressure rises until the right ventricle fails. The only effective treatment is lung transplantation.

The alveolar wall capillary network is the main exchange system of the pulmonary circulation. In resting adults, the pulmonary capillary bed contains about 75 ml of blood, spread out in a vast array of thin-walled, interconnecting vessels. During exercise, capillary blood volume increases as the microvessels are recruited and distended by the increased pressure and flow. Capillary volume during heavy exercise approaches the maximal anatomic volume (about 200 ml). The average thickness of the capillary walls is 0.1 μm, which, together with the attenuated type 1 alveolar epithelium, minimizes the path of oxygen diffusion between alveolar gas and the hemoglobin in the circulating red blood cells. The total capillary surface area for gas exchange, as mentioned earlier, is about 70 m^2 (40 times body surface area).

Under most conditions, capillary volume is approximately equal to the stroke volume of the right ventricle. Thus, at rest, red blood cells that enter the pulmonary capillaries remain there for 0.75 second, which is more than adequate time for O_2 and CO_2 to equilibrate between alveolar gas and blood. During strenuous exercise, when cardiac output is three times the resting value, the rise in pulmonary arterial pressure recruits more alveolar wall capillaries. Capillary volume may double, which gives plenty of time for O_2 and CO_2 to equilibrate, despite the increased blood flow.

The total blood volume of the pulmonary circulation (main pulmonary artery to left atrium) is 500 ml, which is about 10% of the total circulating blood volume. The lung is 40% to 50% blood by weight; this fraction is larger than that for any other organ. The vascular volume, except for the blood in the capillaries, is distributed almost equally between the arterial and venous vessels. The large vascular volume serves as a capacitance reservoir (buffer) for the left atrium. If venous return to the right ventricle changes, the left ventricle diastolic filling does not change appreciably for two to three cardiac cycles.

During normal breathing, the filling of the right and left ventricles is not synchronous. As pleural pressure becomes more subatmospheric during inspiration (see Chapter 33), the right ventricle receives more blood than the left ventricle because the pressure gradient for blood to flow from the periphery back to the heart (venous return) is increased. At the same time, the left ventricle ejects less blood than the right ventricle because the left ventricle is contained within a chamber (thorax) with a lower pressure than that of the systemic arteries, which are surrounded by the higher atmospheric pressure. During expiration, the opposite occurs.

■ *Pressure, Resistance, and Pressure-Flow Curves*

The pressures in the pulmonary circulation of a normal resting adult are compared with those in the systemic circulation in Fig. 34-1. The pressure in the pulmonary artery (Table 34-1) is about one seventh of that in the aorta. Furthermore, left atrial pressure is higher than right atrial pressure (see also Fig. 24-21). At a normal resting cardiac output (Q) of 5 L/min, a mean pulmonary arterial pressure ($\bar{P}pa$) of 19 cm H_2O, and a mean left atrial pressure ($\bar{P}la$) of 11 cm H_2O, the **pulmonary vascular resistance (PVR)** is very low relative to the systemic resistance; *PVR is less than 10% of that in the systemic vascular bed.*

A useful view of pulmonary hemodynamics is obtained by measuring the changes in driving pressure (Ppa − Pla) across the pulmonary vasculature as cardiac output varies. The resultant graphs are called **pressure-flow** curves. Two representative curves of different physiological conditions are shown schematically in Fig. 34-2. Vascular resistance is represented on a pressure-flow curve by the slope of the line from the origin to a given point on the curve. Unlike the measurement of compliance (see Chapter 33), vascular resistance is *not* the slope (tangent) of the curve itself.

■ **Table 34-1** Pressures in the pulmonary circulation of normal, resting, supine adult humans

	mm Hg	*cm H_2O*
Pulmonary artery*		
Systolic/diastolic	24/9	33/11
Mean	14	19
Arterioles		
Mean	12	16
Capillaries		
Mean	10.5	14
Venules		
Mean	9	12
Left atrium		
Mean	8	11

*The pulmonary arterial and left atrial pressures are measured at cardiac catheterization; the former directly, the latter by wedging the arterial catheter in a branch of the pulmonary artery.

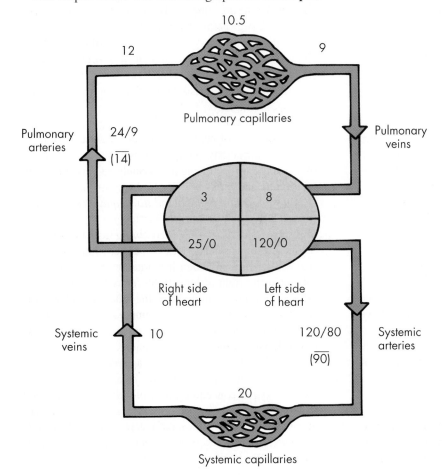

■ **Fig. 34-1** Schematic representation of the phasic and mean pressures within the systemic and pulmonary circulations in a normal, resting human adult lying supine (dorsal recumbency). The units are millimeters of mercury (mm Hg) for easy comparison. The driving pressure in the systemic circuit (Pao − Pra) = 90 − 3 = 87 mm Hg, whereas the driving pressure in the pulmonary circuit (Ppa − Pla) = 14 − 8 = 6 mm Hg. As cardiac output must be the same in both circuits in the steady state because they are in series, the resistance to flow through the lungs is less than 10% that of the rest of the body. Note also that the pressures in the left heart chambers are higher than those in the right heart. Any congenital openings between the right and left sides of the heart favor left-to-right flow.

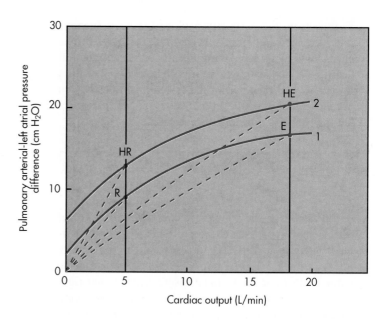

■ **Fig. 34-2** Representative pressure-flow curves that might be obtained in the human pulmonary circulation. Curve *1* is the normal sea level curve, with point *R* the resting condition and point *E* steady-state exercise. The slopes of the dashed lines from the origin to the points on the curve represent pulmonary vascular resistance. Curve *2* shows the effects of acute alveolar hypoxia. Curve *2* lies above curve *1,* meaning that there is increased resistance at any given flow, such as points *HR* and *HE* representing rest and exercise during hypoxia.

The shape of the pulmonary pressure-flow curve is due to the greater distensibility (higher compliance) of the pulmonary vessels at low rather than high distending pressures. As in the systemic veins, the collagen fibers in the adventitia of the resistance vessels stiffen the vessels as the transmural pressure rises. On the normal pressure-flow curve (curve 1 in Fig. 34-2), the resistance during exercise *(E)* is less than at rest *(R)*. Alveolar hypoxia (curve 2 in Fig. 34-2) causes vasoconstriction, and therefore the driving pressure (and consequently the resistance) is greater at any given flow.

■ *Pulmonary Blood Flow*

Although the Fick equation is still the primary reference for measuring cardiac output, several quicker methods are also used, all of which are based on what is known as the *indicator dilution principle* (see Chapter 23).

■ *Shunts between Right and Left Sides of the Heart*

Right-to-left shunt. An important functional test of the adequacy of the pulmonary circulation is to determine what fraction of the cardiac output effectively flows through pulmonary capillaries (exchanges with alveolar gas) and what fraction bypasses the lungs to enter the systemic arteries without becoming oxygenated. The latter fraction is called the **venous admixture** and includes true anatomic shunts.

A small amount of venous admixture is normal, because some venous blood enters the left atrium and ventricle by way of the bronchopulmonary venous anastomoses and the intracardiac thebesian veins. *Right-to-left shunts always reduce systemic arterial oxygen tension and concentration.*

In some diseases such as **bronchiectasis,** a chronic infectious airway disease, or **lung tumors,** which receive their blood supply from the bronchial circulation, flow through the overgrown bronchial circulation may rise to 10% to 20% of cardiac output. In certain congenital anomalies, the right-to-left anatomic shunt may be 50% of cardiac output. Functionally, however, uneven $\dot{V}/Q$ accounts for much more shunting than do anatomic shunts. Fig. 34-3 shows a large right-to-left shunt through an unventilated lung.

If one thinks of venous admixture as a stream of blood being continuously pumped around the body without delivering any O_2 or picking up any CO_2, then venous admixture must reduce the efficiency of gas exchange. *Venous admixture is the blood flow equivalent of wasted ventilation.*

Left-to-right shunt. Blood flowing from the left to the right side of the heart does not affect systemic arterial oxygen tension, although it markedly affects the Po_2 of blood in the right atrium, right ventricle, or pulmonary artery. In a left-to-right shunt, the left ventricular output represents the systemic flow plus the shunt flow; that is, pulmonary blood flow exceeds systemic blood flow by the volume of flow through the shunt.

In a person with a left-to-right cardiac shunt, cardiac catheterization characteristically reveals a step increase in the oxygen concentration of blood somewhere in the right side of the heart. Determining which chamber first shows the increase allows the location of the shunt to be identified and its size estimated on the basis of the change in Po_2.

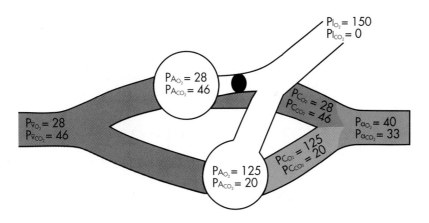

$P_{I_{O_2}} = 150$
$P_{I_{CO_2}} = 0$

$P_{A_{O_2}} = 28$
$P_{A_{CO_2}} = 46$

$P_{\bar{v}_{O_2}} = 28$
$P_{\bar{v}_{CO_2}} = 46$

$P_{c_{O_2}} = 28$
$P_{c_{CO_2}} = 46$

$P_{a_{O_2}} = 40$
$P_{a_{CO_2}} = 33$

$P_{A_{O_2}} = 125$
$P_{A_{CO_2}} = 20$

$P_{c_{O_2}} = 125$
$P_{c_{CO_2}} = 20$

■ **Fig. 34-3**   Schema of venous admixture (right-to-left shunt). Notice the marked decrease in arterial P_{O_2} compared with P_{CO_2}. The (A − a) P_{O_2} is 85 mm Hg.

Right-to-left shunts (venous admixture) commonly occur in pulmonary diseases and in some forms of congenital heart disease. Left-to-right shunts are much less common and are usually associated with congenital heart disease. They occur, although rarely, in congenital pulmonary disease and indicate a bizarre misalignment of the vascular anatomy of the lung.

■ *Distribution of Blood Flow*

The normal pressures in the aorta (120/80, mean 90 mm Hg) refer to pressures at the level of the heart (Fig. 34-1). Gravity, however, affects pressure by 0.74 mm Hg/cm body height. In a standing adult human (175 cm tall), systemic arterial pressure is 130 mm Hg higher in the feet than in the head.

The effects of gravity are relatively greater (in proportion to the total range of pressures) in the pulmonary circulation than in the systemic circulation, because the pressures in the pulmonary circulation are much lower than in the systemic circulation. The normal upright adult lung at total lung capacity (TLC) is about 30 cm high. The average pressures shown in Table 34-1 are valid only at the level of the heart. When lung volume is at TLC, the bottom of the lung is about 15 cm below the left atrium. For each 1 cm below the left atrium, the pulmonary arterial pressure increases by 1 cm H_2O. At the bottom of the lung in the costodiaphragmatic recess, the pulmonary arterial pressure is 34 cm H_2O and pulmonary venous pressure 26 cm H_2O. Although the higher pressures toward the bottom of the lung do not change the driving pressure (8 cm H_2O), they do change the transmural distending pressure. The higher transmural pressure toward the bottom of the lung distends the blood vessels and decreases the resistance to flow. Thus, flow is greater toward the bottom of the lung because the resistance is less, not because the driving pressure is greater.

This pressure pattern is important because changes in pulmonary arterial pressure affect the distribution of blood flow over the height of the lung. As arterial pressure rises, relatively more flow occurs toward the top of the lung. The effect is readily predicted on the basis of the distensibility of the lung vessels. This effect is illustrated in Fig. 34-4, which is a graphic consequence of Fig. 32-8.

The pressure in the microvessels near the bottom of the lung is much higher than that near the top. Such increases in hydrostatic pressure favor fluid filtration. Patients with high left atrial pressure as a consequence of congestive heart failure tend to accumulate interstitial fluid (pulmonary edema) at the bottom of the lung first.

■ *Alveolar and Extra-Alveolar Vessels*

Pulmonary blood vessels may be divided into two groups, according to how pleural pressure affects their transmural pressures during breathing. In Fig. 32-8, the extra-alveolar vessels are represented by the arteries and veins, whereas the alveolar vessels are mainly the capillaries, which are very thin-walled soft tubes. The pressure outside the alveolar vessels is the alveolar pressure, which is ordinarily equal to the atmospheric pressure. The pressure outside the extra-alveolar vessels, however, is less than the alveolar pressure, and it is similar to pleural pressure (−5 cm H_2O at functional reserve capacity [FRC]), as described in Chapter 33. When the lung expands and pleural pressure falls, the pressure outside the extra-alveolar vessels falls relative to alveolar pressure. This fall in pressure causes the extra-alveolar vessels to enlarge during inspiration, which increases pulmonary blood volume.

Alveolar pressure does not vary much with breathing. In the upper part of the lung, where the effective venous pressure falls below the alveolar pressure, the transmural pressure across the small veins becomes compressive at the point where the veins leave the alveolar region. As the

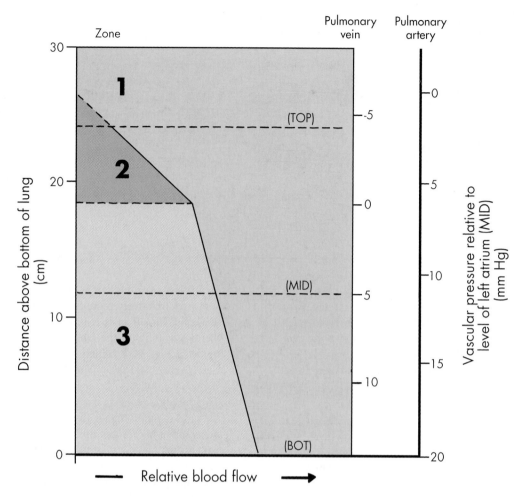

■ **Fig. 34-4**   Distribution of flow in the normal upright human lung at rest at functional reserve capacity (FRC). The *TOP* of the lung is 24 cm (left-hand ordinate) above the bottom *(BOT)*. At the level of the left atrium *(MID)*, left atrial and pulmonary arterial mean pressures are 5 and 12 mm Hg, respectively, as shown on the two parallel scales along the right-hand ordinate. Note that these pressures are less than those in the supine resting individual (Fig. 34-1) because gravity causes blood to pool below the heart level, which reduces cardiac output and the pulmonary vascular distending pressure. Most of the lung is in zone 3, because pulmonary venous pressure does not fall below 0 (atmospheric pressure) for those regions that are less than 18 cm above the *BOT*. Zone 2 occurs in the upper 6 cm. Arterial pressure does not fall below the alveolar pressure. In zone 2, flow is regulated by the alveolar pressure, which compresses the outflow from the alveolar microvessels. In zone 3, although the driving pressure is constant, flow continues to increase toward the bottom of the lung because of the passive distention of the vessels by the increasing vascular pressure.

blood vessels are compressed, vascular resistance at that point increases. The effect is similar to the dynamic compression of the large airways described in Chapter 33.

The uneven distribution of blood flow caused by gravity is usually divided into three zones, depending on the relative values of pulmonary arterial, venous, and alveolar pressures. The effect of gravity on blood flow distribution is shown in Fig. 34-4. In zone 1, flow is zero because pulmonary arterial pressure (Ppa) is less than alveolar pressure (PA). In zone 3, flow is high, and it changes with distance down the lung because of the increasing transmural pressure. In zone 2, the alveolar pressure (PA) exceeds the pulmonary venous pressure (Ppv). The transmural pressure of these vessels is negative; that is, Ppv − PA < 0. Any small veins exposed to alveolar pressure are compressed at the outflow end of the alveolar compartment.

Although all three zones can exist in the human lung, pulmonary arterial pressure is normally high enough so that the zone 1 condition of no flow does not prevail. Also, the condition described for zone 2 is limited to the upper third of the lung, because the pulmonary venous pressure is normally well above the alveolar pressure in the lower two thirds of the lung.

During mechanical ventilation, alveolar pressure is artificially increased, because positive pressure is applied to the airway opening. The amount of lung in zone 2 increases, as alveolar pressure rises relative to pulmonary venous pressure. The rise in alveolar pressure increases resistance to blood flow in that zone. Intensive care physicians must be sure that positive-pressure ventilation does not decrease cardiac output nor increase a$\dot{V}$/Q imbalance.

When pulmonary vascular pressures are increased, the distribution of blood flow over the height of the lung is more uniform. Thus, during strenuous exercise, blood flow distribution is nearly uniform throughout the lung. The $\dot{V}$/Q distribution therefore improves, which tends to increase Pa_{O_2}.

■ Regulation of Pulmonary Blood Flow

■ Longitudinal Distribution of Resistance

As noted, the resistance to blood flow in the pulmonary arteries and arterioles is much less than that in the systemic circulation, where arterioles and small arteries contribute 75% of the total resistance. In a person breathing normally, the alveolar wall capillaries contribute up to 40% of the total resistance, the arteries about 50%, and the veins about 10%. In the systemic circulation, capillary resistance is trivial.

A small pressure decrease (a few centimeters of H_2O) in the systemic capillaries represents a substantial quantity in the pulmonary circulation. In Table 34-1 the average pressure difference (Ppa − Pla) across the lung is $19 - 11 = 8$ cm H_2O. An approximately 3 cm H_2O pressure drop (37% of the total) occurs in the alveolar wall capillaries. This pressure drop depends on the dimensions and distensibility of the alveolar wall capillary network, because the dimensions of the capillaries are not actually regulated. The fraction of resistance within the alveolar wall vessels is sensitive to the lung volume (less at low volume), to the blood flow rate (less at high flow), and to the vascular distending pressure (greater at low pressure).

■ Passive Regulation

When humans exercise submaximally, cardiac output may rise threefold. This increase in blood flow is accommodated by the pulmonary circulation without an equivalent rise in pulmonary vascular driving pressure. This accommodation occurs because of **recruitment** and **distention** of microvessels by the increasing transmural pressure in the very small vessels (arterioles, capillaries, and venules). As already noted, the volume of blood in the pulmonary capillaries during exercise may double,

and the contribution of the capillaries to total resistance substantially decreases. When the flow increases three-fold, the driving pressure across the lungs may increase only about 50%. Therefore, the calculated PVR must have decreased by 50%.

■ Active Regulation

Although the passive effects of pressure on the distensible pulmonary vascular bed are prominent, active regulation does occur under physiological and pathological conditions. The small amount of smooth muscle in the small arteries is adequate to alter PVR substantially. Furthermore, the smooth muscle may undergo marked hypertrophy in certain pathological conditions.

Many naturally occurring substances affect the vasomotor tone of pulmonary arterial or venous vessels. Constrictors include reduced PA_{O_2}, thromboxane A_2, α-adrenergic catecholamines, histamine, angiotensin, several prostaglandins, neuropeptides, leukotrienes, serotonin, endothelin, and increased Pco_2. Dilators include increased PA_{O_2}, prostacyclin, nitric oxide, β-adrenergic catecholamines, acetylcholine, bradykinin, and dopamine.

Effect of alveolar oxygen tension on pulmonary blood flow. The partial pressure of oxygen in the alveoli is the critical factor that governs the pulmonary circulation minute by minute. The Po_2 in the air spaces is far more important than is the oxygen tension within the mixed venous blood. The reason PA_{O_2} is so important is that the small, muscular pulmonary arteries are surrounded by the alveolar gas of the terminal respiratory units they subserve (Fig. 32-9). Oxygen diffuses through the thin alveolar walls into the smooth muscle cells. Ordinarily, PA_{O_2} is high (100 mm Hg), and hence the smooth muscle cells of the microvessels near the alveolar walls are bathed in the highest oxygen tensions of any organ. This fact has become the basis for the most reasonable hypothesis about how reduced PA_{O_2} (alveolar hypoxia) controls PVR.

In the lung, as alveolar oxygen tension falls, the nearby arterioles tend to constrict. Conversely, in the systemic circulation, low oxygen tension relaxes the local resistance vessels, which permits the vessels to dilate passively (see Chapter 28). *The response of pulmonary vascular smooth muscle to decreased Po_2 is opposite to that of systemic vascular smooth muscle.*

The low Po_2 acts directly on the vascular smooth muscle cells. *The physiological importance of this action is that, as alveolar oxygen tension falls in a given region of the lung, local vascular resistance rises and blood flow is diverted to other parts of the lung.* Furthermore, small changes in local resistance may shift blood flow markedly without any significant effect on overall PVR, provided that less than 20% of the volume of lung is involved.

On the other hand, a global reduction in alveolar oxygen tension, such as occurs when one ascends to a high altitude or breathes low oxygen mixtures, increases total PVR. In acute alveolar hypoxia, the resistance may be more than twice the normal value that prevails at sea level. This sustained response occurs in humans and in most mammals who live at high altitudes. The effect of alveolar oxygen tension on PVR is imposed chiefly on the arterioles and small muscular arteries, although the pulmonary veins do constrict in newborn infants.

In many types of lung disease, hypoxic vasoconstriction is a major compensatory factor that tends to restore arterial Po_2 toward normal. However, if a disease process inhibits hypoxic vasoconstriction, Pa_{O_2} may fall because blood flow cannot be shifted away from the poorly ventilated region. This problem occurs in **lobar pneumonia.** An important clinical test of the vasoconstrictor component of pulmonary hypertension is to determine the effect of oxygen inhalation on PVR; if resistance falls, the hypertension must be partially reversible.

The evolution of animal life is exactly suited to the amount of oxygen in our atmosphere (21% at sea level). A level of 0% oxygen is lethal within several minutes. Too much oxygen is also disastrous; for example, breathing 100% oxygen for long periods of time causes severe lung injury with edema, and it is generally fatal within 3 to 5 days. Injury is probably mediated by the large increase in the rate of oxygen radical production. In premature newborns, supplemental oxygen can cause a permanent blindness known as **retrolental fibroplasia,** unless care is taken to ensure that arterial Po_2 is not elevated.

Effect of thromboxane and prostacyclin on pulmonary blood flow. Thromboxane A$_2$, a product of cell membrane arachidonic acid metabolism, is an important vasoconstrictor. Thromboxane A$_2$ is one of the most powerful known constrictors of pulmonary arterial and venous smooth muscle. It is produced in the pulmonary circulation in several types of acute lung injury. Many cells, particularly macrophages, but also leukocytes and endothelial cells, produce and release thromboxane. As with oxygen, the effect is localized mainly to the region where the thromboxane is released, because the half-time of thromboxane inactivation in blood is only several seconds.

Prostacyclin (prostaglandin I$_2$) is another product of arachidonic acid metabolism. It is a potent vasodilator as well as an inhibitor of platelet activation. Endothelial cells are probably the chief source of this substance. However, little thromboxane or prostacyclin is produced normally.

Nitric oxide (NO) is another potent endogenous vasodilator that has a very localized effect. If any NO diffuses into circulating blood, it immediately and irreversibly binds to the heme iron in hemoglobin (see Chapter 35). Thus, its action is strictly localized to the vascular bed in which it is produced. Interest in the clinical use of NO has increased in recent years. NO has great potential for selective pulmonary vasodilation, because it can be delivered by inhalation.

■ *Bronchial Circulation*

The bronchial arteries supply water and nutrients to the mucosal cells and glands of the airways down to and including the terminal bronchioles. They also nourish the pleura, interlobular septal supporting tissues, and pulmonary arteries and veins. The bronchial circulation does not normally supply the terminal respiratory unit, which receives nutrients via the pulmonary circulation.

The pressure in the main bronchial arteries is the same as that in the aorta, and therefore the driving pressure is high regardless of body position. Although bronchial blood flow is less than 1% of cardiac output, this flow is adequate for the portion of the lung tissue it serves.

About half of the bronchial blood flow returns to the right side of the heart via bronchial veins that empty into the azygos or hemiazygos veins before they enter the right atrium. The remainder flows through small bronchopulmonary anastomoses (<100 μm in diameter) into the pulmonary veins and thereby contributes to the normal venous admixture (right-to-left shunt).

When the pulmonary circulation is obstructed (as in pulmonary thrombosis or embolism), the bronchial arteries dilate and may develop connections with pulmonary arterial vessels. When this occurs, the blood that flows through the alveolar capillaries is systemic arterial blood, which takes up little oxygen from the alveolar gas but may give up CO_2 because the alveolar CO_2 is low. The bronchial circulation keeps the lung alive when the pulmonary blood flow is shut off.

The bronchial circulation conditions the inspired air, especially under circumstances in which air bypasses the upper air passages, such as when one breathes through the mouth during exercise. The inhaled air is warmed and humidified in the upper air passages by heat and water evaporation from the lung. The heat and water come ultimately from the pulmonary (99%) and bronchial (1%) circulations. Hence, water does not evaporate from the alveolar surfaces.

The bronchial, but not the pulmonary, circulation has **angiogenic potential** after the lung stops growing in late adolescence. As injuries to the lung are repaired, the new growth is supplied by vessels that bud from the bronchial microvessels. The difference in angiogenic potential between the bronchial and pulmonary circulation is manifest even though the bronchial and pulmonary vessels are very close anatomically. Bronchial vascular growth must also be considered in the treatment of lung cancer. No matter where a tumor originates (metastatic or local), it always develops a bronchial blood supply as it grows. Localized therapy (such as microemboli to cut off the tumor blood supply, or infusions of toxic chemicals) is directed into the bronchial circulation that supplies the tumor to achieve the best results.

■ *Matching Ventilation to Perfusion*

■ *Ventilation and Perfusion*

In the ideal lung, the ventilation/perfusion ($\dot{V}/Q$) of every lung unit is the same. However, not even healthy normal people have ideal lungs, which is why the normal systemic arterial oxygen partial pressure ranges between 85 and 100 mm Hg. This narrow range of partial pressures suggests that the distribution of $\dot{V}/Q$ is well regulated. The concept of matching gas (ventilation) and blood (perfusion) for successful O_2 and CO_2 exchange is central to an understanding of gas exchange. *Inequalities of the distribution of $\dot{V}/Q$ ratios are the most common cause of inefficient O_2 and CO_2 exchange.*

If resting normal alveolar ventilation, $\dot{V}_A$, is 4.2 L/min and pulmonary blood flow, Q, is 5 L/min, the normal $\dot{V}/Q = 4.2/5.0 = 0.84$ (no units). These values, together with the normal $\dot{V}_{CO_2}$, yield the normal $Pa_{O_2} = 100$ mm Hg and $Pa_{CO_2} = 40$ mm Hg when R = 0.80, according to the alveolar gas and alveolar air equations in Chapter 32. In exercise, $\dot{V}/Q$ rises. For example, during maximal steady-state exercise, $\dot{V}_{O_2}$ may reach 1500 ml/min (six times resting) with $\dot{V}_A = 26$ L/min and Q = 15 L/min, and hence $\dot{V}/Q = 1.7$. If the respiratory exchange ratio remains at 0.80, the arterial blood gases remain essentially normal. Thus, in order to interpret the overall lung $\dot{V}/Q$ ratio, it is necessary to know the respiratory exchange ratio, R, and the steady-state oxygen consumption, $\dot{V}_{O_2}$, as well as the alveolar ventilation.

$\dot{V}/Q$ mismatching is generally expressed in terms of its effect on the alveolar-arterial P_{O_2} difference. The effect on CO_2 is parallel but much smaller. The main cause of CO_2 retention is hypoventilation.

The matching of ventilation to perfusion is important clinically. In patients with cardiopulmonary disease, the most frequent cause of systemic arterial hypoxemia is neither hypoventilation nor venous admixture (right-to-left shunt); it is an uneven matching of alveolar ventilation and alveolar blood flow.

Two extreme instances of $\dot{V}/Q$ mismatching have already been introduced: wasted ventilation (see Chapter 32) and venous admixture (earlier in this chapter). In the following sections, we look at these extreme conditions in more detail.

■ *Wasted Ventilation*

Wasted ventilation may occur clinically when a large blood clot (pulmonary embolism) obstructs a branch of the pulmonary artery. In Fig. 32-14, the blood flow to the upper lung is cut off. If compensatory changes in ventilation do not occur and if half of the blood flow and alveolar ventilation went to each lung before the obstruction, then after the occlusion all of the blood flow is diverted to the lower lung. However, half of the ventilation still goes to each lung. Clearly, in this situation, the ventilation to the unperfused lung is wasted, because it fails to oxygenate any of the mixed venous blood. The overall efficiency of lung ventilation is decreased, because more than half the power used in breathing moves air that serves no useful purpose.

The $\dot{V}/Q$ ratio of the upper lung is infinite because the denominator (blood flow) equals zero (2.1/0), but what is the $\dot{V}/Q$ ratio of the perfused lung? It cannot be the normal value of 0.84 because that lung receives its normal portion of alveolar ventilation but all of the cardiac output. Its $\dot{V}/Q$ ratio is 2.1/5.0 = 0.42.

Fortunately, compensatory changes begin almost immediately and tend to shift ventilation from the useless lung to the functional one. This shift brings the $\dot{V}/Q$ back toward its normal value. If this compensation did not occur, the Pa_{CO_2} would increase (hypoventilation) and Pa_{O_2} would decrease.

■ *Venous Admixture*

Venous admixture is shown schematically in Fig. 34-3. In this example, the upper lung receives no ventilation but still has its normal blood flow. Clearly, hypoxemia will result, because 50% of cardiac output is shunted. The $\dot{V}/Q$ of the unventilated lung = 0/2.5 = 0; thus, a right-to-left shunt is equivalent to a $\dot{V}/Q$ ratio equal to zero.

On the other hand, ventilation of the lower lung has doubled relative to its blood flow. The $\dot{V}/Q$ of that lung = 4.2/2.5 = 1.68. The situation in this lung is clearly hyperventilation, by the definition in Chapter 32. Thus, the blood that leaves this lung via the pulmonary veins will have a decreased P_{CO_2} and an increased P_{O_2}. However, when the P_{O_2} is near 100 mm Hg, the slope of the HbO_2 equilibrium curve is flat (see Fig. 32-2). The important result is that increased blood flow through a ventilated lung cannot compensate for the low P_{O_2} of the shunt through the unventilated lung. Therefore, Pa_{O_2} will decrease, sometimes substantially. The effect is much less for P_{CO_2}, which explains why physicians measure overall lung performance by measuring the (A-a) P_{O_2} difference.

■ *Other Ventilation/Perfusion Distributions*

If wasted ventilation (Q = 0; $\dot{V}/Q = \infty$) and left-to-right shunt ($\dot{V}_A = 0$; $\dot{V}/Q = 0$) represent the extremes of $\dot{V}/Q$

mismatching, then all other possible $\dot{V}/Q$ ratios must lie between them.

As noted at the beginning of this section, the $\dot{V}/Q$ distribution throughout the normal lung is not homogeneous. Some lung units are overventilated and some are underventilated. Fig. 34-5 shows the distribution of $\dot{V}/Q$ in a normal human adult. The average normal value (0.84) is shown as the thin vertical line. The $\dot{V}/Q$ ratios are shown on the X axis. The logarithmic X-axis scale is used to show the wide range of $\dot{V}/Q$ ratios that may be encountered in diseased lungs.

An elegant way to measure the $\dot{V}/Q$ distribution experimentally in the lung is the multiple inert gas procedure, in which six inert gases of differing gas-to-blood solubility ratios are infused intravenously until a steady state of lung gas elimination is established. From the infused and expired partial pressures of each gas, the most likely pattern of $\dot{V}/Q$ distribution is then computed. This test is not done clinically, however, because it is invasive, time consuming, and expensive. Clinically, doctors measure only the $(A - a) \, P_{O_2}$ difference.

Any deviation of $\dot{V}/Q$ from the ideal value impairs the efficiency of O_2 and CO_2 transfer. In other words, such deviations increase the differences between alveolar and arterial gas tension, especially that for oxygen.

■ Distribution of Ventilation

If the normal lung is not uniformly ventilated, what mechanisms contribute to the nonuniformity? Regional nonuniform ventilation, top to bottom in the upright human lung, is mainly due to gravity. This type of nonuniformity probably disappears in astronauts in space. Local nonuniform ventilation among terminal respiratory units is caused by variable airway resistance (R) or compliance (C), and it may be described by the time constant ($\tau = R \times C$).

■ Regional Ventilation Distribution

Each level of lung is suspended from, and supported by, the lung above it; that is, the lung does not "sit" on the diaphragm nor "hang" from the trachea, even when the subject is in the upright position. Ultimately, the force that maintains lung support is transmitted through the layer of pleural liquid between the lung and the chest wall. As the mass of lung that must be supported increases, the weight of the lung pulling down or away from the chest wall increases. Thus, pleural pressure decreases. If pleural pressure is decreased, static translung pressure ($P_L = P_A - P_{pl}$) must be increased.

Consequently, the alveoli are expanded more near the top of the lung. Indeed, the relative alveolar volume par-

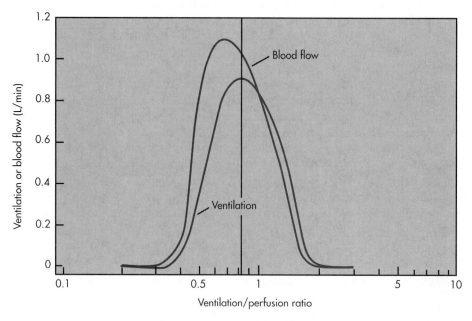

■ **Fig. 34-5** Normal human $\dot{V}/Q$ distribution curves. The ordinate refers to blood flow or ventilation (L/min). Their quotient is the ventilation/perfusion ratio shown on the abscissa on a logarithmic scale. The range of $\dot{V}/Q$ in the normal lung is 0.3 to 1.2; the overall normal $\dot{V}/Q = 0.84$ as shown by the vertical line.

allels the compliance curve of the lung. Fig. 34-6 shows the end-expiratory volume of two lung units, one near the top and one near the bottom, at three locations along the pressure-volume curve.

Over the normal tidal volume range, the differences in regional ventilation are small, because the slope of the pressure-volume curve is nearly constant. Hence, the gravitational effect on the regional distribution of ventilation is less than expected. Nevertheless, the lower portion of the lung tends to be ventilated more because the end-expiratory volume (FRC) is less, and the compliance is slightly greater than at the top of the lung (Fig. 34-6, *middle*).

Regional distribution of ventilation is affected by body position. The effect is less when one is supine than when one is prone. As previously discussed, in this supine position, abdominal pressure pushes the diaphragm cephalad. This displacement affects the FRC of all units, but especially those near the diaphragm.

After one takes a single maximal inspiration of pure O_2, the regional distribution of ventilation in large part determines the slope of the expired alveolar nitrogen plateau (Fig. 34-7), because the better ventilated alveoli tend to empty first (the "first in, first out" rule). This rule is the basis of a simple and useful pulmonary function test (the **single-breath nitrogen test**) to assess the uniformity of ventilation distribution.

■ *Local Ventilation Distribution*

An uneven distribution of ventilation that does not depend on gravity is associated with varying alveolar time constants ($\tau = R \times C$). Evidence suggests that local variations in ventilation distribution are important, even in the normal lung. In other words, resistance and compliance differences among terminal respiratory units vary substantially on both functional and anatomic grounds.

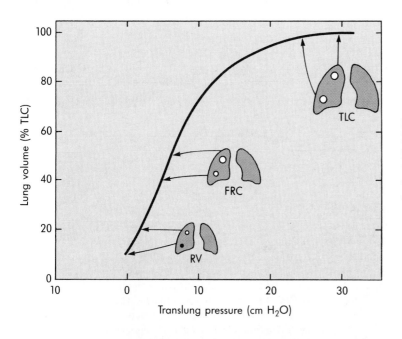

■ **Fig. 34-6**   Regional distribution of lung volume. Because of suspension of the lung from top to bottom, pleural pressure and translung pressure, PL, of units at the top will be greater than those at the bottom. The effect is greatest at residual volume *(RV)*, is less at *FRC*, and disappears at total lung capacity *(TLC)*.

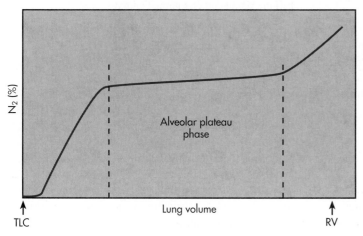

■ **Fig. 34-7**   The single-breath nitrogen washout curve is a simple useful pulmonary function test of regional ventilation distribution. It clearly shows that not all lung units have equal V̇/Q. The well-ventilated units (short time constant) empty faster than less well ventilated units (long time constant). The portion of the curve up to the vertical dashed line represents the washout of dead space air mixed with alveolar gas. The long alveolar plateau rises slowly (<2%) if ventilation distribution is relatively uniform, as shown here. The final phase, after the second vertical line, shows very late, slowly emptying alveoli. This phase is accentuated with age.

Because it is not related to gravity, this type of nonuniformity does not disappear in astronauts in space.

Fig. 34-8 illustrates the varying time constant concept. A longer time constant means slower ventilation of a lung unit. Thus, a unit with increased resistance, increased compliance, or both will take longer to fill, when other factors are constant. Furthermore, a decrease in compliance of a unit decreases its absolute volume at any given translung pressure.

As pointed out in Chapter 33, breathing is a dynamic process, so that ventilation time is important even in subjects at rest. At the normal breathing rate of 12/min, inspiratory time is about 2 seconds and expiratory time about 3 seconds. These times may not be long enough for every terminal respiratory unit to achieve a steady state, as described in the section on intrinsic PEEP (see Chapter 33).

Fig. 34-8 shows the behavior of three units: one is normal, one has twice the airway resistance of the others, and one has half the compliance of the others. The graph shows the time course of filling of the three units during a normal 2-second inspiration. The normal unit, N, and the low compliance unit reach a new steady state, although the volume of the less distensible unit is reduced. The unit with increased R reaches only 80% of its predicted steady-state value. If inspiration were prolonged, the high-resistance unit would also eventually fill to its steady-state level.

■ *Distribution of Perfusion*

■ *Regional Blood Flow Distribution*

Gravity affects the regional distribution of blood flow in the lung by affecting the transmural distending pressure of the vessels and the relative arterial, venous, and alveolar pressures (review the three lung zones shown in Fig. 34-4). However, in normal upright humans at rest, the gravitational effects on pulmonary blood flow are small but not insignificant. As we have seen, most of the lung is in zone 3, where the blood flow gradient is not as large as in zone 2 (Fig. 34-4).

■ *Local Perfusion Distribution*

An uneven distribution of blood flow to terminal respiratory units, not related to gravity, is important. One component of this uneven distribution is related to anatomy (geometry); that is, the diameter, length, and branching angles of the vessels to each unit vary. This factor is not affected by large changes in blood flow. The second component is the variation in local alveolar oxygen tension. This component affects the arterial resistance to the various lung units by altering vasomotor tone. Normally, the hypoxic vasoconstrictor effect is minimal; it probably acts on the lower $\dot{V}/Q$ regions to divert flow to the better-ventilated lung units.

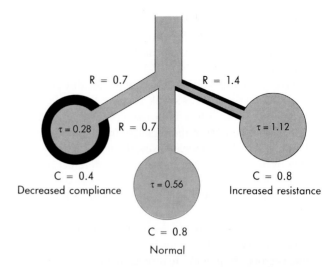

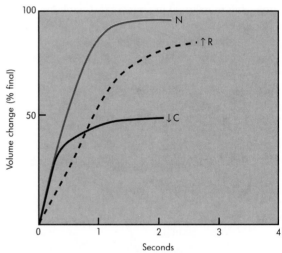

■ **Fig. 34-8** Examples of local regulation of ventilation due to variation of resistance *(R)* or compliance *(C)* of individual lung units. In the upper schema, the normal lung has a time constant, τ, of 0.56 second. This unit reaches 97% of final equilibrium in 2 seconds, the normal inspiratory time, as shown in the lower graph. The unit at the right has a twofold increase in resistance; hence, its time constant is doubled. That unit fills more slowly and reaches only 80% equilibrium during a normal breath. The unit is underventilated. The unit on the left has reduced compliance (stiff), which acts to reduce its time constant. This unit fills faster than the normal unit but receives only half the ventilation of a normal unit.

■ *Effect of $\dot{V}/Q$ Mismatching*

Local $\dot{V}/Q$ ratios. No simple test is available to assess the distribution of $\dot{V}/Q$ ratios in the lung. Therefore, the effect of mismatching of ventilation to perfusion is examined in a general way by determining the alveolar-to-arterial difference in oxygen tension $(A - a) Po_2$. Normally, blood that leaves units near the bottom of the lung has a lower Po_2 and consequently a lower So_2 than does the blood that leaves units near the top. The reason for this difference is that the flow is greater but the ventilation is less to units near the bottom than to those near the top of the lung.

Increasing Pa_{O_2} above normal does not have much effect on arterial oxygen saturation or concentration, because the HbO_2 equilibrium curve is so flat at Po_2 values greater than 70 mm Hg (see Fig. 32-2). When $\dot{V}/Q$ mismatching occurs, the arterial Po_2 will always be less than the ideal value. However, in some lung diseases, the change in Po_2 can be very large.

Normally, venous admixture caused by mixed venous blood that bypasses the lung (anatomic shunt) is only 1% to 2% of cardiac output, whereas the $\dot{V}/Q$ mismatch contribution is equivalent to a venous admixture of 4% to 5%. Thus, the normal systemic arterial Po_2 in humans breathing air at sea level is not 100 mm Hg. The value is generally between 85 and 90 mm Hg; $(A - a) Po_2 = 10$ to 15 mm Hg. An $(A - a) Po_2$ difference less than 20 mm Hg is considered normal.

Although arterial Po_2 may be submaximal as a consequence of the $\dot{V}/Q$ distribution that prevails even in normal subjects, the effect on arterial oxygen saturation is trivial. Sa_{O_2} is 96.9% when $Pa_{O_2} = 90$ mm Hg; that is, the saturation is about 0.5% less than the ideal saturation of 97.4%.

> Very sick patients may have $(A - a) Po_2$ differences of 60 mm Hg when they breathe ordinary air; that is, their arterial O_2 tension is only 40 mm Hg. However, some of these hypoxemic patients may function surprisingly well. People who live at high altitudes and who are well acclimatized may also have $Pa_{O_2} = 40$ mm Hg. They carry on many normal activities, even active sports!

■ Compensation for $\dot{V}/Q$ Mismatching

Obviously, the extreme conditions represented in Figs. 32-14 and 34-3 are unstable. Wasted ventilation is enormous in the former and wasted blood flow is enormous in the latter. As a result, Pa_{CO_2} and Pa_{O_2} are adversely affected.

Fortunately, various compensatory mechanisms can alleviate some of the $\dot{V}/Q$ mismatch. Initially, the increased Pa_{CO_2} invokes centrally mediated (brain controlled) increases in ventilation. However, the increase in total ventilation is inadequate, because the wasted ventilation fraction is not affected (see Fig 32-14).

Local compensatory factors are more important. When ventilation is wasted, the local Pco_2 falls. The decreased local Pco_2 lowers the hydrogen ion concentration, $[H^+]$, around the associated airway smooth muscle. The fall in $[H^+]$ leads to airway constriction and a shift of ventilation away from the terminal respiratory units with high $\dot{V}/Q$ ratios. This kind of compensation can be very effective, depending on the size of the affected lung unit.

If blood flow is reduced to a terminal respiratory unit, the local alveolar cell metabolism will be affected. The most notable change is that the production or release of surfactant is decreased, which increases the alveolar surface tension. An increase in the air-liquid interfacial tension reduces the unit's compliance, and its FRC volume decreases. This response is an effective compensatory mechanism for severely underperfused units. However, it is slow to develop compared with the very fast changes in total ventilation (seconds) and in local airway tone (seconds to minutes) that are induced by changes in Pco_2.

The effectiveness of hypoxic vasoconstriction in shifting flow away from an underventilated unit depends on the fraction of the lung that is involved. If the vessels are constricted to only a small fraction (<20%) of the mass, then shifting flow away from the underventilated units is very effective because the vasoconstriction has little impact on overall pulmonary hemodynamics; that is, pulmonary arterial pressure is not increased.

When a large fraction of the lung (>20%) is involved, hypoxic vasoconstriction increases the pulmonary arterial pressure. The extreme case is global alveolar hypoxia (as in high altitudes), in which pulmonary arterial pressure may be doubled. The large increase in pulmonary arterial pressure actually improves the $\dot{V}/Q$ distribution, because the pressure rise tends to even out the normal gravitational maldistribution of blood flow.

■ Summary

1. In normal humans, pulmonary vascular resistance is only about 10% of that in the systemic circulation.

2. When blood flows from the systemic veins to the systemic arteries without being fully oxygenated (right-to-left shunt), the systemic arterial oxygen tension and concentration decrease.

3. In left-to-right shunts, pulmonary blood flow is increased, but the systemic arterial oxygen tension and concentration and the systemic blood flow are normal.

4. The distribution of pulmonary blood flow is affected by gravity over the height of the air-filled lung because the pulmonary arterial and left atrial pressures are normally low, and the vessels are distensible or collapsible. Three flow conditions are possible: zone 1, no flow; zone 2, flow is regulated by compression of microvessels at the outflow from the alveolar walls; and zone 3, flow depends on driving pressure, vascular geometry, and smooth muscle tone.

5. Although passive regulation of pulmonary blood flow distribution predominates normally, active regulation may become very important. The main regulator is alveolar oxygen tension.

6. Alveolar hypoxia produces an immediate and sustained local increase in vascular resistance by causing the small pulmonary arteries to constrict.

7. Thromboxane is a powerful constrictor and prostacyclin a powerful dilator of the pulmonary vasculature.

8. The bronchial circulation nourishes the walls of the airways and blood vessels; it warms and humidifies incoming air; and it supplies substrate to airway glands, mucosa, and smooth muscle.

9. The distribution of ventilation/perfusion ratios among terminal respiratory units is not uniform even in the normal lung and may be very nonuniform in disease. The limiting ratios are wasted ventilation and venous admixture.

10. Ventilation is distributed nonuniformly in the lung on regional (gravitational) and local (nongravitational) bases. Regional distribution predominates in the normal upright human. Local factors that affect ventilation distribution to each terminal respiratory unit are its resistance and compliance, whose product is the time constant.

11. Blood flow is distributed nonuniformly in the lung on regional (gravitational) and local (nongravitational) bases. The main local factor that affects perfusion distribution is the alveolar oxygen tension in the small lung units. Compensatory hypoxic vasoconstriction is very effective, provided that the amount of lung tissue involved is less than 20% of lung mass.

12. The overall effect of ventilation/perfusion distribution can be judged by determining the alveolar-arterial oxygen tension difference, which is normally 10 to 15 mm Hg.

■ *Self-Study Problems*

1. When the pulmonary arterial flow to a lung region is blocked, as by an embolus, the region may survive on its bronchial flow. Why does the affected lung region continue to expire CO_2 but not take up significant O_2?

2. Cite three conditions under which inhaled nitric oxide may not relieve an increased pulmonary vascular resistance. Explain why each condition prevents a response.

3. What congenital defects underlie left-to-right shunts that increase P_{O_2} first in the (1) right atrium, (2) right ventricle, (3) pulmonary artery?

■ *Bibliography*

Journal articles

Archer SL, Huang J, Peterson D, Weir EK: A redo-based O_2 sensor in rat pulmonary vasculature, *Circ Res* 73:1100, 1993.

Bhattacharya J, Staub NC: Direct measurement of microvascular pressures in the isolated perfused dog lung, *Science* 210:327, 1980.

Deffenbach ME, Charan NB, Lakshminarayan S, Butler J: The bronchial circulation: small, but a vital attribute of the lung, *Am Rev Respir Dis* 135:463, 1987.

Furchgott RF, Vanhoutte PM: Endothelium-derived relaxing and contracting factors, *FASEB J* 3:2007, 1989.

Hyman AL, Spannhake EW, Kadowitz PJ: Prostaglandins and the lung, *Am Rev Respir Dis* 117:111, 1978.

Lenfant C: Measurement of ventilation/perfusion distribution with alveolar arterial differences, *J Appl Physiol* 18:1090, 1963.

Milic-Emili J et al: Regional distribution of inspired gas in the lung, *J Appl Physiol* 21:749, 1966.

Mitzner W: Resistance of the pulmonary circulation, *Clin Chest Med* 4:127, 1983.

Neonatal Inhaled Nitric Oxide Study Group: Inhaled nitric oxide in full-term and nearly full-term infants with hypoxic respiratory failure, *N Engl J Med* 336:597, 1997

Weir K, Archer SL: The mechanism of acute hypoxic pulmonary vasoconstriction: the tale of two channels, *FASEB J* 9:183, 1995.

West JB, Collery CT, Naimark A: Distribution of blood flow in isolated lung: relation to vascular and alveolar pressures, *J Appl Physiol* 19:713, 1964.

West JF: Ventilation-perfusion relationships, *Am Rev Respir Dis* 116:919, 1977.

Books and monographs

Forster RE II, Dubois AB, Briscoe WA, Fisher AB: *The lung: physiologic basis of pulmonary function tests,* ed 3, Chicago, 1986, Mosby–Year Book.

Grover RF, Wagner WW, McMurtry JR, Reeves JT: *Pulmonary circulation.* In: *Handbook of physiology, the cardiovascular system,* sect 3, vol III, Bethesda, Md, 1984, American Physiological Society.

Harris P, Heath D: *The human pulmonary circulation,* ed 2, Edinburgh, 1978, Churchill Livingstone.

Nunn JF: *Applied respiratory physiology,* ed 3, London, 1987, Butterworths.

Transport of Oxygen and Carbon Dioxide: Tissue Oxygenation

The central problem that had to be solved in the evolution of large multicellular animals was how to get oxygen and its metabolite carbon dioxide into and out of the cells of the body. Diffusion is too slow at distances greater than about 100 μm (0.1 mm). Therefore, respiratory and circulatory systems have evolved to provide efficient tissue oxygenation regardless of body size. However, despite this solution, several problems involving oxygen transport may still occur. **Hypoxic hypoxia** refers to inadequate O_2 uptake into blood as it passes through the lungs (e.g., in severe chronic obstructive pulmonary disease). **Stagnant hypoxia** refers to inadequate blood flow to an organ (e.g., in arteriosclerotic peripheral vascular disease). **Anemic hypoxia** means inadequate blood oxygen-carrying capacity (e.g., when hemoglobin is inactivated by carbon monoxide). Finally, **histotoxic hypoxia** refers to interference with mitochondrial respiration (e.g., in cyanide poisoning, which blocks the respiratory enzyme chain).

■ *Oxygen Transport*

One liter of plasma holds only 3 ml O_2 in physical solution when the arterial P_{O_2} is 100 mm Hg. This situation would represent the most extreme state of anemic hypoxia. If O_2 transport in blood depended on dissolved oxygen to sustain normal resting oxygen consumption of 250 ml/min, cardiac output would have to be 80 L/min, even if all the oxygen in the blood could be extracted. Fortunately, red blood cells contain the iron-containing red protein hemoglobin. Hemoglobin, at its normal concentration of 150 g/L, permits whole blood to carry 65 times more oxygen than does plasma when the P_{O_2} is 100 mm Hg.

■ *The Hemoglobin-Oxygen Equilibrium Curve*

Fig. 35-1 shows the relationship (the HbO_2 equilibrium curve) between the oxygen concentration of hemoglobin and oxygen partial pressure of normal human blood at

37° C and a hydrogen ion concentration [H^+] of 36 nmol/L (36×10^{-9} mol/L; pH = 7.40). The curve shows the percentage oxygen saturation as a function of P_{O_2}. However, the curve gives little information about oxygen transport. To interpret the equilibrium curve, it is necessary to know more about the rates of the chemical reactions between O_2 and Hb within erythrocytes and the concentration of hemoglobin in blood.

■ *Hemoglobin, the Oxygen Carrier Protein*

Hemoglobin consists of four O_2-binding heme molecules (iron-containing porphyrin rings). Each heme group is combined with one globin (protein) chain. The molecular weight of hemoglobin is 66,500. Three important physiological properties characterize the chemical binding between hemoglobin and O_2:

1. Hemoglobin combines reversibly with O_2. The term **hemoglobin** (Hb) refers to the unoxygenated form; the oxygen-containing form is called **oxyhemoglobin** (HbO_2). The iron in the four heme pigments is in the ferrous (Fe^{++}; reduced) state. When arterial blood is 90% saturated, some of the Hb molecules bind four oxygens, and some bind less than four. The ratio of the oxygen bound to Hb to the total amount that can be bound is defined as the **oxygen saturation** (S_{O_2}). The maximal amount of O_2 that can be bound to Hb ($S_{O_2} = 100\%$) per unit of blood is called its **oxygen capacity.**

2. Molecular oxygen associates with or dissociates from hemoglobin within milliseconds, even when the hemoglobin is densely packed in red blood cells. This fast reaction is critical for O_2 transport, because blood remains in the exchange capillaries less than 1 second.

3. The shape of the HbO_2 equilibrium curve is sigmoid (S-shaped), which reflects the molecular interaction among the four heme groups. When oxygen is bound to three hemes, the remaining

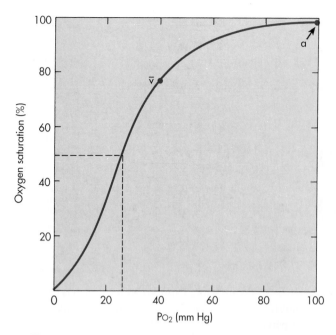

■ **Fig. 35-1**   The normal hemoglobin-oxygen (HbO₂) equilibrium curve. It relates oxygen partial pressure (abscissa) and fractional saturation of hemoglobin in erythrocytes (ordinate). The P50 (*intersection of dashed lines*) is used to compare the curves under different conditions or among different hemoglobins. The normal arterial (*a*) and mixed venous (*v̄*) blood points are indicated.

heme group's oxygen-binding capacity is greatly enhanced (i.e., it has an increased affinity for oxygen). The shape of the curve indicates that the loading of O_2 in the lungs (PA_{O_2} = 100 mm Hg) and the unloading of O_2 in the systemic tissue capillaries ($P\bar{c}_{O_2}$ = 55 mm Hg) are maximized. The functional significance of the flat upper portion of the curve is that the arterial oxygen saturation does not change much until Pa_{O_2} has decreased to about 70 mm Hg (hypoxic hypoxia). The HbO₂ equilibrium curve may be modified by a number of physiological or pathological factors. The curve can be affected in two ways: a shift in its position or a change in its shape. A change in the shape of the curve indicates a much greater interference with O_2 transport than does a shift in the curve.

Although the normal hemoglobin concentration in blood is 150 g/L, anemic individuals have a lower hemoglobin concentration (anemic hypoxia). In chronic anemia, the circulating hemoglobin concentration may be less than 50 g/L. Even then, people with an insidious development of anemia (e.g., slow gastrointestinal bleeding) may complain only of slight tiredness at day's end or an inability to do much exercise. Blood loss, as in menstruation, is the most common cause of mild anemia in women. It is normal for women of child-bearing age to have a hemoglobin concentration of 135 g/L. **Iron deficiency anemia** is

usually caused by a dietary problem and is easily treated in most patients. **Pernicious anemia** is usually due to a problem with the absorption of vitamin B_{12} in the small intestine.

■ *Oxygen Transport in Blood*

If a person's **hematocrit** (the fraction of blood that consists of red blood cells) is less than 30%, the anemia is usually associated with a disease that affects the turnover of red blood cells (the normal lifespan of circulating red blood cells is 120 days). The hematocrit affects the viscosity of blood as it flows through small vessels (see Chapter 25). An extreme condition is the complete absence of red blood cells; this condition is incompatible with human life. The other extreme is severe **polycythemia** (many red blood cells), as in **chronic mountain sickness,** in which the hematocrit may approach a maximal value of 80%.

The power (work per unit time) requirement for the heart to transport the normal quantity of oxygen is at a minimum when the hematocrit is in the range of 40% to 50%. When the hematocrit is less than 30% (low O_2 capacity) or greater than 55% (high viscosity), the heart must work much harder to pump adequate quantities of blood to meet the oxygen needs of the tissues.

Mountain climbers once believed that adapting to high altitude before attempting record climbs was beneficial because the O_2 capacity of blood increased. However, a German team demonstrated that hemodilution by bleeding did not impair the ability of climbers, and that the diluted blood flowed better through the skin and thereby markedly decreased the incidence of frostbite. Doctors remove blood to reduce blood viscosity in selected clinical conditions (e.g., to improve skin blood flow in patients with diabetic ulcers). On the other hand, transfusions of packed red cells ("blood doping") had a brief and illegal popularity, both in race horses and in human runners. The rationale for this practice was that the increased oxygen-carrying capacity would enhance O_2 transport and give performers a competitive edge. However, the increased blood viscosity was found to increase the work of the heart, and performance did not improve.

■ *Factors Affecting the HbO₂ Equilibrium Curve*

The standard HbO₂ equilibrium curve shown in Fig. 35-1 applies precisely only under the following conditions: human hemoglobin type A, hydrogen ion concentration $[H^+]$ = 40 nmol/L (pH = 7.40), P_{CO_2} = 40 mm Hg, temperature $= 37°$ C and 2,3-diphosphoglycerate concentration [2,3-DPG] $= 15$ $\mu mol/g$ Hb.

When the value of any of the last four factors ([H+], P_{CO_2}, temperature, [2,3-DPG]) increases, the affinity of hemoglobin for oxygen decreases. The standard way to describe the effect is in terms of P50 (P_{O_2} that yields 50% saturation). P50 increases when any of the above factors increases, as shown by the black dashed curve in Fig. 35-2. The entire HbO_2 curve is shifted proportionally to the right of the standard curve. The change is in the position of the curve, not its shape.

Conversely, when the value of any of the four factors falls (Fig. 35-2, *solid black curve*), the affinity of hemoglobin for oxygen increases and P50 decreases. The entire HbO_2 curve is shifted to the left. Again, the change is in the position of the curve, not its shape. An easy to remember rule about the relationship between P50 and the Hb affinity for O_2 is: *when Hb affinity for O_2 changes, the P50 changes in the opposite direction.*

The hydrogen ion, H+, has a greater affinity for deoxygenated hemoglobin than for oxyhemoglobin. Increased [H+] reduces the O_2 affinity of oxyhemoglobin. When carbon dioxide (CO_2), the principal metabolic acid, diffuses into systemic capillary blood, it forms carbonic acid. The H+ concentration increases, which in turn decreases the hemoglobin O_2 affinity.

The temperature effect is such that increased temperature favors dissociation and decreased temperature favors association of O_2 with Hb.

The compound 2,3-DPG is present in red blood cells in high concentration relative to that in other cells, because mature red blood cells (which have no mitochondria) respire by anaerobic metabolism (glycolysis), and 2,3-DPG is produced as a side reaction. 2,3-DPG binds to hemoglobin more strongly than to oxyhemoglobin and thereby reduces its affinity for oxygen. The concentration of 2,3-DPG increases in chronic hypoxemia (decreased Pa_{O_2}) and when blood [H+] decreases (increased pH), whereas the concentration of 2,3-DPG decreases in stored blood.

> One of the factors that favor oxygen flow across the placenta is that the hemoglobin (type F) of the fetus is not affected by 2,3-DPG. Therefore, the HbO_2 equilibrium curve for a fetus indicates a greater O_2 affinity (left shifted) than does the curve for its mother's hemoglobin (type A). Furthermore, the Hb concentration in the blood of a fetus is greater (up to 200 g/L) than in the mother's blood. Thus, the fetus's arterial blood has nearly the same O_2 concentration as its mother's blood, even though the arterial P_{O_2} of the fetus is less than 40 mm Hg.

Normally, shifts in [H+], P_{CO_2}, temperature, and [2,3-DPG] are small. For example, venous blood has a higher P_{CO_2} (46 mm Hg) and [H+] (42 nmol/L; pH = 7.38) than does arterial blood (P_{CO_2} = 40 mm Hg and [H+] = 40

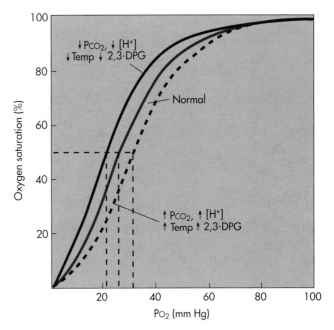

■ **Fig. 35-2** Changes of the hydrogen ion concentration [H+], CO_2, temperature, and 2,3-diphosphoglycerate concentration affect the affinity of O_2 for hemoglobin in the directions indicated by the black dashed curve (decreased affinity; shift to the right) and the solid black curve (increased affinity; shift to the left). A horizontal lightly dashed line at S_{O_2} = 50% is also shown. Affinity changes are quantified by their effect on P50. The curves are all of the same shape—only their positions have shifted.

nmol/L [pH = 7.40]). Therefore, the HbO_2 curve of mixed venous blood lies slightly to the right of the curve of arterial blood. The P50 increases from 26 to 29 mm Hg. Fig. 35-3 compares the HbO_2 equilibrium curves of arterial and mixed venous blood. At the mixed venous P_{O_2} = 40 mm Hg, the shift of the curve unloads almost 10% more O_2 without any further decrease in P_{CO_2}, and thereby an adequate P_{O_2} difference is maintained for oxygen diffusion.

■ *Comparison of Myoglobin with Hemoglobin*

Separately, each of the four globin chains with its heme group of hemoglobin combines with one molecule of O_2 in a manner similar to that of myoglobin, which is the single-chain heme pigment in skeletal muscle cells (molecular weight 16,500 daltons). The myoglobin-oxygen equilibrium curve (MbO_2) lies to the left of the HbO_2 equilibrium curve. The shape (hyperbola) of the myoglobin curve is also different, because each molecule has only one heme group, and therefore molecular interactions cannot take place among the heme groups. The HbO_2 and MbO_2 equilibrium curves are compared in Fig. 35-4. Because of the low P_{O_2} at which myoglobin binds O_2, the myoglobin is unsuited for O_2 transport. However,

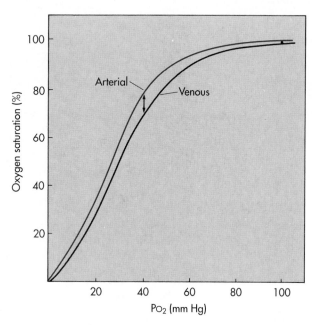

■ **Fig. 35-3**   Normal arterial and venous HbO_2 equilibrium curves. In the lung, the effect of the shift to the left caused by decreased hydrogen ion concentration enhances oxygen uptake. In the systemic capillaries, significant O_2 unloading begins at about $Po_2 = 70$ mm Hg and continues until the red cells leave the capillaries at $Po_2 = 40$ mm Hg. The rising $[H^+]$ concentration caused by the entry of CO_2 shifts the curve to the right, enhancing oxygen dissociation. The $P50$ of the arterial curve is 26 mm Hg; the $P50$ of the venous curve is 29 mm Hg.

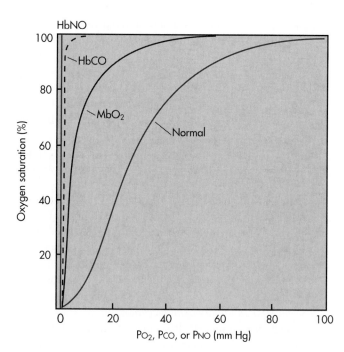

■ **Fig. 35-4**   Comparison among the saturation curves of hemoglobin for oxygen, the normal skeletal muscle oxygen carrier protein myoglobin (MbO_2), and two toxic gases, carbon monoxide (CO) and nitric oxide (NO). The $P50$ of myoglobin is about 5 mm Hg, which is close to the normal intracellular Po_2 of muscle. CO hemoglobin has a $P50$ of 0.4 mm Hg; NO hemoglobin has a $P50$ of about 0.001 mm Hg.

this molecule is useful for storing O_2 temporarily in skeletal muscle cells, where the Po_2 is normally low and within the range over which myoglobin is only partly saturated. The half saturation partial pressure ($P50$) of oxymyoglobin (5 mm Hg) is a reasonable estimate of the Po_2 in the mitochondria of resting skeletal muscle cells.

■ *Carbon Monoxide and Nitric Oxide: Two Pathological Ligands of Hemoglobin*

Fig. 35-4 also shows the equilibrium curve for two pathological hemoglobins: carbon monoxide hemoglobin (HbCO) and nitric oxide hemoglobin (HbNO). O_2, CO, and NO are specific **ligands** for the ferrous iron in hemoglobin, because each is able to donate two electrons to form coordinate covalent bonds. CO has more than 250 times the **affinity** (binding stability) for Hb than does oxygen. Therefore CO associates with hemoglobin more readily than does oxygen and it does not dissociate unless the Pco is very low.

CO is produced when hemoglobin is catabolized in the liver. Because humans degrade almost 1% of their red blood cells daily, they produce considerable CO and HbCO. Fortunately, the CO is steadily removed in the

expired air, because the $P_{ACO} = 0$ normally. Circulating HbCO rarely exceeds 1% to 2% of total hemoglobin.

Cigarette smokers and people who drive in heavy urban traffic may have high levels of HbCO in their blood. Several hours are required for the body to rid itself of the excess CO.

Nitric oxide (NO) binds to hemoglobin 200,000 times more strongly than does oxygen and 1000 times more strongly than does CO. Any endothelial NO that diffuses into the flowing blood is bound by hemoglobin irreversibly. Even when Pno is less than 0.001 mm Hg, hemoglobin will bind it until no more NO is available. Although NO toxicity is a rare form of poisoning, physicians who advise long-term inhalation of NO to reverse pulmonary hypertension must consider its cumulative toxicity. Fig. 35-4 shows that the equilibrium curve for HbNO is a vertical line, parallel to the Y axis.

■ *Position of the HbO_2 Curve and O_2 Transport*

A shift to the right (decreased O_2 affinity) of the HbO_2 equilibrium curve indicates that the quantity of oxygen that can be taken up at any $P_{A_{O_2}}$ is reduced as blood flows through the lung capillaries. However, because the HbO_2 equilibrium curve is nearly flat when P_{O_2} is above 70 mm Hg, the arterial oxygen concentration is not affected much by interventions that shift the curve to the right. A shift to the right of the HbO_2 equilibrium curve, however, indicates that the quantity of oxygen that can be dissociated (released) from blood is enhanced as it flows through the systemic tissue capillaries. This enhancement has the beneficial effect of increasing the delivery of oxygen at a given P_{O_2}. The rising P_{CO_2} and $[H^+]$ in systemic capillary blood is reflected by a slight shift to the right (P_{50} increases by 3 mm Hg). The small vertical arrow in Fig. 35-3 shows the difference in O_2 delivery when the HbO_2 curve shifts to the right because of the chemical differences between arterial and venous blood.

Conversely, a shift to the left (which denotes an increased O_2 affinity) indicates that the binding of oxygen by hemoglobin is increased at any specified partial pressure. This increase in oxygen binding enhances the uptake of oxygen in the pulmonary capillaries.

In the systemic capillaries, however, a leftward shift would not be helpful, because it indicates that the amount of oxygen that can be unloaded is decreased at any given P_{O_2}. This condition could lead to tissue hypoxia (insufficient O_2 for aerobic metabolism), unless it is compensated by an increased blood flow.

Effects of Blood Oxygen Capacity

Breathing affects $P_{A_{O_2}}$, whereas other factors (dietary iron, vitamin B_{12}, the hormone erythropoietin) regulate blood hemoglobin concentration. The usual HbO_2 equilibrium curve (Fig. 35-1), in which the ordinate represents O_2 saturation, does not show changes in blood O_2 capacity. To show such changes in capacity, we must let the Y axis represent the absolute concentration of oxygen (ml O_2/L).

The dark-colored line in Fig. 35-5 represents the normal blood O_2 content as a function of P_{O_2}. The light-colored line shows how a 50% reduction in the hemoglobin concentration (to 75 g Hb/L) would affect the equilibrium curve. On the O_2 concentration versus P_{O_2} graph, the anemia curve is moved down, reflecting the reduction in O_2 capacity. However, on a saturation versus P_{O_2} graph, the HbO_2 equilibrium curve would be identical for the normal condition (100% [Hb]) and for the 50% [Hb] condition.

Thus, the saturation versus P_{O_2} graph shows that the arterial P_{O_2} and P_{50} are not affected by a 50% reduction in Hb concentration. The mixed venous P_{O_2}, however, is reduced from 40 mm Hg to about 26 mm Hg, as long as cardiac output remains constant. Of course, cardiac output does not really remain constant as anemia becomes more severe. People with severe anemia compensate for the lower blood O_2 capacity by increasing cardiac output.

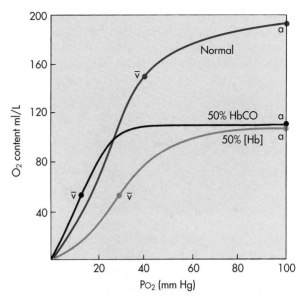

■ Fig. 35-5   Comparison of oxygen content curves under three conditions shows why HbCO is so toxic to the oxygen transport system. Fifty percent [Hb] represents a reduction in circulating hemoglobin by half; 50% HbCO represents binding of half the circulating hemoglobin with CO. The 50% [Hb] and 50% HbCO curves show the same decreased oxygen content in arterial blood. However, CO has a profound effect in lowering venous P_{O_2}. The arterial (a) and mixed venous ($\overline{v}$) points at constant cardiac output are indicated.

The heart accomplishes this increased output with only modest increases in left ventricular power output, because the blood viscosity is diminished as the hematocrit is reduced (see Chapter 25).

Shape of the HbO_2 Curve and O_2 Transport

Changes in the shape of the HbO_2 curve almost always denote deleterious effects on oxygen transport, because the shape change indicates an increase in the affinity of hemoglobin for O_2. Under this condition, the unloading of oxygen in systemic capillaries must occur at a lower P_{O_2}, and therefore tissue P_{O_2} decreases.

CO poisoning is the most common clinical example of an acute reduction in the ability of blood to carry O_2. Fig. 35-5 (*black curve*) shows how 50% HbCO in a person with a normal hemoglobin concentration of 150 g/L affects oxygen transport. The arterial P_{O_2} is normal, but the blood oxygen concentration is reduced to about the same level as for the anemia example (50% [Hb]). If this effect were the only one caused by CO, it would not be any worse than anemia. However, the HbCO line shows that the mixed venous P_{O_2} has moved far to the left. The reason for the very low $P\overline{v}_{O_2}$ is that when CO binds tightly to two of the four heme groups in each hemoglobin molecule, the affinity of hemoglobin for O_2 is disturbed and the heme group interaction is destroyed. The affinity of CO for Hb is so much greater than that of O_2 (Fig. 35-4) that, even at very low concentrations of CO in alveolar gas, the quantity of HbCO in the blood will be substantial.

As mentioned earlier, NO binds to hemoglobin far more tightly than CO. The HbNO equilibrium curve in Fig. 35-4 is a vertical line parallel with the Y axis. The P_{50} of HbNO is less than 0.001 mm Hg—1000 times less than the P_{50} of HbO_2. The combination is essentially irreversible, and it lasts for the lifetime of the red blood cell (120 days).

Fortunately, NO is not a common contaminant of air. Tiny amounts of NO are produced by internal combustion engines, but they are inactivated by catalytic converters. NO is an oxygen radical. It reacts with air to produce various oxides of nitrogen, of which the brown, irritant gas nitrogen dioxide (NO_2), is the main product. Unlike CO, NO_2 can be easily detected. NO in tiny quantities (< 100 ppm; $P_{N_2} < 0.1$ mm Hg) is being evaluated as a therapy in various types of pulmonary hypertension. Obviously, physicians are concerned about the effects of NO on blood oxygen transport. To date, the amounts of HbNO formed have been minuscule; most of the NO is converted to inactive forms in the lung tissue.

■ *Defects in Hemoglobin*

Several genetic variants of hemoglobin exist, some of which adversely affect the HbO_2 equilibrium curve. Normal adult human hemoglobin is type A or A_2.

The most common variant is **fetal hemoglobin (HbF),** which is the major hemoglobin in the fetus. It is normally replaced soon after birth by hemoglobin A. As mentioned earlier, HbF is beneficial to the fetus, whose arterial P_{O_2} is low (< 40 mm Hg).

Another variant is **hemoglobin S (HbS),** which crystallizes into long rods when P_{O_2} is low and [H^+] is increased. The rods distort the shape of the flexible red blood cells into a characteristic sickle shape. The resultant disease is known as **sickle cell anemia.** Although HbS binds O_2 in a manner similar to that in which HbA binds O_2, red blood cells that contain HbS have more 2,3-DPG, and consequently the HbO_2 curve is shifted to the right.

The problem in sickle cell disease is not so much with oxygen transport, but with the physical obstruction of microvessels when the red blood cells change shape and then tangle and form microemboli. Anemia caused by a shortened red cell lifespan also occurs. **Sickle cell trait** (one HbS and one HbA gene) occurs

principally in black Africans. In Africa, sickling may have conferred an evolutionary advantage. Sickling destroys malarial parasites that reside in red blood cells. Malaria is endemic in many parts of equatorial Africa. Sickle cell disease (two HbS genes) is a very serious problem, not compatible with longevity, although newer treatments can prevent most sickling crises.

In most genetic variants of hemoglobin the heme-heme interaction is destroyed. This interaction normally gives hemoglobin its great functional value. The equilibrium curves are hyperbolic, as is that of MbO_2, which indicates these forms of hemoglobin are useless for O_2 transport. If these variant Hb forms constitute a substantial fraction of the circulating hemoglobin, they are lethal, either in utero or shortly after birth.

Another factor that affects the HbO_2 equilibrium is the oxidation of the heme iron from its functional ferrous state (Fe^{++}; reduced) to the nonfunctional ferric state (Fe^{+++}). Normally, reducing enzymes present in erythrocytes keep Hb in its ferrous form. However, certain compounds (nitrates and sulfates) can increase the oxidized hemoglobin content and cause a condition known as **methemoglobinemia.** Oxidized hemoglobin does not bind or transport oxygen.

■ *Erythropoietin Regulation of Red Blood Cell Production*

Erythropoietin is a hormone produced by the kidney in response to decreased renal oxygen delivery. Both hemoglobin concentration and Pa_{O_2} can modulate erythropoietin secretion. When oxygen delivery to the kidney declines—even slightly—renal cortical interstitial cells produce and secrete erythropoietin, which goes to the bone marrow and stimulates erythropoiesis. The regulation is so finely tuned that circulating hemoglobin concentration is normally very stable.

What possible oxygen sensing mechanism can detect small changes in oxygen transport? *Erythropoietin production appears to be regulated by the local concentration of oxygen radicals in the cortex of the kidney.* Evidence suggests that O_2-sensing mechanisms are located in organs that have high oxygen delivery rates relative to their metabolism. Both lung and kidney share this characteristic, as does the carotid body (see Chapter 28). Renal cortical blood flow is high and the tissue P_{O_2} is also high. Both hypoxic hypoxia and anemic hypoxia lower the renal cortical Pt_{O_2} and stimulate erythropoietin production.

In the anemia associated with chronic renal failure, the circulating hemoglobin concentration may be 50 g/L, because of inadequate renal output of erythropoietin. Exactly why the interstitial cells stop producing the hormone is not known; the interstitial cells may have been destroyed by the disease process. When the patient is treated with erythropoietin, the blood oxygen level often improves dramatically.

■ *Oxygen Diffusion*

The two critical steps in oxygen transport from ambient air to the tissue mitochondria are (1) diffusion from the alveolar gas phase to the red blood cells in the lung capillaries and (2) diffusion from the systemic capillaries to the mitochondria in the cells of the peripheral tissues.

■ *Oxygen Diffusion across the Alveolocapillary Barrier*

In subjects at rest or under stress, the time it takes for red blood cells to move through the capillaries is nearly always adequate for the P_{O_2} in the red blood cells to come into equilibrium with the P_{O_2} in the alveolar gas. In other words, diffusion is not rate limiting. The pulmonary capillary blood volume is about equal to the stroke volume of the right ventricle; thus, red blood cells have the time of about one cardiac cycle for gas exchange.

Inert gases (e.g., nitrogen, anesthetic gases) equilibrate between alveolar gas and pulmonary capillary blood very rapidly (several milliseconds). The reason why oxygen is transferred at a slower rate than these gases is that the mixed venous blood (50 ml/L) has an enormous unfilled capacity for O_2 . In other words, the "effective" solubility of oxygen in blood is markedly increased by hemoglobin. Although the rate of the chemical reaction $Hb + O_2 \rightarrow HbO_2$ is rapid (milliseconds), equilibration is significantly delayed because of the low solubility of O_2 in the water within the alveolar wall tissue and plasma.

For respiratory gases, the diffusion equation is:

$$\dot{V}_{O_2} = \frac{D \times A\,(P_{A_{O_2}} - P_{c_{O_2}})}{L^2} \qquad (35\text{-}1)$$

where $\dot{V}_{O_2}$ is the volume flow of gas by diffusion (oxygen consumption); D is the diffusivity, a number dependent on the molecular size and solubility of the gas; A is the effective alveolar surface area across which the diffusion occurs; and L is the path length (squared) along which the diffusion occurs. The O_2 partial pressure difference is the driving force. The mean oxygen pressure in the pulmonary capillary blood ($P_{c_{O_2}}$) is a complex function, not only of the rate of diffusion across the air-blood barrier but also of the process of diffusion and chemical reaction that occurs when oxygen penetrates the red blood cells and chemically reacts with hemoglobin.

One example of a true diffusion limitation for oxygen arises when a person exercises strenuously (increased oxygen demand) while breathing air with a low oxygen content (alveolar hypoxia). Under these conditions, the driving pressure for oxygen diffusion ($P_{A_{O_2}} - P_{c_{O_2}}$) is reduced, while the oxygen demand ($\dot{V}_{O_2}$) and the cardiac output are increased.

■ *Oxygen Diffusion to the Mitochondria*

At the second critical point in the O_2 transport chain, namely, in the peripheral tissues, the diffusion conditions are not very favorable. *Tissue diffusion is the true rate-limiting process.*

The diffusion equation that applies to the peripheral tissues is slightly different from that which applies to the lungs:

$$\dot{V}_{O_2} = \frac{D \times A\,(P_{c_{O_2}} - P_{t_{O_2}})}{L^2} \qquad (35\text{-}2)$$

where A is now the systemic capillary surface area and L is the path length from the capillaries to the mitochondria. $P_{c_{O_2}}$ and $P_{t_{O_2}}$ are the mean systemic capillary P_{O_2} and the mean tissue P_{O_2}, respectively.

Arterial blood enters the systemic capillaries at a P_{O_2} of 100 mm Hg. However, $P_{c_{O_2}}$ must be substantially less than 100 mm Hg before any significant quantity of O_2 dissociates from hemoglobin. Thus, the mean capillary P_{O_2} is about 55 mm Hg; this value is closer to 40 mm Hg (venous blood) than to 100 mm Hg (arterial blood). The force that drives oxygen diffusion to the tissue cells depends on the partial pressure difference between the capillary blood and the most distant mitochondria. Fortunately, mitochondria can carry out oxidative metabolism when $P_{t_{O_2}}$ is as low as 1 mm Hg.

Under normal resting conditions, $P_{t_{O_2}}$ usually exceeds 5 mm Hg, which means that all mitochondria are receiving adequate oxygen. A reasonable estimate of mean resting $P_{t_{O_2}}$ is about 10 mm Hg. Tissue oxygen tension decreases progressively not only along the length of the capillaries but also in the radial direction away from each capillary.

The most important factor that affects tissue O_2 diffusion is the length of the path over which oxygen must travel to reach the tissue cells (Fig. 35-6). In the left ventricular myocardium, a vital tissue that requires a large oxygen supply per unit mass, the capillaries are about 25 μm apart—the width of one muscle fiber. Thus, from each capillary, oxygen must diffuse outward within a tissue cylinder with a radius of about 13 μm.

This may not seem to be a great distance, but it is ten times farther than across the alveolocapillary barrier. Also, because the diffusion rate is inversely related to the path length squared (L^2) (see equations 35-1 and 35-2)

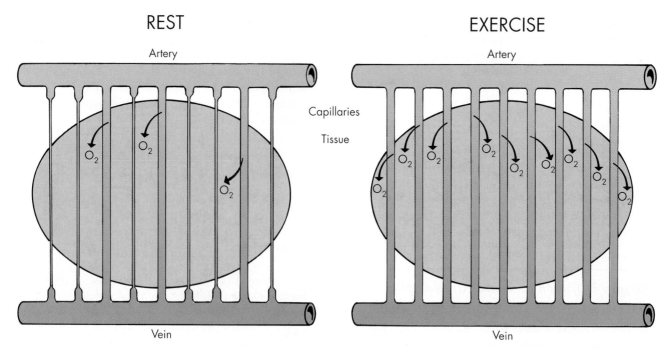

■ Fig. 35-6   Tissue oxygen transport is sensitive not only to capillary Po$_2$ but also to the distance over which oxygen must diffuse to reach all mitochondria. In skeletal muscle, there are about three times as many capillaries as required for adequate oxygenation under rest conditions. During strenuous exercise, all of the capillaries are perfused, thereby markedly decreasing the distance over which oxygen must diffuse to reach the mitochondria.

the same number of oxygen molecules require about 100 times longer to diffuse the 13 μm from the capillary to the farthest heart muscle mitochondrion than from the alveolar gas phase to the surface of the red cells in the pulmonary capillaries. In addition, mitochondria along the way extract oxygen from the blood, so that tissue Po$_2$ falls in a complex manner. In brain cortex, the capillaries are about 36 μm apart; in resting skeletal muscle, they are about 80 μm apart.

The most effective way for the body to improve oxygen delivery to tissue cells is to decrease the diffusion path length by recruiting more capillaries. This process also increases the surface area of the capillaries across which oxygen diffuses. Capillaries are recruited in skeletal muscle, where functional capillary density increases threefold during strenuous exercise (Fig. 35-6).

Although the rate of oxygen dissociation from hemoglobin is slower than the rate of association, the Po$_2$ of venous blood leaving an organ is very close to the Po$_2$ of the end-capillary blood under most conditions.

Cyanide poisoning is the classic example of a respiratory chain poison. It blocks electron flow from cytochrome a and a$_3$ to O$_2$. Other toxins, such as sodium azide (N$_3^-$), the pesticide rotenone, and the antibiotic antimycin A, work at different points along the electron transport chain. The effects of such poisons are very difficult to treat. Administering a high level of inspired oxygen has little effect. When exposure to the toxins is high, death occurs quickly, even though the venous blood is as well saturated with oxygen as the arterial blood.

■ *Tissue Oxygen Extraction*

The mean difference between arterial and venous oxygen concentration at rest is 50 ml O$_2$/L. More important, the net O$_2$ transport occurs only in arterial blood—from the alveolar capillaries to the systemic capillaries (Fig. 35-7). The remaining HbO$_2$ (150 ml O$_2$/L) serves as an O$_2$ reserve for use in emergencies (transient states of inadequate blood flow) and to maintain the Po$_2$ of systemic capillary blood at a level sufficiently high to drive adequate O$_2$ diffusion to the tissues.

Under maximal steady-state exercise conditions, a threefold increase in cardiac output may be associated with a sixfold increment in oxygen consumption. The steady-state mixed venous oxygen saturation does not often fall below 50% (P$\bar{\text{v}}_{\text{O}_2}$ = 29 mm Hg). However, the O$_2$ saturation in venous blood from some muscle groups may be less than 50% in strenuous exercise, especially in exhausting or non–steady-state conditions.

The normal myocardium extracts a large quantity of oxygen per volume of blood even at rest; that is, the coronary venous oxygen saturation is about 50% (see Chapter 30). Increases in oxygen demand by the heart are met almost entirely by an increase in coronary blood flow.

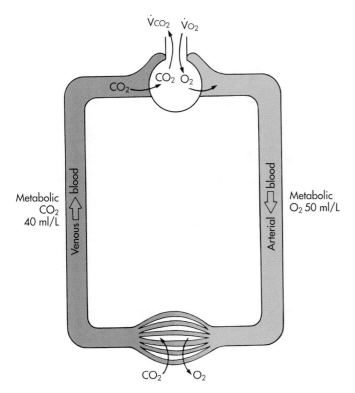

■ Fig. 35-7   Scheme of oxygen and carbon dioxide transport in blood. Metabolic O_2 transport occurs only in arterial blood; metabolic CO_2 transport occurs only in venous blood. The numbers shown for $\dot{V}O_2$ and $\dot{V}CO_2$ are for 1 L of blood. Their ratio is the respiratory exchange ratio, R, which at rest is about 0.80.

■ Carbon Dioxide Transport

■ CO₂ Concentration in Blood

One of the chief products of cellular metabolism is the volatile carbonic acid H_2CO_3, which is excreted mainly through the lungs as CO_2. The other important metabolic products are water, heat, and "fixed" or nonvolatile acids. Breathing also contributes to water and heat exchange, as mentioned in earlier chapters.

As Fig. 35-7 shows, metabolic CO_2 is carried by venous blood to the lung, where it is eliminated in the expired gas. The total amount of CO_2 thus transported, $\dot{V}CO_2$, averages 200 ml/min in a resting adult, but it may increase sixfold during steady-state exercise.

The basal secretion of carbonic acid in 24 hours is staggering. It is 200 ml/min × 60 min/hr × 24 hr/day = 288,000 ml/day. That is almost 13 moles of CO_2! A mole of CO_2 weighs 44 g, which brings the daily weight of expired CO_2 to 44 × 13 = 572 g—more than half a kilogram. If a person retained all that acid, he or she would die.

Normally, the quantity of CO_2 transported per liter of cardiac output is 36 ml (5 L/min × 36 ml/L = 200

■ Table 35-1   Transport of CO_2 per liter of normal human blood

PCO_2,	mm Hg	Arterial 36	Mixed venous 46	$a - \bar{v}$ difference 6
Dissolved,	ml/L	25	29	4
Carbamino,	ml/L	24	38	14
HCO_3^-,	ml/L	433	455	22
TOTAL,	ml/L	482	522	40

ml/min) (Table 35-1). At a normal $PaCO_2$ of 40 mm Hg, the total CO_2 concentration in arterial blood is about 480 ml/L, and in mixed venous blood it is about 520 ml/L. The large amount of CO_2 in blood and other body liquids is required for the maintenance of the hydrogen ion concentration, $[H^+]$, of the internal environment (see Chapter 44). Although metabolic CO_2 transport and hydrogen ion regulation occur simultaneously, and CO_2 and H^+ interact in venous blood, it is sometimes useful to think of them as two independent physiological processes.

■ Mechanisms of CO₂ Transport by Blood

As CO_2 is formed in cells, it increases the tissue PCO_2 above the PCO_2 of the arterial blood that enters the capillaries. The normal mean resting Pt_{CO_2} is about 50 mm Hg. CO_2, which is 20 times more soluble in water than is oxygen (αCO_2, 37° C = 0.7 ml/[L × mm Hg]), diffuses from the cells along its partial pressure gradient into the capillary blood. As Table 35-1 and Fig. 35-8 show, CO_2 is carried in blood in three forms; as **dissolved CO_2** (a tiny fraction of which is converted to carbonic acid $[H_2CO_3]$), as **bicarbonate ion** (HCO_3^-), and as a form bound to hemoglobin and plasma proteins (**carbamino-CO_2**). The mechanism of CO_2 transport is complex, but it is important to understand it.

Dissolved CO_2 is hydrated to form carbonic acid:

$$CO_2 + H_2O \leftrightarrow H_2CO_3 \qquad (35\text{-}3)$$

By physiological standards, this reaction is slow (it takes many seconds) in tissue liquid or plasma. However, it is markedly accelerated (microseconds) inside the red blood cell because of the enzyme **carbonic anhydrase.** Carbonic anhydrase is present in red blood cells but is virtually absent in plasma and interstitial liquid (Fig. 35-8). The equilibrium shown in equation 35-3 is normally far to the left; that is in the direction of dissolved CO_2. Thus, very little carbonic acid is in solution in body liquids.

As carbonic acid is formed, it rapidly dissociates into ions:

$$H_2CO_3 \leftrightarrow H^+ + HCO_3^- \qquad (35\text{-}4)$$

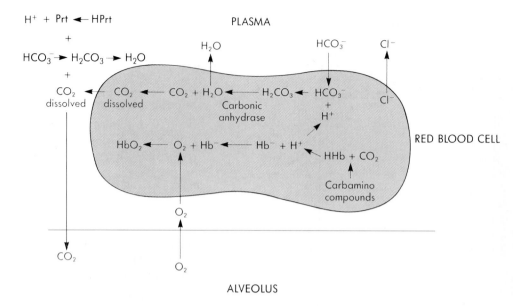

■ **Fig. 35-8** CO_2 exchange between the lung and blood in the pulmonary capillaries. The chemical reactions among O_2, CO_2, Hb, Cl^-, and H_2O are shown for O_2 uptake and CO_2 excretion. In the systemic tissues, these processes occur in reverse.

This reaction is spontaneous and very fast. It would not proceed far, however, unless the H^+ ions produced were removed from the reaction site. The hydrogen ions are removed from solution by combining chemically with the enormous amount of hemoglobin and, to a lesser extent, with the plasma proteins.

The newly formed bicarbonate ions diffuse out of the red blood cells into plasma in exchange for Cl^-, because the red blood cell membrane is permeable to both molecules. Thus, the total CO_2 reaction may be written as

$$CO_2 + H_2O \rightarrow H^+ + HCO_3^-$$

$$H^+ + Hb \rightarrow HHb \qquad (35\text{-}5)$$

The reaction proceeds rapidly in the direction of HCO_3^- formation, when CO_2 is added to systemic capillary blood.

Fig. 35-9 shows the CO_2 equilibrium curve of blood. Over the range of P_{CO_2} that is generally encountered in humans, the relationship is nearly linear, and this is very different from the HbO_2 equilibrium curve. Two lines are shown, because the CO_2 equilibrium curve is significantly affected by the oxygen saturation of hemoglobin; deoxygenated hemoglobin is a weaker acid (less dissociated into H^+ and Hb^- ions) than is oxygenated hemoglobin. As hemoglobin becomes deoxygenated in the systemic capillaries, its ability to bind with CO_2 (to form carbamino-CO_2) is increased.

The fact that the CO_2 equilibrium curve is nearly linear, whereas the HbO_2 equilibrium is markedly curvilinear over the useful ranges of P_{CO_2} and P_{O_2}, respectively, partially explains why the $(A - a)$ P_{O_2} is much greater than that for CO_2, when ventilation and perfusion are mismatched.

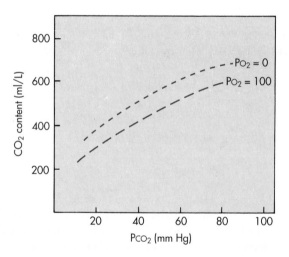

■ **Fig. 35-9**   Blood CO_2 equilibrium curves (arterial and venous). Venous blood can transport more CO_2 than arterial blood at any given P_{CO_2}. Compared with the hemoglobin-oxygen equilibrium curve, the CO_2 curves are essentially straight lines between P_{CO_2} of 20 and 80 mm Hg.

■ *Summary*

1. Hemoglobin quickly and reversibly binds with oxygen. The oxygen capacity of normal human blood (150 g Hb/L) is 200 ml O_2/L.

2. The position of the hemoglobin-oxygen (HbO_2) equilibrium curve is well suited for the loading of oxygen in the lungs and for unloading it in systemic capillaries.

3. Normal physiological factors that affect the HbO_2 curve include hydrogen ion concentration [H^+], P_{CO_2}, temperature, and the concentration of 2,3-diphosphoglycerate in red blood cells. Increases in any of these factors shift the position of the HbO_2 curve to the right, and thereby decrease hemoglobin affinity for oxygen.

4. A 3 mm Hg shift to the right (decreased affinity) occurs as blood passes through systemic capillaries, because P_{CO_2} and hydrogen ion concentrations increase. This shift increases O_2 unloading in the systemic capillaries. A 3 mm Hg shift to the left occurs in the lung, which favors O_2 uptake by blood.

5. The shape of the HbO_2 equilibrium curve indicates that in the systemic capillaries, hemoglobin releases large quantities of oxygen as P_{O_2} falls below 70 mm Hg.

6. The shape of the curve is affected by carbon monoxide (CO), which has 250 times greater affinity for hemoglobin than does oxygen. Even at very low concentrations, CO combines avidly with hemoglobin, interferes with oxygen binding, and destroys heme group interactions.

7. Nitric oxide (NO) binds to hemoglobin more avidly than does CO, but it is an unstable radical and is quickly converted to other oxides of nitrogen, especially to nitrogen dioxide.

8. Treatment of pulmonary hypertension by inhaled NO shows some promise.

9. The circulating hemoglobin concentration is closely regulated by the hormone erythropoietin, which is produced in the renal cortex when the P_{O_2} and oxygen-carrying capacity of systemic arterial blood decrease.

10. The current favored theory of erythropoietin regulation is that it occurs by means of oxygen radicals.

11. The transport of oxygen between body compartments is governed by diffusion at a rate that depends on the P_{O_2} gradient. The principal diffusion limitation for oxygen is from the systemic capillaries through several microns of interstitial liquid to the mitochondria of the respiring cells.

12. Carbon dioxide (CO_2) is produced by aerobic metabolism in mitochondria, diffuses into systemic capillary blood, and is transported to the lungs, where it diffuses into alveolar gas and is exhaled.

13. CO_2 combines with water to produce carbonic acid. In red blood cells, the enzyme carbonic anhydrase catalyzes this reaction. Once formed, carbonic acid dissociates instantly into hydrogen ions and bicarbonate ions. The hydrogen ions are removed by combining chemically with the enormous amount of hemoglobin within the red blood cells. The bicarbonate ions diffuse out of the red blood cells in exchange for chloride ions.

■ Self-Study Problems

1. Explain why normal people can function very effectively even when their systemic arterial P_{O_2} is only 40 mm Hg (e.g., hypoxic hypoxia of high altitude), which is the same tension found in normal mixed venous blood.

2. Several long automobile tunnels (Japan, Denmark, English Channel) have been opened since 1980. If the traffic in these tunnels is heavy, the average speed might be 40 miles per hour. What problems of oxygen transport may occur? How hazardous would a traffic stoppage be? Should people with severe lung disease be allowed to drive through the tunnel? What problems might confront maintenance workers in the tunnel?

3. Discuss whether edema-filled alveoli constitute a diffusion defect (the barrier is too thick) or a ventilation/perfusion problem (the alveoli are full of liquid). If the alveolar-arterial oxygen partial pressure difference was found to be 300 mm Hg while the subject was breathing oxygen for 10 minutes, what would you conclude about the mechanism of the arterial hypoxemia?

4. Describe how the oxygen supply to skeletal muscle is regulated at rest and during vigorous exercise.

5. Various drugs can antagonize the carbonic anhydrase in circulating red blood cells. What changes might you expect in the blood or in the body if you studied a person before and after such a substance had been taken? Distinguish between early (non–steady-state) events and steady-state events.

■ Bibliography

Journal articles

Crowell JW, Smith EE: Determinants of the optimal hematocrit, *J Appl Physiol* 22:501, 1967.

Staub NC: Alveolar arterial oxygen tension due to diffusion, *J Appl Physiol* 18:673, 1963.

Staub NC: The emerging role of the microcirculation in clinical medicine, *J Lab Clin Med* 98:311, 1981.

Wasserman K, Whipp BJ: Exercise physiology in health and disease, *Am Rev Respir Dis* 112:219, 1975.

Books and monographs

Comroe JH Jr: *Physiology of respiration*, ed 2, Chicago, 1974, Mosby–Year Book.

Murray JF: *The normal lung*, ed 2, Philadelphia, 1986, WB Saunders.

Nunn JF: *Applied respiratory physiology*, ed 3, London, 1987, Butterworths.

Schmidt RF, Thews G: *Human physiology* (English ed), Berlin, 1983, Springer.

Control of Breathing

The control of breathing can be summarized by this statement: *both the rate and depth of breathing are regulated so that Pa_{CO_2} is maintained close to 40 mm Hg.* In Chapter 32, we assumed that arterial (a) and alveolar (A) carbon dioxide (CO_2) tensions were ordinarily equal ($Pa_{CO_2} = PA_{CO_2}$). In this chapter we continue this assumption and use these terms interchangeably. Just as the alveolar ventilation equation (Chapter 32) implies, it is PA_{CO_2}—and not PA_{O_2}—that is controlled. When PA_{CO_2} is regulated, PA_{O_2} is automatically set (alveolar gas equation, Chapter 32) to an appropriate value that depends on the ambient partial pressure of oxygen and the health of the lungs ($\dot{V}/Q$ distribution).

The Pa_{CO_2}-sensitive mechanism is the main controller of breathing. It operates on a breath-by-breath basis as we go about our daily activities, so that we scarcely ever think about our breathing patterns. However, the Pa_{CO_2} controller can be overridden in systemic arterial hypoxemia (e.g., acclimatization to living at high altitude) by a Pa_{O_2}-sensitive controller. This controller takes over when arterial oxygen tension decreases below 60 mm Hg ($Sa_{O_2} = 91\%$). When the arterial oxygen tension drops to this level, the oxygen supply to the tissue mitochondria might be impaired because the oxygen diffusion gradient between capillaries and tissue is reduced (see equation 35-2). The Pa_{O_2}-sensitive controller prevents this dangerous effect of hypoxia.

■ *Central Organization of Breathing*

■ *Types of Control*

Two separate, but overlapping, patterns are involved in breathing. These patterns are the **metabolic** (automatic) control pattern and the **behavioral** (voluntary) control pattern. Metabolic breathing is concerned with oxygen delivery to the mitochondria. In addition, because metabolic breathing affects PA_{CO_2}, which in turn affects the concentration of hydrogen ions, this type of breathing is involved in acid-base balance. Metabolic breathing can be briefly overridden. However, within a minute or so, the metabolic control system reasserts its authority.

The metabolic **controller** (Fig. 36-1) lies in the brainstem, which also houses many other primitive automatic control systems. The neurons responsible for inspiration and expiration were previously thought to be located in separate brainstem centers. However, the organization is now conceived to be less specific.

Surrounding and scattered throughout the brainstem is a loose network of interneurons known as the **reticular activating system,** which modulates the brainstem controller by affecting the state of alertness (wakefulness) of the brain. Neurons in the suprachiasmatic nucleus (see Chapter 16) may also be involved. Sleeping and waking follow diurnal and lunar cycles (circadian rhythms).

Less is known about the behavioral control of the respiratory system. It is known, however, that higher brain center controllers in the thalamus and cerebral cortex are involved in behavioral control. Behavioral control is used to coordinate breathing in relation to the many complex, volitional motor activities that make use of the lungs and chest walls; one example is swallowing. Newborns can breathe and swallow simultaneously, but they lose this ability after several months.

Observations of patients with neurologic disorders often give important insights into the control of breathing. From these observations, a number of pathways that carry the cortical and thalamic descending axons to the primary brainstem controllers have been located. Various ablation, stimulation, and recording techniques have been used to explore the brain and to locate breathing control areas. At least two regions in the brainstem function as intrinsic breathing controllers: the **medullary respiratory area** and the **pneumotaxic center** in the pons (anterior brainstem). The brainstem provides nearly complete basic regulation. Even when the medulla is separated from the rest of the brain, the pattern of breathing is essentially normal.

The precise anatomic and functional organization of the respiratory neurons in the medulla continues to be refined. Two separate neuronal networks in the medulla appear to be crucial (Fig. 36-1). These networks include neuronal groups in the **nucleus tractus solitarius,** located dorsally near the exit of the ninth cranial nerve, and in the **nucleus retroambiguus,** a ventral group of neurons that extend rostrally from the first cervical spinal segment to the caudal border of the pons.

The dorsal group of neurons discharge mainly during inspiration. The ventral group contains neurons that are excited during both inspiration and expiration. Motor neurons from both the ventral and dorsal groups direct the respiratory activity of the muscles of the rib cage, diaphragm, and abdomen.

Efferent fibers from the dorsal and ventral motor groups cross over and travel contralaterally in the dorsolateral columns of the spinal cord (pyramidal tracts) to reach the motor neurons that contract the breathing muscles. The fiber tracts for voluntary control of breathing are located separately in the dorsomedial columns (extrapyramidal path).

Afferent nerve fibers from the peripheral chemoreceptors, baroreceptors, and pulmonary mechanoreceptors synapse with the neurons of the dorsal motor group. All the cranial nerves except olfactory (I) and optic (II) nerves enter the brainstem, where they are intimately associated with the primary respiratory neurons.

The mechanism by which the medullary neuron networks cause the switch between inspiration and expiration is not completely clear. Most of the evidence supports the concept that *rhythmic breathing depends on a continuous (tonic) inspiratory drive from the dorsal motor group, and on intermittent (phasic) expiratory inputs from the cerebrum, thalamus, cranial nerves, and ascending spinal cord sensory tracts.* Thus, breathing results from the reciprocal inhibition of interconnected neuronal networks.

Breathing is so automatic that we forget how fine-tuned it must be to allow for so many activities. **Ondine's curse** is a rare disease in which the patient must remember to breathe. The basis for **Ondine's curse** lies in the separation between automatic and voluntary control paths. Discrete lesions in the pyramidal tracts may eliminate rhythmic activity in the muscles of breathing but may leave voluntary breathing intact. A person with Ondine's curse can continue to breathe as long as he or she does not fall asleep.

One of the most common causes of death in the first few months of life is **sudden infant death syndrome (SIDS).** In this syndrome, parents find their baby dead in its crib for no apparent reason, except that it stopped breathing.

A network of neurons in the pons (**pneumotaxic center**) influences the switching between inspiration and expiration. When the pneumotaxic center is inactivated, inspiration becomes greatly prolonged. This pattern is called **apneusis** (prolonged inspiration that lasts tens of seconds).

Thoracic **mechanoreceptors,** chiefly stretch receptors in the walls of the airways, are crucial in setting the

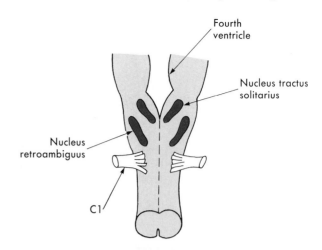

■ **Fig. 36-1**   The metabolic controller of breathing is located in the medulla (the most primitive portion of the brain). The neurons are mainly in two ill-defined areas called the *nucleus tractus solitarius* and the *nucleus retroambiguus.* In addition to breathing control, these nuclei subserve cardiovascular control functions. The reticular activating system (*not shown*) surrounds the nuclei, connecting with them and with higher brain centers to control the state of alertness.

breathing frequency. These stretch receptors are stimulated by lung inflation and deflation. The afferent impulses travel up the vagus nerves and affect the duration of inspiration and expiration. Neurons in the ventral motor group are excited by lung inflation. Stretch receptor input therefore mainly influences inspiration. Interruption of the stretch receptor traffic by cutting or cooling the vagus nerves prolongs inspiration (Fig. 36-2).

By artificially inflating the lung at different times in the breathing cycle, the effect of lung volume changes on the timing of inspiration and expiration can be demonstrated. For example, inflation of the lung when the phrenic nerve is active can terminate inspiration. The effect of lung inflation on the respiratory pattern depends on the volume of gas introduced; more volume is required early in inspiration to terminate inspiration, but less volume is required late in inspiration. After vagotomy, lung inflation does not affect the duration of inspiration. The input from the lung's stretch receptors has less influence when the subject is conscious than when he or she is asleep.

The timing of inspiration and expiration is automatically modulated under most conditions. For example, when the resistance to inspiration is increased, the decreased rate of lung expansion leads to prolonged inspiration. Hence, more time is available for gas to enter the lung and a constant tidal volume can be maintained, as in an attack of asthma.

The increased lung volume (functional residual capacity) of people with chronic obstructive pulmonary disease (mainly expiratory obstruction) slows the rate of

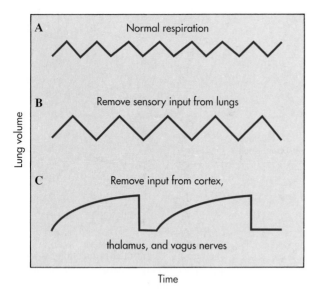

■ **Fig. 36-2**   Some patterns of breathing. **A,** Normal breathing at about 15/min in man. **B,** The effect of removing sensory input from various lung receptors (mainly stretch) is to lengthen each breathing cycle and to increase tidal volume so that alveolar ventilation is little affected. **C,** When input from the cerebral cortex and thalamus are also eliminated together with vagal blockade, the result is prolonged inspiratory activity broken after several seconds by brief expirations (apneusis).

breathing. These patients take quick inspirations followed by long slow expirations, so that dynamic expiratory airway compression is minimized (see Chapter 33). Stimulation of the stretch receptors in the lung and chest wall by the greater lung volume delays the onset of the next inspiratory effort.

The following operational model (Fig 36-3) synthesizes the brainstem mechanisms that generate the respiratory rhythm:

1. Signals from the central and peripheral chemoreceptors impinge on a pool of inspiratory neurons (pool A; dorsal motor group). These neurons send their main axons to the spinal motor neurons involved with breathing and increase their activity (induce inspiratory muscle contraction). Consequently, the time course of the increase in dorsal motor group activity is matched by changes in tidal volume. Increased input from various chemoreceptors (described later in this chapter) also increases the neural activity.
2. The central inspiratory activity stimulates another pool of neurons (pool B; ventral motor group in Fig. 36-3), which is probably also located in the nucleus tractus solitarius. In addition, pool B receives signals from pulmonary stretch receptors via the vagus nerves. As the lung expands, the stretch receptor signals increase and are added to the pool's input. Signals from stretch receptors in the chest wall ascend in the spinal cord. This activity also impinges on pool B.

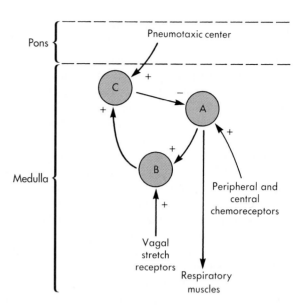

■ **Fig. 36-3**   The basic wiring diagram of the brainstem ventilatory controller. The signs on the main outputs *(arrows)* of the neuron pools indicate whether the outputs are excitatory (+) or inhibitory (−). Pool A provides tonic inspiratory stimuli to the muscles of breathing. Pool B is stimulated by pool A and provides additional stimulation to the muscles of breathing, and pool B stimulates pool C. Other brain centers feed into pool C (inspiratory cutoff switch), which sends inhibitory impulses to pool A. Afferent information (feedback) from various sensors acts at different locations: chemoreceptors act on pool A, and intrapulmonary sensory fibers act via the vagus nerves on pool B. A pneumotaxic center in the anterior pons receives input from the cerebral cortex, and it modulates the pool C group.

3. Pool B in turn activates pool C. Pool C is called the "inspiratory cutoff switch" because its output inhibits the main inspiratory neurons in pool A. When excitation reaches a critical level in pool C, the activity of pool A is extinguished and expiration begins.
4. An increase in chemoreceptor activity raises the cutoff switch threshold and enhances central inspiratory activity. Ablation of the pneumotaxic center in the pons also raises the cutoff switch threshold.

This model of breathing pattern generation (i.e., tonic inspiratory activity that is inhibited only when sufficient sensory signals are received) is attractive because no intrinsic cyclic neuronal activity has been found. The model also integrates the effects of changes in arterial blood CO_2 and O_2 levels (chemoreceptor activity) and of certain reflex stimuli into various normal and abnormal breathing patterns.

Cortical and thalamic centers modulate the function of the respiratory controller. As mentioned above, projections from the cerebral motor cortex that subserve behavioral (volitional) control descend to the respiratory neurons in the brainstem via the dorsomedial tracts and to the spinal motor neurons via the dorsolateral corticospinal tracts, which are located in the dorsolateral columns.

■ *Spinal Integration*

Descending nerve impulses from the brain reach various segments of the spinal cord, where they are integrated with intrasegmental and intersegmental activity to modulate the membrane potentials of the spinal motor cells. This modulation leads to rhythmic increases and decreases in the excitability of these motor cells (Fig. 36-3).

Excitation and inhibition of respiratory muscles involve segmental interneuronal networks and descending influences. For example, inhibition of antagonist muscles takes place through interneurons that connect the motor neurons of inspiratory and expiratory muscles. Stretch of intercostal muscles or electrical stimulation of dorsal roots in thoracic segments T9 to T12 excites intercostal and phrenic motor neurons and causes the thoracic cavity to expand. In contrast, stimuli to segments T1 to T8 inhibit phrenic motor neuron activity and terminate inspiration.

Spinal reflexes are important in breathing because they augment muscle force within the same breath, when respiratory resistance is increased or compliance is decreased. Spinal motor neuron reflexes that involve the intercostal muscle are especially beneficial to the newborn. The baby's cartilaginous rib cage is very compliant and needs to be stabilized during inspiration so that the subatmospheric pleural pressure does not suck the rib cage inward. Intercostal muscle stretch receptors sense the inward movement of the rib cage as a decrease in pleural pressure during inspiration. The nerves activated by these receptors cause the neurons to stimulate contraction in muscles that oppose the distortion.

■ *Chemoreceptor Control of Breathing*
■ *Carbon Dioxide*

In humans, the central chemoreceptors are located at or near the ventrolateral surface of the medulla, between the origins of the seventh and tenth cranial nerves (Fig. 36-4). These central chemoreceptors account for about 75% of the CO_2-induced increases in ventilation, and they respond to changes in the hydrogen ion concentration ($[H^+]$) of the surrounding brainstem interstitial fluid. The peripheral chemoreceptors (the carotid bodies) account for the remaining 25% of the CO_2-induced increases in ventilation.

Both central and peripheral chemoreceptors respond in proportion to the level of Pa_{CO_2}. Elevations of Pa_{CO_2} up to 100 mm Hg cause a linear increase in ventilation (Fig. 36-5). In a healthy, awake human subject, hyperventilation may drastically lower arterial carbon dioxide tension, but it rarely causes **apnea** (cessation of breathing). On the other hand, in anesthetized animals and humans, artificial hyperventilation may produce apnea. This difference is explained by nonspecific environmental stimuli (noise, light, or touch) that maintain the reticular activating system in a condition of alertness.

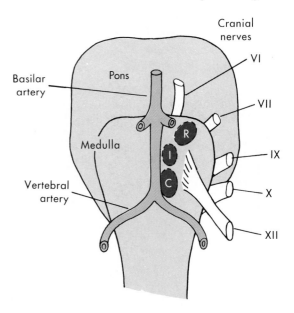

■ **Fig. 36-4** The locations of the three CO_2 ($[H^+]$)-sensitive areas on the ventrolateral medulla. The receptor cells are not actually at the surface but are close to it. *R*, *I*, and *C* refer to the rostral, intermediate, and caudal receptor areas, respectively.

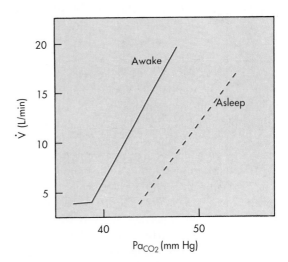

■ **Fig. 36-5** Dose-response curves for ventilation as a function of arterial P_{CO_2}. Sensitivity is defined as the slope of the line and the extrapolated intercept on the abscissa. The normal operating point is at $\dot{V}_E = 5$ L/min and $Pa_{CO_2} = 40$ mm Hg. The extrapolated intercept of about 35 mm Hg does not occur because other stimuli keep us breathing. However, when the reticular activating system is turned off, as during sleep *(dashed line)*, the ventilatory response to P_{CO_2} is decreased (reduced slope), and apnea occurs at about 40 mm Hg.

Sensitivity to CO_2 is quantified as the slope of the line that relates ventilation to Pa_{CO_2} (Figs. 36-5 and 36-6). Although inspired CO_2 quickly equilibrates with arterial blood and with the brain, considerable time is required for ventilation to reach its final steady state, because adjustments of various hydrogen ion buffer systems take place very slowly because of the blood-brain barrier (see Chapter 11). In normal individuals, the average acute

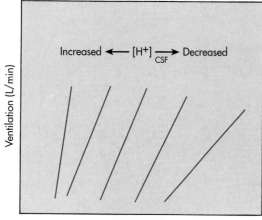

■ Fig. 36-6   The ventilatory response to P_{CO_2} is affected by the hydrogen ion concentration, [H⁺], of the cerebrospinal fluid *(CSF)* and brainstem interstitial liquid. When a subject is in chronic metabolic acidosis (e.g., diabetic acidosis), the [H⁺] CSF is increased and the ventilatory response to inspired P_{CO_2} is increased (steeper slope). Conversely, when a subject is in chronic metabolic alkalosis (a relatively uncommon condition), the [H⁺] CSF is decreased and the ventilatory response to inspired P_{CO_2} is decreased (reduced slope). The positions of the response lines are also shifted, indicating altered response thresholds.

ventilatory response to adding CO_2 to the inspired air is about 2.5 L/(mm Hg × min). The CO_2 response varies considerably among individuals owing to differences in body size, age, sex, genetic make-up, or personality.

The effects of long-term increases or decreases in arterial [H⁺] (chronic metabolic acidosis and alkalosis, respectively) on the ventilatory response to CO_2 are shown in Fig. 36-6. At any level of Pa_{CO_2}, ventilation is greater when acidosis prevails and less when alkalosis prevails. When fixed acid (e.g., HCl or H_2SO_4) is injected directly into the blood, the increased [H⁺] immediately stimulates the carotid body chemoreceptors. Hence, ventilation increases and Pa_{CO_2} decreases. The diffusion of CO_2 out of the cerebral interstitial fluid occurs much faster than does any of the brain's compensatory mechanisms. Thus, the cerebral interstitial fluid initially becomes alkaline (↓ [H⁺]) when ventilation increases, and therefore central chemoreceptor activity diminishes (reduced CO_2 sensitivity as shown in Fig. 36-6). Over many hours, the brain [H⁺] increases and ventilation rises toward a new steady state.

As noted previously, the carotid bodies (peripheral chemoreceptors) contribute about 25% to the total ventilatory response to CO_2. Because the peripheral chemoreceptors react rapidly to changes in inspired CO_2, their response to hypercapnia can be evaluated by measuring the immediate change in ventilation that occurs in the first few breaths after an abrupt change in inspired CO_2 concentration.

■ The Influence of Brain Blood Flow on Breathing

The P_{CO_2} of brain interstitial fluid also depends on cerebral blood flow, because the brain cells produce CO_2, just as do other cells. However, brain metabolism is fairly constant, and hence the rate of CO_2 production is constant. When cerebral blood flow rises, the interstitial fluid P_{CO_2} falls, but not below the arterial P_{CO_2}. Because hypercapnia increases cerebral blood flow (see Chapter 30), the effects of CO_2 on the cerebral vessels also influence the relationship between ventilation and Pa_{CO_2}.

■ Oxygen

Although CO_2 is the main controlled variable in breathing, oxygen can also become important in the control of breathing when the arterial P_{O_2} decreases sufficiently. Oxygen sensors in the carotid body are then stimulated, and ventilation increases. The relationship between Pa_{O_2} and ventilation is hyperbolic, as shown in Fig. 36-7, *A*. However, if the carotid bodies are removed, hypoxia depresses breathing, because the fall in brain P_{O_2} depresses the neuronal activity in the brainstem. This effect of hypoxia resembles that of most cells in the central nervous system.

The carotid body response to hypoxia is an emergency switch that is activated in severe hypoxia. As Fig. 36-7, *A* shows, hypoxia is a stronger stimulus when arterial P_{CO_2} is elevated. Thus, **asphyxia** (hypercapnia plus hypoxia) stimulates the drive to breathe much more than does hypoxia alone.

A decrease in oxygen radicals may be the biochemical trigger that activates the carotid body chemoreceptors when Pa_{O_2} decreases. The normal P_{O_2} of carotid body tissue apparently maintains sufficient concentrations of activated oxygen species to silence the afferent impulse activity over the carotid body nerve.

■ Factors That Affect the Responses to CO_2 and O_2

In most tissues, hypoxia acts as a depressant. In the brain, hypoxia inhibits cerebral arterial vascular tone and thereby increases brain blood flow. As mentioned above, an increased blood flow lowers brain P_{CO_2} somewhat, and thus depresses breathing.

Hypoxia accentuates the effects of hypercapnia and acidosis on peripheral chemoreceptor activity. This interaction is especially important in mediating the immediate increase in ventilation that occurs when blood [H⁺] is increased (Fig. 36-7, *B*). *Hypercapnia enhances the ventilatory response to hypoxia.* If a constant P_{CO_2} is not maintained when gases low in oxygen are inhaled, the ventilatory response to hypoxia is attenuated by the accompanying decrease in Pa_{CO_2}, as predicted by the

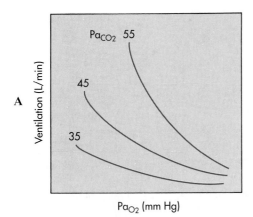

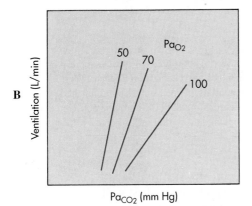

■ **Fig. 36-7** The effects of hypoxia (**A**) and hypercapnia (**B**) on ventilation as the other respiratory gas partial pressure is varied. **A,** At a given Pa_{CO_2}, ventilation increases more and more as Pa_{CO_2} decreases. When Pa_{CO_2} is allowed to decrease (the normal condition) during hypoxia, there is little stimulation of breathing until Po_2 falls below 60 mm Hg. The hypoxic response is mediated through the carotid body chemoreceptors. **B,** The sensitivity of the ventilatory response to CO_2 is enhanced by hypoxia.

alveolar ventilation equation (Fig. 36-7, *A*). This effect, of course, is the normal response to hypoxia.

Arterial Po_2 and Pco_2 rise and fall by 2 to 3 mm Hg during each breathing cycle, as alveolar volume and pulmonary capillary blood flow change. The change in arterial oxygen tension is trivial, but the changing arterial carbon dioxide tension affects the carotid bodies. The absolute level of Pco_2 and its rate of change are both involved in stimulating breathing. Thus, carotid body nerve activity is enhanced by increasing tidal volume, even when the mean level of Pa_{CO_2} is unchanged.

The central nervous system may modify the sensitivity of the peripheral chemoreceptors to alterations in Po_2 and the range of O_2 tensions over which they respond. Changes in sympathetic nervous activity alter carotid body blood flow, which is one way to affect the oxygen tension that surrounds the carotid body cells. Thus, decreases in carotid body blood flow increase its sensitivity to hypoxia.

Chronic hypoxemia, which can occur in people fully acclimatized to high altitude, depresses the ventilatory response to hypoxia. The respiratory depression may be due to adaptation of the peripheral chemoreceptors or the breathing controllers in the central nervous system.

■ *Mechanical Control of Breathing*

■ *Sensory Receptors in the Lungs*

Sensory receptors in the lungs and airways, as in other hollow viscera, are stimulated by irritation of the mucosa or by changes in distending pressure. Afferent sensory traffic travels to the brainstem via the vagus nerves. About 90% of the axons in the vagus nerves are sensory, and most of the sensory axons come from the lungs.

There are three types of pulmonary receptors: (1) stretch receptors located within the smooth muscle layer of the extrapulmonary airways; (2) irritant receptors that ramify among airway epithelial cells and whose distribution is similar to that of the stretch receptors; and (3) unmyelinated C fibers situated in the lung interstitium and alveolar walls. Receptors of the first type serve a regulatory function; the last two types are protective receptors.

The stretch receptors are excited by an increase in bronchial transmural pressure, and they adapt slowly to a sustained stimulus. As the lung is inflated, these receptors act to inhibit inspiration and promote expiration. They are responsible for the **Hering-Breuer reflex,** which produces apnea in response to large lung inflations and augments expiratory muscle contraction. The Hering-Breuer reflex is weak in adult humans but is strong in newborn infants.

Irritant receptor and C-fiber receptor neurons rapidly adapt when subjected to a sustained stimulus. Irritant receptors are stimulated chemically by various noxious agents, such as nitrogen dioxide, sulfur dioxide, ammonia, and inhaled antigens (pollens).

Industrial and environmental gases or particles may cause pulmonary symptoms or disease. Workers affected include farm workers (**silo fillers' disease),** various metal processing workers, and firefighters. Living downwind from a chemical plant can lead to widespread urban exposures when certain chemicals (e.g., chlorine, ammonia, or sulfuric acid) are released.

The irritant receptors can also be stimulated mechanically by lung inflation, increases in airflow (a sudden rapid inspiration of dry or cold air is often followed by a cough), particles impinging on the bronchial surfaces, or changes in bronchial smooth muscle tone (as in an acute asthma attack).

Irritant receptor stimulation causes cough, bronchoconstriction, mucus secretion, apnea, and glottal closure followed by rapid, shallow breathing. In addition to the primary defense mechanism of cough, this pattern of defensive breathing limits penetration of potentially harmful substances into the lung and thereby prevents these substances from reacting with the gas exchange surfaces.

The C fibers also participate in an intrabronchial axon-reflex that releases neuropeptides in the bronchial sub-mucosa and causes localized vasodilation and increased venular leakiness. Thus, activation of this reflex causes the mucosa to swell owing to vascular congestion and edema.

Bronchiolitis, most often caused by the **respiratory syncytial virus,** occurs mainly in children under the age of 2 years. The bronchioles do not normally contribute much to overall airway resistance, but when edema develops they can narrow and close. This reaction leads to **dyspnea** (difficulty in breathing), lung hyperinflation, and **cyanosis** (lowered arterial and venous oxygen saturation).

The irritant receptors may also improve lung compliance by initiating the periodic sighs (large breaths) that occur during normal breathing. These sighs expand the alveolar surface area and replenish the surfactant molecules. The chemical mediators (histamine, leukotriene C_4, or bradykinin) released in the lung during allergic reactions also stimulate irritant receptors. The augmentation of inspiratory activity and increases in breathing frequency produced by irritant receptor excitation may enhance ventilation during asthmatic attacks when the work of breathing is greatly increased.

C fibers may also be excited by distortion of the lung's interstitium, which occurs, for example, during edema, and by several chemicals, including antihistamine and capsaicin (the active irritant in pepper). Intense stimulation of C fibers causes laryngeal closure and apnea, followed by rapid, shallow breathing. Such stimulation may be responsible for **tachypnea** (rapid breathing) seen in patients with pulmonary emboli, lung edema, or pneumonia.

■ Receptors in the Chest Wall

As in other skeletal muscles, the muscles of breathing (the diaphragm, intercostal muscles, and anterior abdominal wall) develop force that depends on their initial length (preload) and on the force that opposes shortening (afterload). The preload varies with posture; the afterload varies with the effort required by chest wall expansion and by the resistance to airflow. The receptors in the chest wall modify motor nerve discharge to the breathing muscles through reflexes at the spinal cord level. In this manner, the receptors help minimize ventilation changes.

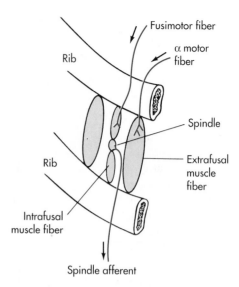

■ **Fig. 36-8** The intercostal muscle spindle and its innervation. The motor nerve (fusiform fiber) has its origin in the small γ motor neurons of the ventral horns in the spinal cord. The afferent neurons travel to the cord and participate in segmental, intersegmental, and central reflex control of posture and breathing.

The receptors in the chest wall include the joint, tendon, and muscle spindle receptors. These receptors are generally connected to large myelinated fibers. Because these receptors can sense effort, they are different from the intrinsic lung stretch receptors. Joint receptor activity varies with the extent and speed of rib movement. Tendon organs in the intercostal muscles and the diaphragm monitor the force of muscle contraction and tend to inhibit inspiration. Muscle spindles are abundant in the intercostal and abdominal wall muscles but scarce in the diaphragm. The spindles help coordinate breathing during changes in posture and speech. They also help stabilize the rib cage when breathing is impeded by increases in airway resistance or by decreases in lung compliance.

Fig. 36-8 shows the operation of the intercostal muscle spindle and its neural connections. Spindles are located on intrafusal muscle fibers, which are aligned in parallel with the main muscle bundles that elevate the ribs. Motor innervation of the intercostal muscles originates in ventral horn motor neurons. The intrafusal fibers, on the other hand, are innervated by γ motor neurons (see also Chapter 12).

Some of the muscle spindle receptors fire phasically with breathing, that is, impulse activity is increased during inspiration and inhibited during expiration. Other fusimotor fibers are tonically active. Without phasic activity, spindle discharge would decrease when the extrafusal fibers in the external intercostal muscles contract during inspiration. Simultaneous activation of fusimotor and motor neurons causes the spindles to be under continuous stretch during inspiration. This constant stretch enhances the contribution made by the intercostal muscles to breathing. When inspiratory movements are impeded (increased afterload), afferent activity from the chest wall sensory axons increases. This increase in afferent activity in turn increases inspiratory muscle force and helps preserve tidal volume within the same breath.

Spindle afferent fibers project to the cerebral cortex and provide the information that allows conscious perception of respiratory movements. The sensation of breathlessness (exertional dyspnea) during or after exhausting exercise or in various lung diseases may result from an imbalance in the demand for muscle shortening and the actual degree of shortening, as reflected by spindle afferent activity.

■ *Respiratory Failure*

Lung disease frequently interferes with the ventilatory responses to changes in the arterial tensions of CO_2 and O_2. The interference may be due to increased work of breathing, decreased efficiency of gas exchange, impaired chest wall muscle function, or reduced central drive in response to chemical or mechanical stimuli.

Normally, the reserve power of the diaphragm and chest wall muscles is enormous. However, people with severe impairment of chest wall muscle function may develop **respiratory failure.** In respiratory failure, ventilation cannot keep up with O_2 demand. According to the alveolar ventilation equation, Pa_{CO_2} must rise. Patients with the poorest chemosensitivity are the most likely to develop elevated Pa_{CO_2} (CO_2 retention).

■ *Abnormal Breathing Patterns*

Breathing is normally a smooth, cyclic process, but in some diseases of the central nervous system episodes of apnea recur. **Cheyne-Stokes breathing** is a manifestation of instability of ventilatory control in which tidal volume waxes and wanes cyclically in association with recurrent periods of apnea (Fig. 36-9). Blood concentrations of O_2 and CO_2 fluctuate markedly during Cheyne-Stokes breathing. It may appear during hypoxia, during sleep, or immediately after voluntary hyperventilation.

Cheyne-Stokes breathing is caused by a delay in information transfer (feedback) to the central and peripheral chemoreceptors. This breathing pattern occurs when the transit time around the circulation is prolonged; that is, when cardiac output is reduced, as in congestive heart failure.

In **Biot's breathing,** periods of normal breathing are interrupted by sudden periods of apnea. The mechanism for this pattern is unclear; it may be a variant of Cheyne-Stokes breathing. It occurs in patients with central nervous system diseases, especially meningitis.

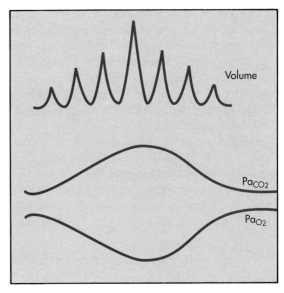

■ Fig. 36-9 In Cheyne-Stokes breathing, tidal volume and consequently arterial blood gases wax and wane. Generally, Cheyne-Stokes breathing is a sign of vasomotor instability, particularly low cardiac output.

Grossly irregular breathing occurs in some patients with medullary lesions and occasionally in persons with absent responses to chemical stimuli (primary alveolar hypoventilation).

Increased breathing with hypocapnia occurs in diseases that excite irritant receptors or lung C fibers (asthma and pulmonary embolism) or that cause metabolic acidosis. In diabetic coma, this form of hyperventilation is called **Kussmaul breathing.**

Apneustic breathing, with its prolonged inspiratory pauses, has already been discussed.

Hyperventilation is also a symptom of the psychiatric disorder **hysteria,** which is also called **neurocirculatory asthenia.** The disorder involves anxiety-induced behavioral control mechanisms. The hypocapnia evoked by the hyperventilation induces cerebral vasoconstriction, which is sometimes sufficient to cause fainting from inadequate cerebral blood flow.

■ *Sleep*

In alert, conscious humans, stimuli from the environment act reflexly via brain centers to affect breathing, as we have previously described. Even when the chemical drive is weak, such stimuli help to sustain breathing, because alertness augments the environmental stimuli.

The state of alertness fluctuates even in awake subjects (boredom, day dreaming). However, the fluctuations are more pronounced during sleep, and they may markedly affect breathing. The neural and biochemical mechanisms that produce sleep involve an excitatory and inhibitory interplay among various areas of the brain. The suprachiasmatic and reticular activating systems are both shut down during sleep.

Sleep is divided into two main stages: a slow-wave stage and a rapid eye movement (REM) stage. Dreaming occurs during the latter stage (see also Chapter 16). Each stage is associated with characteristic changes in respiratory, central nervous system, muscular, and cardiovascular activity.

◼ *Regulation of Breathing during Sleep*

As sleep begins, the level of environmental stimulation is reduced and cerebral influences on the medullary controllers are withdrawn. Consequently, ventilation decreases and arterial P_{CO_2} rises during slow-wave sleep. Systemic blood pressure and heart rate decrease, hypercapnic ventilatory responses are attenuated, and the CO_2 response curve is shifted to the right (reduced sensitivity and threshold), as shown in Fig. 36-5.

REM sleep is divided into phasic and tonic stages. In tonic REM sleep, breathing remains regular, but tidal volume may decrease. In addition, the ventilatory response to inspired CO_2 is further reduced, but the ventilatory response to hypoxia is maintained. External stimuli and changes in blood gas tensions are less effective in producing arousal in REM sleep than in slow-wave sleep. Phasic REM sleep is associated with irregular breathing patterns, because the intrinsic activity of higher brain centers dominates respiratory neuron activity.

The activity of the upper airway muscles also decreases during sleep. Ventilation and the adequacy of gas exchange also depend on the caliber of the upper airways. These airways (nose, pharynx, and larynx) are convoluted and semirigid, but they include movable structures. During inspiration, the pressure within the upper airways and the extrathoracic trachea becomes slightly subatmospheric. This slight pressure drop tends to collapse the soft structures of the nasopharynx (uvula and soft palate) and to displace the tongue posteriorly. Consequently, upper airway caliber is reduced and resistance to airflow increases. Snoring, a mainly inspiratory noise, ensues. These effects are counterbalanced by the actions of the upper airway muscles, which enlarge and stiffen the various structures. In awake subjects, all of these muscles are tonically active. In sleep, however, the activity of the upper airway muscles is markedly reduced.

Various neural reflexes modulate breathing during sleep. Mechanical stimulation of the airways in animals in either slow-wave or REM sleep elicits reflex responses that differ from those observed in the awake state. For example, laryngeal stimulation during wakefulness produces coughing, but it causes apnea during REM sleep. Irritant and stretch reflexes not only affect the activity of chest wall muscles but also influence the muscles of the upper airway. The excitation of pulmonary stretch receptors by lung inflation can markedly reduce the level of activity of the vocal cord abductor and tongue protrusor muscles.

The phasic and tonic activity of skeletal muscle decreases during sleep, particularly in the REM stage. The loss of activity in upper airway muscles during sleep is far greater than the loss of activity of the diaphragm. Because of the relative loss of tone in the upper airway, the negative airway pressure created by the diaphragm during inspiration may be sufficient to occlude the upper airway.

◼ *Sleep Apnea*

Apneic periods occur during sleep in about one third of normal individuals. They are particularly frequent among men of all ages, but they are also common in elderly women. Apnea may last for more than 10 seconds and may be associated with reductions in arterial oxygen saturation to 75% or less (Pa_{O_2} < 40 mm Hg). These periods of apnea occur during all stages of sleep but are most common in the lighter stages of slow-wave and REM sleep.

Sleep apneas have been classified into two distinct categories: **central** and **obstructive** (Fig. 36-10). Central apnea is characterized by a cessation of all breathing efforts; pleural pressure does not oscillate and electrical activity is absent in the phrenic nerves that activate the diaphragm. In obstructive apnea, airflow ceases despite persistent breathing efforts, because the upper airway is obstructed. **Snoring,** a major sleep disorder, is an early manifestation of partial inspiratory obstruction of the upper airway. Arousal is an important element in terminating sleep apnea. Arousal may result from chemoreceptor excitation by hypoxia and hypercapnia.

Breathing disturbances that occur during sleep may be primary factors in certain diseases. In patients with such disturbances, prolonged and frequent obstructive apneas occur. The recurrent periods of hypoxia and hypercapnia may lead to polycythemia, right-sided heart failure, and pulmonary hypertension.

◼ *Exercise*

The ability to exercise depends on the capacity of the cardiovascular and respiratory systems, acting in concert, to increase O_2 delivery to the tissues and to remove the excess CO_2 (see also Chapter 31). Only the respiratory adaptations are considered here.

■ Respiratory Adaptations to Exercise

Because of the low resistance and great distensibility of the vascular bed of the lung, the increase in blood flow during exercise is accompanied by only a moderate increase in pulmonary vascular pressure. During exercise, more capillaries are recruited, and the area available for gas diffusion increases, although the time spent by red blood cells in the capillaries is somewhat decreased. The alveolar-arterial Po_2 difference decreases slightly from the resting value in moderate exercise, reflecting the more uniform distribution of ventilation/perfusion ratios associated with the rise in pulmonary arterial pressure. However, as exercise intensifies, the Po_2 difference begins to widen as the non–steady state develops (which occurs when the anaerobic threshold is exceeded or with exhaustion).

As tidal volume rises, inspiratory pleural pressure becomes more subatmospheric. Hence, the airways distend, which increases the anatomic dead space. However, the physiological dead space decreases because of the improvement in ventilation/perfusion matching.

The ventilatory adjustments that take place during exercise are geared to its intensity and duration. During very brief intense exercise, as in the 100-meter dash, breathing is frequently suspended until the end of the exercise. With prolonged exercise, however, ventilation is elevated above the resting level, and it increases even more as exercise becomes more strenuous.

Acid-base balance is normal during steady-state exercise (up to about a sixfold increase in oxygen consumption), because O_2 delivery to the tissue mitochondria is adequate to meet all energy requirements. However, further increases in the level of exercise cause cells to use a combination of aerobic metabolism and anaerobic glycolysis. The lactic acid formed during glycolysis diffuses into the blood and increases the H^+ ion concentration, as shown in Fig. 36-11. The level of work at which a sustained metabolic acidosis (an increase in $[H^+]$) begins to develop is called the **anaerobic threshold** (Fig. 36-11). The level of the anaerobic threshold is higher in athletes than in untrained subjects.

When the level of exercise is below the anaerobic threshold, ventilation is linearly related to both CO_2 production and O_2 consumption (Fig. 36-11). Arterial Po_2, Pco_2, and pH are virtually unchanged from rest, although venous values are markedly altered (see Chapter 35).

The rise in arterial $[H^+]$ that occurs when the level of exercise exceeds the anaerobic threshold stimulates the carotid body. Ventilation increases out of proportion to the rise in O_2 consumption. Thus, because of the hyperventilation that results from the increased blood lactic acid level at very high work intensities, Pa_{CO_2} falls and Pa_{O_2} rises.

■ Mechanism of Exercise Hyperpnea

The increase in total and alveolar ventilation is the most important respiratory adjustment in exercise. Exercise

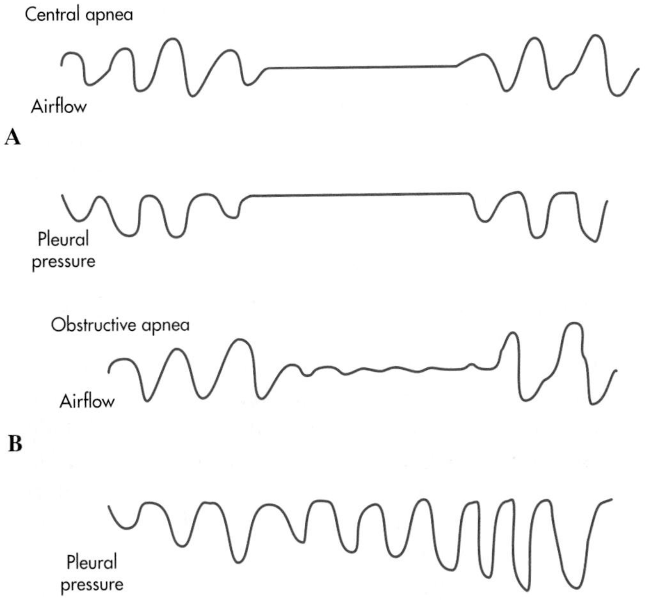

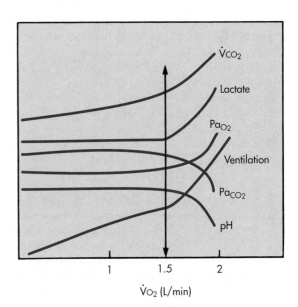

■ **Fig. 36-11** Some important metabolic changes that occur during exercise. The anaerobic threshold is marked by the sudden change in the measured variables, which is due mainly to the developing lactic acidosis as anaerobic glycolysis takes over more and more of the muscle energy supply caused by the relative failure of the body to supply sufficient oxygen to the muscles at the rate demanded by the level of exercise.

■ **Fig. 36-10** The two main types of sleep apnea. **A,** Central apnea is characterized by no attempt to breathe, as demonstrated by no pleural pressure oscillations. **B,** In obstructive sleep apnea, the pleural pressure oscillations increase as CO_2 rises. This indicates that airflow resistance is very high owing to upper airway obstruction.

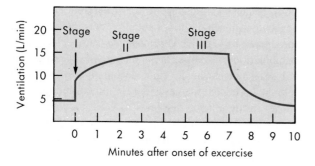

■ **Fig. 36-12**   The three stages of exercise: I, onset; II, transient period of adjustment; III, the steady state.

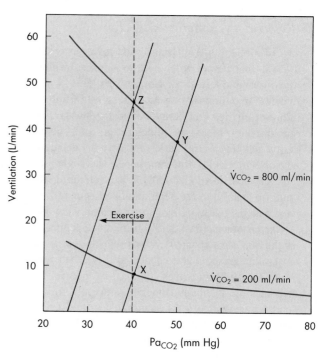

■ **Fig. 36-13**   Shifts of CO_2–ventilation response line between rest and exercise. On the basis of the CO_2 response line at rest (*X*), Pco_2 ought to intercept the exercise CO_2 production curve at *Y*, if the CO_2 response is unchanged. However, the response is shifted toward greater sensitivity *(Z)*, which maintains Pa_{CO_2} at 40 mm Hg. Ventilation has increased without any apparent rise in Pa_{CO_2}.

increases ventilation in distinct stages (Fig. 36-12). In stage I, ventilation increases abruptly; in stage II, ventilation increases more gradually; in stage III, ventilation remains constant. Both neural and chemical factors regulate ventilation during exercise. From 3 to 4 minutes are required after the beginning of moderate exercise before a new steady rate of ventilation is reached; with strenuous exercise, it may take longer. Preliminary warm-up reduces the time required to reach the new plateau.

The brain receives sensory inputs from various sources, and these inputs stimulate ventilation during exercise. These sources include (1) cardiovascular mechanoreceptors in the systemic or pulmonary circulations, (2) temperature changes that affect central or peripheral chemoreceptors, (3) mechanoreceptors in muscle, (4) receptors that monitor blood gas concentration and metabolic activity in muscle, and (5) receptors that monitor blood gas concentrations in the mixed venous blood. Ventilation may also be increased by general environmental stimulation of the central nervous system. It is not known which of the above-mentioned signals mediates the tight coupling of ventilation to metabolic rate. Despite large changes in CO_2 production and O_2 consumption during exercise, the steady-state arterial Po_2 and Pco_2 partial pressure remain remarkably constant. Hence, stimulation of chemoreceptors alone by changes in arterial blood gases cannot account for exercise hyperpnea (see Chapter 31).

Fig. 36-13 illustrates the response of the central controller to increasing Pa_{CO_2} at rest ($\dot{V}co_2$ = 200 ml/min) and in moderately heavy exercise ($\dot{V}co_2$ = 800 ml/min). If the exercise-induced change in ventilation were caused by the ventilatory drive from the newly produced CO_2 that accumulates in the bloodstream, the response line would intersect the curve for the higher CO_2 production at point *Y*. This point defines the elevation in arterial Pco_2 that would occur during exercise, if CO_2 were the only factor responsible for the hyperpnea. The fact that Pa_{CO_2} is essentially unchanged during steady-state exercise indicates that some factor sensitive to metabolic rate has increased the rate and depth of breathing. The effect of this metabolic factor is reflected by a shift in the CO_2 response line (see point *Z* in Fig. 36-13).

As mentioned above, the Pa_{CO_2} ([H^+]) fluctuates with breathing and produces corresponding fluctuations in peripheral chemoreceptor discharge. The oscillations of carotid body activity are greater during exercise because of the increased level of metabolic activity and the larger tidal volumes. These increases in metabolic activity and tidal volume may represent the additional drive that maintains ventilation in proportion to metabolic rate.

■ *Respiratory Effects of High Altitude*

As the altitude increases, the barometric pressure decreases (Fig. 36-14), although the relation is not linear. As an individual ascends from sea level to high altitude, Pa_{O_2} falls, as expressed by the alveolar gas equation. The resultant hypoxemia elicits a variety of compensatory responses. Some of these responses occur quickly, while others develop gradually.

The initial hyperventilation that occurs at high altitude is caused by stimulation of the peripheral chemoreceptors, mainly the carotid bodies. The increase in ventilation reduces arterial Pco_2 and [H^+]. These decreases in arterial Pco_2 and [H^+] in turn reduce the excitation of central chemoreceptors and thus limit the increase in ventilation.

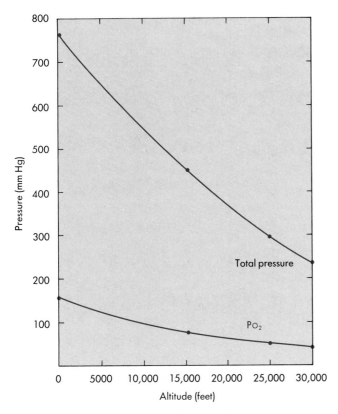

■ **Fig. 36-14** Barometric pressure and P_{O_2} fall exponentially as one ascends to high altitude (abscissa). The $F_{I_{O_2}}$ remains constant at 21%.

When a person has been at high altitude for 2 or 3 days, ventilation increases steadily as part of the acclimatization process. The increase in ventilation occurs, in part, by the following mechanisms: (1) the renal excretion of sodium bicarbonate reduces plasma HCO_3^- concentration and returns the blood [H^+] toward normal; (2) the HCO_3^- concentration is decreased in brain interstitial fluid, probably by a metabolic process that moves sodium ions from the brain interstitial fluid into the blood (reducing the strong ion difference that normally maintains plasma bicarbonate); and (3) a modest amount of anaerobic metabolism occurs in the hypoxic brain—this metabolic change permits lactate ions to substitute for the reduced bicarbonate ions.

Another important alteration that occurs at high altitude is an increase in sensitivity of the ventilatory response to CO_2 (steepening of the slope of the CO_2–ventilation response curve), as in Fig. 36-7, *B*. Consequently, the threshold for a stimulatory effect occurs at a lower P_{CO_2}.

People who live at high altitudes and who are chronically hypoxic slowly lose some of their ventilatory response to hypoxia. Hypoxic desensitization is more likely to occur when chronic exposure to hypoxia begins in infancy.

A similarly blunted response to hypoxia is found in patients who are hypoxemic due to a type of congenital heart disease in which blood is shunted from the right to the left side of the heart. Whether the blunted ventilatory response is caused by some depressant effect of chronic hypoxia on the central nervous system or whether it originates at the peripheral chemoreceptors is not clear.

Exposure to high altitude also increases the hemoglobin concentration (hematocrit) and consequently augments the blood oxygen-carrying capacity. The increase in red blood cell production is caused by increased secretion of erythropoietin from the kidney (see also Chapter 40). This hormone accelerates red cell production in the bone marrow. During exposure to high altitude, the concentration of 2,3-diphosphoglycerate also rises in the red blood cell. The increased 2,3-diphosphoglycerate concentration decreases the affinity of hemoglobin for O_2 (see Chapter 35). The P_{50} of the blood is shifted to the right, which improves delivery of oxygen at a high P_{O_2} in the systemic capillaries. Thus, three mechanisms (increased blood O_2 capacity, a right-shifted HbO_2 equilibrium curve, and increased Pa_{CO_2}) conspire to maintain oxygen transport to the systemic tissue cells in the face of long-term hypoxia.

Occasionally, tolerance of high altitude disappears completely and serious symptoms develop, such as ventilatory depression, polycythemia, and heart failure. This intolerance to altitude (**chronic mountain sickness**) is relieved by descent to a lower altitude or by administration of oxygen. Once a person develops chronic mountain sickness he or she should no longer live at altitude.

■ *Effect of Age on Breathing*
■ *The Newborn*

One of the first changes that must occur after birth is the transformation of the liquid-filled fetal lung to one containing air. High distending forces are needed in the first few breaths to overcome the high surface tension that opposes alveolar expansion with air. With successful air inflation, more alveolar surfactant is recruited into the air-liquid interface, so that functional residual capacity stabilizes and the work of breathing is diminished.

The ability of the newborn to maintain air in the lungs also depends on how well the rib cage can resist the collapsing forces produced by contraction of the diaphragm (**paradoxical breathing**). In premature infants, the rib cage is very pliable and surfactant production may be poor. A 2-kg premature baby born at 36 weeks (a month early) is in a better condition than a 1-kg infant born at 28 weeks, before surfactant production begins. Both the soft rib cage and high surface tension increase the danger of lung collapse. Over the last 30 years, survival rates of premature babies have increased significantly. Corticosteroid-induced lung maturation, positive-pressure breathing, and artificial alveolar surfactant instillation are three of the more dramatic advances that have contributed to these increased survival rates.

Pulmonary vascular resistance is very high in the fetus, because the vessels are constricted and contain as much smooth muscle as systemic vessels (see also Chapter 30). Less than 10% of cardiac output passes through the fetal pulmonary capillaries.

Breathing may be irregular at birth, particularly in the premature infant. The patterns of breathing range from regular to frequent apneic episodes. In preterm infants, apnea is predominantly central; that is, breathing movements are absent. Responsiveness to CO_2 is less well developed in the immature infant.

As a defense mechanism against hypoxia, premature babies may reduce their basal metabolism. Therefore, increasing the environmental temperature above the neutral temperature (34° to 35° C) increases their metabolism and is counterproductive. Preterm babies and normal birth-weight babies respond to a reduction in inspired O_2 concentrations with a transient increase in ventilation for approximately 1 minute, followed by a sustained depression. This biphasic response to hypoxemia is explained by initial stimulation of the peripheral chemoreceptors, followed by an overriding depression of the brainstem respiratory controllers.

Changes in lung volume reflexly alter the timing of breathing more in newborns than in adults. A small but sustained increase in lung volume in newborns shuts off inspiration, prolongs expiration, and decreases the breathing frequency, via the Hering-Breuer reflex. Conversely, lung deflation reflexly increases the respiratory rate via stimulation of lung deflation receptors.

Pulmonary irritant reflexes have been elicited in the neonate; direct stimulation of the lining of the tracheal wall augments breathing efforts.

■ *The Elderly*

Pulmonary performance declines after age 30. The changes proceed at a variable rate that depends both on the aging process and on the extent of exposure to noxious agents in the environment (cigarette smoking is the chief hazard). As lung elasticity decreases, the transpulmonary pressure at a given lung volume decreases (i.e., lung compliance increases). Thus, the bronchi, particularly in the dependent portions of the lung, collapse at higher lung volumes (see Chapter 33). These changes account for the elevated functional residual capacity in the elderly.

As subjects age, the chest wall stiffens because of structural changes in the rib cage. Thus, compliances of lung and chest wall change in opposite directions. As muscle strength decreases in the elderly, vital capacity

and forced expiratory flow rates decrease. In addition, the internal surface area of the lung decreases as the alveoli become wider and shallower due to the loss of elastic fibers in the alveolar walls and alveolar ducts.

Ventilation/perfusion ratios become more variable with advancing age, and as a result arterial P_{O_2} falls about 3 mm Hg per decade. The arterial P_{CO_2}, however, is still regulated at 40 mm Hg, but the ventilatory responses to both hypercapnia and hypoxia are reduced.

■ *Summary*

1. Two main types of control regulate breathing. Metabolic (automatic) control is concerned with oxygen delivery and acid-base balance (Pa_{CO_2}). Behavioral (voluntary) control is related to coordinated activities in which breathing may be temporarily suspended or altered.

2. The respiratory control system consists of a central controller (driver) located in the brainstem (medulla and pons), an effector (mainly the muscles of the chest wall but also the smooth muscle of the airways), and various sensors that report back to the central controller the results of the intended action.

3. The modern view of the brainstem controller is that it contains a tonically active inspiratory neuron pool, which receives input from various sensors. The summed sensory input generally inhibits inspiratory activity. Higher centers regulate behavioral breathing by temporarily overriding the brainstem pattern generator.

4. The sensory component includes central chemoreceptors (on or near the surface of the medulla); peripheral chemoreceptors (carotid bodies); and proprioceptors (lung stretch, irritant, and C-fiber receptors; plus diaphragm, intercostal, and abdominal muscle spindles, and tendon and joint organs).

5. The medullary receptors are most sensitive to Pa_{CO_2}. The initial ventilatory response to CO_2 is large and occurs rapidly.

6. The peripheral chemoreceptors (carotid bodies) are sensitive to reduced arterial oxygen tension or to reduced carotid body blood flow. The normal response to hypoxia is scarcely manifested until Pa_{O_2} decreases substantially.

7. Irritant receptors in the large airways protect the delicate alveolar surfaces from particles, chemical vapors, and physical factors, mainly by inducing cough.

8. C-fiber receptors in the terminal respiratory units are stimulated by distortion of the alveolar walls (lung congestion or edema).

9. Many factors influence ventilation in exercise; the main controlled variable is Pa_{CO_2}.

10. Sleep is a complex phenomenon consisting of several phases during which breathing control varies. The sensitivity to both CO_2 and O_2 is diminished, possibly because the reticular activating system is depressed.

11. Acute and chronic hypoxia affect breathing differently, because of slow adjustments in cerebrospinal fluid $[H^+]$, which alter CO_2 sensitivity.

12. Control of breathing in the newborn and elderly is different from control in young healthy adults. Special features characterize breathing control in newborns and the elderly.

■ *Self-Study Problems*

1. In what physical activities is breathing an integral component?

2. Why is the anatomic location of the carotid body favorable?

3. Severe hemorrhage increases peripheral vasoconstriction and heart rate. Why does it cause rapid breathing?

4. Children may threaten to hold their breath until they die. Normally, why is this impossible?

■ *Bibliography*

Journal articles

Coleridge HM, Coleridge JCG: Pulmonary reflexes: neural mechanisms of pulmonary defense, *Annu Rev Physiol* 56:69, 1994.

Dempsey JA, Vidruk EH, Mitchell GS: Pulmonary control systems in exercise: update, *Fed Proc* 44:2260, 1985.

Euler C von: On the central pattern generator for the basic breathing rhythmicity, *J Appl Physiol* 55:1647, 1983.

Haddad GG, Jiang C: O_2-sensing mechanisms in excitable cells: role of plasma membrane K^+ channels, *Annu Rev Physiol* 59:23, 1997.

Long S, Duffin J: The neuronal determinants of respiratory rhythm, *Prog Neurobiol* 27:101, 1986.

Lydic R: State-dependent aspects of regulatory physiology, *FASEB J* 1:6, 1987.

Mitchell RA, Burger AJ: Neural regulation of respiration, *Am Rev Respir Dis* 111:206, 1975.

Pack AI: Sensory inputs to the medulla, *Annu Rev Physiol* 43:73, 1981.

Richter DW: Generation and maintenance of the respiratory rhythm, *J Exp Biol* 100:93, 1982.

Schiaefke ME: Central chemosensitivity: a respiratory drive, *Rev Physiol Biochem Pharmacol* 90:171, 1981.

Wasserman K, Whipp BJ: Exercise physiology in health and disease, *Am Rev Respir Dis* 112:219, 1975.

Whipp BJ, Ward SA: Cardiopulmonary coupling during exercise, *J Exp Biol* 100:175, 1982.

Books and monographs

Comroe JH Jr: *Physiology of respiration*, ed 2, Chicago, 1974, Mosby–Year Book.

Nunn FJ: *Applied respiratory physiology*, ed 3, London, 1987, Butterworths.

Phillipson EA: *Sleep disorders*. In Murray JF, Nadel JA, editors: *Textbook of respiratory medicine*, ed 2, Philadelphia, 1994, WB Saunders, p 2301.

THE GASTROINTESTINAL SYSTEM

Howard C. Kutchai

CHAPTER

37

Gastrointestinal Motility

The gastrointestinal system consists of the gastrointestinal tract and associated glandular organs that produce secretions. The major structures of the gastrointestinal tract are the mouth, pharynx, esophagus, stomach, duodenum, jejunum, ileum, colon, rectum, and anus. The duodenum, jejunum, and ileum make up the small intestine. Associated glandular organs include the salivary glands, liver, gallbladder, and pancreas.

The major physiological functions of the gastrointestinal system are to digest foodstuffs and absorb nutrient molecules into the bloodstream. The gastrointestinal system carries out these functions by motility, secretion (see Chapter 38), digestion, and absorption (see Chapter 39). **Motility** refers to the movements that mix and circulate the gastrointestinal contents and propel them along the length of the tract. Gastrointestinal contents are usually propelled in the orthograde (forward) direction; that is, away from the mouth and toward the anus. Retrograde (backward) propulsion does occur, however; vomiting is a notable example. **Secretion** refers to the processes by which the glands associated with the gastrointestinal tract release water and substances into the tract. **Digestion** is defined as the processes by which food and large molecules are chemically degraded to produce smaller molecules that can be absorbed across the wall of the gastrointestinal tract. **Absorption** refers to the processes by which nutrient molecules are absorbed by cells that line the gastrointestinal tract and enter the bloodstream.

■ *Structure of the Gastrointestinal Tract*

The structure of the gastrointestinal tract varies greatly from region to region, but common features exist in the overall organization of the tissue. Fig. 37-1 depicts the general layered structure of the gastrointestinal tract wall.

The **mucosa** is the innermost layer of the gastrointestinal tract. It consists of an **epithelium,** the **lamina propria,** and the **muscularis mucosae.** The epithelium is a single layer of specialized cells that lines the lumen of the gastrointestinal tract. The nature of the epithelium varies greatly from one part of the digestive tract to another. The lamina propria consists largely of loose connective tissue that contains collagen and elastin fibrils. The lamina propria is rich in several types of glands and contains lymph nodules and capillaries. The muscularis mucosae is the thin, innermost layer of intestinal smooth muscle. The mucosal folds and ridges are caused by contractions of the muscularis mucosae.

The next layer is the **submucosa.** The submucosa consists largely of loose connective tissue with collagen and elastin fibrils. In some regions of the gastrointestinal tract, glands are present in the submucosa. The larger nerve trunks and blood vessels of the intestinal wall lie in the submucosa.

The next layer, the **muscularis externa,** typically consists of two substantial layers of smooth muscle cells: an inner circular layer and an outer longitudinal layer. In humans and most mammals, the circular layer of the small intestine is subdivided into an **inner dense circular layer,** which consists of smaller, more closely packed cells, and an **outer circular layer.** Contractions of the muscularis externa mix and circulate the contents of the lumen and propel them along the gastrointestinal tract.

The wall of the gastrointestinal tract contains many interconnected neurons. The submucosa contains a dense network of nerve cells in the submucosa called the **submucosal plexus (Meissner's plexus).** The prominent **myenteric plexus (Auerbach's plexus)** is located between the circular and longitudinal smooth muscle layers. These **intramural plexuses,** together with the other neurons of the gastrointestinal tract, constitute the **enteric nervous system.** The enteric nervous system helps to integrate the motor and secretory activities of the gastrointestinal system. If the sympathetic and parasympathetic nerves to the gut are cut, many motor and secretory activities continue, because these processes are directly controlled by the enteric nervous system.

The **serosa,** or **adventitia,** is the outermost layer of the gastrointestinal tract. This layer consists mainly of connective tissue covered with a layer of squamous mesothelial cells.

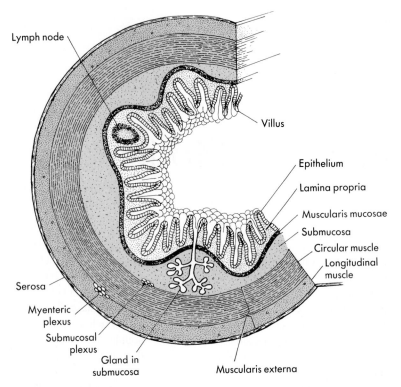

■ Fig. 37-1   The general organization of the layers of the gastrointestinal tract. (Redrawn from Ham AW: *Histology,* ed 3, Philadelphia, 1957, JB Lippincott.)

■ *Regulation of Gastrointestinal Tract Functions*

The functions of the gastrointestinal tract are regulated and coordinated by hormones, paracrine agonists, and neurons. Hormones are produced by endocrine cells and are released into the blood to reach their target cells via the circulation. Paracrine agonists are released by cells in the vicinity of the target cells and reach the target cells by diffusion. Regulation may be classified as **endocrine, paracrine,** or **neurocrine,** depending on the cell type that produces the regulatory substance and the route of delivery of the substance to the target cell.

Much of the hormonal and neural regulation of gastrointestinal functions is intrinsic to the gastrointestinal tract. In **intrinsic regulation,** both the cells that regulate and the cells that respond reside in the gastrointestinal tract. However, some hormonal and neural regulation of gastrointestinal functions is **extrinsic.** These extrinsic regulatory mechanisms are mediated by endocrine cells that are located outside the gastrointestinal tract and by neurons whose cell bodies are located in the central nervous system or in prevertebral and paravertebral sympathetic ganglia. These overlapping layers of hormonal and neural control allow for subtle and precise control of gastrointestinal functions.

■ *Gastrointestinal Hormones*

Endocrine cells are located in the mucosa or submucosa of the stomach and the intestine, as well as in the pancreas. These endocrine cells produce an array of hormones (Table 37-1). Some of these hormones act on secretory cells located in the wall of the gastrointestinal tract, in the pancreas, or in the liver to alter the rate or the composition of their secretions (see Chapter 38). Other hormones act on smooth muscle cells in specific segments of the gastrointestinal tract, on gastrointestinal sphincters, or on the musculature of the gallbladder (see Chapter 37).

■ *Paracrine Mediators in the Gastrointestinal Tract*

Paracrine substances regulate the secretory and motor functions of the gastrointestinal tract. For example, histamine is released from cells in the wall of the stomach. The substance is a key physiological agonist of hydrochloric acid (HCl) secretion by gastric parietal cells.

Other paracrine agonists are released by cells of the extensive **gastrointestinal immune system.** The mass of

■ Table 37-1   Gastrointestinal hormones

Location of endocrine cells that produce the hormone	Hormone
Stomach	Gastrin
	Somatostatin
Duodenum or jejunum	Secretin
	Cholecystokinin (CCK)
	Motilin
	Gastric inhibitory peptide (GIP)
	Somatostatin
Pancreatic islets	Insulin
	Glucagon
	Pancreatic polypeptide
	Somatostatin
Ileum or colon	Enteroglucagon
	Peptide YY
	Neurotensin
	Somatostatin

Gastrin, CCK, secretin, GIP, and motilin have been shown to have physiological roles in the gastrointestinal system. The physiological roles of the other hormones listed remain to be explained.

cells with immune function in the gastrointestinal tract is approximately equal to the combined mass of immunocytes (immune cells) in the rest of the body. The gastrointestinal immune system secretes antibodies in response to specific food antigens and mounts an immunologic defense against many pathogenic microorganisms.

The components of the gastrointestinal immune system include cells in mesenteric lymph nodes, Peyer's patches in the wall of the intestine, and immunocytes that reside in the mucosa and submucosa (Fig. 37-2). Mucosal and submucosal immunocytes include intraepithelial lymphocytes, B and T lymphocytes, plasma cells, mast cells, macrophages, and eosinophils. These immune cells secrete **inflammatory mediators** such as histamine, prostaglandins, leukotrienes, cytokines, and others. Once released, these mediators diffuse to secretory and smooth muscle cells in the gastrointestinal tract, where they affect their activities and modulate the function of neurons in the gastrointestinal tract. The gastrointestinal immune system is involved in some of the most troublesome gastrointestinal disorders, such as **celiac disease, inflammatory bowel disease,** and **Crohn's disease.**

■ *Innervation of the Gastrointestinal Tract*

Sympathetic innervation. *Sympathetic innervation of the gastrointestinal tract is mainly via postganglionic adrenergic fibers whose cell bodies are located in **pre-vertebral** and **paravertebral** ganglia* (Fig. 37-3). The celiac, superior and inferior mesenteric, and hypogastric plexuses provide sympathetic innervation to various segments of the gastrointestinal tract. Activation of the sym-

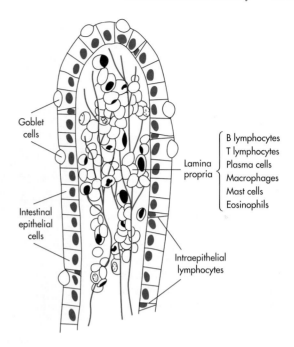

■ Fig. 37-2   A small intestinal villus showing intraepithelial lymphocytes and various immunocytes in the lamina propria. (Redrawn from Kagnoff MF: *Immunology and inflammation of the gastrointestinal tract.* In Sleisenger MH, Fordtran JS, editors: *Gastrointestinal disease,* ed 5, Philadelphia, 1993, WB Saunders.)

pathetic nerves usually inhibits the motor and secretory activities of the gastrointestinal system. *Most of the sympathetic fibers do not directly innervate structures in the gastrointestinal tract but rather terminate on neurons in the intramural plexuses.* Some vasoconstrictor sympathetic fibers directly innervate blood vessels of the gastrointestinal tract. Other sympathetic fibers innervate glandular structures in the wall of the gut.

Although stimulation of the sympathetic input to the gastrointestinal tract inhibits motor activity of the muscularis externa, it induces contraction of the muscularis mucosae and some sphincters. The inhibitory effect of the sympathetic nerves on the muscularis externa does not result from direct action on the smooth muscle cells, because few sympathetic nerve endings lie in the muscularis externa. Rather, the sympathetic nerves influence neural circuits in the enteric nervous system; these circuits provide input to the smooth muscle cells. The sympathetic nerves may reinforce this effect by reducing blood flow to the muscularis externa. Other fibers that travel with the sympathetic nerves may be cholinergic; still others release neurotransmitters that remain to be identified.

Parasympathetic innervation. Parasympathetic innervation of the gastrointestinal tract down to the level of the transverse colon is provided by branches of the vagus nerves (Fig. 37-3). The remainder of the colon, the rectum, and the anus receive parasympathetic fibers from

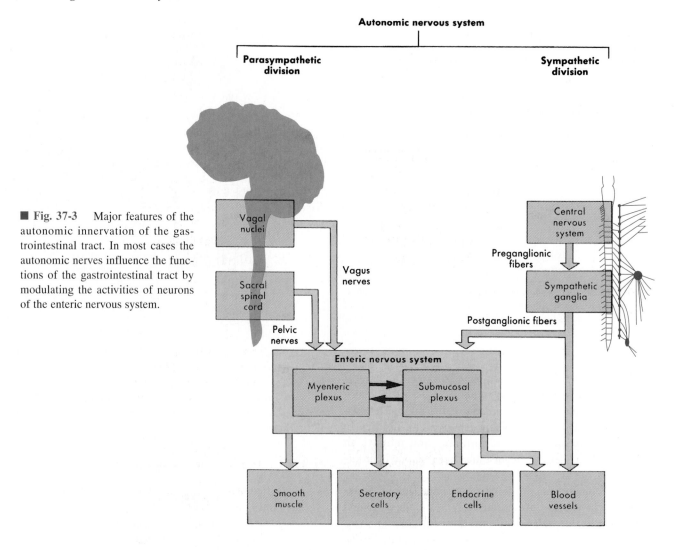

■ **Fig. 37-3**   Major features of the autonomic innervation of the gastrointestinal tract. In most cases the autonomic nerves influence the functions of the gastrointestinal tract by modulating the activities of neurons of the enteric nervous system.

the pelvic nerves. These parasympathetic fibers are preganglionic and predominantly cholinergic. Other fibers that travel in the vagus nerve and its branches release other transmitters, some of which have not been identified. The parasympathetic fibers terminate predominantly on the ganglion cells in the intramural plexuses. The ganglion cells then directly innervate the smooth muscle and secretory cells of the gastrointestinal tract. Excitation of parasympathetic nerves usually stimulates the motor and secretory activities of the gastrointestinal tract.

The enteric nervous system. The myenteric and submucosal plexuses are the best-defined plexuses in the wall of the gastrointestinal tract (Fig. 37-4). These two plexuses are networks of nerve fibers and ganglion cell bodies. Interneurons in the plexuses connect afferent sensory fibers with efferent neurons to smooth muscle and secretory cells, and thereby form reflex arcs that are located wholly within the gastrointestinal tract wall. Consequently, the myenteric and submucosal plexuses can coordinate activity in the absence of extrinsic innervation of the gastrointestinal tract. Axons of plexus neu-

rons innervate gland cells in the mucosa and submucosa, smooth muscle cells in the muscularis externa and muscularis mucosae, and intramural endocrine and exocrine cells.

About 10^8 neurons—about the same number contained in the spinal cord—reside in the gastrointestinal tract. These gastrointestinal neurons constitute the semiautonomous enteric nervous system. In addition to motor neurons that innervate muscle and secretory cells and blood vessels in the gastrointestinal tract, the enteric nervous system also contains numerous sensory receptors and interneurons. Sensory neurons that respond to mechanical deformation, particular chemical stimuli, pain, and temperature have been identified. The myenteric and submucosal plexuses give rise to bundles of nerve fibers that form nonganglionated plexuses, such as the **mucosal plexus** and the **deep muscular plexus.**

The extrinsic innervation of the gastrointestinal tract, via sympathetic and parasympathetic nerves, projects primarily onto the neurons of the myenteric and submucosal plexuses to excite or inhibit particular plexus neurons. In this way, the extrinsic innervation influences the motor

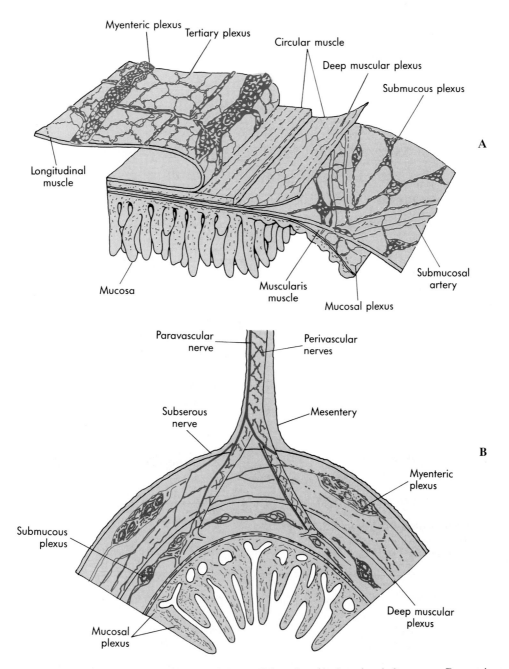

■ **Fig. 37-4** Major neural plexuses of the small intestine. (**A,** Seen in whole mounts; **B,** seen in transverse section.) The two ganglionated plexuses are the myenteric and submucosal plexuses. Fibers originating in the myenteric and submucosal plexuses form the nonganglionated plexuses: the tertiary plexus (which innervates the longitudinal layer of muscularis externa), the deep muscular plexus (which supplies the inner dense circular muscle), and the mucosal plexus. Neurons and neuronal processes are shown in color. (Redrawn from Furness JB, Costal M: *Neuroscience* 5:1, 1980.)

and secretory functions of the gastrointestinal tract via the enteric nervous system. However, much of the regulation of gastrointestinal activities is effected by the enteric nervous system, independent of sympathetic or parasympathetic input.

Reflex control. Afferent fibers in the gastrointestinal tract provide the afferent limbs of both **local** and **central reflex arcs** (Fig. 37-5). **Chemoreceptor** and **mechanoreceptor** endings are present in the mucosa and

muscularis externa. The cell bodies of many of these sensory receptors are located in the myenteric and submucosal plexuses. The axons of some of these receptor cells synapse with other cells in the plexuses to mediate local reflex activity. Other sensory receptors send signals back to the central nervous system. The complex afferent and efferent innervation of the gastrointestinal tract allows for fine control of secretory and motor activities by intrinsic and extrinsic reflex arcs.

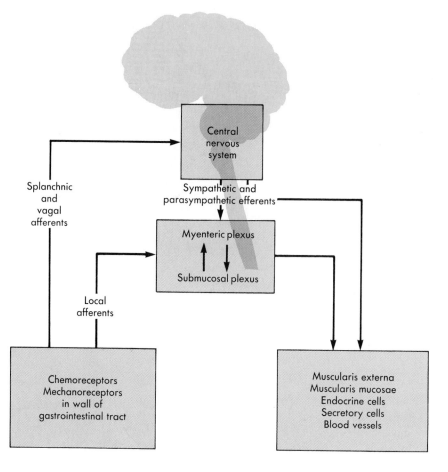

■ **Fig. 37-5**   Local and central reflex pathways in the gastrointestinal system.

■ *Gastrointestinal Smooth Muscle*

■ *Properties of Gastrointestinal Smooth Muscle Cells*

The smooth muscle cells of the gastrointestinal tract are long (about 500 μm in length) and slender (5 to 20 μm across). The cells are arranged in bundles that are separated and defined by connective tissues (see Chapter 19).

■ *Electrophysiology of Gastrointestinal Smooth Muscle*

Resting membrane potential. The resting membrane potential of gastrointestinal smooth muscle cells ranges from approximately −40 to −80 mV. The electrogenic Na^+, K^+-ATPase (see Chapter 2) contributes significantly to the resting membrane potential in gastrointestinal smooth muscle. In guinea pig taeniae coli, for example, almost one half of the resting membrane potential results from the electrogenicity of the Na^+, K^+-ATPase.

Slow waves. In most other excitable tissues, the resting membrane potential remains rather constant. In gastrointestinal smooth muscle, the resting membrane potential characteristically varies or oscillates (Fig. 37-6). These oscillations are called **slow waves** (they are also known as the **basic electrical rhythm**). The frequency of

slow waves varies from about 3 per minute in the stomach to 12 per minute in the duodenum.

Slow waves are generated by **interstitial cells.** These cells are located in a thin layer between the longitudinal and circular layers of the muscularis externa. Interstitial cells have properties of both fibroblasts and smooth muscle cells. Their long processes form gap junctions with longitudinal and circular smooth muscle cells. These gap junctions enable the slow waves to be conducted rapidly to both muscle layers. Because gap junctions electrically couple the smooth muscle cells of both longitudinal and circular layers, the slow wave spreads throughout the smooth muscle of each segment of the gastrointestinal tract.

The amplitude and, to a lesser extent, the frequency of the slow waves can be modulated by the activity of intrinsic and extrinsic nerves and by hormones and paracrine substances. In general, sympathetic nerve activity decreases the amplitude of the slow waves or abolishes them completely, whereas stimulation of parasympathetic nerves increases the size of the slow waves.

If the peak of the slow wave exceeds the cell's threshold to fire action potentials, one or more action potentials may be triggered during the peak of the slow wave (Fig. 37-6). The action potentials enhance contractile force of the smooth muscle.

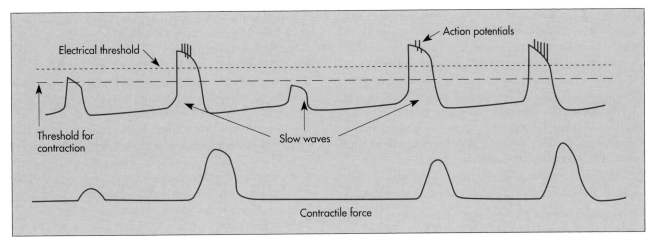

■ **Fig. 37-6**   Contraction of small intestinal smooth muscle occurs when the depolarization caused by the slow wave exceeds a *threshold for contraction*. When depolarization of a slow wave exceeds the *electrical threshold*, a burst of action potentials occurs. The action potentials elicit a much stronger contraction than occurs in the absence of action potentials. The contractile force increases with increasing number of action potentials. (Modified from Sarna SK: *In vivo myoelectric activity: methods, analysis and interpretation.* In Wood JD, editor: *Handbook of physiology*, sect 6, *The gastrointestinal system*, vol 1, pt. 2, Bethesda, Md, 1989, American Physiological Society.)

Action potentials. Action potentials in gastrointestinal smooth muscle are more prolonged (10 to 20 msec) than those of skeletal muscle and have little or no overshoot. The rising phase of the action potential is caused by ion flow through channels that conduct both Ca^{++} and Na^+ and are relatively slow to open. Ca^{++} that enters the cell during the action potential helps to initiate contraction (see Chapter 19).

When the membrane potential of gastrointestinal smooth muscle reaches the electrical threshold, typically near the peak of a slow wave, a train of action potentials (1 to 10/sec) is fired (Fig. 37-6). The extent of depolarization of the cells and the frequency of action potentials are enhanced by some hormones and paracrine agonists and by compounds liberated from excitatory nerve endings. Inhibitory hormones and neuroeffector substances hyperpolarize the smooth muscle cells and may diminish or abolish action potential spikes.

Relationship between membrane potential and tension. Slow waves that are not accompanied by action potentials elicit weak contractions of the smooth muscle cells (Fig. 37-6). Much stronger contractions are evoked by the action potentials that are intermittently triggered near the peaks of the slow waves. The greater the frequency of action potentials that occur at the peak of a slow wave, the more intense is the contraction of the smooth muscle. Because smooth muscle cells contract rather slowly (about one tenth as fast as skeletal muscle cells), the individual contractions caused by each action potential in a train do not cause distinct twitches; rather, they sum temporally to produce a smoothly increasing level of tension (Fig. 37-6).

Between trains of action potentials the tension developed by gastrointestinal smooth muscle falls, but not to zero. This nonzero resting, or baseline, tension of smooth muscle is called **tone**. The tone of gastrointestinal smooth muscle is altered by neuroeffectors, hormones, paracrine substances, and drugs.

Electrical coupling between smooth muscle cells. Neighboring cells are described as "well coupled electrically" if a charge in the membrane potential of one cell spreads rapidly, and with little decrease, to the adjacent cell. The smooth muscle cells of the circular layer are better coupled than are those of the longitudinal layer. The cells of the circular layer are joined by frequent gap junctions that allow the spread of electrical current from one cell to another (see Chapter 4).

■ *Neural Control of Gastrointestinal Activities*

Control of the contractile and secretory activities of the gastrointestinal tract involves the central nervous system, the enteric nervous system, and hormones and paracrine substances. The autonomic nervous system typically only modulates the patterns of muscular and secretory activity; these activities are controlled more directly by the enteric nervous system.

■ *Neuromuscular Interactions*

The neurons of the intramural plexuses send axons to the smooth muscle layers, and each axon may branch extensively to innervate many smooth muscle cells. Neuromuscular interactions in the gastrointestinal tract do not involve true neuromuscular junctions with specialization of the postjunctional membrane, as occurs at neuromuscular junctions in skeletal muscle (see Chapter 4).

The circular smooth muscle layer of the muscularis externa is heavily innervated by excitatory and inhibitory motor nerve terminals that are closely associated with the plasma membranes of the smooth muscle cells of this layer. In contrast, longitudinal smooth muscle cells are much less richly innervated by the neurons of the intrinsic plexuses than are the circular layer cells, and the neuromuscular contacts are not as intimate.

■ Sympathetic and Parasympathetic Control of Gastrointestinal Function

The major types of sympathetic and parasympathetic input to the gastrointestinal tract are summarized in Table 37-2. Most sympathetic and parasympathetic fibers project not onto muscle or gland cells in the gastrointestinal tract, but rather onto neurons of the enteric nervous system. Exceptions include the direct sympathetic innervation of gastrointestinal blood vessels.

Afferent fibers are abundant in the sympathetic and parasympathetic nerves to the gastrointestinal tract. These fibers carry signals from chemosensitive and mechanosensitive nerve endings in the wall of the gastrointestinal tract. The cell bodies of the afferent fibers in the sympathetic nerves are located primarily in dorsal root ganglia. The cell bodies of the afferent fibers in the branches of the vagus nerves are located in the nodose ganglion and in the solitary nucleus, whereas cell bodies of the afferent fibers in the pelvic nerves are located in sacral dorsal root ganglia.

The reflex control of gastrointestinal function effected by autonomic sensory and efferent fibers provides a central level of control that overlies and influences the local reflex control by the enteric nervous system. The central reflex pathways are clearly required for coordination of the activities of gastrointestinal regions that are located far away from one another. An example of this long-range control is the gastrocolic reflex: increased motor and secretory activity in the colon is coordinated with increased contractile and secretory activity in the stomach.

■ The Enteric Nervous System

As previously stated, the plexuses that make up the enteric nervous system function as a semiautonomous nervous system that controls the motor and secretory activities of the digestive system. Fig. 37-4 depicts the myenteric and submucosal plexuses and their locations in the wall of the intestine. Both plexuses consist of ganglia that are interconnected by tracts of fine, unmyelinated nerve fibers. Some neurons in the ganglia (Table 37-3) are sensory neurons; the sensory endings of these neurons are located in the gastrointestinal tract. Some of the neurons in the enteric ganglia are effector neurons that send axons to smooth muscle cells of the circular or longitudinal layers and muscularis mucosae, to secretory

■ Table 37-2   Extrinsic neurons of the gastrointestinal tract

Neural pathway	Function
In motor pathways	Sympathetic motility-inhibiting neurons
	Sympathetic vasoconstrictor neurons
	Sympathetic secretomotor-inhibiting neurons
	Vagal inputs to enteric excitatory pathways
	Vagal inputs to enteric inhibitory pathways
	Pelvic nerve inputs to enteric excitatory and inhibitory pathways and to enteric vasodilator pathways
	Vagal inputs promoting gastrin and acid secretion
In sensory pathways	Mechanoreceptor neurons
	Chemoceptive neurons
	Nociceptive neurons

The cell bodies of efferent neurons are in vagal nuclei, sympathetic ganglia, or the sacral spinal cord. The cell bodies of sensory neurons are in vagal nuclei or in dorsal root ganglia. (Adapted from Costa M, Furness JB: In Makhlouf GM, editor: *Handbook of physiology*, sect 6, *The gastrointestinal system*, vol II, *Neural and endocrine biology*, Bethesda, Md, 1989, American Physiological Society.)

■ Table 37-3   Neurons of the enteric nervous system

Type of neuron	Function
Motor neurons	Enteric excitatory motor neurons
To muscle	Enteric inhibitory motor neurons
To arterioles	Enteric vasodilator neurons
To epithelia	Enteric secretomotor neurons (cholinergc and noncholinergic)
	Motor neurons to gastric parietal cells
	Motor neurons to gastrointestinal endocrine cells
Sensory neurons	Distention (stretch)-sensitive neurons
Associative neurons	Chemoceptive neurons
Intestinofugal neurons	Interneurons in motility vasomotor and secretomotor pathways
	Neurons with cell bodies in enteric ganglia and terminals in prevertebral ganglia

The cell bodies of these neurons are in myenteric or submucosal ganglia. (Adapted from Costa M, Furness JB: In Makhlouf GM, editor: *Handbook of physiology*, sect 6, *The gastrointestinal system*, vol II, *Neural and endocrine biology*, Bethesda, Md, 1989, American Physiological Society.)

cells of the gastrointestinal tract, or to gastrointestinal blood vessels. Many of the neurons in the enteric ganglia are interneurons; these neurons form part of the neuronal network that integrates the sensory input to the ganglia and formulates the output of the effector neurons.

Neuromodulatory substances. Most of the neurotransmitters and neuromodulatory substances that function in the central nervous system (see Chapter 4) also function in the gastrointestinal tract. Table 37-4 lists some of the neuroactive substances present in the gastrointestinal tract and summarizes current knowledge about the functions of these substances in gastrointestinal control.

Table 37-5 shows the quantitative distribution of neuroactive substances, or biochemical markers of these substances, in neurons of the myenteric and submucosal ganglia of guinea pig small intestine. The distribution of neuroactive substances in myenteric neurons differs from their distribution in submucosal neurons. Enteric neurons often contain more than one putative neurotransmitter or neuromodulator, and *these neurons may release more than one neuroactive substance in response to stimulation.* The combination of neuroactive substances present in a particular neuron correlates with the morphology and function of the neuron and with its projections.

■ **Table 37-4**   Substances that may be neurotransmitters or neuromodulators in the enteric nervous system

Substance	Location and role
Acetylcholine (ACh)	Primary excitatory transmitter to muscle, to intestinal epithelium, to parietal cells, to some gut endocrine cells, and at neuroneuronal synapses
Adenosine triphosphate (ATP)	Probably contributes to transmission from enteric inhibitory muscle motor neurons
γ-Aminobutyric acid (GABA)	Present in different populations of neurons, depending on species and region Does not appear to be a primary neurotransmitter
Calcitonin gene–related peptide (CGRP)	Present in some secretomotor neurons and interneurons Role unknown
Cholecystokinin (CCK)	Present in some secretomotor neurons and in some interneurons May contribute to excitatory transmission Generally excites muscle
Dynorphin (DYN) and dynorphin-related peptides	Present in secretomotor neurons, interneurons, and motor neurons to muscle Does not appear to be a primary transmitter
Enkephalin (ENK) and enkephalin-related peptides	Present in interneurons and muscle motor neurons In most regions these substances probably provide feedback inhibition of transmitter release
Galanin	Present in secretomotor neurons, descending interneurons, and inhibitory motor neurons in human intestine Role unknown
Gastrin-releasing peptide (GRP) (mammalian bombesin)	Excitatory transmitter to gastrin cells Also found in nerve fibers to muscle and in interneurons, where its roles are not known
Neuropeptide Y	Present in secretomotor neurons, where it appears to inhibit secretion of water and electrolytes Also present in interneurons and inhibitory muscle motor neurons
Nitric oxide (NO)	A cotransmitter from enteric inhibitory muscle motor neurons Possible transmitter at neuroneuronal synapses
Norepinephrine	Noradrenergic nerve fibers in the intestine are not strictly enteric: they are of sympathetic origin Major roles are to inhibit motility in nonsphincter regions, to contract the muscle of the sphincters, to inhibit secretomotor reflexes, and to act as vasoconstrictor neurons to enteric arterioles
Serotonin (5-HT)	Appears to participate in excitatory neuroneuronal transmission
Somatostatin	Despite its widespread distribution in enteric neurons, no clearly defined roles have been established
Tachykinins (substance P, neurokinin A, neuropeptide K, and neuropeptide γ)	Excitatory transmitters to muscle; and are cotransmitters with ACh May contribute to excitatory neuroneuronal transmission
Vasoactive intestinal peptide (VIP) (and peptide histidine isoleucine [PHI])	Excitatory transmitter from secretomotor neurons Possibly a transmitter of enteric vasodilator neurons Contributes to transmission from enteric inhibitory muscle motor neurons

Modified from Furness JB et al: *Trends Neurosci* 15:66, 1992.

■ **Table 37-5**   Neurochemically identified nerve cell bodies in myenteric ganglia of guinea pig small intestine

Myenteric ganglia about 10,000 neurons/cm length	
Neurochemical	*Proportion (%)*
Aromatic amine handling	0.5
Acetylcholinesterase	High
Calcium-binding protein	30
Cholecystokinin	6
Calcitonin gene–related peptide	2
Choline acetyltransferase	High
Dynorphin	49
Enkephalin	51
Gastrin-releasing peptide	19
Monoamine oxidase B	10
Neuropeptide Y	28
Nitric oxide (NO)	10
Somatostatin	6
Substance P	37
Vasoactive intestinal peptide	39

Submucosal ganglia about 7000 neurons/cm length	
Neurochemical	*Proportion (%)*
Dynorphin/galanin/vasoactive intestinal peptide	45
Choline acetyltransferase/ cholecystokinin/calcitonin gene–related peptide/ (galanin)/neuropeptide Y/somatostatin	20
Choline acetyltransferase/ substance P	11
Choline acetyltransferase	14
NO synthase	10
Aromatic amine handling	11

Adapted from Costa M, Furness JB: In Makhlouf GM, editor: *Handbook of physiology*, sect 6, *The gastrointestinal system*, vol II, *Neural and endocrine biology*, Bethesda, Md, 1989, American Physiological Society.

Functions of enteric neurons. The types of neurons in the enteric nervous system and their major functions are summarized in Table 37-3.

Myenteric neurons. Most neurons in myenteric ganglia are motor neurons. The motor neurons in myenteric ganglia include both excitatory and inhibitory neurons. These neurons project to the smooth muscle cells of the muscularis externa. The myenteric ganglia also contain sensory neurons and interneurons. About one third of neurons in myenteric ganglia are sensory. Other myenteric neurons project to neurons in submucosal ganglia or to mucosal effectors.

Excitatory motor neurons release **acetylcholine** onto **muscarinic receptors** on the smooth muscle cells; they also release **substance P.** Inhibitory motor neurons release **VIP (vasoactive intestinal polypeptide)** and **NO (nitric oxide).** Most myenteric interneurons release acetylcholine onto **nicotinic receptors** on motor neurons or on other interneurons.

Submucosal neurons. Most neurons in submucosal ganglia regulate glandular, endocrine, and epithelial cell secretion. Stimulatory secretomotor neurons release acetylcholine and VIP onto gland cells or epithelial cells. The submucosal ganglia also have numerous sensory neurons. These neurons are the afferent limbs of the secretomotor reflexes. Most of the sensory neurons respond to chemical stimuli or to mechanical deformation of the mucosa. Submucosal interneurons release acetylcholine onto other neurons in submucosal ganglia or project to myenteric ganglia. Submucosal ganglia also contain vasodilator neurons that release acetylcholine and/or VIP onto submucosal blood vessels.

Intrinsic reflexes. All of the component cells of an **intrinsic reflex** are located in the wall of the gastrointestinal tract. Numerous intrinsic reflexes control the motor and secretory activities of each segment of the gastrointestinal tract. A well-characterized intrinsic reflex is shown in Fig. 37-7. *Localized mechanical or chemical stimulation of the intestinal mucosa elicits contraction above (oral to) and relaxation below (anal to) the point of stimulation.*

■ *Chewing (Mastication)*

Although chewing is sometimes a voluntary behavior it is more frequently a reflex behavior. Chewing performs several functions. It lubricates food by mixing it with salivary mucus. If the food contains starch, salivary amylase, an enzyme that breaks down starch, is added to the food during chewing. Finally, chewing mechanically chops food into smaller pieces so that it can be swallowed and propelled more easily, and more readily mixed with the digestive secretions of the stomach and duodenum.

■ *Swallowing*

Swallowing can be initiated voluntarily, but thereafter it is almost entirely under reflex control. The swallowing reflex is a rigidly ordered sequence of events that propels food from the mouth to the stomach. This reflex also inhibits respiration and prevents the entrance of food into the trachea (Fig. 37-8) during swallowing. *The afferent limb of the swallowing reflex begins when touch receptors, most notably those near the opening of the pharynx, are stimulated.* Sensory impulses from these receptors are transmitted to an area in the medulla and lower pons called the **swallowing center.** Motor impulses travel from the swallowing center to the musculature of the pharynx and upper esophagus via various cranial nerves and to the remainder of the esophagus by vagal motor neurons.

Swallowing can be divided into three phases: oral, pharyngeal, and esophageal.

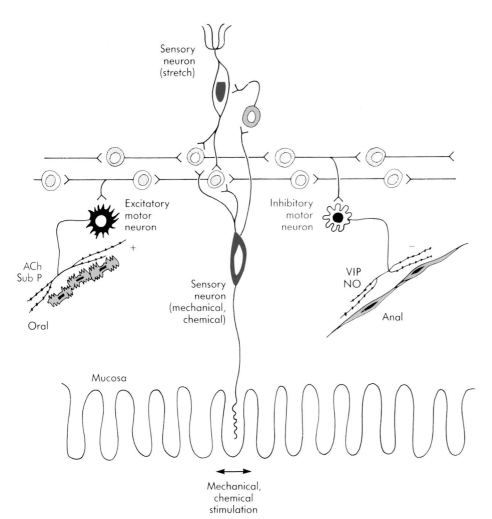

■ **Fig. 37-7** Localized mechanical or chemical stimulation of the intestinal mucosa typically elicits contraction above and relaxation below the point of stimulation. This figure depicts the enteric neuronal circuitry responsible for this reflex behavior. In the center of the figure are two sensory neurons: a stretch-sensitive neuron in the muscle layer *(white cytoplasm, colored nucleus)* and mechanosensitive or chemosensitive neuron *(colored cytoplasm, white nucleus)* with its receptive ending in the mucosa. Stimulation of either of these sensory neurons results in activation of ascending *(oral)* excitatory pathways and descending *(anal)* inhibitory pathways to circular muscle *(cm)*. *ACh,* Acetylcholine; *Sub P,* substance P; *VIP,* vasoactive intestinal peptide; *NO,* nitric oxide. (Courtesy of Dr. Terence K. Smith.)

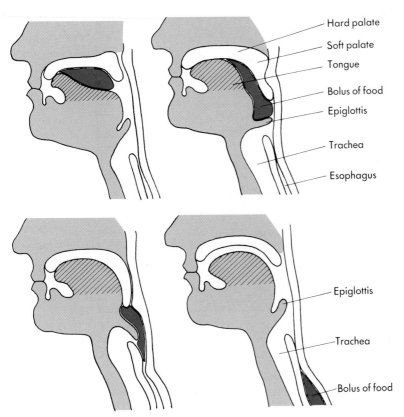

■ **Fig. 37-8** Major events involved in the swallowing reflex. (Modified from Johnson LR: *Gastrointestinal physiology,* ed 2, St Louis, 1981, Mosby–Year Book.)

■ *Oral Phase*

The **oral,** or **voluntary, phase,** of swallowing is initiated when the tip of the tongue separates a bolus of food from the mass of food in the mouth. First the tip of the tongue, and later the more posterior portions of the tongue, press against the hard palate. The action of the tongue moves the bolus upward and then backward into the mouth. The bolus is forced into the pharynx, where it stimulates the touch receptors that initiate the swallowing reflex.

■ *Pharyngeal Phase*

The **pharyngeal phase** of swallowing involves the following sequence of events, which occurs in less than 1 second:

1. The soft palate is pulled upward and the palatopharyngeal folds move inward toward one another. These movements prevent reflux of food into the nasopharynx and open a narrow passage through which food moves into the pharynx.
2. The vocal cords are pulled together and the larynx is moved forward and upward against the epiglottis.

These actions prevent food from entering the trachea and help to open the upper esophageal sphincter.

3. The **upper esophageal sphincter (UES)** relaxes to receive the bolus of food (Fig. 37-9). The superior constrictor muscles of the pharynx then contract strongly to force the bolus deeply into the pharynx.
4. A **peristaltic wave** is initiated with contraction of the pharyngeal superior constrictor muscles, and the wave moves toward the esophagus (Figs. 37-8 and 37-9). This wave forces the bolus of food through the relaxed UES.

During the pharyngeal stage of swallowing, respiration is also reflexly inhibited.

■ *Esophageal Phase*

The **esophageal phase** of swallowing is controlled mainly by the swallowing center. After the bolus of food passes the UES, a reflex action causes the sphincter to constrict. A peristaltic wave, which is called **primary peristalsis,** then begins just below the UES. This wave travels at approximately 3 to 5 cm/sec, and traverses the

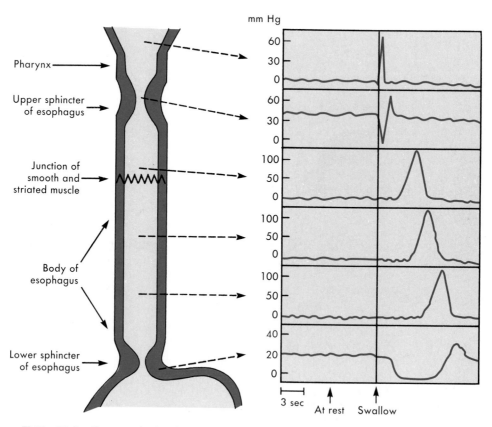

■ **Fig. 37-9** Pressures in the pharynx, esophagus, and esophageal sphincters during swallowing. Note the reflex relaxation of the upper and lower esophageal sphincters and the timing of their relaxation. (Redrawn from Christensen J: In Christensen J, Wingate DL, editors: *A guide to gastrointestinal motility,* Bristol, UK, 1983, John Wright & Sons.)

entire esophagus in less than 10 seconds (Fig. 37-9). Primary peristalsis is controlled by the swallowing center. If the primary peristalsis is insufficient to clear the esophagus of food, distention of the esophagus initiates another peristaltic wave, called **secondary peristalsis.** This peristaltic wave begins above the site of distention and moves downward. Input from esophageal sensory fibers to the central and enteric nervous systems modulates both primary and secondary esophageal peristalsis.

■ *Esophageal Function*

■ *Function, Structure, and Innervation of the Esophagus*

After food is swallowed, the esophagus functions as a conduit to move the food from the pharynx to the stomach. In the upper third of the esophagus, both the inner

circular and the outer longitudinal muscle layers are striated. In the lower third, the muscle layers are composed entirely of smooth muscle cells. The middle third contains both skeletal and smooth muscles. Thus, the esophagus contains a gradient of muscle, from all skeletal at the top to all smooth at the bottom.

The esophageal musculature, both striated and smooth, is mainly innervated by branches of the vagus nerve. Somatic motor fibers of the vagus nerve form motor endplates on the striated muscle fibers. Visceral motor nerves are preganglionic parasympathetic fibers that synapse primarily on the nerve cells of the myenteric plexus. *Neurons of the myenteric plexus directly innervate the smooth muscle cells of the esophagus and communicate with one another.* The neural circuits that control esophageal motility are schematized in Fig. 37-10.

The **UES** and the **lower esophageal sphincter (LES)** prevent the entry of air and gastric contents, respectively,

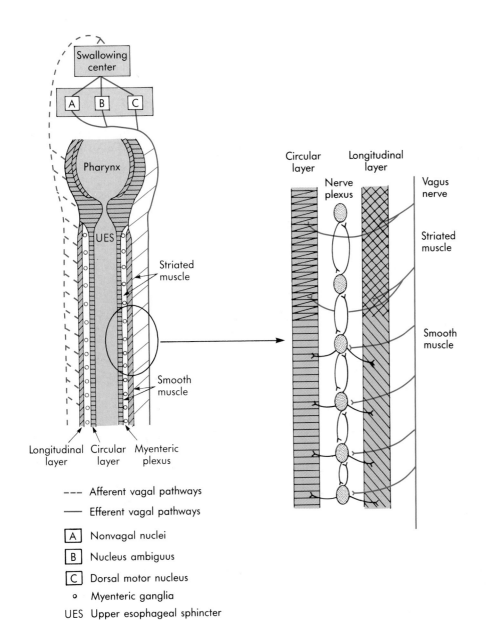

■ **Fig. 37-10** Local and central neural circuits involved in the control of esophageal motility. *Left,* Motor neurons reach the esophagus in branches of the vagus nerves, and sensory feedback to the swallowing center is carried by vagal afferent fibers. *Right,* Enlarged view of the circled region of the esophagus to show vagal somatic motor neurons that innervate the striated muscle of the pharynx and upper esophagus, and vagal visceral motor neurons that innervate the smooth muscle of the lower esophagus. Note that the visceral motor neurons terminate predominantly on neurons of the myenteric plexus. *UES,* Upper esophageal sphincter. (Adapted from Johnson LR: *Gastrointestinal physiology,* ed 5, St Louis, 1997, Mosby–Year Book.)

- - - Afferent vagal pathways

——— Efferent vagal pathways

A Nonvagal nuclei

B Nucleus ambiguus

C Dorsal motor nucleus

o Myenteric ganglia

UES Upper esophageal sphincter

into the esophagus. The LES opens with the initiation of esophageal peristalsis (Fig. 37-9). The opening of the LES is mediated by impulses in branches of the vagus nerve. In the absence of esophageal peristalsis, the sphincter remains tightly closed to prevent reflux of the gastric contents, which would cause esophagitis and the sensation known as "heartburn."

Reflux is particularly problematic because the pressure in the thoracic esophagus is close to intrathoracic pressure, which is almost always less than intraabdominal pressure. The difference between intraabdominal and intrathoracic pressures increases during each inspiration (see Chapter 33). In addition, because the crura of the diaphragm wrap around the esophagus at the level of the LES, contraction of the diaphragm helps to increase the pressure in the LES with each inspiration. In individuals with weakness of the diaphragm, and particularly in those with **hiatal hernia,** esophagitis may be caused by increased reflux.

cholinergic. The relaxation of the sphincter that occurs in response to primary peristalsis in the esophagus is primarily mediated by vagal fibers that inhibit the circulatory muscle of the LES. Although the inhibitory neurotransmitter is not known with certainty, it is thought that VIP and NO mediate this relaxation of the LES.

In some individuals, the sphincter fails to relax sufficiently during swallowing to allow food to enter the stomach. This condition is known as **achalasia.** Therapy for achalasia involves either mechanically dilating or surgically weakening the LES or administering drugs that inhibit its tone. In individuals with **diffuse esophageal spasm,** prolonged and painful contraction of the lower part of the esophagus occurs after swallowing, instead of the normal esophageal peristaltic wave. In individuals with **incompetence of the LES,** gastric juice can move back up into the lower esophagus and erode the esophageal mucosa.

■ Lower Esophageal Sphincter

Control of LES tone. The resting pressure in the LES is about 20 mm Hg. The tonic contraction of the circular musculature of the sphincter is regulated by nerves, both intrinsic and extrinsic, and by hormones and neuromodulators. A significant fraction of this basal tone in this sphincter is mediated by vagal cholinergic nerves. Stimulation of sympathetic nerves to the sphincter also causes the LES to contract.

Relaxation of the LES. The intrinsic and extrinsic innervation of the LES is both excitatory and inhibitory (Fig. 37-11). Vagal excitatory fibers are predominantly

■ Gastric Motility

The major functions of gastric motility are (1) to allow the stomach to serve as a reservoir for the large volume of food that may be ingested at a single meal, (2) to break food into smaller particles and mix food with gastric secretions so that digestion can begin, and (3) to empty gastric contents into the duodenum at a controlled rate.

Fig. 37-12 shows the major anatomic subdivisions of the stomach. *The fundus and the body of the stomach can accommodate volume increases as large as 1.5 L without a great increase in intragastric pressure;* this phenomenon is called **receptive relaxation.** Because the contractions of the fundus and body are normally weak, much of

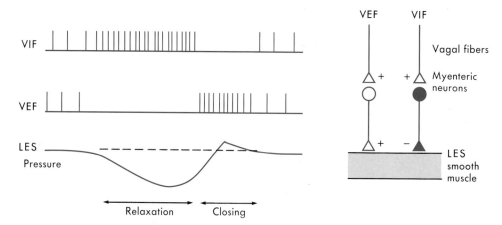

■ **Fig. 37-11**   The lower esophageal sphincter (LES) is innervated by both vagal excitatory fibers (VEF) and vagal inhibitory fibers (VIF). Relaxation of the LES is associated with an increased frequency of action potentials in VIF and decreased frequency of action potentials in VEF. Reciprocal changes occur when the sphincter regains its resting tone. (Adapted from Miolan JP, Roman C: *J Physiol Paris* 74:709, 1978.)

the gastric contents remains relatively unmixed for long periods. *The fundus and the body thus serve the reservoir functions of the stomach. In the antrum, however, contractions are vigorous.* These contractions break the food down into smaller pieces and mix the food thoroughly with gastric juice. At this point, the partly digested food is a semisolid mass called *chyme.* The antral contractions "feed" the chyme in small squirts into the duodenal bulb. *Several mechanisms adjust the rate of gastric emptying so that chyme is not delivered to the duodenum too rapidly.* The physiological mechanisms that underlie gastric motility are discussed below.

■ Structure and Innervation of the Stomach

The basic structure of the gastric wall follows the general scheme presented in Fig. 37-1. The circular muscle layer of the muscularis externa is more prominent than the longitudinal layer. The muscularis externa of the fundus and the body of the stomach is relatively thin. In contrast, the muscularis externa of the antrum is considerably thicker, and it increases in thickness toward the pylorus. In the antrum and pylorus, the inner layer of obliquely oriented muscle cells is incomplete.

The stomach is richly innervated by extrinsic nerves and by the neurons of the enteric nervous system. Axons from the cells of the intramural plexuses innervate smooth muscle and secretory cells.

Parasympathetic innervation is supplied by the vagus nerves, while sympathetic innervation is provided by the celiac plexus. In general, parasympathetic nerves stimulate gastric smooth muscle motility and gastric secretions, whereas sympathetic activity inhibits these functions. Numerous sensory afferent fibers leave the stomach in the vagus nerves; some of these fibers travel with sympathetic nerves. Other sensory neurons are the afferent links between sensory receptors and the intramural plexuses of the stomach. Some of these afferent fibers relay information about intragastric pressure, gastric distention, intragastric pH, or pain.

■ Responses to Gastric Filling

When a wave of esophageal peristalsis begins, a reflex causes the LES to relax. This relaxation of the LES is followed by *receptive relaxation of the fundus and body of the stomach.* The stomach will also relax if it is filled directly with gas or liquid. The nerve fibers in the vagi are a major efferent pathway for reflex relaxation of the stomach. The vagal fibers that mediate this response may release VIP and/or NO as their transmitters.

■ Mixing and Emptying of Gastric Contents

The muscle layers in the fundus and body are thin; weak contractions characterize these parts of the stomach. As a result, the contents of the fundus and the body settle into layers based on the density of the contents. Gastric contents may remain unmixed for as long as 1 hour after eating. *Fats tend to form an oily layer on top of the other gastric contents. Consequently, fats are emptied later than are the other gastric contents.* Liquids can flow around the mass of food contained in the body of the stomach and are emptied more rapidly into the duodenum (Fig. 37-13). Solid food is emptied more slowly. Large or indigestible particles are retained in the stomach for even longer periods.

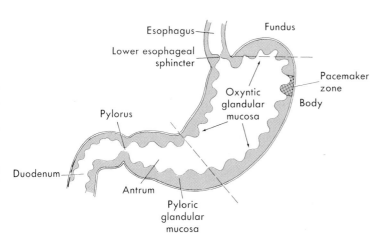

■ **Fig. 37-12** The major anatomic subdivisions of the stomach.

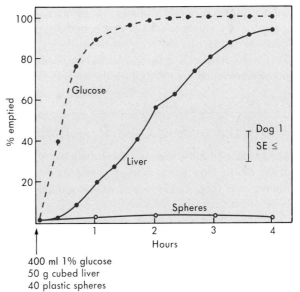

■ **Fig. 37-13** Rates of emptying of different meals from dog stomach. A solution (1% glucose) is emptied faster than a digestible solid (cubed liver). An indigestible solid (7-mm plastic spheres) remains in the stomach until the contractile phase of the migrating myoelectric complex occurs. (Redrawn from Hinder RA, Kelly KA: *Am J Physiol* 233:E335, 1977.)

When food enters the stomach, gastric contractions begin. These contractions usually begin in the middle of the body of the stomach and travel toward the pylorus. They increase in force and velocity as they approach the gastroduodenal junction. Thus, *the major mixing activity occurs in the antrum of the stomach.* The contents of the antrum are mixed rapidly and thoroughly with gastric secretions as a result of these forceful, rapid contractions. As each peristaltic wave reaches the pylorus, the pyloric sphincter snaps shut, so that the stomach empties in small squirts, one for each peristaltic wave. The rapid contraction of the terminal antrum also propels the chyme back into the antrum; this movement is called **retropulsion.** Retropulsion is particularly effective at mixing and breaking down gastric contents.

■ *Fed versus Fasted State*

After an individual eats, the antrum contracts about three times per minute. As discussed later, the rate of gastric emptying is regulated by feedback mechanisms that diminish the force of antral contractions and enhance contraction of the pyloric sphincter.

In a fasted animal, a different pattern of antral contractions occurs. The antrum is quiescent for 75 to 90 minutes, after which a brief period (5 to 10 minutes) of intense electrical and motor activity occurs. *This activity is characterized by strong contractions of the antrum with a relaxed pylorus.* During this period, even large chunks of material that remain from the previous meal are emptied from the stomach. This period of intense contractions is followed by 75 to 90 minutes of quiescence. This cycle of contractions in the stomach is part of a pattern of contractile activity that periodically sweeps from the stomach to the terminal ileum during fasting. This cyclic contractile activity is known as the **migrating myoelectric complex (MMC)** (discussed later).

■ *Electrical Activity and Gastric Contractions*

The gastric peristaltic waves occur at about the frequency of the gastric slow waves that are generated by a **pacemaker zone** (Fig. 37-12) located near the middle of the body of the stomach. These waves are conducted toward the pylorus. In humans, the frequency of slow waves is about three per minute.

The gastric slow wave is triphasic (Fig. 37-14), and its shape resembles the action potentials in cardiac muscle. However, the gastric slow wave lasts about 10 times longer than does the cardiac action potential, and it does not overshoot.

Gastric smooth muscle contracts when the depolarization during the slow wave exceeds the threshold for contraction (Fig. 37-14). The greater the extent of depolarization and the longer the muscle cell remains depo-

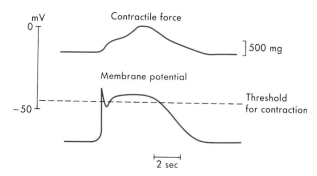

■ **Fig. 37-14**   Relationship between contraction of smooth muscle of dog stomach *(upper tracing)* and intracellularly recorded slow wave *(lower tracing)*. Note the triphasic shape of the slow wave in gastric smooth muscle. Contraction occurs when the depolarizing phase of the slow wave exceeds the threshold for contraction, even though there are no action potential spikes on the plateau of the slow wave. When action potentials occur, a much stronger contraction is elicited. (Redrawn from Szurszewski J: *Electrical basis for gastrointestinal motility.* In Johnson LR, editor: *Physiology of the gastrointestinal tract,* New York, 1981, Raven Press.)

larized above the threshold, the greater is the force of contraction. In the gastric antrum, action potential spikes frequently occur during the plateau phase (Fig. 37-15). *The contraction that results from these action potentials is much stronger* than a contraction that occurs in the absence of action potentials. Acetylcholine and the hormone **gastrin** stimulate gastric contractility by increasing the amplitude and duration of the plateau phase of the gastric slow wave. Norepinephrine has the opposite effect.

■ *Gastroduodenal Junction*

The pylorus separates the gastric antrum from the first part of the **duodenum,** the **duodenal bulb.** The pylorus functions as a sphincter. The circular smooth muscle of the pylorus forms two ringlike thickenings that are followed by a connective tissue ring that separates the pylorus from the duodenum.

The electrical rhythm of the duodenum is 10 to 12 slow waves per minute, which is much faster than the three per minute of the stomach. The electrical activity of the duodenal bulb is influenced by the basic electrical rhythms of both the stomach and the postbulbar duodenum. The bulb thus contracts somewhat irregularly. However, the contractions of the antrum and duodenum are coordinated; when the antrum contracts, the duodenal bulb is often relaxed.

The essential functions of the gastroduodenal junction are (1) *to allow the carefully regulated emptying of gastric contents* at a rate consistent with the ability of the duodenum to process the chyme and (2) *to prevent regurgitation of duodenal contents* back into the stomach.

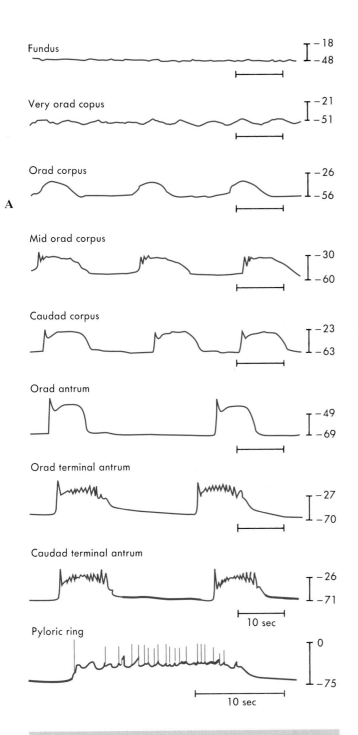

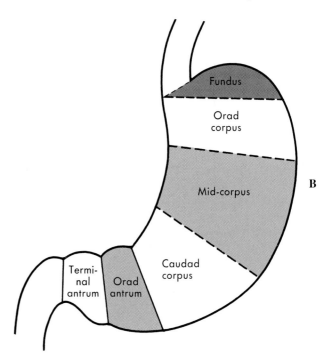

A

B

■ **Fig. 37-15** Intracellular recordings (**A**) of the electrical activity in smooth muscle cells of isolated strips of various regions (**B**) of a dog's stomach. Note that slow waves are absent in the fundus and weak in the orad corpus, and gain in strength and definition toward the antrum. Only in the terminal antrum and pylorus do action potential spikes occur on the plateaus of the slow waves. Action potential spikes are associated with stronger contractions. In the intact stomach, the slow waves in the different parts of the stomach have the same frequency because they are driven by the same pacemaker. In these records, the intrinsic slow wave frequency differs in the isolated strips of muscle. (Redrawn from Szurszewski J: *Electrical basis for gastrointestinal motility*. In Johnson LR, editor: *Physiology of the gastrointestinal tract*, New York, 1981, Raven Press.)

Excitatory cholinergic vagal fibers stimulate constriction of the sphincter. Inhibitory vagal fibers release another transmitter, probably **VIP** or **NO,** that relaxes the sphincter. The hormones **cholecystokinin (CCK), gastrin, gastric inhibitory peptide (GIP),** and **secretin** all promote constriction of the pyloric sphincter and thereby slow gastric emptying.

■ *Regulation of Gastric Emptying*

The emptying of gastric contents is regulated by both neural and hormonal mechanisms. The duodenal and jejunal mucosa contain receptors that sense acidity, osmotic pressure, certain fats and fat digestion products, and peptides and amino acids (Fig. 37-16). The chyme that leaves the stomach is usually hypertonic, and it becomes even more hypertonic because of the action of the digestive enzymes in the duodenum. *Gastric empty-*

The gastric mucosa is highly resistant to acid, but it may be damaged by bile. The duodenal mucosa has the opposite properties. Thus, if gastric emptying is too rapid, a **duodenal ulcer** may develop. On the other hand, regurgitation of duodenal contents may contribute to **gastric ulcers.** Gastric ulcers may be exacerbated when gastric emptying is slower than normal.

The pylorus is densely innervated by both vagal and sympathetic nerve fibers. Sympathetic fibers increase the constriction of the pyloric sphincter. Vagal fibers are both excitatory and inhibitory to pyloric smooth muscle.

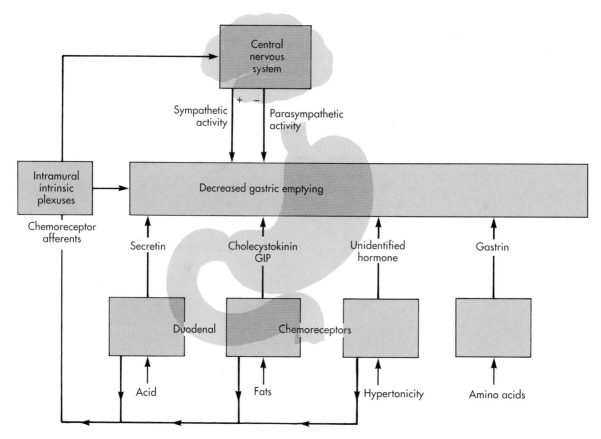

■ **Fig. 37-16** Duodenal stimuli elicit neural and hormonal inhibition of gastric emptying. *GIP,* Gastric inhibitory peptide.

ing is slowed by hypertonic solutions in the duodenum, by duodenal pH below 3.5, and by the presence of amino acids and peptides in the duodenum. The presence of fatty acids or monoglycerides (products of fat digestion) in the duodenum also dramatically decreases the rate of gastric emptying. As a result of these mechanisms:

1. The rate at which fat is emptied into the duodenum does not exceed the rate at which the fat can be emulsified by the bile acids and lecithin of the bile.
2. Acid is not dumped into the duodenum more rapidly than it can be neutralized by pancreatic and duodenal secretions and by other mechanisms.
3. The rates at which the other components of chyme enter the small intestine do not exceed the rate at which the small intestine can process those components.

The slowing of gastric emptying in response to the different components of the duodenal contents is mediated by neural and hormonal mechanisms:

1. *Acid in the duodenum.* In response to acid in the duodenum, the force of gastric contractions promptly decreases and duodenal motility increases. This response has neural and hormonal components. The presence of acid in the duodenum releases **secretin,** which diminishes the rate of gastric emptying by inhibiting antral contractions and by stimulating contraction of the pyloric sphincter (Fig. 37-17).
2. *Fat-digestion products.* The presence of fat-digestion products in the duodenum and jejunum decreases the rate of gastric emptying. This response results partly from the release of **CCK** from the duodenum and jejunum. CCK decreases the rate of gastric emptying. The presence of fatty acids in the duodenum and jejunum releases another hormone, **GIP,** that also decreases the rate of gastric emptying.
3. *Osmotic pressure of duodenal contents.* Hyperosmotic solutions in the duodenum and jejunum slow the rate of gastric emptying. This response has both neural and hormonal components. Hypertonic solutions in the duodenum release an unidentified hormone that slows the rate of gastric emptying.
4. *Peptides and amino acids in the duodenum.* Peptides and amino acids release **gastrin** from **G cells** located in the antrum of the stomach and the duodenum. Gastrin increases the strength of antral contractions and increases constriction of the pyloric sphincter; the net effect of these actions usually diminishes the rate of gastric emptying. Release of GIP and CCK is also promoted by the

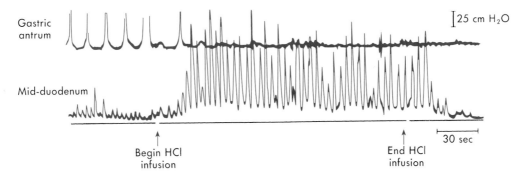

■ Fig. 37-17 Effect of instilling 100 mM hydrochloric acid (HCl) at 6 ml/min into the duodenum of a dog. Contractile activity of the gastric antrum *(upper tracing)* is inhibited, and contractions of the mid-duodenum *(lower tracing)* are stimulated. (Redrawn from Brink BM et al: *Gut* 6:163, 1965.)

presence of peptides and amino acids in the duodenum; these hormones also contribute to a decreased rate of gastric emptying in response to amino acids in the duodenum.

In some patients with **duodenal ulcers,** the effectiveness of the mechanisms that release hormones from the duodenum may be diminished. As a result of this malfunction, the rate of gastric emptying or of gastric acid secretion is abnormally high. In normal individuals, instillation of acid into the duodenum via a nasogastric tube dramatically decreases the rate and force of contractions of the gastric antrum. However, in some patients with duodenal ulcer, this response to acid in the duodenum is markedly diminished.

■ *Vomiting*

Vomiting is the expulsion of gastric (and sometimes duodenal) contents from the gastrointestinal tract via the mouth. Vomiting is often preceded by a feeling of nausea, a rapid or irregular heartbeat, dizziness, sweating, pallor, and dilation of the pupils. It is usually preceded by **retching,** in which gastric contents are forced up into the esophagus but do not enter the pharynx.

Vomiting is a reflex behavior controlled and coordinated by a **vomiting center** in the medulla oblongata (Fig. 37-18). Many areas in the body have receptors that provide afferent input to the vomiting center. *Distention of the stomach and duodenum is a strong stimulus that elicits vomiting. Tickling the back of the throat, painful injury to the genitourinary system, dizziness, and certain other stimuli can bring about nausea and vomiting.*

Certain chemicals, called **emetics,** can also elicit vomiting. Some emetics stimulate receptors in the stomach, or more often in the duodenum. **Ipecac,** a commonly used emetic, stimulates duodenal receptors. Other emetics (e.g., **apomorphine**) act on receptors in the floor of the fourth ventricle, in an area known as the **chemore-**ceptor trigger zone. The chemoreceptor trigger zone lies on the blood side of the blood-brain barrier, and thus it can be reached by most blood-borne substances.

When the vomiting reflex is initiated, the sequence of events is the same regardless of the stimulus that initiates the reflex. Early events in the vomiting reflex include a wave of **reverse peristalsis** that sweeps from the middle of the small intestine to the duodenum. The pyloric sphincter and the stomach relax to receive intestinal contents. A forced inspiration then occurs against a closed glottis. This inspiration decreases intrathoracic pressure, while a lowering of the diaphragm that also occurs during this inspiration increases intra-abdominal pressure. The forced inspiration is followed by a forceful contraction of abdominal muscles, which sharply elevates intra-abdominal pressure and drives gastric contents into the esophagus. The LES relaxes reflexly to receive the gastric contents, and the pylorus and antrum contract. *When a person retches, the UES remains closed and prevents vomiting.* When the respiratory and abdominal muscles relax, the esophagus is emptied by secondary peristalsis into the stomach. Often, a series of stronger and stronger retches precedes vomiting.

When a person vomits, the rapid propulsion of gastric contents into the esophagus is accompanied by a reflex relaxation of the UES. **Vomitus** is projected into the pharynx and mouth. Entry of vomitus into the trachea is prevented by movement of the vocal cords closer together, closure of the glottis, and inhibition of respiration.

■ *Motility of the Small Intestine*

The small intestine makes up about three fourths of the length of the human gastrointestinal tract. It is about 5 m in length, and chyme typically takes 2 to 4 hours to traverse it.

The first 5% or so of the small intestine is the duodenum, which has no mesentery and has a characteristic histology that distinguishes it from the rest of the small

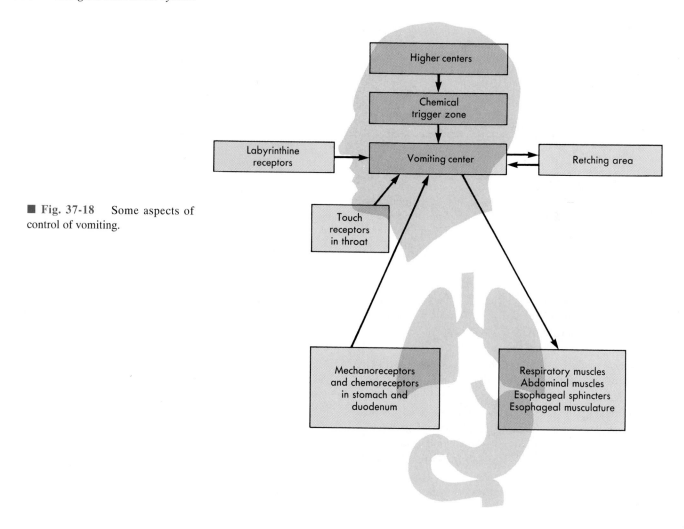

■ **Fig. 37-18** Some aspects of control of vomiting.

intestine. The remaining small intestine is divided into the **jejunum** and the **ileum.** The jejunum is more proximal and occupies about 40% of the length of the small bowel. The ileum is the remaining distal part of the small intestine.

The small intestine, particularly the duodenum and jejunum, is the site where most digestion and absorption take place. The movements of the small intestine mix chyme with digestive secretions, bring fresh chyme into contact with the absorptive surface of the microvilli, and propel chyme toward the colon.

The most frequent type of movement of the small intestine is called **segmentation.** Segmentation (Fig. 37-19) is characterized by closely spaced contractions of the circular muscle layer. These contractions divide the small intestine into small neighboring segments. In rhythmic segmentation, the sites of the circular contractions alternate, so that an individual segment of gut contracts and then relaxes. *Segmentation effectively mixes chyme with digestive secretions* and brings fresh chyme into contact with the mucosal surface.

In contrast to segmentation, **peristalsis** is the progressive contraction of successive sections of circular smooth muscle. The contractions move along the gastrointestinal

tract in an orthograde direction. Peristaltic waves occur in the small intestine but usually involve only a short length of intestine. As in other parts of the digestive tract, the slow waves of the smooth muscle cells determine the timing of intestinal contractions.

■ *Electrical Activity of Small Intestinal Smooth Muscle*

Regular slow waves occur all along the small intestine. The frequency is highest (11 to 13 per minute in humans) in the duodenum but declines along the length of the small intestine (to a minimum of eight or nine per minute in humans) in the terminal part of the ileum. The slow waves may or may not be accompanied by bursts of action potential spikes (Fig. 37-20). When action potentials occur, they elicit strong smooth muscle contractions that cause the major mixing and propulsive movements of the small intestine. Because action potential bursts are localized to short segments of the intestine, they are responsible for the highly localized contractions of the circular smooth muscle that cause segmentation.

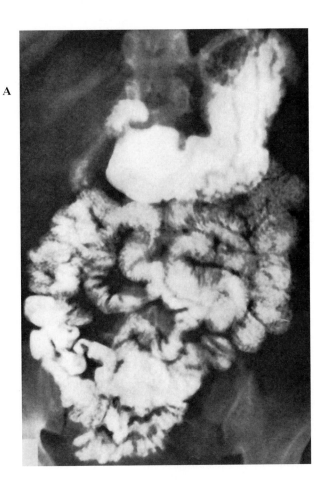

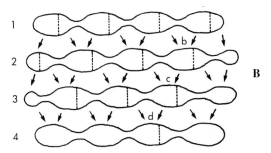

■ **Fig. 37-19**　**A,** X-ray view showing the stomach and small intestine filled with barium contrast medium in a normal individual. Note that segmentation of the small intestine divides its contents into ovoid segments. **B,** The sequence of segmental contractions in a portion of the cat's small intestine. Lines *1* to *4* indicate successive patterns in time. The dotted lines indicate where contractions will occur next. The arrows show the direction of chyme movement. (**A** from Gardner EM et al: *Anatomy, a regional study of human structure,* ed 4, Philadelphia, 1975, WB Saunders. **B** redrawn from Cannon WB: *Am J Physiol* 6:251, 1902.)

Slow waves

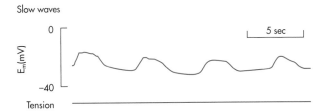

The basic electrical rhythm of the small intestine is entirely intrinsic; that is, it is independent of extrinsic innervation. The frequency of the action potential spike bursts that elicit strong contractions depends on the excitability of the smooth muscle cells of the small intestine. The excitability of the smooth muscle cells is in turn influenced by circulating hormones, the autonomic nervous system, and the enteric neurons. Although direct control of intestinal motility resides in the intramural plexuses, the parasympathetic and sympathetic innervation of the small intestine modulates contractile activity. *Excitability is enhanced by parasympathetic nerves and is inhibited by sympathetic nerves, and both autonomic divisions act via the intramural plexuses.* These modulating extrinsic neural circuits are essential for certain long-range intestinal reflexes (discussed later).

Slow waves and prepotentials that give rise to action potentials

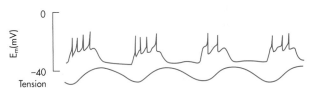

■ **Contractile Behavior of the Small Intestine**

Contractions of the duodenal bulb mix the chyme with pancreatic and biliary secretions, and they propel the chyme along the duodenum. Contractions of the duodenal bulb typically occur after contractions of the gastric antrum. This sequence helps prevent regurgitation of duodenal contents back into the stomach.

Slow waves and prepotentials that fail to give rise to action potentials

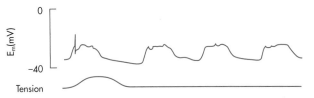

■ **Fig. 37-20**　Electrical and contractile activity of isolated longitudinal muscle of rabbit jejunum. The upper tracing in each panel is the transmembrane electrical potential difference (millivolts), and the lower tracing shows contractile tension. Under the conditions shown, the tissue contracts only in response to action potentials. The greater the number of action potentials, the stronger is the contraction. (Redrawn from Bortoff A: *Am J Physiol* 201:203, 1961.)

Segmentation is the most frequent type of movement by the small intestine (Fig. 37-19). The maximal rate of segmental contractions is the same as the frequency of slow waves: eleven or twelve per minute in the duodenum and eight or nine per minute in the ileum. In some individuals, the frequency of segmental contractions is fairly constant. In others, periods of segmentation are interrupted by brief periods of relative quiescence.

Short-range peristalsis also occurs in the small intestine, although much less frequently than does segmentation. The relatively low rate of net propulsion of chyme in the small intestine allows time for digestion and absorption.

The importance of the slow rate of propulsion in the small intestine can be demonstrated by treatment of patients with agents that alter small intestinal motility. Administration of **codeine** and other **opiates** markedly reduces the frequency and the volume of stools. This effects results from a decrease in small intestinal motility; this diminished motility in turn increases the transit time of the jejunal contents. The longer transit time allows salts, water, and certain nutrients to be more completely absorbed in the small intestine, so that the volume of contents that enters the colon is less than normal. Treatment with **castor oil,** a potent laxative, causes the opposite effects. Castor oil contains hydroxy fatty acids that stimulate small intestinal motility and decrease small intestinal transit time. Hence, salts and water are delivered to the colon at a rate that overwhelms the ability of the colon to absorb them, and diarrhea results.

■ Intestinal Reflexes

When a bolus of material is placed in the small intestine, *the intestine typically contracts behind the bolus and relaxes ahead of it* (Fig. 37-7). This response is known as the **law of the intestine.** This action propels the bolus in an orthograde direction, as does a peristaltic wave.

Certain intestinal reflexes can occur along a considerable length of the gastrointestinal tract. These long-range reflexes depend on the function of both intrinsic and extrinsic nerves.

Overdistention of one segment of the intestine relaxes the smooth muscle in the rest of the intestine. This response is known as the **intestinointestinal reflex.**

The stomach and the terminal part of the ileum interact in a reflex called the **gastroileal reflex**. In this response, elevated secretory and motor functions of the stomach increase the motility of the terminal part of the ileum and accelerate the movement of material through the **ileocecal sphincter.**

■ Migrating Myoelectric Complex

The contractile behavior of the small intestine previously discussed is characteristic of the period after ingestion of a meal. In a fasted individual or some hours after the processing of a previous meal, the motility of the small intestine follows a different pattern. In this "fasting" pattern, *bursts of intense electrical and contractile activity are separated by longer quiescent periods.* Like the similar pattern that occurs in the stomach during fasting, these bursts of activity in the small intestine and the intervening long periods of quiescence are called the **migrating myoelectric complex (MMC).** An MMC is propagated from the stomach to the terminal ileum.

In humans, the MMC repeats every 75 to 90 minutes (Fig. 37-21). At about the time that one MMC reaches the distal ileum, a new MMC begins in the stomach.

The strongest contractions of both stomach and small-intestine MMCs are more vigorous and more propulsive than are the contractions that occur in the fed individual. These intense contractions sweep the small bowel clean and empty its contents into the colon. Thus, the MMC has been termed the "housekeeper of the small intestine."

The MMC also inhibits the migration of colonic bacteria into the terminal ileum. Individuals with weak or absent MMC contractions may be susceptible to bacterial overgrowth in the ileum. Substances released by the bacteria may stimulate secretion of NaCl and water by the epithelium of the small intestine and cause diarrhea.

■ Contractile Activity of the Muscularis Mucosae

Sections of the muscularis mucosae of the small intestine contract irregularly at an average rate of about three contractions per minute. These contractions alter the pattern of ridges and folds of the mucosa, mix the luminal contents, and bring different parts of the mucosal surface into contact with freshly mixed chyme. The villi of the small intestine also contract irregularly, especially in the proximal part of the small intestine. These contractions help to empty the central lacteals of the villi and increase intestinal lymph flow.

■ Emptying the Ileum

The **ileocecal sphincter,** also known as the **ileocecal valve,** separates the terminal end of the ileum from the **cecum,** the first part of the colon (Fig. 37-22). Normally, this sphincter is closed. However, short-range peristalsis in the terminal part of the ileum relaxes the sphincter and allows a small amount of chyme to squirt into the cecum. Distention of the

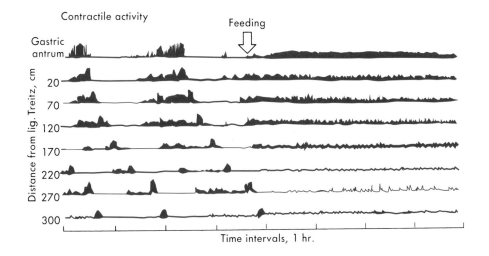

Contractile activity

Feeding

■ **Fig. 37-21** Contractile activity in the stomach and small intestine of a fasting dog, showing the characteristic pattern of the migrating myoelectric complex. The ligament of Treitz marks the border between the duodenum and the jejunum. (From Itoh Z, Sekiguchi T: Interdigestive motor activity in health and disease, *Scand J Gastroenterol Suppl* 82:121, 1983.)

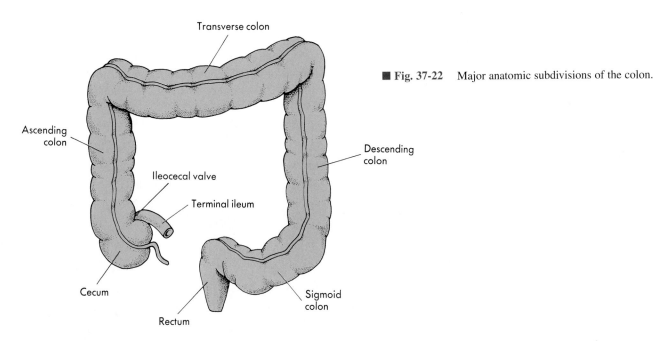

■ **Fig. 37-22** Major anatomic subdivisions of the colon.

distal ileum promotes peristalsis in the ileum and thus the opening of the ileocecal sphincter. Distention of the cecum causes the ileocecal sphincter to close. The ileocecal sphincter normally permits ileal chyme to enter the colon at a rate that allows the colon to absorb most of the salts and water in the chyme. The opening and closing of the ileocecal sphincter are coordinated mainly by the neurons of the intramural plexuses. The extrinsic innervation plays a role in longer-range control of the ileocecal sphincter, such as occurs in the gastroileal reflex.

■ *Motility of the Colon*

The colon receives 500 to 1500 ml of chyme per day from the ileum. Most of the salts and water that enter the colon are absorbed; the feces normally contain only about 50 to

100 ml of water each day. Colonic contractions mix the chyme and circulate it across the mucosal surface of the colon. As the chyme becomes semisolid, this mixing resembles a kneading process. *Normally, the progress of colonic contents is slow,* about 5 to 10 cm per hour at most.

One to three times daily a wave of contraction, called **mass movement,** occurs in the colon. A mass movement differs from a peristaltic wave because the contracted segments remain contracted for some time. Mass movements push the contents within a significant length of colon in an orthograde direction.

■ *Structure and Innervation of the Colon*

The major subdivisions of the colon, or large intestine, are the **cecum**, the **ascending colon**, the **transverse** colon, the **descending colon**, the **sigmoid colon**, the **rectum**, and the **anal canal** (Fig. 37-22).

The structure of the wall of the large intestine follows the general plan of the gastrointestinal tract presented earlier in this chapter. However, the colon has some characteristic features. The longitudinal muscle layer of the muscularis externa is concentrated into three bands, called the **taeniae coli.** The longitudinal muscle layer located between the taeniae coli is thin. In contrast, the longitudinal muscle of the rectum and anal canal is substantial and continuous.

Parasympathetic innervation of the cecum and the ascending and transverse colon is via branches of the vagus nerve; that of the descending and sigmoid colon, the rectum, and the anal canal is via the **pelvic nerves** from the sacral spinal cord. The parasympathetic fibers end mainly on neurons of the intramural plexuses. Sympathetic fibers innervate the proximal part of the large intestine via the **superior mesenteric plexus,** the distal part of the large intestine via the **inferior mesenteric** and **superior hypogastric plexuses,** and the rectum and anal canal via the **inferior hypogastric plexus.**

Stimulation of the sympathetic nerves stops colonic movements. Stimulation of the vagal nerves causes segmental contractions of the proximal part of the colon. Stimulation of the pelvic nerves causes expulsive movements of the distal colon and sustained contraction of some segments.

The anal canal is usually kept closed by the internal and external sphincters. The **internal anal sphincter** is a thickening of the *circular smooth muscle* of the anal canal. The **external anal sphincter** is more distal and consists entirely of **striated muscle.** The external anal sphincter is innervated by *somatic motor fibers* via the pudendal nerves. *This innervation allows the anal sphincter to be controlled both by reflexes and voluntarily.*

■ *Motility of the Cecum and Proximal Colon*

Most contractions of the cecum and proximal part of the large intestine are segmental, and they are more effective at mixing and circulating the colonic contents than at propelling them. The mixing action facilitates absorption of salts and water by the mucosal epithelium.

Localized segmental contractions divide the colon into neighboring ovoid segments, called **haustra** (Fig. 37-23). Thus, segmentation in the colon is known as **haustration.** The most dramatic difference between haustration and the segmentation that occurs in the small intestine is the regularity of the haustra and the large length of the large intestine involved in haustration at one time. The structural basis for the haustral pattern may be the localized thickenings that occur in the circular muscle of the colon. Haustral contractions, which can increase the local luminal pressure by 10 to 50 mm Hg, result in back-and-forth mixing of luminal contents.

In the proximal colon, "antipropulsive" patterns predominate. Reverse peristalsis and segmental propulsion toward the cecum both take place. Consequently, chyme is retained in the proximal colon, and this retention facilitates the absorption of salts and water.

■ *Motility of the Central and Distal Colon*

Normally, a mass movement fills the central and distal parts of the colon with semisolid feces. Segmental haustral contractions knead the feces and thus facilitate the absorption of remaining salts and water. Mass movements then sweep the feces toward the rectum.

■ *Control of Colonic Motility*

As in other segments of the gastrointestinal tract, the intramural plexuses directly control the contractile behavior of the colon, while the extrinsic innervation plays a modulating role. Enteric stimulatory motor neurons use acetylcholine and substance P as neurotransmitters; inhibitory enteric motor neurons release VIP and NO onto colonic smooth muscle cells. The extrinsic autonomic

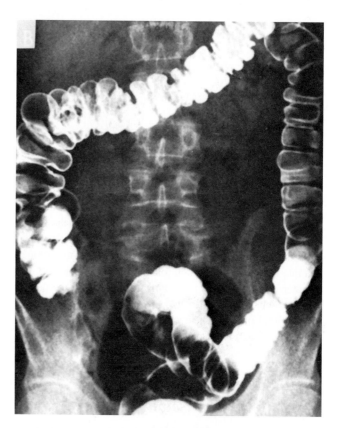

■ **Fig. 37-23** X-ray image showing a prominent haustral pattern in the colon of a normal individual. (From Keats TE: *An atlas of normal roentgen variants,* ed 2, Chicago, 1979, Mosby–Year Book.)

nerves to the colon modulate the control of colonic motility by the enteric nervous system. The **defecation reflex** (discussed later) is an exception, because *it requires the function of the spinal cord via the pelvic nerves.*

■ *Electrophysiology of the Colon*

Circular muscle. The colon contains two classes of rhythm-generating cells. Interstitial cells near the inner border of the circular muscle produce regular slow waves with a frequency of about six per minute. The slow waves have high amplitude and their shape resembles that of gastric slow waves. Interstitial cells near the outer border of the circular muscle produce **myenteric potential oscillations.** These oscillations are low in amplitude and much higher in frequency than the slow waves.

The circular muscle of the colon does not usually fire action potentials. Contractile agonists, such as acetylcholine released from excitatory enteric motor neurons, enhance contractions by increasing the *duration of some of the slow waves.* These longer slow waves elicit contractions of the circular muscle (Fig. 37-24).

Longitudinal muscle. Longitudinal colonic muscle displays myenteric potential oscillations. In contrast to the circular smooth muscle, however, the longitudinal muscle cells fire occasional action potentials at the peaks of the myenteric potential oscillations. The action potentials elicit contraction of the longitudinal muscle. Contractile agonists increase the frequency of action potentials.

■ *Reflex Control of Colonic Motility*

Distention of one part of the colon causes a relaxation in other parts of the colon. This **colonocolonic reflex** is mediated partly by the sympathetic fibers that supply the colon. Another reflex that functions in the colon is the **gastrocolic reflex.** After a meal enters the stomach, the reflex causes the motility of proximal and distal colon and the frequency of mass movements to increase. The gastrocolic reflex depends on the autonomic innervation to the colon; hormones such as CCK and gastrin may also be involved.

■ *The Rectum and Anal Canal*

The rectum is usually empty, or nearly so. The rectum is more active in segmental contractions than is the sigmoid colon, so that the rectal contents tend to move in a retrograde direction into the sigmoid colon. The anal canal is kept tightly closed by the anal sphincters. Just before

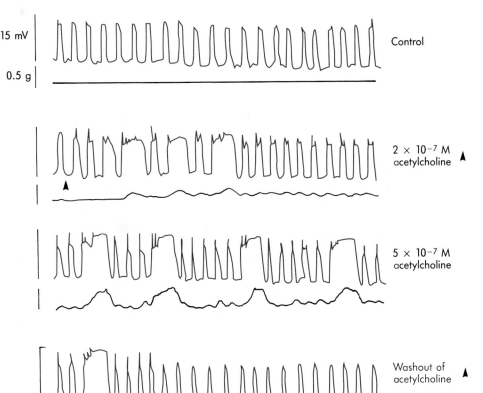

■ **Fig. 37-24** Effects of acetylcholine, a contractile agonist, on electrophysiological and contractile behavior of circular smooth muscle cells of canine colon. In each panel the top trace *(color)* is the membrane potential recording and the bottom trace *(black)* is the contractile response. Superfusion of the preparation with acetylcholine causes somewhat irregular lengthening of the slow waves. The longer slow waves elicit contractions. (Redrawn from Huizenga JD, Chang G, Diamant NE, El-Sharkaway TY: *J Pharmacol Exp Ther* 231:692, 1984.)

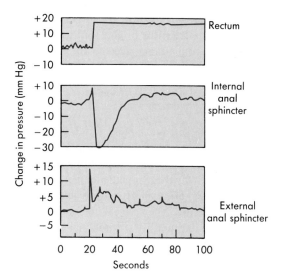

■ **Fig. 37-25**   Responses of internal and external anal sphincters to prolonged distention of the rectum. Note that the responses of the sphincters are transient. (Redrawn from Shuster MM et al: *Bull Johns Hopkins Hosp* 116:79, 1965.)

defecation, a mass movement in the sigmoid colon causes the rectum to fill. *It is the filling of the rectum that brings about reflex relaxation of the internal anal sphincter and reflex constriction of the external anal sphincter* (Fig. 37-25) *and causes the urge to defecate.* Persons who lack functional motor nerves to the external anal sphincter defecate involuntarily when the rectum is filled. The reflex reactions of the sphincters to rectal distention are transient. If defecation is postponed, the sphincters regain their normal tone, and the urge to defecate temporarily subsides.

In **Hirschsprung's disease,** also known as **congenital megacolon,** enteric neurons are congenitally absent from part of the colon. Usually, only the internal anal sphincter and a short length of colon proximal to it lack enteric neurons, but larger segments of the colon may be affected. In a normal person, filling of the rectum by a mass movement leads to reflex relaxation of the distal rectum and the internal anal sphincter. In the absence of enteric neurons, this reflex relaxation does not occur. As a result, functional obstruction of the distal colon and dilation of the colon above the obstruction occur.

■ *Defecation*

When the circumstances are appropriate, an individual may voluntarily relax the external anal sphincter to allow defecation to proceed. Highly propulsive contractions of the descending and sigmoid colon are part of the defecation reflex. Defecation is a complex behavior that involves both reflex and voluntary actions. *The integrating center for the reflex action is in the sacral spinal cord, and it is modulated by higher centers.* The principal efferent pathways are cholinergic parasympathetic fibers in the pelvic nerves. The role of the sympathetic nervous system is not significant in normal defecation.

Voluntary actions are also important in defecation. The external anal sphincter is voluntarily held in the relaxed state. Intra-abdominal pressure is elevated to aid in expulsion of feces. Evacuation is normally preceded by a deep breath, which moves the diaphragm downward. The glottis then closes, and contractions of the respiratory muscles on full lungs elevate both intrathoracic and intra-abdominal pressure. Contractions of the muscles of the abdominal wall further increase intra-abdominal pressure, which may be as great as 200 cm H$_2$O. This increase in pressure helps to force feces through the relaxed sphincters. The muscles of the pelvic floor relax, allowing the floor to drop. This activity helps to straighten out the rectum and prevent rectal prolapse.

■ *Summary*

1. The gastrointestinal tract has a characteristic layered structure that consists of mucosa, submucosa, muscularis externa, and serosa; this structure varies somewhat in different parts of the tract.

2. The gastrointestinal tract receives both sympathetic and parasympathetic innervation. Autonomic nerves influence the motor and secretory activities of the gastrointestinal tract and regulate the caliber of blood vessels of the gastrointestinal tract.

3. Contractions of the smooth muscle of the muscularis externa mix and propel the contents of the gastrointestinal tract.

4. Gastrointestinal smooth muscle cells are electrically coupled. Their resting membrane potential oscillates in a rhythm characteristic of each segment of the gastrointestinal tract. The membrane potential oscillations, called slow waves, control the timing and force of contractions of gastrointestinal smooth muscle.

5. The nerve plexuses of the gastrointestinal tract constitute the enteric nervous system. This system contains about the same number of neurons as are present in the spinal cord. The enteric nervous system contains motor neurons, sensory neurons, and interneurons.

6. Enteric sensory neurons function as the afferent arms of enteric reflex arcs by which the enteric nervous system controls most of the motor and secretory activities of the gastrointestinal tract. The autonomic nervous

system modulates the activities of the enteric nervous system.

7. Swallowing is a reflex coordinated by a swallowing center in the medulla and pons. The swallowing reflex is initiated by touch receptors in the pharynx. This reflex involves a series of ordered and coordinated motor impulses to the muscles of the pharynx, upper esophageal sphincter, esophageal striated muscle, esophageal smooth muscle, and lower esophageal sphincter.

8. Contractions of the stomach mix food with gastric juice and mechanically break the food down into smaller pieces. Gastric emptying is closely regulated. This regulation ensures that gastric contents are not emptied into the duodenum at a rate faster than the duodenum and jejunum can neutralize gastric acid and process the chyme.

9. Hormonal and neural mechanisms initiated by the presence of acid, fats, peptides, amino acids, and hypertonicity in the duodenum regulate gastric emptying.

10. Segmentation is the major contractile activity of the small intestine. Segmental contractions mix and circulate intestinal contents, but they are not very propulsive. The slow rate of transport of intestinal contents allows adequate time for digestion and absorption.

11. In a fasted individual, a different pattern of motility, called the migrating myoelectric complex (MMC), occurs. The MMC is characterized by 75- to 90-minute periods of quiescence, interrupted by periods of vigorous and intensely propulsive contractions that last 3 to 6 minutes. The MMC sweeps the stomach and the small intestine clear of any debris left from the previous meal.

12. In the proximal colon, antipropulsive contractions predominate, which allows time for absorption of salts and water.

13. In the transverse and descending colon, haustral contractions mix and knead colonic contents to facilitate extraction of salts and water. Mass movements that occur in the colon one to three times daily sweep colonic contents toward the anus.

14. Filling the rectum with feces initiates the defecation reflex. The integrating center for the defecation reflex is in the sacral spinal cord, and the pelvic nerves are the principal motor pathway that regulates the actions of the distal colon, the rectum, the anal canal, and the internal anal sphincter in defecation. Both reflex and voluntary activities are involved in defecation.

■ Self-Study Problems

1. Briefly summarize control of the motor and secretory activities of the gastrointestinal tract by the enteric nervous system and by the sympathetic and parasympathetic innervation.

2. What are slow waves? What are the relationships among slow waves, action potentials, and contractions of gastrointestinal smooth muscle?

3. Describe the regulation of gastric emptying by chemical stimuli in the duodenum.

4. Contrast the contractile behavior of the small intestine of a fed individual with that of a fasted person.

5. Describe the normal motility of the colon.

■ *Bibliography*
Journal articles

Bornstein JC, Furness JB: Correlated electrophysiological and histochemical studies of submucous neurons and their contribution to understanding enteric neural circuits, *J Auton Nerv Syst* 25:1, 1988.

Bornstein JC, Furness JB, Smith TK, Trussell DC: Synaptic responses evoked by mechanical stimulation of the mucosa in morphologically characterized myenteric neurons of the guinea-pig ileum, *J Neurosci* 11:505, 1991.

Bywater RAB, Taylor GS, Furukawa K: The enteric nervous system in the control of motility and secretion, *Digest Dis* 5:193, 1987.

Costa M, Brookes S, Steele P, Vickers J: Chemical coding of neurons in the gastrointestinal tract, *Adv Exp Med Biol* 298:17, 1991.

Furness JB, Bornstein JC, Murphy R, Pompolo S: Roles of peptides in the enteric nervous system, *Trends Neurosci* 15:66, 1992.

Furness JB et al: Correlated functional and structural analysis of enteric neural circuits, *Arch Histol Cytol* 52 (suppl):161, 1989.

Hara Y, Kubota Y, Szurszewski JH: Electrophysiology of smooth muscle of the small intestine of some mammals, *J Physiol* 372:501, 1986.

Lang IM: Digestive tract motor correlates of vomiting and nausea, *Can J Physiol Pharmacol* 68:242, 1990.

Langton P et al: Spontaneous electrical activity of interstitial cells of Cajal isolated from canine proximal colon, *Proc Natl Acad Sci USA* 86:7280, 1989.

Sanders KM: Ionic mechanisms of electrical rhythmicity in gastrointestinal smooth muscles, *Annu Rev Physiol* 54:439, 1992.

Smith TK, Bornstein JC, Furness JB: Distension-evoked ascending and descending reflexes in the circular muscle of guinea-pig ileum: an intracellular study, *J Auton Nerv Syst* 29: 203, 1990.

Smith TK, Bornstein JC, Furness JB: Interactions between reflexes evoked by distension and mucosal stimulation: electrophysiological studies of guinea-pig ileum, *J Auton Nerv Syst* 34:69, 1991.

Smith TK, Reed JB, Sanders KM: Interaction of two electrical pacemakers in muscularis of canine proximal colon, *Am J Physiol* 252:C290, 1987.

Wood JD: Enteric neurophysiology, *Am J Physiol* 247:G585, 1984.

Books and monographs

Christensen J, Wingate DL, editors: *A guide to gastrointestinal motility,* Bristol, UK, 1983, John Wright & Sons.

Conklin JL, Christensen J: *Motor functions of the pharynx and esophagus.* In Johnson RL, editor: *Physiology of the gastrointestinal tract,* ed 3, New York, 1994, Raven Press.

Davenport HW: *Physiology of the digestive tract,* ed 5, Chicago, 1985, Mosby–Year Book.

Furness JB, Bornstein JC: *The enteric nervous system and its extrinsic connections.* In Yamada T, editor: *Textbook of gastroenterology,* vol 1, Philadelphia, 1991, JB Lippincott.

Furness JB, Costa M: *The enteric nervous system,* Edinburgh, 1987, Churchill Livingstone.

Gabella G: *Structure of muscles and nerves in the gastrointestinal tract.* In Johnson RL, editor: *Physiology of the gastrointestinal tract,* ed 3, New York, 1994, Raven Press.

Grundy D: *Gastrointestinal motility: the integration of physiological mechanisms,* Lancaster, UK, 1985, MTP Press.

Kamm MA, Lennard-Jones JE, editors: *Gastrointestinal transit,* Petersfield, UK, 1991, Wrightson Biomedical Publishing.

Makhlouf GM, editor: *Handbook of physiology,* sect 6, *The gastrointestinal system,* vol II, *Neural and endocrine biology,* Bethesda, Md, 1989, American Physiological Society.

Makhlouf GM: *Neuromuscular function of the small intestine.* In Johnson RL, editor: *Physiology of the gastrointestinal tract,* ed 3, New York, 1994, Raven Press.

Mayer EM: *The physiology of gastric storage and emptying.* In Johnson RL, editor: *Physiology of the gastrointestinal tract,* ed 3, New York, 1994, Raven Press.

Sanders KM, Smith TK: *Electrophysiology of colonic smooth muscle.* In Wood JD, editor: *Handbook of physiology,* sect 6, *The gastrointestinal system,* vol I, Bethesda, Md, 1989, American Physiological Society.

Wood JD: *Electrical and synaptic behavior of enteric neurons.* In Wood JD, editor: *Handbook of physiology,* sect 6, *The gastrointestinal system,* vol I, Bethesda, Md, 1989, American Physiological Society.

Gastrointestinal Secretions

This chapter deals with the glandular secretion of fluids and compounds that have important functions in the digestive tract. The secretions of the **salivary glands, gastric glands, exocrine pancreas,** and **liver** are considered. The composition and digestive function of each section are discussed, and the regulation of secretory processes is emphasized.

Digestive secretions are released from glands by the action of specific effector substances on the secretory cells. These effector substances may be classified as neurocrine, endocrine, or paracrine (see Chapter 5).

A substance that stimulates a particular cell to secrete is called a **secretagogue.** Although secretagogues are numerous, only a few signal transduction mechanisms (discussed in Chapter 5) mediate secretion.

■ *Secretion of Saliva*

In humans, the salivary glands produce about 1 L of saliva each day. Saliva lubricates food to make swallowing easier, and it also facilitates speaking.

In people who lack functional salivary glands, **xerostomia** (dry mouth), **dental caries,** and infections of the buccal mucosa are prevalent. Saliva contains **secretory immunoglobulins** (antibodies) directed against microorganisms in the mouth, and lysozyme that hydrolyzes a major component of bacterial outer membranes. In the absence of antibodies and lysozyme, organisms that cause buccal infections and dental caries proliferate. The basic pH of saliva also helps prevent dental caries.

■ *Functions of Saliva*

Mucins, which are glycoproteins produced by the submaxillary and sublingual glands, lubricate food so that it may be more readily swallowed. The major digestive function of saliva is carried out by the enzyme **salivary amylase,** which breaks down starch. Salivary amylase has the same specificity as the α-amylase of pancreatic juice (see Chapter 39); it reduces starch to oligosaccharide molecules. The optimal pH for salivary amylase is about 7, but it is active between pH 4 and 11. After mixing with food in the mouth, amylase continues to break down starch in the mass of food in the stomach. Its action is terminated only when the contents of the antrum are mixed with enough gastric acid to lower the pH to less than 4. More than half the starch in a well-chewed meal may be reduced to small oligosaccharides by the action of salivary amylase. However, because of the efficiency with which pancreatic α-amylase digests starch in the small intestine, starch is well absorbed even in the absence of salivary amylase.

Other components of saliva are present in smaller amounts. These components include RNAase, DNAase, lysozyme, lactoperoxidase, lingual lipase, kallikrein, and secretory immunoglobulin A (IgA).

■ *Structure of Salivary Glands*

In humans, the **parotid glands,** the largest salivary glands, are entirely serous. The watery secretion from these glands lacks mucins. The **submaxillary** and **sublingual glands** are mixed mucous and serous glands, and they secrete a more viscous saliva that contains mucins. Many smaller salivary glands are present in the oral cavity. The microscopic structure of a mixed salivary gland is depicted in Fig. 38-1. **Serous acinar cells** are located in the **secretory endpieces** (also called **acini**). Serous acinar cells have apical **zymogen granules** that contain salivary amylase and perhaps other salivary proteins also (Fig. 38-2). **Mucous acinar cells** secrete glycoprotein mucins into the saliva. **Intercalated ducts** drain the acinar fluid into larger ducts, the **striated ducts,** which empty into still larger **excretory ducts** (Fig. 38-1). A single large duct brings the secretions of each major gland into the mouth.

The production of saliva by a salivary gland begins in the secretory endpieces, which elaborate a fluid called

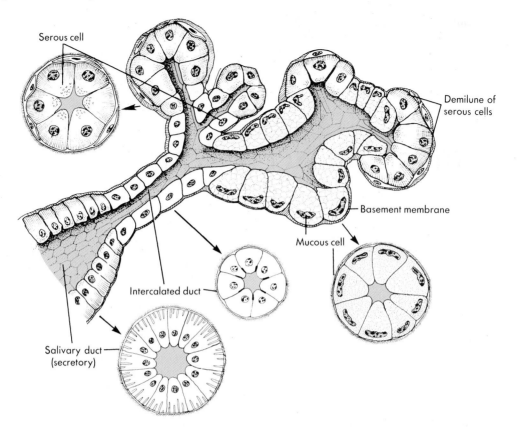

■ **Fig. 38-1**   Structure of the human submandibular gland, as seen with the light microscope. (Redrawn after Braus H: *Anatomie des Menschen,* Berlin, 1934, Julius Springer.)

■ **Fig. 38-2**   Schematic representation of the cellular morphology of a secretory endpiece of a serous salivary gland. Colored circles represent zymogen granules. Upon stimulation, the contents of zymogen granules are released by exocytosis into the lumen of the acinus. (Redrawn from Young JA, van Lennep LW: *Morphology of salivary glands,* London, 1978, Academic Press.)

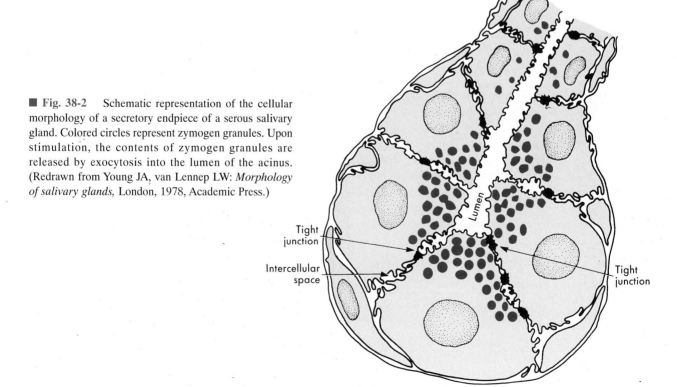

the **primary secretion.** The cells that line the ducts modify this primary secretion to produce saliva.

■ *Metabolism and Blood Flow of Salivary Glands*

The salivary glands produce a prodigious flow of saliva. The maximal rate of saliva production in humans is about 1 ml/min/g of gland; *at this rate, the glands are producing their own weight in saliva each minute!* Salivary glands have a high rate of metabolism and a high blood flow; both are proportional to the rate of saliva formation. *The blood flow to maximally secreting salivary glands is approximately 10 times that of an equal mass of actively contracting skeletal muscle.* Stimulation of the parasympathetic nerves to salivary glands increases blood flow by dilating the vasculature of the glands. **Vasoactive intestinal polypeptide (VIP)** and **acetylcholine** are released from parasympathetic nerve terminals in the salivary glands; both of these compounds contribute to vasodilation during secretory activity.

■ *Secretion of Saliva*

Ionic composition of saliva. *In humans, saliva is always hypotonic to plasma.* As shown in Fig. 38-3, salivary concentrations of Na^+ and Cl^- are less than those of plasma. The greater the secretory flow rate, the higher is the tonicity of the saliva; at maximal flow rates, the tonicity of saliva in humans is about 70% of that of plasma. The pH of saliva from resting glands is slightly acidic. During active secretion, however, the saliva becomes basic, and its pH increases to near 8. The increase in pH that accompanies saliva secretion is partly caused by an increase in bicarbonate concentration with increasing flow rate. Except at the lowest salivary flow rates, the concentration of bicarbonate in saliva is greater than the plasma concentration of bicarbonate. The concentration of K^+ in saliva is always much greater than its concentration in plasma. When salivary flow rates are very low, salivary K^+ levels are high.

Secretion of water and electrolytes. A **two-stage model of salivary secretion** (Fig. 38-4) postulates that

1. The secretory endpieces, perhaps with the participation of intercalated ducts, produce a **primary secretion** that is isotonic to plasma. The amylase concentration of this primary secretion and the rate at which it is secreted vary with the level and type of stimulation. However, the electrolyte composition of the secretion is fairly constant. Levels of Na^+, K^+, HCO_3^-, and Cl^- are close to plasma levels.

2. The excretory ducts, and probably the striated ducts also, modify the primary secretion by extracting Na^+ and Cl^- from, and adding K^+ and HCO_3^- to, the saliva. The ducts only modify the composition of the primary secretion; they do not add to the volume of saliva.

Because the ducts remove more Na^+ and Cl^- ions from saliva than they add K^+ and HCO_3^-, saliva becomes progressively more hypotonic as it flows through the ducts. The faster the flow rate of the saliva through the striated and excretory ducts, the closer to isotonicity it becomes.

Secretion of salivary amylase. As noted previously, serous acinar cells have zymogen granules (Fig. 38-2) that contain salivary amylase. These granules are located in the apical cytoplasm of these cells. When the gland is stimulated to secrete, the zymogen granules fuse with the plasma membrane and release their contents into the lumen of the secretory endpiece by exocytosis.

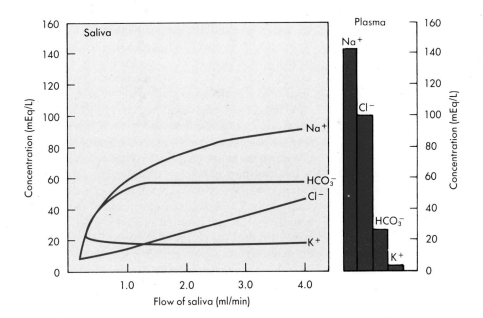

■ **Fig. 38-3** Average composition of parotid saliva as a function of the salivary flow rate. Saliva is hypotonic to plasma at all flow rates, but the tonicity increases with increasing flow rate. The bicarbonate level in saliva exceeds that in plasma, except at very low flow rates. (Redrawn from Thaysen JH et al: *Am J Physiol* 178:155, 1954.)

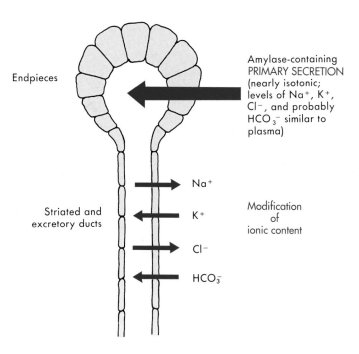

Endpieces

Amylase-containing
PRIMARY SECRETION
(nearly isotonic;
levels of Na$^+$, K$^+$,
Cl$^-$, and probably
HCO$_3^-$ similar to
plasma)

Na$^+$

Striated and
excretory ducts

K$^+$

Modification
of
ionic content

Cl$^-$

HCO$_3^-$

■ **Fig. 38-4**   Schematic representation of the two-stage model of salivary secretion. The primary secretion, containing salivary amylase and electrolytes at concentrations similar to those in plasma, is produced by the acinar cells. The striated and excretory ducts modify the composition of saliva by absorbing Na$^+$ and Cl$^-$ and secreting K$^+$ and HCO$_3^-$.

■ *Neural Control of Salivary Gland Function*

The primary physiological control of the salivary glands is by the parasympathetic nervous system. In contrast, the control of most other gastrointestinal secretions is primarily hormonal. Excitation of either sympathetic or parasympathetic nerves to the salivary glands stimulates salivary secretion, but the effects of the parasympathetic nerves are stronger and more long-lasting. Interruption of the sympathetic nerves does not disrupt salivary gland function. If the parasympathetic supply is interrupted, however, salivation is severely impaired and the salivary glands atrophy.

Sympathetic fibers to the salivary glands stem from the superior cervical ganglion. Preganglionic parasympathetic fibers come via branches of the facial and glossopharyngeal nerves (cranial nerves VII and IX, respectively). These fibers form synapses with postganglionic neurons in ganglia in or near the salivary glands. The acinar cells and ducts are supplied with parasympathetic nerve endings.

Parasympathetic stimulation increases the synthesis and secretion of salivary amylase and mucins, enhances the transport activities of the ductular epithelium, greatly increases blood flow to the glands, and stimulates glandular metabolism and growth.

The increase in salivary secretion that results from stimulation of sympathetic nerves is transient. Sympathetic stimulation constricts blood vessels, which causes a decrease in salivary gland blood flow.

Stimulation of both sympathetic and parasympathetic, causes contraction of myoepithelial cells that surround the acini. This contraction serves to empty the acinar contents into the ducts and thus augments salivary flow.

■ *Ionic Mechanisms of Salivary Secretion*

Ion transport in ductular cells. Fig. 38-5 shows a simplified model of ion transport processes in the epithelial cells of excretory ducts and probably of striated ducts also. The Na$^+$, K$^+$-ATPase located in the basolateral membrane of the epithelial cell maintains the electrochemical potential gradients of Na$^+$ and K$^+$ that power most of the other ionic transport processes of the cell. In the apical membrane, the parallel operation of Na$^+$, H$^+$, Cl$^-$, HCO$_3^-$, and H$^+$, K$^+$ exchangers results in the absorption of Na$^+$ and Cl$^-$ from the luminal fluid and the secretion of K$^+$ and HCO$_3^-$ into the lumen. The impermeability of the ductular epithelium to water prevents the ducts from absorbing too much water by osmosis.

As noted, both parasympathetic and sympathetic stimulation each increase the flow rate of saliva. This increase in flow rate is mediated partly by the inhibition of Na$^+$ absorption across the luminal membrane of the epithelial cells.

Ion transport in acinar cells. Fig. 38-6 shows a simplified view of the mechanisms of ion secretion in serous acinar cells. The basolateral membrane of the cell contains the Na$^+$, K$^+$-ATPase and an Na$^+$, K$^+$, 2 Cl$^-$ cotransporter that uses the energy of the Na$^+$ gradient to power the active uptake of K$^+$ and Cl$^-$. Cl$^-$ and bicarbonate leave the acinar cell to enter the luminal fluid via an electrogenic anion channel located in the apical membrane of the acinar cell. Acinar cell fluid secretion is strongly

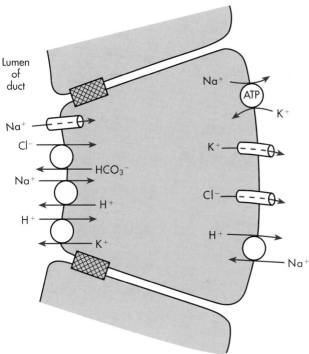

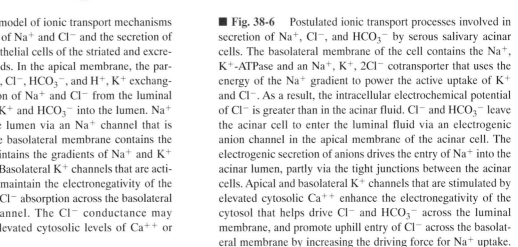

■ **Fig. 38-5**   Postulated model of ionic transport mechanisms involved in the absorption of Na^+ and Cl^- and the secretion of K^+ and HCO_3^- by the epithelial cells of the striated and excretory ducts of salivary glands. In the apical membrane, the parallel operation of Na^+, H^+, Cl^-, HCO_3^-, and H^+, K^+ exchangers results in the absorption of Na^+ and Cl^- from the luminal fluid and the secretion of K^+ and HCO_3^- into the lumen. Na^+ is also absorbed from the lumen via an Na^+ channel that is blocked by amiloride. The basolateral membrane contains the Na^+, K^+-ATPase that maintains the gradients of Na^+ and K^+ and Na^+, H^+ exchangers. Basolateral K^+ channels that are activated by increased Ca^{++} maintain the electronegativity of the cytosol that helps to drive Cl^- absorption across the basolateral membrane via a Cl^- channel. The Cl^- conductance may increase in response to elevated cytosolic levels of Ca^{++} or cyclic AMP.

■ **Fig. 38-6**   Postulated ionic transport processes involved in secretion of Na^+, Cl^-, and HCO_3^- by serous salivary acinar cells. The basolateral membrane of the cell contains the Na^+, K^+-ATPase and an Na^+, K^+, $2Cl^-$ cotransporter that uses the energy of the Na^+ gradient to power the active uptake of K^+ and Cl^-. As a result, the intracellular electrochemical potential of Cl^- is greater than in the acinar fluid. Cl^- and HCO_3^- leave the acinar cell to enter the luminal fluid via an electrogenic anion channel in the apical membrane of the acinar cell. The electrogenic secretion of anions drives the entry of Na^+ into the acinar lumen, partly via the tight junctions between the acinar cells. Apical and basolateral K^+ channels that are stimulated by elevated cytosolic Ca^{++} enhance the electronegativity of the cytosol that helps drive Cl^- and HCO_3^- across the luminal membrane, and promote uphill entry of Cl^- across the basolateral membrane by increasing the driving force for Na^+ uptake. The anion conductance of the apical membrane is increased in response to elevation of cytoplasmic Ca^{++} or cyclic AMP.

enhanced in response to elevations of intracellular Ca^{++} concentration.

■ *Cellular Control of Salivary Secretion: Signal Transduction Mechanisms*

Control mechanisms in ductular cells. The ducts of salivary glands respond to both cholinergic and adrenergic agonists by increasing the rates of secretion of K^+ and HCO_3^-.

Control mechanisms in serous acinar cells. Acetylcholine, norepinephrine, substance P, and **VIP** are released in salivary glands by specific nerve terminals.

Each of these neuroeffectors increases the secretion of salivary amylase and the flow of saliva.

These neuroeffector substances act mainly by elevating the intracellular concentration of cyclic AMP (cAMP) or by increasing the concentration of Ca^{++} in the cytosol (Fig. 38-7). Acetylcholine, substance P, and norepinephrine acting on α receptors increase the cytosolic concentration of Ca^{++} in the serous acinar cells. In contrast, norepinephrine acting on β receptors and VIP elevate the cAMP concentration in acinar cells. Agonists that elevate cAMP concentration in serous acinar cells elicit a secretion that is rich in amylase; agonists that mobilize Ca^{++} elicit a secretion that is more voluminous but that has a lower concentration

■ **Fig. 38-7**   The cellular mechanisms whereby norepinephrine *(Norepi),* acetylcholine *(ACh),* and substance P evoke salivary secretion. Norepinephrine acting on α-adrenergic receptors, acetylcholine, and substance P increases intracellular Ca^{++}. Norepinephrine acting on β-adrenergic receptors increases intracellular levels of cyclic AMP *(cAMP).* Effectors that increase cellular cAMP elicit a primary secretion that is richer in amylase than is the secretion evoked by agents that increase intracellular Ca^{++}. Substances that increase intracellular Ca^{++} produce a greater volume of acinar cell secretion than do agonists that increase intracellular cAMP. (Modified from Peterson OH. In Johnson RL, editor: *Physiology of the gastrointestinal tract,* New York, 1981, Raven Press.)

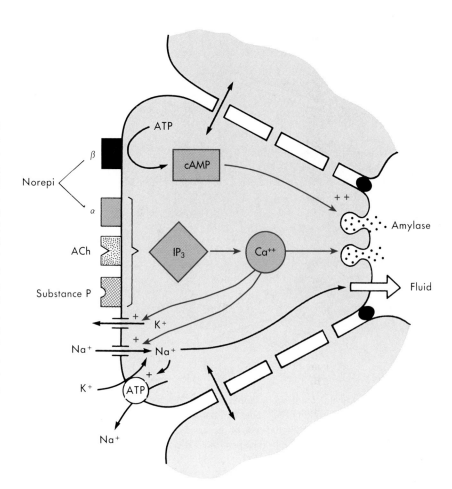

of amylase. Ca^{++} mobilizing agonists may also elevate the concentration of cyclic GMP (cGMP), which may mediate the trophic effects evoked by these agonists.

■ *Gastric Secretion*

The stomach serves several functions. It functions as a reservoir that allows the ingestion of a large meal. Later, the stomach empties its contents (now called *chyme)* into the duodenum at a controlled rate consistent with the ability of the duodenum and small intestine to process the chyme.

The major secretions of the stomach are hydrochloric acid (HCl), pepsins, intrinsic factor, mucus, and bicarbonate. HCl kills most ingested microorganisms. HCl also catalyzes the cleavage of inactive pepsinogens to active **pepsins.** In addition, HCl provides a low pH environment, which is required for the action of pepsins in digesting proteins and peptides. **Intrinsic factor,** a glycoprotein, binds vitamin B_{12} and allows it to be absorbed in the ileum. The hormone **gastrin,** released by G cells in the gastric antrum, promotes secretion of HCl and pepsinogens. Mucus and bicarbonate secretions protect the stomach from mechanical and chemical damage.

■ *Structure of the Gastric Mucosa*

The surface of the gastric mucosa (Fig. 38-8) is covered by columnar **epithelial cells** that secrete mucus and an alkaline fluid that protects the epithelium from mechanical injury and gastric acid. The gastric mucosal surface is studded with **gastric pits;** each pit is the opening of a duct into which one or more **gastric glands** empty (Fig. 38-8, *A).* The gastric pits are so numerous that they account for a significant fraction of the total surface area of the gastric mucosa.

The gastric mucosa can be divided into three distinct regions, based on the structures of the glands present. The small **cardiac glandular region,** located just below the lower esophageal sphincter, contains primarily mucus-secreting gland cells. The remainder of the gastric mucosa is divided into the **oxyntic** (acid-secreting) **glandular region,** located above the gastric notch, and the **pyloric glandular region,** below the notch (see Fig. 37-12).

The structure of a gastric gland from the oxyntic glandular region is illustrated in Fig. 38-8, *B.* The surface epithelial cells extend slightly into the duct opening. **Mucous neck cells,** which secrete mucus, are located in the narrow neck of the gland. **Parietal** or **oxyntic cells,** which secrete HCl and **intrinsic factor,** and **chief** or **peptic cells,** which secrete **pepsinogens,** are located deeper

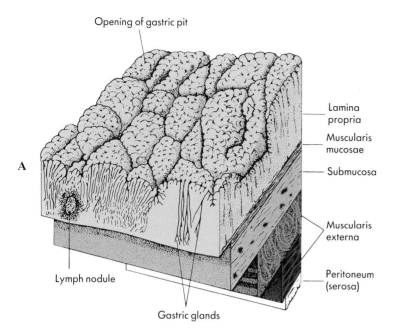

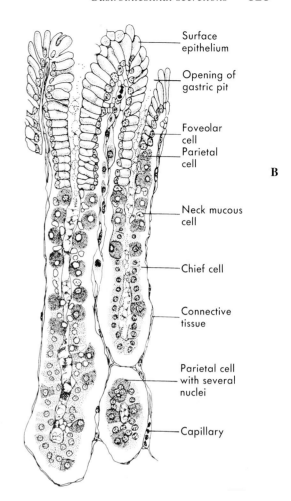

■ **Fig. 38-8** Structure of the gastric mucosa. **A,** Reconstruction of part of the gastric wall. **B,** Two gastric glands from a human stomach. (**A** redrawn from Braus H: *Anatomie des Menschen,* Berlin, 1934, Julius Springer. **B** redrawn from Weis L, editor: *Histology: cell and tissue biology,* ed 5, New York, 1981, Elsevier.)

in the gland. Parietal cells are particularly numerous in glands in the fundus, whereas mucus-secreting cells are more numerous in the glands of the pyloric glandular region. Pyloric glands also contain **G cells,** which secrete the hormone **gastrin.**

The stomach has the remarkable ability to repair damage to its epithelial surface. Surface epithelial cells are exfoliated into the lumen at a considerable rate during normal gastric function. These cells are replaced by mucous neck cells, which then differentiate into columnar epithelial cells and migrate up out of the necks of the glands.

■ *Gastric Acid Secretion*

The fluid secreted into the stomach is called **gastric juice.** Gastric juice is a mixture of the secretions of the surface epithelial cells and the secretions of gastric glands. *Among the important components of gastric juice are HCl, salts, water, pepsins, intrinsic factor, mucus, and bicarbonate.* Secretion of all these components increases after a meal.

Ionic composition of gastric juice. The ionic composition of gastric juice depends on the rate of secretion. Fig. 38-9 shows that the higher the secretory rate, the higher is the concentration of hydrogen ions. At lower

secretory rates, $[H^+]$ decreases and $[Na^+]$ increases. $[K^+]$ is always higher in gastric juice than in plasma. Consequently, prolonged vomiting may lead to hypokalemia. At all rates of secretion, Cl^- is the major anion of gastric juice. At high rates of secretion, gastric juice resembles an isotonic solution of HCl. Gastric HCl converts pepsinogens to active pepsins (see below) and provides an acid pH at which pepsins are active.

The high acidity of gastric juice kills most ingested microorganisms. Individuals who have low rates of gastric acid secretion, either because of disease or because they are taking medications that suppress HCl secretion, are more susceptible to infection by ingested pathogens and may have bacterial overgrowth in the stomach or upper small intestine.

Rate of secretion of gastric acid. The rate of gastric acid secretion varies considerably among individuals. In humans, basal (unstimulated) rates of gastric acid production typically range from about 1 to 5 mEq/hr. During maximal stimulation, HCl production rises to 6 to 40 mEq/hr. The total number of parietal cells in the stomachs of normal individuals varies greatly, and this variation is partly responsible for the wide range of basal and stimulated rates of HCl secretion.

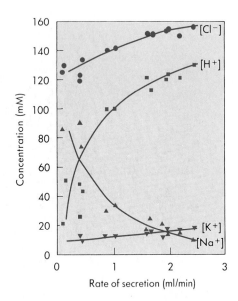

■ **Fig. 38-9**   Concentrations of ions in gastric juice as a function of the rate of secretion in a normal young person. At low flow rates, gastric juice is hypotonic to plasma. At high flow rates, gastric juice approaches isotonicity and contains predominantly H^+ and Cl^- (Redrawn from Davenport HW: *Physiology of the digestive tract,* ed 5, Chicago, Mosby–Year Book; and adapted from Nordgren B: *Acta Physiol Scand* 58(suppl 202):1, 1963.)

Morphologic changes that accompany gastric acid secretion. Parietal cells have a distinctive ultrastructure (Fig. 38-10). Branching **secretory canaliculi** course through the cytoplasm and are connected by a common outlet to the cell's luminal surface. Microvilli line the surfaces of the secretory canaliculi. The cytoplasm of unstimulated parietal cells contains numerous tubules and vesicles, which together are called the **tubulovesicular system.** The membranes of the tubulovesicles contain the transport proteins responsible for secretion of H^+ and Cl^- into the lumen of the gland.

In order to secrete HCl, parietal cells must undergo a morphologic change that is prompted by stimulation. When parietal cells are stimulated to secrete HCl (Fig. 38-10, *B*), tubulovesicular membranes fuse with the plasma membrane of the secretory canaliculi. *This extensive membrane fusion greatly increases the number of HCl-pumping sites available at the surface of the secretory canaliculi.*

Cellular mechanisms of gastric acid secretion. When parietal cells are secreting gastric acid at the maximal rate, H^+ is pumped against a concentration gradient that is about 1 million-fold: about pH 7 in the parietal cell cytosol to about pH 1 in the lumen of the gastric gland. Also, because the lumen of the stomach is electronegative by 30 to 80 mV relative to the serosa, Cl^- enters the gastric lumen against both chemical and electrical potential differences. Energy is required for transport of both H^+ and Cl^- into gastric juice.

The apical membrane of the parietal cell (the membrane that lines the secretory canaliculus) contains an H^+, K^+-ATPase, which exchanges H^+ for K^+. This ATPase (Fig. 38-11) is the primary H^+ pump. Both H^+ and K^+ are pumped against their electrochemical potential gradients. The H^+, K^+-ATPase is closely related to the Na^+, K^+-ATPase of plasma membranes and the Ca^{++}-ATPase of sarcoplasmic reticulum membranes.

Drugs that specifically inhibit the H^+, K^+-ATPase have recently been developed. Substituted benzimidazoles, such as **omeprazole,** are inactive at neutral pH. At a low pH, however, they are converted to a form that reacts with sulfhydryl groups on the H^+, K^+-ATPase. This reaction inactivates its enzymatic and ion pumping activities. Because the inactivation of H^+, K^+-ATPase by omeprazole is irreversible, the drug should be administered only once daily.

When H^+ is pumped out of the parietal cell (Fig. 38-12), an excess of HCO_3^- is left behind. HCO_3^- flows down its electrochemical gradient across the basolateral plasma membrane. *The protein that mediates HCO_3^- efflux, called the Cl^-, HCO_3^- countertransporter, also transports Cl^- in the opposite direction. Thus, Cl^- moves against its electrochemical potential gradient into the cell. The energy for this active transport of Cl^- comes from the downhill movement of HCO_3^- across the basolateral membrane.* As a result of the combined action of the H^+,K^+-ATPase and the Cl^-, HCO_3^- countertransporter, Cl^- is concentrated in the cytoplasm of the parietal cell. The Cl^- leaves the parietal cell at the apical membrane via an electrogenic anion channel.

Stimulation of the parietal cell to secrete H^+ and Cl^-. Histamine, acetylcholine, and gastrin are the three physiological agonists of HCl secretion by parietal cells. Histamine elevates the intracellular concentration of cAMP, while acetylcholine and gastrin elevate the intracellular Ca^{++} concentration.

The basolateral membranes of parietal cells contain two types of K^+ channels (Fig. 38-12). One type of K^+ channel is activated by cAMP; the other type is activated by Ca^{++}. Activation of the basolateral K^+ channels hyperpolarizes the cell and thereby increases the driving force for Cl^- to leave the cell. Cl^- leaves the cell through the electrogenic Cl^- channels in the apical membrane on the boundary of the secretory canaliculus. The K^+ channels also mediate the efflux of K^+ that accumulates in the parietal cell via the activity of the H^+, K^+-ATPase.

The conductance of the electrogenic Cl^- channels of the apical membrane is dramatically increased by elevated cAMP concentrations and by hyperpolarization of the cell. In addition, cAMP and Ca^{++} prompt the insertion of more Cl^- channels into the luminal membrane and promote the fusion of cytosolic tubovesicles with the membrane of the secretory canaliculi. This latter process

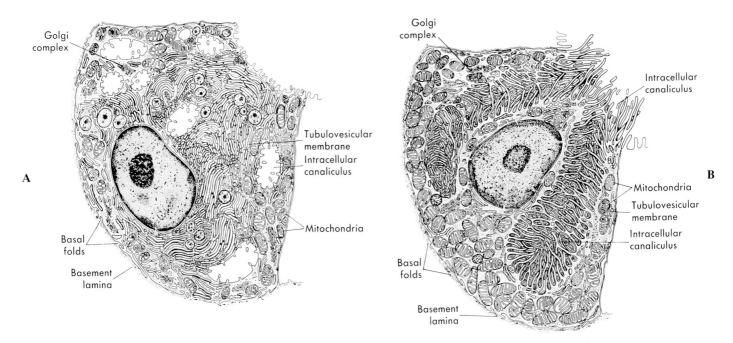

■ **Fig. 38-10** **A,** Drawing of a resting parietal cell with cytoplasm full of tubulovesicles and an internalized intracellular canaliculus. **B,** An acid-secreting parietal cell. Tubulovesicles have fused with the membrane of the intracellular canaliculus, which is now open to the lumen of the gland and lined with abundant, long microvilli. (Redrawn after Ito S. In Johnson RL, editor: *Physiology of the gastrointestinal tract,* New York, 1981, Raven Press.)

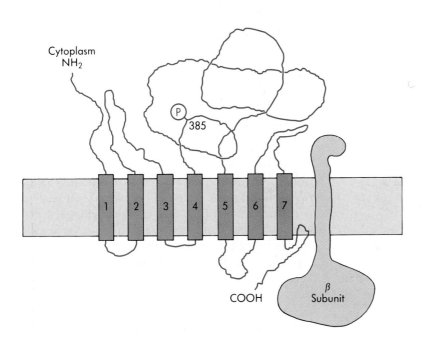

■ **Fig. 38-11** Model of the structure of the H^+, K^+-ATPase. This ion-transporting ATPase is present in the tubovesicular membrane and in the membrane that bounds the secretory canaliculus. This protein pumps H^+ into the lumen of the secretory canaliculus in exchange for K^+ taken into the parietal cell. The phosphorylation site, aspartate 385, is identified. The β subunit is a glycoprotein that may function similarly to the β subunit of the Na^+, K^+-ATPase. (Modified from Rabon EC, Reuben MA: *Annu Rev Physiol* 52:321, 1990.)

increases the number of H^+, K^+-ATPase molecules in the canalicular membrane (Fig. 38-10).

■ *Secretion of Pepsins*

Pepsins, often collectively called **pepsin,** are a group of proteases secreted by the chief cells of the gastric glands. *Pepsins are secreted as inactive proenzymes called*

pepsinogens. Pepsinogens are contained in membrane-bound zymogen granules in the chief cells. Zymogen granules release their contents by exocytosis when the chief cells are stimulated to secrete.

Pepsinogens are converted to active pepsins by the cleavage of acid-labile linkages. The lower the pH, the more rapid is this conversion. Pepsins also act proteolytically on pepsinogens to form more pepsins. Pepsins are most proteolytically active at a pH of 3 and below. Pepsins

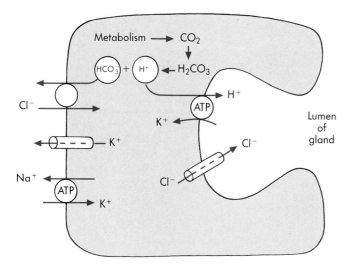

■ **Fig. 38-12** Postulated model of the major ionic transport processes involved in the secretion of H^+ and Cl^- by parietal cells. Cl^- enters the cell across the basolateral membrane against an electrochemical gradient. Cl^- entry is powered by the downhill efflux of HCO_3^-. The high level of HCO_3^- in the cytosol is generated by the extrusion of H^+ across the luminal membrane. H^+ is pumped into the secretory canaliculus by the H^+, K^+-ATPase. Cl^- enters the canalicular fluid by an electrogenic ion channel. The Cl^- conductance of the luminal membrane is increased in response to increased cytosolic Ca^{++} and cyclic AMP. The conductance of basolateral K^+ channels is also enhanced by the second messengers, and K^+ efflux through these channels increases the electronegativity of the cytosol and increases the driving force for efflux of Cl^- across the apical membrane.

may digest as much as 20% of the protein in a typical meal. When the duodenal contents are neutralized, pepsins are inactivated irreversibly by the neutral pH.

■ *Secretion of Intrinsic Factor*

Intrinsic factor, a glycoprotein secreted by the parietal cells of the stomach, is required for the normal absorption of vitamin B$_{12}$ (see Chapter 39). Intrinsic factor is released in response to the same stimuli that elicit the secretion of HCl by parietal cells. *Secretion of intrinsic factor is the only gastric function that is essential for human life.*

■ *Secretion of Mucus and Bicarbonate*

Mucus and bicarbonate protect the surface of the stomach from the effects of HCl and pepsins.

Secretion of mucus. Secretions that contain glycoprotein **mucins** are viscous and sticky and are collectively termed **mucus.** Mucins are secreted by mucous neck cells located in the necks of gastric glands and by the surface epithelial cells of the stomach. Mucus is stored in large granules in the apical cytoplasm of mucous neck

cells and surface epithelial cells, and is released by exocytosis.

Gastric mucins are about 80% carbohydrate by weight and consist of four similar monomers of about 500,000 daltons each that are linked together by disulfide crosslinks (Fig. 38-13). These tetrameric mucins form a sticky gel that adheres to the surface of the stomach. However, this gel is subject to proteolysis by pepsins, which cleave bonds near the center of the tetramers. This process releases fragments that do not form gels, and thus dissolves the protective mucus layer. Maintenance of the protective mucus layer requires continuous synthesis of new tetrameric mucins to replace those mucins that are cleaved by pepsins.

Mucus is secreted at a significant rate in the resting stomach. Secretion of mucus is stimulated by some of the same stimuli that enhance acid and pepsinogen secretion, especially by acetylcholine released from parasympathetic nerve endings near the gastric glands. If the gastric mucosa is mechanically deformed, neural reflexes are evoked that enhance mucus secretion.

Secretion of bicarbonate. The surface epithelial cells also secrete a watery fluid that contains Na^+ and Cl^- concentrations similar to those of plasma, but with higher K^+ and HCO_3^- concentrations than those of plasma. Bicarbonate is entrapped by the viscous mucus that coats the surface of the stomach. *The high HCO_3^- concentration makes the mucus layer alkaline,* and thus the mucus secreted by the resting mucosa lines the stomach with a sticky, viscous, alkaline coat. When food is eaten, the rates of secretion of both mucus and of HCO_3^- increase. The maximal rate of bicarbonate secretion is about 10% of the maximal rate of HCl secretion. Bicarbonate secretion is enhanced by acetylcholine released from nerve endings near the surface epithelial cells.

The gastric mucosal barrier. *The protective mucus gel that forms on the luminal surface of the stomach, and alkaline secretions entrapped within it, constitute a **gastric mucosal barrier** that prevents damage to the mucosa by gastric contents* (Fig. 38-14). The mucus gel layer, which is about 0.2 mm thick, effectively separates the bicarbonate-rich secretions of the surface epithelial cells from the acidic contents of the gastric lumen. Thus, the mucus allows the pH of the epithelial cells to be maintained at nearly neutral pH, despite a luminal pH of about 2. Mucus also slows the diffusion of acid and pepsins to the epithelial cell surface. *The protection of the gastric epithelium depends on both mucus and HCO_3^- secretion; neither mucus alone nor HCO_3^- alone can hold the pH at the epithelial cell surface near neutral.*

The gastric mucosal barrier of a normal individual can protect the stomach even when rates of secretion of HCl and pepsins are elevated. If the secretion of either HCO_3^- or mucus is suppressed, however, the gastric mucosal barrier is compromised, and the effects of acid and pepsin on the surface of the stomach may produce **gastric ulcers.**

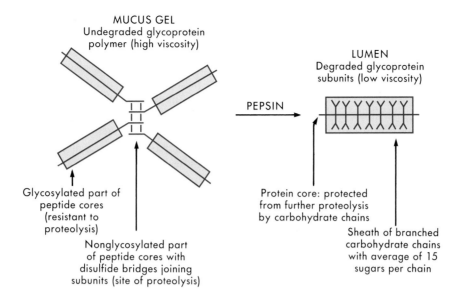

■ **Fig. 38-13** Schematic depiction of the structure of gastric mucins before and after hydrolysis by pepsin. Intact mucins are tetramers of four similar monomers of about 500,000 daltons each that are attached by disulfide cross-links. Each monomer is largely covered by carbohydrate side chains that protect it from proteolytic degradation. The tetrameric mucins form a sticky gel that adheres to the surface of the stomach. The central portion of the mucin tetramer, near the disulfide cross-links, is more susceptible to proteolytic digestion. Pepsins cleave bonds near the center of the tetramers to release fragments about the size of monomers; these fragments do not form gels, so that proteolysis dissolves the gel. (Redrawn from Allen A: *Br Med Bull* 34:28, 1978.)

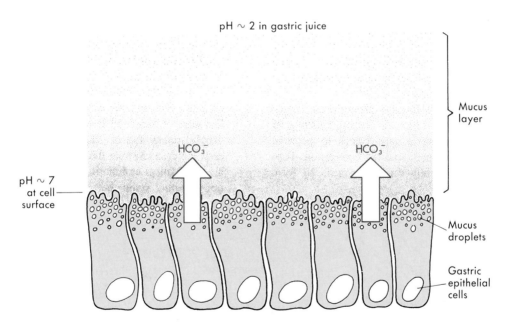

■ **Fig. 38-14** The protection provided to the mucosal surface of the stomach by the bicarbonate-containing mucus layer is known as the gastric mucosal barrier. In man, the mucus layer is about 0.2 mm thick. Buffering by the bicarbonate-rich secretions of the surface epithelial cells, and the restraint to convective mixing caused by the high viscosity of the mucus layer, allow the pH at the cell surface to remain near 7, whereas the pH in the gastric juice in the lumen is 1 to 2.

Aspirin and other **nonsteroidal anti-inflammatory agents** inhibit secretion of both mucus and HCO_3^-; prolonged use of these drugs may damage the mucosal surface and produce **gastritis** or even gastric ulcers. α-Adrenergic agonists diminish HCO_3^- secretion. This effect may play a role in the pathogenesis of **stress ulcers;** chronically elevated levels of circulating epinephrine may suppress HCO_3^- secretion sufficiently to decrease protection of the epithelial cell surface.

■ *Control of Gastric Acid Secretion*

Control of HCl secretion at the level of the parietal cell. Acetylcholine, histamine, and **gastrin** are the three physiological agonists of HCl secretion. Each of these secretagogues binds to a distinct class of receptors on the plasma membrane of the parietal cell and directly stimulates the parietal cell to secrete HCl (Fig. 38-15). Acetylcholine is released near parietal cells by cholinergic nerve terminals. Gastrin, a hormone, is produced by G cells in the mucosa of the gastric antrum and the duodenum, and reaches parietal cells via the bloodstream. Histamine, a paracrine agonist, is released from cells in the gastric mucosa and diffuses to the parietal cells. Thus, the control of HCl secretion provides an example of regulation by all three types of control mechanisms—neurocrine, endocrine, and paracrine—that regulate gastrointestinal secretions.

Cellular mechanisms of parietal cell agonists. The receptors on the parietal cell membrane for acetylcholine, gastrin, and histamine, as well as the intracellular second messengers by which these secretagogues act, are shown in Fig. 38-15. Histamine, acetylcholine, and gastrin potentiate one another's actions on the parietal cell.

Histamine is a major physiological mediator of HCl secretion. Antagonists of H$_2$ histamine receptors, such as **cimetidine,** block a large portion of the acid secretion elicited by any of the known secretagogues.

Histamine is synthesized and stored in **enterochromaffin-like (ECL) cells,** which are present in the gastric muscosa. When stimulated by acetylcholine or gastrin, the ECL cells release histamine, which diffuses to nearby parietal cells to stimulate HCl secretion. Gastrin is not as potent as acetylcholine or histamine indirectly stimulating parietal cells to release HCl. Cimetidine can greatly reduce the physiological response to elevated blood levels of gastrin. Thus, a major component of the response to gastrin may result from gastrin-stimulated release of histamine.

Histamine binding to H$_2$ receptors on parietal cell plasma membranes activates adenylyl cyclase and elevates the cytosolic concentration of cAMP. These events stimulate HCl secretion by activating basolateral K$^+$ channels and apical Cl$^-$ channels; they also cause more H$^+$, K$^+$-ATPase molecules and Cl$^-$ channels to be inserted into the apical plasma membrane (Fig. 38-12).

Acetylcholine binds to M$_3$ muscarinic receptors and opens Ca^{++} channels in the apical plasma membrane. Acetylcholine also elevates the intracellular Ca^{++} concentration by promoting release of Ca^{++} from intracellular stores. An elevated intracellular Ca^{++} concentration enhances HCl secretion by activating basolateral K$^+$ channels and by causing more H$^+$, K$^+$-ATPase molecules and Cl$^-$ channels to be inserted into the apical plasma membrane.

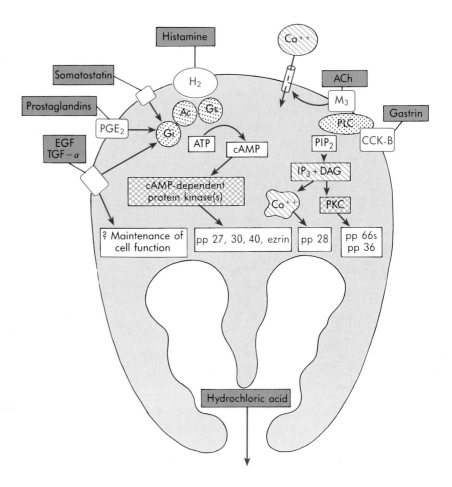

■ **Fig. 38-15** Signal transduction mechanisms of secretagogues and antagonists of acid secretion by parietal cells. Acetylcholine *(ACh)* binds to M$_3$ muscarinic receptors. Histamine acts via H$_2$ histamine receptors. Gastrin binds to CCK-B/gastrin receptors. Acetylcholine and gastrin act to open Ca^{++} channels and to release Ca^{++} from intracellular stores in order to increase cytosolic free Ca^{++}. Histamine activates adenylyl cyclase and increases intracellular levels of cyclic AMP *(cAMP)*. The secretagogues activate protein kinase C, cAMP-dependent protein kinase, and Ca^{++}-calmodulin–dependent kinases. Some of the proteins that are phosphorylated by the kinases are shown; the signaling functions of these phosphoproteins remain to be elucidated. Certain inhibitors of acid secretion, such as somatostatin, prostaglandins of the E class, and epidermal growth factor *(EGF)*, inhibit adenylyl cyclase and lower the cytosolic level of cAMP. *PLC,* Phospholipase C; *PKC,* protein kinase C; *TGF,* transforming growth factor. (Redrawn from Chew CS: *Curr Opin Gastroenterol* 7:856, 1991.)

Gastrin enhances acid secretion by binding to CCK-B receptors to elevate the intracellular Ca^{++} concentration. **Proglumide** is an antagonist of the binding of gastrin to CCK-B receptors.

Before the availability of cimetidine and other H$_2$ receptor blockers, gastric and duodenal ulcers were resistant to drug therapy. Consequently, surgical treatments of ulcers were among the most common surgical operations performed. H$_2$ receptor blockers revolutionized therapy for gastric and duodenal ulcer disease and for most other disorders related to hypersecretion of gastric acid. Surgical interventions are now rarely necessary. These drugs can dramatically reduce secretion of HCl, and they have few side effects.

Endogenous antagonists of acid secretion. **Somatostatin, prostaglandins** of the E and I series, and **epidermal growth factor (EGF)** act on parietal cells to inhibit HCl secretion by inhibiting adenylyl cyclase and decreasing the cAMP concentration (Fig. 38-15). A prostaglandin analog, called **misoprostol,** suppresses acid secretion in this way.

Somatostatin, released from D cells near the bases of gastric glands, is probably a physiological regulator of acid secretion by parietal cells. Somatostatin may also inhibit release of histamine by ECL cells.

In vivo control of acid secretion rate. When the stomach has been empty for several hours, HCl is secreted at a basal rate, which is approximately 10% of the maximal rate. After a meal, the stomach promptly increases the rate of acid secretion. There are three phases of increased acid secretion in response to food: the **cephalic phase,** elicited before food reaches the stomach; the **gastric phase,** elicited by the presence of food in the stomach; and the **intestinal phase,** elicited by mechanisms that originate in the duodenum and upper jejunum (Table 38-1).

The cephalic phase. The cephalic phase of gastric secretion is elicited by the sight, smell, and taste of food. Cephalic phase secretion is entirely mediated by branches of the vagus nerves. Vagal fibers then stimulate enteric neurons that are predominantly cholinergic, and it is these enteric neurons that directly elicit cephalic phase

secretion. Acetylcholine released from these neurons directly stimulates parietal cells to secrete HCl. Indirectly, acetylcholine stimulates acid secretion by releasing gastrin from G cells in the antrum and duodenum, and by releasing histamine from ECL cells in the gastric mucosa.

The low pH in the antrum of the stomach inhibits HCl secretion by directly inhibiting parietal cells and by evoking inhibitory neural reflexes. In the absence of food in the stomach to buffer the acid secreted, the pH of the antral contents falls rapidly during the cephalic phase. The rate of acid secretion during the cephalic phase may be 40% of the maximal rate, but because of the inhibitory mechanisms evoked by low pH in the antrum, the amount of acid secreted is small.

The brain may also influence gastric acid secretion by other mechanisms, but their physiological importance remains uncertain. Low glucose levels in cerebral blood, which occur, for example, during insulin-induced hypoglycemia, stimulate gastric acid secretion. Certain neuropeptides present in brain neurons, when injected into cerebrospinal fluid, stimulate or inhibit gastric secretion of HCl.

The gastric phase. The gastric phase of gastric secretion is elicited by the presence of food in the stomach. The principal stimuli are distention of the stomach and the presence of amino acids and peptides that result from the actions of pepsins. Most of the acid secreted in response to a meal is secreted during the gastric phase.

Distention of either the body or the antrum of the stomach stimulates mechanoreceptors in the gastric wall. These mechanoreceptors are the afferent arms of local and central reflexes. Both the local and central reflexes are largely cholinergic. The central reflexes have their afferent and efferent fibers in the vagus nerves; thus, they are called **vagovagal reflexes.** Activation of these local and central reflexes causes acetylcholine to be released onto parietal cells, which directly stimulates them to secrete HCl, and onto antral G cells, which are stimulated to release gastrin.

The presence of amino acids and peptides in the antrum elicits HCl secretion by causing G cells in the antrum to release gastrin. Intact proteins do not have this effect. Other ingested substances that may enhance gas-

■ **Table 38-1**   Major mechanisms for stimulation of gastric acid secretion

Phase	*Stimulus*	*Pathway*	*Stimulus to parietal cell*
Cephalic	Chewing, swallowing	Vagus nerve to	
		1. Parietal cells	Acetylcholine
		2. G cells	Gastrin
Gastric	Gastric distention	Local and vagovagal reflexes to	
		1. Parietal cells	Acetylcholine
		2. G cells	Gastrin
Intestinal	Protein digestion products in duodenum	1. Intestinal G cells	Gastrin
		2. Intestinal endocrine cells	Entero-oxyntin

Modified from Johnson LR, editor: *Gastrointestinal physiology,* ed 3, St Louis, 1985, Mosby–Year Book.

tric acid secretion include calcium ions, caffeine, and alcohol. Gastric distention enhances the effects of chemical stimuli of HCl secretion.

Secretion of HCl elicited by any of the mechanisms just described is effectively blocked by bathing the mucosal surface with a solution that has a pH of 2 or less. Once the buffering capacity of the gastric contents is saturated, gastric pH falls rapidly and inhibits further acid release. *In this way, the acidity of gastric contents regulates itself.* The mechanisms for this self-regulation stem from the antrum. Low pH in the antrum inhibits HCl secretion by parietal cells by evoking local inhibitory reflexes, by directly inhibiting parietal cell secretion, and by inhibiting the release of gastrin from G cells.

The intestinal phase. The presence of chyme in the duodenum brings about neural and endocrine responses that *first stimulate and later inhibit acid secretion by the stomach.* Early in gastric emptying, when the pH of gastric chyme is greater than 3, stimulation predominates. Later, when the buffer capacity of gastric chyme is exhausted and the pH of chyme emptied into the duodenum falls to less than 3, inhibition prevails. Tables 38-1 and 38-2 summarize the major mechanisms that stimulate and inhibit gastric acid secretion.

STIMULATION OF SECRETION. Gastric secretion is enhanced by distention of the duodenum and by the presence of protein digestion products (peptides and amino acids) in the duodenum. Duodenal distention increases gastric acid secretion by means of vagovagal reflexes that stimulate parietal cells and G cells in the gastric antrum. Peptides and amino acids stimulate G cells in the duodenum and proximal jejunum to release gastrin. In addition, amino acids and peptides that are absorbed in the duodenum and jejunum are carried in the blood to the gastric antrum, where they enhance gastrin release by G cells.

In addition, protein digestion products prompt the release of the hormone *entero-oxyntin* from the duodenum. This poorly characterized hormone also stimulates gastric acid secretion.

INHIBITION OF SECRETION. Several different mechanisms that operate during the intestinal phase inhibit gastric secretion (Table 38-2). These mechanisms are evoked by the presence of acid, fat digestion products, and hypertonicity in the duodenum and proximal part of the jejunum.

Acid solutions in the duodenum inhibit gastric acid by parietal cells via enteric and vagovagal reflexes. Acid solutions in the duodenum also release the hormone **secretin** into the bloodstream. Secretin inhibits gastric acid by inhibiting gastrin release by G cells and by decreasing the response of parietal cells to secretagogues. Acid in the duodenal bulb releases another hormone, **bulbogastrone,** which inhibits acid secretion by the parietal cells.

Products of triglyceride digestion in the duodenum and proximal part of the jejunum release two hormones, **gastric inhibitory peptide (GIP)** and **cholecystokinin (CCK),** that inhibit acid secretion by parietal cells.

Hyperosmotic solutions in the duodenum release an unidentified hormone that inhibits gastric acid secretion. Hormones that are released from the intestine and affect gastric secretions are called **enterogastrones.**

■ *Gastric and Duodenal Ulcers*

Ulceration of the gastric or duodenal mucosa occurs in many individuals. The term **peptic ulcer disease** includes both gastric and duodenal ulcers. Among the mechanisms that may contribute to ulcer formation are diminished effectiveness of the gastric mucosal barrier, hypersecretion of acid, and infection by ***Helicobacter pylori*** bacteria.

Diminished effectiveness of the gastric mucosal barrier, and formation of gastric ulcers, may result from long-term treatment with nonsteroidal anti-inflammatory agents. These agents reduce the rates of secretion of mucus and bicarbonate.

Hypersecretion of acid may contribute to formation of duodenal ulcers. In **Zollinger-Ellison syndrome,** a gastrin-secreting tumor results in increased HCl secretion and in the formation of duodenal ulcers.

Helicobacter pylori infection is responsible for nearly all cases of gastric and duodenal ulcers that are not related to medication. H. pylori has the highly unusual ability to thrive in an acid environment. The bacteria contain large amounts of urease, an enzyme that cat-

---

■ **Table 38-2**   Major mechanisms for inhibition of gastric acid secretion

Region	Stimulus	Mediator	Inhibit gastrin release	Inhibit acid secretion
Antrum	Acid (pH <3.0)	None, direct	+	
Duodenum	Acid	Secretin	+	+
		Bulbogastrone	+	+
		Nervous reflex		+
Duodenum and jejunum	Hyperosmotic solutions	Unidentified enterogastrone		+
	Fatty acids, monoglycerides	Gastric inhibitory peptide	+	+
		Cholecystokinin		+
		Unidentified enterogastrone		+

Modified from Johnson LR, editor: *Gastrointestinal physiology,* ed 3, St Louis, 1985, Mosby–Year Book.

alyzes the conversion of urea to ammonia and CO_2. Ammonia helps to buffer the acid surrounding the bacteria. *H. pylori* colonizes the mucus layer of the stomach and duodenum. It does not actually invade the mucosa; rather, it causes damage by secreting proteins that evoke both cellular and humoral immune responses. The invasion of the mucosa by macrophages and other immunocytes results in **chronic superficial gastritis,** which frequently leads to ulcer disease.

The stomachs of approximately 40% of all individuals are infected with *H. pylori!* Most of these people may have chronic superficial gastritis that causes no intolerable symptoms. In other individuals, *H. pylori* causes more severe gastritis or ulcerations. Chronic severe gastritis caused by *H. pylori* has been implicated in many gastric cancers (Fig. 38-16).

Most duodenal ulcers are also associated with *H. pylori* infection of the stomach. Duodenal ulcer patients are often hypersecretors of HCl; this hypersecretion may be partly attributed to diminished sensitivity to inhibition of HCl secretion by secretin released from the duodenum.

Antibiotic therapy is part of the recommended treatment of gastric or duodenal ulcer disease in *H. pylori*–infected patients. In addition, drugs that suppress HCl secretion are administered, because suppression of HCl secretion renders *H. pylori* more sensitive to antibiotics. Treatment with **omeprazole** or H_2-receptor antagonists without antibiotics reduces the population of *H. pylori* and promotes healing of ulcers. When administration of blockers of acid secretion is discontinued, however, *H. pylori* again flourishes, and ulcers recur in almost all cases.

■ *Pepsinogen Secretion*

Most of the agents that stimulate parietal cells to secrete acid also release pepsinogens from chief cells (Fig. 38-17). Thus, *the rates of release of acid and pepsinogens from the gastric glands are highly correlated.* Acetylcholine is a potent stimulus for the chief cells to release pepsinogens. Gastrin also directly stimulates chief cells. Acid in contact with the gastric mucosa stimulates pepsinogen release by a local neural reflex.

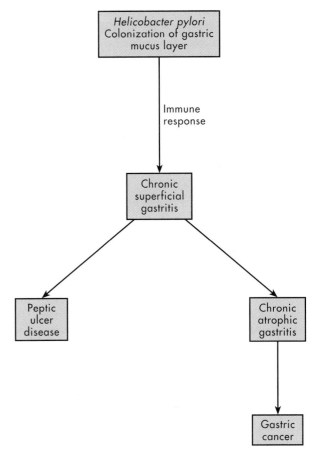

■ **Fig. 38-16**   Diseases caused by infection of the gastric mucosal surface by *Helicobacter pylori*. Most individuals whose stomachs are infected with the bacterium have chronic superficial gastritis. It is not known why in certain people this condition progresses to peptic ulcer disease, to more severe gastritis, or to gastric cancer.

■ **Fig. 38-17**   Cellular mechanisms of agonists that elicit pepsinogen secretion by chief cells. Secretin, vasoactive intestinal polypeptide *(VIP)*, and β-adrenergic agonists act via receptors that increase the intracellular level of cyclic AMP *(cAMP)*. Acetylcholine *(ACh)*, gastrin, and cholecystokinin *(CCK)* act by the inositol phosphate pathway to increase intracellular $[Ca^{++}]$. The mechanism whereby H^+ ions potentiate secretion of pepsinogens remains to be elucidated. *PK-A,* Protein kinase A; *PK-C,* protein kinase C; *PL-C,* phospholipase C; *DAG,* diacyclglycerol; *IP₃,* inositol trisphosphate. (Modified from Hershey SJ: In *Handbook of physiology,* sect 6, vol III, *The gastrointestinal system,* Bethesda, Md, 1989, American Physiological Society.)

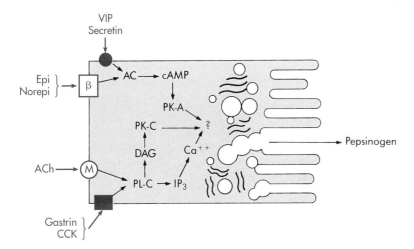

Secretin and CCK, which are released by the duodenal mucosa, also stimulate chief cells to secrete pepsinogens.

■ Pancreatic Secretion

The human pancreas weighs less than 100 g, yet each day it secretes 1 kg (10 times its mass) of pancreatic juice. The pancreas is unusual in that it serves both endocrine and exocrine secretory functions. *The exocrine juice is composed of an **aqueous component** and an **enzyme component**.* The aqueous component *is rich in bicarbonate and helps to neutralize duodenal contents. The enzyme component contains enzymes for digesting carbohydrates, proteins, and fats.* Both neural and hormonal signals control pancreatic exocrine secretion. These signals are triggered mainly by the presence of acid and digestion products in the duodenum. *Secretin chiefly elicits secretion of the aqueous component, whereas CCK stimulates the secretion of pancreatic enzymes.*

■ Structure and Innervation of the Pancreas

The structure of the exocrine pancreas resembles that of the salivary glands (Figs. 38-1 and 38-2). The pancreas contains microscopic, blind-ended tubules that are surrounded by polygonal acinar cells and are organized into lobules. The primary function of these lobules, or acini, is to secrete the enzyme component of pancreatic juice. The tiny ducts that drain the acini are called **intercalated ducts.** The intercalated ducts empty into somewhat larger **intralobular ducts** (Fig. 38-18). All of the intralobular ducts of a particular lobule then drain into a single **extralobular duct;** this duct in turn empties into still larger ducts. These larger ducts converge into a main duct that enters the duodenum along with the **common bile duct.**

*The endocrine portion of the pancreas is composed of cells that reside in the **islets of Langerhans.*** Although islet cells account for less than 2% of the volume of the pancreas, their hormones play an essential role in regulating metabolism. **Insulin, glucagon, somatostatin,** and **pancreatic polypeptide** are the hormones that are released from cells of the islets of Langerhans (see Chapter 47). Each of these hormones, when administered intravenously, influences the exocrine secretion of the pancreas, but the exact physiological roles of these effects remain to be established.

The pancreas is supplied by branches of the celiac and superior mesenteric arteries. The portal vein drains the pancreas. The acini and islets are supplied by separate capillary networks. Some of the capillaries that supply the islets converge into venules, which then branch to form a second capillary bed around the acini.

The pancreas is innervated by branches of the vagus nerve. Vagal fibers form synapses with cholinergic neurons that lie within the pancreas; these neurons innervate both acinar and islet cells. Postganglionic sympathetic nerves from the celiac and superior mesenteric plexuses innervate pancreatic blood vessels. *Secretion of pancreatic juice is stimulated by parasympathetic activity and inhibited by sympathetic activity.*

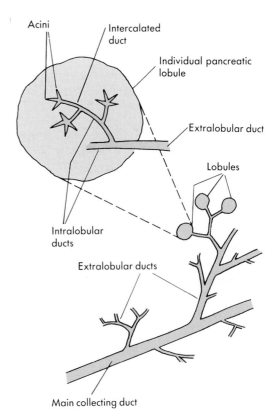

■ Fig. 38-18   Duct system of the pancreas. (Redrawn from Swanson CH, Solomon AK: *J Gen Physiol* 62:407, 1973.)

■ Aqueous Component of Pancreatic Juice

The **aqueous component** of pancreatic juice is produced principally by the columnar epithelial cells that line the pancreatic ducts. Pancreatic juice is nearly isotonic to plasma at all rates of flow. The Na^+ and K^+ concentrations of pancreatic juice are similar to those in plasma. HCO_3^- (at levels well above those in plasma) and Cl^- are the major anions contained in pancreatic juice. The HCO_3^- concentration varies from approximately 70 mEq/L at low rates of secretion to more than 130 mEq/L at high secretory rates (Fig. 38-19). Cl^- concentrations vary reciprocally with HCO_3^- concentrations.

The aqueous component secreted by the duct cells is slightly hypertonic to plasma, and its HCO_3^- concentration is high. As the secretion flows through the ducts, water moves into the ducts across the epithelium and makes the pancreatic juice isotonic. In addition, some HCO_3^- is exchanged for Cl^- (Fig. 38-20) as the pancreatic juice makes its way through the ducts.

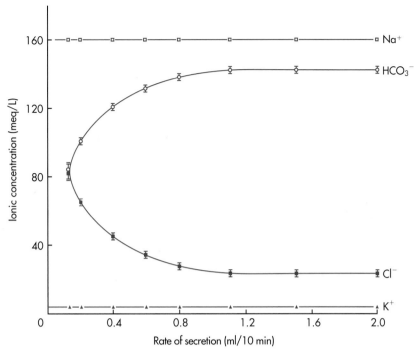

■ Fig. 38-19 Concentrations of the major ions in the pancreatic juice of anesthetized cats as functions of the secretory flow rate. Secretion was stimulated by intravenous administration of secretin. (Redrawn from Case RM, Harper AA, Scratcherd T: *J Physiol (Lond)* 201:335, 1969.)

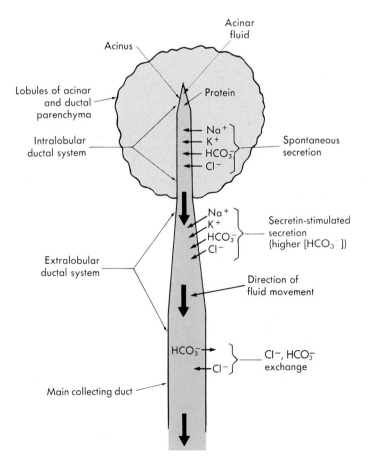

■ Fig. 38-20 Locations of important transport processes involved in the elaboration of pancreatic juice. Acinar fluid is isotonic and resembles plasma in its concentrations of Na^+, K^+, Cl^-, and HCO_3^-. The secretion of acinar fluid and the proteins it contains is stimulated by cholecystokinin and acetylcholine. A spontaneous secretion that is produced by the *intralobular* ducts has higher concentrations of K^+ and HCO_3^- than does plasma. The hormone secretin stimulates water and electrolyte secretion by the cells that line the *extralobular* ducts. The secretin-stimulated secretion is still richer in HCO_3^- than the spontaneous secretion. (Adapted from Swanson CH, Solomon AK: *J Gen Physiol* 62:407, 1973.)

Under resting conditions, the aqueous component is produced primarily by the intercalated and other intralobular ducts. *When secretion is stimulated by secretin, however, the additional aqueous component is made primarily by the extralobular ducts* (Fig. 38-20). The secretin-stimulated fluid secreted by the extralobular ducts has a higher bicarbonate concentration than does the fluid spontaneously secreted by the intralobular ducts.

A current model of the cellular mechanisms whereby extralobular ducts secrete a bicarbonate-rich fluid is shown in Fig. 38-21. Bicarbonate in the blood that perfuses the pancreas, rather than bicarbonate that is produced by the duct epithelial cell, is the major source of the bicarbonate that is secreted into the lumen of the extralobular duct.

■ *Enzyme Component of Pancreatic Juice*

*The secretions of the acinar cells make up the **enzyme component** of pancreatic juice.* The fluid that is secreted by the acinar cells resembles plasma in its tonicity and in the concentrations of various ions; a current view of the ionic transport mechanisms involved is shown in Fig. 38-22. The cells of the intercalated ducts may also contribute to these secretions.

The enzyme component of pancreatic juice contains enzymes that are important for the digestion of all the major classes of foodstuffs (Table 38-3). If pancreatic enzymes are absent, the absorption of lipids, proteins, and carbohydrates is abnormal.

The proteases contained in pancreatic juice are

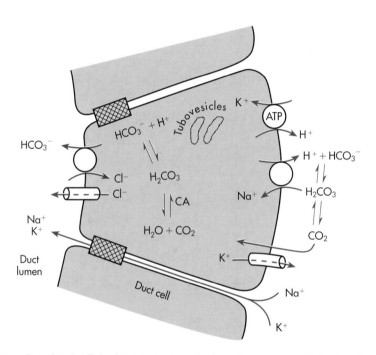

■ Fig. 38-21 Postulated cellular ion transport mechanisms for secretion of bicarbonate-rich fluid by epithelial cells of pancreatic extralobular ducts. Blood is the principal source of the bicarbonate secreted into the duct lumen. Blood perfusing the ducts is acidified by Na^+, H^+ exchangers and H^+, K^+-ATPases in the basolateral membrane, resulting in formation of CO_2 from blood bicarbonate. CO_2 diffuses into the ductular epithelial cell, where its hydration to form H_2CO_3 is catalyzed by carbonic anhydrase *(CA)*. Dissociation of H_2CO_3 to H^+ and HCO_3^-, together with extrusion of H^+ across the basolateral membrane, produces a high intracellular $[HCO_3^-]$. HCO_3^- flows down its electrochemical potential gradient across the luminal membrane via the Cl^-, HCO_3^- exchanger. Cl^- is recycled back into the lumen by the electrogenic Cl^- channels in the luminal membrane. Na^+ enters the luminal fluid by flowing through the tight junctions in response to the negative electrical potential in the lumen that is produced by electrogenic Cl^- transport. Efflux of K^+ through basolateral K^+ channels maintains the intracellular electronegativity that is part of the driving force for the transport of Cl^- and HCO_3^- across the luminal membrane. Secretin, the most important physiological agonist, elevates intracellular cyclic AMP, which dramatically increases the open time of the luminal Cl^- channel. In addition, cAMP probably activates basolateral K^+ channels and promotes the insertion of more H^+, K^+-ATPase molecules into the basolateral membrane. Calcium mobilizing agonists, such as acetylcholine and CCK, open Ca^{++}-activated K^+ channels in the basolateral membrane, and in this way mildly enhance secretion when acting alone and markedly potentiate the effects of secretin.

secreted in an inactive zymogen form. The major pancreatic proteases are **trypsin, chymotrypsin,** and **carboxypeptidase.** The zymogen forms in which they are secreted are **trypsinogen, chymotrypsinogen,** and **procarboxypeptidase,** respectively. Trypsinogen is specifically activated by **enteropeptidase** (also called **enterokinase**), which is secreted by the duodenal mucosa. Trypsin then activates trypsinogen, chymotrypsinogen, and procarboxypeptidase. **Trypsin inhibitor,** a protein present in pancreatic juice, prevents the premature activation of proteolytic enzymes in the pancreatic ducts.

Pancreatic juice also contains an α-amylase that is secreted in active form. Like salivary amylase, **pancreatic amylase** cleaves starch molecules into oligosaccharides. In addition, pancreatic juice contains a number of lipid-digesting enzymes, or **lipases.** Among the major pancreatic lipases are **triacylglycerol hydrolase, cholesterol ester hydrolase,** and **phospholipase A_2.** Pancreatic juice also contains **ribonuclease** and **deoxyribonuclease.** The digestive functions of these pancreatic enzymes are discussed in Chapter 39.

The pancreatic enzymes are stored in **zymogen granules** located in the apical cytoplasm of the acinar cells. In response to secretagogues, the contents of the zymogen granule are released by exocytosis into the lumen of the acinus. Acinar cells that have been depleted of zymogen granules can also secrete enzymes; the details of this secretory mechanism remain unclear.

Cl^- enters the acinar lumen via electrogenic Cl^- channels in the apical plasma membranes of the acinar cells (Fig. 38-22) and the ductular epithelial cells (Fig. 38-21). The primary molecular defect in **cystic fibrosis** is a mutation in the gene that encodes this Cl^- channel. As a result of this mutation, the number of Cl^- channels inserted into the plasma membrane is drastically reduced. The decreased transport of Cl^- into the acinar and duct lumens impairs the transport of both Na^+ and water. Consequently, in cystic fibrosis, the acini and ducts of the pancreas and the small airways of the lung become clogged with mucus. As a result, the acinar cells and duct system of the pancreas are destroyed, and chronic infections of the lungs can occur. In infants with cystic fibrosis, the pancreatic exocrine function is irreversibly damaged in utero. Because of the almost complete absence of pancreatic enzymes, infants with cystic fibrosis frequently have severe digestive difficulties, especially in the digestion and absorption of fats.

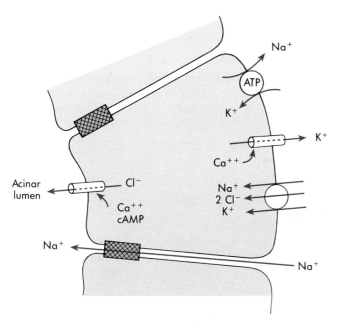

■ **Fig. 38-22** Postulated ionic mechanisms for secretion of NaCl-rich fluid by the pancreatic acinar cells and perhaps by the cells of the intercalated ducts also. The basolateral membrane has an electroneutral transporter that uses the energy of the Na^+ gradient to take up 1 Na^+ along with 1 K^+ and 2 Cl^-; the latter two ions are transported into the cell against their electrochemical potential gradients. Cl^- leaves the cell across the luminal membrane via a Cl^- channel that is activated by cyclic AMP *(cAMP)* and Ca^{++}. Na^+ enters the lumen via the leaky tight junctions between adjacent acinar cells. The basolateral membrane has Ca^{++}-activated K^+ channels. Ca^{++}-mobilizing agonists thus hyperpolarize the cell and thereby increase the force for luminal Cl^- efflux and for basolateral Na^+-driven Cl^- entry.

■ Regulation of Secretion of Pancreatic Juice

Stimulation of the vagal branches to the pancreas enhances secretion of pancreatic juice, whereas activation of sympathetic fibers inhibits pancreatic secretion, partly by decreasing blood flow to the pancreas. The hormones secretin and CCK, which are released from the duodenal

■ **Table 38-3** Some of the proteins of human pancreatic juice

Protein	Molecular weight	Mass proportion (%)
α-Amylase	54,800	5.3
Triacyglycerol hydrolase	50,500	0.7
Phospholipase A_2	17,500	—
Colipase 1	—	—
Colipase 2	—	—
Procarboxypeptidase A1	46,000	16.8
Procarboxypeptidase A2	47,000	8.1
Procarboxypeptidase B1	47,000	4.4
Procarboxypeptidase B2	47,000	2.9
Trypsinogen 1	28,000	23.1
Trypsinogen 2	26,000	—
Trypsinogen 3	26,700	16.0
Chymotrypsinogen	29,000	1.7
Proelastase 1	30,500	3.1
Proelastase 2	30,500	1.2

Based on data from Scheele G et al: *Gastroenterology* 80:461, 1981.

mucosa, stimulate secretion of the aqueous and enzyme components, respectively. Because the production of the aqueous and enzyme components of pancreatic juice is separately controlled (Fig. 38-20), the protein content of the juice varies from less than 1% to as much as 10%.

Like the secretion of gastic HCl, the secretion of pancreatic juice is released during three phases: the cephalic phase, the gastric phase, and the intestinal phase.

The cephalic phase. Sham feeding* induces the secretion of a low volume of pancreatic juice with a high protein content. Vagal impulses stimulate pancreatic secretion during the cephalic phase. In addition, gastrin released from the mucosa of the gastric antrum in response to vagal impulses stimulates pancreatic secretion during this phase. Although gastrin is a member of the same class of peptides as CCK, it is about half as potent a pancreatic secretagogue as is CCK.

The gastric phase. During the gastric phase of secretion, distention of the stomach elicits vagovagal reflexes that induce the pancreas to secrete a small volume of pancreatic juice with high enzyme concentration. Furthermore, gastrin, released in response to gastric distention and to the presence of amino acids and peptides in the antrum of the stomach, also enhances pancreatic secretion.

The intestinal phase. In the intestinal phase of secretion, certain components of the chyme in the duodenum and upper jejunum evoke pancreatic secretion. Acid in

the chyme elicits the secretion of a large volume of pancreatic juice with a low enzyme concentration. *The hormone **secretin** is the major mediator of this response to acid.* Released by cells in the mucosa of the duodenum and upper jejunum in response to acid in the lumen, secretin directly stimulates pancreatic ductular epithelial cells to secrete the bicarbonate-rich aqueous component of the pancreatic juice.

The presence of peptides and certain amino acids in the duodenum elicits the secretion of pancreatic juice that is rich in enzyme components. Fatty acids and monoglycerides in the duodenum also elicit secretion of protein-rich pancreatic juice. *The hormone CCK, which is released by cells in the duodenum and upper jejunum in response to these digestion products, is the most important physiological mediator of the enzyme component of pancreatic juice.*

CCK potentiates the stimulatory effect of secretin on the ducts. Furthermore, secretin potentiates the effect of CCK on acinar cells.

Enteropancreatic vagovagal reflexes also enhance pancreatic secretion during the intestinal phase; vagotomy significantly reduces the secretion of pancreatic juice.

■ *Cellular Mechanisms of Secretagogues and Inhibitors*

Acinar cells. Acinar cells have receptors for several secretagogues; a simplified representation of these receptors is shown in Fig. 38-23. Occupation of receptors for CCK/gastrin, acetylcholine, and substance P, stimulates the hydrolysis of inositol phospholipids and elevates the

---

*In humans, food is chewed but not swallowed. In animals, a hole in the esophagus is connected to the skin, so that food that is swallowed does not reach the stomach. Sham feeding thus evokes only cephalic phase events and not gastric or intestinal phase components.

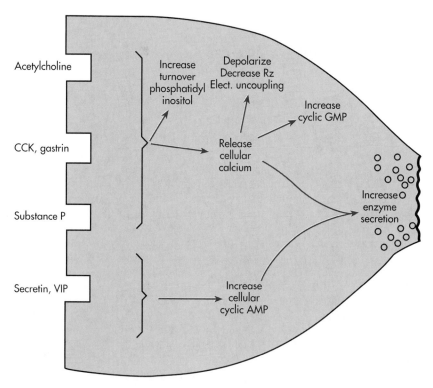

■ **Fig. 38-23** Representation of the cellular mechanisms of action of secretagogues on pancreatic acinar cells. Acetylcholine, CCK, and gastrin (the last two acting on the same receptor class) and substance P activate inositol lipid hydrolysis and mobilize intracellular Ca^{++}. Secretin and VIP act to enhance adenylyl cyclase activity and increase intracellular levels of cyclic AMP.

intracellular Ca⁺⁺ concentration. The calcium-mobilizing agonists also increase the concentration of cGMP. Although cGMP is not directly involved in enhancing secretion, it may promote growth and maintenance of acinar cells. Receptors for secretin and VIP stimulate adenylyl cyclase and increase the cellular concentrations of cAMP. Secretagogues that increase cAMP potentiate the effects of those that elevate intracellular Ca⁺⁺ concentrations, and vice versa. Somatostatin inhibits acinar cell secretions by inhibiting adenylyl cyclase and reducing the cAMP concentration.

Extralobular duct epithelial cells. The principal physiological agonist of pancreatic duct cell secretion, secretin, stimulates the extralobular duct cells to secrete by elevating the intracellular concentration of cAMP. VIP also has this effect on duct cells. VIP-containing neurons are present in the pancreas, but their physiological role has not been established. CCK elevates the intracellular Ca⁺⁺ concentration and potentiates the effects of secretion, but CCK alone is a weak secretagogue. Acetylcholine is not an effective agonist for the duct epithelial cells.

Other regulatory substances. Somatostatin, glucagon, and pancreatic polypeptide—all released from pancreatic islet cells—inhibit secretion by extralobular ducts; the physiological significance of these effects is uncertain. Insulin, insulin-like growth factors, and EGF potentiate enzyme synthesis and secretion. They also have the trophic effects of increasing cellular metabolism and maintaining differentiated functions of the exocrine pancreas.

■ Functions of the Liver and Gallbladder

■ Structure of the Liver

The histologic appearance of the liver is shown in Fig. 38-24. Each liver **lobule** is organized around a **central vein.** At the periphery of the lobule, blood enters the **sinusoids** from branches of the **portal vein** and the **hepatic artery** (see also Chapter 30). In the sinusoids, blood flows toward the center of the lobule between plates of **hepatocytes** that are one or two cells thick. Because of the large fenestrations between the endothelial cells that line the sinusoids, each hepatocyte is in direct contact with sinusoidal blood. The intimate contact of a large portion of the hepatocyte surface with blood accounts in part for the liver's ability to clear the blood of certain classes of compounds. **Biliary canaliculi** lie between adjacent hepatocytes. These canaliculi drain into bile ducts at the periphery of the lobule.

■ Functions of the Liver

The liver performs many vital functions. It is essential in regulating metabolism, synthesizing proteins and other molecules, storing vitamins and iron, degrading hormones, and inactivating and excreting drugs and toxins.

The liver regulates the metabolism of carbohydrates, lipids, and proteins. Liver and skeletal muscle are the two major sites of glycogen storage in the body. When the level of glucose in the blood is high, some of this glucose is converted to glycogen, which is deposited in the liver. When the blood glucose level is low, glycogen in the liver is broken down to glucose (**glycogenolysis),** and the glucose is then released into the blood. The liver thus helps to maintain a relatively constant blood glucose level. The liver is also the major site of **gluconeogenesis,** the conversion of amino acids, lipids, or simple carbohydrates (e.g., lactate) into glucose. Carbohydrate metabolism by the liver is regulated by several hormones (see Chapters 46 and 47).

The liver is also centrally involved in lipid metabolism. As described in Chapter 39, absorbed lipids leave the intestine in **chylomicrons** in the lymph. Lipoprotein lipase on the endothelial cell surface of blood vessels hydrolyzes some of the triglycerides in the chylomicrons and releases glycerol and fatty acids. The glycerol and fatty acids are then taken up by **adipocytes.** What remains from this processing of chylomicrons are **chylomicron remnants** rich in cholesterol. These remnants are taken up by hepatocytes and degraded. Hepatocytes also synthesize and secrete **very-low-density lipopro-**

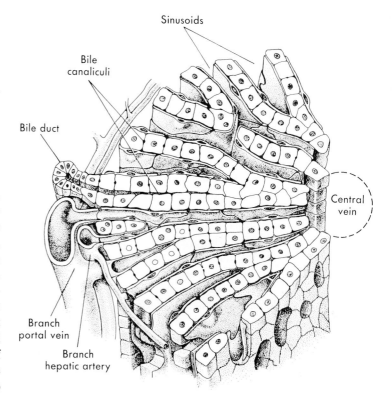

■ **Fig. 38-24** Diagrammatic representation of a hepatic lobule. A central vein is located in the center of the lobule, with plates of hepatocytes disposed radially. Branches of the portal vein and hepatic artery are located on the periphery of the lobule, and blood from both perfuses the sinusoids. Peripherally located bile ducts drain the bile canaliculi that run between the hepatocytes.(Adapted from Bloom W, Fawcett DW: *A textbook of histology,* ed 10, Philadelphia, 1975, WB Saunders.)

teins **(VLDLs).** VLDLs are then converted to the other types of serum lipoproteins (such as high-density lipoproteins and low-density lipoproteins). These lipoproteins are the major sources of cholesterol and triglycerides that supply most other tissues of the body. *Bile is the only route of excretion of cholesterol. Hepatocytes are thus a principal source of cholesterol in the body, and they are the major site of excretion of cholesterol. Thus, hepatocytes play a central role in the regulation of serum cholesterol levels.*

> Because carbohydrate utilization is impaired in **diabetes mellitus,** β oxidation of fatty acids provides a major source of energy for the body (see Chapter 46). In the liver, the oxidation of fatty acids produces acetoacetate, β-hydroxybutyrate, and acetone. These three compounds are called **ketone bodies.** Ketone bodies are released from hepatocytes and carried in the circulation to other tissues, where they are metabolized. The levels of ketone bodies in the urine and blood can indicate the severity of diabetic acidosis.

The liver is also centrally involved in protein metabolism. When proteins are broken down (catabolized), amino acids are deaminated to form **ammonia** (NH_3). Ammonia cannot be further broken down by most tissues, and toxic levels of ammonia may therefore result. Ammonia is dissipated by conversion to **urea,** which takes place mainly in the liver. The liver also synthesizes all the nonessential amino acids. In addition, *the liver synthesizes all the major plasma proteins,* including the plasma lipoproteins, albumins, globulins, fibrinogens, and other proteins involved in blood clotting.

The liver stores certain substances important in metabolism. *Next to hemoglobin in red blood cells, the liver is the most important storage site for iron. Some vitamins, most notably A, D, and B_{12}, are also stored in the liver.* Hepatic storage protects the body from transient deficiencies of these vitamins.

The liver transforms and excretes many hormones, drugs, and toxins. These substances are frequently converted to inactive forms by reactions that occur in hepatocytes. The smooth endoplasmic reticulum of hepatocytes contains a variety of enzymes and cofactors that are responsible for the chemical transformation of many substances. Other enzymes in the endoplasmic reticulum catalyze the conjugation of many compounds with glucuronic acid, glycine, or glutathione. The transformations that occur in the liver render many compounds more water soluble so that they are more readily excreted by the kidneys. Some liver metabolites are secreted into the bile.

■ *Bile*

*The hepatic function most important to the digestive tract is the secretion of **bile.*** Bile, produced by hepatocytes, contains **bile acids, cholesterol, phospholipids,** and **bile pigments.** All of these constituents are secreted by hepatocytes into the bile canaliculi, along with an isotonic fluid that resembles plasma in its electrolyte concentrations. The bile canaliculi merge into ever larger ducts and finally into a single large bile duct. The epithelial cells that line the bile ducts secrete a watery, bicarbonate-rich fluid that contributes to the volume of bile leaving the liver.

The secretory function of the liver resembles that of the exocrine pancreas. In both organs, the major parenchymal cell type produces a primary secretion that contains the substances that carry out the main digestive function of the organ. In both the liver and the pancreas, the primary secretion is isotonic to plasma, and the levels of Na^+, K^+, and Cl^- are close to plasma levels. The primary secretion of both pancreas and liver is stimulated by CCK. The epithelial cells that line the duct systems of these organs modify the primary secretion. When stimulated by secretin, the ductular epithelial cells contribute an aqueous secretion with a high bicarbonate concentration.

Between meals, bile is diverted into the **gallbladder.** *The gallbladder epithelium extracts salts and water from the stored bile, concentrating the bile acids fivefold to twentyfold.* After an individual eats, the gallbladder contracts and empties its concentrated bile into the duodenum. *The most potent stimulus for emptying of the gallbladder is CCK.* From 250 to 1500 ml of bile enter the duodenum each day.

Bile acids **emulsify** lipids and thereby increase the surface area available to lipolytic enzymes. Bile acids then form **mixed micelles** (see Chapter 39) with the products of lipid digestion. Micelles increase the transport of the products of lipid digestion to the brush border surface, thereby enhancing the absorption of lipids by the epithelial cells. The epithelial cells actively absorb bile acids, mainly in the terminal ileum. Only about 10% to 20% of bile acids escapes absorption and is excreted. Bile acids that return to the liver are avidly taken up by hepatocytes, which rapidly resecrete them during the course of digestion. The entire bile acid pool is recirculated two or more times in response to a typical meal. This recirculation of the bile is known as the **enterohepatic circulation** (Fig. 38-25). Approximately 20% of the bile acid pool is excreted in the feces each day and is replenished by hepatic synthesis of new bile acids.

> Bile acids lost into the feces are the only significant mechanism of cholesterol excretion. Treatment with drugs that block the reabsorption of bile acids in the ileum promotes the synthesis of new bile acids from cholesterol. These drugs can be used to lower the level of cholesterol in the blood.

Fraction of bile secreted by hepatocytes

Bile acids. Bile acids make up about 65% of the dry weight of bile. Other important compounds secreted by the hepatocytes into the bile include phospholipids (about 20%), cholesterol (about 4%), proteins (about 5%), and bilirubin and related bile pigments (about 0.3%).

Bile acids are synthesized by the hepatocytes from cholesterol (Fig. 38-26), from which they acquire their steroid nucleus. The major bile acids synthesized by the liver are called **primary bile acids.** These are **cholic acid** (3-hydroxyl groups) and **chenodeoxycholic acid** (2-hydroxyl groups). The presence of the carboxyl and hydroxyl groups makes the bile acids much more water soluble than the cholesterol from which they are synthesized.

The bacteria that normally colonize in the digestive tract dehydroxylate bile acids to form **secondary bile acids.** The major secondary bile acids are **deoxycholic acid** (from dehydroxylation of cholic acid) and **lithocholic acid** (from dehydroxylation of chenodeoxycholic acid). Bile contains both primary and secondary bile acids.

Bile acids are normally conjugated with glycine or taurine. The glycine or taurine is linked by a peptide bond between the carboxyl group of an unconjugated bile acid and the amino group of glycine or taurine (Fig. 38-26, *bottom*). At the near neutral pH of the gastrointestinal tract, conjugated bile acids are more completely ionized, and are thus more water soluble, than are unconjugated bile acids. Conjugated bile acids are present almost entirely as salts of various cations (mostly Na+) and are often called **bile salts.**

The steroid nucleus of bile acids is almost planar. In solution, the polar (hydrophilic) groups of bile acids—the hydroxyl groups, the carboxyl moiety of glycine or taurine, and the peptide bond—are arranged on one side of the molecule (Fig. 38-27, *A*). *This arrangement makes the bile acid molecule amphipathic,* that is, having both hydrophilic and hydrophobic domains. Because they are amphipathic, bile acids tend to form molecular aggregates, called **micelles,** in a solution. In a bile acid micelle, the hydrophobic side of the bile acid faces inside and away from water, and the hydrophilic surface faces outward toward the water. Bile acid micelles form when the concentration of bile acids exceeds a certain limit, called the **critical micelle concentration.** Above this concentration, any additional bile acid will join the micelles and not form a molecular solution. Normally, the bile acid concentration in bile is much greater than the critical micelle concentration.

Phospholipids and cholesterol in bile. Hepatocytes also secrete phospholipids, especially **lecithins,** into bile. Cholesterol is also secreted into the bile, thus constituting the major route for cholesterol excretion. Hepatocytes secrete phospholipids and cholesterol into the bile canaliculi as lipid bilayer vesicles. The secretory mechanism involves exocytosis.

Because the lipid vesicles are greatly outnumbered by bile acid micelles, phospholipids and cholesterol mole-

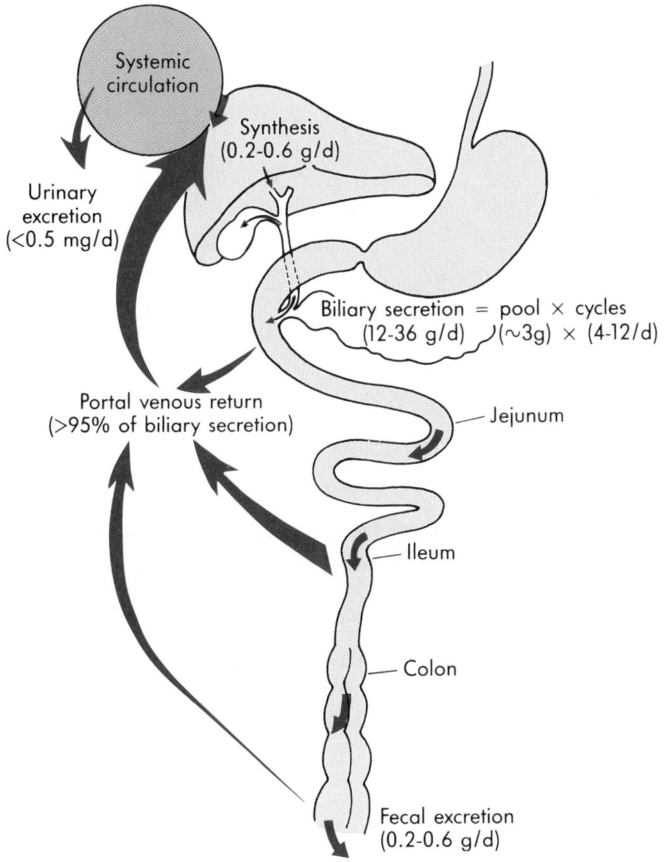

■ **Fig. 38-25** Representation of key components of the enterohepatic circulation of bile acids in normal humans. Bile is dumped into the duodenum by contractions of the gallbladder. In the small intestine, bile acids first emulsify dietary fat and then form mixed micelles with the products of fat digestion. In the terminal ileum, bile acids are reabsorbed. Bile acids return to the liver in the portal blood, where they are avidly taken up by hepatocytes and resecreted into bile. (Redrawn from Carey MC, Cahalane MJ. In Arias IM et al: *The liver: biology and pathobiology,* ed 2, New York, 1988, Raven Press.)

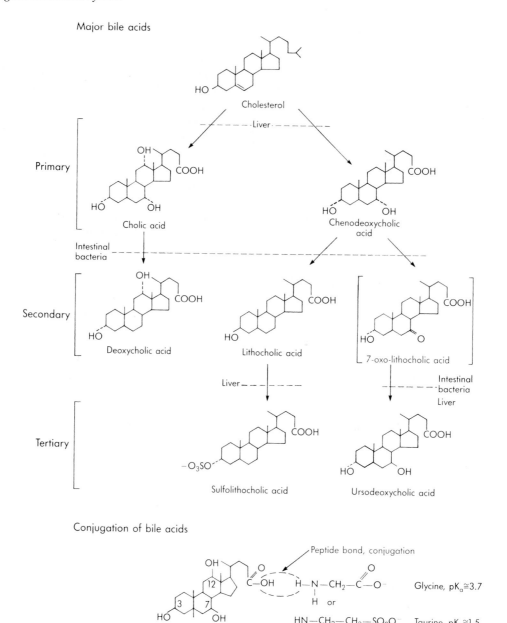

Major bile acids

Conjugation of bile acids

■ **Fig. 38-26** Structures and sites of conversion of major primary, secondary, and tertiary bile acids in human bile. At the bottom of the figure, the conjugation of cholic acid with glycine or taurine is shown. (Redrawn from Carey MC, Cahalane MJ. In Arias IM et al: *The liver: biology and pathobiology,* ed 2, New York, 1988, Raven Press.)

cules partition into the bile acid micelles (Fig. 38-27, *B*), and the lipid vesicles gradually disappear. In the small intestine, the products of triglyceride digestion (2-monoglycerides and free fatty acids) and fat-soluble vitamins partition into these mixed micelles. The more phospholipid that is present, the greater is the amount of cholesterol that can be solubilized in the micelles.

If more cholesterol is present in the bile than can be solubilized in the micelles, bile is said to be **supersaturated** with cholesterol, and crystals of cholesterol tend

to form in the bile. Cholesterol crystals in bile aid in the formation of **cholesterol gallstones** (the most common variety) in the duct system of the liver or (more often) in the gallbladder. Normal individuals tend to secrete bile that is supersaturated in cholesterol only at night; the bile of individuals with cholesterol gallstones tends to be supersaturated with cholesterol throughout the entire day.

Bile pigments. When aging red blood cells are degraded in reticuloendothelial cells, the porphyrin moi-

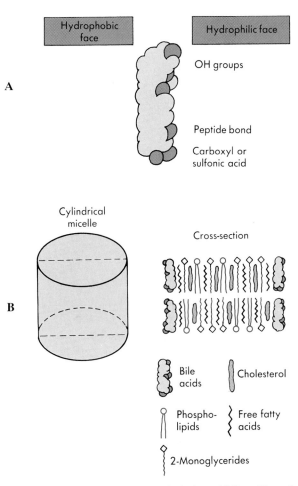

A

Hydrophobic face   Hydrophilic face

OH groups

Peptide bond

Carboxyl or sulfonic acid

Cylindrical micelle

Cross-section

B

Bile acids

Cholesterol

Phospho-lipids

Free fatty acids

2-Monoglycerides

■ **Fig. 38-27** Schematic depiction of bile acids and mixed micelles. **A,** A bile acid molecule in solution. The molecule is amphipathic; it has a hydrophilic face and a hydrophobic face. The amphipathic nature of bile acids is the key to their ability to emulsify lipids and to form mixed micelles with the products of lipid digestion. **B,** A model of the structure of a bile acid–lipid mixed micelle.

ety of hemoglobin is converted to **bilirubin.** Bilirubin is released into the plasma, where it is bound to albumin. Hepatocytes efficiently remove bilirubin from blood in the sinusoids and conjugate it with one or two glucuronic acid molecules. The resultant **bilirubin glucuronides** are then secreted into the bile, probably by an adenosine triphosphate (ATP)–dependent transport protein in the canalicular membrane. Bilirubin is yellow and contributes to the color of bile.

Colonic bacteria convert bilirubin to urobilinogen, some of which is absorbed into the blood. A fraction of the urobilinogen is excreted in urine; the remainder is taken up by hepatocytes and resecreted into bile.

Secretion of the bile duct epithelium. The epithelial cells that line the bile ducts secrete an aqueous secretion that accounts for about 50% of the total volume of the bile. This aqueous secretion is isotonic and contains Na^+ and K^+ at concentrations similar to those of plasma. However, the concentration of HCO_3^- is greater and the concentration of Cl^+ is less than in plasma. *The secretory activity of the bile duct epithelium is specifically stimulated by secretin.*

■ *Cellular Mechanisms of Bile Secretion*

Secretion of bile acids. As is the case for all epithelia, the apical plasma membrane of the hepatocyte (the membrane that faces the bile canaliculus) contains a different transport protein composition than does the basolateral plasma membrane (the membrane that faces the sinusoidal blood). As shown in Fig. 38-28, multiple transport mechanisms are located in the hepatocyte plasma membrane for uptake of bile acids, both conjugated and unconjugated, from the sinusoidal blood.

In hepatocyte cytosol, bile acids are mostly bound to **bile acid–binding proteins.** These binding proteins prevent the concentrated bile acids from disrupting the membranes of hepatocyte organelles. Almost all deconjugated bile acids are reconjugated with glycine or taurine. Some of the secondary bile acids are rehydroxylated to primary bile acids.

Bile acids are secreted into the lumen of the secretory canaliculus, probably by facilitated transporters that are protein mediated and are located in the apical membrane. Bile acids move into bile down concentration and electrical potential gradients; the cytosol is about 35 mV negative to the lumen. The concentration gradient is maintained partly because the bile acids form micelles in the canaliculi. The formation of micelles keeps the concentration of bile acids in true solution quite low (equal to the critical micelle concentration). The bile acid transporters in the canalicular membrane are not yet well characterized.

Secretion of water and electrolytes into bile. Water and electrolytes are present in the bile canaliculi in concentrations that equal those of plasma. The osmotic pressure of bile acids and other molecules secreted by the hepatocytes causes water to flow into the canaliculi via the leaky tight junctions that join the hepatocytes. The electrolytes are brought along by solvent drag. In addition, ionic secretory processes in the hepatocyte may contribute electrolytes to the canalicular bile.

The bile duct epithelial cells secrete a bicarbonate-rich fluid into the duct lumen. The major ion transport processes are probably similar to those of the cells that line the pancreatic extralobular ducts (Fig. 38-21), and the mechanism of secretin stimulation of secretion is probably the same as in pancreatic ducts.

■ *Bile Concentration and Storage in the Gallbladder*

Between meals, the tone of the **sphincter of Oddi,** which guards the entrance of the common bile duct into the duodenum, is high. Thus, most bile flow is diverted into the

■ **Fig. 38-28**   Postulated mechanisms for uptake and secretion of bile acids by hepatocytes. In blood, both conjugated and unconjugated bile acids are bound to proteins, principally albumin. Hepatocytes effectively remove most bile acids from portal blood. Conjugated bile acids are taken up across the basolateral membranes of hepatocytes by an Na^+, bile acid cotransport protein and by an Na^+-independent mechanism. Unconjugated bile acids are taken up by simple diffusion and by a transport protein that exchanges bile acids for inorganic anions. In the cytosol of hepatocytes, most bile acids are bound to bile acid–binding proteins. The canalicular membrane contains an ATP-dependent bile acid transporter that is capable of transporting bile acids into the canalicular lumen against large concentration gradients. Na^+, Cl^-, and water are believed to enter canalicular bile via the leaky tight junctions that join the hepatocytes.

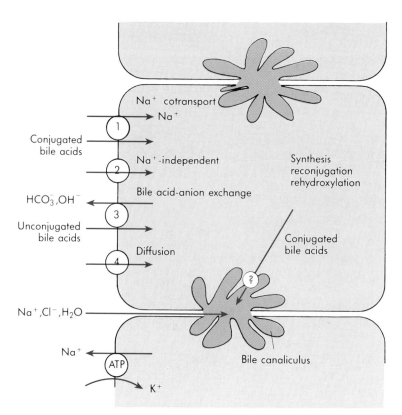

gallbladder. The gallbladder is a small organ, with a capacity of 15 to 60 ml in humans. Between meals, this volume of bile may be secreted by the liver. The gallbladder concentrates the bile by absorbing Na^+, Cl^-, HCO_3^-, and water from the bile, increasing the bile acid concentration fivefold to twentyfold. The active transport of Na^+ is the primary active process in the concentrating action of the gallbladder.

Because of its high rate of water absorption, the gallbladder serves as a model for water and electrolyte transport by epithelia connected by tight junctions. The **standing osmotic gradient mechanism** for fluid absorption was first proposed for the gallbladder (Fig. 38-29). Investigators noted that during fluid reabsorption by the gallbladder, the lateral intercellular spaces between the epithelial cells were large and swollen. When fluid transport was blocked, the intercellular spaces almost disappeared. These observations suggested that the intercellular spaces are a major route of fluid flow during absorption.

In the standing osmotic gradient mechanism, the active transport of Na^+ into the lateral intercellular spaces is the primary active transport process. Na^+, K^+-ATPase molecules are concentrated in the basolateral membrane near the mucosal (apical) end of the intercellular channels. Cl^+ and HCO_3^- are also transported into the intercellular space to preserve electroneutrality. The hypertonic concentration of NaCl near the apical end of the intercellular space causes the osmotic flow of water into the intercellular space from the gallbladder lumen and from adjacent

epithelial cells. Water distends the intercellular channels, and the fluid flows down the intercellular space toward the basement membrane. Ions and water then move across the basement membrane of the epithelium and are carried away in the blood.

■ *Emptying of the Gallbladder*

Emptying of the gallbladder begins several minutes after the start of a meal. Intermittent contractions of the gallbladder force bile through the partially relaxed sphincter of Oddi. During the cephalic and gastric phases of digestion, gallbladder contraction and relaxation of the sphincter are mediated by cholinergic fibers in the vagus nerves and by gastrin released from the stomach. Stimulation of sympathetic nerves to the gallbladder and duodenum inhibits emptying of the gallbladder.

The highest rate of gallbladder emptying occurs during the intestinal phase of digestion; the strongest stimulus for the emptying is CCK. CCK reaches the gallbladder via the circulation, and it causes strong contractions of the gallbladder and relaxation of the sphincter of Oddi. Substances that mimic the actions of CCK in promoting gallbladder emptying (such as gastrin) are called **cholecystagogues.** Gastrin has the same sequence of five amino acids at its C terminus as does CCK; however, gastrin is about half as potent a cholecystagogue as CCK. Nevertheless, gastrin-induced gallbladder contractions occur during the cephalic and gastric phases of digestion.

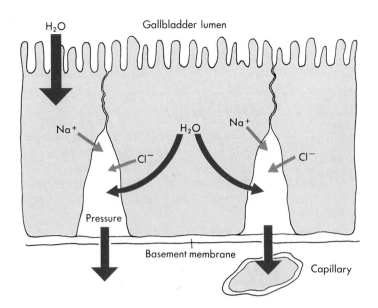

■ **Fig. 38-29** Water absorption from the gallbladder by the standing osmotic gradient mechanism. Na^+, K^+-ATPase molecules are especially concentrated in the basolateral membrane near the mucosal (apical) end of the intercellular channels. Cl^- and HCO_3^- are also transported into the intercellular space, probably because of the electrical potential created by electrogenic Na^+ transport. The high ion concentration near the apical end of the intercellular space causes the fluid there to be hypertonic. This produces an osmotic flow of water from the lumen via adjacent cells into the intercellular space. Water distends the intercellular channels because of increased hydrostatic pressure. As a result of water flow from adjacent cells, the fluid becomes less hypertonic as it flows down the intercellular channel, so that the fluid is essentially isotonic when it reaches the serosal (basal) end of the channel. Ions and water move across the basement membrane of the epithelium and are carried away by the capillaries.

Under normal circumstances, the rate of gallbladder emptying is sufficient to keep the concentration of bile acids in the duodenum above the critical micelle concentration.

■ *Intestinal Absorption of Bile Acids and Their Enterohepatic Circulation*

The functions of bile acids in emulsifying dietary lipid and in forming mixed micelles with the products of lipid digestion are discussed in Chapter 39. Normally, by the time chyme reaches the terminal part of the ileum, dietary fat is almost completely absorbed. Bile acids are then absorbed. *Transport mechanisms are present in the brush border of the terminal ileum for uptake of both conjugated and unconjugated bile acids.* Conjugated bile acids can be taken up against a large concentration gradient. Because bile acids are also lipid soluble, they can be taken up by simple diffusion as well. Bacteria in the terminal part of the ileum and colon deconjugate bile acids and also dehydroxylate them to produce secondary bile acids. Both deconjugation and dehydroxylation lessen the polarity of bile acids, thereby enhancing their lipid solubility and their absorption by simple diffusion.

Typically, about 0.2 to 0.6 g of bile acids escape absorption and are excreted in the feces each day. This quantity is 15% to 35% of the total bile acid pool, which is normally replenished by synthesis of new bile acids by the liver.

Bile acids, whether absorbed by active transport or by simple diffusion, are transported away from the intestine in the portal blood, mostly bound to albumin in plasma. In the liver, hepatocytes avidly extract the bile acids from the portal blood. *In a single pass through the liver, the portal blood is almost completely cleared of bile acids.*

Bile acids in all forms, primary and secondary, both conjugated and deconjugated, are taken up by the hepatocytes. The hepatocytes reconjugate almost all the deconjugated bile acids and rehydroxylate some of the secondary bile acids. These bile acids are secreted into the bile along with newly synthesized bile acids (Fig. 38-28).

■ *Control of Bile Acid Synthesis and Secretion*

The rate of return of the bile acids to the liver affects the rate of synthesis and secretion of bile acids. *Bile acids in the portal blood stimulate the uptake and resecretion of bile acids by the hepatoctyes but inhibit the synthesis of new bile acids* (Fig. 38-30). The stimulation of secretion is called the **choleretic effect** of bile acids; substances that enhance bile acid secretion are called **choleretics.** So powerful is the stimulus to resecrete the returning bile acids that the entire pool of bile acids (1.5 to 31.5 g) recirculates twice in response to a typical meal. In response to a meal with a very high fat content, the bile acid pool may recirculate five or more times.

■ *Gallstones*

Cholesterol is essentially insoluble in water. When bile contains more cholesterol than can be solubilized in the bile acid–phospholipid micelles, crystals of cholesterol form in the bile. Such bile is said to be **supersaturated** with cholesterol. The formation of cholesterol gallstones in supersaturated bile was discussed previously on p 640.

Bile pigment gallstones are the other major class of gallstones; their main constituent is the calcium salt of unconjugated bilirubin. Conjugated bilirubin is quite

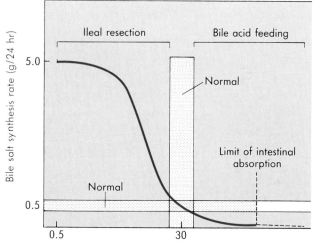

Fig. 38-30 A reciprocal relationship exists between the rates of de novo synthesis of bile acids by hepatocytes and the rate of secretion of bile acids. When bile acids return to the liver in the portal blood, synthesis is inhibited and the energy of the hepatocyte is used to reprocess and secrete the returning bile acids. Removal of the distal ileum decreases the rate of return of bile acids in the portal blood, resulting in a much greater rate of synthesis of bile acids. Feeding bile acids results in increased levels of bile acids in portal blood and in greater inhibition of bile acid synthesis. (Redrawn from Carey MC, Cahalane MJ. In Arias IM et al: *The liver: biology and pathobiology,* ed 2, New York, 1988, Raven Press.)

soluble and does not form insoluble calcium salts in bile. In liver disease, bile may contain elevated levels of unconjugated bilirubin, because hepatocytes are deficient in forming the glucuronides of bilirubin. Individuals with liver disease have an increased likelihood of forming bile pigment stones.

Intestinal Secretions

The mucosa of the intestine, from the duodenum through the rectum, produces secretions that contain mucus, electrolytes, and water. The total volume of intestinal secretions is about 1500 ml/day. The mucus in the secretions protects the mucosa from mechanical damage. The nature of the secretions and the mechanisms that control secretion vary in different segments of the intestine.

Duodenal Secretions

The duodenal submucosa contains branching glands that produce a secretion rich in mucus. The duodenal epithelial cells also produce a small amount of duodenal secre-

tions. The duodenal secretion contains mucus and an aqueous component that does not differ significantly from plasma in its concentrations of the major ions.

Secretions of the Small Intestine

Goblet cells, which lie among the columnar epithelial cells of the small intestine, secrete mucus. During normal digestion, an aqueous secretion is produced by the epithelial cells at a rate only slightly less than the rate of fluid absorption by the small intestine (see Chapter 39).

Secretions of the Colon

The secretions of the colon are smaller in volume but richer in mucus than are the small intestinal secretions. The mucus is produced by numerous goblet cells in the colonic mucosa. The aqueous component of colonic secretions is rich in K^+ and HCO_3^-. Colonic secretion is stimulated by mechanical irritation of the mucosa and by activation of cholinergic pathways to the colon. Stimulation of sympathetic nerves to the colon decreases the rate of colonic secretion.

Summary

1. The epithelial cells that line the gastrointestinal tract and the cells of various glands associated with the gastrointestinal tract produce secretions that contain water, electrolytes, proteins, and other substances.

2. The gastrointestinal secretions are regulated by intrinsic and extrinsic neurons, hormones, and paracrine mediators.

3. Salivary glands produce a hypotonic fluid that contains bicarbonate and potassium concentrations in excess of plasma levels. Saliva contains an α-amylase that begins the digestion of starch. Mucus in saliva lubricates food. Parasympathetic nerves are the key regulators of salivary secretion.

4. The stomach serves as a reservoir for ingested food and empties gastric contents into the duodenum at a regulated rate. Parietal cells secrete HCl and intrinsic factor into the stomach. Chief cells secrete pepsinogens.

5. The regulation of HCl secretion in the stomach involves extrinsic and intrinsic nerves, and acetylcholine is the major stimulatory neurotransmitter. Gastrin, a hormone released by G cells in the gastric antrum and in the duodenum, and histamine, a paracrine agonist released by ECL cells in the stomach, are also important physiological agonists of HCl secretion.

6. HCl catalyzes the conversion of pepsinogens to active pepsins. Pepsins convert a significant fraction of ingested protein to oligopeptides.

7. Mucus and bicarbonate secretions form the gastric mucosal barrier that protects the epithelial cells of the stomach from the effects of HCl and pepsins.

8. The pancreas produces a bicarbonate-rich fluid that contains enzymes essential for the digestion of carbohydrates, proteins, and fats. Pancreatic acinar cells produce the enzyme component of pancreatic juice; the intralobular and extralobular ducts secrete much of the aqueous component (water and electrolytes) of pancreatic juice.

9. Cholecystokinin (CCK) is the major physiological agonist of pancreatic acinar cell secretion of the enzyme component. Secretin is the major stimulus for secretion of bicarbonate-rich fluid by the extralobular ducts of the pancreas. CCK and secretin are hormones released by cells in the duodenum and jejunum in response to the presence of fat digestion products and acid, respectively.

10. The liver produces and the gallbladder concentrates a secretion called bile. Bile is a bicarbonate-rich fluid that contains bile acids, bile pigments, phospholipids, cholesterol, and numerous other components. Bile acids play a vital role in the digestion and absorption of lipids.

11. Hepatocytes are responsible for secreting the organic components of bile. The cells of the bile ducts secrete a bicarbonate-rich fluid. CCK is a major secretagogue for secretion by the hepatocytes. Secretin stimulates the bile ducts to produce their bicarbonate-rich fluid.

12. Bile acids are absorbed in the terminal ileum and return to the liver in the portal vein. Hepatocytes rapidly clear the blood of bile acids and resecrete them. Bile acids in the portal blood are a powerful stimulus to the hepatocytes to resecrete bile acids. The bile acid pool may be recirculated two to five times in response to a single meal. The secretion, return, and resecretion of bile acids is known as the enterohepatic circulation of bile acids.

■ Self-Study Problems

1. Describe the "two-stage model" of salivary secretion.

2. Which cells of the stomach have important secretory functions? What do they secrete?

3. Summarize the control of gastric acid secretion during the cephalic, gastric, and intestinal phases.

4. Describe the secretion of pancreatic juice in the absence and in the presence of secretin.

5. Describe the functions of hepatocytes and duct cells in bile secretion.

■ *Bibliography*

Journal articles

Allen A, Garner A: Mucus and bicarbonate secretion in the stomach and their possible role in mucosal protection, *Gut* 21:249, 1980.

Blaser MJ: The bacteria behind ulcers, *Sci Am* 274:104, 1996.

Chew CS: CCK, carbachol, gastrin, histamine, and forskolin increase [Ca]$_i$ in gastric glands, *Am J Physiol* 250:G312, 1986.

Chew CS: Intracellular mechanisms in control of acid secretion, *Curr Opin Gastroenterol* 7:856, 1991.

El-Omer EM et al: *Helicobacter pylori* infection and abnormalities of gastric secretion in patients with duodenal ulcer disease, *Gastroenterology* 109:681, 1995.

Gerber JG, Payne NA: The role of gastric secretagogues in regulating gastric histamine release in vivo, *Gastroenterology* 102:403, 1992.

Jensen RT, Gardner JD: The cellular basis of action of gastrointestinal peptides, *Adv Cyclic Nucleotide Protein Phosphorylation Res* 17:375, 1984.

Putney JW Jr: Identification of cellular activation mechanisms associated with salivary secretion, *Annu Rev Physiol* 48:75, 1986.

Rabon EC, Reuben MA: The mechanism and structure of the gastric H, K-ATPase, *Annu Rev Physiol* 52:321, 1990.

Raeder M: The origin and subcellular mechanisms causing pancreatic bicarbonate secretion, *Gastroenterology* 103:1674, 1992.

Raufman J-P: Gastric chief cells: receptors and signal transduction mechanisms, *Gastroenterology* 102:699, 1992.

Reuss L: Ion transport across gallbladder epithelium, *Physiol Rev* 69:503, 1989.

Shamburek RD, Schubert ML: Control of gastric acid secretion, *Gastroenterol Clin North Am* 21:527, 1992.

Walsh JH: Peptides as regulators of gastric acid secretion, *Annu Rev Physiol* 50:41, 1988.

Williams JA: Regulatory mechanisms in pancreas and salivary acini, *Annu Rev Physiol* 46:361, 1984.

Books and monographs

Allen A, editor: *Mechanisms of mucosal protection in the upper gastrointestinal tract,* New York, 1984, Raven Press.

Argent BE, Case RM: *Pancreatic ducts: cellular mechanisms and control of bicarbonate secretion.* In Johnson LR, editor: *Physiology of the gastrointestinal tract,* ed 3, New York, 1994, Raven Press.

Arias IM et al: *The liver: biology and pathobiology,* ed 2, New York, 1988, Raven Press.

Cook DI, Van Lennep EW, Roberts ML, Young JA: *Secretion by the major salivary glands.* In Johnson LR, editor: *Physiology of the gastrointestinal tract,* ed 3, New York, 1994, Raven Press.

Davenport HW: *Physiology of the digestive tract,* ed 5, Chicago, 1982, Mosby–Year Book.

Feldman M: *Gastric secretion.* In Sleisenger M, Fordtran JS, editors: *Gastrointestinal diseases,* ed 5, Philadelphia, 1993, WB Saunders.

Flemström G: *Gastric and duodenal secretion of mucus and bicarbonate.* In Johnson LR, editor: *Physiology of the gastrointestinal tract,* ed 3, New York, 1994, Raven Press.

Forte JG, Soll AH: *Cell biology of hydrochloric acid secretion.* In *Handbook of physiology,* sect 6, *The gastrointestinal system,* vol III, Bethesda, Md, 1989, American Physiological Society.

Go VLW et al, editors: *The pancreas: biology, pathobiology, and disease,* ed 2, New York, 1993, Raven Press.

Gorelick FS, Jamieson JD: *The pancreatic acinar cell: structure-function relationships.* In Johnson LR, editor: *Physiology of the gastrointestinal tract,* ed 3, New York, 1994, Raven Press.

Hernandez DE, Glavin GB, editors: *Neurobiology of stress ulcers, Ann NY Acad Sci,* vol 299, New York, 1990, New York Academy of Sciences.

Hersey SJ: *Gastric secretion of pepsins.* In Johnson LR, editor: *Physiology of the gastrointestinal tract,* ed 3, New York, 1994, Raven Press.

Hoffman AF: *Biliary secretion and excretion: the hepatobiliary components of the enterohepatic circulation of bile acids.* In Johnson LR, editor: *Physiology of the gastrointestinal tract,* ed 3, New York, 1994, Raven Press.

Sachs G: *The gastric H, K-ATPase: regulation and structure/function of the acid pump of the stomach.* In Johnson LR, editor: *Physiology of the gastrointestinal tract,* ed 3, New York, 1994, Raven Press.

Scharschmidt BF: *Bilirubin metabolism, bile formation, and gallbladder and bile duct function.* In Sleisenger MH, Fordtran JS, editors: *Gastrointestinal disease,* ed 5, Philadelphia, 1993, WB Saunders.

Siegers C-P, Watkins JB III, editors: *Biliary excretion of drugs and other chemicals,* New York, 1991, Gustav Fischer Verlag.

Soll AH, Berglindh T: *Receptors that regulate gastric acid secretory function.* In Johnson LR, editor: *Physiology of the gastrointestinal tract,* ed 3, New York, 1994, Raven Press.

Tavoloni N, Berk PD, editors: *Hepatic transport and bile secretion,* New York, 1993, Raven Press.

Yule DI, Williams JA: *Stimulus-secretion coupling in the pancreatic acinus.* In Johnson LR, editor: *Physiology of the gastrointestinal tract,* ed 3, New York, 1994, Raven Press.

CHAPTER

39

Digestion and Absorption

Most nutrients cannot be absorbed by the epithelial cells that line the gastrointestinal tract in the forms in which they are ingested. **Digestion** refers to the processes by which ingested molecules are converted to forms that can be absorbed by gastrointestinal tract epithelial cells. In digestion, ingested molecules are cleaved into smaller ones by reactions catalyzed by enzymes in the lumen or on the luminal surface of the gastrointestinal tract. **Absorption** refers to the processes by which molecules are transported through the epithelial cells that line the gastrointestinal tract to enter the blood or lymph draining that region of the tract.

■ *Digestion and Absorption of Carbohydrates*

■ *Carbohydrates in the Diet*

Plant starch, **amylopectin,** is the major source of carbohydrate in most human diets. *Humans have no nutritional requirement for carbohydrate per se, but it is usually the principal source of calories.* Amylopectin is a high-molecular-weight ($>10^6$), branched molecule of glucose monomers. Another, smaller source of dietary starch is **amylose.** Amylose has a lower molecular weight ($<10^5$) than amylopectin, and it is a linear α-1,4 linked polymer of glucose. **Cellulose,** the major component of dietary fiber, is an α-1,4 linked glucose polymer. Intestinal enzymes cannot hydrolyze β-glycosidic linkages; thus, cellulose and other molecules with β-glycosidic linkages remain undigested. **Glycogen** is a branched animal starch. The amount of glycogen ingested varies widely among cultures and among individuals within a given culture. **Sucrose** and **lactose** are the principal dietary disaccharides; **glucose** and **fructose** are the major monosaccharides.

■ *Digestion of Carbohydrates*

The structure of a branched starch molecule is depicted in Fig. 39-1. Starch is a polymer of glucose, and it consists of chains of glucose units linked by α-1,4 glycosidic bonds. The α-1,4 chains have branch points formed by α-1,6 linkages, and thus the starch molecule is highly branched.

The digestion of starch begins in the mouth with the action of the α-**amylase,** formerly known as **ptyalin,** which is contained in salivary secretions. This enzyme catalyzes the hydrolysis of the internal α-1,4 links of starch, but it cannot hydrolyze the α-1,6 branching links or the terminal α-1,4 linkages. The α-amylase secreted by the pancreas has the same specificity. The principal products of α-amylase digestion of starch are shown in Fig. 39-1. The action of the salivary α-amylase continues until the food in the stomach is mixed with gastric acid, which inactivates the enzyme. Although considerable amounts of starch may be digested by the salivary α-amylase, this enzyme is not required for complete digestion and absorption of starch. After the salivary α-amylase is inactivated by gastric acid, no further processing of carbohydrate occurs in the stomach.

The α-amylase secreted by the pancreas is highly active. Both salivary and pancreatic α-amylases produce the same products, but the total activity of the pancreatic enzyme is considerably greater than that of the salivary amylase. Pancreatic α-amylase is most concentrated in the duodenum. Within 10 minutes after entering the duodenum, starch is almost completely converted to maltose, maltotriose, α-1,4 linked malto-oligosaccharides (from four to nine glucose units long), and α-limit dextrins (Fig. 39-1), which contain five to nine glucose monomers.

Further digestion of these oligosaccharides is accomplished by enzymes (called **oligosaccharidases**) that reside in the brush border membrane of the epithelium of the duodenum and jejunum (Fig. 39-2). The major brush border oligosaccharidases are **lactase,** which splits lactose into glucose and galactose; **sucrase,** which splits sucrose into fructose and glucose; α-**dextrinase** (also called **isomaltase**), which "debranches" the α-limit dextrins by cleaving the α-1,6 linkages at the branch points; and **glucoamylase**, which breaks malto-oligosaccharides down into single glucose units.

The activity of these four brush border oligosaccharidases is highest in the duodenum and upper jejunum. Their activity gradually declines through the rest of the small intestine. The digestion of α-limit dextrins proceeds with the sequential removal of glucose monomers from the nonreducing ends. The branch points of the oligosaccharides are cleaved by α-dextrinase (Fig. 39-3).

Sucrase and α-dextrinase are noncovalently associated subunits of a single protein. After this protein is inserted into the brush border membrane, it is cleaved into two separate polypeptides to form the two different enzymes.

■ *Absorption of Carbohydrates*

Of all the divisions of the gastrointestinal tract, the duodenum and upper jejunum have the highest capacity to absorb sugars. The capacities of the lower jejunum and ileum are progressively less. The only dietary monosaccharides that are well absorbed are glucose, galactose, and fructose.

Glucose and galactose are actively taken up by the brush border epithelial cells by a well-characterized transport protein (see Chapter 1) called **SGLT1** (for **sodium-glucose transport protein 1**). As its name implies, SGLT1 uses the energy of the Na⁺ gradient to actively transport glucose and galactose into the intestinal epithelial cells. Glucose and galactose compete for entry; most other sugars are not effective competitors. The active entry of glucose and galactose into the intestinal epithelial cells is stimulated by the presence of Na⁺ in the lumen. Similarly, the entry of Na⁺ into the epithelial cell across the brush border membrane is stimulated by glucose or galactose in the lumen. SGLT1 transports two Na⁺ ions and one glucose or galactose molecule across the brush border membrane. The electrochemical potential gradient for Na⁺ is created by Na⁺, K⁺-ATPase pumps

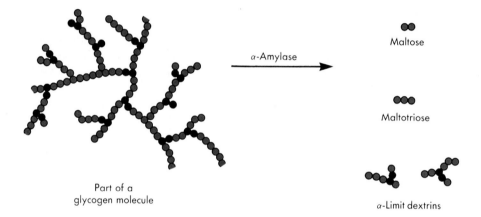

■ **Fig. 39-1**   Structure of a branched starch molecule and the action of α-amylase. The colored circles represent glucose monomers linked by α-1,4 linkages. The black circles represent glucose units linked by α-1,6 linkages at the branch points. The α-1,6 linkages and terminal α-1,4 bonds cannot be cleaved by α-amylase.

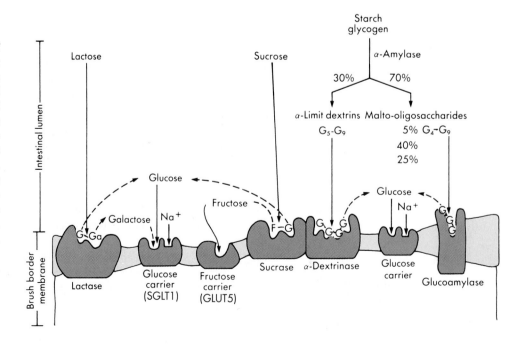

■ **Fig. 39-2**   Functions of the major brush border oligosaccharidases. The glucose, galactose, and fructose molecules released by enzymatic hydrolysis are then transported into the epithelial cell by specific transport carrier proteins. The glucose-galactose transporter is also known as SGLT1 and the fructose transporter as GLUT5. *G*, Glucose; *Ga*, galactose; *F*, fructose. (From Gray GM: *N Engl J Med* 292:1225, 1975.)

present in the basolateral plasma membranes of the intestinal epithelial cells.

Glucose and galactose leave the intestinal epithelial cell at the basal and lateral plasma membranes via facilitated transport, and they then diffuse into the mucosal capillaries. Fig. 39-4 summarizes major features of glucose and galactose absorption. The transport protein responsible for efflux of glucose and galactose across the basolateral membrane is **GLUT2.** GLUT2, a member of the family of monosaccharide facilitated transporters, is also present in liver, kidney, and pancreatic islet cells.

Fructose is not a substrate for the brush border glucose-galactose transporter. The facilitated transport of fructose across the brush border plasma membrane is mediated by a separate transport protein called **GLUT5.** GLUT5 is present only in the brush border plasma membrane of mature intestinal epithelial cells. GLUT5 is rather specific for fructose; fructose transport is not inhibited by glucose, galactose, or most other sugars. Fructose crosses the basolateral membrane of the intestinal epithelial cells via the same GLUT2 transporters used by glucose and galactose.

SGLT1, GLUT2, and GLUT5 are expressed in mature intestinal epithelial cells near the tips of the villi, but they are not present in immature intestinal epithelial cells in the crypts of Lieberkühn.

Absorption of carbohydrate from different food sources. The extent of absorption of the different forms of dietary carbohydrate—monosaccharides, disaccharides, and starch—varies in the human small intestine. Monosaccharides and disaccharides in the diet are completely absorbed in the small intestine. Dietary starch, however, is not completely absorbed. In healthy humans fed a test meal that contains 20 or 60 g of starch, about 6% to 10% escapes absorption in the small intestine. This quantity of starch is passed on to the colon, where it

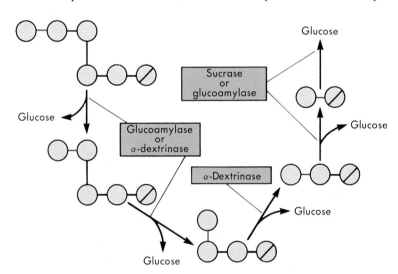

■ **Fig. 39-3** Cleavage of an α-limit dextrin by the oligosaccharidases of the brush border plasma membrane. Glucose monomers are removed in sequence, beginning at the nonreducing end of the molecule. Note the overlapping specificities of glucoamylase and α-dextrinase and of sucrase and glucoamylase. α-Dextrinase (isomaltase) is the only enzyme that cleaves the α-1,6 linkages at the branch points of the α-limit dextrins. (From Gray GM: *Carbohydrate absorption and malabsorption.* In Johnson RL, editor: *Physiology of the gastrointestinal tract,* New York, 1981, Raven Press.)

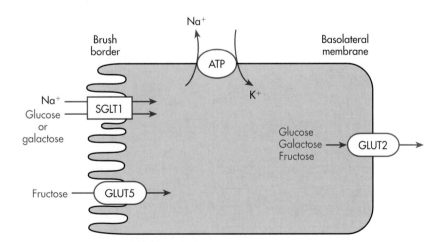

■ **Fig. 39-4** Absorption of glucose, galactose, and fructose in the upper small intestine. Glucose and galactose enter the epithelial cell at the brush border against a concentration gradient via the SGLT1 transport protein; the Na^+ gradient provides the energy for monosaccharide entry. Facilitated transport of fructose across the brush border membrane is mediated by GLUT5. Glucose, galactose, and fructose leave the cell at the basolateral membrane by facilitated transport via a common transporter, GLUT2.

serves as an excellent carbon source for colonic bacteria. The failure to completely absorb carbohydrate from starch is normal and is not associated with any untoward symptoms.

The rate and extent of absorption of starch may vary with the starch-containing foodstuff (Table 39-1). Starch-containing foods that are more rapidly absorbed result in a greater rate and quantity of insulin release from the pancreas.

■ *Carbohydrate Malabsorption Syndromes*

Malabsorption of carbohydrates is usually caused by a deficiency in one of the oligosaccharidases of the brush border.

Lactose malabsorption syndrome is a common disorder caused by a deficiency of lactase in the brush border of the duodenum and jejunum. As a result of this deficiency, undigested lactose cannot be absorbed and is instead passed on to the colonic bacteria, which avidly metabolize the lactose. The bacteria release gas and metabolic products that enhance colonic motility. Individuals with this disorder are said to be **lactose intolerant.** The symptoms of this disorder (and of the other carbohydrate malabsorption syndromes) are intestinal distention, borborygmi (gurgling noises in the intestine), flatulence, and diarrhea.

■ **Table 39-1**   Absorption of glucose from various carbohydrate-containing foods

Food	Glycemic index
Glucose	100
Carrots	92
Corn flakes	80
Rice, white	72
Potatoes, raw	70
Bread, white	69
Shredded wheat	67
Bananas	62
Corn	59
Pear	51
All-Bran	51
Spaghetti	50
Potatoes, sweet	48
Orange	40
Apple	39
Beans, navy	31
Beans, kidney	29
Sausages	28

Healthy adult men and women were fed amounts of the various food listed sufficient to provide 50 g of carbohydrate. Their blood glucose levels were followed for 2 hours after eating the carbohydrate. For each substance the amount of glucose that appeared in the blood over the 2 hours, expressed as a percentage of the increased amount of glucose in the blood in the 2 hours after eating 50 g of glucose, is called the **glycemic index.** Data are the means of 5 to 10 individuals. (Based on data from Jenkins DJA et al: *Am J Clin Nutr* 34:362, 1981.)

More than 50% of the adults in the world are lactose intolerant. This condition may be genetically determined. In Asian societies, lactose intolerance among adults is almost universal. Most northern European adults, on the other hand, are lactose tolerant. A large proportion of African-American adults are lactose intolerant. Many lactose-intolerant adults simply do not drink milk or eat certain milk products, and they therefore avoid the symptoms without being aware that they have the disorder. The presence of lactose in the diet may induce a higher level of intestinal lactase activity than would be present in the absence of dietary lactose.

Congenital lactose intolerance is rare. Infants with this disorder are deficient in jejunal lactase and have diarrhea when they are fed breast milk or formula containing lactose. The resultant dehydration and electrolyte imbalance are life threatening. Such infants must be fed a formula that contains sucrose or fructose instead of lactose.

Sucrase-isomaltase deficiency is characterized by very low levels of sucrase and isomaltase activity in the small intestinal brush border. This deficiency is an autosomal recessive, inherited disorder that results in intolerance to ingested sucrose or starch. About 10% of Greenland's Eskimos and as many as 0.2% of North Americans have sucrase-isomaltase deficiency. In this disorder, either the synthesis of the single protein that carries out both sucrase and isomaltase activities is suppressed or the protein is destroyed by antibodies. Individuals with sucrase-isomaltase deficiency do well on diets low in sucrose and starch.

Glucose-galactose malabsorption syndrome is a very rare hereditary disorder caused by a missense mutation in SGLT1, the brush border active transport protein for glucose and galactose. Ingestion of glucose, galactose, or starch leads to flatulence and severe diarrhea. Fructose is well tolerated and can be fed to infants with this disorder. The brush border oligosaccharidases are normal in this disease.

All these disorders can be diagnosed with the **oral sugar tolerance test.** In this procedure, the patient is given an oral dose of the sugar in question, and the levels of that sugar in the patient's blood and feces are monitored. If the patient is intolerant of the administered sugar, diarrhea will ensue. The sugar will fail to appear in the blood but will appear in the feces. In suspected oligosaccharidase deficiency, the definitive test involves sampling the jejunal mucosa and assaying it for the deficient enzyme.

■ *Digestion and Absorption of Proteins*

The amount of dietary protein varies greatly among cultures and even among individuals within a culture. In poor societies, an adult may find it difficult to obtain the amount of protein (0.5 to 0.7 g/day/kg of body weight) required to balance normal catabolism of proteins.

Children find it even more difficult to get the relatively greater amounts of protein they require to sustain normal growth. In wealthier societies, chiefly in industrially developed countries, a typical individual ingests protein far exceeding the nutritional requirement.

In addition to ingested protein, the gastrointestinal tract must also process the 10 to 30 g of protein per day contained in digestive secretions and a similar amount of protein in exfoliated epithelial cells. *In normal humans, essentially all ingested protein is digested and absorbed.* Most of the protein in digestive secretions and exfoliated epithelial cells is also digested and absorbed. The small amount of protein present in the feces is derived principally from colonic bacteria, exfoliated cells, and proteins in mucous secretions of the colon. In humans, ingested protein is almost completely absorbed by the time the meal has traversed the jejunum.

Digestion of Proteins

Digestion in the stomach. The chief cells of the stomach secrete the inactive protein **pepsinogen,** which is converted by hydrogen ions to the active enzyme, **pepsin.** The extent to which pepsin hydrolyzes dietary protein is significant but highly variable. At most, pepsin reduces only about 15% of dietary protein to amino acids and small peptides. However, the duodenum and small intestine have such a high capacity to process protein that the total absence of pepsin does not impair the digestion and absorption of dietary protein.

Digestion in the duodenum and small intestine. It is the proteases secreted by the pancreas that play the major role in protein digestion. The most important of these proteases are **trypsin, chymotrypsin, carboxypeptidases A and B, and elastase.** These enzymes are present in inactive, proenzyme forms in the pancreatic juice. The enzyme **enteropeptidase** (also called **enterokinase**), which is secreted by the mucosa of the duodenum and jejunum, converts trypsinogen to trypsin. Trypsin acts autocatalytically to activate trypsinogen, and it also converts the other proenzymes to the active enzymes (Fig. 39-5). Within the duodenum, all the pancreatic proteases are highly active, and they rapidly convert dietary protein to small peptides. About 50% of the ingested protein is digested and absorbed in the duodenum.

The brush border of the duodenum and the small intestine also contains a number of peptidases. These peptidases are integral membrane proteins whose active sites face the intestinal lumen. The proximal jejunum contains the highest amounts of these brush border enzymes. These enzymes reduce the peptides produced by pancreatic proteases to oligopeptides and amino acids. The brush border peptidases include **aminopeptidases,** which cleave single amino acids from the N terminals of peptides; **dipeptidases,** which cleave dipeptides to amino acids; and **dipeptidyl aminopeptidases,** which cleave a dipeptide from the N-terminal end of a peptide. Fig. 39-6 illustrates some major proteases and peptidases present in the small intestine.

The principal products of protein digestion by pancreatic proteases and brush border peptidases are small peptides and amino acids. The small peptides (primarily dipeptides, tripeptides, and tetrapeptides) are produced in concentrations about three or four times higher than those of the single amino acids. As discussed below, small peptides and amino acids are transported across the brush border plasma membrane into intestinal epithelial cells. Small peptides are then hydrolyzed by peptidases in the cytosol of the epithelial cells; consequently, single amino acids and a few dipeptides appear in the portal blood. These cytosolic peptidases are more abundant than the brush border peptidases, and they are particularly active against dipeptides and tripeptides, which are transported with high efficiency across the brush border membrane. The brush border peptidases, on the other hand, are mainly active against peptides of four or more amino acids.

Absorption of the Products of Protein Digestion

Absorption of intact proteins and large peptides. Intact proteins and large peptides are not absorbed by humans to an extent that is nutritionally significant. Small amounts of luminal proteins are taken up by the M cells of the mucosal immune system. In ruminants and rodents, but not in humans, the neonatal intestine has a high capacity for the specific absorption by receptor-mediated endocytosis of immune proteins present in colostrum. This absorption is vital in the development of normal immune competence in ruminants and rodents.

Absorption of small peptides. After the breakdown of proteins by pancreatic proteins and brush border peptidases, the dipeptides and tripeptides produced are trans-

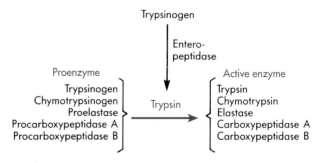

■ **Fig. 39-5** Conversion of inactive proenzymes of pancreatic juice to active enzymes by the action of trypsin. Trypsinogen of pancreatic juice is proteolytically converted to active trypsin by enteropeptidase (also known as enterokinase) secreted by the epithelial cells of the duodenum and jejunum. Trypsin then activates the other proenzymes of pancreatic juice as shown.

ported across the brush border membrane. The rate of transport of these small peptides usually exceeds the rate of transport of individual amino acids. In the experiments shown in Fig. 39-7, glycine was absorbed by the human jejunum less rapidly as a single amino acid than it was as glycylglycine or glycylglycylglycine.

A single membrane transport system with broad specificity is probably responsible for the absorption of small peptides. This transport system apparently has a high affinity for dipeptides and tripeptides but very low affinities for peptides of four or more amino acid residues. The transport system is stereospecific, and it prefers peptides of the physiological L-amino acids. The affinity of the system is higher for peptides of amino acids with bulky side chains. The transport of dipeptides and tripeptides is powered by the electrochemical potential difference of H^+ across the membrane (Fig. 39-8) and is thus a secondary active process. The jejunum is more active than the ileum in uptake of dipeptides and tripeptides. The total amount of each

amino acid that enters jejunal epithelial cells in the form of dipeptides or tripeptides is greater than the amount that enters as the single amino acid.

Most of the small peptides that enter the intestinal epithelial cells are cleaved to single amino acids in the cell and absorbed into the blood as single amino acids. However, recent evidence suggests that a small, but significant, amount of dipeptides and tripeptides is transported into the blood by a peptide transporter in the basolateral membrane; this transporter remains poorly characterized.

Absorption of amino acids. The ileum is more active in the uptake of single amino acids than is the jejunum; as observed in the previous section, the opposite order applies to small peptides. Amino acids are transported across the brush border plasma membrane into the epithelial cell via certain specific amino acid transport systems. Transport of amino acids out of the epithelial cell across the basolateral membrane occurs primarily by a different set of transporters. Some of the transporters in

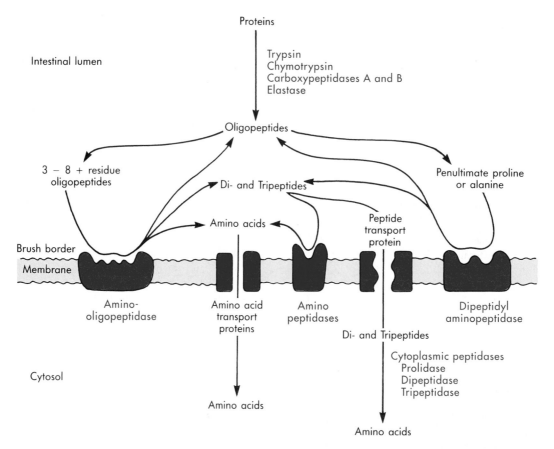

■ **Fig. 39-6**   The hierarchy of proteases and peptidases that functions in the small intestine. The pancreatic proteases convert dietary proteins to oligopeptides. Brush border peptidases then convert the oligopeptides to amino acids (about 70%) and dipeptides and tripeptides (about 30%). The amino acids are taken up across the brush border membrane by amino acid transporters and the small peptides by a peptide transporter. In the cytosol of the enterocyte, dipeptides and tripeptides are cleaved to single amino acids. (Modified from Van Dyke RW: *Mechanisms of digestion and absorption of food.* In Sleisenger MH, Fordtran JS, editors: *Gastrointestinal disease,* ed 4, Philadelphia, 1989, WB Saunders.)

both membranes depend on the Na⁺ gradient (as previously described for glucose and galactose absorption), whereas other transport systems are independent of Na⁺. The basolateral membrane, however, is less highly differentiated than is the brush border membrane. The amino acid transporters present in the basolateral membrane occur in many nonepithelial cells, whereas the amino acid transporters in the brush border membrane are mostly unique to epithelial cells.

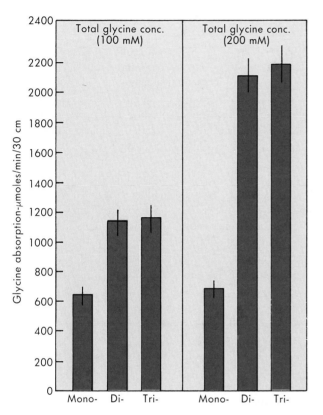

■ **Fig. 39-7** Glycine is absorbed more rapidly by the human small intestine in the form of diglycine or triglycine than as free glycine. (From Adibi SA, Morse EL: *J Clin Invest* 60:1008, 1977.)

For some amino acids, simple diffusion may be a significant pathway across both brush border and basolateral membranes. The more hydrophobic the amino acid and the larger its concentration gradient across the membrane, the greater is the importance of diffusion.

Brush border membrane. Current knowledge of amino acid transporters present in the brush border plasma membrane is summarized in Table 39-2. Of the seven transporter types present, five depend on the Na⁺ gradient and catalyze secondary active uptake of amino acids. Two transporters are independent of Na⁺, and their uptake of amino acids is mediated by facilitated transport.

The basolateral membrane. The five classes of amino acid transporters present in the basolateral membrane are listed in Table 39-3. The three transporters that are independent of the Na⁺ gradient are primarily responsible for efflux of amino acids into the blood. The two Na⁺-dependent systems mediate active uptake of amino acids across the basolateral membrane; these transporters serve to provide amino acids for protein synthesis in the epithelial cells during interdigestive periods.

There are no known basolateral transporters of acidic amino acids. Glutamine, glutamate, and aspartate are among the fuels preferred by intestinal epithelial cells. Most of the glutamine, glutamate, and aspartate that enter the cells across the brush border are probably shunted to the pathways of energy metabolism, and these amino acids are not transported across the basolateral membrane into the blood.

■ *Defects of Amino Acid Absorption*

Hartnup's disease is a rare hereditary disorder that involves defective renal and intestinal transport of neutral amino acids. Neutral amino acids are present in the urine. Hartnup's disease is probably caused by defects in the B system of the epithelial cells of the small intestine and the proximal renal tubule.

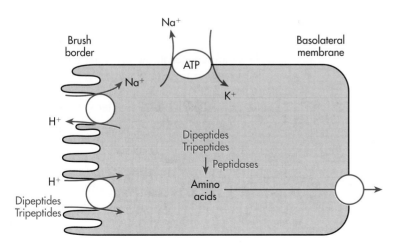

■ **Fig. 39-8** A wide variety of dipeptides and tripeptides is taken up across the brush border plasma membrane by a single type of H⁺- powered secondary active transport protein. The H⁺ gradient is created by Na⁺, H⁺ exchangers in the brush border membrane. In the epithelial cell cytosol, peptidases cleave most of the dipeptides and tripeptides to single amino acids, which leave the cell at the basolateral membrane by facilitated transport.

■ **Table 39-2** Amino acid transporters of the brush border plasma membrane of the upper small intestine

Transporter type	Preferred substrates
Na$^+$-dependent	
B	Neutral amino acids
B$^{0,+}$	Neutral amino acids, basic amino acids, and cystine
IMINO	Imino acids (proline and hydroxy-proline)
X$^-_{AG}$	Acidic amino acids
β	β amino acids (taurine is the most important natural substrate)
Independent of Na$^+$	
b$^{0,+}$	Neutral amino acids, basic amino acids, cystine
y$^+$	Basic amino acids

■ **Table 39-3** Amino acid transporters of the basolateral plasma membrane of the upper small intestine

Transporter type	Preferred substrates
Na$^+$-dependent	
A	Neutral amino acids, imino acids
ASC	Small neutral amino acids, especially alanine, serine, and cystine
Independent of Na$^+$	
asc	Same as for ASC
y$^+$	Basic amino acids
L	Larger and hydrophobic neutral amino acids

Cystinuria is a disorder characterized by the presence of cystine in the urine. This disease appears to be caused by a defect in either B$^{0,+}$ or b$^{0,+}$ transporters in the brush border membrane of the epithelial cells of the small intestine and the renal proximal tubule.

Prolinuria is a rare disorder that involves defective renal and intestinal reabsorption of proline. Proline and hydroxyproline are present in the urine. Prolinuria appears to be caused by a defect in the IMINO system in the epithelial cell brush border plasma membrane of the small intestine and the renal proximal tubule.

Because the epithelial cells are still capable of absorbing dipeptides and tripeptides, neither Hartnup's disease, cystinuria, nor prolinuria results in malnutrition.

■ Intestinal Absorption of Salts and Water

Normally, humans absorb almost 99% of the water and ions contained in ingested food and gastrointestinal secretions. The net movement of water and ions is normally from the lumen to the blood. In most cases, this net movement represents the difference between the large unidirectional movements from lumen to blood and from blood to lumen.

■ Absorption of Water

Typically, about 2 L of water is ingested each day, and approximately 7 L/day is contained in the gastrointestinal secretions (Fig. 39-9). Only about 50 to 100 ml/day of water is lost in the feces. The gastrointestinal tract thus typically absorbs almost 9 L/day.

Very little net absorption of water occurs in the duodenum. In fact, water is usually added to the chyme to bring it to isotonicity. Chyme delivered from the stomach is often hypertonic. The action of digestive enzymes creates still more osmotic activity. The duodenum is highly permeable to water, and very large fluxes of water occur from lumen to blood and from blood to lumen. Usually, the net flux is from blood to lumen owing to the hypertonicity of the chyme.

Large net water absorption occurs in the small intestine; the jejunum is more active than the ileum in absorbing water. The net absorption that occurs in the colon is relatively small, about 400 ml/day. However, the colon can absorb water against a larger osmotic pressure difference than can the rest of the gastrointestinal tract. Fig. 39-9 summarizes the handling of water by the gastrointestinal tract.

■ Absorption of Na$^+$

Na$^+$ is absorbed along the entire length of the intestine (Table 39-4). *As is the case with water, net absorption is the result of large, unidirectional fluxes of Na$^+$ from blood to lumen and from lumen to blood.* The unidirectional fluxes are greater in the proximal gut than in the distal intestine because the brush border surface area is greater per unit length in the jejunum. This ratio diminishes toward the ileum and is smaller still in the colon. Therefore, the amount of Na$^+$ flux that occurs in the intestine correlates with the amount of surface area. The tight junctions between epithelial cells are leakiest in the duodenum and upper jejunum, somewhat tighter in the ileum, and quite tight in the colon. Hence, the paracellular fluxes of water and electrolytes diminish along the length of the intestine.

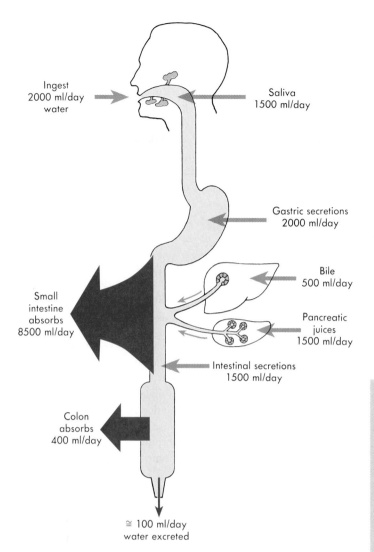

Na⁺ crosses the brush border membrane down an electrochemical gradient, and it is actively extruded from epithelial cells by the Na⁺, K⁺-ATPase in the basal and lateral plasma membrane. Normally, the contents of the small intestine are isotonic to plasma. Luminal contents have about the same Na⁺ concentration as does plasma, so that Na⁺ absorption normally takes place in the absence of a significant concentration gradient. Na⁺ absorption is active, however, and can occur against a small electrochemical potential difference for Na⁺.

The net rate of absorption of Na⁺ is highest in the jejunum. Here, Na⁺ absorption is enhanced by the presence of glucose, galactose, and neutral amino acids in the lumen. These substances and Na⁺ cross the brush border membrane on the same transport proteins. Na⁺ moves down its electrochemical potential gradient and provides the energy for moving the sugars (glucose and galactose) and neutral and acidic amino acids into the epithelial cells against a concentration gradient. Thus, Na⁺ enhances the absorption of sugars and amino acids, and vice versa.

The ability of glucose to enhance the absorption of Na⁺, and hence of Cl⁻ and water, is exploited in **oral rehydration therapy** for **cholera** and other secretory diarrheas. When patients with cholera drink a solution that contains glucose, NaCl, and other constituents, the absorption of glucose, salt, and water helps to counteract the secretory fluxes of salt and water that would otherwise dehydrate the patient. Despite its simplicity, oral rehydration therapy is a major advance because of its impact on world health.

The net rate of Na⁺ absorption in the ileum is smaller. Na⁺ absorption is only slightly stimulated by sugars and amino acids. The ileum can absorb Na⁺ against a larger electrochemical potential than can the jejunum.

In the colon, Na⁺ is normally absorbed against a large electrochemical potential difference. Sodium concentrations in the luminal contents can be as low as 25 mM, compared with about 120 mM in the plasma.

■ Fig. 39-9 Overall fluid balance in the human gastrointestinal tract. About 2 L of water is ingested each day, and 7 L of various secretions enters the gastrointestinal tract. Of this total of 9 L, 8.5 L is absorbed in the small intestine. About 500 ml is passed on to the colon, which normally absorbs 80% to 90% of the water presented to it. (Redrawn from Vander AJ, Sherman JH, Luciano DS: *Human physiology,* ed 6, New York, 1994, McGraw-Hill.)

■ Table 39-4   Transport of Na⁺, K⁺, Cl⁻, and HCO₃⁻ in the small and large intestines

Segment of intestine	Na⁺	K⁺	Cl⁻	HCO₃⁻
Jejunum	Actively absorbed; absorption enhanced by sugars, neutral amino acids	Passively absorbed when concentration rises because of absorption of water	Absorbed	Absorbed
Ileum	Actively absorbed	Passively absorbed	Absorbed, some in exchange for HCO₃⁻	Secreted, partly in exchange for Cl⁻
Colon	Actively absorbed	Net secretion occurs when (K⁺) concentration in lumen <25 mM	Absorbed, some in exchange for HCO₃⁻	Secreted, partly in exchange for Cl⁻

■ *Absorption of Cl⁻ and HCO₃⁻*

In the proximal duodenum, HCO₃⁻ is secreted into the lumen. In the jejunum, both Cl⁻ and HCO₃⁻ are absorbed in large amounts. At the end of the jejunum, most of the HCO_3^- in the hepatic and pancreatic secretions has been absorbed. In the ileum, Cl^- is absorbed, but HCO_3^- is normally secreted. If the HCO_3^- concentration in the lumen of the ileum exceeds about 45 mM, the flux from lumen to blood exceeds that from blood to lumen, and net absorption occurs. *In the colon, the transport of these ions is qualitatively similar to that in the ileum, in that Cl⁻ is absorbed and bicarbonate is usually secreted.*

■ *Absorption of K⁺*

As with the other ions, the net movement of potassium across the intestinal epithelium represents the difference between large unidirectional fluxes from lumen to blood and from blood to lumen. *In the jejunum and in the ileum, the net flux of K⁺ is from lumen to blood.* As the volume of intestinal contents is reduced by the absorption of water, K^+ is concentrated. This action provides a driving force for the movement of K^+ across the intestinal mucosa and into the blood. Evidence for active transport of K^+ in the small intestine is lacking. *In the colon, K⁺ may be either secreted or absorbed.* Net secretion occurs when the luminal concentration is less than about 25 mM; above 25 mM, net absorption occurs. Under most circumstances, net secretion of K^+ takes place in the colon; the secretory process is active (Table 39-4).

Most of the absorption of K^+ in the small intestine is caused by the absorption of water, which increases the K^+ concentration in the lumen. Hence, significant K^+ loss may occur in diarrhea. If diarrhea is prolonged, the K^+ level in the extracellular fluid compartment of the body falls. Because maintenance of normal extracellular levels of K^+ is important to many body functions, especially those of the heart and other muscles, life-threatening consequences such as **cardiac dysrhythmias** may ensue with a decrease in K^+. Infants with prolonged diarrhea are particularly susceptible to **hypokalemia** (low plasma K^+).

■ *Routes of Salt and Water Absorption by the Intestine*

The tight junctions. The epithelial cells that line the intestine are connected to their neighbors by tight junctions near their luminal surfaces. The tight junctions are leakiest in the duodenum, a little tighter in the jejunum, tighter still in the ileum, and tightest in the colon.

Transcellular versus paracellular transport. Because tight junctions are leaky, some fraction of the water and ions that traverse the intestinal epithelium passes between, rather than through, the epithelial cells. Transmucosal movement achieved by passing through tight junctions and the lateral intercellular spaces of an epithelium is called **paracellular transport.** Passage through the epithelial cells is termed **transcellular transport.**

Because the tight junctions in the duodenum are very leaky, a major portion of the large unidirectional fluxes of water and ions that takes place in the duodenum occurs via the paracellular pathway. The proportions of water or a particular ion that pass through the transcellular and paracellular routes are determined by the relative permeabilities of the two pathways for a particular substance. Even in the ileum, where the junctions are much tighter than in the duodenum, the paracellular pathway contributes more to the total ionic conductance of the mucosa than does the transcellular pathway.

Villous versus crypt cells. The highly differentiated epithelial cells near the tips of the villi are specialized for absorption of water and ions, whereas the less differentiated cells in the crypts produce net secretion of water and ions.

■ *Ion Transport by Intestinal Epithelial Cells*

The movement of water across the intestinal epithelium is secondary to the movement of ions and other solutes. In all regions of the intestine, the basolateral plasma membrane contains the Na⁺, K⁺-ATPase. As a result of the active extrusion of Na⁺ ions from the cytoplasm by the Na⁺, K⁺-ATPase, the electrochemical potential of Na⁺ in the cytoplasm is much less than that in the luminal fluid. Na⁺ enters the epithelial cell by moving down this large electrochemical potential gradient. Membrane transport proteins of the epithelial cells couple the influx of Na⁺ to the secondary active transport of sugars, amino acids, and other ions.

Ion transport in the jejunum. In the jejunum (Fig. 39-10) net absorption of Na⁺, Cl⁻, and HCO₃⁻ occurs. Na⁺ enters the epithelial cell at the brush border via the nutrient-coupled, Na⁺-powered transporters (electrogenic) and via the Na⁺, H⁺ exchanger. Na⁺ is extruded from the cell across the basolateral membrane by the Na⁺, K⁺-ATPase. Absorption of both Cl⁻ and HCO₃⁻ is powered by the slight luminal electronegativity generated by Na⁺ uptake at the brush border and by the concentration of luminal ions that occurs as a result of the large net absorption of water in the jejunum.

Acidification of the jejunal contents by gastric acid and by the Na⁺,H⁺ exchanger pushes the bicarbonate/carbonic acid equilibrium toward carbonic acid, which is in equilibrium with CO_2 and water. CO_2 is highly diffusible and is readily absorbed across the mucosa and into the blood. Most of the HCO_3^- dumped into the duodenum in bile and pancreatic juice is absorbed by this mechanism.

Ion transport in the ileum. In the ileum (Fig. 39-11), net absorption of Na^+ and Cl^- occurs by mechanisms that are similar to those in the jejunum. However, the Na^+-powered nutrient transporters are less numerous than in the jejunum. Net secretion of HCO_3^- in exchange for absorption of Cl^- occurs via an **anion exchanger** in the brush border membrane. HCO_3^- enters the epithelial cells across the basolateral membrane by Na^+-powered secondary active transport. *Note that the coupled operation of the Na^+, H^+ exchanger and the Cl^-, HCO_3^- transporter of the luminal membrane results in the absorption of NaCl and the secretion of H_2CO_3.* In both jejunum and ileum, K^+ is concentrated by absorption of water; the elevated K^+ concentration drives net absorption of K^+, predominantly through the tight junctions.

Ion transport processes in the colon. In the colon, net absorption of Na^+ and Cl^- and net secretion of HCO_3^- occur by mechanisms similar to those in the ileum. In the colon, however, entry of Na^+ across the brush border membrane occurs via an electrogenic Na^+ channel (Fig. 39-12). Because the tight junctions of the colon are so tight, electrogenic Na^+ transport produces an electrical potential of about 30 mV (lumen negative) across the mucosa. This potential drives the net secretion of K^+ into the lumen, mostly through the tight junctions. In the distal colon, active absorption of K^+ and secretion of H^+ is powered by an H^+, K^+-ATPase that resembles the gastric H^+ pump.

The tight junctions in all regions of the intestine are more permeable to cations than to anions. The large electronegativity in the lumen of the colon causes K^+ to flow from the intercellular spaces to the lumen via the tight junctions. This process may be the major mechanism for the net secretion of K^+ that usually occurs in the colon. Facilitated transport of K^+ from cytoplasm to intestinal lumen across the luminal plasma membrane may also occur in the colon.

■ *The Mechanism of Water Absorption*

As noted, the absorption of water depends on the absorption of ions, principally Na^+ and Cl^-. Under normal circumstances, water absorption in the small intestine occurs in the absence of an osmotic pressure difference between the luminal contents and the blood in the intestinal capillaries. Water absorption by the colon typically proceeds against an osmotic pressure gradient. Water is absorbed by a mechanism known as standing gradient osmosis (see Fig. 38-29). The major features of the standing gradient osmotic mechanism are described in Chapter 38.

Because most water absorption takes place in the absence of a transmucosal osmotic pressure difference, the absorption of the end products of digestion, particularly sugars and amino acids, is important in water

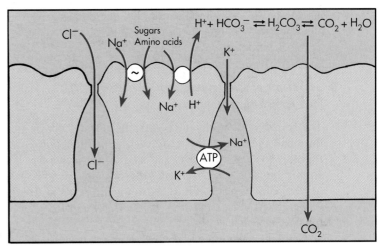

■ **Fig. 39-10**   Summary of major ion transport processes that occur in the jejunum.

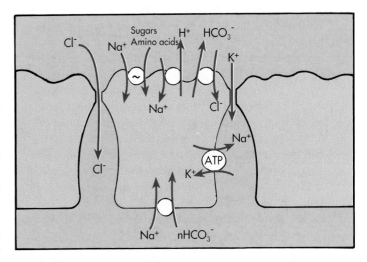

■ **Fig. 39-11**   Summary of major ion transport processes that occur in the ileum.

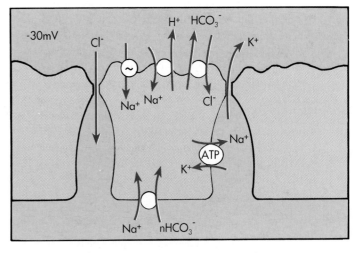

■ **Fig. 39-12**   Summary of major ion transport processes that occur in the colon.

absorption. The absorption of sugars and amino acids allows more water to be absorbed.

■ *Secretion of Electrolytes and Water by Cells in Lieberkühn's Crypts*

The normal net absorption of electrolytes and water by the small intestine is the result of large unidirectional fluxes from lumen to blood and from blood to lumen. *Mature epithelial cells near the tips of the villi are active in net absorption, whereas more immature cells in Lieberkühn's crypts function as net secretors of electrolytes and water.*

A current view of the ionic transport mechanisms that function in the crypt cells is shown in Fig. 39-13. In this model, Cl^- is actively taken up at the basolateral plasma membrane by the $Na^+, K^+, 2Cl^-$ cotransporter (see Chapter 1). This transporter uses the electrochemical potential difference of Na^+ to actively transport Cl^- and K^+ into the cell. Cl^- leaves the cell at the luminal membrane via an electrogenic Cl^- channel. Na^+ is transported into the lumen, driven by the net luminal electronegativity produced by the electrogenic Cl^- secretion into the lumen. Efflux of K^+ via K^+ channels in the basolateral membrane prevents K^+ from accumulating in the cytosol of the crypt cell and maintains an electrical potential difference (cytosol negative) across the luminal and basolateral membranes. This potential difference contributes to the electrochemical driving force for efflux of Cl^- across the luminal membrane and for basolateral influx of Na^+ (and thus of Cl^- also).

The amount of time that the luminal Cl^- channel remains open is enhanced by cyclic AMP (cAMP), and basolateral K^+ channels are activated by Ca^{++} or by elevated cAMP. Thus, net secretion by the crypt cells is enhanced by agonists that elevate intracellular AMP (e.g., prostaglandins and vasoactive intestinal peptide [VIP]) and by Ca^{++}-mobilizing agonists (e.g., acetylcholine). The effects of agonists that elevate AMP are potentiated by agonists that increase cytosolic Ca^{++}, and vice versa.

In secretory diarrheal diseases, such as **cholera,** the secretion of Cl^-, Na^+, and water into the intestinal lumen by the cells in Lieberkühn's crypts is specifically elevated. Cholera is caused by the cholera toxin that is produced by the bacterium *Vibrio cholerae.* **Cholera toxin** permanently activates adenylyl cyclase, and thereby elevates the concentration of cAMP in the crypt cells. cAMP activates the brush border Cl^- channels and thereby prolongs the secretion of Cl^- (and therefore also of Na^+ and water). Cholera patients may produce up to 20 L/day of watery stool. Such patients are likely to die unless they are promptly and adequately rehydrated.

The luminal Cl^- channel in the cells in Lieberkühn's crypts is the same protein that is defec-

tive in **cystic fibrosis (CF).** CF is by far the most common autosomal recessive disorder; about 1 in 20 American adults are CF carriers. Animal experiments show that CF carriers, who have one normal and one defective copy of the gene for the Cl^- channel, suffer much less severe diarrhea in response to cholera than do normal individuals. Because cholera and related secretory diarrheas are the major causes of death in children in areas that lack adequate sanitation, the resistance of CF carriers to secretory diarrheas may explain the unusual prevalence of this mutation.

■ *Physiological Regulation of Salt and Water Absorption*

The control of net absorption of electrolytes and water by epithelial cells near the villous tips and of net secretion of water and electrolytes by cells in the crypts of Lieberkühn is complex. Rates of absorption and secretion of electrolytes and water are influenced by hormones; sympathetic, parasympathetic, and enteric nervous systems; and cells of the gastrointestinal immune system. Moreover, interactions among these regulatory pathways are also important in the control of secretion and absorption.

Hormones, paracrine agonists, and substances released from neurons in the wall of the gastrointestinal tract regulate the absorption and secretion of water and electrolytes by intestinal epithelial cells. Some of these regu-

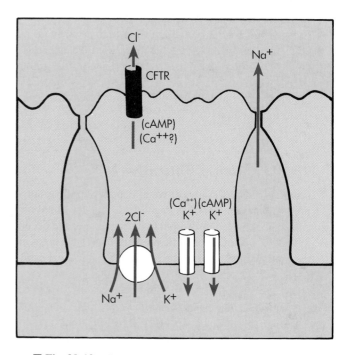

■ **Fig. 39-13**   Ion transport pathways involved in secretion of Cl^-, Na^+, and water by the epithelial cells in Lieberkühn's crypts in the small intestine. CFTR, Cystic fibrosis transmembrane regulator.

latory substances, and the cells that release them, are listed in Table 39-5.

Endocrine control of absorption and secretion. Some of the hormones that influence absorption and secretion of electrolytes and water are released by cells in the wall of the gastrointestinal tract; others come from endocrine cells located elsewhere in the body. Among the hormones that can influence intestinal absorption and secretion are mineralocorticoids, glucocorticoids, catecholamines, somatostatin, and enkephalins.

Aldosterone increases net absorption of water and electrolytes in the colon. The principal action of aldosterone on the colonic epithelial cell is to stimulate the synthesis of the luminal electrogenic Na^+ channel. As a result of this synthesis, the number of Na^+, K^+-ATPase molecules also increases in the basolateral membrane of these cells.

Glucocorticoids stimulate electrolyte and water absorption in both the small and large intestines. This stimulation is most likely the result of an increase in the number of Na^+, K^+-ATPase molecules in the basolateral membranes of enterocytes.

Epinephrine acts on α-receptors on epithelial cells to increase electroneutral NaCl absorption in the ileum and to suppress secretory fluxes. Epinephrine also acts at the level of the submucosal ganglia to inhibit secretomotor outflow to epithelial cells.

Somatostatin stimulates electrolyte and water absorption in the ileum and colon and inhibits secretion. In intestinal epithelial cells, somatostatin appears to act by decreasing cellular levels of cAMP. The ability of somatostatin to decrease secretion by crypt cells has led to the use of somatostatin analogs to treat secretory diarrheas. Somatostatin may also act on enteric neurons to suppress secretomotor outflow to enterocytes.

Opioids act on δ-receptors in the intestine to stimulate salt and water absorption. Opioids act on other receptor subtypes to inhibit intestinal motility. Both of these effects may contribute to the antidiarrheal effects of opioids.

Neural regulation of absorption and secretion. Most of the direct innervation of intestinal epithelial cells comes from neurons of the enteric nervous system, especially from the submucosal ganglia. The predominant influences of parasympathetic and sympathetic neurons occur via their influences on the activities of enteric neurons. Neural reflexes, both extrinsic and intrinsic to the gastrointestinal tract, regulate the absorptive and secretory activities of intestinal epithelial cells.

Enteric nervous system. Epithelial cells are innervated by secretomotor neurons, predominantly from submucosal ganglia, but also from the myenteric ganglia. This innervation stimulates net secretion. An array of mucosal reflexes controls and coordinates the neural outflow from the enteric nervous system to intestinal epithelial cells. *Submucosal secretomotor neurons release acetylcholine and/or VIP onto epithelial cells to stimulate secretion.* In contrast, enteric neurons that inhibit secretion by intestinal epithelial cells have not been found.

In addition to those already mentioned, other neurotransmitters, putative transmitters, and neuromodulators are present in enteric neurons, and these neuroactive substances may influence absorption and secretion. They may directly act on epithelial cells, or they may exert their influences at the level of the submucosal ganglia to stimulate or inhibit outflow from secretomotor neurons.

Reflexes in the enteric nervous system modulate secretomotor outflow from submucosal ganglia to intestinal epithelial cells. Some of these reflexes are elicited by luminal stimuli, such as distention of the gut lumen; stroking the mucosal surface; or the presence in the

■ **Table 39-5** Endogenous substances that influence intestinal absorption and secretion of water and electrolytes

Source	Stimulate net secretion	Stimulate net absorption
Mucosal epithelial cells	Serotonin Gastrin Neurotensin	Somatostatin
Lamina propria cells (non-neural, especially immunocytes)	Arachidonic acid metabolites Histamine Active oxidants Platelet-activating factor Bradykinin	?
Enteric neurons	Acetylcholine Serotinon VIP Substance P	Norepinephrine Neuropeptide Y
Blood	VIP Calcitonin Prostaglandins Atrial natriuretic peptides	Epinephrine Corticosteroids Mineralocorticoids Angiotensin

Adapted from Chang EB, Rao MC: *Intestinal water and electrolyte transport: mechanisms of physiological and adaptive responses.* In Johnson LR, editor: *Physiology of the gastrointestinal tract,* ed 3, New York, 1994, Raven Press.
VIP, Vasoactive intestinal peptide.

lumen of glucose, acid pH, bile salts, ethanol, cholera toxin, or an antigen to which the gastrointestinal immune system has been previously sensitized. All of these stimuli evoke reflex stimulation of secretion. Most of these stimuli also enhance propulsive motility in the stimulated gut segment. These actions demonstrate the interplay between neural control of secretion and motility.

Parasympathetic nervous system. The enteric nervous system is heavily innervated by parasympathetic fibers, to both myenteric and submucosal ganglia. *Stimulation of the parasympathetic fibers diminishes absorptive fluxes and enhances secretion.* Parasympathetic fibers do not directly innervate epithelial cells to a significant degree. Parasympathetic tone apparently contributes to basal rates of secretion. Cholinergic input to the interneurons and secretomotor neurons, especially in the submucosal plexus, enhances secretomotor outflow to epithelial cells and perhaps to other mucosal effector cells also.

Sympathetic nervous system. Stimulation of sympathetic nerves to the gut enhances net absorption. Chemical ablation of the sympathetic nerves diminishes absorption. In addition, diabetic autonomic neuropathy causes decreased sympathetic outflow to the intestine and contributes to "diabetic diarrhea."

Some adrenergic fibers directly innervate epithelial cells, where norepinephrine acts on α receptors to enhance absorption. Sympathetic input to the enteric nervous system diminishes the secretomotor outflow by enteric neurons, especially in the submucosal ganglia, to epithelial cells. Norepinephrine, acting on α receptors, has multiple effects on neurons of submucosal ganglia. These effects decrease the secretomotor outflow to epithelial cells. Somatostatin, another transmitter known to stimulate absorption, is coreleased with norepinephrine at some nerve terminals.

Catecholamines and α-adrenergic agents can strongly inhibit intestinal secretion evoked by cholera toxin, dibutyryl cAMP, VIP, 5-hydroxytryptamine, and many other potent secretagogues.

Regulation of absorption and secretion by the gastrointestinal immune system. The cells of the gastrointestinal immune system contain numerous mediators that influence gastrointestinal salt and water transport. Most of these compounds enhance net secretion of water and electrolytes. The mediators include histamine, serotonin, prostaglandins and thromboxanes, leukotrienes, platelet-activating factor, adenosine, reactive oxygen species, nitric oxide, and endothelin. The cells that contain these mediators include mast cells, phagocytes, lymphocytes, basophils, neutrophils, endothelial cells, and fibroblasts.

Primed mast cells play a central role in the gastrointestinal response to an antigen. A primed mast cell is one that carries antibody on its surface. When the antibody "recognizes" its particular antigen, the mast cell degranulates and releases many different mediators. Several of these mediators induce hypersecretion of salts and water by the epithelial cells as well as hypermotility. Mast cells

also release cytokines that recruit other mucosal immune cells to the response. These cells may then also release secretagogues.

Mediators released from mast cells and other gastrointestinal immunocytes evoke secretion in two ways: they (1) directly affect intestinal epithelial cells to stimulate secretion and/or inhibit absorption and (2) act on enteric neurons to increase the activity in secretomotor circuits. Histamine and prostaglandins appear to be key mediators of the effects on enteric neurons.

In addition to acting as targets of the immune mediators, enteric neurons modulate the release of these mediators from mast cells and influence the function of other gastrointestinal immunocytes. Neurons that release substance P onto mast cells stimulate degranulation of the mast cells and contribute to neurogenic inflammation and to secretion of water and electrolytes.

Inhibition of absorption and promotion of secretion of water and electrolytes by inflammatory mediators may play a key role in the secretory diarrhea of **inflammatory bowel disease, Crohn's disease,** and other intestinal immune disorders.

Pathophysiological Alterations of Salt and Water Absorption

The general causes of abnormalities in the absorption of salts and water include (1) deficiency of a normal ion transport system; (2) abnormal absorption of a nonelectrolyte (nutrient), which results in osmotic diarrhea; (3) hypermotility of the intestine, which leads to abnormally rapid flow of intestinal contents past the absorptive epithelium; and (4) an enhanced rate of net secretion of water and electrolytes by the intestinal mucosa. Examples of each of these classes of abnormalities follow.

Deficiency of a normal ion transport system. In **congenital chloride diarrhea,** the Cl^-, HCO_3^- exchange transport system in the brush border plasma membrane of the ileum and colon is missing or grossly deficient. As a result, chloride absorption is severely impaired. Impairment of chloride absorption leads to a type of diarrhea in which the stools contain an unusually high chloride concentration; the concentration of Cl^- in the stool exceeds the sum of the concentrations of Na^+ and K^+. In addition, because the Na^+, H^+ exchanger continues to operate, H^+ is eliminated in the feces without HCO_3^- to neutralize it. The net loss of H^+, with retention of HCO_3^-, contributes to metabolic alkalosis.

Abnormal absorption of a nutrient. In any of the carbohydrate malabsorption syndromes, the sugar that is retained in the lumen of the small intestine increases the osmotic pressure of the luminal contents. Water is also retained as a result, and an increased volume of chyme is passed on to the colon. The increased volume flow may overwhelm the ability of the colon to absorb electrolytes and water, and pronounced diarrhea results. In addition, the high level of carbohydrates provides a medium that supports increased growth and metabolism of colonic bacteria. The increased production of CO_2 by colonic bacteria contributes to gaseousness and borborygmi, and certain products of bacterial metabolism inhibit absorption of electrolytes by the colonic epithelium.

Hypermotility of the intestine. The causes of hypermotility of the intestine are not well understood. Hypermotility of the small intestine may deliver electrolytes and water to the colon at faster rates than they can be absorbed by the colonic epithelial cells. Hypermotility of the colon may result in the elimination of feces before the maximal amount of salts and water can be extracted from them. Hypermotility may add to other factors that cause diarrhea. In cases of fat malabsorption, colonic bacteria metabolize lipids and produce certain waste products, such as hydroxylated fatty acids, that enhance the motility of the colon and inhibit salt and water absorption by the colonic epithelium.

Enhanced secretion of water and electrolytes. Increased secretion of water and electrolytes is an important mechanism in serious diarrheal diseases. As mentioned previously, immature epithelial cells in Lieberkühn's crypts normally function to secrete Na^+, Cl^-, and H_2O. When the secretory activities of the crypt cells are elevated, the unidirectional secretory flux may exceed the unidirectional absorptive flux, so that net secretion prevails. Cholera, discussed previously, is perhaps the best understood type of secretory diarrhea. Other agents that elevate cAMP in intestinal epithelial cells also lead to secretion of water and electrolytes.

VIP, which is present in certain enteric neurons and also circulates as a hormone, elevates cAMP in intestinal epithelial cells. Certain individuals with islet cell tumors of the pancreas suffer from a watery diarrhea known as **pancreatic cholera.** In this disorder, elevated plasma levels of VIP cause secretory diarrhea.

The epithelial cells of the crypts of the small intestine are also stimulated to secrete electrolytes and water by elevated intracellular Ca^{++} concentrations (Fig. 39-13). Acetylcholine, serotonin, substance P, and neurotensin elicit intestinal secretion of water and electrolytes by increasing the concentration of intracellular Ca^{++}. All these agents are present in intrinsic neurons of the intestinal wall and thus may contribute to diarrhea in certain pathological situations.

■ *Absorption of Calcium*

Calcium ions are actively absorbed by all segments of the intestine. The duodenum and jejunum are especially active and can concentrate Ca^{++} against a greater than tenfold concentration gradient. The rate of absorption of Ca^{++} is much greater than that of any other divalent ion, but still 50 times slower than Na^+ absorption.

The ability of the intestine to absorb Ca^{++} is regulated. Animals that receive a calcium-deficient diet increase their ability to absorb Ca^{++}. Animals that receive high-calcium diets are less able to absorb Ca^{++}. Intestinal absorption of Ca^{++} is markedly stimulated by vitamin D. Parathyroid hormone stimulates intestinal absorption of Ca^{++} by promoting release of the active form of vitamin D from the kidney.

Most Ca^{++} absorption occurs through the intestinal epithelial cells, but significant absorption also takes place across tight junctions via the paracellular pathway. This absorption is driven by the elevated concentration of Ca^{++} in the intestinal lumen that results from the absorption of water.

■ *Cellular Mechanism of Calcium Absorption*

The brush border membrane. Cellular mechanisms of Ca^{++} absorption by the epithelial cells of the small intestine are depicted in Fig. 39-14. Ca^{++} moves through Ca^{++} channels down its electrochemical potential gradient across the brush border membrane into the cytosol. A protein, called the **intestinal membrane calcium-binding protein (IMCal),** may bind Ca^{++} at the inner face of the brush border membrane.

Epithelial cell cytosol. The cytosol of the intestinal epithelial cells contains a protein called **calbindin,** an essential component of Ca^{++} absorption. Calbindin is also known as the **intestinal calcium binding protein (CaBP).** In mammals, calbindin has a molecular weight of about 9000 and binds two calcium ions with high affinity. As discussed below, the level of calbindin in an epithelial cell correlates well with its capacity to absorb Ca^{++}. Calbindin allows large amounts of Ca^{++} to traverse the cytosol, and binding of Ca^{++} to calbindin prevents concentrations of free Ca^{++} ions that are high enough to form insoluble salts with intracellular anions.

Ca^{++} is also transported through the cytosol of intestinal epithelial cells in membrane vesicles. Vesicular Ca^{++} is released across the basolateral membrane by exocytosis. Calbindin also promotes Ca^{++} transport via the vesicular pathway.

The basolateral membrane. The basolateral plasma membrane contains two transport proteins that can eject Ca^{++} from the cell against its electrochemical potential gradient. A **Ca^{++}-ATPase** in the basolateral membrane, a primary active transport protein, splits ATP and uses the energy to transport Ca^{++}. The Na^+, Ca^{++} exchanger present in the basolateral membrane uses the energy of the Na^+ gradient to extrude Ca^{++} by secondary active transport. The Na^+, Ca^{++} exchanger is more effective when intracellular Ca^{++} concentrations are high, whereas the Ca^{++}-ATPase is the major mechanism for Ca^{++} extrusion when intracellular concentrations of Ca^{++} are low. Ca^{++}

■ **Fig. 39-14** Cellular mechanisms of Ca++ absorption in the small intestine. Ca++ crosses the brush border plasma membrane via Ca++ channels. In the cytosol of the enterocyte, Ca++ is bound to calbindin. Ca++ is extruded across the basolateral membrane by a Ca++, ATPase and an Na+, Ca++ exchange mechanism. Some Ca++ is transported through the cytosol in membrane vesicles and released at the basolateral membrane by exocytosis. *IMCal,* Intestinal membrane calcium-binding protein.

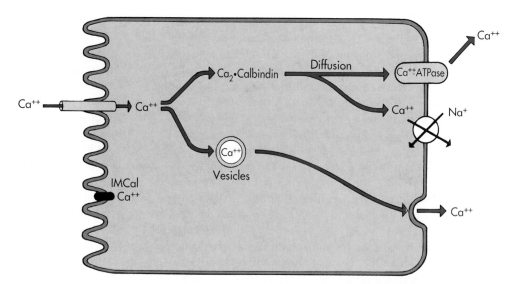

itself, bound to calmodulin, stimulates the activity of the Ca++-ATPase, as does phosphorylation of the Ca++-ATPase by cAMP-dependent protein kinase.

■ *Actions of Vitamin D*

Vitamin D is essential for normal levels of calcium absorption by the intestine (see also Chapter 48).

> In **rickets,** a disease caused by vitamin D deficiency, the rate of absorption of Ca++ is very low, and thus the amount of Ca++ available for bone growth is also low. In children with rickets, bone growth is abnormal. Because of the failure to deposit normal amounts of calcium salts in the bone matrix, bones are softer and more flexible than normal. These changes contribute to the characteristic "bow-legged" appearance of children with rickets.

Fig. 39-15 illustrates the effects of administration of vitamin D on intestinal absorption of Ca++ by chicks with rickets. Vitamin D stimulates each phase of absorption of Ca++ by the epithelium of the small intestine: passage across the brush border membrane, traversal of the cytosol, and active extrusion across the basolateral membrane. Like other steroid hormones, vitamin D exerts its major effects by binding to nuclear receptors and stimulating the synthesis of messenger RNA that encodes particular proteins. The protein synthesized as a result of vitamin D_3 stimulation is cytosolic calbindin. The calbindin level correlates well with the capacity of the small intestine to absorb Ca++. Vitamin D also increases the level of the brush border–associated calbindin, which may promote transport of Ca++ across the brush border plasma membrane. In addition, vitamin D increases the level of the basolateral Ca++-ATPase that actively pumps calcium out of the enterocyte.

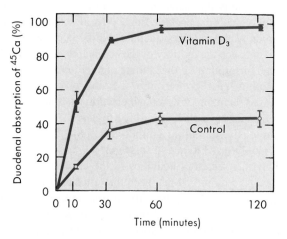

■ **Fig. 39-15** Effects of vitamin D_3 on absorption of Ca++ by chick duodenum. Control animals were fed a diet deficient in vitamin D *(lower curve).* *Upper curve,* Ca++ absorption by animals fed the same diet but administered vitamin D_3 24 hours before the experiment. (Redrawn from Wasserman RH: *J Nutr* 77:69, 1962.)

■ *Absorption of Iron*

A typical adult in Western societies ingests about 15 to 20 mg of iron daily. Only 0.5 to 1 mg of iron is absorbed by normal adult men, and 1 to 1.5 mg is absorbed by premenopausal adult women. Iron depletion, caused by hemorrhage, for example, increases iron absorption. Growing children and pregnant women also absorb increased amounts of iron. Iron deficiency is common, even in economically developed countries, and is the most prevalent nutrient deficiency in the world.

Iron absorption is limited because iron tends to form insoluble salts with anions, such as hydroxide, phosphate, and bicarbonate, that are present in intestinal secretions. Iron also tends to form insoluble complexes with other substances commonly present in food, such as phytate, tannins, and the fiber of cereal grains. These iron complexes are more soluble at low pH. Therefore,

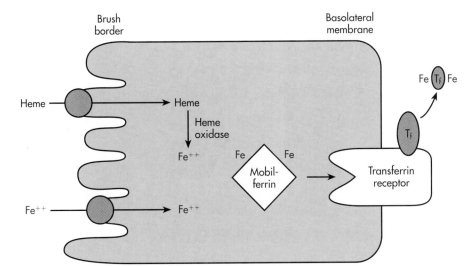

Brush border

Basolateral membrane

■ **Fig. 39-16** Current view of the mechanism of iron absorption by the epithelial cells of the small intestine. Fe⁺⁺ is bound and transported across the brush border plasma membrane by a specific transport protein. Heme is taken up by a separate facilitated transport system. In the cytosol, iron is released from heme. Fe⁺⁺ in the cytosol is bound to mobilferrin. Fe⁺⁺ is transported across the basolateral plasma membrane by transferrin (Tf) receptors that bind transferrin on the extracellular surface and transfer Fe⁺⁺ to transferrin.

hydrochloric acid (HCl) secreted by the stomach enhances iron absorption, whereas iron absorption is commonly low in individuals deficient in acid secretion. Ascorbate effectively promotes iron absorption. Ascorbate forms a soluble complex with iron, thereby preventing iron from forming insoluble complexes. Ascorbate also reduces Fe^{+++} to Fe^{++}. The tendency of Fe^{++} to form insoluble complexes is much less than that of Fe^{+++}, and partly for this reason, Fe^{++} is absorbed much better than is Fe^{+++}.

Heme iron is relatively well absorbed; about 20% of ingested heme is absorbed. Proteolytic enzymes release heme groups from proteins in the intestinal lumen. Heme is probably taken up by facilitated transport by the epithelial cells that line the upper small intestine. In the epithelial cell, iron is split from the heme by reactions that involve **heme oxygenase.** No intact heme is transported into the portal blood. The heme oxygenase reaction is the rate-limiting step in the absorption of heme iron.

■ *Cellular Mechanism of Inorganic Iron Absorption*

Our understanding of the mechanisms of absorption of inorganic or nonheme iron is incomplete; a provisional model is depicted in Fig. 39-16. Duodenal epithelial cells are principally responsible for absorption of nonheme iron. The brush border plasma membrane contains transport proteins that bind Fe^{++} and transport it into the duodenal epithelial cells; Fe^{+++} is not transported. Brush border receptors for **lactoferrin,** an iron-binding protein in milk, also exist. In the epithelial cell, Fe^{++} is bound to a cytosolic iron-binding protein called **mobilferrin.** Mobilferrin may function in a way analogous to calbindin, namely, to receive Fe^{++} from the brush border transporter, to prevent Fe^{++} from forming insoluble complexes with intracellular anions, and to facilitate the diffusion of Fe^{++} through the cytosol.

At the basolateral membrane, **transferrin receptors** bind plasma transferrin. These receptors apparently mediate the transfer of Fe^{++} from mobilferrin in the cytosol to transferrin on the extracellular face of the basolateral membrane. The Fe^{++}-transferrin complex is then released to the extracellular fluid and diffuses into the blood. The transport of Fe^{++} across the basolateral membrane is the rate-limiting step in its absorption; the rate of transport is limited by the number of transferrin receptors present in the basolateral membrane.

■ *Regulation of Iron Absorption*

Iron absorption is regulated in accordance with the body's need for iron. In chronic iron deficiency or after hemorrhage, the duodenum and jejunum increase their capacity to absorb iron. The intestine also protects the body from the consequences of absorbing too much iron. However, the excretion of iron is limited. Thus, the absorption of more iron than is needed may lead to iron overload.

Iron overload can result from chronic ingestion of large amounts of absorbable iron. This condition is common in certain African tribes that regularly consume a home-brewed beer with a high iron content. In the genetic disorder called **idiopathic hemochromatosis,** an excessive amount of iron is absorbed from a diet that is normal in iron content.

An important mechanism for preventing excess absorption of iron is the almost irreversible binding of iron to **ferritin** in the intestinal epithelial cell. *Iron bound to ferritin is not available for transport into the plasma* (Fig. 39-17) but is instead lost into the intestinal lumen and excreted in the feces when the intestinal epithelial cell exfoliates. The amount of apoferritin present in the intestinal epithelial cells determines how much iron can be trapped in this nonabsorbable pool.

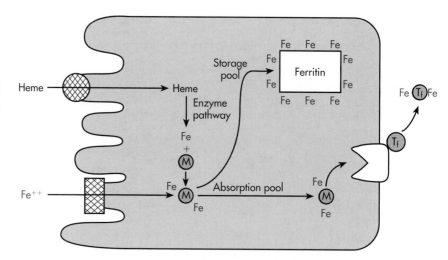

■ **Fig. 39-17**   In the enterocytes of the upper small intestine, iron bound to mobilferrin *(M)* is available for transport across the basolateral membrane. Iron bound to ferritin is, however, unavailable for absorption and is lost into the lumen when the cell is exfoliated.

After a hemorrhage, the capacity of the duodenum and jejunum to absorb iron increases, with a time lag of 3 to 4 days. During this time, the intestinal epithelial cells migrate from their sites of formation in Lieberkühn's crypts to the tips of the villi, where they are most involved in absorptive activities.

The mechanisms that alter the capacity of the epithelial cells to absorb iron are incompletely understood. The iron-absorbing capacity of the epithelial cells may be programmed when the cells are in Lieberkühn's crypts. High levels of Fe^{++} in the intestinal epithelial cells promote translation of the messenger RNA that encodes apoferritin, and they diminish the stability of the message for the basolateral transferrin receptor. In an iron-replete individual, levels of apoferritin are high and the amount of transferrin receptor is low. Thus, irreversible iron storage is enhanced, while the rate of Fe^{++} absorption is decreased. In iron deficiency, levels of ferritin are low and the amount of transferrin receptor is high, so that less storage and more absorption of Fe^{++} occurs.

■ *Absorption of Other Ions*

■ *Magnesium*

Magnesium is absorbed along the entire length of the small intestine. About half of the normal dietary intake of magnesium is absorbed. The largest portion of Mg^{++} absorption takes place in the ileum; a smaller portion is absorbed in the duodenum. The colon absorbs a still smaller, but significant, portion of Mg^{++}. The rate of Mg^{++} absorption is not adjusted in response to dietary loads.

The cellular mechanisms of Mg^{++} absorption are not well understood. Much Mg^{++} absorption may occur by the paracellular pathway, and it may be driven by the concentration of Mg^{++} in the lumen when water is absorbed.

■ *Phosphate*

Like magnesium, phosphate is also absorbed all along the small intestine. From highest to lowest capacity for phosphate absorption per centimeter of length of the gastrointestinal tract, the order is duodenum > jejunum > ileum. Because both the length of the duodenum and its transit time are short, the jejunum is responsible for the largest portion of phosphate absorption. In response to low levels of serum phosphate, the intestinal capacity to absorb phosphate increases. This response depends on vitamin D, but the mechanisms by which vitamin D enhances phosphate absorption are not well understood. Phosphate crosses the brush border plasma membrane largely by Na^+-powered secondary active transport. Phosphate leaves the cell by moving down its electrochemical potential gradient across the basolateral membrane by means of facilitated transport.

■ *Copper*

Approximately 50% of the copper ingested in the diet is absorbed, mainly in the jejunum. When dietary copper is low, the fraction of ingested copper that is absorbed increases. The cellular mechanisms of copper absorption and excretion are not well understood, but protein-mediated transport and oxidative metabolism of the intestinal epithelial cells may be involved in copper transport. Copper is secreted in the bile bound to certain bile acids, and most of this copper is lost in the feces. In individuals who fail to secrete sufficient amounts of copper in the bile, the body's copper pool grows and copper accumulates in certain tissues.

■ *Absorption of Water-Soluble Vitamins*

Most water-soluble vitamins can be absorbed by simple diffusion if taken in sufficiently high doses. Nevertheless, specific transport mechanisms are important in the normal absorption of most water-soluble vitamins. Several water-soluble vitamins are taken up across the brush border membrane by Na^+-powered secondary active transport processes. Table 39-6 summarizes current knowledge about these transport mechanisms.

■ **Table 39-6**   Intestinal absorption of vitamins

Vitamin	Species	Site of absorption	Transport mechanism	Maximal absorptive capacity in humans (per day)	Dietary requirement in humans (per day)
Ascorbic acid (C)	Humans, guinea pig	Ileum	Active*	>5000 mg	<50 mg
Biotin	Hamster	Upper small intestine	Active*	?	?
Choline	Guinea pig, hamster	Small intestine	Facilitated	?	?
Folic acid					
Pteroylglutamate	Rat	Jejunum	Facilitated	>1000 μg/dose	100-200 μg
5-Methyltetrahydrofolate	Rat	Jejunum	Diffusion		
Nicotinic acid	Rat	Jejunum	Facilitated*	?	10-20 mg
Pantothenic acid		Small intestine	?	?	(?) 10 mg
Pyridoxine (B$_6$)	Rat, hamster	Small intestine	DIffusion	>50 mg/dose	1-2 mg
Riboflavin (B$_2$)	Humans, rat	Jejunum	Facilitated	10-12 mg/dose	1-2 mg
Thiamin (B$_1$)	Rat	Jejunum	Active*	8-14 mg	≈1 mg
Vitamin B$_{12}$	Humans, rat, hamster	Distal ileum	Active*	6-9 μg	3-7 μg

Data from Matthews DM. In Smyth DH, editor: *Intestinal absorption,* vol 4B: *Biomembranes,* London, 1974, Plenum Press; and Rose RC: *Annu Rev Physiol* 42:157, 1980.

*Na$^+$-powered secondary active transport.

■ *Absorption of Vitamin B$_{12}$*

A specific transport process has also been implicated in the absorption of vitamin B$_{12}$. The dietary requirement for B$_{12}$ is fairly close to the maximal absorption capacity for the vitamin. In the absence of sufficient vitamin B$_{12}$, the maturation of red blood cells slows and **pernicious anemia** ensues. Because of its medical importance, considerable research has focused on the absorption of vitamin B$_{12}$. Enteric bacteria synthesize vitamin B$_{12}$ and other B vitamins, but the colonic epithelium lacks specific mechanisms for their absorption.

Storage in the liver. The liver contains a large store of vitamin B$_{12}$ (2 to 5 mg). Vitamin B$_{12}$ is normally present in the bile (0.5 to 5 μg daily), but about 70% of this vitamin B$_{12}$ is normally reabsorbed. Because only about 0.1% of the store is lost daily, the store will last for 3 to 6 years even if absorption totally ceases.

Gastric phase. Most of the vitamin B$_{12}$ present in food is bound to proteins. During the gastric phase of digestion, the low pH in the stomach and the digestion of proteins by pepsin release free vitamin B$_{12}$. The free vitamin B$_{12}$ is rapidly bound to a number of vitamin B$_{12}$–binding glycoproteins called **R proteins.** R proteins are present in saliva and in gastric juice, and bind vitamin B$_{12}$ tightly over a wide pH range. The R proteins of saliva and gastric juice have molecular weights near 60,000 and are closely related to transcobalamins I, II, and III.

Intrinsic factor (IF) is a vitamin B$_{12}$–binding protein that is secreted by the gastric parietal cells. IF is a glycoprotein that contains 15% carbohydrate and has a molecular weight of about 45,000. The rate of IF secretion usually parallels the rate of HCl secretion. IF binds vitamin B$_{12}$ with less affinity than do the R proteins. Thus, in the

stomach, most of the vitamin B$_{12}$ released from food is bound by R proteins.

Intestinal phase. During the intestinal phase of digestion, pancreatic proteases begin degradation of the complexes between R proteins and cobalamins. This degradation greatly lowers the affinities of the R proteins for cobalamins, so that cobalamins are transferred to IF. IF and IF-cobalamin complexes resist digestion by pancreatic proteases. As described later, the normal mechanism for absorption involves brush border receptors for IF-cobalamin complexes. These receptors do not recognize the R protein–cobalamin complexes. Thus, in pancreatic insufficiency, when R proteins are not degraded, cobalamins remain bound to R proteins. These complexes are not available for absorption, and therefore vitamin B$_{12}$ deficiency may ensue.

Absorption of vitamin B$_{12}$. Fig. 39-18 summarizes the mechanism of vitamin B$_{12}$ absorption. The normal absorption of cobalamins depends on the presence of IF. When IF binds vitamin B$_{12}$, IF undergoes a conformational change that favors the formation of dimers; each dimer binds two vitamin B$_{12}$ molecules. The brush border plasma membranes of the epithelial cells of the ileum contain a receptor protein that recognizes and binds the IF-B$_{12}$ dimer. Free IF does not compete for binding, and the receptor does not recognize free cobalamins. Binding to the receptor is required for uptake of vitamin B$_{12}$ into the cell. It is likely that the IF-B$_{12}$ complex is taken up into the ileal epithelial cell across the brush border plasma membrane.

After the uptake of the IF-B$_{12}$ complex, vitamin B$_{12}$ is slowly transported through the epithelial cell and into the blood. Vitamin B$_{12}$ does not appear in the blood until 4 hours after it is ingested, and the peak B$_{12}$ level in plasma

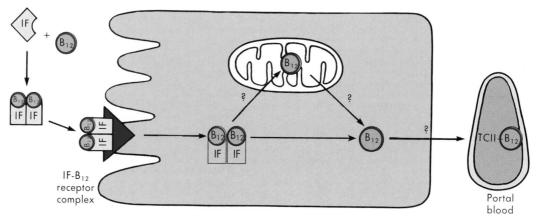

■ **Fig. 39-18**   Postulated mechanism of vitamin B$_{12}$ absorption by epithelial cells of the ileum.

occurs 6 to 8 hours after a meal. The reason for this delay is not well understood, but for much of the lag period B$_{12}$ may be located predominantly in the mitochondria of the epithelial cells.

The exit of vitamin B$_{12}$ from the cells of the ileal epithelium is even less understood than its entry. Facilitated or active transport is presumably involved. Most of the B$_{12}$ that is absorbed appears in the portal blood bound to **transcobalamin II,** a globulin. Transcobalamin II is synthesized in the liver, but the ileal epithelium also makes this protein. The transcobalamin II–B$_{12}$ complex is rapidly cleared from the portal blood by the liver by means of receptor-mediated endocytosis.

Absorption in the absence of IF. In the complete absence of IF, about 1% to 2% of an ingested load of B$_{12}$ will be absorbed. If large doses of vitamin B$_{12}$ are taken (about 1 mg/day), enough B$_{12}$ can be absorbed to treat pernicious anemia. The IF-independent mechanism shows no maximal absorptive capacity, does not appear to be limited to the ileum, and shows a much shorter lag time (about 1 hour) than IF-dependent absorption.

In the absence of sufficient levels of vitamin B$_{12}$, the maturation of red cells slows and anemia results. **Pernicious anemia** is caused by atrophy of the gastric mucosa, with almost complete inability to secrete HCl, pepsin, and IF. Most patients with pernicious anemia have serum antibodies against parietal cells. However, it is not clear whether the antibodies cause the disease or are the response to gastric damage from some other cause.

Pernicious anemia in childhood is rare and has three forms: (1) an **autoimmune type of pernicious anemia** with characteristics just described; (2) **congenital IF deficiency,** in which pepsin and acid secretion are normal but IF secretion is deficient; and (3) **congenital vitamin B$_{12}$** malabsorption syndrome, in which gastric function and levels of IF are normal, but B$_{12}$ absorption is deficient owing to a defect in the ileal IF-B$_{12}$ receptors.

■ *Digestion and Absorption of Lipids*

The primary lipids of a normal diet are triglycerides. The diet contains smaller amounts of sterols, sterol esters, and phospholipids (Fig. 39-19). Because lipids are only slightly soluble in water, each stage of their processing poses special problems to the gastrointestinal tract. In the stomach, lipids tend to separate out into an oily phase. In the duodenum and small intestine, lipids are emulsified with the aid of bile acids. The large surface area of the emulsion droplets allows access of the water-soluble lipolytic enzymes to their substrates. The digestion products of lipids form small molecular aggregates, known as **micelles,** with the bile acids. The micelles are small enough to diffuse among the microvilli and allow absorption of the lipids from molecular solution at the intestinal brush border. The digestion and absorption of lipids are more complex than for any other class of nutrients and are more frequently subject to malfunction.

■ *Digestion of Lipids in the Stomach*

Because fats tend to separate out into an oily phase that sits on top of the gastric contents, they are emptied from the stomach later than the other gastric contents. Any tendency to form emulsions with phospholipids or other natural emulsifying agents is inhibited by the high acidity of the stomach. Fat in the duodenum strongly inhibits gastric emptying. This inhibition ensures that the fat is not emptied from the stomach more rapidly than it can be accommodated by the duodenal mechanisms that provide for emulsification and digestion.

Significant hydrolysis of triglycerides occurs in the stomach. The enzymes responsible for lipid hydrolysis in the stomach are known as **preduodenal lipases.** These enzymes operate most effectively at acid pHs. In rats, the principal preduodenal lipase is **lingual lipase,** which is produced by glands under the circumvallate papillae of the tongue. In humans, lingual lipase is only a minor

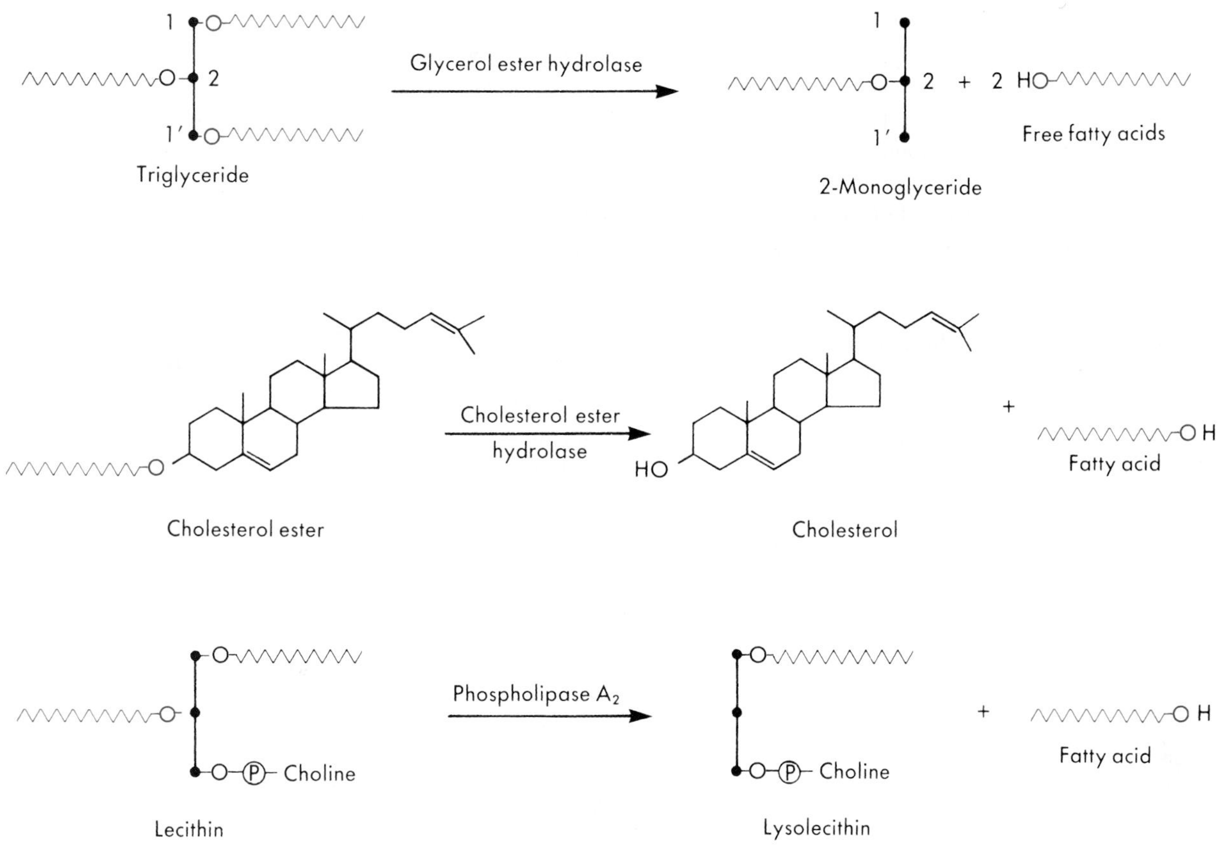

■ **Fig. 39-19** Action of major pancreatic lipases. The cleavage of lipids by glycerol ester hydrolase (pancreatic lipase), cholesterol ester hydrolase, and phospholipase A_2 is illustrated. *P*, Phosphate.

component of preduodenal lipase; the major component is **gastric lipase** produced by gland cells in the fundus of the stomach. Normally, the amount of pancreatic lipase is so great that the absence of preduodenal lipase does not cause malabsorption of triglycerides. However, when pancreatic lipase is grossly deficient or pancreatic lipase is inactive because of high acidity in the upper small intestine (e.g., in Zollinger-Ellison syndrome), the hydrolysis of triglycerides by gastric lipase may be essential for digestion and absorption of triglycerides.

■ *Digestion of Lipids in the Duodenum and Jejunum*

The lipolytic enzymes of the pancreatic juice are water-soluble molecules and thus have access to the lipids only at the surfaces of the fat droplets. The surface area available for digestion is increased many thousand times by emulsification of the lipids. Bile acids themselves are rather poor emulsifying agents. However, with the aid of lecithin, which is present in high concentration in the bile, the bile acids emulsify dietary fats. The emulsion droplets are about 1 μm in diameter and have a large surface area on which the digestive enzymes can work.

Pancreatic lipolytic enzymes. *Pancreatic juice contains the major lipolytic enzymes responsible for digestion of lipids* (Fig. 39-19). The most important digestive enzymes are **glycerol ester hydrolase, colipase, cholesterol ester hydrolase,** and **phopholipase A.**

Glycerol ester hydrolase (also called simply **pancreatic lipase**) cleaves the 1 and 1′ fatty acids from a triglyceride to produce two free fatty acids and one 2-monoglyceride. Glycerol ester hydrolase of pancreatic juice has a molecular weight of about 50,000 and is rather specific for triglycerides. Pancreatic lipase has very low activity against triglycerides in molecular solution, but it is very active on droplets or emulsions of triglycerides. The enzyme operates at the interface between the aqueous phase and the triglyceride-containing oil phase. The activity of pancreatic lipase is proportional to the surface area of the oil phase. The amount of pancreatic lipase present in samples of duodenal contents can hydrolyze the average daily intake of triglyceride in 1 to 2 minutes.

Pancreatic lipase is essentially completely inactivated by bile salts at physiological concentrations. However, a protein of 10,000 molecular weight, known as **colipase,** present in pancreatic juice can relieve the inactivation of lipase by bile salts. Bile salts inhibit the activity of pancreatic lipase by binding to the surface of triglyceride-containing oil droplets, and thereby they prevent the pancreatic lipase from binding. Colipase displaces bile salts from the surface of oil droplets. One pancreatic lipase molecule then binds to each colipase molecule. The resultant lipase-colipase complex then cleaves the 1 and 1′ fatty acids from triglycerides at the surface of the oil droplet.

Cholesterol ester hydrolase (cholesterol esterase) cleaves the ester bond in a cholesterol ester to yield one fatty acid and free cholesterol. Cholesterol esterase is probably identical to a nonspecific enzyme, known as **nonspecific lipase** or **nonspecific esterase,** that cleaves fatty acid ester linkages in a variety of lipid substrates. In humans, nonspecific lipase has a molecular weight of about 100,000. The enzyme forms dimers in the presence of bile salts, and in this form it is protected from proteolytic digestion. The dimeric enzyme hydrolyzes fatty acids from cholesterol esters, lysophospholipids, triglycerides, 2-monoglycerides, and fatty acyl esters of vitamins A, D, and E. The total activity of nonspecific lipase in pancreatic juice is small compared with the activity of pancreatic lipase.

Phospholipase A$_2$ cleaves the ester bond at the 2 position of a glycerophosphatide to yield, in the case of phosphatidylcholine, one fatty acid and one lysophosphatidylcholine. Phospholipase A$_2$ is secreted as a proenzyme by the pancreas. Tryptic cleavage of the proenzyme activates phospholipase A$_2$ against phospholipids emulsified by bile salts. Phospholipase A$_2$ is a highly stable protein with a molecular weight of 14,000, and it requires calcium ions for activity. Neither phospholipase A$_2$ nor pancreatic lipase appreciably cleaves the fatty acyl ester linkage at the number 1 position of a phospholipid. Therefore, lysophosphatides are the principal form in which phospholipids are absorbed.

The formation of micelles. Bile acids form micelles with the products of fat digestion, especially 2-monoglycerides. The micelles are multimolecular aggregates, about 5 nm in diameter, and they contain about 20 to 30 molecules. The hydrophobic acyl chains of 2-monoglycerides and lysophosphatides tend to be in the interior of the micelle, and the more polar portions tend to face the surrounding water (see Fig. 38-27). Bile acids are flat molecules that have a polar and a nonpolar face. Much of the surface of the micelles is covered with bile acids, with the nonpolar face of the bile acid toward the lipid interior of the micelle and the polar face toward the outside. Extremely hydrophobic molecules, such as long-chain fatty acids, cholesterol, and certain fat-soluble vitamins, tend to partition into the interior of the micelle. Micelles contain almost no intact triglyceride.

Bile acids must be present at a certain minimal concentration, called the **critical micelle concentration,** before micelles will form. Conjugated bile acids have a much lower critical micelle concentration than unconjugated forms. Normally, bile acids are present in the duodenum at concentrations greater than the critical micelle concentration.

Lipids and lipid digestion products in the micelles exchange rapidly with lipid digestion products in the aqueous solution surrounding the micelle. In this way, micelles keep the aqueous solution that surrounds them saturated with 2-monoglycerides, various fatty acids, cholesterol, and lysophosphatides. These lipids are present in the aqueous solution at low concentrations because of their limited water solubility.

■ *Absorption of the Products of Lipid Digestion*

The function of micelles in lipid absorption. Mixed micelles are important in the absorption of the products of lipid digestion and in the absorption of most other fat-soluble molecules (such as the fat-soluble vitamins). Micelles are small enough to diffuse among the microvilli that form the brush border. The presence of micelles tends to keep the aqueous solution that contacts the brush border plasma membrane saturated with fatty acids, 2-monoglycerides, cholesterol, and other micellar contents. *Thus, the huge surface area of the brush border is made available for the absorption of the micellar contents* (Fig. 39-20).

Uptake of lipids by intestinal epithelial cells. The duodenum and jejunum are most active in fat absorption, and most ingested fat is absorbed by the midjejunum. The fat present in normal stools is not ingested fat (which is completely absorbed), but fat from colonic bacteria and exfoliated intestinal epithelial cells. Cholesterol is absorbed more slowly than most of the other constituents of the micelles. Therefore, as the micelles progress down the small intestine, they become enriched in cholesterol.

Role of the unstirred layer. Free fatty acids, 2-monoglycerides, and the other products of lipid digestion cross the brush border plasma membrane so rapidly that this step does not limit the rate of their uptake. *The main limitation to the rate of lipid uptake by the epithelial cells of the upper small intestine is the diffusion of the mixed micelles through an unstirred layer* (or diffusion boundary layer) on the luminal surface of the brush border plasma membrane (Fig. 39-20). Partly because the surface of the intestinal mucosa is convoluted, the fluid in immediate contact with the epithelial cell surface is not readily mixed with the bulk of the luminal contents. The effective thickness of this unstirred layer ranges from 200 to 500 μm. Nutrients present in the well-mixed contents of the intestinal lumen must diffuse through the unstirred layer to reach the brush border plasma membrane. A concentration gradient exists across the unstirred layer, with micelles and lipid digestion products in lower concentration at the brush border surface than in the well-mixed contents of the lumen. A pH gradient also exists across the unstirred layer: the fluid in immediate contact with the brush border plasma membrane is about 1 pH unit more acidic than the bulk luminal contents. The lower pH at the brush border surface may enhance absorption of

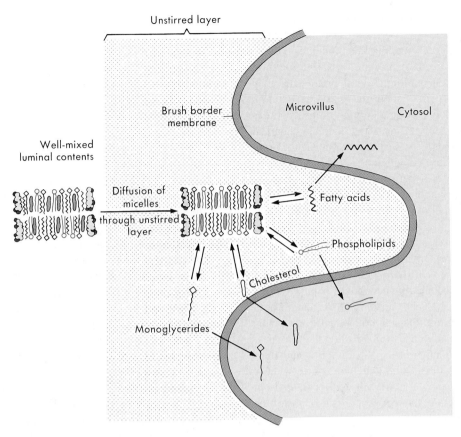

■ Fig. 39-20 Lipid absorption in the small intestine. Mixed micelles of bile acids and lipid digestion products diffuse through the unstirred layer and among the microvilli. As digestion products are absorbed from free solution by the enterocytes, more digestion products partition out of the micelles. The ability of micelles to diffuse among the microvilli makes the whole surface of the brush border available for lipid absorption. Transport proteins mediate the facilitated transport of fatty acids and cholesterol across the brush border plasma membrane. In the cytosol of the epithelial cell, fatty acids are bound to fatty acid–binding protein and cholesterol is bound to sterol carrier proteins.

fatty acids, because protonated fatty acids are more lipid soluble than ionized ones.

Transport of lipids across the brush border membrane. Because of their high lipid solubility, the fatty acids, 2-monoglycerides, cholesterol, and lysolecithin can simply diffuse across the brush border membrane. Nevertheless, transport proteins in the brush border membrane have been shown to mediate the uptake of long-chain fatty acids and cholesterol.

Cholesterol esterase is bound to the luminal surface of the brush border plasma membrane of the upper small intestine. Hydrolysis of cholesterol esters in such close proximity to the membrane may promote cellular uptake of cholesterol. A protein in the brush border membrane mediates facilitated transport of cholesterol.

A specific protein in the brush border plasma membrane facilitates the transport of long-chain fatty acids. This protein is called **MVM-FABP,** for **microvillous membrane fatty acid–binding protein.** MVM-FABP uses the energy of the Na+ gradient to power the secondary active uptake of long-chain fatty acids. MVM-FABP may also mediate the uptake of lysophospholipids.

■ *Handling of Lipids Inside the Intestinal Epithelial Cell*

Cytosolic lipid transport proteins. Two classes of fatty acid–binding proteins exist in the cytosol of epithelial cells of the upper small intestine. These proteins are known as **I-FABP** and **L-FABP.** I-FABP was first isolated from intestine, and L-FABP was first found in liver. I-FABP binds long-chain fatty acids. L-FABP has a broader specificity and binds cholesterol, monoglycerides, and lysophosphatides as well as fatty acids.

Two isoforms of sterol carrier proteins, **SCP-1** and **SCP-2,** are also present in epithelial cell cytosol. These proteins bind cholesterol and other sterols.

Binding of lipids to intracellular binding proteins may prevent lipids from forming oil droplets in the cytosol.

The binding proteins apparently function to transport lipid digestion products from the brush border plasma membrane to the smooth endoplasmic reticulum.

Resynthesis of lipids in the smooth endoplasmic reticulum. The products of lipid digestion are carried by the binding proteins to the smooth endoplasmic reticulum. In the smooth endoplasmic reticulum, which becomes engorged with lipid after a meal, considerable chemical reprocessing of lipids occurs (Fig. 39-21). The 2-monoglycerides are re-esterified with fatty acids at the 1 and 1' carbons to re-form triglycerides. Lysophospholipids are reconverted to phospholipids. Cholesterol is re-esterified substantially, although some free cholesterol remains. The processing of 2-monoglycerides and lysophospholipids is essentially complete. The intestinal epithelial cells are also capable of some synthesis of new lipids.

Chylomicron formation and transport. The reprocessed lipids, along with new lipids that are synthesized in the epithelial cell, accumulate in the smooth endoplasmic reticulum. Phospholipids tend to cover the external surfaces of these lipid droplets, with their hydrophobic acyl chains in the fatty interior and their polar head groups toward the aqueous exterior. These lipid droplets are known as **pre-chylomicrons.** About 10% of their surface is covered by apolipoproteins of the A, B, and C classes.

Pre-chylomicrons are transferred from the smooth endoplasmic reticulum to the Golgi apparatus of the intestinal epithelial cells. Further processing of the pre-chylomicrons occurs in the Golgi apparatus. The lipid droplets, now known as **chylomicrons,** are ejected from the cell by exocytosis and enter the lateral intercellular spaces (Fig. 39-21). Chylomicrons are too large to traverse the basement membrane that invests the mucosal capillaries. However, they do enter the lacteals, which have sufficiently large fenestrations for the chylomicrons to pass through. Chylomicrons leave the intestine with the lymph, primarily via the thoracic duct, and flow into the venous circulation.

In certain disorders, lipids are malabsorbed and chylomicrons do not appear in intestinal lymph. In such diseases, intestinal epithelial cells become engorged with lipid, and few chylomicrons are exported. In **abetalipoproteinemia,** apo-B is missing from serum lipoproteins. It was previously thought that a deficiency of apo-B was responsible for the lipid malabsorption, but it is now known that apo-B is present in intestinal epithelial cells in this disorder. The molecular defect responsible for the failure to produce and release chylomicrons in abetalipoproteinemia remains to be elucidated. In **chylomicron storage disease,**

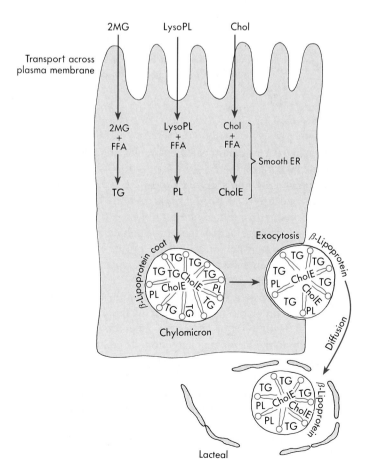

■ **Fig. 39-21** Lipid resynthesis occurs in the smooth endoplasmic reticulum (ER) of intestinal epithelial cells of the small intestine. Resynthesized lipids accumulate in chylomicrons. Chylomicrons are coated with phospholipids and apolipoproteins and are exported by exocytosis. Chylomicrons enter the lacteals and leave the intestine in the lymph. *FFA,* Free fatty acid; *2MG,* 2-monoglyceride; *TG,* triglyceride; *LysoPL,* lysophospholipid; *PL,* phospholipid; *Chol,* cholesterol; *CholE,* cholesterol ester.

chylomicrons appear to mature normally in the Golgi apparatus, but the Golgi apparatus fails to release the chylomicrons by exocytosis.

Chylomicrons are approximately spherical and vary greatly in size (60 to 750 nm). When large amounts of lipid are being absorbed, large chylomicrons are formed; when little lipid is being absorbed, the chylomicrons tend to be small. Triglycerides account for about 90% of the mass of chylomicrons. Phospholipids, mainly biliary phospholipids, cover about 80% of the surface of the chylomicrons and account for about 5% of their mass. Apolipoproteins cover the remaining 20% of the chylomicron surface. Cholesterol and cholesterol esters are present in the triglyceride-rich core of the particles; each of these substances makes up about 1% of the chylomicron mass.

Many, but not all, of the apoproteins associated with chylomicrons in intestinal lymph are synthesized by intestinal epithelial cells. Hepatocytes are the other major source of apolipoproteins.

When fat is absent from the intestine, the intestinal epithelial cells of the upper small intestine do not form chylomicrons, but they do synthesize **very-low-density lipoproteins (VLDLs)** and release them into intestinal lymph. VLDLs are smaller and more dense than chylomicrons. Compared with chylomicrons, VLDLs have much less triglyceride (60% of VLDL mass) and much more protein (about 10% of VLDL mass).

■ *Absorption of Bile Acids*

Absorption of dietary lipids is typically complete when these substances reach the midjejunum. Bile acids, by contrast, are absorbed largely in the terminal part of the ileum. As for other fat-soluble substances, the unstirred layer is an important barrier to bile acid absorption. Bile acids cross the brush border plasma membrane by two routes: by an active transport process and by simple diffusion (Fig. 39-22). The active process is secondary active transport, powered by the Na⁺ gradient across the brush border membrane. Conjugated bile acids are the principal substrates for active absorption; unconjugated bile acids have poor affinity for the transporter. However, because unconjugated bile acids are less polar than conjugated bile acids, they are better absorbed by simple diffusion. The fewer hydroxyl groups on a bile acid, the poorer substrate the bile acid is for active absorption and the more nonpolar is the bile acid. For these reasons, dehydroxylation of bile acids by enteric bacteria to form secondary bile acids enhances absorption of bile acids by diffusion.

Other aspects of the absorption of bile acids are less well understood. Bile acids may be bound to proteins, which remain to be identified, in intestinal epithelial cells. The process by which bile acids traverse the basolateral plasma membrane of the enterocyte has not been characterized.

Absorbed bile acids are carried away from the intestine in the portal blood, mostly bound to albumins. Hepatocytes avidly extract bile acids, essentially clearing the bile acids from the blood in a single pass through the liver. In the hepatocytes, most deconjugated bile acids are reconjugated, and some secondary bile acids are rehydroxylated. The reprocessed bile acids, together with newly synthesized bile acids, are secreted into bile.

■ *Malabsorption of Lipids*

Malabsorption of lipids occurs more frequently than malabsorption of proteins or carbohydrates. Among the general causes of lipid malabsorption are bile deficiency, pancreatic insufficiency, and the intestinal mucosal atrophy that occurs in some disease states.

In cases of **bile deficiency** and **pancreatic insufficiency,** the levels of bile acids and lipolytic enzymes,

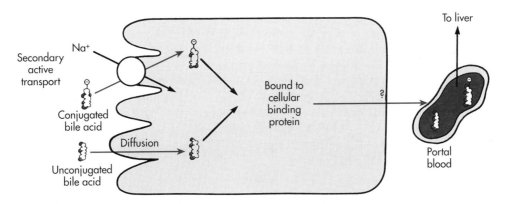

■ **Fig. 39-22**   Absorption of bile acids by epithelial cells of the terminal ileum. Bile acids are absorbed both by simple diffusion and by Na⁺-powered secondary active transport. Conjugated bile acids are absorbed avidly by active transport. Unconjugated bile acids are absorbed chiefly by simple diffusion. In the cytosol of the epithelial cells, bile acids are bound to specific binding proteins. The mechanisms of transport of bile acids across the basolateral membrane remain to be elucidated.

respectively, must be severely reduced before serious malabsorption occurs. In both bile deficiency and pancreatic insufficiency, the quantity of fecal fat is roughly proportional to the quantity ingested.

Even in the complete absence of bile acids, significant hydrolysis of triglyceride occurs. The rate of absorption of fatty acids from triglycerides may be 50% of normal. Cholesterol, cholesterol esters, and fat-soluble vitamins are much less water soluble than are fatty acids, and their absorption is grossly deficient in the absence of bile acids.

In the complete absence of pancreatic lipases, all lipid classes are poorly absorbed. This problem probably occurs because 2-monoglycerides and lysophosphatides (products of the action of pancreatic lipases) are required for the formation of mixed micelles with bile acids.

In **tropical sprue** and **gluten enteropathy,** the intestinal epithelium is flattened and the density of microvilli is decreased. Lipid malabsorption in these diseases is probably a consequence of the marked decrease in the surface area available for lipid absorption.

■ *Absorption of Fat-Soluble Vitamins*

Because of their solubility in nonpolar environments, the fat-soluble vitamins (A, D, E, and K) partition into the mixed micelles formed by the bile acids and lipid digestion products. Fat-soluble vitamins enter the intestinal epithelial cell by diffusing across the brush border plasma membrane. The presence of bile acids and lipid digestion products enhances the absorption of fat-soluble vitamins. In the intestinal epithelial cell, the fat-soluble vitamins enter the chylomicrons and leave the intestine in the lymph. In the absence of bile acids, a significant portion of the ingested load of a fat-soluble vitamin may be absorbed and leave the intestine in the portal blood.

■ *Summary*

1. The α-amylases of saliva and pancreatic juice cleave branched starch into maltose, maltotriose, and α-limit dextrins. These digestion products are then reduced to glucose molecules by glucoamylase and isomaltase, carbohydrate-digesting enzymes on the brush border plasma membrane.

2. The brush border also contains the disaccharidases sucrase and lactase that cleave sucrose and lactose into monosaccharides. These cleavage products are transported into the epithelial cell by the monosaccharide transport proteins of the brush border membrane, the glucose-galactose transporter and the fructose transporter.

3. Protein digestion begins in the stomach with the action of pepsins. The pancreatic proteases rapidly cleave proteins in the duodenum and jejunum to oligopeptides. Peptidases on the brush border membrane reduce oligopeptides to single amino acids and to dipeptides and tripeptides.

4. Amino acids are taken into the epithelial cell by an array of amino acid–transporting proteins in the brush border membrane. Dipeptides and tripeptides are taken up by a brush border peptide transport protein with broad specificity.

5. A typical human ingests 2 L of water per day, and about 7 L enters the gastrointestinal tract in gastrointestinal secretions. About 99% of the water presented to the gastrointestinal tract is absorbed; approximately 100 ml of water escapes into feces each day. The absorption of water is powered by the absorption of ions and nutrients, predominantly in the small intestine.

6. The mature epithelial cells at the tips of small intestinal villi are active in absorption of water and electrolytes. Cells in Lieberkühn's crypts are net secretors of water and ions. The net absorption that usually occurs in the small intestine is the resultant of much larger absorptive and secretory fluxes. In secretory diarrheal diseases, such as cholera, the secretory fluxes in the crypt cells increase and the absorptive fluxes in cells at the villous tips are inhibited.

7. Calcium is actively absorbed in the small intestine. Vitamin D stimulates the absorption of Ca^{++} by enhancing the synthesis of cytosolic calbindin, a Ca^{++}-binding protein. Ca^{++} is transported across the basolateral membrane by the Ca^{++}-ATPase and the Na^+, Ca^{++} exchange protein. The capacity of the intestinal epithelial cells to absorb Ca^{++} is regulated in accordance with the body's need for Ca^{++}.

8. About 5% of the ingested inorganic iron is absorbed by the small intestine; approximately 20% of heme iron is absorbed. The brush border membrane of small intestinal epithelial cells has transport proteins that bind Fe^{++} and transport it into the cytosol. In the cytosol of the intestinal epithelial cell, some of the Fe^{++} is bound to mobilferrin and some is bound to ferritin.

9. Iron bound to ferritin is unavailable for absorption and is lost into the feces when the cell is exfoliated. Fe^{++} bound to mobilferrin is passed on to transferrin receptors in the basolateral membrane. The transferrin receptors bind transferrin on the extracellular face of the basolateral membrane and transfer Fe^{++} across the membrane to transferrin. Absorbed iron appears in the portal blood bound to transferrin.

10. Most water-soluble vitamins are taken up by specific transporters in the small intestinal brush border membrane. Vitamin B_{12} is bound to R proteins in saliva and gastric juice. When R proteins are digested, vitamin B_{12} is bound by intrinsic factor (IF). Receptors on the ileal brush border membrane recognize the IF-B_{12} complex and allow vitamin B_{12} to be absorbed by the ileal epithelial cell. Vitamin B_{12} appears in the plasma bound to transcobalamin II. Pernicious anemia is caused by a deficiency of IF.

11. Triglyceride is the principal dietary lipid. Lipids form droplets in the stomach and are emulsified in the duodenum by bile acids. Emulsification greatly increases the surface area available for the action of lipases of the pancreatic juice.

12. The products of triglyceride digestion, 2-monoglycerides and fatty acids, form mixed micelles with bile acids. Cholesterol, fat-soluble vitamins, and other lipids partition into the micelles. Mixed micelles are small enough to diffuse among the microvilli. Thus, the micelles greatly enhance the brush border surface area available for lipid absorption.

13. In the epithelial cell, triglycerides and phospholipids are resynthesized and packaged along with other lipids into chylomicrons. Chylomicrons are coated with phospholipids and apolipoproteins and released at the basolateral membrane by exocytosis. Chylomicrons leave the intestine in the lymphatic vessels and the thoracic duct.

■ *Self-Study Problems*

1. What are the mechanisms for absorption of monosaccharides by intestinal epithelial cells?

2. Describe the digestion of peptides in the lumen of the small intestine, on the brush border of the small intestine, and in the small intestinal epithelial cells.

3. How do the intestinal epithelial cells at the tips of the villi differ from those in the crypts of Lieberkühn in their transport of electrolytes and water? Describe the cellular ion transport mechanisms in the crypt cells.

4. Describe the cellular mechanisms of Ca^{++} absorption in the small intestine.

5. Describe the cellular mechanisms that diminish iron absorption when iron levels are high and that increase iron absorption in an iron-depleted individual.

6. What is the rate-limiting step in the intestinal absorption of the products of lipid digestion? How are the products of lipid digestion absorbed across the brush border plasma membrane?

■ *Bibliography*
Journal articles

Binder HJ: The pathophysiology of diarrhea, *Hosp Pract* 19:107, 1984.

Caspary WF: Physiology and pathophysiology of intestinal absorption, *Am J Clin Nutr* 55:S299, 1992.

Cheeseman CI: Molecular mechanisms involved in regulation of amino acid transport, *Prog Biophys Mol Biol* 55:71, 1991.

Cooke HJ: Neuroimmune signaling in regulation of intestinal transport, *Am J Physiol* 266:G167, 1994.

Eastwoood MA: The physiological effect of dietary fiber: an update, *Annu Rev Nutr* 12:19, 1992.

Gray GM: Starch digestion and absorption in nonruminants, *J Nutr* 122:172, 1992.

Hediger MA, Coady MJ, Ikeda TS, Wright EM: Expression cloning and cDNA sequencing of the Na^+/glucose co-transporter, *Nature* 330:379, 1987.

Jenkins DJA et al: Glycemic index of foods: a physiological basis for carbohydrate exchange, *Am J Clin Nutr* 34:362, 1981.

Nemere I: Vesicular calcium transport in chick intestine, *J Nutr* 122:657, 1992.

Seetharam B, Alpers DH: Absorption and transport of cobalamin (vitamin B_{12}), *Annu Rev Nutr* 2:343, 1982.

Stephen AM, Haddad AC, Phillips SF: Passage of carbohydrate into the colon: direct measurements in humans, *Gastroenterology* 85:589, 1983.

Stremmel W: Uptake of fatty acids by jejunal mucosal cells is mediated by a fatty acid binding membrane protein, *J Clin Invest* 82:2001, 1988.

Thomson ABR, Keelan M, Garg ML, Clandinin MT: Intestinal aspects of lipid absorption: in review, *Can J Physiol Pharmacol* 67:179, 1989.

Thurnhofer H, Hauser H: Uptake of cholesterol by small intestinal brush border membrane is protein mediated, *Biochemistry* 29:2142, 1990.

Turk E, et al: Glucose/galactose malabsorption caused by a defect in the Na^+/glucose cotransporter, *Nature* 350:354, 1991.

Wasserman et al: Intestinal calcium transport and calcium extrusion processes at the basolateral membrane, *J Nutr* 122:662, 1992.

Books and monographs

Alpers DH: *Digestion and absorption of carbohydrates and proteins*. In Johnson LR, editor: *Physiology of the gastrointestinal tract*, ed 3, New York, 1994, Raven Press.

Barrett KE, Dharmsathaphorn K: *Secretion and absorption: small intestine and colon*. In Yamada T, editor: *Textbook of gastroenterology*, vol 1, Philadelphia, 1991, JB Lippincott.

Binder HJ, Sandle GI: *Electrolyte transport in the mammalian colon*. In Johnson LR, editor: *Physiology of the gastrointestinal tract*, ed 3, New York, 1994, Raven Press.

Chang EB, Rao MC: *Intestinal water and electrolyte transport: mechanisms of physiological and adaptive responses*. In Johnson LR, editor: *Physiology of the gastrointestinal tract*, ed 3, New York, 1994, Raven Press.

Civitelli R, Avioli LV: *Calcium, phosphate, and magnesium absorption*. In Johnson LR, editor: *Physiology of the gastrointestinal tract*, ed 3, New York, 1994, Raven Press.

Cooke HJ, Reddix RA: *Neural regulation of intestinal electrolyte transport.* In Johnson LR, editor: *Physiology of the gastrointestinal tract,* ed 3, New York, 1994, Raven Press.

Davenport HW: *Physiology of the digestive tract,* ed 5, Chicago, 1982, Mosby–Year Book.

Davidson NO: *Cellular and molecular mechanisms of small intestinal lipid transport.* In Johnson LR, editor: *Physiology of the gastrointestinal tract,* ed 3, New York, 1994, Raven Press.

Field M: *Intestinal ion transport mechanisms.* In Field M , editor: *Diarrheal diseases,* New York, 1991, Elsevier.

Ganapathy V, Brandsch M, Leibach FH: *Intestinal transport of amino acids and peptides.* In Johnson LR, editor: *Physiology of the gastrointestinal tract,* ed 3, New York, 1994, Raven Press.

Gray GM: *Dietary protein processing: intraluminal and enterocyte surface events.* In Field M, Frizzell RA, editors: *Handbook of physiology,* sect 6, *The gastrointestinal system,* vol IV, Bethesda, Md, 1991, American Physiological Society.

Greenberger NJ: *Gastrointestinal disorders: a pathophysiologic approach,* ed 3, Chicago, 1986, Mosby–Year Book.

Hoffman AF: *Intestinal absorption of bile acids and biliary constituents.* In Johnson LR, editor: *Physiology of the gastrointestinal tract,* ed 3, New York, 1994, Raven Press.

Johnson LR, editor: *Gastrointestinal physiology,* ed 5, St Louis, 1996, Mosby–Year Book.

Matthews DM: Protein absorption: *development and present state of the subject,* New York, 1991, Wiley- Liss.

Rose RC: *Intestinal transport of water-soluble vitamins.* In Field M, Frizzell RA, editors: *Handbook of physiology,* sect 6, *The gastrointestinal system,* vol IV, Bethesda, Md, 1991, American Physiological Society.

Rucker RB, Lönnderdal B, Keen CL: *Intestinal absorption of nutritionally important trace elements.* In Johnson LR, editor: *Physiology of the gastrointestinal tract,* ed 3, New York, 1994, Raven Press.

Sellin JH: *Intestinal electrolyte absorption and secretion,* In Sleisenger MH, Fordtran JS, editors: *Gastrointestinal disease,* ed 5, Philadelphia, 1993, WB Saunders.

Sullivan SK, Field M: *Ion transport across mammalian small intestine.* In Field M, Frizzell RA, editors: *Handbook of physiology,* sect 6, *The gastrointestinal system,* vol IV, Bethesda, Md, 1991, American Physiological Society.

Tso P: *Intestinal lipid absorption.* In Johnson LR, editor: *Physiology of the gastrointestinal tract,* ed 3, New York, 1994, Raven Press.

Wright EM et al: *Intestinal sugar transport.* In Johnson LR, editor: *Physiology of the gastrointestinal tract,* ed 3, New York, 1994, Raven Press.

THE KIDNEY

Bruce A. Stanton
Bruce M. Koeppen

Elements of Renal Function

■ *Overview of Renal Function*

The kidneys are both excretory and regulatory organs. By excreting water and solutes, the kidneys rid the body of excess water and waste products. They also regulate the volume and composition of the body fluids within a very narrow range, despite wide variations in the intake of food and water. Because of the kidneys' homeostatic role, the tissues and cells of the body are able to carry out their normal functions in a relatively constant environment.

The kidneys have several major functions, including
- Regulation of body fluid osmolality and volumes
- Regulation of electrolyte balance
- Regulation of acid-base balance
- Excretion of metabolic products and foreign substances
- Production and secretion of hormones

The control of body fluid osmolality is important for the maintenance of normal cell volume in all tissues of the body. Control of the volume of the body fluids is necessary for normal function of the cardiovascular system. The kidneys, working in concert with components of the cardiovascular, endocrine, and central nervous systems, accomplish these tasks by regulating the excretion of water and NaCl.

The kidneys play an essential role in regulating the amount of several important inorganic ions in the body, including Na^+, K^+, Cl^-, HCO_3^-, H^+, Ca^{++}, and $Po_4^{\equiv}$. To maintain appropriate balance, the excretion of these electrolytes must be equal to their daily intake. If intake of an electrolyte exceeds its excretion, the amount of this electrolyte in the body increases and the individual is said to be in positive balance for that electrolyte. Conversely, if excretion of an electrolyte exceeds its intake, its amount in the body decreases, and the individual is in negative balance for that electrolyte. For many electrolytes the kidneys are the sole or primary route by which they are excreted.

Another important role of the kidneys is the regulation of acid-base balance. Many of the metabolic functions of the body are exquisitely sensitive to pH. Thus, the pH of the body fluids must be maintained within narrow limits. The pH is maintained by buffers within the body fluids and by the coordinated action of the lungs, liver, and kidneys.

The kidneys also excrete a number of end products of metabolism that are no longer needed by the body. These waste products include urea (from amino acids), uric acid (from nucleic acids), creatinine (from muscle creatine), end products of hemoglobin metabolism, and metabolites of hormones. The kidneys eliminate these substances from the body at a rate that matches their production. Thus, the kidneys regulate hormone concentrations within the body fluids. The kidneys also eliminate foreign substances from the body, such as drugs, pesticides, and other chemicals ingested in food.

Finally, the kidneys are important endocrine organs that produce and secrete renin, calcitriol, and erythropoietin. **Renin** activates the renin-angiotensin-aldosterone system, which helps regulate blood pressure and sodium and potassium balance. **Calcitriol,** a metabolite of vitamin D_3, is necessary for normal reabsorption of Ca^{++} by the gastrointestinal tract and for its deposition in bone (see also Chapter 48). In patients with renal disease, the kidneys' ability to produce calcitriol is impaired, and levels of this hormone are reduced. As a result, Ca^{++} reabsorption by the intestine is decreased. This reduced intestinal Ca^{++} reabsorption contributes to the abnormalities in bone formation seen in patients with chronic renal disease. Another consequence of many kidney diseases is a reduction in erythropoietin production and secretion. **Erythropoietin** stimulates red blood cell formation by the bone marrow. Decreased erythrocyte production is a cause of the anemia seen in chronic renal failure.

In the following chapters, various aspects of these important renal functions are considered. Where information is available, these functions are considered at several levels of organization: whole kidney, single nephron, cell, membrane, and transport protein.

■ *Functional Anatomy of the Kidneys*

Structure and function are closely linked in the kidneys. Consequently, an appreciation of the gross anatomic and histologic features of the kidneys is necessary to understand their function.

■ *Gross Anatomy*

The kidneys are paired organs that lie on the posterior wall of the abdomen behind the peritoneum on either side of the vertebral column. In the adult human, each kidney weighs between 115 and 170 g and is approximately 11 cm in length, 6 cm in width, and 3 cm thick.

The gross anatomic features of the human kidney are illustrated in Fig. 40-1. The medial side of each kidney contains an indentation through which pass the renal artery and vein, nerves, and pelvis. If a kidney were cut in half, two regions would be evident: an outer region called the **cortex** and an inner region called the **medulla.** The cortex and medulla are composed of **nephrons** (the functional units of the kidney), blood vessels, lymphatics, and nerves. The medulla in the human kidney is divided into 8 to 18 conical masses, the **renal pyramids.** The base of each pyramid originates at the corticomedullary border and the apex terminates in a **papilla,** which lies within a **minor calyx.** Minor calyces collect the urine from each papilla. The numerous minor calyces expand into two or three open-ended pouches, the **major calyces.** The major calyces in turn feed into the pelvis. The **pelvis** represents the upper expanded region of the ureter, which carries urine from the pelvis to the urinary bladder. The walls of the calyces, pelvis, and ureters contain smooth muscle that contracts to propel the urine toward the **urinary bladder.**

The blood flow to the two kidneys is equal to about 25% (1.25 L/min) of the cardiac output in resting individuals. However, the kidneys constitute less than 0.5% of the total body weight. As illustrated in Fig. 40-2 *(left panel)*, the renal artery branches to form progressively the **interlobar artery,** the **arcuate artery,** the **interlobular artery** (cortical radial artery), and the **afferent arteriole,** which leads into the **glomerular capillary network** (i.e., **glomerulus).** The glomerular capillaries come together to form the **efferent arteriole,** which leads into a second capillary network, the **peritubular capillaries,** which supply blood to the nephron. The vessels of the venous system run parallel to the arterial vessels and branch progressively to form the **interlobular vein** (cortical radial vein), the **arcuate vein,** the **interlobar vein,** and the **renal vein,** which courses beside the ureter.

■ **Fig. 40-1**   Structure of the human kidney, cut to show internal structures. (Modified from Marsh DJ: *Renal physiology,* New York, 1983, Raven Press.)

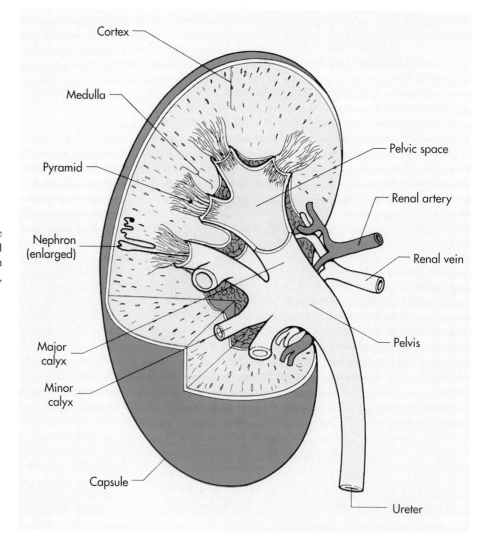

Cortex

Medulla

Pyramid

Nephron (enlarged)

Major calyx

Minor calyx

Capsule

Pelvic space

Renal artery

Renal vein

Pelvis

Ureter

■ *Ultrastructure of the Nephron*

*The functional unit of the kidneys is the **nephron**.* Each human kidney contains approximately 1.2 million nephrons, which are hollow tubes composed of a single cell layer (Fig. 40-2, *right panel*). The nephron consists of (1) a renal corpuscle, (2) a proximal tubule, (3) a loop of Henle, (4) a distal tubule, and (5) a collecting duct system.* The renal corpuscle consists of glomerular capillaries and Bowman's capsule. The **proximal tubule** initially forms several coils followed by a straight segment that descends toward the medulla. The next segment is

Henle's loop, which consists of the straight part of the proximal tubule, the descending thin limb (which ends in a hairpin turn), the ascending thin limb (only in nephrons with long loops of Henle), and the **thick ascending limb.** Near the end of the thick ascending limb, the nephron

---

*The organization of the nephron is actually more complicated than presented here. However, for simplicity and clarity of presentation in subsequent chapters, the nephron is divided into five segments. For details on the subdivisions of the five nephron segments, consult the references by Kriz and Bankir, Kriz and Kaissling, and Tisher and Madsen. The collecting duct system is not actually part of the nephron, but for simplicity we consider the collecting duct system part of the nephron.

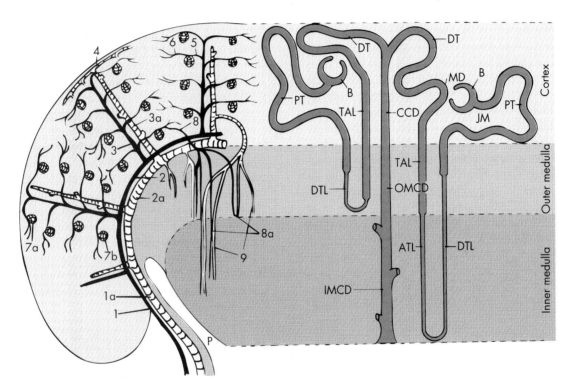

■ **Fig. 40-2** *Left panel,* Organization of the vascular system of the human kidney (not drawn to scale). The course and distribution of the intrarenal blood vessels are depicted; peritubular capillaries are not shown. The renal artery branches to form interlobar arteries *(1)*, which give rise to arcuate arteries *(2)*. Arcuate arteries lead to interlobular arteries *(3)*, which radiate toward the renal capsule and branch to form afferent arterioles *(5)*. Afferent arterioles branch to form glomerular capillary networks (i.e., glomeruli: *7a, 7b,*) which then coalesce to form efferent arterioles *(6)*. The efferent arterioles of the superficial nephrons form capillary networks (not shown) that suffuse the cells in the cortex. The efferent arterioles of the juxtamedullary nephrons divide into descending vasa recta *(8)*, which form capillary networks that supply blood to the outer and inner medulla *(8a)*. Blood from the peritubular capillaries enters, consecutively, the stellate vein *(4)*, interlobular vein *(3a)*, arcuate vein *(2a)*, and interlobar vein *(1a)*. Blood from the ascending vasa recta *(9)* enters the interlobular and arcuate veins. *P,* Pelvis. (Modified from Kriz W, Bankir L: A standard nomenclature for structures of the kidney, *Am J Physiol* 254:F1, 1988.) *Right panel,* Organization of the human nephron (not drawn to scale). A superficial nephron is illustrated on the left and a juxtamedullary nephron *(JM)* on the right. *B,* Bowman's capsule; *DT,* distal tubule; *PT,* proximal tubule; *CCD,* cortical collecting duct; *TAL,* thick ascending limb; *DTL,* descending thin limb; *OMCD,* outer medullary collecting duct; *ATL,* ascending thin limb; *IMCD,* inner medullary collecting duct; *MD,* macula densa. The loop of Henle includes the straight portion of the *PT,* and the *DTL, ATL,* and *TAL.* (Modified from Koushanpour E, Kriz W: *Renal physiology: principles, structure, and function,* ed 2, New York, 1986, Springer-Verlag; and Kriz W, Bankir L: A standard nomenclature for structures of the kidney, *Am J Physiol* 254:F1,1988.)

passes between its afferent and efferent arterioles. This short segment of the thick ascending limb is called the **macula densa.** The **distal tubule** begins a short distance beyond the macula densa and extends to the point in the cortex where two or more nephrons join to form the **cortical collecting duct.** The cortical collecting duct enters the medulla and becomes the **outer medullary collecting duct,** and then the **inner medullary collecting duct.**

Each nephron segment consists of cells that are uniquely suited to perform specific transport functions (Fig. 40-3). Proximal tubule cells have an extensively amplified apical membrane (the urine side of the cell) called the **brush border;** only cells in the proximal tubule have this brush border. The basolateral membrane (the blood side of the cell) of proximal tubule cells is highly invaginated. These invaginations contain many mitochondria. In contrast, cells of the descending thin limb and ascending thin limb of Henle's loop have poorly developed apical and basolateral surfaces and only a few mitochondria. The cells of the thick ascending limb and the distal tubule have abundant mitochondria and extensive infoldings of the basolateral membrane. The collecting duct is composed of two cell types: **principal cells** and **intercalated cells.** Principal cells have a moderately invaginated basolateral membrane and contain few mitochondria. Intercalated cells have a high density of mitochondria. The final segment of the nephron, the inner medullary collecting duct, is composed of inner medullary collecting duct cells. Cells of the inner medullary collecting duct have poorly developed apical and basolateral surfaces and few mitochondria.

There are two types of nephrons: **superficial** and **juxtamedullary** (Fig. 40-2, *right panel*). The renal corpuscle of each superficial nephron is located in the outer region of the cortex. Its loop of Henle is short, and its efferent arteriole branches into peritubular capillaries that surround the nephron segments of its own and adjacent nephrons. This capillary network conveys oxygen and important nutrients to the nephron segments, delivers substances to the nephron for secretion (i.e., the movement of a substance from the blood into the tubular fluid), and serves as a pathway for the return of reabsorbed water and solutes to the circulatory system. A few species, including man, also possess very short superficial nephrons whose loops of Henle never enter the medulla.

The renal corpuscle of each juxtamedullary nephron is located in the region of the cortex next to the medulla (Fig. 40-2, *right panel*). The juxtamedullary nephrons differ anatomically from superficial nephrons in two important ways: (1) the loop of Henle is longer and extends deeper into the medulla and (2) the efferent arteriole forms not only a network of peritubular capillaries, but also a series of vascular loops called the **vasa recta.** As illustrated in Fig. 40-2 *(left panel)*, the vasa recta descend into the medulla, where they form capillary networks that surround the collecting ducts and ascending limbs of Henle's loop. The blood returns to the cortex in the ascending vasa recta. *Although less than 0.7% of the renal blood flow enters the vasa recta, these vessels perform many important functions, including conveying oxygen and important nutrients to nephron segments, delivering substances to the nephron for secretion, serving as a pathway for the return of reabsorbed water and solutes to the circulatory system, and concentrating and diluting the urine.*

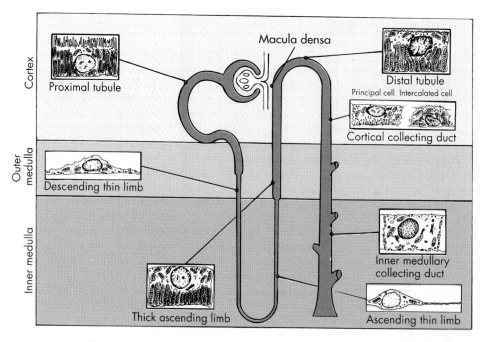

■ **Fig. 40-3**   Diagram of a nephron, including the cellular ultrastructure.

Ultrastructure of the Renal Corpuscle

The first step in urine formation begins with the passive movement of a plasma ultrafiltrate, an essentially protein-free fluid, from the glomerular capillaries into Bowman's space. To appreciate the process of ultrafiltration, one must understand the anatomy of the renal corpuscle. The glomerulus consists of a network of capillaries supplied by the afferent arteriole and drained by the efferent arteriole (Figs. 40-4 to 40-7). During embryologic development, the glomerular capillaries press into the closed end of the proximal tubule, forming the Bowman's capsule of a renal corpuscle. The capillaries are covered by epithelial cells, called **podocytes,** which form the **visceral layer** of Bowman's capsule (Figs. 40-4 to 40-7). The visceral cells face outward at the vascular pole (i.e., where the afferent and efferent arterioles enter and exit Bowman's capsule) to form the parietal layer of Bowman's capsule. The space between the visceral layer and the parietal layer is called **Bowman's space,** which, at the urinary pole (i.e., where the proximal tubule joins Bowman's capsule) of the glomerulus, becomes the lumen of the proximal tubule.

The **endothelial cells** of glomerular capillaries are covered by a **basement membrane,** which is surrounded by podocytes (Figs. 40-6). The capillary endothelium, basement membrane, and foot processes of podocytes form the so-called **filtration barrier** (Figs. 40-4 to 40-7). The endothelium is fenestrated (i.e., it contains 700 Å holes where $1Å = 10^{-10}$ m) and is freely permeable to water; to small solutes such as sodium, urea, and glucose; and even to small proteins, but it is not permeable to cells. Because endothelial cells express negatively charged glycoproteins on their surface, they can retard the filtration of large anionic proteins (see p 690). The basement membrane, which is a porous matrix of extracellular proteins including type IV collagen, laminin, fibronectin, and other negatively charged proteins, is an important filtration barrier to plasma proteins. The podocytes, which are **endocytic** (i.e., the process of endocytosis allows materials to enter the cell without passing through the membrane), have long, finger-like processes that completely encircle the outer surface of the capillaries (Fig. 40-7). The processes of the podocytes interdigitate to cover the basement membrane and are separated by gaps, called **filtration slits.** Each filtration slit is bridged by a thin diaphragm, which contains pores with dimensions of 40×140 Å. Therefore, the filtration slits retard the filtration of some proteins and

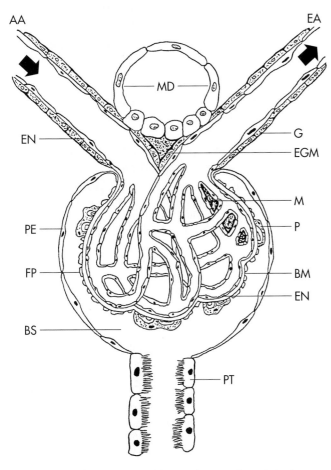

■ **Fig. 40-4** Anatomy of the renal corpuscle and the juxtaglomerular apparatus. The latter is composed of the (1) macula densa of the thick ascending limb, (2) extraglomerular mesangial cells, and (3) renin-producing granular cells of the afferent and efferent arterioles. *AA,* Afferent arteriole, *EA,* efferent arteriole; *G,* granular cell of the afferent and efferent arterioles; *MD,* macula densa; *BM,* basement membrane; *FP,* foot processes of the podocyte; *P,* podocyte cell body (visceral cell layer); *M,* mesangial cells between capillaries; *EGM,* extraglomerular mesangial cells between the afferent and efferent arterioles; *EN,* endothelial cell; *PT,* proximal tubule cell; *BS,* Bowman's space; *PE,* parietal epithelium. (Modified from Koushanpour E, Kriz W: *Renal physiology: principles, structure, and function,* ed 2, New York, 1986, Springer-Verlag.)

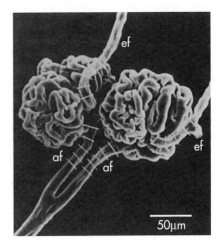

■ **Fig. 40-5** Scanning electron micrograph of interlobular artery; afferent arteriole *(af);* efferent arteriole *(ef);* and glomerulus. The white bars on the afferent and efferent arterioles indicate that they are about 15 to 20 mm in diameter. (From Kimura K et al: *Am J Physiol* 259:F936, 1990.)

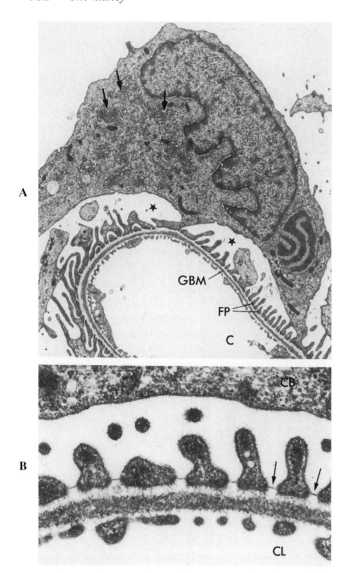

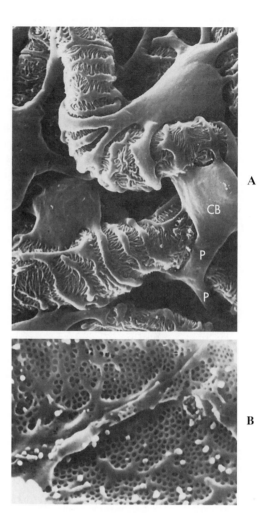

■ **Fig. 40-6** **A,** Electron micrograph of a podocyte surrounding a glomerular capillary. The cell body of the podocyte contains a large nucleus with three indentations. Cell processes of the podocyte form the interdigitating foot processes *(FP)*. The arrows in the cytoplasm of the podocyte indicate the well-developed Golgi apparatus. *C,* Capillary lumen; *GBM,* glomerular basement membrane. Stars indicate Bowman's space. (Magnification ~5700 ×.) **B,** Electron micrograph of the filtration barrier of a glomerular capillary. *CL,* Capillary lumen; *CB,* cell body of a podocyte. The filtration barrier is composed of three layers: the endothelium, the basement membrane, and the foot processes of the podocytes. Note the diaphragm bridging the floor of the filtration slits *(arrows)*. (Magnification ~42,700 ×.) (Courtesy of Kriz W, Kaissling B: *Structural organization of the mammalian kidney.* In Seldin DW, Giebisch G, editors: *The kidney: physiology and pathophysiology,* ed 2, New York, 1992, Raven Press.)

■ **Fig. 40-7** **A,** Scanning electron micrograph showing the outer surface of glomerular capillaries. This is the view that would be seen from Bowman's space. Processes *(P)* of podocytes run from the cell body *(CB)* toward the capillaries where they ultimately split into foot processes. Interdigitation of the foot processes creates the filtration slits. (Magnification ~2,500 ×.) **B,** Scanning electron micrograph of the inner surface (blood side) of a glomerular capillary. This view would be seen from the lumen of the capillary. The fenestrations of the endothelial cells are seen as small 700-Å holes. (Magnification ~12,000 ×.) (Courtesy of Kriz W, Kaissling B: *Structural organization of the mammalian kidney.* In Seldin DW, Giebisch G, editors: *The kidney: physiology and pathophysiology,* ed 2, New York, 1992, Raven Press.)

macromolecules that pass through the endothelium and basement membrane. *Because the endothelium, basement membrane, and filtration slits contain negatively charged glycoproteins, some molecules are held back on the basis of size and charge.* For molecules with an effective molecular radius between 20 and 42 Å, cationic molecules are filtered more readily than anionic molecules (see p 690).

The **nephrotic syndrome** is produced by a variety of disorders and is characterized by an increase in the permeability of the glomerular capillaries to proteins. The augmented permeability results in an increase in urinary protein excretion **(proteinuria).** Thus, the appearance of proteins in the urine can indicate kidney disease. Individuals with the nephrotic syndrome may also develop edema and hypoalbuminemia as a result of the proteinuria.

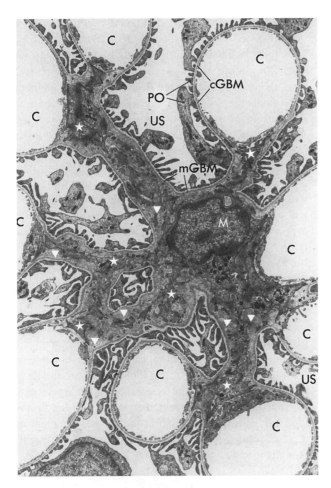

■ **Fig. 40-8** Electron micrograph of the mesangium, the area between glomerular capillaries containing mesangial cells. *C,* Glomerular capillaries; *cGBM,* capillary glomerular basement membrane surrounded by foot processes of podocytes *(PO)* and endothelial cells; *mGBM,* mesangial glomerular basement membrane surrounded by foot processes of podocytes and mesangial cells; *M,* mesangial cell that gives rise to several processes, some marked by stars; *US,* urinary space. Note the extensive extracellular matrix surrounded by mesangial cells (marked by *triangles*). (Magnification ~4,100 ×.) (From Kriz W, Kaissling B: *Structural organization of the mammalian kidney.* In Seldin DW, Giebisch G, editors: *The kidney: physiology and pathophysiology,* ed 2, New York, 1992, Raven Press.)

cells or **Goormaghtigh cells**). Extraglomerular mesangial cells exhibit phagocytic activity.

> Mesangial cells are involved in the development of immune complex–mediated glomerular disease. Because the glomerular basement membrane does not completely surround the glomerular capillaries (Fig. 40-8), immune complexes can enter the mesangial area without crossing the glomerular basement membrane. Accumulation of immune complexes induces the infiltration of inflammatory cells into the mesangium and prompts the production of cytokines and autocoids by cells in the mesangium. These cytokines and autocoids enhance the inflammatory response, which can lead to cell scarring and eventually obliterate the glomerulus.

■ *Ultrastructure of the Juxtaglomerular Apparatus*

The structures of the juxtaglomerular apparatus include (1) the macula densa of the thick ascending limb, (2) the extraglomerular mesangial cells, and (3) the renin-producing **granular cells** of the afferent and efferent arterioles (Fig. 40-4). The cells of the macula densa represent a morphologically distinct region of the thick ascending limb. This region passes through the angle formed by the afferent and efferent arterioles of the same nephron. The cells of the macula densa contact the extraglomerular mesangial cells and the granular cells of the afferent and efferent arterioles. Granular cells of the afferent and efferent arterioles are modified smooth muscle cells that manufacture, store, and release **renin.** Renin is involved in the formation of **angiotensin II** and ultimately in the secretion of **aldosterone** (see Chapters 43 and 51). The juxtaglomerular apparatus is one component of an important feedback mechanism (i.e., **tubuloglomerular feedback mechanism**) that is involved in the autoregulation of renal blood flow and of the glomerular filtration rate.

■ *Innervation of the Kidney*

Renal nerves help regulate renal blood flow, glomerular filtration rate, and salt and water reabsorption by the nephron. The nerve supply to the kidneys consists of sympathetic nerve fibers that originate mainly in the celiac plexus. There is no parasympathetic innervation. Adrenergic fibers that innervate the kidneys release norepinephrine and dopamine. The adrenergic fibers lie adjacent to the smooth muscle cells of the major branches of the renal artery (interlobar, arcuate, and interlobular arteries) and the afferent and efferent arterioles. Moreover, the renin-producing granular cells of the afferent and efferent arterioles are innervated by sympathetic

Another important component of the renal corpuscle is the **mesangium,** which consists of **mesangial cells** and the **mesangial matrix** (Fig. 40-8). Mesangial cells are similar in structure to monocytes. They surround glomerular capillaries, provide structural support for the glomerular capillaries, secrete the extracellular matrix, exhibit phagocytic activity, and secrete prostaglandins and cytokines. Because they also contract and are adjacent to glomerular capillaries, mesangial cells may influence the glomerular filtration rate by regulating blood flow through glomerular capillaries or by altering the capillary surface area. Mesangial cells located outside the glomerulus (between the afferent and efferent arterioles) are called **extraglomerular mesangial cells (or lacis**

nerves. Renin secretion is stimulated by increased sympathetic activity. Nerve fibers also innervate the proximal tubule, loop of Henle, distal tubule, and collecting duct; activation of these nerves enhances sodium reabsorption by these nephron segments.

■ Anatomy and Physiology of the Lower Urinary Tract

■ Gross Anatomy and Histology

Once urine leaves the renal calyces and renal pelvis, it flows through the **ureters** and enters the **urinary bladder,** where it is stored (Fig. 40-9). The ureters are muscular tubes 30 cm long. They enter the bladder on its posterior aspect near the base, above the bladder neck. The bladder is composed of two parts: the **fundus** or body, which stores urine, and the **neck,** which is funnel shaped and connects with the **urethra.** The bladder neck, which is 2 to 3 cm long, is also called the posterior urethra. In females, the posterior urethra is the end of the urinary tract and the point where urine exits the body. In males, urine flows through the posterior urethra into the anterior urethra, which extends through the penis. Urine leaves the urethra through the external meatus.

The renal calyces, pelvis, ureter, and urinary bladder are lined with a transitional epithelium composed of several layers of cells: basal columnar cells, intermediate cuboidal cells, and superficial squamous cells. This epithelium is surrounded by spiral and longitudinal smooth muscle fibers. The bladder is also lined with a transitional epithelium that is surrounded by smooth muscle fibers, called the **detrusor muscle.** Detrusor mus-

cle fibers are arranged at random. They do not form layers except close to the bladder neck, where the fibers form three layers: inner longitudinal, middle circular, and outer longitudinal. Muscle fibers in the bladder neck form the **internal sphincter.** This is not a true sphincter but a thickening of the bladder wall formed by converging muscle fibers. *The internal sphincter is not under conscious control.* Its inherent tone prevents emptying of the bladder until appropriate stimuli trigger urination. The urethra passes through the **urogenital diaphragm,** which contains a layer of skeletal muscle called the **external sphincter.** This muscle is under voluntary control and can be used to prevent or interrupt urination, especially in males. In females, the external sphincter is poorly developed; thus, it is less important in voluntary bladder control. The smooth muscle cells in the lower urinary tract are electrically coupled, exhibit spontaneous action potentials, contract when stretched, and are under autonomic control.

The walls of the ureters, bladder, and urethra are highly folded and therefore very distensible. In the bladder and urethra, these folds are called **rugae.** As the bladder fills with urine, the rugae flatten and the volume of the bladder increases with very little change in intravesical pressure. Bladder volume can increase from a minimum of 10 ml after urination to 400 ml, yet pressure changes only 5 cm H_2O, which illustrates the highly compliant nature of the bladder.

■ Innervation of the Bladder

Innervation of the bladder and urethra is important in controlling urination. The smooth muscle of the bladder

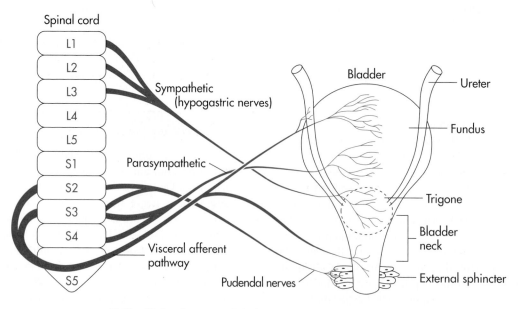

■ Fig. 40-9   Anatomy of the lower urinary tract and its innervation.

neck receives sympathetic innervation from the hypogastric nerves. α-Adrenergic receptors, located mainly in the bladder neck and the urethra, cause contraction. Stimulation of these receptors induces closure of the urethra and thus facilitates storage of urine. Sacral parasympathetic fibers (muscarinic) innervate the body of the bladder and cause a sustained bladder contraction. Sensory fibers of the pelvic nerves (visceral afferent pathway) also innervate the fundus. These sensory fibers carry input from receptors that detect bladder fullness, pain, and temperature sensation. The sacral pudendal nerves innervate the skeletal muscle fibers of the external sphincter; excitatory impulses cause the external sphincter to contract.

■ *Passage of Urine from the Kidney to the Bladder*

Renal calyces stretch as they collect urine. Stretching promotes their inherent pacemaker activity. Pacemaker activity generates action potentials, which initiate a peristaltic contraction. The peristaltic wave begins in the calyces, spreads to the pelvis and along the length of the ureter, and passes along the smooth muscle syncytium. This process thereby forces urine from the renal pelvis toward the bladder. The ureters are innervated with sensory nerve fibers (pelvic nerves).

Nephrolithiasis (kidney stones) is a common medical problem: 5% to 10% of Americans develop kidney stones sometime in their life. Most stones (80%-90%) are composed of calcium salts. The remaining stones are composed of uric acid, magnesium-ammonium acetate, or cysteine. Stones are formed by crystallization in a supersaturated urinary milieu. When the ureter is blocked with a kidney stone, reflex constriction of the ureter around the stone elicits severe flank pain.

■ *Micturition*

Micturition is the process of emptying the urinary bladder. Two processes are involved: (1) progressive filling of the bladder until the pressure rises to a critical value and (2) a neuronal reflex called the **micturition reflex,** which empties the bladder. The micturition reflex is an automatic spinal cord reflex. However, it can be inhibited or facilitated by centers in the brainstem and the cerebral cortex.

Filling of the bladder stretches the bladder wall and triggers a reflex initiated by stretch receptors, causing the bladder wall to contract. Sensory signals from the bladder fundus enter the spinal cord via pelvic nerves and return directly to the bladder through parasympathetic

fibers in the same nerves. Stimulation of parasympathetic fibers causes intense stimulation of the detrusor muscle. The smooth muscle in the bladder is a syncytium; accordingly, stimulation of the detrusor also causes the muscle cells in the neck of the bladder to contract. Because the muscle fibers of the bladder outlet are oriented both longitudinally and radially, contraction opens the bladder neck and allows urine to flow through the posterior urethra. A voluntary relaxation of the external sphincter, achieved by cortical inhibition of the pudendal nerve, permits the flow of urine through the external meatus. Voluntary relaxation of the external sphincter is required for urine to flow through it, and may be the event that initiates micturition. Interruption of the hypogastric sympathetic nerves and the pudendal nerves to the lower urinary tract does not alter the micturition reflex. In contrast, destruction of the parasympathetic nerves results in complete bladder dysfunction.

■ *Assessment of Renal Function*

The coordinated actions of the nephron's various segments determine the amount of a substance that appears in the urine. This represents three general processes: (1) glomerular filtration, (2) reabsorption of the substance from the tubular fluid back into the blood, and (3) (in some cases) secretion of the substance from the blood into the tubular fluid. The first step in the formation of urine by the kidneys is the production of an ultrafiltrate of plasma across the glomerulus. The process of glomerular filtration and the regulation of glomerular filtration rate and renal blood flow are discussed next. The concept of **renal clearance,** which is the theoretical basis of measurements of glomerular filtration rate and renal blood flow, is presented in the following section. Reabsorption and secretion are discussed in subsequent chapters.

Knowledge of the **glomerular filtration rate (GFR)** is essential in evaluating the severity and course of **kidney disease.** The GFR is equal to the sum of the filtration rates of all the functioning nephrons. Thus, GFR is an index of kidney function. A fall in GFR generally means that disease is progressing, whereas an increase in GFR generally suggests recovery.

■ *Renal Clearance*

The concept of renal clearance is based on the **Fick principle** (mass balance or conservation of mass) (see also Chapter 23). Fig. 40-10 illustrates the various factors required to describe the mass balance relationships of a kidney. The renal artery is the single input source to the kidney, whereas the renal vein and ureter constitute the

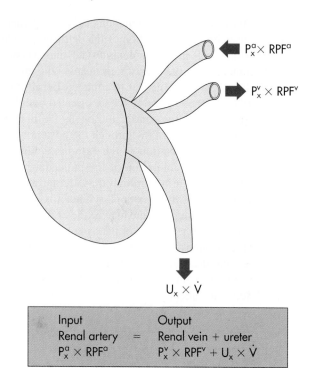

■ **Fig. 40-10**   Mass balance relationships for the kidney. See text for definition of symbols.

two output routes. The following equation defines the mass balance relationship:

$$P^a_x \times RPF^a = (P^v_x \times RPF^v) + (U_x \times \dot{V}) \qquad (40\text{-}1)$$

where P^a_x and P^v_x are the concentrations of substance x in the renal artery and renal vein plasma, respectively; RPF^a and RPF^v are the renal plasma flow rates in the artery and vein, respectively; U_x is the concentration of x in the urine; and $\dot{V}$ is the urine flow rate. This relationship permits the quantification of the amount of x excreted in the urine versus the amount returned to the systemic circulation in the renal venous blood. Thus, for any substance that is neither synthesized nor metabolized, the amount that enters the kidneys is equal to the amount that leaves the kidneys in the urine plus the amount that leaves the kidneys in the renal venous blood.

The principle of renal clearance emphasizes the excretory function of the kidney; it considers only the rate at which a substance is excreted into the urine, and not its rate of return to the systemic circulation in the renal vein. Therefore, in terms of mass balance (equation 40-1), the urinary excretion rate of x ($U_x \times \dot{V}$) is proportional to the plasma concentration of x (P^a_x).

$$P^a_x \sim U_x \times \dot{V} \qquad (40\text{-}2)$$

To equate the urinary excretion rate of x to its renal arterial plasma concentration, one must determine the rate at which x is removed from the plasma by the kidneys. This removal rate is the clearance (C_x):

$$P^a_x \times C_x = U_x \times \dot{V} \qquad (40\text{-}3)$$

If equation 40-3 is rearranged, and if the concentration of x in the renal artery plasma (P_x) is assumed to be identical to its concentration in a plasma sample from any peripheral blood vessel, the following relationship is obtained:

$$C_x = \frac{U_x \times \dot{V}}{P_x} \qquad (40\text{-}4)$$

Clearance has the dimensions of volume/time, and it represents a volume of plasma from which all the substance has been removed and excreted into the urine per unit of time. This last point is best illustrated by considering the following example.

If a substance is present in the urine at a concentration of 100 mg/ml, and the urine flow rate is 1 ml/min, the excretion rate for this substance is calculated as:

$$\text{excretion rate} = U_x \times \dot{V} =$$
$$(100 \text{ mg/ml}) \times (1 \text{ ml/min}) = 100 \text{ mg/min} \quad (40\text{-}5)$$

If this substance is present in the plasma at a concentration of 1 mg/ml, its clearance according to equation 41-4 is:

$$C_x = \frac{U_x \dot{V}}{P_x} = \frac{100 \text{ mg/min}}{1 \text{ mg/ml}} = 100 \text{ ml/min} \qquad (40\text{-}6)$$

That is, 100 ml of plasma will be completely cleared of substance x each minute. The definition of clearance as a volume of plasma from which all the substance has been removed and excreted into the urine per unit time is somewhat misleading. The volume of plasma in this equation is not a real volume of plasma; rather, it is an idealized volume.* Nevertheless the concept of clearance is important because it can be used to measure the GFR and renal plasma flow and to determine whether a substance is reabsorbed or secreted along the nephron.

■ *Glomerular Filtration Rate: Clearance of Inulin*

Inulin is a polymer of fructose (molecular weight about 5000) that can be used to measure the GFR. It is not produced by the body and therefore must be administered intravenously. Inulin is freely filtered across the glomerulus into Bowman's space and is neither reabsorbed, secreted, nor metabolized by the cells of the nephron. Accordingly, *the amount of inulin excreted in the urine per minute equals the amount of inulin filtered at the glomerulus each minute* (Fig. 40-11):

$$\text{amount filtered} = \text{amount excreted}$$
$$\text{GFR} \times P_{in} = U_{in} \times \dot{V} \qquad (40\text{-}7)$$

where GFR is the glomerular filtration rate, P_{in} and U_{in} are the plasma and urine concentrations of inulin, and $\dot{V}$

---

*For most substances cleared from the plasma by the kidneys, only a portion is actually removed and excreted in a single pass through the kidneys.

is the rate of urine flow. If equation 40-7 is solved for the GFR:

$$GFR = U_{in} \times \frac{\dot{V}}{P_{in}} \qquad (40\text{-}8)$$

This equation is in the same form as that for clearance (see equation 40-4). *Thus, determining the clearance of inulin provides a means for determining the GFR.*

Inulin is not the only substance that can be used to measure GFR. Any substance that meets the following criteria will serve as an appropriate marker for the measurement of GFR. The substance must

1. Be freely filtered across the glomerulus into Bowman's space.
2. Not be reabsorbed or secreted by the nephron.
3. Not be metabolized or produced by the kidney.
4. Not alter GFR.

Whereas inulin is used extensively in experimental studies, the need to administer it intravenously limits its clinical use. Consequently, **creatinine** is used to estimate GFR in clinical practice. Creatinine is a byproduct of skeletal muscle creatine metabolism. It is produced at a relatively constant rate, and the amount produced is proportional to the muscle mass. Because creatinine is produced endogenously, an intravenous infusion is unnecessary. However, creatinine is not a perfect substance to use to measure GFR, because a small amount is secreted by the organic cation secretory system in the proximal tubule (see Chapter 41). The error introduced by this secretory component is approximately 10%. Thus, the amount of creatinine excreted in the urine exceeds the amount expected from filtration alone by 10%. However, the method used to quantitate the plasma creatinine concentration overestimates the true value by 10%. Consequently, the two errors cancel, and *in most clinical situations* **creatinine clearance** *provides a reasonably accurate measure of GFR.*

As illustrated in Fig. 40-11, not all the inulin (or any substance used to measure GFR) that enters the kidney in the renal arterial plasma is filtered at the glomerulus. Likewise, not all the plasma entering the kidney is filtered.* The portion of plasma that is filtered is termed the **filtration fraction** and is determined as:

$$\text{filtration fraction} = \frac{GFR}{RPF} \qquad (40\text{-}9)$$

where, again, RPF is renal plasma flow. Under normal conditions, the filtration fraction averages 0.15 to 0.20. *This means that only 15% to 20% of the plasma that enters the glomerulus is actually filtered.* The remaining 80% to 85% continues on through the glomerulus

---

*Nearly all the plasma that enters the kidney in the renal artery passes through the glomerulus. Approximately 10% does not.

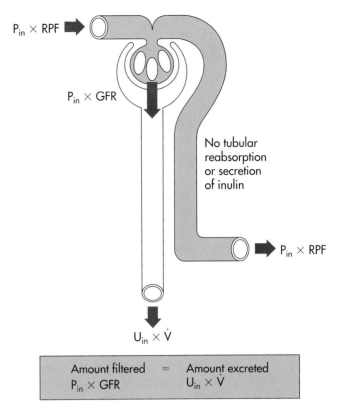

Amount filtered　=　Amount excreted
$P_{in} \times GFR$　　$U_{in} \times \dot{V}$

■ **Fig. 40-11**　Renal handling of inulin. Inulin is freely filtered across the glomerulus and is neither reabsorbed, secreted, nor metabolized by the nephron. P_{in}, Plasma inulin concentration; *RPF*, renal plasma flow; *GFR*, glomerular filtration rate; U_{in}, urinary concentration of inulin; $\dot{V}$, urine flow rate. Note that all inulin entering the kidney in the renal artery is not filtered at the glomerulus (normally 15% to 20% of plasma and inulin is filtered). The portion that is not filtered is returned to the systemic circulation in the renal vein.

into the efferent arterioles and peritubular capillaries, and is finally returned to the systemic circulation in the renal vein.

A fall in GFR may be the first and only clinical sign of kidney disease. Thus, measuring GFR is important when kidney disease is suspected. For example, a 50% loss of functioning nephrons will reduce the GFR only by approximately 20% to 30%. The decline in GFR is not 50% because the remaining nephrons compensate. Because measurements of GFR are cumbersome, kidney function is usually assessed in the clinical setting by measuring plasma [creatinine] (P_{cr}), which is inversely related to GFR (Fig. 40-12). However, as Fig. 40-12 shows, GFR must decline substantially before an increase in P_{cr} can be detected in a clinical setting. For example, a fall in GFR from 120 to 100 ml/min is accompanied by an increase in P_{cr} from 1.0 to 1.2 mg/dl. This does not appear to be a significant change in P_{cr}, yet GFR has actually fallen by almost 20%.

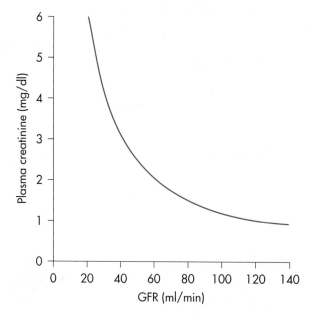

■ **Fig. 40-12** Relationship between GFR and plasma creatinine concentration. As with inulin, the amount of creatinine filtered is essentially equal to the amount excreted (i.e., amount filtered = amount excreted, thus, GFR × P_{cr} = U_{Cr} × $\dot{V}$). Because production of creatinine is constant, excretion must be constant to maintain creatinine balance. Thus, if GFR falls from 120 to 60 ml/min, P_{cr} must increase from 1 to 2 mg/dl to keep the filtration of creatinine and thus its excretion equal to the production rate.

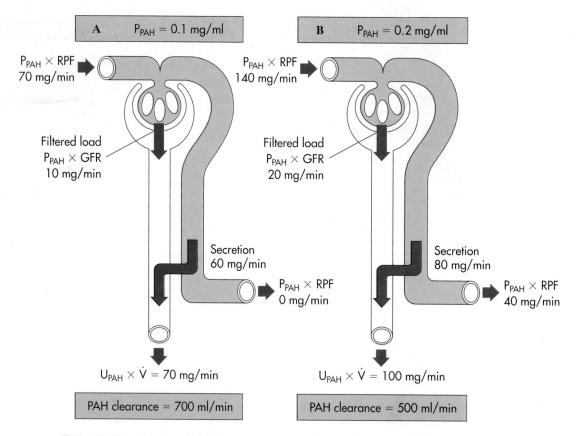

■ **Fig. 40-13** Renal handling of PAH at two different plasma concentrations *(P_{PAH})*. **A,** The P_{PAH} is less than the value that would lead to saturation of the PAH secretory mechanism (i.e., <80 mg/min). **B,** The elevated P_{PAH} delivers more PAH to the secretory mechanism than can be secreted (i.e., >80 mg/min). In both cases the RPF is 700 ml/min and the GFR is 100 ml/min. U_{PAH}, Urine PAH concentration; $\dot{V}$, urine flow rate. The clearance of PAH is calculated from equation 40-4.

■ *Renal Plasma Flow: Clearance of PAH*

P-Aminohippuric acid (PAH) is an organic anion filtered across the glomerulus that can be used to measure RPF (Fig. 40-13). As with inulin, PAH is not produced in the body and therefore must be infused intravenously. PAH is an organic anion that is excreted into the urine by the processes of glomerular filtration and tubular secretion. For our discussion it is sufficient to know that the PAH secretory mechanism in the proximal tubule has a maximal rate of approximately 80 mg/min. Delivery of PAH to the peritubular capillaries at a rate less than 80 mg/min will cause virtually all the PAH to be secreted into the tubular fluid, and thus little PAH will remain in the renal vein plasma. When the plasma PAH concentration is low and the secretory mechanism is not overwhelmed (generally at plasma [PAH] below 0.12 mg/ml), the clearance of PAH can be used to measure the renal plasma flow. However, when the PAH secretory mechanism is overwhelmed, the clearance of PAH cannot be used to measure RPF. Fig. 40-14 shows the renal handling of PAH in terms of whole kidney mass balance and illustrates why, when PAH delivery to the peritubular capillaries is less than about 80 mg/min, PAH clearance is a reliable estimate of the RPF. The amount of PAH that arrives at the kidneys per minute is simply the product of the plasma PAH concentration (P^a_{PAH}) and RPF. Because all the PAH is excreted into the urine (when PAH delivery to the peritubular capillaries is less than about 80 mg/min), and none is returned to the systemic circulation via the renal vein, the following mass balance relationship holds true:

$$RPF \times P^a_{PAH} = U_{PAH} \times \dot{V} \qquad (40\text{-}10)$$

where U_{PAH} is urine PAH concentration and $\dot{V}$ is the rate of urine flow. Rearranging and solving for RPF, the following equation is obtained:

$$RPF = \frac{U_{PAH} \times \dot{V}}{P^a_{PAH}} \qquad (40\text{-}11)$$

This equation conforms to the general clearance equation (equation 40-4). *Thus, at low plasma PAH concentrations, the PAH clearance is equal to the RPF.* At high plasma PAH concentrations, however, the PAH secretory mechanism will be saturated, and a significant amount of PAH will appear in the renal venous blood. Thus, at high plasma PAH concentrations, equations 40-10 and 40-11 do not hold, and the clearance of PAH does not equal the RPF.

The relationship between PAH clearance and RPF described here is idealized. Even at plasma PAH concentrations that do not exceed the capability of the secretory mechanism, some PAH still appears in the renal venous blood. The reason for this is related to the anatomy of the nephron and of the renal blood vessels. The PAH secretory mechanism is located in the proximal tubule. The PAH entering the peritubular capillaries

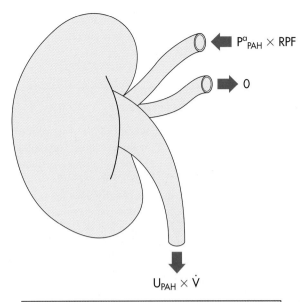

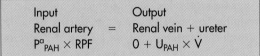

■ **Fig. 40-14** Mass balance relationships for the use of PAH clearance to measure the renal plasma flow *(RPF)*. P^a_{PAH}, Plasma PAH concentration; U_{PAH}, urine PAH concentration; $\dot{V}$, urine flow rate.

surrounding proximal tubules is secreted. However, some capillaries perfuse the medulla (i.e., vasa recta), the renal capsule, and parts of the renal hilum instead of forming peritubular capillaries. Thus, the PAH in this plasma cannot be secreted, and this PAH will be returned to the systemic circulation in the renal vein plasma. Because clearance of PAH does not provide an accurate measure of RPF (i.e., it underestimates the true value by approximately 10%), we refer to the clearance of PAH as providing a measure of the **effective renal plasma flow (ERPF):** effective in the sense that this measure represents plasma flow past those portions of the nephron that can effectively secrete PAH.

The clearance of PAH can also be used to estimate the renal blood flow (RBF). Normally, the plasma fraction of blood accounts for 50% to 60% of the blood volume, and the cells account for the remainder. To determine what fraction of the blood is composed of cells, we measure the **hematocrit (HCT).** Normally the HCT is in the range of 0.40 to 0.50. Once the HCT is known, the renal blood flow can be calculated as follows:

$$RBF = \frac{RPF}{1 - HCT} \qquad (40\text{-}12)$$

Thus, if the HCT of an individual is 0.40 and the RPF is 700 ml/min, RBF is 1167 ml/min (i.e., RBF = (700/(1 − 0.4) = 1167 ml/min). However, measurement of RPF provides little useful information and is rarely performed in clinical situations. Kidney function is usually assessed by measuring plasma creatinine concentration (P_{cr}), which, as discussed above, is inversely related to GFR (Fig. 40-12).

■ Glomerular Filtration

In normal adults, the GFR averages 90 to 140 ml/min for males and 80 to 125 ml/min for females. Thus, in a 24-hour period, as much as 180 L/day of plasma is filtered at the glomerulus. After age 30 GFR declines with age. However, this decline in GFR usually does not adversely affect the kidneys' excretory function, nor their ability to maintain fluid, electrolyte, and acid-base balance.

The first step in the formation of urine is the production of an ultrafiltrate of the plasma at the glomerulus. The ultrafiltrate is devoid of cellular elements and is essentially protein free. The concentrations of salts and of organic molecules, such as glucose and amino acids, are similar in the plasma and ultrafiltrate. Ultrafiltration is driven by Starling forces (see Chapter 27) across the glomerular capillaries, and changes in these forces alter the GFR. GFR and RPF are normally held within narrow ranges by a phenomenon called **autoregulation** (see also Chapter 28). This section reviews the composition of the glomerular filtrate, the dynamics of its formation, and the relationship between RPF and GFR. In addition, the factors that contribute to the autoregulation of GFR and RBF are discussed.

■ Determinants of Ultrafiltrate Composition

The unique structure of the glomerular filtration barrier (capillary endothelium, basement membrane, and filtration slits of the podocytes) determines the composition of the plasma ultrafiltrate. The glomerular filtration barrier restricts the filtration of molecules on the basis of size and electrical charge (Fig. 40-15). In general, neutral molecules with a radius less than 20 Å are filtered freely, molecules larger than 42 Å are not filtered, and molecules between 20 and 42 Å are filtered to various degrees. For example, serum albumin, an anionic protein that has an effective molecular radius of 35.5 Å, is filtered poorly: approximately 7 grams of albumin are filtered each day.* Because albumin is reabsorbed avidly by the proximal tubule, however, almost none appears in the urine.

Fig. 40-15 illustrates how electrical charge affects the filtration of macromolecules (e.g., dextrans) by the glomerulus. **Dextrans** are a family of exogenous polysaccharides that are manufactured in various molecular weights. They can be in an electrically neutral form or have negative (polyanionic) charges or positive (polycationic) charges. As the size (i.e., effective molecular radius) of a dextran increases, the rate at which it is filtered decreases. For any given molecular radius, cationic molecules are more readily filtered than are anionic molecules. The reduced filtration of anionic molecules is explained by the presence of negatively charged glycoproteins on the surface of all components of the glomerular filtration barrier. These charged glycoproteins repel similarly charged molecules. Because most plasma proteins are negatively charged, the negative charge on the filtration barrier restricts the filtration of proteins that have a molecular radius of 20 to 42 Å.

> The importance of the negative charges on the filtration barrier in restricting filtration of plasma proteins is shown in Fig. 40-16. Removal of negative charges

---

*Approximately 50,000 g/day of albumin passes through the glomeruli. Therefore, the filtration of 7 g/day represents approximately 0.01% of the albumin that passes through the glomeruli. This is well below the filtration fraction for substances that are freely filtered (15%-20%).

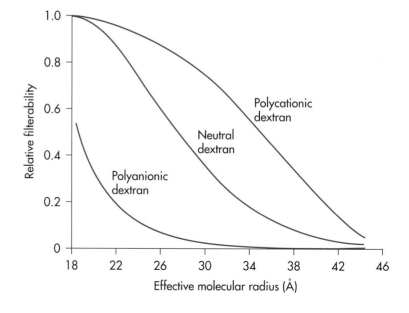

■ **Fig. 40-15** Influence of size and electrical charge of dextran on its filterability. A value of one indicates that it is filtered freely, whereas a value of zero indicates that it is not filtered. The filterability of dextrans between approximately 20 and 42 Å depends on charge. Dextrans larger than 42 Å are not filtered, regardless of charge, and polycationic dextrans and neutral dextrans smaller than 20 Å are freely filtered.

from the filtration barrier causes proteins to be filtered solely on the basis of their effective molecular radius. Hence, at any molecular radius between approximately 20 and 42 Å, the filtration of polyanionic proteins will exceed the filtration that prevails in the normal state (in which the filtration barrier has anionic charges). In a number of glomerular diseases, the negative charge on the filtration barrier is reduced because of immunologic damage and inflammation. As a result, filtration of proteins is increased, and proteins appear in the urine (**proteinuria**).

■ *Dynamics of Ultrafiltration*

The forces responsible for the glomerular filtration of plasma are the same as those involved in fluid exchange across all capillary beds (see Chapter 27). Ultrafiltration occurs because Starling forces (i.e., hydrostatic and oncotic pressures) drive fluid from the lumen of glomerular capillaries, across the filtration barrier, and into Bowman's space (Fig. 40-17). The hydrostatic pressure in the glomerular capillary (P_{GC}) is oriented to promote the movement of fluid from the glomerular capillary into Bowman's space. Because the reflection coefficient (σ) for proteins across the glomerular capillary is essentially 1, the glomerular ultrafiltrate is essentially protein free and the oncotic pressure in Bowman's space (π_{BS}) is near zero. Therefore, P_{GC} is the only force that favors filtration. Filtration is opposed by the hydrostatic pressure in Bowman's space (P_{BS}) and the oncotic pressure in the glomerular capillary (π_{GC}).

The Starling forces across the glomerular capillary are difficult to measure, and only estimates have been made for humans. As shown in Fig. 40-17, a net ultrafiltration pressure (P_{UF}) of 17 mm Hg exists at the afferent end of the glomerulus, whereas at the efferent end the P_{UF} is 8 mm Hg (where $P_{UF} = P_{GC} - P_{BS} - \pi_{GC}$). Two additional points concerning Starling forces and this pressure change are important. First, P_{GC} decreases slightly along the length of the capillary because of the resistance to flow in the capillary. Second, π_{GC} increases along the length of the glomerular capillary: because water is filtered and protein is retained in the glomerular capillary, the protein concentration in the capillary rises and π_{GC} increases.

The GFR is proportional to the sum of the Starling forces that exist across the capillaries [$(P_{GC} - P_{BS}) - \sigma(\pi_{GC} - \pi_{BS})$] times the ultrafiltration coefficient, K_f:

$$GFR = K_f [(P_{GC} - P_{BS}) - \sigma(\pi_{GC} - \pi_{BS})] \quad (40\text{-}13)$$

The K_f is the product of the intrinsic permeability of the glomerular capillary and the glomerular surface area available for filtration. The rate of glomerular filtration is considerably greater in glomerular capillaries than in systemic capillaries, mainly because the K_f is approximately 100 times higher in glomerular capillaries. Furthermore, in addition, the hydrostatic pressure within the glomerular capillaries is approximately twice as high as that in systemic capillaries.

The GFR can be altered by changing K_f or by changing any of the Starling forces. In normal individuals GFR is regulated by alterations in P_{GC} that are mediated primarily by changes in glomerular arteriolar resistance. P_{GC} is affected in three ways.

1. Changes in afferent arteriolar resistance: A fall in resistance increases P_{GC} and GFR, whereas an increase in resistance decreases P_{GC} and GFR.
2. Changes in efferent arteriolar resistance: A fall in resistance reduces P_{GC} and GFR, whereas an increase in resistance elevates P_{GC} and GFR.

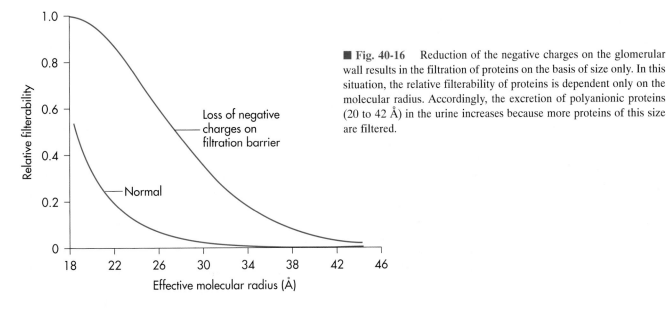

■ **Fig. 40-16** Reduction of the negative charges on the glomerular wall results in the filtration of proteins on the basis of size only. In this situation, the relative filterability of proteins is dependent only on the molecular radius. Accordingly, the excretion of polyanionic proteins (20 to 42 Å) in the urine increases because more proteins of this size are filtered.

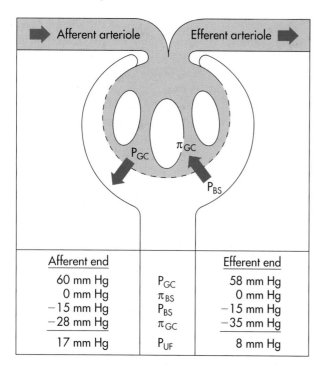

Afferent end		Efferent end
60 mm Hg	P_{GC}	58 mm Hg
0 mm Hg	π_{BS}	0 mm Hg
−15 mm Hg	P_{BS}	−15 mm Hg
−28 mm Hg	π_{GC}	−35 mm Hg
17 mm Hg	P_{UF}	8 mm Hg

■ **Fig. 40-17** Schematic representation of an idealized glomerular capillary and the Starling forces across the glomerular capillary. P_{UF}, Net ultrafiltration pressure; P_{GC}, glomerular capillary hydrostatic pressure; P_{BS}, Bowman's space hydrostatic pressure; π_{GC}, glomerular capillary oncotic pressure; π_{BS}, Bowman's space oncotic pressure. The reflection coefficient (σ) for protein across the glomerular capillary is 1.

3. Changes in renal arteriolar pressure. An increase in blood pressure transiently increases P_{GC} (which enhances GFR), whereas a decrease in blood pressure transiently decreases P_{GC} (which reduces GFR).

Pathological conditions and drugs may also affect GFR. A reduction in GFR in disease states is most often due to decreases in K_f because of the loss of filtration surface area. GFR also changes in pathophysiological conditions owing to changes in P_{GC}, π_{GC}, and P_{BS}.

1. Changes in K_f. Increased K_f enhances GFR, whereas decreased K_f reduces GFR. Some kidney diseases reduce K_f by decreasing the number of filtering glomeruli (i.e., surface area). Some drugs and hormones that dilate the glomerular arterioles also increase K_f. Similarly, drugs and hormones that constrict the glomerular arterioles also decrease K_f.

2. Changes in P_{GC}. In situations where mean arterial pressure falls (i.e., hemorrhage), GFR declines because P_{GC} falls. As discussed above, a reduction in P_{GC} is caused by a decline in renal arterial pressure, an increase in afferent arteriolar resistance, or a decrease in efferent arteriolar resistance.

3. Changes in π_{GC}. An inverse relationship exists between π_{GC} and GFR. Alterations in π_{GC} result from changes in protein synthesis outside the kidneys. In addition, protein loss in the urine caused by some renal diseases can lead to a decrease in plasma protein concentration and thus π_{GC}.

4. Changes in P_{BS}. Increased P_{BS} reduces GFR, whereas decreased P_{BS} enhances GFR. Acute obstruction of the urinary tract (e.g., a kidney stone occluding the ureter) increases P_{BS}.

■ *Renal Blood Flow*

In resting subjects, the blood flow to the kidneys (about 1.25 L/min) is equal to about 25% of the cardiac output. However, the kidneys constitute less than 0.5% of total body weight. Blood flow through the kidneys serves several important functions, including:

1. Indirectly determining the GFR.
2. Modifying the rate of solute and water reabsorption by the proximal tubule.
3. Participating in the concentration and dilution of the urine.
4. Delivering oxygen, nutrients, and hormones to the cells of the nephron and returning carbon dioxide and reabsorbed fluid and solutes to the general circulation.
5. Delivering substrates for excretion in the urine.

The blood flow through any organ may be represented by the following equation:

$$Q = \Delta P/R \qquad (40\text{-}14)$$

where Q equals blood flow, ΔP equals mean arterial pressure minus venous pressure for that organ, and R equals the resistance to flow through that organ (see also Chapter 25). Accordingly, RBF is equal to the pressure difference between the renal artery and the renal vein divided by the renal vascular resistance:

$$RBF = \frac{\text{aortic pressure renal venous pressure}}{\text{renal vascular resistance}} \qquad (40\text{-}15)$$

Because the afferent arteriole, the efferent arteriole, and the interlobular artery are the major resistance vessels in the kidney, they determine renal vascular resistance. The kidneys, like most organs, regulate their blood flow by adjusting the vascular resistance in response to changes in arterial pressure. As shown in Fig. 40-18, these adjustments are so precise that blood flow remains relatively constant as arterial blood pressure changes between 90 and 180 mm Hg. GFR is also regulated over the same range of arterial pressures. The phenomenon that allows this relatively constant maintenance of RBF and GFR, **autoregulation** (see also p 690 and Chapter 28), is achieved by changes in vascular resistance, primarily within the afferent arterioles of the kidneys.

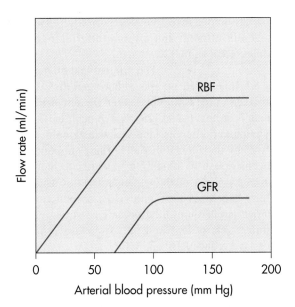

■ **Fig. 40-18** Relationships between arterial blood pressure and renal blood flow *(RBF)* and glomerular filtration rate *(GFR)*. Autoregulation allows RBF and GFR to remain relatively constant as blood pressure changes from 90 to 180 mm Hg.

Because both GFR and RBF are regulated over the same range of pressures, and because RPF is an important determinant of GFR, it is not surprising that the same mechanisms regulate both flows.

Two mechanisms are responsible for autoregulation of RBF and GFR: one mechanism that responds to changes in arterial pressure, and another that responds to changes in the flow rate of tubular fluid. Both regulate the tone of the afferent arteriole. The pressure-sensitive mechanism, or **myogenic mechanism,** is related to an intrinsic property of vascular smooth muscle: the tendency to contract when it is stretched (see also Chapter 28). Accordingly, when arterial pressure rises and the renal afferent arteriole is stretched, the smooth muscle contracts. Because the increase in the resistance of the arteriole offsets the increase in pressure, RBF, and therefore GFR, remain constant (i.e., RBF is constant if the ratio of ΔP/R is kept constant, see equation 40-14).

The second mechanism responsible for autoregulation of GFR and RBF is the flow-dependent mechanism known as **tubuloglomerular feedback** (Fig. 40-19). This mechanism involves a feedback loop in which the flow of tubular fluid (or some other factor, such as the rate of NaCl reabsorption, which increases in direct proportion to flow) is sensed by the macula densa of the juxtaglomerular apparatus (JGA). The JGA sends a signal that affects afferent arteriolar resistance, and thus GFR. When GFR increases and causes the flow of tubular fluid at the macula densa to rise, the JGA sends a signal that causes vasoconstriction to return RBF and GFR to normal levels. In contrast, when GFR and tubular flow

past the macula densa decrease, the JGA sends a signal causing RBF and GFR to increase to normal levels. The signal affects RBF and GFR mainly by changing the resistance of the afferent arteriole, but the mediator for this effect is controversial. The major unknowns about tubuloglomerular feedback concern the variable that is sensed at the macula densa and the effector substance that alters the resistance of the afferent arteriole. It has been suggested that the macula densa senses flow-dependent changes in NaCl reabsorption. The effector mechanism may be adenosine, which constricts the afferent arteriole (in contrast to its vasodilator effect on most other vasculature beds); adenosine triphosphate (ATP), which selectively vasoconstricts the afferent arteriole; or even a metabolite of arachidonic acid. Nitric oxide (NO), a vasodilator produced by the macula densa, may also play a role in tubuloglomerular feedback, but it is not essential for autoregulation. The macula densa may release both a vasoconstrictor and a vasodilator (e.g., NO) that oppose each other's action at the level of the afferent arteriole.

Because animals engage in many activities that can change arterial blood pressure, mechanisms that maintain RBF and GFR relatively constant despite changes in arterial pressure are highly desirable. Alterations in GFR influence water and solute excretion (the reason is discussed in the next chapter). If RBF and GFR were to rise or fall suddenly in proportion to changes in blood pressure, urinary excretion of fluid and solute would also change suddenly. Such changes in water and solute excretion, without comparable alterations in intake, would alter fluid and electrolyte balance. Accordingly, autoregulation of GFR and RBF is an effective means for uncoupling renal function from arterial pressure, and ensures that fluid and solute excretion remain constant. Three points concerning autoregulation should be made:

1. Autoregulation is absent below arterial pressures of 90 mm Hg.
2. Autoregulation is not perfect; RBF and GFR do change slightly as arterial blood pressure varies.
3. Despite autoregulation, several hormones, GFR and RBF can change under appropriate conditions (Table 40-1).

Individuals with **renal artery stenosis** (a narrowing of the artery lumen), caused by atherosclerosis, for example, can have an elevated systemic blood pressure mediated by stimulation of the renin-angiotensin system (see Chapter 42 for details). The pressure in the artery proximal to the stenosis is increased, but pressure is normal or reduced distal to the stenosis. Autoregulation plays an important role in maintaining RBF, P_{GC}, and GFR in the presence of this stenosis. The administration of drugs to lower systemic blood pressure also lowers pressure distal to the stenosis; accordingly, RBF, P_{GC}, and GFR fall.

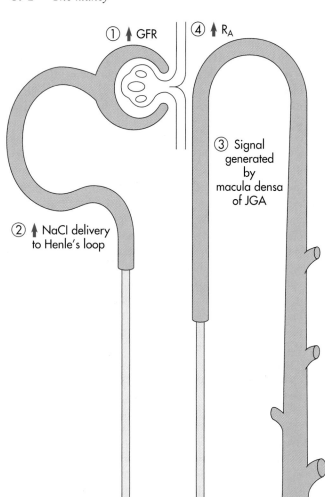

① ↑ GFR

④ ↑ R_A

③ Signal generated by macula densa of JGA

② ↑ NaCl delivery to Henle's loop

■ **Fig. 40-19**   Tubuloglomerular feedback. An increase in GFR *(1)* increases NaCl delivery to the loop of Henle *(2)*, which is sensed by the macula densa and converted into a signal *(3)*, This signal increases R_A *(4:* the resistance of the afferent arteriole), which decreases GFR. *JGA,* Juxtaglomerular apparatus.

■ *Regulation of Renal Blood Flow and Glomerular Filtration Rate*

Several factors and hormones have a major effect on RBF and GFR (Table 40-1). As discussed in the previous section, the myogenic mechanism and tubuloglomerular feedback play key roles in maintaining RBF and GFR. *Sympathetic nerves, angiotensin II, prostaglandins, NO, endothelin, bradykinin, and perhaps adenosine exert the major control over RBF and GFR.* The physiological and pathophysiological roles of the other hormones discussed below are under investigation. Fig. 40-20 shows how changes in afferent and efferent arteriolar resistance modulate RBF and GFR.

Sympathetic nerves. The afferent and efferent arterioles are innervated by sympathetic neurons; however, sympathetic tone is minimal when the circulating blood volume is normal (see p 729). Norepinephrine is released by sympathetic nerves, and circulating epinephrine is secreted by the adrenal medulla. These substances cause vasoconstriction by binding to α_1-adrenoceptors, which are located mainly on the afferent arterioles. This binding thereby decreases RBF and GFR. A reduction in the effective circulating blood volume or strong emotional stimuli, such as fear and pain, activate sympathetic nerves and reduce RBF and GFR.

Because **hemorrhage** decreases arterial blood pressure, it activates the sympathetic nerves to the kidneys via the baroreceptor reflex (Fig. 40-21). Norepinephrine causes intense vasoconstriction of the afferent and efferent arterioles, and thereby decreases RBF and GFR. The rise in sympathetic activity also increases the release of epinephrine and angiotensin II, which causes further vasoconstriction and a fall in RBF. The rise in the vascular resistance of the kidney and other vascular beds increases total peripheral resistance. The resultant increased blood pressure (BP = cardiac output × total peripheral resistance) offsets the fall in mean arterial blood pressure caused by hemorrhage (see also Chapter 31). Hence, this system works to preserve arterial pressure at the expense of maintaining a normal RBF and GFR. Importantly, although autoregulatory mechanisms can prevent the effects of changes in arterial pressure on RBF and GFR, sympathetic nerves and angiotensin II have important salutary effects on RBF and GFR.

Angiotensin II. Angiotensin II is produced systemically and within the kidney. It constricts the afferent and efferent arterioles* and decreases RBF and GFR (see Chapter 42 for details on the renin-angiotensin system). Fig. 40-21 shows how norepinephrine, epinephrine, and angiotensin II act together to decrease RBF and GFR, as would occur, for example, with hemorrhage.

Angiotensin converting enzyme (ACE) degrades and thereby inactivates bradykinin and converts angiotensin I, an inactive hormone, to angiotensin II. Thus, ACE increases angiotensin II levels and decreases bradykinin levels. Drugs called **ACE inhibitors,** which reduce systemic blood pressure in

---

*The efferent arteriole is more sensitive to angiotensin II than is the afferent arteriole. Therefore, with low concentrations of angiotensin II, constriction of the efferent arteriole predominates. However, with high concentrations of angiotensin II, constriction of both afferent and efferent arterioles occurs.

■ Table 40-1   Major hormones that influence GFR and RBF

	Stimulus	*Effect on GFR*	*Effect on RBF*
Vasoconstrictors			
Sympathetic nerves	↓ ECV	↓	↓
Angiotensin II	↓ ECV, renin	↓	↓
Endothelin	Shear stress, angiotensin II, bradykinin, epinephrine	↓	↓
Vasodilators			
Prostaglandins (PGI$_2$, PGE$_2$)	↓ ECV, shear stress, angiotensin II	NC	↑
Nitric oxide	Shear stress, acetylcholine, histamine, bradykinin, adenosine triphosphate	↑	↑
Bradykinin	Prostaglandin, ↓ angiotensin converting enzyme	↑	↑

ECV, Effective circulating volume (see p 729).

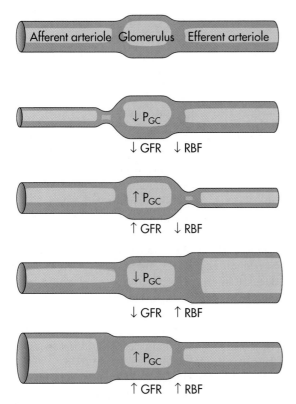

■ **Fig. 40-20**   Relationship between selective changes in the resistance of either the afferent arteriole or efferent arteriole and RBF and GFR. Constriction of either the afferent or efferent arteriole increases resistance. According to equation 40-14 (Q = ΔP/R), an increase in resistance (R) will decrease flow, Q (i.e., RBF). Dilation of either the afferent or efferent arteriole will increase flow (i.e., RBF). Constriction of the afferent arteriole decreases P$_{GC}$ (because less of the arterial pressure is transmitted to the glomerulus) and thereby reduces GFR. In contrast, constriction of the efferent arteriole elevates P$_{GC}$ and thus increases GFR. Dilation of the afferent arteriole increases P$_{GC}$, because more of the arterial pressure is transmitted to the glomerulus, and thereby increases GFR. In contrast, dilation of the efferent arteriole decreases P$_{GC}$ and thus decreases GFR. (Modified from Rose BD, Rennke HG: *Renal pathophysiology: the essentials,* Baltimore, 1994, Williams & Wilkins.)

patients with hypertension, reduce angiotensin II levels and elevate bradykinin levels. These effects lower systemic vascular resistance, reduce blood pressure, and decrease renal vascular resistance. ACE inhibitors therefore increase RBF and GFR (see Chapter 42).

Prostaglandins. Prostaglandins may not regulate RBF or GFR in healthy, resting people. However, during pathophysiological conditions, such as hemorrhage, prostaglandins (PGI$_2$, PGE$_2$) are produced locally within the kidneys and increase RBF without changing GFR. Prostaglandins increase RBF by dampening the vasoconstrictor effects of sympathetic nerves and angiotensin II. This effect of prostaglandins prevents severe and potentially harmful vasoconstriction and renal ischemia. Prostaglandin synthesis is stimulated by decreased effective circulating volume and stress (e.g., surgery, anesthesia), angiotensin II, and sympathetic nerves.

Nitric oxide.   NO, an endothelium-derived relaxing factor, plays an important vasodilatory role in normal conditions, and counteracts vasoconstriction produced by angiotensin II and catecholamines. An increase in shear force acting on endothelial cells in the arterioles, as well as a number of hormones (including acetylcholine, histamine, bradykinin, and ATP), increase the production of NO. This increased NO production causes vasodilation of the afferent and efferent arterioles in the kidneys. In addition, NO decreases total peripheral resistance, and inhibition of NO production increases blood pressure.

*Abnormal production of NO is observed in individuals with **diabetes mellitus** and **hypertension**.* Excess NO production in diabetes may be responsible for the glomerular hyperfiltration and damage of the glomerulus that are characteristic of this disease. Elevated NO levels increase glomerular capillary pressure secondary to a fall in afferent arteriolar resis-

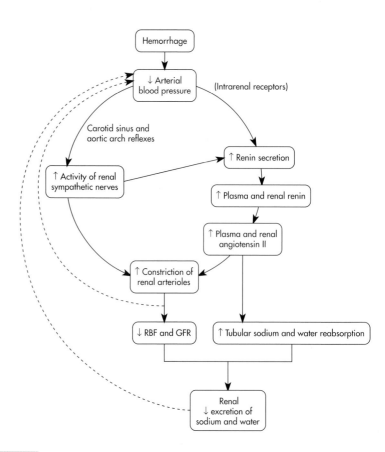

■ **Fig. 40-21**   Pathway by which hemorrhage activates renal sympathetic nerve activity and stimulates angiotensin II production. (Modified from Vander AJ: *Renal physiology,* ed 2, New York, 1980, McGraw-Hill.)

tance. The ensuing hyperfiltration is thought to cause glomerular damage. The normal response to an increase in dietary salt intake includes stimulation of NO production, which maintains blood pressure. In some individuals, NO production may not increase appropriately in response to an increase in salt intake, and therefore blood pressure rises.

Endothelin. Endothelin is a potent vasoconstrictor secreted by endothelial cells of renal vessels, mesangial cells, and distal tubular cells in response to angiotensin II, bradykinin, epinephrine, and shear stress. Endothelin causes profound vasoconstriction of the afferent and efferent arterioles and decreases GFR and RBF. Although this potent vasoconstrictor may not influence GFR and RBF in normal resting subjects, endothelin production is elevated in a number of glomerular disease states (e.g., renal disease associated with diabetes mellitus).

Bradykinin. Kallikrein is a proteolytic enzyme produced in the kidneys. Kallikrein cleaves circulating kininogen to bradykinin, which is a vasodilator that acts by stimulating the release of NO and prostaglandins. Bradykinin increases GFR and RBF.

Adenosine. Adenosine is produced within the kidneys and causes vasoconstriction of the afferent arteriole, thereby reducing RBF and GFR. As previously mentioned, adenosine may play a role in tubuloglomerular feedback.

Atrial natriuretic peptide (ANP). ANP secretion by the heart rises with hypertension and expansion of extra-cellular fluid volume, causing vasodilation of the afferent arteriole and vasoconstriction of the efferent arteriole. The net effect of ANP is therefore to produce a modest increase in GFR with little change in RBF.

ATP. Various cells release ATP into the renal interstitial fluid. ATP has dual effects on GFR and RBF. Under some conditions, ATP constricts the afferent arteriole, reduces RBF and GFR, and may play a role in tubuloglomerular feedback. In contrast, in other situations, ATP may stimulate NO production and increase GFR and RBF.

Glucocorticoids. Administration of therapeutic doses of glucocorticoids increases GFR and RBF.

Histamine. Local release of histamine may play a role in modulating RBF in the normal state and during inflammation and injury. Histamine increases RBF without elevating GFR by decreasing the resistance of the afferent and efferent arterioles.

Dopamine. The proximal tubule produces the vasodilator hormone dopamine. Dopamine has several actions within the kidney, such as increasing RBF and inhibiting renin secretion.

As shown in Fig. 40-22, endothelial cells are important in regulating the resistance of the afferent and efferent arterioles by producing a number of paracrine hormones, including NO, PGI_2, endothelin, and angiotensin II. These hormones regulate contraction or relaxation of smooth muscle cells in afferent and efferent arterioles or mesangial cells. Shear stress, acetylcholine, histamine, bradykinin, and ATP stimulate the

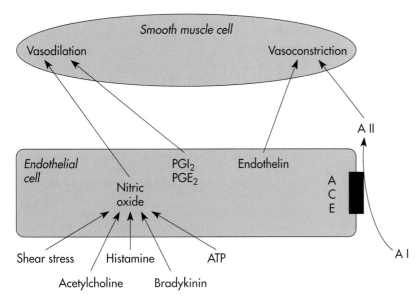

■ **Fig. 40-22**   Examples of interactions of endothelial cells with smooth muscle or mesangial cells. *ACE,* Angiotensin converting enzyme; *AI,* angiotensin I; *AII,* angiotensin II; *PGI₂,* prostaglandin I₂; *PGE₂,* prostaglandin E₂. (Modified from Navar LG et al: *Physiol Rev* 76:425, 1996.)

production of NO, which increases GFR and RBF. Angiotensin converting enzyme (primarily on the surface of endothelial cells lining the afferent arteriole and glomerular capillaries) converts angiotensin I to angiotensin II, which decreases GFR and RBF. Angiotensin II may also be produced in juxtaglomerular cells and proximal tubular cells. PGI_2 and PGE_2 secretion by endothelial cells, stimulated by sympathetic nerve activity or angiotensin II, increases GFR and RBF. Finally, endothelin release from endothelial cells decreases GFR and RBF.

■ *Summary*

1. The functional unit of the kidney is the nephron. Each nephron consists of a renal corpuscle, proximal tubule, loop of Henle, distal tubule, and collecting duct.

2. The renal corpuscle is composed of glomerular capillaries and Bowman's capsule.

3. The juxtaglomerular apparatus is one component of an important feedback mechanism that regulates renal blood flow and glomerular filtration rate. The juxtaglomerular apparatus consists of the macula densa, the extraglomerular mesangial cells, and the renin-producing granular cells in the afferent arteriole.

4. The lower urinary tract consists of the ureters, bladder, and urethra. Micturition is the process of emptying the urinary bladder. The micturition reflex is an automatic spinal cord reflex. However, it can be inhibited or facilitated by centers in the brainstem and cortex.

5. The rate of glomerular filtration is calculated by measuring the clearance of inulin or creatinine. Changes

in GFR can be monitored by measuring the plasma creatinine concentration.

6. Effective renal plasma flow is determined by the clearance of ᴘ-aminohippuric acid (PAH).

7. Starling forces across the glomerular capillaries provide the driving force for the ultrafiltration of plasma from the glomerular capillaries into Bowman's space.

8. The glomerular ultrafiltrate is devoid of cellular elements and contains very little protein, but otherwise is identical to plasma. Proteins with a molecular radius smaller than 20 Å are readily filtered, proteins between 20 and 42 Å are filtered at rates that depend on size and charge (anionic proteins are less readily filtered), and proteins with a molecular radius greater than 42 Å are not filtered.

9. Renal blood flow (1.25 L/min) is about 25% of cardiac output, yet the kidneys constitute less than 0.5% of total body weight. RBF determines the GFR; modifies solute and water reabsorption by the proximal tubule; participates in concentration and dilution of the urine; delivers oxygen, nutrients, and hormones to the cells of the nephron; returns carbon dioxide and reabsorbed fluid and solutes to the general circulation; and delivers substrates for excretion in the urine.

10. Autoregulation allows RBF and GFR to remain constant despite changes in arterial blood pressure between 90 and 180 mm Hg. Autoregulation is achieved by changes in renal vascular resistance mediated by the myogenic reflex and tubuloglomerular feedback.

11. Sympathetic nerves, angiotensin II, prostaglandins, NO, endothelin, bradykinin, and perhaps adenosine exert the most control over RBF and GFR.

■ *Self-Study Problems*

1. A drug that completely inhibits the reabsorption of glucose by the kidney is administered. The following data are obtained to assess this drug's effect on the clearance of glucose. Fill in the missing data.

Before drug

Plasma [inulin]:	1 mg/ml
Plasma [glucose]:	1 mg/ml
Inulin excretion rate:	100 mg/min
Glucose excretion rate;	0 mg/min
Inulin clearance:	_____ ml/min
Glucose clearance:	_____ mlmin

After drug

Plasma [inulin]:	1 mg/ml
Plasma [glucose]:	1 mg/ml
Inulin excretion rate:	100 mg/min
Glucose excretion rate;	_____ mg/min
Inulin clearance:	_____ ml/min
Glucose clearance:	_____ ml/min

How do you explain the change in glucose excretion and clearance seen with this drug?

2. What is the functional significance of the juxta-glomerular apparatus?

3. An individual receives a knife wound to the spinal cord at the level of the twelfth thoracic vertebra. After recovery, his legs are paralyzed and he has no sensation below the waist. With regard to urinary bladder function, he has no sensation of bladder fullness and is incontinent (i.e., unable to control micturition). Studies of his bladder function show spontaneous contractions of the detrusor muscle, especially as the bladder fills with urine. How do you explain this individual's urinary bladder function?

4. Finding which of the following substances in the urine would indicate damage to the glomerular ultrafiltration barrier? Explain why.
   A. Red blood cells
   B. Glucose
   C. Sodium
   D. Proteins

5. Explain how hormones (e.g., sympathetic agonists, angiotensin II, and prostaglandins) change renal blood flow.

■ *Bibliography*

Journal articles

Kriz W, Bankir L: A standard nomenclature for structures of the kidney, *Am J Physiol* 254:F1, 1988.

Navar LG et al: Paracrine regulation of the renal microcirculation, *Physiol Rev* 76(2):425-536, 1996.

Raji L, Bayliss C: Glomerular actions of nitric oxide, *Kidney Int* 48:20-32, 1995.

Toto RD: Conventional measurement of renal function utilizing serum creatinine, creatinine clearance, inulin and para-aminohippuric acid clearance, *Curr Opin Nephrol Hypertens* 4(6):505-509, 1995.

Umans JG, Levi R: Nitric oxide in the regulation of blood flow and arterial pressure, *Ann Rev Physiol* 57:771-790, 1995.

Books and monographs

Arendshorst WJ, Navar LG: *Renal circulation and glomerular hemodynamics.* In Schrier RW, Gottschalk CW, editors: *Diseases of the kidney,* ed 5, Boston, 1993, Little, Brown.

Bradley WE: *Physiology of the urinary bladder.* In Walsh PC, Gittes RF, Perlmutter AD, Stamey TA, editors: *Campbell's urology,* ed 5, Philadelphia, 1986, WB Saunders.

Dworkin LD, Brenner BM: *Biophysical basis of glomerular filtration.* In Seldin DW, Giebisch G, editors: *The kidney: physiology and pathophysiology,* ed 2, New York, 1992, Raven Press.

Dworkin LD, Brenner BM: *The renal circulation.* In Brenner BM, editor: *The kidney,* ed 5, Philadelphia, 1996, WB Saunders.

Carlson JA, Harrington JT: *Laboratory evaluation of renal function.* In Schrier RW, Gottschalk CW, editors: *Diseases of the kidney,* ed 5, Boston, 1993, Little, Brown.

Fanestil DD: *Compartmentation of body water.* In Narins RG, editor: *Clinical disorders of fluid and electrolyte metabolism,* ed 5, New York, 1994, McGraw-Hill.

Kriz W, Kaissling B: *Structural organization of the mammalian kidney.* In Seldin DW, Giebisch G, editors: *The kidney: physiology and pathophysiology,* ed 2, New York, 1992, Raven Press.

Maddox DA, Brenner BM: *Glomerular ultrafiltration.* In Brenner BM, editor: *The kidney,* ed 5, Philadelphia, 1996, WB Saunders.

Rose BD: *Clinical physiology of acid-base and electrolyte disorders,* ed 4, New York, 1994, McGraw-Hill .

Schuster VL, Seldin DW: *Renal clearance.* In Seldin DW, Giebisch G, editors: *The kidney: physiology and pathophysiology,* ed 2, New York, 1992, Raven Press.

Tanagho EA: *Anatomy of the genitourinary tract.* In Tanagho EA, McAnich JW, editors: *Smith's general urology,* ed 14, Norwalk, Conn, 1995, Appleton & Lange.

Tisher CC, Madsen KM: *Anatomy of the kidney.* In Brenner BM, editor: *The kidney,* ed 5, Philadelphia, 1996, WB Saunders.

Tucker MS, Stafford SJ: *Disorders of micturition.* In Schrier RW, Gottschalk CW, editors: *Diseases of the kidney,* ed 5, Boston, 1993, Little, Brown.

Ulfendahl HR, Wolgast M: *Renal circulation and lymphatics.* In Seldin DW, Giebisch G, editors: *The kidney: physiology and pathophysiology,* ed 2, New York, 1992, Raven Press.

Solute and Water Transport along the Nephron: Tubular Function

Formation of urine involves three basic processes:

- Ultrafiltration of plasma by the glomerulus
- Reabsorption of water and solutes from the ultrafiltrate
- Secretion of selected solutes into the tubular fluid

Although 180 L of essentially protein-free fluid is filtered by the human glomeruli each day,* less than 1% of the filtered water and NaCl, and variable amounts of the other solutes, are excreted in the urine (Table 41-1). By the processes of reabsorption and secretion, the renal tubules modulate the volume and composition of the urine (Table 41-2). Consequently, the tubules precisely control the volume, osmolality, composition, and pH of the intracellular and extracellular fluid compartments.

The first part of this chapter defines basic transport mechanisms used by kidney cells to reabsorb and secrete solutes. Then, NaCl and water reabsorption and some of the factors and hormones that regulate reabsorption are discussed. Details on acid-base transport; K^+, Ca^{++}, and P_i transport; and their regulation are provided in Chapters 43 and 44.

■ General Principles of Membrane Transport

Solutes may be transported across cell membranes by passive mechanisms, by active transport mechanisms, or by endocytosis. In mammals, solute movement occurs by both passive and active mechanisms, whereas *all water movement is passive* (see Box 41-1).

*The normal glomerular filtration rate (GFR) averages 127-184 L/day in women and 140-197 L/day in men. Thus, the volume of the ultrafiltrate represents a volume 10 times that of the extracellular fluid volume. For simplicity, throughout the remainder of this book, we will assume that the GFR is 180 L/day.

■ **Table 41-1**   Filtration, excretion, and reabsorption of water, electrolytes, and solutes

Substance	Measure	Filtered	Excreted	Reabsorbed	% Filtered load reabsorbed
Water	L/day	180	1.5	178.5	99.2
Na^+	mEq/day	25,200	150	25,050	99.4
K^+	mEq/day	720	100	620	86.1
Ca^{++}	mEq/day	540	10	530	98.2
HCO_3^-	mEq/day	4320	2	4318	99.9+
Cl^-	mEq/day	18,000	150	17,850	99.2
Glucose	mmol/day	800	0	800	100.0
Urea	g/day	56	28	28	50.0

The filtered amount of any substance is calculated by multiplying the concentration of that substance in the ultrafiltrate by the glomerular filtration rate (GFR); for example, the filtered load of Na^+ is calculated as $[Na^+]$ultrafiltrate (140 mEq/L) $\times$ GFR (180 L/day) = 25,200 mEq/day.

■ **Table 41-2**   Composition of urine

Substance	Concentration
Na^+	50-130 mEq/L
K^+	20-70 mEq/L
NH_4^+	30-50 mEq/L
Ca^{++}	5-12 mEq/L
Mg^{++}	2-18 mEq/L
Cl^-	50-130 mEq/L
P_i	20-40 mEq/L
Urea	200-400 mM
Creatinine	6-20 mM
pH	5.0-7.0
Osmolality	500-800 mOsm/kg H_2O
Glucose*	0
Amino acids*	0
Protein*	0
Blood*	0
Ketones*	0
Leukocytes*	0
Bilirubin*	0

Modified from Valtin HV: *Renal physiology*, ed 2, Boston, 1983, Little, Brown.

*These values represent average ranges. Asterisks indicate that the presence of these substances in freshly voided urine is measured with dipstick reagent strips. These small strips of plastic contain reagents that change color in a semiquantitative manner in the presence of specific compounds. Water excretion ranges between 0.5 and 1.5 L/day.

■ *Passive Mechanisms*

Passive movement of a solute across a membrane develops spontaneously and does not require direct expenditure of metabolic energy. In **passive transport (diffusion),** uncharged solutes move from an area of higher concentration to an area of lower concentration (i.e., down their chemical concentration gradient). Additionally, because ions are charged, the passive diffusion of ions is affected by the electrical potential difference (i.e., electrical gradient) across cell membranes and across the renal tubules. Cations (Na^+, K^+, and so forth) move to the negative side of the membrane, whereas anions (Cl^-, HCO_3^-, and so forth) move to the positive side of the membrane. Diffusion of lipid-soluble substances, such as the gases O_2, CO_2, and NH_3, occurs across the lipid bilayer of plasma membranes. Diffusion of water **(osmosis)** occurs through channels in the cell membrane and is driven by osmotic pressure gradients. When water is reabsorbed across tubule segments, the solutes dissolved in the water are also carried along with the water. This process, called **solvent drag,** can account for a substantial amount of solute reabsorption across the proximal tubule.

In **facilitated diffusion,** transport depends on the interaction of the solute with a specific protein in the membrane that facilitates movement of the solute across the membrane. In a broad application, the term facilitated diffusion describes several different types of membrane transporters. For example, one form of facilitated diffusion is the diffusion of ions (such as Na^+ and K^+) across membranes. These ions move through water-filled channels created by proteins that span the plasma membrane. Another example is the movement of a single molecule across the membrane by means of a transport protein **(uniport),** as occurs with urea and glucose.*

---

*Some authors restrict the term *facilitated diffusion* to this type of transport, and use as the classic example the glucose uniporter that brings glucose into a wide variety of cells (e.g., skeletal muscle cells).

A third form of facilitated diffusion is **coupled transport,** in which two or more solutes move across a membrane by interacting with a specific transport protein. Coupled transport of two or more solutes in the same direction is mediated by a **symport mechanism.** Examples of symport mechanisms in the kidneys include Na^+-glucose, Na^+-amino acid, and Na^+-phosphate symporters in the proximal tubule and $1Na^+$-$1K^+$-$2Cl^-$ symport in the thick ascending limb of Henle's loop. Coupled transport of two or more solutes in opposite directions is mediated by an **antiport mechanism.** For example, Na^+-H^+ antiporter in the proximal tubule mediates Na^+ reabsorption and H^+ secretion. With coupled transporters, at least one of the solutes is usually transported against its chemical (and electrical) gradient. The energy for this uphill movement is derived from the passive downhill movement of at least one of the other solutes into the cell. For example, in the proximal tubule, operation of the Na^+-H^+ antiporter in the cell's apical membrane causes H^+ to move against its electrochemical gradient out of the cell into the tubular lumen. This uphill movement of H^+ is driven by the movement of Na^+ from the tubular lumen into the cell down its electrochemical gradient. The uphill movement of H^+ is termed **secondary active transport** because the movement of H^+ is not directly coupled to the hydrolysis of adenosine triphosphate (ATP) (see below). Instead, the energy is derived from the gradient of the other coupled ion (in this example, Na^+).

■ *Active Mechanisms*

Transport is active if it is coupled directly to energy derived from metabolic processes (i.e., consumes ATP). In **active transport,** solutes usually move from an area of lower concentration to an area of higher concentration. In the kidney, *the most prevalent active transport mechanism is the Na^+, K^+-ATPase* (or sodium pump). Located in the basolateral membrane, the Na^+, K^+-ATPase is composed of several proteins. Together these proteins actively move Na^+ out of the cell and move K^+ into the cell. Other active transport mechanisms in the kidneys include the H^+-ATPase, H^+, K^+-ATPase, and Ca^{++}-ATPase. H^+-ATPase and H^+, K^+-ATPase are responsible for H^+ secretion in the collecting duct system (see Chapter 44). The Ca^{++}-ATPase is responsible for Ca^{++} movement from the cytoplasm into the blood (see Chapter 43).

Endocytosis is another form of active transport. In **endocytosis,** a section of the plasma membrane invaginates. The portions around this invagination then engulf the substance being transported. Once the substance is engulfed, the membrane completely pinches off and forms a vesicle in the cytoplasm. Endocytosis is an important mechanism for reabsorbing small proteins and macromolecules by the proximal tubule and for the retrieval of water channels from the apical membrane of collecting duct cells. Because endocytosis requires ATP, it is a form of active transport.

■ *General Principles of Transepithelial Solute and Water Transport*

Renal cells are held together by **tight junctions** (Fig. 41-1). The tight junctions separate the apical membranes from the basolateral membranes. Below the tight junctions, the cells are separated by lateral intercellular spaces. A useful way to visualize the renal epithelium is to consider a six-pack of soda: the soda cans are the cells and the plastic holder represents the tight junctions.

In the nephron, a substance can be reabsorbed or secreted through cells (the transcellular pathway) or between cells (the paracellular pathway) (Fig. 41-1). Na^+ reabsorption by the proximal tubule is a good example of transport by the **transcellular pathway.** Na^+ reabsorp-

tion in this nephron segment depends on the operation of Na^+, K^+-ATPase (Fig. 41-1). Na^+, K^+-ATPase is located exclusively in the basolateral membrane. This pump moves Na^+ out of the cell into the blood and moves K^+ into the cell. Thus, Na^+, K^+-ATPase lowers intracellular Na^+ concentration and increases intracellular K^+ concentration. Because intracellular $[Na^+]$ is low (12 mEq/L) and the $[Na^+]$ in tubular fluid is high (145 mEq/L), Na^+ moves across the apical cell membrane down a chemical concentration gradient from the tubular lumen into the cell. Na^+, K^+-ATPase, sensing the addition of Na^+ to the cell, is stimulated to increase the rate of Na^+ extrusion into the blood. This action returns intracellular Na^+ to normal levels. Transcellular Na^+ reabsorption by the proximal tubule is thus a two-step process:

1. Na^+ moves across the apical membrane into the cell down an electrochemical gradient established by Na^+, K^+-ATPase.
2. Na^+ moves across the basolateral membrane against an electrochemical gradient via Na^+, K^+-ATPase.

The reabsorption of Ca^{++} and K^+ across the proximal tubule is a good example of **paracellular transport.**

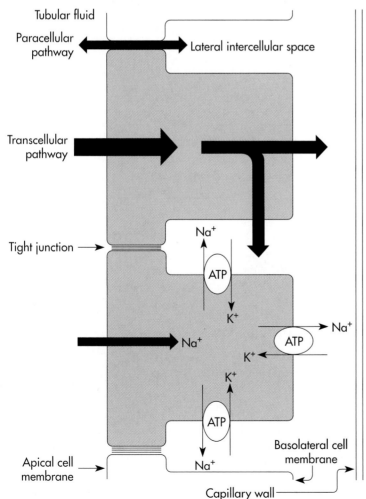

■ **Fig. 41-1** Paracellular and transcellular transport pathways in the proximal tubule. See text for details. *ATP,* Adenosine triphosphate.

Some of the water reabsorbed across the proximal tubule crosses the paracellular pathway. Some solutes dissolved in this water (in particular Ca++ and K+) are carried along with the reabsorbed fluid and are reabsorbed by the process of solvent drag.

■ *NaCl, Solute, and Water Reabsorption along the Nephron*

In a quantitative sense, the reabsorption of NaCl and water represents the major function of the nephrons (approximately 25,000 mEq/day of Na+ and 179 L/day of water are reabsorbed; Table 41-1). In addition, the transport of many other important solutes is linked either directly or indirectly to Na+ reabsorption. In the following sections, we discuss the NaCl and water transport properties of each nephron segment and its regulation by hormones and other factors.

■ *Proximal Tubule*

The proximal tubule reabsorbs approximately 67% of the filtered water, Na+, Cl− , K+, and other solutes. In addition, the proximal tubule reabsorbs virtually all the glucose and amino acids filtered by the glomerulus. *The key element in proximal tubule reabsorption is the Na+, K+-ATPase in the basolateral membrane.* The reabsorption of every substance, including water, is linked in some way to the operation of Na+, K+-ATPase.

Na+ reabsorption. Na+ is reabsorbed by different mechanisms in the early (first half) and late (second half) segments of the proximal tubule. In the early segment, Na+ is reabsorbed primarily with HCO₃⁻ and a number of organic molecules (e.g., glucose, amino acids, Pᵢ, lactate). By contrast, in the second half of the proximal tubule, Na+ is reabsorbed mainly with Cl⁻. This difference exists because of differences in Na+ transport systems present in the early and late segments of the proxi-

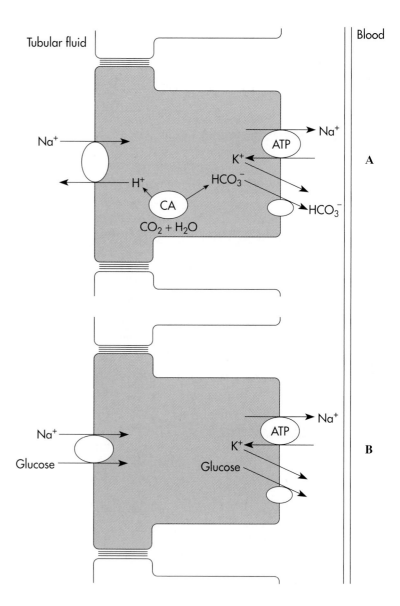

■ **Fig. 41-2** Na+ transport processes in the first half of the proximal tubule. The transport mechanisms depicted in **A** and **B** are present in all cells in the first half of the proximal tubule. They are separated into different cells to simplify the discussion. **A,** The operation of the Na+-H+ antiporter in the apical membrane and the Na+, K+-ATPase and the HCO₃⁻ transporter in the basolateral membrane mediate NaHCO₃ reabsorption. CO₂ and H₂O combine inside the cells to form H+ and HCO₃⁻ in a reaction facilitated by the enzyme carbonic anhydrase *(CA)*. **B,** The operation of the Na+-glucose transporter in the apical membrane, in conjunction with the Na+, K+-ATPase and the glucose transporter in the basolateral membrane, mediate Na+-glucose reabsorption. Na+ reabsorption is also coupled with other solutes, including amino acids, Pᵢ, and lactate. Reabsorption of these solutes is mediated by Na+-amino acid, Na+-Pᵢ, and Na+-lactate symporters located in the apical membrane and the Na+, K+-ATPase and the amino acid, Pᵢ, and lactate transporters in the basolateral membrane.

mal tubule, and because of differences in the composition of tubular fluid at these sites.

As illustrated in Fig. 41-2, in the early segment of the proximal tubule, Na^+ uptake into the cell is coupled with either H^+ or organic solutes. Na^+ entry into the cell across the apical membrane is mediated by specific symporter and antiporter proteins, and not by diffusion through channels. For example, Na^+ entry is coupled with the pumping of H^+ out of the cell by the Na^+-H^+ antiporter (Fig. 41-2, *A*). H^+ secretion results in $NaHCO_3$ reabsorption (see also Chapter 44). Na^+ also enters proximal cells by several symporter mechanisms, including Na^+-glucose, Na^+-amino acid, Na^+-P_i, and Na^+-lactate symporters (Fig. 41-2, *B*). The glucose (and other organic solutes) that enters the cell with Na^+ leaves the cell across the basolateral membrane by passive transporter mechanisms. Any Na^+ that enters the cell across the apical membrane leaves the cell and enters the blood via the Na^+, K^+-ATPase. *In brief, in the early segment of the proximal tubule, the reabsorption of Na^+ is coupled to that of HCO_3^- and a number of organic molecules.* Reabsorption of many organic molecules is so avid in this segment that they are almost completely removed from the tubular fluid (Fig. 41-3). The reabsorption of $NaHCO_3$ and Na^+-organic solutes across the proximal tubule establishes a transtubular osmotic gradient that provides the driving force for the passive reabsorption of water by osmosis. Because more water than Cl^- is reabsorbed in the early segment of the proximal tubule, the Cl^- concentration in tubular fluid rises along the length of the early proximal tubule (Fig. 41-3).

In the second half of the proximal tubule, Na^+ is primarily reabsorbed with Cl^- across both the transcellular and paracellular pathways (Fig. 41-4). Na^+ is reabsorbed with Cl^- rather than with organic solutes or HCO_3^- as the accompanying anion. This occurs because the cells lining the late proximal tubule have different Na^+ transport mechanisms from those in the early proximal tubule. Furthermore, the tubular fluid that enters the late proximal tubule contains very little glucose and amino acids but has a high concentration of Cl^- (140 mEq/L) compared with that in the early proximal tubule (105 mEq/L). The high Cl^- concentration is due to the preferential reabsorption of Na^+ with HCO_3^- and organic solutes in the early proximal tubule (Fig. 41-2).

The mechanism of transcellular Na^+ reabsorption in the late proximal tubule is shown in Fig. 41-4. Na^+ enters the cell across the luminal membrane by the parallel operation of Na^+-H^+ and one or more Cl^- anion antiporters. Because the secreted H^+ and anion combine in the tubular fluid and reenter the cell, the operation of the Na^+-H^+ and Cl^- anion antiporters is equivalent to NaCl uptake from tubular fluid into the cell. Na^+ leaves the cell by the action of Na^+, K^+-ATPase, and Cl^- leaves the cell by the action of a KCl symport protein in the basolateral membrane.

NaCl is also reabsorbed across the late proximal tubule by a paracellular route. *Paracellular NaCl reabsorption occurs because the rise in $[Cl^-]$ in the tubular fluid in the early proximal tubule creates a concentration gradient of Cl^- (140 mEq/L in the tubule lumen and 105 mEq/L in the interstitium). This concentration gradient favors the diffusion of Cl^- from the tubular lumen across the tight junctions into the lateral intercellular space.* Movement of the negatively charged Cl^- causes the tubular fluid to become positively charged relative to the blood. This positive transepithelial voltage causes the diffusion of positively charged Na^+ out of the tubular fluid

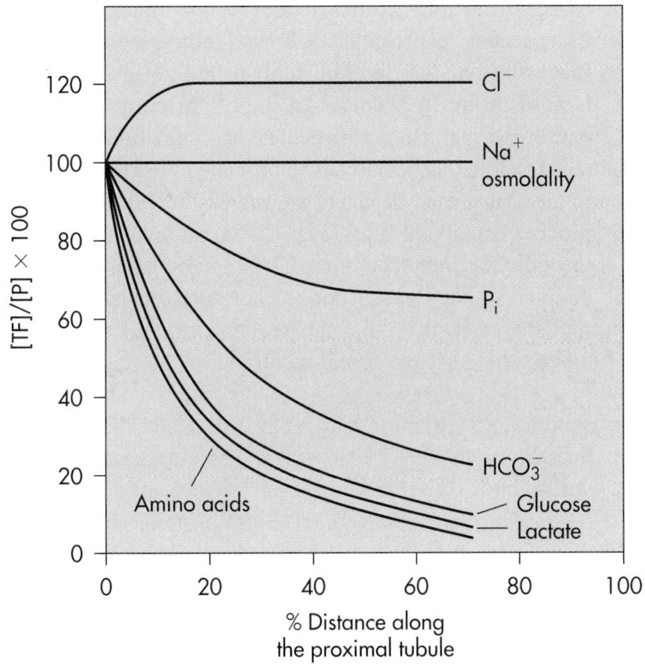

■ Fig. 41-3   Concentration of solutes in tubular fluid as a function of length along the proximal tubule. [TF] is the concentration of the substance in tubular fluid; [P] is the concentration of the substance in plasma. Values above 100 indicate that relatively less of the solute than water was reabsorbed; values below 100 indicate that relatively more of the substance than water was reabsorbed. (Modified from Vander AJ: *Renal physiology*, ed 4, New York, 1991, McGraw-Hill.)

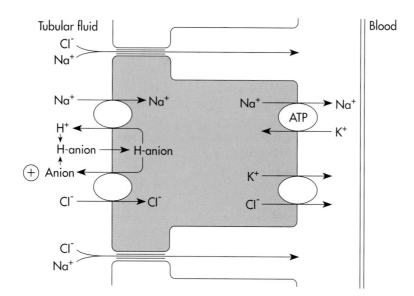

■ **Fig. 41-4**   Na⁺ transport processes in the second half of the proximal tubule. Na⁺ and Cl⁻ enter the cell across the apical membrane by the operation of parallel Na⁺-H⁺ and Cl⁻-anion antiporters. More than one Cl⁻ anion antiporter may be involved in this process, but only one is depicted here. The secreted H⁺ and anion combine in the tubular fluid to form an H⁺-anion complex that can recycle across the plasma membrane. Accumulation of H⁺-anion in tubular fluid establishes an H⁺-anion concentration gradient that favors H⁺-anion recycling across the apical plasma membrane into the cell. Inside the cell H⁺ and the anion dissociate and recycle back across the apical plasma membrane. The net result is NaCl uptake across the apical membrane. The anion may be OH⁻, formate (HCO$_2$⁻), oxalate⁻, HCO$_3$⁻, or sulfate. The lumen-positive transepithelial voltage (indicated by the plus sign inside the circle in the tubular lumen) is generated by the diffusion of Cl⁻ (lumen-to-blood) across the tight junction. The high [Cl⁻] of tubular fluid provides the driving force for Cl⁻ diffusion.

across the tight junction into the blood. Thus, in the late proximal tubule, some Na⁺ and Cl⁻ is reabsorbed across the tight junctions by passive diffusion. The reabsorption of NaCl establishes a transtubular osmotic gradient that provides the driving force for the passive reabsorption of water by osmosis (as described below).

In summary, reabsorption of Na⁺ and Cl⁻ in the proximal tubule occurs across the paracellular pathway and across the transcellular pathway. Approximately 17,000 mEq of the 25,200 mEq of NaCl filtered each day is reabsorbed in the proximal tubule (~67% of the filtered load). Of this, two thirds is transported across the transcellular pathway, while the remaining one third is transported across the paracellular pathway (Tables 41-3 and 41-4).

Water reabsorption.   The proximal tubule reabsorbs 67% of the filtered water (Fig. 41-5). *The driving force for water reabsorption is a transtubular osmotic gradient established by solute reabsorption (i.e., NaCl, Na⁺-glucose, and so forth).* The reabsorption of Na⁺ along with organic solutes HCO$_3$⁻ and Cl⁻ from the tubular fluid into the lateral intercellular spaces reduces the osmolality of the tubular fluid and increases the osmolality of the lateral intercellular space. Because the proximal tubule is highly permeable to water, water will flow by osmosis

across both the tight junctions and the proximal tubular cells. Accumulation of fluid and solutes within the lateral intercellular space increases the hydrostatic pressure in this compartment. This increased hydrostatic pressure forces fluid and solutes to move into the capillaries. Thus, water reabsorption follows solute reabsorption in the proximal tubule. The reabsorbed fluid is slightly hyperosmotic to plasma. An important consequence of osmotic water flow across the proximal tubule is that some solutes, especially K⁺ and Ca⁺⁺, are carried along in the reabsorbed fluid and are thereby reabsorbed by the process of solvent drag (Fig. 41-5). The reabsorption of virtually all organic solutes, Cl⁻, other ions, and water is coupled to Na⁺ reabsorption. Therefore, changes in Na⁺ reabsorption influence the reabsorption of water and other solutes by the proximal tubule.

Fanconi's syndrome is a renal disease that is either hereditary or acquired. It results from an impaired ability of the proximal tubule to reabsorb amino acids, glucose, and low-molecular-weight proteins. Because other segments of the nephron cannot reabsorb these solutes, Fanconi's syndrome causes an increase in the excretion of amino acids, glucose, P$_i$, and low-molecular-weight proteins in the urine.

Tubular fluid

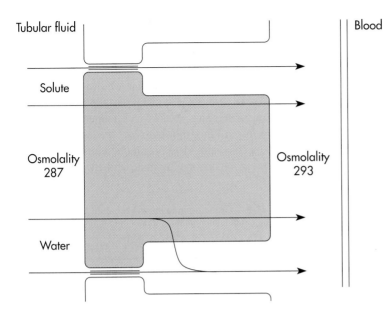

Blood

■ **Fig. 41-5** Routes of water and solute reabsorption across the proximal tubule. Transport of solutes, including Na⁺, Cl⁻, and organic solutes, into the lateral intercellular space increases the osmolality of this compartment, which establishes the driving force for osmotic water reabsorption across the proximal tubule. This occurs because some Na⁺, K⁺-ATPase and some transporters of organic solute, HCO₃⁻, and Cl⁻, are located on the lateral cell membranes and deposit these solutes between cells. Furthermore, some NaCl also enters the lateral intercellular space by diffusion across the tight junction (i.e., paracellular pathway). An important consequence of osmotic water flow across the transcellular and paracellular pathways in the proximal tubule is that some solutes, especially K⁺ and Ca⁺⁺, are carried along in the reabsorbed fluid and are thereby reabsorbed by the process of solvent drag.

■ **Table 41-3**   NaCl transport along the nephron

Segment	Percentage filtered reabsorbed	Mechanism of Na⁺ entry across the apical membrane	Major regulatory hormones
Proximal tubule	67%	Na⁺-H⁺ exchange, Na⁺-cotransport with amino acids and organic solutes, Na⁺/H⁺-Cl⁻/anion exchange Paracellular	Angiotensin II Norepinephrine Epinephrine Dopamine
Loop of Henle	25%	1Na⁺-1K⁺-2Cl⁻ symport	Aldosterone
Distal tubule	~4%	NaCl symport	Aldosterone
Late distal tubule and collecting duct	~3%	Na⁺ channels	Aldosterone Atrial natriuretic peptide Urodilatin

■ **Table 41-4**   Water transport along the nephron

Segment	Percentage of filtered load reabsorbed	Mechanism of water reabsorption	Hormones that regulate water permeability
Proximal tubule	67%	Passive	None
Loop of Henle	15%	DTL only; passive	None
Distal tubule	0%	No water reabsorption	None
Late distal tubule and collecting duct	~8%-17%	Passive	ADH, ANP*

*ANP inhibits the ADH-stimulated water permeability.
ADH, Antidiuretic hormone; *ANP,* atrial natriuretic peptide.

Protein reabsorption. Proteins filtered by the glomerulus are also reabsorbed in the proximal tubule. As mentioned previously, peptide hormones, small proteins, and even small amounts of larger proteins, such as albumin, are filtered by the glomerulus. The glomerulus filters only a small amount of proteins (the concentration of proteins in the ultrafiltrate is only 40 mg/L). However, the amount of protein filtered per day is significant because the GFR is so high:

filtered protein = GFR × [protein] in the ultrafiltrate
filtered protein = 180 L/day × 40 mg/L = 7.2 g/day

Protein reabsorption in the proximal tubule begins when the proteins are partially degraded by enzymes on the surface of the proximal tubule cells. These partially degraded proteins are taken into the cell by endocytosis. Once they are inside the cell, enzymes digest the proteins and peptides into their constituent amino acids. Amino acids then exit the cell across the basolateral membrane and return to the blood. Normally, this mechanism reabsorbs virtually all of the protein filtered and hence the urine is essentially protein free. However, because the mechanism is easily saturated, if the amount of protein filtered increases, protein will appear in the urine.

Disruption of the glomerular filtration barrier to proteins will increase the filtration of proteins and result in **proteinuria** (the appearance of protein in the urine). Proteinuria is frequently seen with kidney disease.

During routine urinalysis, it is not abnormal to find traces of protein in the urine. Protein in the urine can be derived from two sources: (1) filtration and incomplete reabsorption by the proximal tubule and (2) synthesis by the thick ascending limb of Henle's loop. Cells in the thick ascending limb produce **Tamm-Horsfall glycoprotein** and secrete the protein into the tubular fluid. Because the mechanism for protein reabsorption is upstream of the thick ascending limb (i.e., proximal tubule), the secreted Tamm-Horsfall glycoprotein appears in the urine.

Organic anion and organic cation secretion. In addition to reabsorbing solutes and water, cells of the proximal tubule secrete organic cations and organic anions (Tables 41-5 and 41-6 present a partial listing). Many of these organic anions and cations are end products of metabolism that circulate in the plasma. The proximal tubule also secretes numerous exogenous organic compounds, including P-aminohippuric acid (PAH), drugs such as penicillin, and pollutants. Many of these organic compounds can be bound to plasma proteins and are not readily filtered. Therefore, excretion by filtration alone eliminates only a small portion of these potentially toxic substances from the body. Such substances are also secreted from the peritubular capillaries into the tubular fluid. These secretory mechanisms are very powerful and remove virtually all organic anions and cations from the plasma entering the kidneys. Hence, these substances are removed from the plasma by both filtration and secretion.

An example of organic anion secretion is PAH transport across the proximal tubule (Fig. 41-6). This secretory pathway has a maximal transport rate, has a low specificity (i.e., it transports a variety of organic anions), and is responsible for the secretion of all organic anions listed in Table 41-5. PAH is taken into the cell across the basolateral membrane, against its chemical gradient, in exchange for α-ketoglutarate (αKG) via a PAH-αKG antiport mechanism. αKG accumulates inside the cells via the metabolism of glutamate and by an Na^+-αKG

■ **Table 41-5**   Some organic anions secreted by the proximal tubule

Endogenous anions	Drugs
Cyclic adenosine monophosphate (cAMP)	Acetazolamide
Bile salts	Chlorothiazide
Hippurates	Furosemide
Oxalate	Penicillin
Prostaglandins	Probenecid
Urate	Salicylate (aspirin)
	Hydrochlorothiazide
	Bumetanide

■ **Table 41-6**   Some organic cations secreted by the proximal tubule

Endogenous cations	Drugs
Creatinine	Atropine
Dopamine	Isoproterenol
Epinephrine	Cimetidine
Norepinephrine	Morphine
	Quinine
	Amiloride
	Procainamide

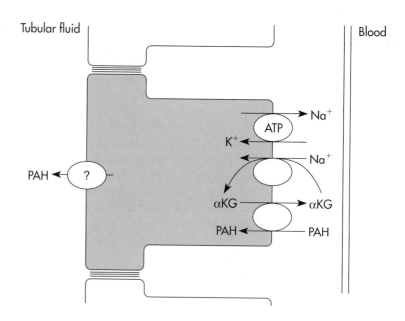

■ **Fig. 41-6**   Organic anion secretion (e.g., P-aminohippuric acid [PAH]) across the proximal tubule. PAH enters the cell across the basolateral membrane by a PAH-α-ketoglutarate (αKG) antiport mechanism. The uptake of αKG into the cell, against its chemical gradient, is driven by the movement of Na^+ into the cell. The αKG recycles across the basolateral membrane. PAH leaves the cell across the apical membrane down its chemical concentration gradient by an unknown mechanism.

symporter, also present in the basolateral membrane. Thus, PAH uptake into the cell against its electrochemical gradient is coupled to the exit of αKG out of the cell down its chemical gradient; this activity is generated by the Na$^+$-αKG antiport mechanism and the metabolism of glutamate. The resultant high intracellular concentration of PAH provides the driving force for PAH exit across the luminal membrane into the tubular fluid via a PAH-anion antiporter (Fig. 41-6).

Because all organic anions compete for the same transporter, elevated plasma levels of one anion inhibit the secretion of the others. For example, infusing PAH can produce a reduction of penicillin secretion by the proximal tubule. Because the kidneys are responsible for eliminating penicillin, the infusion of PAH into individuals receiving penicillin reduces urinary penicillin excretion, and thereby extends the biological half-life of the drug. In World War II, when penicillin was in short supply, hippurates were given with the penicillin to extend the drug's therapeutic effect.

Fig. 41-7 illustrates the mechanism of organic cation (OC$^+$) transport across the proximal tubule. Organic cations are taken into the cell, across the basolateral membrane, by a mechanism that involves facilitated diffusion. This uniport mechanism is driven by the magnitude of the voltage difference (negative potential) across the basolateral membrane. Organic cation transport across the luminal membrane into the tubular fluid is mediated by an OC$^+$-H$^+$ antiporter. Because the transport mechanisms for organic cation secretion are nonspecific, several cations compete for the transport pathway (Table 41-6).

The histamine H$_2$-antagonist **cimetidine** is used to treat gastric ulcers. Cimetidine is secreted by the organic cation pathway in the proximal tubule. It reduces the urinary excretion of the antiarrhythmic drug **procainamide** (also an organic cation), by competing with procainamide for the secretory pathway. Note that coadministration of organic cations can increase the plasma concentration of both drugs to levels much higher than those seen when the drugs are given alone. This increase can lead to drug toxicity.

■ *Henle's Loop*

Henle's loop reabsorbs approximately 25% of the filtered NaCl and K$^+$. Ca^{++} and HCO$_3^-$ are also reabsorbed in the loop of Henle (see Chapters 43 and 44 for more details). This reabsorption occurs almost exclusively in the thick ascending limb. By comparison, the ascending thin limb has a much lower reabsorptive capacity, and the descending thin limb does not reabsorb significant amounts of solutes. The loop of Henle reabsorbs approximately 15% of the filtered water. Water reabsorption occurs exclusively in the descending thin limb. *The ascending limb is impermeable to water.*

The key element in solute reabsorption by the thick ascending limb is the Na$^+$, K$^+$-ATPase in the basolateral membrane (Fig. 41-8). As with reabsorption in the proximal tubule, the reabsorption of every solute by the thick ascending limb is in some way linked to Na$^+$, K$^+$-ATPase. This pump maintains a low intracellular [Na$^+$]. This low [Na$^+$] provides a favorable chemical gradient for the movement of Na$^+$ from the tubular fluid into the cell. The movement of Na$^+$ across the apical membrane

Tubular fluid

Blood

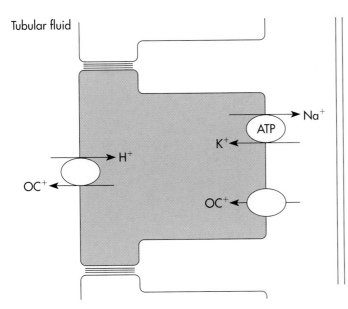

■ **Fig. 41-7** Organic cation secretion *(OC$^+$)* across the proximal tubule. OC$^+$ enters the cell across the basolateral membrane by facilitated diffusion. The uptake of OC$^+$ into the cell, against its chemical gradient, is driven by the cell-negative potential difference. OC$^+$ leaves the cell across the apical membrane in exchange with H$^+$ by an OC$^+$-H$^+$ antiport mechanism.

into the cell is mediated by the 1Na+-1K+-2Cl− symporter, which couples the movement of 1Na+ with 1K+ and 2Cl−. Using the potential energy released by the downhill movement of Na+ and Cl−, this symport drives the uphill movement of K+ into the cell. An Na+-H+ antiporter in the apical cell membrane also mediates Na+ reabsorption as well as H+ secretion (HCO3− reabsorption) in the thick ascending limb (Chapter 44 contains details of HCO3− reabsorption by the thick ascending limb). Na+ leaves the cell across the basolateral membrane via the action of Na+, K+-ATPase, and K+, Cl− and HCO3− leave the cell across the basolateral membrane by separate pathways.

The voltage across the thick ascending limb is important in the reabsorption of several cations. The tubular fluid is positively charged relative to the blood because of the unique location of transport proteins in the apical and basolateral membranes. *Two points are important here: (1) increased salt transport by the thick ascending limb increases the magnitude of the positive charge in the lumen and (2) this voltage is an important driving force for the reabsorption of several cations, including Na+, K+, and Ca++ across the paracellular pathway* (Fig. 41-8). Thus, salt reabsorption across the thick ascending limb occurs by transcellular and paracellular pathways.

Fifty percent of solute transport is transcellular and 50% is paracellular. Because the thick ascending limb is impermeable to water, reabsorption of NaCl and other solutes reduces the osmolality of tubular fluid to less than 150 mOsm/Kg H2O.

Inhibition of the 1Na+-1K+-2Cl− symporter in the thick ascending limb by loop diuretics, such as **furosemide,** inhibits NaCl reabsorption by the thick ascending limb and thereby increases urinary NaCl excretion. Furosemide also inhibits K+ and Ca++ reabsorption by reducing the lumen-positive voltage, which drives the paracellular reabsorption of these ions. Thus, furosemide also increases urinary K+ and Ca++ excretion. Furosemide also increases water excretion by reducing the osmolality of the interstitial fluid in the medulla. Water reabsorption by the descending thin limb of Henle's loop is passive and driven by the osmotic gradient between the tubular fluid in the descending thin limb (which is ~290 mOsm/kg H2O at the beginning of the limb) and the interstitial fluid (which is ~1200 mOsm/kg H2O in the medulla). Thus, a reduction of the osmolality of the interstitial fluid will reduce water reabsorption and thereby increase excretion.

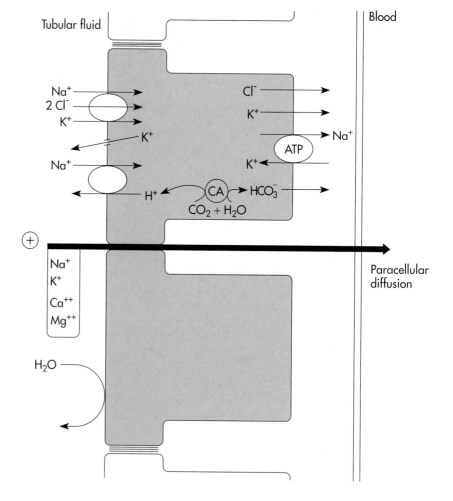

■ **Fig. 41-8** Transport mechanisms for NaCl reabsorption in the thick ascending limb of Henle's loop. The positive charge in the lumen plays a major role in driving passive paracellular reabsorption of cations. *CA,* Carbonic anhydrase.

■ *Distal Tubule and Collecting Duct*

The distal tubule and the collecting duct reabsorb approximately 7% of the filtered NaCl, secrete variable amounts of K+ and H+, and reabsorb a variable amount of water (~8%-17%). Water reabsorption depends on the plasma concentration of ADH. The initial segment of the distal tubule (early distal tubule) reabsorbs Na+, Cl−, and Ca++, and is impermeable to water (Fig. 41-9). NaCl entry into the cell across the apical membrane is mediated by a Na+-Cl− symporter (Fig. 41-9). Na+ leaves the cell via the action of Na+, K+-ATPase, and Cl− leaves the cell by diffusion via channels. NaCl reabsorption is reduced by **thiazide diuretics,** which inhibit the Na+-Cl− symporter. Thus, the dilution of the tubular fluid begins in the thick ascending limb and continues in the early distal tubule.

The last segments of the distal tubule (late distal tubule) and of the collecting duct are composed of two cell types, **principal cells** and **intercalated cells.** As shown in Fig. 41-10, *principal cells reabsorb Na+ and water and secrete K+. Intercalated cells either secrete H+ (reabsorb HCO$_3$−) or secrete HCO$_3$− and thus are important in regulating acid-base balance (Chapter 44 contains details on H+ and HCO$_3$− secretion by intercalated cells). Intercalated cells also reabsorb K+.* Both Na+ reabsorption and K+ secretion by principal cells depend on the activity of the Na+, K+-ATPase in the basolateral membrane (Fig. 41-10). By maintaining a low cell [Na+], this pump provides a favorable chemical gradient for the movement of Na+ from the tubular fluid into the cell. Because Na+ enters the cell by diffusion through Na+-selective channels in the apical membrane,[*] the neg-

---

[*]Recently, cDNA clones for the renal Na+ channel (i.e., Epithelial Na+ Channel, or ENaC) have been isolated. ENaC is composed of three subunits: α, β, and γ, and all three subunits are required to form functional Na+ channels.

ative charge inside the cell facilitates Na+ entry. Na+ leaves the cell across the basolateral membrane and enters the blood via the action of Na+, K+-ATPase. This sodium reabsorption generates a lumen-negative charge across the late distal tubule and collecting duct. Cells in the collecting duct reabsorb significant amounts of Cl−, probably across the paracellular pathway. Reabsorption of Cl− is driven by the voltage differences across the late distal tubule and collecting duct.

> **Liddle's syndrome** is a rare genetic disorder characterized by an increase in the extracellular fluid volume (ECFV), which causes an increase in blood pressure (i.e., hypertension). Liddle's syndrome is caused by mutations in the genes that encode either the β or γ subunit of ENaC.[*] These mutations cause Na+ channels to become overactive. Inappropriately high rates of renal Na+ absorption occur, which lead to an increase in the ECFV (see Chapter 42). **Pseudohypoaldosteronism type I (PHA1)** is an uncommon and inherited disorder characterized by an increase in Na+ excretion, a reduction in ECFV, and hypotension. PHA1 is due to mutations in the genes encoding the γ subunit of ENaC. These mutations inactivate the channel, resulting in inappropriately low rates of renal Na+ absorption, which reduces the ECFV.

K+ is secreted from the blood into the tubular fluid by principal cells in two steps (Fig. 41-10). First, K+ uptake across the basolateral membrane occurs via the action of Na+, K+-ATPase. In the second step, K+ leaves the cells by passive diffusion. Because the [K+] inside the cells is high (150 mEq/L) and the [K+] in tubular fluid is low (~10 mEq/L), K+ diffuses down its concentration gradient across the apical cell membrane into the tubular fluid. Although the negative potential inside the cells tends to retain K+ within the cell, the electrochemical gradient

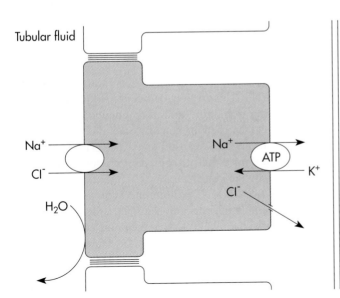

Tubular fluid   Blood

■ **Fig. 41-9** Transport mechanism for Na+ and Cl− reabsorption in the early segment of the distal tubule. This segment is impermeable to water. See text for details.

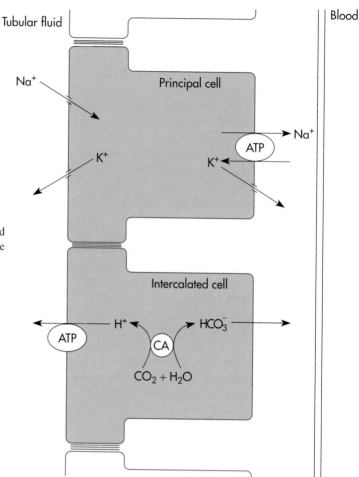

Tubular fluid

Blood

Na⁺

Principal cell

Na⁺

ATP

K⁺

K⁺

Intercalated cell

ATP

H⁺

HCO_3^-

CA

$CO_2 + H_2O$

■ **Fig. 41-10**   Transport pathways in principal cells and intercalated cells of the distal tubule and collecting duct. See text for details. *CA,* Carbonic anhydrase.

across the apical membrane favors K⁺ secretion from the cell into the tubular fluid. Additional details of K⁺ secretion and its regulation are considered in Chapter 43. The mechanism of K⁺ reabsorption by intercalated cells is not completely understood but is thought to be mediated by an H⁺, K⁺-ATPase located in the apical cell membrane (see Chapter 43).

Amiloride is a diuretic that inhibits Na⁺ reabsorption by the distal tubule and collecting duct by directly inhibiting Na⁺ channels in the luminal cell membrane. Amiloride also inhibits Cl⁻ reabsorption indirectly: inhibition of Na⁺ reabsorption reduces the magnitude of the negative charge in the lumen, which is the driving force for paracellular Cl⁻ reabsorption. Because amiloride reduces the negative charge in the lumen, it also acts to inhibit K⁺ secretion. By inhibiting K⁺ secretion across the distal tubule and collecting duct, amiloride reduces the amount of K⁺ excreted in the urine. Consequently, amiloride is frequently referred to as a **K⁺-sparing diuretic**. It is most often used in patients who excrete too much K⁺ in their urine.

■ *Regulation of NaCl and Water Reabsorption*

Several hormones and factors regulate NaCl reabsorption. Table 41-7 summarizes, for each hormone, the major stimulus for secretion, the nephron site of action, and the effect on transport. Angiotensin II, aldosterone, ANP, urodilatin, epinephrine, and norepinephrine released by sympathetic nerves are the most important hormones that regulate NaCl reabsorption and thereby urinary NaCl excretion. However, other hormones (including dopamine and glucocorticoids), Starling forces, and the phenomenon of glomerulotubular balance also influence NaCl reabsorption. ADH is the only major hormone that directly regulates the amount of water excreted by the kidneys.

Angiotensin II. The hormone angiotensin II has a potent stimulating effect on NaCl and water reabsorption in the proximal tubule. A decrease in the **effective circulating volume (ECV)** activates the renin-angiotensin-aldosterone system (discussed in Chapter 42), thereby increasing plasma angiotensin II concentration.

■ Table 41-7   Hormones that regulate NaCl and water absorption

Hormone	Major stimulus	Nephron site of action	Effect on transport
Angiotensin II	↑ Renin	PT	↑ NaCl and H_2O reabsorption
Aldosterone	↑ Angiotensin II, ↑ $[K^+]_p$	TAL, DT/CD	↑ NaCl and H_2O reabsorption*
ANP	↑ BP, ↑ ECV	CD	↓ H_2O and NaCl reabsorption
Urodilatin	↑ BP, ↑ECV	CD	↓ H_2O and NaCl reabsorption
Sympathetic nerves	↓ ECV	PT, TAL, DT/CD	↑ NaCl and H_2O reabsorption*
Dopamine	↑ ECV	PT	↓ H_2O and NaCl reabsorption
ADH	↑ P_{osm}, ↓ ECV	DT/CD	↑ H_2O reabsorption*

*All the hormones listed act within minutes, except aldosterone, which exerts its action on NaCl reabsorption with a delay of 1 hour. *PT*, Proximal tubule; *TAL*, thick ascending limb; *DT/CD*, distal tubule and collecting duct; *ECV*, effective circulating volume; *BP*, blood pressure; $[K^+]_p$, plasma $[K^+]$; P_{osm}, plasma osmolality. The asterisks indicate that the effect on H_2O reabsorption does not include the TAL. ↓ indicates a decrease and ↑ indicates an increase.

Aldosterone. Aldosterone is synthesized by the glomerulosa cells of the adrenal cortex. It stimulates NaCl reabsorption by the thick ascending limb of Henle's loop and the distal tubule and collecting duct. Aldosterone also stimulates K^+ secretion by the distal tubule and collecting duct (see Chapter 42). *The two most important stimuli for aldosterone secretion are an increase in angiotensin II concentration and an increase in plasma [K^+].* By its stimulation of NaCl reabsorption in the collecting duct, aldosterone also increases water reabsorption by this nephron segment.

Some individuals with an expanded ECF volume and elevated blood pressure are treated with drugs that inhibit angiotensin converting enzyme (**ACE inhibitors**, e.g., **captopril**). These drugs lower fluid volume and blood pressure. Inhibition of ACE blocks the degradation of angiotensin I to angiotensin II and thereby lowers plasma angiotensin II levels (see Chapter 42). The decline in plasma angiotensin II concentration has three effects: (1) NaCl and water reabsorption by the proximal tubule falls; (2) aldosterone secretion falls, which reduces NaCl reabsorption in the distal tubule and collecting duct; and (3) because angiotensin is a potent vasoconstrictor, the systemic arterioles dilate and arterial blood pressure falls. In addition, ACE degrades the vasodilating hormone bradykinin; ACE inhibitors therefore increase the concentrations of bradykinin. Thus, ACE inhibitors decrease the ECF volume and the arterial blood pressure by promoting renal NaCl and water excretion and by depressing total peripheral resistance.

Atrial natriuretic peptide and urodilatin. ANP and urodilatin are encoded by the same gene and have very similar amino acid sequences. **ANP** is a 28-amino acid hormone secreted by the cardiac atria. Its secretion is stimulated by a rise in blood pressure and an increase in the effective circulating volume. ANP reduces blood pressure by decreasing total peripheral resistance and by enhancing urinary NaCl and water excretion. The hormone also inhibits NaCl reabsorption by the medullary portion of the collecting duct, inhibits ADH-stimulated water reabsorption across the collecting duct, and reduces the secretion of ADH from the posterior pituitary.

Urodilatin is a 32-amino acid hormone that differs from ANP by the addition of four amino acids to the aminoterminus. Urodilatin is secreted by the distal tubule and collecting duct and is not present in the systemic circulation; thus, urodilatin influences only the function of the kidneys. Urodilatin secretion is stimulated by a rise in blood pressure and an increase in the effective circulating volume. It inhibits NaCl and water reabsorption across the medullary portion of the collecting duct. Urodilatin is a more potent natriuretic and diuretic hormone than ANP because ANP entering the kidneys in the blood is degraded by a neutral endopeptidase that has no effect on urodilatin.

Sympathetic nerves. Catecholamines released from sympathetic nerves (norepinephrine) and the adrenal medulla (epinephrine) stimulate NaCl and water reabsorption by the proximal tubule, the thick ascending limb of Henle's loop, the distal tubule, and the collecting duct. Activation of sympathetic nerves, (e.g., after hemorrhage or due to a decrease in the effective circulating volume) stimulates NaCl and water reabsorption by the proximal tubule, the thick ascending limb of Henle's loop, the distal tubule, and the collecting duct.

Dopamine. Dopamine, a catecholamine, is released from dopaminergic nerves in the kidneys and may also be synthesized by cells of the proximal tubule. The action of dopamine is opposite to that of norepinephrine and epinephrine. Dopamine secretion is stimulated by an increase in the effective circulating volume, and it directly inhibits NaCl and water reabsorption in the proximal tubule.

Antidiuretic hormone. *Antidiuretic hormone is the most important hormone that regulates water balance* (see Chapters 42 and 49). This hormone is secreted by the posterior pituitary in response to an increase in plasma osmolality or a decrease in the effective circulating volume.

ADH increases the permeability of the collecting duct to water. Also, because an osmotic gradient exists across the wall of the collecting duct, ADH increases water reabsorption by the collecting duct (see Chapter 42 for details). ADH has little effect on urinary NaCl excretion.

Starling forces. Starling forces (see also Chapters 27 and 40) regulate NaCl and water reabsorption across the proximal tubule (Fig. 41-11). As described above, Na$^+$, Cl$^-$, HCO$_3^-$, amino acids, glucose, and water are transported into the intercellular space of the proximal tubule. Starling forces between this space and the peritubular capillaries facilitate the movement of the reabsorbed substances into the capillaries. Starling forces that favor this movement are the capillary oncotic pressure (π_c) and the hydrostatic pressure in the intercellular space (P$_i$). The opposing Starling forces are the interstitial oncotic pressure (π_i) and the capillary hydrostatic pressure (P$_c$). Normally, the sum of the Starling forces favors movement of solute and water from the intercellular space into the capillary. However, some of the solutes and fluid that enter the lateral intercellular space leak back into the proximal tubular fluid. Starling forces do not affect transport by the loop of Henle, distal tubule, and collecting duct, because these segments are less permeable to water than is the proximal tubule.

A number of forces can alter the Starling forces across the peritubular capillaries surrounding the proximal tubule. For example, dilation of the efferent arteriole increases the hydrostatic pressure in the peritubular capillaries (P$_c$), whereas constriction of the efferent arteriole decreases P$_c$. An increase in P$_c$ inhibits solute and water reabsorption by increasing the back leak of NaCl and water across the tight junction, whereas a decrease in P$_c$ stimulates reabsorption by decreasing back leak across the tight junction.

The oncotic pressure in the peritubular capillary is partly determined by the rate of formation of the glomerular ultrafiltrate. For example, if one assumes a constant plasma flow in the afferent arteriole, then as less ultrafiltrate is formed (i.e., as GFR decreases), the plasma proteins become less concentrated in the plasma that enters the efferent arteriole and peritubular capillary. Hence, the peritubular oncotic pressure decreases. The peritubular oncotic pressure is directly related to the filtration fraction (FF = GFR/RPF). A fall in FF, because of a decrease in GFR at constant RPF, decreases the peritubular capillary oncotic pressure. This in turn increases the back flux of NaCl and water from the lateral intercellular space into the tubular fluid, and thereby decreases net solute and water reabsorption across the proximal tubule. An increase in FF has the opposite effect.

The importance of Starling forces in regulating solute and water reabsorption by the proximal tubule is underscored by the phenomenon of **glomerulotubular (G-T) balance.** Spontaneous changes in GFR markedly alter the filtered load of sodium (filtered load = GFR × [Na$^+$]). Without rapid adjustments in Na$^+$ reabsorption to counter the changes, urinary Na$^+$ excretion would fluctuate widely and disturb the Na$^+$ balance of the whole body. However, spontaneous changes in GFR do not alter Na$^+$ balance because of the phenomenon of G-T balance. *When body Na$^+$ balance is normal, G-T balance refers to the simultaneous increase in Na$^+$ and water reabsorption as a result of an increase in GFR and filtered load of Na$^+$. Thus, a constant fraction of the filtered Na$^+$ and water is reabsorbed from the proximal tubule despite variations in GFR.* The net result of G-T balance is to reduce the impact of GFR changes on the amount of Na$^+$ and water excreted in the urine.

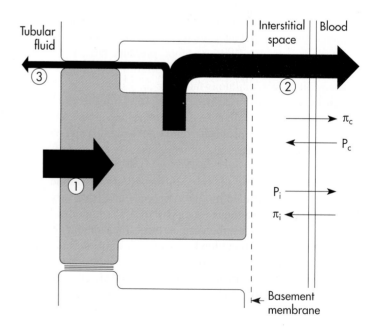

■ **Fig. 41-11**   Routes of solute and water transport across the proximal tubule and the Starling forces that modify reabsorption. *1,* Solute and water are reabsorbed across the apical membrane and then cross the lateral cell membrane. Some solute and water reenter the tubule fluid (arrow labeled *3*), and the remainder enters the interstitial space and then flows into the capillary (arrow labeled *2*). The width of the arrows is directly proportional to the amount of solute and water moving by the pathways labeled *1* to *3*. Starling forces across the capillary wall determine the amount of fluid flowing through pathways *2* versus *3*. Transport mechanisms in the apical cell membranes determine the amount of solute and water entering the cell (pathway *1*). π_c, Capillary oncotic pressure; P_c, capillary hydrostatic pressure; π_i, interstitial fluid oncotic pressure; P_i, interstitial hydrostatic pressure. Thin arrows across the capillary wall indicate the direction of water movement in response to each force.

Two mechanisms are responsible for G-T balance. One is related to the oncotic and hydrostatic pressures between the peritubular capillaries and the lateral intercellular space (i.e., Starling forces). For example, an increase in GFR (at constant RPF) raises the protein concentration in the glomerular capillary plasma above normal. This protein-rich plasma leaves the glomerular capillaries, flows through the efferent arteriole, and enters the peritubular capillaries. The increased oncotic pressure in the peritubular capillaries augments the movement of solute and fluid from the lateral intercellular space into the peritubular capillaries. This action increases net solute and water reabsorption by the proximal tubule.

The second mechanism responsible for G-T balance is initiated by an increase in the filtered load of glucose and amino acids. As discussed earlier in this chapter, the reabsorption of Na$^+$ in the early proximal tubule is coupled to that of glucose and amino acids. The rate of Na$^+$ reabsorption therefore depends in part on the filtered load of glucose and amino acids. As GFR and the filtered load of glucose and amino acids increase, Na$^+$ and water reabsorption also rise.

In addition to G-T balance, another mechanism minimizes changes in the filtered load of Na$^+$. As discussed earlier in this chapter, an increase in GFR (and thus in the amount of Na$^+$ filtered by the glomerulus) activates the tubuloglomerular feedback mechanism. This action returns GFR and the filtration of Na$^+$ to normal values. Thus, spontaneous changes in GFR (e.g., those caused by changes in posture and blood pressure) increase the amount of Na$^+$ filtered for only a few minutes. Until GFR returns to normal values, the mechanisms that underlie G-T balance maintain urinary Na$^+$ excretion constant and thereby maintain Na$^+$ homeostasis.

■ *Summary*

1. The four major segments of the nephron (proximal tubule, Henle's loop, distal tubule, and collecting duct) determine the composition and volume of the urine by the processes of selective reabsorption of solutes and water and selective secretion of solutes.

2. Tubular reabsorption allows the kidneys to retain those substances that are essential and to regulate their levels in the plasma by altering the degree to which they are reabsorbed. The reabsorption of Na$^+$, Cl$^-$, other anions, and organic solutes together with water constitutes the major function of the nephron. Approximately 25,200 mEq of Na$^+$ and 179 L of water are reabsorbed each day. The proximal tubule cells reabsorb 67% of the glomerular ultrafiltrate, and cells of the loop of Henle reabsorb about 25% of the filtered NaCl and about 15% of the filtered water. The distal segments of the nephron (distal tubule and collecting duct system) have a more limited reabsorptive capacity. However, the final adjustments in the composition and volume of the urine, and most of the regulation by hormones and other factors, occur in distal segments.

3. Secretion of substances into tubular fluid is a means for excreting various byproducts of metabolism. It also eliminates exogenous organic anions and bases (e.g., drugs) and pollutants from the body. Many organic compounds are bound to plasma proteins and are therefore unavailable for ultrafiltration. Secretion is thus their major route of excretion in the urine.

4. Various hormones (including angiotensin II, aldosterone, ADH, ANP, and urodilatin), sympathetic nerves, dopamine, and Starling forces regulate NaCl reabsorption by the kidneys. ADH is the major hormone that regulates water reabsorption.

■ *Self-Study Problems*

1. Consider the amount of water and NaCl filtered and reabsorbed by the kidneys each day. What does this tell you about the amount of energy (ATP) expended by the kidneys? Could this explain why the blood flow is so high relative to the size of the kidneys?

2. Compare and contrast passive and active transport.

3. Describe the mechanisms and pathways of Na$^+$, glucose, amino acid, Cl$^-$, and water reabsorption by the proximal tubule. Which pathways occur in the first phase of reabsorption and which occur in the second phase? How do Starling forces affect solute and water reabsorption?

4. Describe how Na$^+$ and Cl$^-$ are reabsorbed by the thick ascending limb of Henle's loop. If a diuretic that inhibits NaCl reabsorption (e.g., furosemide) in the thick ascending limb were given to an individual, what would happen to water reabsorption by this segment?

5. What is glomerulotubular balance? What is the physiological importance of this phenomenon? What would happen to Na$^+$ balance if glomerulotubular balance did not exist?

■ *Bibliography*

Journal articles

Aronson PS: 1994 Homer W. Smith Award. From flies to physiology—accidental findings along the trail of renal NaCl transport, *J Am Soc Nephrol* 12:2001-2013, 1995

Benos DJ et al: Diversity and regulation of amiloride-sensitive Na$^+$ channels, *Kidney Int* 49:1632-1637, 1996.

Canessa CM et al: Amiloride-sensitive epithelial Na$^+$ channel is made of three homologous subunits, *Nature* 367:463-467, 1994.

Forssmann W-G: Urodilatin: a renal natriuretic peptide, *Nephron* 69:211-222, 1995.

Hansson JH et al: Hypertension caused by a truncated epithelial sodium channel γ subunit: genetic heterogeneity of Liddle syndrome, *Nat Genet* 11:76-82, 1995.

Murer H, Biber J: Renal sodium-phosphate cotransport, *Curr Opin Nephrol Hypertens* 3:504-510, 1994.

Pritchard JB, Miller DS: Mechanisms mediating renal secretion of organic anions and cations, *Physiol Rev* 73:765-796, 1993.

Strautnieks SS, Thompson RJ, Gardiner RM, Chung E: A novel splice-site mutation in the γ subunit of the epithelial sodium channel gene in three pseudohypoaldosteronism type 1 families, *Nat Genet* 13:248-250, 1996.

Warnock DG, Bubien JK: Liddle syndrome: clinical and cellular abnormalities, *Hosp Pract* 29:95-105, 1994.

Books and monographs

Berry CA, Ives HE, Rector FC Jr: *Renal transport of glucose, amino acids, sodium, chloride and water*. In Brenner BM, editor: *The kidney*, ed 5, Philadelphia, 1996, WB Saunders.

Kershaw D, Wiggins RC: *Proteinuria*. In Shayman JA, editor: *Renal pathophysiology*, Philadelphia, 1995, JB Lippincott.

Koeppen BK, Stanton BA: *Sodium chloride transport: distal nephron*. In *The kidney: physiology and pathophysiology*, ed 2, New York, 1992, Raven Press.

Prichard JB, Miller DS: *Proximal tubular transport of organic anions and cations*. In Seldin DW, Giebisch G, editors: *The kidney: physiology and pathophysiology*, ed 2, New York, 1992, Raven Press.

Silbernagel S: *Tubular transport of amino acids and small peptides*. In Windhager EE, editor: *Handbook of physiology*, sect 8: *Renal physiology*, Vol II, New York, 1992, Oxford University Press.

Control of Body Fluid Osmolality and Volume

The kidneys maintain the osmolality and volume of the body fluids within a narrow range by regulating the excretion of water and NaCl, respectively. This chapter discusses the regulation of renal water excretion (urine concentration and dilution) and NaCl excretion. As an introduction to this material, we will review the normal volume and composition of the various body fluid compartments.

■ *The Body Fluid Compartments*

■ *Volumes of Body Fluid Compartments*

Water accounts for approximately 60% of body weight. Individual water content varies with the amount of adipose tissue; the greater the amount of adipose tissue, the smaller is the fraction of body weight attributable to water. Water content of the body also varies with age. In the newborn infant, water constitutes about 75% of body weight. This amount decreases to the adult value of 60% by the age of 1 year.

As illustrated in Fig. 42-1, **total body water** is distributed between two major compartments, which are separated by the cell membrane. The **intracellular fluid (ICF)** compartment is the larger compartment; it contains approximately two thirds of total body water. The remaining one third is contained in the **extracellular fluid (ECF)** compartment. Expressed as percentages of body weight, the volumes of total body water, ICF, and ECF can be estimated as*:

$$\text{total body water} = 0.6 \times (\text{body weight})$$
$$\text{ICF} = 0.4 \times (\text{body weight}) \qquad (42\text{-}1)$$
$$\text{ECF} = 0.2 \times (\text{body weight})$$

---

*In these and all subsequent calculations, it is assumed that 1 L of fluid (e.g., ICF and ECF) has a mass of 1 kg. This assumption allows interconversion between units of osmolality and volume.

The ECF compartment is subdivided into **interstitial fluid (ISF)** and **plasma;** these compartments are separated by the capillary wall. The interstitial fluid, which represents the fluid surrounding the cells in the various tissues of the body, comprises three fourths of the ECF volume. Included in this compartment is water contained within bone and dense connective tissue. The plasma volume represents the remaining one fourth of the ECF.

■ *Composition of Body Fluid Compartments*

The concentrations of the major cations and anions in the ECF and ICF are listed in Table 42-1. Na^+ is the major cation of the ECF, and Cl^- and HCO_3^- are the major anions. Because these compartments are separated only by the capillary wall, which is freely permeable to small ions, the ionic composition of the two major compartments of the ECF (interstitial fluid and plasma) is similar. *The major difference between the composition of the ISF and that of plasma is that the plasma contains significantly more protein.* Although the presence of protein in the plasma can affect the distribution of cations and anions across the capillary wall by the Gibbs-Donnan effect (see Chapter 2), this effect is normally quite small, and the ionic composition of the interstitial fluid and plasma can be considered identical.

Because of its abundance, Na^+ (and its attendant anions Cl^- and HCO_3^-) is the major determinant of the osmolality of the ECF. Accordingly, a rough estimate of the ECF osmolality can be obtained by simply doubling the sodium concentration ($[Na^+]$). For example, if the plasma $[Na^+]$ is 145 mEq/L, the osmolality of plasma and thus of the body fluids can be estimated as follows:

$$\text{plasma osmolality} = 2 \times (\text{plasma } [Na^+]) = 290 \text{ mOsm/kg } H_2O \qquad (42\text{-}2)$$

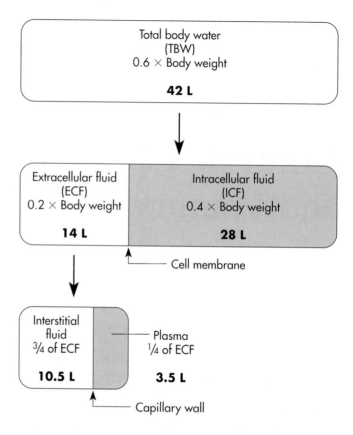

■ Fig. 42-1 Relationship between the volumes of the major body fluid compartments. The actual values shown are calculated for a 70-kg individual.

■ Table 42-1 Distribution of some cations and anions between extracellular fluid (ECF) and intracellular fluid (ICF)

		ECF	ICF
Na^+	(mEq/L)	145	12
K^+	(mEq/L)	4	150
Ca^{++}	(mEq/L)	5	0.001
Cl^-	(mEq/L)	105	5
HCO_3^-	(mEq/L)	25	12
P_i	(mEq/L)	2	100
pH		7.4	7.1

The ICF concentrations are estimates from skeletal muscle, and include amounts bound to intracellular proteins and free within the cytosol. Intracellular phosphate (P_i) is primarily in the form of organic molecules (e.g., adenosine triphosphate [ATP]).

The normal plasma osmolality ranges from approximately 285 to 295 mOsm/kg H_2O. Because water is in osmotic equilibrium across the capillary wall and the plasma membrane of cells, measuring the plasma osmolality also provides a measure of the osmolality of the ECF and ICF.

In clinical situations, a more accurate estimate of the plasma osmolality is obtained by also considering the contribution of glucose and urea to plasma osmolality. Accordingly, plasma osmolality can be estimated as follows:

$$\text{plasma osmolality} = 2 \, (\text{plasma} \, [Na^+]) \, + \, \frac{[\text{glucose}]}{18} + \frac{[\text{urea}]}{2.8} \quad (42\text{-}3)$$

The glucose and urea concentrations are expressed in units of milligrams per deciliter (if we divide glucose by 18 and urea by 2.8, we can convert from the units of mg/dl to mmol/L and thus to mOsm/kg H_2O).* This estimation of plasma osmolality is especially useful when dealing with patients who have an elevated plasma [glucose] secondary to **diabetes mellitus,** and in patients with **chronic renal failure,** whose plasma [urea] is elevated. However, urea and glucose are not "effective osmoles" in the determination of the effect of changes in plasma osmolality on shifts of fluid between the ICF and ECF.† Therefore, multiplying the plasma [Na^+] by two provides the best estimate of the effective osmolality of the plasma. This effective osmolality is most important in determining the impact of changes in body fluid osmolality on ICF and ECF volumes.

In contrast to ECF, the [Na^+] of ICF is low. K^+ is the predominant cation of this compartment. This asymmetric distribution of Na^+ and K^+ across the plasma membrane is maintained by the activity of the ubiquitous Na^+, K^+-ATPase. By its action, Na^+ is pumped out of the cell in exchange for K^+. The anion composition of ICF also

---

*The [urea] in plasma is measured as the portion of nitrogen in the urea molecule, or blood urea nitrogen (BUN).
†A solute can exert an osmotic pressure only if it does not cross the cell membrane; such solutes are termed *effective osmoles*. Because urea and glucose freely cross many cell membranes, they are considered *ineffective osmoles*.

differs markedly from that of ECF; [Cl⁻] and [HCO₃⁻] of ICF are lower than those of ECF. The major ICF anions are phosphates, organic anions, and protein.

■ *Fluid Exchange between Body Fluid Compartments*

Water moves freely between the various body fluid compartments. Two forces determine this movement: hydrostatic pressure and osmotic pressure. **Hydrostatic pressure** is generated by the pumping of the heart (and the effect of gravity on the column of blood in the vessels). The **osmotic pressure** of the plasma proteins (oncotic pressure) is an important determinant of fluid movement across capillary walls (see Chapter 27), whereas osmotic pressure differences between the ICF and ECF are responsible for fluid movement across cell membranes. Because the plasma membranes of cells are highly permeable to water, a change in the osmolality of either ICF or ECF results in the rapid movement of water between these compartments. Thus, except for transient changes, the ICF and ECF compartments are in osmotic equilibrium.

In contrast to the movement of water, the movement of ions across cell membranes is variable and depends on the presence of specific membrane transporters. Consequently, a useful starting point in analyzing the fluid exchange between ICF and ECF under pathophysiological conditions is to assume that appreciable shifts of ions between the compartments do not occur. This assumption about the movement of fluids between ICF and ECF is outlined in the fluid shift analysis on the right.

To illustrate this approach, consider what happens when solutions containing various amounts of NaCl are added to the ECF.*

Example 1: addition of isotonic NaCl to ECF. Addition of an isotonic NaCl solution (e.g., intravenous infusion of 0.9% NaCl: osmolality ≈ mOsm/kg H₂O)† to the ECF will increase the volume of this compartment by the volume of fluid administered. Because this fluid has the same osmolality as ECF, and therefore also ICF, no driving force for fluid movement exists between these compartments, and the volume of the ICF will not change. Although Na⁺ can cross cell membranes, it is effectively restricted to the ECF by the activity of the Na⁺, K⁺-ATPase, which is present in all cells. Therefore,

---

*Fluids are usually administered intravenously. When electrolyte solutions are infused by this route, rapid (i.e., minutes) equilibration occurs between plasma and interstitial fluid, because of the high permeability of the capillary wall to water and electrolytes. Thus, these fluids are essentially added to the entire ECF.

†0.9% NaCl solution has a concentration of 154 mEq/L. Because NaCl does not dissociate completely (i.e., 1.88 osmoles/mole), the osmolality of this solution is 290 mOsm/kg H₂O, or essentially iso-osmotic to the body fluids. Because NaCl is an effective osmole, a 0.9% solution is also isotonic.

Principles for analysis of fluid shifts between ICF and ECF

- The volumes of the various body fluid compartments can be estimated in the normal adult by the following:

(0.4 × body weight)

Total body water
(0.6 × body weight)

Intracellular fluid

(0.75 × ECF)

Interstitial fluid

Extracellular fluid

(0.2 × body weight)

Plasma

(0.25 × ECF)

- All exchanges of water and solutes with the external environment occur through the ECF (e.g., intravenous infusion, intake, or loss via the gastrointestinal tract). Changes in ICF are secondary to fluid shifts between ECF and ICF. Fluid shifts occur only if perturbation of the ECF alters its osmolality.

- Except for brief periods (seconds to minutes) ICF and ECF are in osmotic equilibrium. A measurement of plasma osmolality provides a measure of both ECF and ICF osmolality.

- For the sake of simplification, it can be assumed that equilibration between ICF and ECF occurs only by movement of water, and not by movement of osmotically active solutes.

- Conservation of mass must be maintained. This principle is especially important in situations in which either water and/or solutes are added to or excreted from the body.

---

no net movement of the infused NaCl into the cells occurs.

Example 2: addition of hypotonic NaCl to ECF. Addition of a hypotonic NaCl solution to ECF (e.g., intravenous infusion of 0.45% NaCl: osmolality ≈ 145 mOsm/kg H₂O) will decrease the osmolality of this compartment and causes water to move into the ICF. After osmotic equilibration is reached, the osmolalities of ICF and ECF will be equal, but lower than before the infusion, and the volume of each compartment will be increased. The increase in ECF volume will be greater than the increase in ICF volume.

Example 3: addition of hypertonic NaCl to ECF. Addition of a hypertonic NaCl solution to ECF (e.g., intravenous infusion of 3% NaCl: osmolality ≈ 1000 mOsm/kg H₂O) will increase the osmolality of this compartment and cause water to move out of cells. After osmotic equilibration is reached, the osmolality of ECF and ICF will be equal. The volume of ECF will be increased, while that of ICF will be decreased. The increase in ECF volume includes the volume of the infused solution, plus the volume of fluid that shifts out of ICF into ECF.

Intravenous solutions are available in many formulations. The type of fluid administered to a particular patient is dictated by the patient's need. For example, if the patient's vascular volume needs to be increased, a solution containing substances that have low permeability across the capillary wall is infused (e.g., 5% albumin). The oncotic pressure generated by the albumin molecules causes fluid to be retained in the vascular compartment, thus expanding its volume. Expansion of ECF is accomplished most often with isotonic saline solutions (e.g., 0.9% NaCl). As already noted, administration of an isotonic NaCl solution does not generate an osmotic pressure gradient across the plasma membrane of cells. Therefore, the entire volume of infused solution remains in the ECF. Patients whose body fluids are hyperosmotic may need hypotonic solutions. These solutions may be hypotonic NaCl (e.g., 0.45% NaCl or 5% dextrose in water [D5W]). Administration of D5W solution is equivalent to infusion of distilled water, because the dextrose is ultimately metabolized to CO_2 and water. Administration of these fluids increases the volumes of both ICF and ECF. Finally, patients whose body fluids are hypotonic may need hypertonic solutions. These solutions, which are typically NaCl-containing solutions (e.g., 3% and 5% NaCl), will expand the volume of ECF but decrease the volume of ICF. Other constituents, such as electrolytes (e.g., K^+ or drugs), can be added to intravenous solutions to tailor the therapy to the patient's fluid, electrolyte, and metabolic needs.

■ *Control of Body Fluid Osmolality: Urine Concentration and Dilution*

The kidneys are responsible for regulating water balance, and under most conditions are the major route for elimination of water from the body (Table 42-2). Other routes of water loss from the body include evaporation from the cells of the skin and the respiratory passages. Collectively, water loss by these routes is termed **insensible water loss,** because the individual is unaware of its occurrence. Additional water can be lost by the production of sweat. Water loss by this mechanism can increase dramatically in a hot environment, with exercise, or in the presence of fever (Table 42-3). Finally, water can be lost from the gastrointestinal tract. Fecal water loss is normally small but increases with diarrhea. Gastrointestinal water losses can also occur with vomiting.

Water loss in sweat, feces, and evaporation from the lungs and skin is not regulated. In contrast, *the renal excretion of water is tightly regulated to maintain water balance.* The maintenance of water balance requires that water intake precisely match water loss from the body. If intake exceeds losses, positive water balance exists. Conversely, when intake is less than losses, negative water balance exists.

When water intake is low or water losses increase, the kidneys conserve water by producing a small volume of urine that is hyperosmotic with respect to plasma. When water intake is high, a large volume of hypo-osmotic urine is produced. In a normal individual, urine osmolality can vary from approximately 50 to 1200 mOsm/kg H_2O, and the corresponding urine volume can vary from near 18 L/day to 0.5 L/day.

When the maintenance of water balance is disrupted, the body fluid osmolality is altered. These alterations are usually measured by changes in plasma osmolality (P_{osm}). Because the major determinant of plasma osmo-

■ **Table 42-2**   Normal routes of water gain and loss in adults at room temperature (23° C)

Route	ml/day
Water intake	
Fluid*	1200
In food	1000
Metabolically produced from food	300
TOTAL	2500
Water output	
Insensible	700
Sweat	100
Feces	200
Urine	1500
TOTAL	2500

*Fluid intake varies widely for both social and cultural reasons.

■ **Table 42-3**   Effect of environmental temperature and exercise on water loss and intake in adults (in ml/day)

	Normal temperature	Hot weather	Prolonged heavy exercise
Water loss			
Insensible loss:			
Skin	350	350	350
Lungs	350	250	650
Sweat	100	1400	5000
Feces	200	200	200
Urine	1500	1200	500
Total loss	2500	3400	6700
Water intake to maintain water balance	2500	3400	6700

In hot weather and during prolonged heavy exercise, water balance is maintained only if the individual increases water intake to match the increased loss of water in sweat. Decreased water excretion by the kidneys alone is insufficient to maintain water balance.

lality is Na^+ (with its anions Cl^- and HCO_3^-), disorders of water balance will result in alterations in the plasma [Na^+]. When evaluating an abnormal plasma [Na^+] in an individual, it is tempting to suspect a problem in Na^+ balance. However, the problem most often relates to water balance, not Na^+ balance. Changes in Na^+ balance result in alterations in the volume of extracellular fluid, not its osmolality.

In the clinical setting, **hypo-osmolality** (a reduction in plasma osmolality) shifts water into cells, and this process results in cell swelling. Symptoms associated with hypo-osmolality are related primarily to swelling of brain cells. For example, a rapid fall in P_{osm} can alter neurologic function and thereby cause nausea, malaise, headache, confusion, lethargy, seizures, and coma. When P_{osm} is increased (i.e., **hyperosmolality**), water is lost from cells. The symptoms of an increase in P_{osm} are also primarily neurologic, and they include lethargy, weakness, seizures, coma, and even death.

The kidneys control water excretion independently of their ability to control the excretion of a number of other physiologically important substances (e.g., Na^+, K^+, H^+, urea). Indeed, this dual control is necessary for survival, because it allows the kidneys to achieve water balance without upsetting the other homeostatic functions of the kidneys.

The following sections discuss the mechanisms by which the kidneys excrete either hypo-osmotic (dilute) or hyperosmotic (concentrated) urine. The control of antidiuretic hormone (ADH) secretion and its important role in regulating the excretion of water by the kidneys are also explained (see also Chapter 49).

■ *Antidiuretic Hormone*

Antidiuretic hormone (ADH), or vasopressin, acts on the kidneys to regulate the volume and osmolality of the urine. When plasma ADH levels are low, a large volume of urine is excreted (**diuresis**), and the urine is dilute.* When plasma ADH levels are elevated, a small volume of urine is excreted (**antidiuresis**), and the urine is concentrated.

ADH is a small peptide nine amino acids in length. It is synthesized by neuroendocrine cells located within the supraoptic and paraventricular nuclei of the hypothalamus (see also Chapter 49). The synthesized hormone is packaged in granules, which are transported down the axon of the cell and then stored in the nerve terminals located in the neurohypophysis (posterior pituitary). The anatomy of the hypothalamus and pituitary gland is illustrated in Fig. 42-2.

Several factors influence the secretion of ADH by the posterior pituitary. Two physiological regulators of ADH secretion are the osmolality of the body fluids (osmotic) and the volume and pressure of the vascular system (hemodynamic). Other factors that can alter ADH secretion include nausea (stimulates), atrial natriuretic peptide (ANP) (inhibits), and angiotensin II (stimulates). A number of drugs, prescription and nonprescription, also affect ADH secretion. For example, nicotine stimulates ADH secretion, whereas ethanol inhibits its secretion (see also Chapter 49).

Osmotic control of ADH secretion. *A change in the body fluid osmolality is the primary regulator of ADH secretion.* Changes in osmolality as small as 1% are sufficient to significantly alter ADH secretion. Cells involved in sensing changes in body fluid osmolality are located in the hypothalamus but are distinct from those that synthesize ADH.* These cells, called **osmoreceptors,** appear to behave as osmometers, and sense changes in body fluid osmolality by either shrinking or swelling. An important point to know about osmoreceptors is that they respond only to solutes that are **effective osmoles.** For example, urea does not affect the function of the osmoreceptors and is thus an **ineffective osmole.** Elevation of the plasma urea concentration by itself has little effect on ADH secretion.

When the effective osmolality of the body fluids increases, osmoreceptors send signals to the ADH synthesizing cells in the supraoptic and paraventricular nuclei of the hypothalamus, and ADH secretion is stimulated. Conversely, when the effective osmolality of the body fluid is reduced, secretion is inhibited. Because ADH is rapidly broken down in the plasma, circulating levels can be reduced to zero within minutes after secretion is inhibited. As a result, the ADH system can respond rapidly to fluctuations in body fluid osmolality.

Fig. 42-3, *A* illustrates the effect of changes in body fluid osmolality (measured as plasma osmolality) on circulating ADH levels. The **set point** of the system is defined as the plasma osmolality value at which ADH secretion begins to increase. Below this set point, virtually no ADH is released. Above the set point, the slope of the relationship is quite steep, reflecting the sensitivity of this system. The set point varies among individuals and is genetically determined. In healthy adults, the set point varies from 280 to 290 mOsm/kg H_2O. Several physiological factors, such as alterations in blood volume and pressure, can also change the set point, as discussed below. Also, pregnancy is associated with a decrease in the set point.

Hemodynamic control of ADH secretion. A decrease in blood volume or arterial pressure also stimulates ADH secretion. The receptors activated by this response are

---

*Diuresis is a general term for a large urinary output. Output of urine that contains primarily water is called a *water diuresis*.

*The osmoreceptor cells are located outside the blood-brain barrier in the anterior wall of the third ventricle (organum vasculosum of the lamina terminalis, and perhaps also the subfornical organ).

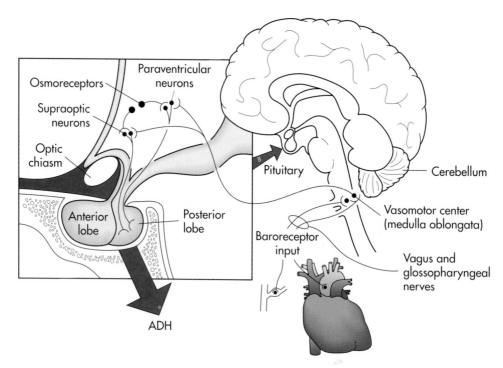

■ Fig. 42-2 Anatomy of the hypothalamus and pituitary gland (midsagittal section) depicting the pathways for antidiuretic hormone (ADH) secretion. Also shown are pathways involved in regulating ADH secretion. Afferent fibers from the baroreceptors are carried in the vagus and glossopharyngeal nerves. The vasomotor center includes the solitary tract nucleus. The closed box gives an expanded view of the hypothalamus and pituitary gland.

located in both the low-pressure (left atrium and pulmonary vessels) and the high-pressure (aortic arch and carotid sinus) sides of the circulatory system (see also Chapters 28 and 29). Because they are located in the high capacitance side of the circulatory system, low-pressure receptors respond to overall vascular volume. High-pressure receptors, on the other hand, respond to arterial pressure. Both groups of receptors are sensitive to stretch of the wall of the structure in which they are located (e.g., cardiac atrial wall, wall of aortic arch) and are thus called **baroreceptors.** Signals from these receptors are carried in afferent fibers of the vagus and glossopharyngeal nerves to the brainstem (solitary tract nucleus of the medulla oblongata), which is part of the center that regulates heart rate and blood pressure (see Chapter 29). Signals are then relayed from the brainstem to the ADH secretory cells of the supraoptic and paraventricular hypothalamic nuclei. Normally, signals from the baroreceptors tonically inhibit ADH secretion. However, when blood volume or arterial pressure decreases, this inhibitory input is overridden and ADH secretion is stimulated. The sensitivity of the baroreceptor system is less than that of the osmoreceptors; a 5% to 10% decrease in blood volume or arterial pressure is required before ADH secretion is stimulated. The baroreceptor system is illustrated in Fig. 42-3, *B*.

Alterations in blood volume or arterial pressure also affect the response to changes in body fluid osmolality

(Fig. 42-3, *C*). With a decrease in blood volume or arterial pressure, the set point shifts to lower osmolality values, and the slope of the relationship is steeper. In an individual with circulatory collapse, the shift in set point allows the kidney to continue to conserve water, even though the water retention will reduce the osmolality of the body fluids. With an increase in blood volume or arterial pressure, the opposite response occurs and the set point shifts to higher osmolality values; the slope of the relationship is therefore decreased.

Inadequate release of ADH from the posterior pituitary results in excretion of large volumes of dilute urine **(polyuria).** To compensate for this loss of water, the individual must ingest large volumes of water **(polydipsia)** to maintain body fluid osmolality constant. If the individual is deprived of water, the body fluids will become hyperosmotic. This condition is called **central diabetes insipidus, neurogenic diabetes insipidus,** or **pituitary diabetes insipidus.** Rarely, central diabetes insipidus is inherited. It occurs more commonly after head trauma, with brain neoplasms, or with brain infections. Individuals with central diabetes insipidus have a urine-concentrating defect that can be corrected by administration of exogenous ADH.

The **syndrome of inappropriate ADH secretion (SIADH)** is a common clinical problem. SIADH is

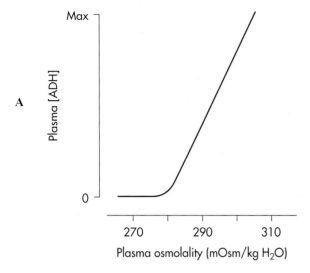

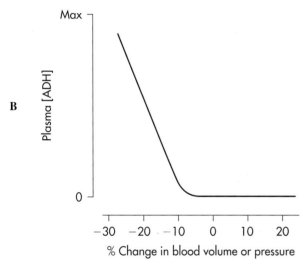

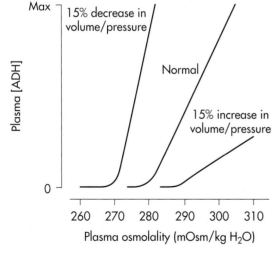

■ **Fig. 42-3** Osmotic and hemodynamic control of ADH secretion. **A,** Effect of changes in plasma osmolality (constant blood volume and pressure) on plasma ADH levels. **B,** Effect of changes in blood volume or pressure (constant plasma osmolality) on plasma ADH levels. **C,** Interactions between osmolar and blood volume and pressure stimuli on ADH secretion.

characterized by plasma ADH levels that are elevated above those expected on the basis of body fluid osmolality and blood volume or arterial pressure (hence the term *inappropriate*). Individuals with SIADH retain water (i.e., reduce renal excretion). If water intake is not reduced in parallel, their body fluids become progressively hypo-osmotic. Characteristically, the urine of these individuals is more concentrated than expected on the basis of the low body fluid osmolality. SIADH can be caused by infections and neoplasms of the brain, drugs (e.g., antitumor agents), pulmonary diseases, and carcinoma of the lung.

ADH actions on the kidney. *The primary action of ADH on the kidneys is to increase the permeability of the collecting duct to water.* It also increases the permeability of the medullary portion of the collecting duct to urea.

The actions of ADH on the water permeability of the collecting duct have been extensively studied. ADH binds to a receptor on the basolateral membrane of the cell. This is called the V$_2$ receptor (vasopressin 2 receptor).* Binding of ADH to this receptor, which is coupled to adenylyl cyclase via a stimulatory G protein (G$_s$), increases the intracellular levels of cyclic adenosine monophosphate (cAMP). The rise in intracellular cAMP activates **protein kinase A,** which prompts the insertion of intracellular vesicles containing **water channels**† into the apical membrane of the cell. These water channels are preformed and reside in vesicles located beneath the cell's apical membrane. When ADH is removed, the water channels return to their original position within the cell, and the apical membrane is once again impermeable to water. The shuttling of water channels into and out of the apical membrane provides a mechanism for rapidly controlling membrane water permeability. Because the basolateral membrane is freely permeable to water, any water that enters the cell through apical membrane water channels exits across the basolateral membrane, resulting in the net absorption of water from the tubule lumen into the peritubular blood.

The collecting ducts of some individuals do not respond normally to ADH. This lack of response can be the result of defects in the ADH receptor, lack of insertion of water channels into the apical membrane, or defective water channels. Regardless of the mechanism,

---

*A different ADH receptor (V$_1$ receptor) is located in blood vessels. This receptor mediates the vasoconstrictor response to ADH. It is this action of ADH that accounts for its alternative name of vasopressin.
†The water channels involved in the collecting duct response to ADH are part of a family of integral membrane proteins called **aquaporins.** The aquaporin-2 channel is inserted into the apical membrane of collecting duct principal cells in response to ADH. Different channels (aquaporin-3 and aquaporin-4) mediate the movement of water across the basolateral membrane of the principal cell. Water movement across the proximal tubule and descending thin limb of Henle's loop is mediated by yet another water channel (aquaporin-1).

these individuals cannot maximally concentrate their urine. Consequently, they suffer from polyuria and polydipsia. This entity is termed **nephrogenic diabetes insipidus** to distinguish it from central diabetes insipidus (see p 720 and Chapter 49). Although nephrogenic diabetes insipidus can be inherited, it is most often caused by other factors such as metabolic disorders (e.g., hypercalcemia) or certain drugs. For example, approximately 30% to 40% of individuals taking the medication lithium for bipolar disorder develop some degree of nephrogenic diabetes insipidus.

ADH also increases the permeability of the terminal portion of the inner medullary collecting duct to urea. The mechanism for urea movement across the inner medullary collecting duct cell is not completely understood, nor is the mechanism by which ADH increases this transport. Urea appears to cross the cell membrane via a specific transport protein. It is likely that ADH increases the permeability of the inner medullary collecting duct to urea by inserting more of these urea transporters into the cell's apical membrane. Increased transport of urea across the basolateral membrane may also occur in response to the action of ADH, again by insertion of additional transporters.

■ *Thirst*

In addition to affecting the secretion of ADH, *changes in plasma osmolality, blood volume, or arterial pressure alter the perception of thirst.* When body fluid osmolality is increased or the blood volume and pressure are reduced, the individual perceives thirst. Of these stimuli, hyperosmolality is the most potent. An increase of only 2% to 3% in plasma osmolality will produce a strong desire to drink, while decreases of 10% to 15% in blood volume and arterial pressure are required to produce the same response.

The neural centers involved in regulating water intake (the thirst center) are located in the anterolateral region of the hypothalamus (subfornical organ and organum vasculosum of the lamina terminalis). Even though they are located in the same region of the hypothalamus, the cells of the thirst center appear to be distinct from the osmoreceptors involved in ADH secretion. However, like the osmoreceptors involved in ADH secretion, thirst center cells respond only to effective osmoles (e.g., NaCl). Even less is known about the pathways involved in the thirst response to decreased blood volume or arterial pressure, but it is believed that the pathways are the same as those involved in regulation of ADH secretion. Angiotensin II, acting on cells of the thirst center (subfornical organ), also evokes the sensation of thirst. Since angiotensin II levels are increased when blood volume and pressure are reduced (see p 732), this effect of angiotensin II contributes to the homeostatic response that restores and maintains the body fluids at their normal volume.

The sensation of thirst is satisfied by the act of drinking even before sufficient water is absorbed from the gastrointestinal tract to correct the plasma osmolality. Oropharyngeal and upper gastrointestinal receptors appear to be involved in this response. However, relief of the thirst sensation via these receptors is short-lived. Thirst is completely satisfied only when the plasma osmolality, blood volume, and arterial pressure are corrected.

The ADH and thirst systems work in concert to maintain water balance. An increase in plasma osmolality invokes drinking and, via ADH action on the kidneys, conservation of water. Conversely, when plasma osmolality is decreased, thirst is suppressed and, in the absence of ADH, renal water excretion is enhanced.

With adequate access to water, the thirst mechanism can prevent the development of hyperosmolality. Indeed, this mechanism is responsible for the polydipsia that occurs in response to the polyuria of both **central and nephrogenic diabetes insipidus.**

Water intake is also influenced by social and cultural factors. Thus, individuals ingest water even in the absence of the thirst sensation. Normally, the kidneys are able to excrete this excess water, since they can excrete up to 18 L/day of urine. However, in some instances the volume of water ingested exceeds the capacity of the kidneys to excrete water. Body fluids then become hypo-osmotic.

The perception of thirst can be influenced by factors other than body fluid osmolality, blood volume, or arterial pressure. As we have noted, angiotensin II is well recognized as promoting the desire to drink.

■ *Renal Mechanisms for Dilution and Concentration of Urine*

Under normal circumstances, the excretion of water is regulated separately from the excretion of solutes (e.g., NaCl). For this separate regulation to occur, the kidneys must excrete urine that is either hypo-osmotic or hyperosmotic with respect to the body fluids. This ability to excrete urine of varying osmolality in turn requires that solute be separated from water at some point along the nephron. As discussed in Chapter 41, reabsorption of solute in the proximal tubule results in the reabsorption of a proportional amount of water. Hence, solute and water are not separated in this portion of the nephron. Moreover, separation does not occur regardless of whether the kidneys excrete dilute or concentrated urine. *Henle's loop, in particular the thick ascending limb, is the major nephron site where the separation of solute and water occurs.* Thus, the excretion of both dilute and concentrated urine requires normal function of Henle's loop.

The production of hypo-osmotic urine is conceptually easy to understand. The nephron must simply reabsorb solute from the tubular fluid and not allow water to follow. As just noted, and as described in greater detail below, reabsorption of solute occurs primarily in the thick ascending limb of Henle's loop. Under appropriate conditions (i.e., in the absence of ADH), the distal tubule and the collecting duct also participate in this process.

The excretion of a hyperosmotic urine is conceptually more difficult to understand. This process requires the removal of water from the tubular fluid, leaving solute behind. Because water can only move passively (driven by an osmotic gradient), the kidneys must generate a hyperosmotic environment that drives water removal from the tubular fluid. Such an environment is generated in the interstitial fluid of the renal medulla. Henle's loop, and especially the thick ascending limb, is critical for generating this hyperosmotic medullary environment. Once this hyperosmotic environment is established in the medullary interstitium, it drives water reabsorption from the collecting duct, and thereby concentrates the urine.

Fig. 42-4 summarizes the essential features of the mechanisms whereby the kidneys excrete either a dilute (*A*) or a concentrated (*B*) urine. First, we consider how the kidneys excrete a dilute urine (**water diuresis**), when ADH levels are low or absent. The following numbers refer to those encircled in Fig. 42-4, *A*.

1. Fluid entering the descending thin limb of Henle's loop from the proximal tubule is iso-osmotic with respect to plasma. This iso-osmotic fluid reflects the essentially iso-osmotic nature of solute and water reabsorption in the proximal tubule (see Chapter 41).
2. The descending thin limb is highly permeable to water but much less so to solutes such as NaCl and urea.* Consequently, as the fluid descends deeper into the hyperosmotic medulla, water is reabsorbed owing to the osmotic gradient that is set up across the descending thin limb. By this process, fluid at the bend of the loop has an osmolality equal to that of the surrounding interstitial fluid. However, while the osmolality of the tubular and interstitial fluids are similar at the bend of the loop, their compositions differ. The tubular fluid [NaCl] is greater than that of the surrounding interstitial fluid, but the [urea] of the tubular fluid is less than that of the interstitial fluid (see p 724).

3. The ascending thin limb is impermeable to water but permeable to NaCl and urea. Consequently, as tubular fluid moves up the ascending limb, NaCl is passively reabsorbed (because tubular fluid [NaCl] > interstitial fluid [NaCl]), while urea passively diffuses into the tubular fluid (because tubular fluid [urea] < interstitial fluid [urea]). The net effect is that the volume of the tubular fluid remains unchanged along the length of the thin ascending limb, but the [NaCl] decreases and the [urea] increases. Overall, the movement of NaCl out of the lumen of the thin ascending limb is greater than the movement of urea into the lumen, and the tubular fluid becomes diluted.
4. The thick ascending limb of Henle's loop is impermeable to water and urea. This portion of the nephron actively reabsorbs NaCl, thereby diluting the tubular fluid. Dilution occurs to such a degree that this segment is often referred to as the **diluting segment** of the kidney. Fluid leaving the thick ascending limb is hypo-osmotic with respect to plasma (approximately 150 mOsm/kg H_2O).
5. The distal tubule and cortical portion of the collecting duct actively reabsorb NaCl but are impermeable to urea. In the absence of ADH, these segments are not permeable to water. Thus, when ADH is absent or present at low levels (i.e., decreased P_{osm}), the distal tubule and the cortical collecting duct are impermeable to water. Accordingly, the osmolality of tubule fluid in these segments is reduced further because NaCl is reabsorbed without water. Fluid entering the cortical portion of the collecting duct is hypo-osmotic with respect to plasma (approximately 100 mOsm/kg H_2O).
6. The medullary collecting duct actively reabsorbs NaCl. Even in the absence of ADH, this segment is slightly permeable to water and urea. Consequently, some urea enters the collecting duct from the medullary interstitium, and a small volume of water is reabsorbed.
7. The urine will have an osmolality of $\approx$ 150 mOsm/kg H_2O and will contain low concentrations of NaCl and urea. The volume of urea excreted can be as much as 18 L/day, or approximately 10% of the glomerular filtration rate (GFR).

Next, we consider how the kidneys excrete a concentrated urine (**antidiuresis**), when P_{osm} and plasma ADH levels are high. The following numbers refer to those encircled in Fig. 42-4, *B*.

1-4. Steps 1 to 4 are similar when either a dilute or a concentrated urine is produced. An important point in understanding how a concentrated urine is produced is that while reabsorption of NaCl by the ascending thin and thick limbs of Henle's loop

---

*Urea is an ineffective osmole for many cells within the body, because it freely crosses the plasma membrane of these cells. However, in many portions of the nephron, urea permeability is quite low (Table 42-4). In these regions of the nephron, urea serves as an effective osmole and causes osmotic water movement.

dilutes the tubular fluid, the reabsorbed NaCl accumulates in the medullary interstitium and raises its osmolality. The accumulation of NaCl in the medullary interstitium is critically important for the production of urine hyperosmotic to plasma, because it provides the osmotic driving force for water reabsorption by the collecting duct. The overall process by which Henle's loop, and in particular the thick ascending limb, generates the hyperosmotic medullary interstitial gradient is termed **countercurrent multiplication.***

5. Owing to NaCl reabsorption by the thick ascending limb of Henle's loop, fluid reaching the collecting duct is hypo-osmotic with respect to the surrounding interstitial fluid. Thus, an osmotic gradient is established across the collecting duct. In the presence of ADH, which increases the water permeability of the collecting duct, water diffuses out of the tubule lumen, and the tubule fluid osmolality increases. This diffusion of water begins the process of urine concentration. The maximal osmolality that the fluid in the cortical collecting duct can attain is approximately 300 mOsm/kg H_2O, which is the osmolality of the surrounding interstitial fluid and plasma. Although the fluid at this point has the same osmolality as that which entered the descending thin limb, its composition has been altered dramatically. Because of NaCl reabsorption by the preceding nephron segments, NaCl accounts for a much smaller portion of the total tubular fluid osmolality. Instead, the tubule fluid osmolality is accounted for by urea (filtered urea, plus urea added in the descending thin and ascending thin limbs of Henle's loop) and other solutes (e.g., K^+, creatinine).

6. The osmolality of the interstitial fluid in the medulla progressively increases from the corticomedullary junction, where it is approximately 300 mOsm/kg H_2O, to the papilla, where it is approximately 1200 mOsm/kg H_2O. Thus, an osmotic gradient exists between tubular fluid and the interstitial fluid along the entire medullary collecting duct. In the presence of ADH, which ren-

ders the medullary collecting duct permeable to water, the osmolality of tubular fluid increases as water is reabsorbed. Because the initial portion of the collecting duct is impermeable to urea, it remains in the tubular fluid, and its concentration in the tubular fluid increases. In the presence of ADH, the urea permeability of the last portion of the medullary collecting duct is increased. Because the urea concentration of the tubular fluid has been increased by water reabsorption in the cortex and outer medulla, its concentration in the tubular fluid is greater than its concentration in the interstitial fluid, and some urea diffuses out of the tubule lumen into the medullary interstitium. The maximal osmolality that the fluid in the medullary collecting duct can attain is equal to that of the surrounding interstitial fluid. The major components of the tubular fluid within the medullary collecting ducts are substances that have either escaped reabsorption or have been secreted into the tubular fluid. Of these, urea is the most abundant.

7. The urine produced when ADH is high has an osmolality of 1200 mOsm/kg H_2O and contains high concentrations of urea and other nonreabsorbed solutes. Because urea in the tubular fluid equilibrates with urea in the medullary interstitial fluid, its concentration in the urine will be similar to that of the interstitium. Urine volume under this condition can be as low as 0.5 L/day.

Table 42-4 summarizes the transport and passive permeability properties of the nephron segments involved in the process of concentrating and diluting the urine. Fig. 42-5 summarizes the volumes of fluid reabsorbed by the different portions of the nephron during the production of either a dilute or a concentrated urine. As illustrated, approximately 10% of the filtered load of water is delivered to the collecting duct. Depending on the plasma ADH concentration, a variable portion of this water is then reabsorbed along the collecting duct, with water excretion ranging from 0.3% to 10% of the filtered load. Note that during antidiuresis, the largest volume of water is reabsorbed in the cortical and outer medullary portions of the collecting duct. A much smaller volume is reabsorbed from the inner medullary collecting duct. This distribution of water reabsorption along the length of the collecting duct (cortex > outer medulla > inner medulla) maintains the hyperosmotic interstitial environment in the inner medulla, which in turn allows maximal urinary concentration. If water reabsorption along the collecting duct were not distributed in this way and a large volume of water were reabsorbed in the inner medulla, the interstitial solutes would be diluted by the added water, interstitial osmolality would decline, and maximal urine concentration would not occur.

Medullary interstitial fluid osmolality. Let us look more closely at the critical role that the interstitial fluid of the renal medulla plays in the way the kidneys handle

---

*The term countercurrent multiplication derives from both the form and function of Henle's loop. Henle's loop consists of two parallel limbs with tubular fluid flowing in opposite directions (countercurrent flow). Fluid flows into the medulla in the descending limb, and out of the medulla in the ascending limb. The ascending limb is impermeable to water and reabsorbs solute from the tubular fluid. Thus, fluid within the ascending limb becomes diluted. This separation of solute and water by the ascending limb is termed the **single effect** of the countercurrent multiplication process. The solute removed from the ascending limb tubular fluid accumulates in the surrounding interstitial fluid and raises its osmolality. Because the descending limb is highly permeable to water, the increased osmolality of the medullary interstitium causes water to be absorbed and thereby concentrates the tubular fluid. The countercurrent flow within the descending and ascending limbs of Henle's loop magnifies, or "multiplies," the osmotic gradient between the tubular fluid in the descending and ascending limbs of Henle's loop.

Water diuresis

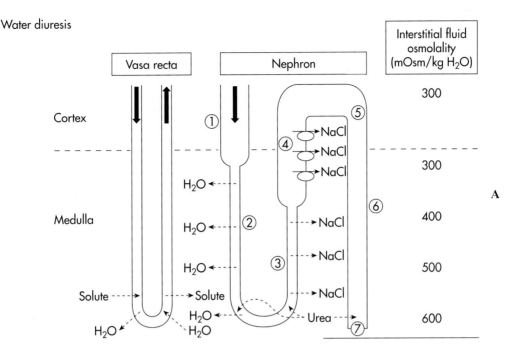

Antidiuresis

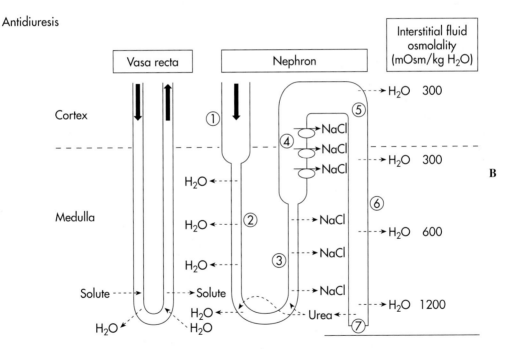

■ **Fig. 42-4**   **A,** Mechanism for the excretion of dilute urine (water diuresis). ADH is absent, and the collecting duct is essentially impermeable to water. Note that the osmolality of the medullary interstitium is reduced during water diuresis. **B,** Mechanism for the excretion of a concentrated urine (antidiuresis). Plasma ADH levels are maximal, and the collecting duct is highly permeable to water. Under this condition, the medullary interstitial gradient is maximal. The circled numbers correlate with the description in the text.

water. The osmotic pressure of this fluid provides the driving force for reabsorbing water from both the descending thin limb of Henle's loop and the collecting duct. The principal components of the medullary interstitial fluid are NaCl and urea, but the concentration of

these solutes is not uniform throughout the medulla (i.e., a gradient exists from cortex to papilla). Other solutes also accumulate in the medullary interstitium (e.g., NH_4^+ and K^+), but the most abundant solutes are NaCl and urea. For simplicity, let us assume that NaCl and urea are

■ **Table 42-4**   Transport and permeability properties of nephron segments involved in urine concentration and dilution

		Passive permeability*			
Tubule segment	*Active transport*	*NaCl*	*Urea*	*H₂O*	*Effect of ADH*
Henle's loop					
Descending thin limb	0	+	+	+++	
Ascending thin limb	0	+++	+	0	
Thick ascending limb	+++	+	0	0	
Distal tubule	+	+	0	0	
Collecting duct					
Cortex	+	+	0	0	↑ H H₂O permeability
Medulla	+	+	++	+	↑ H₂O and urea permeability

*Permeability is proportional to the number of plus signs indicated: +, low permeability; +++, high permeability; 0, impermeable.

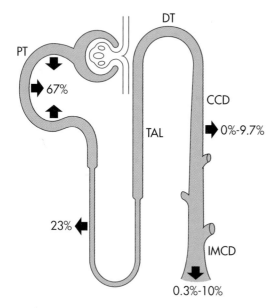

■ **Fig. 42-5**   Segmental water reabsorption. The percentage of the filtered load of water reabsorbed by each nephron segment is indicated. The amount of water reabsorbed by the proximal tubule and Henle's loop is relatively constant regardless of whether dilute or concentrated urine is excreted. The volume of water reabsorbed by the terminal portion of the distal tubule and the collecting duct is controlled by ADH. When ADH is absent, only a small volume of water is reabsorbed, and water excretion can reach 10% of the filtered load. (*Note:* The collecting duct does have limited permeability to water even in the absence of ADH, and therefore some water is actually reabsorbed. However, this volume is small.) Conversely, when ADH levels are maximal, a large volume of water is reabsorbed, and water excretion is less than 1% of the filtered load. *PT,* Proximal tubule; *TAL,* thick ascending limb; *DT,* distal tubule; *CCD,* cortical collecting duct; *IMCD,* inner medullary collecting duct.

the only solutes. At the junction of the medulla with the cortex, the interstitial fluid has an osmolality of approximately 300 mOsm/kg H₂O, with virtually all osmoles attributable to NaCl. The concentrations of both NaCl and urea increase progressively as the tubular fluid moves deeper into the medulla. When a maximally concentrated urine is excreted, the medullary interstitial fluid

osmolality is approximately 1200 mOsm/kg H₂O at the papilla (Fig. 42-4, *B*). Of this value, approximately 600 mOsm/kg H₂O is attributed to NaCl and 600 mOsm/kg H₂O to urea.

The medullary gradient for NaCl is created when NaCl reabsorbed by the nephron segments accumulates in the medulla during the process of countercurrent multiplication. The most important segment in this regard is the ascending limb (thick limb > thin limb) of Henle's loop. Urea accumulation within the medullary interstitium is more complex and occurs most effectively when a hyperosmotic urine is excreted (i.e., antidiuresis). When a dilute urine is produced, especially over extended periods of time, the osmolality of the medullary interstitium declines (compare panels *A* and *B* of Fig. 42-4). This reduced osmolality is almost entirely due to a decrease in the concentration of urea. This decrease in urea concentration reflects washout by the vasa recta (see p 727) and diffusion of urea from the interstitium into the tubular fluid within the medullary portion of the collecting duct (recall that the medullary collecting duct has a significant permeability to urea even in the absence of ADH; see Table 42-4).

Urea is generated by the liver as a result of protein metabolism, and enters the tubular fluid by glomerular filtration. As indicated in Table 42-4, the permeability to urea of most nephron segments involved in urinary concentration and dilution is relatively low, with the exception of the medullary collecting duct (especially in the presence of ADH). As fluid moves along the nephron, and as water is reabsorbed in the collecting duct (i.e., antidiuresis), the urea concentration in the tubular fluid increases. When this urea-rich tubular fluid reaches the medullary collecting duct, where the permeability to urea not only is high but is increased by ADH, urea diffuses down its concentration gradient into the medullary interstitial fluid, where it accumulates. When ADH levels are elevated, the urea within the collecting duct and the interstitium equilibrate. The resultant urea concentration of the urine will be equal to that of the medullary interstitium at the papilla, or approximately 600 mOsm/kg H₂O.

Some of the urea within the interstitium enters the descending thin and ascending thin limbs of Henle's loop. This urea is then trapped in the nephron until it again reaches the medullary collecting duct, where it can reenter the medullary interstitium. Thus, *urea recycles from the interstitium to the nephron, and back into the interstitium. This process of recycling serves to facilitate the accumulation of urea in the medullary interstitium.*

To summarize, the hyperosmotic medullary interstitium is essential for concentrating the tubular fluid within the collecting duct. Because water reabsorption is a passive process driven by an osmotic gradient, the maximal concentration that the urine can attain is equal to that of the medullary interstitium at the papilla (approximately 1200 mOsm/kg H_2O). Since a hyperosmotic medullary interstitium is essential for urine concentration, any condition that reduces this gradient impairs the ability of the kidneys to maximally concentrate the urine.

Individuals on a protein-deficient diet can exhibit a defect in urine-concentrating ability. This inability to maximally concentrate the urine reflects decreased urea levels within the medullary interstitial fluid. When protein intake is inadequate, urea production in the body is decreased. As a result of the decreased production of urea, the urea content, and thus the osmolality, of the medullary interstitium are reduced. Ingestion of adequate amounts of protein restores the medullary interstitial urea gradient.

It is apparent that the concentration of urea in the medullary interstitial fluid plays an important role in determining the osmolality of the urine. When the urea concentration is reduced (i.e., with excretion of dilute urine or reduced protein intake), maximal urine osmolality is reduced in proportion. Conversely, when the urea concentration is increased (i.e., with maximal ADH levels), the urine osmolality increases in parallel. However, urea is an ineffective osmole throughout much of the body, and therefore does not cause water to move between the ICF and ECF. Similarly, urea is not an effective osmole across the medullary collecting duct, because this part of the nephron has a high permeability to urea, especially in the presence of ADH. The role of effective and ineffective osmoles (e.g., urea) in the maintenance of whole body water balance is considered in more detail on p 728. The main point to remember about the role of urea within the medullary interstitium is that urea does not drive water reabsorption from the lumen of the collecting duct into the medullary interstitium. Instead, the urea in the tubular fluid and medullary interstitium equilibrates, especially at the slow tubular flow rates associated with the excretion of a concentrated urine. Thus, urine with a high urea concentration is excreted. It is the medullary interstitial NaCl concentration that is responsible for the reabsorption of water from the medullary collecting duct and thus for the concentration of nonurea solutes (e.g., NH_4^+-salts, K^+-salts, creatinine) in the urine.

Vasa recta function: countercurrent exchange. *The vasa recta, the capillary networks that supply blood to the medulla, are highly permeable to solute and water.* As with Henle's loop, the vasa recta form a parallel set of hairpin loops within the medulla (see Chapter 40). The vasa recta not only bring nutrients and oxygen to the tubules within the medulla, but more importantly remove excess water and solute, which are continuously added to the medullary interstitium by the nephron segments in this region. Note that the ability of the vasa recta to maintain the medullary interstitial gradient is flow dependent. A substantial increase in blood flow through the vasa recta will ultimately dissipate the medullary gradient (i.e., "wash out" the medullary interstitial gradient). Alternatively, if blood flow is reduced, the nephron segments within the medulla will receive inadequate oxygen. Under conditions of reduced blood flow, tubular transport, especially by the thick ascending limb of Henle's loop, is impaired. As a result, the medullary interstitial osmotic gradient cannot be maintained.

■ Assessment of Renal Diluting and Concentrating Ability

Assessment of the dilution and concentration processes involves measurements of urine osmolality and the volume of urine excreted. Urine osmolality ranges from 50 mOsm/kg H_2O to 1200 mOsm/kg H_2O. The corresponding urine volume ranges from 18 L to as little as 0.5 L per day. Note that these ranges are not fixed; rather, they vary from individual to individual.

Traditionally, the handling of water by the kidneys has been quantitated by measuring what has been termed the **free-water clearance.** As noted previously, the central process in the dilution or concentration of urine is the single effect of separating solute from water. Through this separation, the kidneys in a sense, generate a volume of water that is "free of all solute." When the urine is dilute, this **solute-free water** is excreted from the body. When the urine is concentrated, the solute-free water is returned to the systemic circulation. The concept of free-water clearance is merely a means for quantitating the ability of the kidneys to generate solute-free water. The free-water concept follows directly from renal clearance, as described in Chapter 40.

The clearance of total solute (i.e., all osmoles, whether effective or ineffective) from plasma by the kidneys can be calculated as:

$$C_{osm} = \frac{U_{osm} \times \dot{V}}{P_{osm}} \qquad (42\text{-}4)$$

where C_{osm} is the **osmolar clearance,** U_{osm} is the urine osmolality, $\dot{V}$ is the urine flow rate, and P_{osm} is the plasma osmolality. C_{osm} is expressed in units of volume/unit time. Free-water clearance (C_{H_2O}) is then calculated as:

$$C_{H_2O} = \dot{V} - C_{osm} \qquad (42\text{-}5)$$

By rearranging equation 42-3, it should be apparent that:

$$\dot{V} = C_{H_2O} + C_{osm} \qquad (42\text{-}6)$$

In other words, we can divide total urine output ($\dot{V}$) into two hypothetical components. One component contains all the urine solutes and has an osmolality equal to that of plasma (i.e., $U_{osm} = P_{osm}$). This component represents C_{osm}, and represents a volume from which there has been no net separation of solute and water. The second component (C_{H_2O}) is a volume of solute-free water.

When dilute urine is produced, the value of C_{H_2O} is positive, indicating that solute-free water is excreted from the body. When concentrated urine is produced, the value of C_{H_2O} is negative, indicating that solute-free water is retained in the body. By convention, negative C_{H_2O} values are expressed as $T^c_{H_2O}$ (**tubular conservation of water**).

Calculating C_{H_2O} and $T^c_{H_2O}$ can provide important information about the function of those portions of the nephron involved in producing dilute and concentrated urine. *Whether the kidneys excrete or reabsorb free water depends on the presence of ADH.* When ADH is absent or ADH levels are low, solute-free water is excreted. When ADH levels are high, solute-free water is reabsorbed.

The following factors are necessary for the kidneys to excrete a maximal amount of solute-free water (C_{H_2O}):

1. ADH must be absent. Without ADH, the collecting duct does not reabsorb water.
2. The tubular structures, which separate solute from water (i.e., dilute the luminal fluid), must function normally. In the absence of ADH, the following nephron segments can dilute the luminal fluid:
   - Ascending thin limb of Henle's loop
   - Thick ascending limb of Henle's loop
   - Distal tubule
   - Collecting duct
   Because of its high transport rate, the thick ascending limb is quantitatively the most important of these segments involved in the separation of solute and water.
3. An adequate amount of tubular fluid must be delivered to the above nephron sites for maximal separation of solute and water. Factors that reduce delivery (e.g., decreased GFR or enhanced proximal tubule reabsorption) impair the ability of the kidneys to maximally excrete C_{H_2O}.

Similar requirements also apply to the conservation of water by the kidneys ($T^c_{H_2O}$). For the kidneys to conserve water maximally, the following conditions must exist:

1. An adequate amount of tubular fluid must be delivered to those nephron segments in which separation of solute and water occurs. The important segment in the separation of solute and water is the thick ascending limb of Henle's loop. Delivery of tubular fluid to Henle's loop depends in turn on GFR and proximal tubule reabsorption.

2. Reabsorption of NaCl by the nephron segments must be normal; again, the most important segment is the thick ascending limb of Henle's loop.
3. A hyperosmotic medullary interstitium must be present. The interstitial osmolality is maintained by NaCl reabsorption by Henle's loop (conditions 1 and 2) and by effective accumulation of urea. Urea accumulation in turn depends on adequate dietary protein intake.
4. Maximal levels of ADH must be present and the collecting duct must respond normally to ADH.

The concept of free-water clearance as just described does not distinguish between effective and ineffective osmoles, either in the plasma or in the urine. However, urea, which can account for half of total urine osmoles, is not an effective osmole when the movement of water between the ICF and ECF is considered. Accordingly, when one wants to understand how the handling of water by the kidneys contributes to the maintenance of whole body water balance, it is more appropriate to consider only those solutes that are effective osmoles. For plasma (i.e., ECF), the effective osmoles are Na^+ and its attendant anions. For urine, they are the nonurea solutes.

The importance of using effective osmoles in determining the impact of renal water handling on whole body water balance (i.e., body fluid osmolality) is illustrated by the following example. A patient has an elevated plasma [urea], and his plasma [Na^+] is also increased. His total plasma osmolality (including urea) is 320 mOsm/kg H_2O, but his effective plasma osmolality (calculated as $2 \times [Na^+]$) is only 300 mOsm/kg H_2O. His urine osmolality is 600 mOsm/kg H_2O: 300 mOsm/kg H_2O due to urea and 300 mOsm/kg H_2O due to nonurea solutes. His urinary flow rate is 3 L/day.

According to equations 42-4 and 42-5, his total osmolar clearance (C_{osm}) and free-water clearance (C_{H_2O}) are:

$$C_{osm} = \frac{600 \text{ mOsm/kg } H_2O \times 3 \text{ L/day}}{320 \text{ mOsm/kg } H_2O} = 5.6 \text{ L/day} \quad (42\text{-}7)$$

$$C_{H_2O} = 3 \text{ L/day} - 5.6 \text{ L/day} = -2.6 \text{ L/day } (T^c_{H_2O}) \quad (42\text{-}8)$$

Thus, it would appear that the kidneys are conserving 2.6 L/day of solute-free water, which would be an appropriate response to correct the elevated plasma osmolality and hypernatremia. However, when C_{osm} and C_{H_2O} are analyzed from the perspective of effective osmoles, the following results are obtained:

$$C_{osm} = \frac{300 \text{ mOsm/kg } H_2O \times 3 \text{ L/day}}{300 \text{ mOsm/kg } H_2O} = 3 \text{ L/day} \quad (42\text{-}9)$$

$$C_{H_2O} = 3 \text{ L/day} - 3 \text{ L/day} = 0 \text{ L/day} \quad (42\text{-}10)$$

Thus, when viewed from the more appropriate perspective of effective osmoles, it is apparent that the kidneys are not reabsorbing solute-free water, and the patient's kidneys will not correct the hyperosmolality and hypernatremia.

■ *Control of Extracellular Fluid Volume and Regulation of Renal NaCl Excretion*

The major solutes of the ECF are the salts of Na^+. Of these, NaCl is the most abundant. Because NaCl is also the major determinant of the osmolality of ECF, it is commonly assumed that alterations in Na^+ balance disturb ECF osmolality. However, under normal conditions, this is not the case. Changes in Na^+ balance do not normally alter ECF osmolality, because the ADH and thirst systems maintain body fluid osmolality within a narrow range. For example, addition of NaCl to ECF (without water) increases the $[Na^+]$ and osmolality of this compartment (ICF osmolality also increases because of osmotic equilibration with ECF). This increase in osmolality in turn stimulates thirst and the release of ADH from the posterior pituitary. The increased ingestion of water in response to thirst, together with the ADH-induced decrease in water excretion by the kidneys, quickly restores ECF osmolality to normal. However, the volume of ECF increases in proportion to the amount of water ingested, which in turn depends on the amount of NaCl added to ECF. Thus, in the new steady state, addition of NaCl to ECF is equivalent to adding an iso-osmotic solution. Conversely, a decrease in the NaCl content of ECF results in a decrease in the volume of this compartment.

The kidneys are the major route of NaCl excretion from the body. As such, they play an important role in regulating the volume of ECF. *Under normal conditions, the kidneys keep the volume of ECF constant by adjusting the excretion of NaCl to match the amount ingested in the diet.* If ingestion exceeds excretion, ECF volume increases above normal; the opposite occurs if excretion exceeds ingestion.

The typical diet contains approximately 140 mEq/day of Na^+ ($\approx$ 8 g of NaCl), and thus daily Na^+ excretion is also about 140 mEq/day. However, the kidneys can vary the excretion of Na^+ over a wide range. Excretion rates as low as 10 mEq/day can be attained when individuals are placed on a low-salt diet. Conversely, the kidneys can increase their excretion rate to more than 1000 mEq/day when challenged by the ingestion of a high-salt diet. These changes in Na^+ excretion occur with only modest changes in the steady-state Na^+ content of the body.

The response of the kidneys to abrupt changes in NaCl intake typically takes several hours to several days, depending on the magnitude of the change. During this transition period, intake and excretion of Na^+ are not matched as they are in the steady state. Thus, the individual experiences either **positive Na^+ balance** (intake > excretion) or **negative Na^+ balance** (intake < excretion). By the end of the transition period, a new steady state is established and intake once again equals excretion. Provided that the ADH and thirst systems are normal,

alterations in Na^+ balance result in changes in the volume of ECF but not the serum $[Na^+]$ or plasma osmolality. Changes in ECF volume can be monitored by measuring body weight, since 1 L of ECF equals 1 kg of body weight.

The maintenance of Na^+ balance, and thus a constant ECF volume, involves a complex system of sensors and effector signals that act primarily on the kidneys to regulate the excretion of NaCl.* The following sections review the physiology of these Na^+ sensors and explain the various signals involved in the regulation of NaCl excretion. In addition, Na^+ transport by the various portions of the nephron and its regulation are described. Finally, the pathophysiological mechanisms involved in the formation of edema are presented, with emphasis on the role of NaCl handling by the kidneys.

■ *Concept of Effective Circulating Volume*

As noted, Na^+ and its salts are the major constituents of the ECF, and changes in Na^+ balance lead to alterations in ECF volume. Changes in ECF volume can also influence Na^+ balance by altering the amount of NaCl excreted by the kidneys. However, the relationship between ECF volume, renal NaCl excretion, and whole body Na^+ balance is complex, especially in certain pathological conditions. Therefore, to understand the relationship among these factors, one must consider the concept of **effective circulating volume.**

The effective circulating volume is not a measurable and distinct body fluid compartment, and it is defined physiologically not anatomically. *The effective circulating volume refers to the portion of ECF volume that is contained within the vascular system and is "effectively" perfusing the tissues.* In this regard, it reflects, and is dependent on, the volume of and "pressure" within the vascular system. In addition, it is related to cardiac output. However, as illustrated below, the effective circulating volume cannot simply be equated with the volume of fluid within the vascular tree.

In a normal individual, the effective circulating volume varies directly with the volume of ECF and in particular the vascular system (arterial and venous), the arterial blood pressure, and the cardiac output. Thus, a decrease in ECF and vascular volume, arterial pressure, or cardiac output will be sensed by the body as a decrease in effective circulating volume. Conversely, an increase in ECF and vascular volume, arterial pressure, or cardiac output will be sensed as an increase in effective circulating volume.

---

*The absorption of NaCl by the gastrointestinal tract also appears to be influenced by whole body Na^+ balance. With positive Na^+ balance, a reflex reduction in NaCl absorption occurs. Conversely, with negative Na^+ balance, intestinal NaCl absorption is stimulated. These responses are mediated by efferent signals carried in the vagus nerve. This chapter focuses only on the role of the kidneys in the maintenance of Na^+ balance.

ECF volume, vascular volume, arterial blood pressure, and cardiac output all depend on the effective circulating volume, which in turn is related to Na^+ balance. Consequently, the kidneys alter NaCl excretion in response to changes in the effective circulating volume. When the effective circulating volume is decreased, renal NaCl excretion is reduced. This adaptive response restores the effective circulating volume to normal and thereby maintains adequate tissue perfusion. Conversely, an increase in the effective circulating volume results in enhanced renal NaCl excretion, termed **natriuresis.** Again, this is an adaptive response to restore the effective circulating volume to its normal set point.

In a normal individual, Na^+ balance determines the effective circulating volume, the ECF volume, and the vascular volume, which in turn influence arterial blood pressure and cardiac output. However, under some important pathological conditions, the effective circulating volume can vary independently from the ECF and vascular volumes, arterial blood pressure, or even cardiac output. Regardless of the condition, the kidneys adjust their excretion of NaCl in response to perceived changes in the effective circulating volume, and thus how effectively the tissues of the body are perfused.

Patients with **congestive heart failure** frequently have an increase in ECF and vascular volumes, which is manifested as accumulation of fluid in the lungs **(pulmonary edema)** and peripheral tissues **(generalized edema).** This excess fluid is the result of NaCl and water retention by the kidneys. The kidneys' response (i.e., retention of NaCl and water) seems paradoxical, because both the ECF and vascular volumes in such patients are increased. However, the effective circulating volume is decreased in congestive heart failure because of poor cardiac performance, and thus decreased cardiac output. As a result of this decreased effective circulating volume, and by mechanisms described below, the kidneys retain NaCl and water. Hence, the kidneys' response is directed at increasing the effective circulating volume and thereby tissue perfusion. Unfortunately, in the setting of poor cardiac performance, this adaptive response increases ECF volume above its normal set point, and results in the development of pulmonary and generalized edema.

Advanced **hepatic cirrhosis** further illustrates how the effective circulating volume can vary independently of ECF volume, vascular volume, and cardiac output. Patients with advanced hepatic cirrhosis accumulate large volumes of fluid in the peritoneal cavity **(ascites).** This fluid is a component of ECF. These patients' vascular volume is also increased because of pooling of blood in the venous side of the splanchnic circulation (the damaged liver impedes drainage of blood from the splanchnic circulation via the portal vein). Finally, these patients develop multiple **arterio-venous fistulas** throughout the body. These fistulas shunt blood from the arterial to the venous side of the circulation (i.e., bypass the capillary beds) and have the effects of increasing cardiac output but impairing tissue perfusion. Thus, these patients have an increase in ECF volume, vascular volume, and cardiac output. However, their tissues are not effectively perfused. Consequently, the body senses a decreased effective circulating volume, and the kidneys respond by retaining NaCl and water. It is the retention of NaCl and water by the kidneys that results in the increase in ECF volume (i.e., ascites) and vascular volume.

The remaining portions of this section will examine the relationship between the effective circulating volume and renal NaCl excretion in normal adults (i.e., those free of disease). In this setting, changes in the effective circulating volume parallel those of ECF volume, vascular volume, arterial blood pressure, and cardiac output. First, the maintenance of a normal effective circulating volume **(euvolemia)** is reviewed. This is followed by consideration of the renal response to an increase in the effective circulating volume **(volume expansion),** and the renal response to a decrease in the effective circulating volume **(volume contraction).**

■ *Volume Sensing System*

The various sensors involved in monitoring the effective circulating volume are listed in Table 42-5. A number of the sensors are located in the vascular system and monitor its fullness and blood pressure. These are typically called volume receptors; because they respond to stretch, they are also referred to as baroreceptors. The sensors within the liver and central nervous system (CNS) are less well understood and do not seem to be as important as the vascular sensors in monitoring the effective circulating volume.

Vascular low-pressure volume sensors. Baroreceptors are located within the walls of the cardiac atria and pulmonary vessels, and respond to distention of these structures (see also Chapters 28 and 29). Because the low-pressure side of the circulatory system has a high

■ Table 42-5   Volume sensors

  I. Vascular
     A. Low pressure
        1. Cardiac atria
        2. Pulmonary vasculature
     B. High pressure
        1. Carotid sinus
        2. Aortic arch
        3. Juxtaglomerular apparatus of kidneys
 II. Hepatic
III. Central nervous system

capacitance, the atrial and pulmonary vascular sensors respond primarily to the "fullness" of the vascular system, and these baroreceptors send signals to the brainstem (solitary tract nucleus of the medulla oblongata) via afferent fibers in the vagus nerve. The activity of these sensors modulates both sympathetic nerve outflow and ADH secretion. For example, a decrease in filling of the pulmonary vessels and cardiac atria increases sympathetic nerve activity and stimulates ADH secretion. Conversely, distention of these structures decreases sympathetic nerve activity. In general, 5% to 10% changes in blood volume and pressure are necessary to evoke a response.

The cardiac atria possess an additional mechanism related to control of renal NaCl excretion. The myocytes of the atria synthesize and store a peptide hormone, termed **atrial natriuretic peptide (ANP),** that is released when the atria are distended. By mechanisms outlined in subsequent sections, ANP reduces blood pressure and increases the excretion of NaCl and water by the kidneys (see p 734).

Vascular high-pressure volume sensors. Baroreceptors are also present in the arterial side of the circulatory system, located in the wall of the aortic arch, the carotid sinus (see also Chapter 28), and the afferent arteriole of the kidneys. These baroreceptors respond primarily to blood pressure. The aortic arch and carotid baroreceptors also send input to the brainstem (solitary tract nucleus of the medulla oblongata) via afferent fibers in the vagus and glossopharyngeal nerves. The response to this input also involves alterations in sympathetic outflow and ADH secretion. Thus, a decrease in blood pressure will increase sympathetic nerve activity and ADH secretion. An increase in pressure tends to reduce sympathetic nerve activity. The sensitivity of the high-pressure baroreceptors is similar to that of those in the low-pressure side of the vascular system, with 5% to 10% changes in pressure needed to evoke a response.

The **juxtaglomerular apparatus** of the kidneys (see Chapter 40), particularly the afferent arterioles, responds directly to changes in pressure. If perfusion pressure of the afferent arterioles is reduced, renin is released from the myocytes. Renin secretion is suppressed when perfusion pressure is increased. As described in subsequent sections, renin determines blood levels of angiotensin II and aldosterone, both of which play an important role in regulating renal Na+ excretion.

Constriction of a renal artery **(renal artery stenosis)** by an atherosclerotic plaque, for example, reduces perfusion pressure to that kidney. This reduced perfusion pressure is sensed by the afferent arterioles and results in the secretion of renin. The elevated renin levels increase production of angiotensin II, which in turn increases systemic blood pressure by its constrictor effect on arterioles throughout the vascular system.

The increased systemic blood pressure is sensed by the afferent arterioles of the contralateral kidney (i.e., the kidney without stenosis of its renal artery), and renin secretion from that kidney is suppressed.

Hepatic sensors. The liver also contains volume sensors that, although not as important as the vascular sensors in monitoring the effective circulating volume, can modulate renal NaCl excretion. One type of hepatic sensor responds to pressure within the hepatic vasculature and therefore functions in a manner similar to the low- and high-pressure baroreceptors just described. A different type of sensor also appears to exist in the liver; it responds to the concentration of Na+ in the portal vein blood. Afferent signals from both types of sensors are carried to the CNS in the hepatic nerves. These afferent signals are sent to the same region of the brainstem (solitary tract nucleus of the medulla oblongata), where afferent fibers from the low- and high-pressure baroreceptors also converge. Increased pressure within the hepatic vasculature, or an increase in portal vein [Na+], results in a decrease in renal sympathetic nerve activity.* As described subsequently, this decrease in renal sympathetic tone leads to an increase in renal NaCl excretion.

Central nervous system Na+ sensors. Like the hepatic sensors, the CNS sensors are not as important as the vascular sensors in monitoring the effective circulating volume. Nevertheless, alterations in the [Na+] of blood carried to the brain by the carotid arteries, or the [Na+] of the cerebrospinal fluid (CSF), modulate renal NaCl excretion. For example, if the [Na+] in either the carotid artery blood or the CSF is increased, there is a decrease in renal sympathetic nerve activity, which in turn leads to an increase in renal NaCl excretion. The precise location of the Na+ receptors involved in this response is not known, although they are thought to be in the hypothalamus.

■ *Volume Sensor Signals*

The kidneys play an important role in Na+ homeostasis. Both neural and hormonal signals have been identified. These signals are summarized in Table 42-6, as are their effects on renal NaCl and water excretion.

Renal sympathetic nerves. As described in Chapter 40, sympathetic nerve fibers innervate the afferent and efferent arterioles of the glomerulus, as well as nephron cells. With negative Na+ balance (i.e., volume depletion),

---

*The hepatic sensors also appear to be involved in the regulation of gastrointestinal NaCl absorption. For example, when the [Na+] of the portal vein blood is increased, there is a reflex reduction in jejunal NaCl absorption. As noted, the efferent limb of this response is carried in the vagus nerve.

■ **Table 42-6** Signals involved in the control of renal NaCl and water excretion

Renal sympathetic nerves (↑ activity: ↓ NaCl excretion)

↓ Glomerular filtration rte
↑ Renin secretion
↑ Proximal tubule, thick ascending limb of Henle's loop, distal tubule, and collecting duct NaCl reabsorption

Renin-angiotensin-aldosterone (↑ secretion: ↓ NaCl excretion)

↑ Angiotensin II levels stimulate proximal tubule NaCl reabsorption
↑ Aldosterone levels stimulate thick ascending limb of Henle's loop, distal tubule, and collecting duct NaCl reabsorption
↑ ADH secretion

Atrial natriuretic peptide (↑ secretion: ↑ NaCl excretion)

↑ Glomerular filtration rate
↓ Renin secretion
↓ Aldosterone secretion
↓ NaCl and water reabsorption by the collecting duct*
↓ ADH secretion and action of ADH on the collecting duct

ADH (↑ secretion: ↓ H_2O excretion)

↑ H_2O absorption by the collecting duct

*Urodilatin contributes to this effect.

the Na^+ sensors (especially the low- and high-pressure vascular baroreceptors) stimulate renal sympathetic nerve activity. This stimulation has the following effects:

1. The afferent and efferent arterioles are constricted by activation of α-adrenergic receptors. This vasoconstriction (the effect appears to be greater on the afferent arteriole) decreases the hydrostatic pressure within the glomerular capillary lumen, and thereby reduces the GFR. With this decrease in GFR, the filtered load of Na^+ to the nephrons is reduced (filtered load = GFR $\times$ plasma $[Na^+]$).

2. Renin secretion by the cells of the afferent and efferent arterioles is stimulated via activation of β-adrenergic receptors. As described below, renin ultimately increases circulating levels of angiotensin II and aldosterone.

3. NaCl reabsorption along the nephron is directly stimulated via activation of α-adrenergic receptors. Quantitatively, the most important segment influenced by sympathetic nerve activity is the proximal tubule.

The combined effect of these actions contributes to an overall decrease in NaCl excretion, an adaptive response that works to restore euvolemia. Conversely, with positive Na^+ balance (i.e., volume expansion), renal sympathetic nerve activity is reduced. This response generally reverses the effects just described.

Renin-angiotensin-aldosterone system. Smooth muscle cells in the afferent and efferent arterioles are the site of synthesis, storage, and release of **renin.** Three factors play an important role in stimulating renin secretion:

1. *Perfusion pressure.* The afferent arteriole is a high-pressure baroreceptor. When perfusion pressure to the kidneys is reduced, renin secretion is stimulated. Conversely, an increase in perfusion pressure inhibits renin release.

2. *Sympathetic nerve activity.* Activation of the sympathetic nerve fibers innervating the afferent and efferent arterioles results in an increase in renin secretion. Renin secretion is decreased as renal sympathetic nerve activity is decreased.

3. *Delivery of NaCl to the macula densa.* This regulates the GFR by a process called *tubuloglomerular feedback* (see Chapter 40). By this feedback mechanism, increased NaCl delivery to the macula densa results in a decrease in GFR. Conversely, decreased NaCl delivery increases GFR. In addition, the macula densa plays a role in renin secretion. When NaCl delivery to the macula densa is decreased, renin secretion is enhanced. Conversely, an increase in NaCl delivery inhibits renin secretion. This macula densa–mediated secretion of renin does not appear to be involved in the alterations in glomerular hemodynamics that underlie the phenomenon of tubuloglomerular feedback.*

Fig. 42-6 summarizes the essential components of the renin-angiotensin-aldosterone system. Renin alone does not have a physiological function; it functions solely as a proteolytic enzyme. Its substrate is a circulating protein, **angiotensinogen,** which is produced by the liver. Angiotensinogen is cleaved by renin to yield a 10-amino acid peptide, **angiotensin I.** Angiotensin I also has no known physiological function, and is further cleaved to an 8-amino acid peptide, **angiotensin II,** by a converting enzyme **(angiotensin converting enzyme [ACE])** found on the surface of vascular endothelial cells (pulmonary and renal endothelial cells are important sites for the conversion of angiotensin I to angiotensin II). Angiotensin II has several important physiological functions, including

1. Stimulation of aldosterone secretion by the adrenal cortex.

2. Arteriolar vasoconstriction, which increases blood pressure.

3. Stimulation of ADH secretion and thirst.

4. Enhancement of NaCl reabsorption by the proximal tubule.

Angiotensin II is an important secretagogue for **aldosterone** (an increase in plasma $[K^+]$ is the other important stimulus for aldosterone secretion; see Chapter 43.)

---

*It is thought that macula densa–mediated renin secretion may play a role in maintaining systemic arterial pressure under conditions of a reduced vascular volume. For example, when vascular volume is reduced, perfusion of the body tissues (including the kidneys) will decrease. This in turn will result in a decrease in GFR and the filtered load of NaCl. The reduced delivery of NaCl to the macula densa will then stimulate renin secretion, which through angiotensin II (a potent vasoconstrictor) will act to increase blood pressure and thereby maintain tissue perfusion.

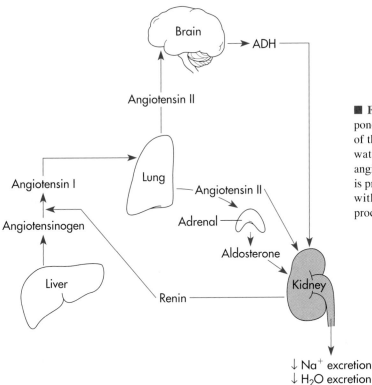

■ **Fig. 42-6** Schematic representation of the essential components of the renin-angiotensin-aldosterone system. Activation of this system results in a decrease in the excretion of Na+ and water by the kidneys. *Note:* Angiotensin I is converted to angiotensin II by angiotensin converting enzyme (ACE), which is present on all vascular endothelial cells. The endothelial cells within the lungs play a significant role in this conversion process. See text for details.

Aldosterone is a steroid hormone produced by the glomerulosa cells of the adrenal cortex (see also Chapter 51). It acts in a number of ways on the kidneys (see also Chapters 43 and 44). With regard to regulation of the effective circulating volume, aldosterone reduces NaCl excretion by stimulating its reabsorption by the thick ascending limb of Henle's loop, the distal tubule, and the collecting duct. The effect of aldosterone on renal NaCl excretion depends primarily on its ability to stimulate Na+ reabsorption in the distal tubule and collecting duct.

The stimulation of Na+ reabsorption by aldosterone in the late portion of the distal tubule and collecting duct has been studied extensively. Aldosterone enters the cell (principal cell) and binds to a cytoplasmic receptor. The hormone-receptor complex enters the nucleus and regulates transcription of messenger ribonucleic acid (mRNA) that encodes for a number of proteins important for Na+ reabsorption by the cell. Although all the intracellular steps involved in the action of aldosterone have not been identified, the net effect on Na+ reabsorption is an increase in Na+ entry into the principal cell across the apical membrane. Na+ exit from the cell across the basolateral membrane is also enhanced. The increase in apical membrane Na+ entry occurs via Na+-selective channels, and the increased exit of Na+ from the cell across the basolateral membrane occurs by the Na+, K+-ATPase. Because the transcellular reabsorption of Na+ by the principal cell generates a lumen-negative transepithelial voltage (see Chapter 41), the enhanced Na+ reabsorption from the luminal fluid increases the magnitude of this

voltage. As a result of the increased magnitude of the transepithelial voltage, the passive movement of Cl− from the lumen to blood via the paracellular pathway is enhanced. Thus, aldosterone increases the reabsorption of NaCl from the tubular fluid. Reduced levels of aldosterone result in a decrease in the amount of NaCl reabsorbed by the principal cell.

Aldosterone also enhances NaCl reabsorption by cells of the thick ascending limb of Henle's loop. The precise cellular mechanisms involved in aldosterone's action on the thick ascending limb cells have not yet been elucidated. However, it is likely that both Na+ entry into the cell (perhaps via the apical membrane 1Na+-1K+-2Cl− symporter) and its extrusion from the cell (via the basolateral membrane Na+, K+-ATPase) is stimulated.

Diseases of the adrenal cortex can alter aldosterone levels and thereby impair the ability of the kidneys to maintain Na+ balance and euvolemia. With decreased secretion of aldosterone **(hypoaldosteronism),** Na+ reabsorption, primarily by the collecting duct, is reduced. The result is a loss of Na+ in the urine. Because urinary Na+ loss can exceed the amount ingested in the diet, negative Na+ balance will ensue, and volume contraction occurs. In response, sympathetic tone is increased, leading to elevated levels of renin, angiotensin II, and ADH. With increased aldosterone secretion **(hyperaldosteronism),** the opposite effects occur. Na+ reabsorption, especially by the collecting duct, is enhanced, resulting in reduced excretion of Na⁺. Consequently, volume expansion results; sympathetic tone is decreased; and levels of renin, angiotensin II, and ADH are decreased. As described below, ANP levels are also elevated in this setting.

As summarized in Table 42-6, *activation of the renin-angiotensin-aldosterone system, as occurs with volume depletion, results in decreased excretion of NaCl by the kidneys.* This system is suppressed with volume expansion, and renal NaCl excretion is therefore enhanced.

Atrial natriuretic peptide. Atrial myocytes produce and store a peptide hormone, atrial natriuretic peptide (ANP), that relaxes vascular smooth muscle and promotes NaCl and water excretion by the kidney.* ANP is released with atrial stretch, as would occur with positive Na⁺ balance and volume expansion. The circulating form of ANP is 28 amino acids in length. In general, ANP actions, as they relate to renal NaCl and water excretion, antagonize those of the renin-angiotensin-aldosterone system. They include the following:

1. Vasodilation of the afferent and vasoconstriction of the efferent arterioles of the glomerulus, increasing GFR and the filtered load of Na⁺.

2. Inhibition of renin secretion by the afferent and efferent arterioles.

3. Inhibition of aldosterone secretion by the glomerulosa cells of the adrenal cortex. ANP reduces aldosterone secretion by two mechanisms: it inhibits renin secretion, thereby reducing angiotensin II–induced aldosterone secretion; and it acts directly on the glomerulosa cells of the adrenal cortex to inhibit aldosterone secretion.

4. Inhibition of NaCl reabsorption by the collecting duct. This effect is due in part to reduced levels of aldosterone; however, ANP also acts directly on the collecting duct cells. Through its second messenger, cyclic guanine monophosphate (cGMP), ANP inhibits Na⁺ channels in the apical membrane of the cell, and thereby NaCl reabsorption. This effect is predominantly in the medullary portion of the collecting duct.

5. Inhibition of ADH secretion by the posterior pituitary and ADH action on the collecting duct. This results in a reduction in water reabsorption by the collecting duct and thus increased excretion of water in the urine.

Taken together, these effects of ANP increase the excretion of NaCl and water by the kidneys. Hypothetically, a reduction in circulating levels of ANP would be expected to decrease NaCl and water excretion. However, no convincing evidence for this effect has been found.

Antidiuretic hormone. As already discussed, with volume depletion, ADH secretion by the posterior pituitary is stimulated. The elevated levels of ADH cause decreased water excretion by the kidneys, which serves to reestablish euvolemia.

■ *Control of Na⁺ Excretion during Euvolemia*

The maintenance of Na⁺ balance and therefore euvolemia requires a precise balance between the amount of NaCl ingested and that excreted from the body. In a euvolemic individual, daily urine NaCl excretion equals daily NaCl intake.

The kidneys can vary the amount of NaCl they excrete over a wide range. Under conditions of salt restriction (e.g., low NaCl diet), virtually no NaCl appears in the urine. Conversely, in individuals who ingest large quantities of salt, renal NaCl excretion can exceed 1000 mEq/day of Na⁺. The kidneys' response to variations in dietary salt intake may take several days. During the transition period, excretion does not match intake, and the individual will be in either positive (intake > excretion) or negative (intake < excretion) Na⁺ balance. When Na⁺ balance is altered during these transition periods, the ECF volume changes in parallel (water excretion, regulated via the ADH system, is also adjusted to keep plasma osmolality constant, resulting in an iso-osmotic change in ECF volume). Thus, with positive balance, volume expansion occurs (detected as an increase in body weight), while with negative balance, volume contraction occurs (detected as a decrease in body weight). Ultimately, renal excretion will reach a new steady state, and euvolemia will be reestablished as NaCl excretion is once again matched to intake. The time course for adjustment of renal NaCl excretion to intake is variable and depends on the magnitude of the change in NaCl intake. Adaptation to large changes in NaCl intake requires a longer time than does the adaptation to small changes in intake.

To comprehend how renal Na⁺ excretion is regulated, the general features of Na⁺ handling along the nephron must be understood. Fig. 42-7 summarizes the contribution of each nephron segment to the reabsorption of the filtered load of Na⁺ under euvolemic conditions (the specific cellular mechanisms of Na⁺ transport are explained in Chapter 41). Most of the filtered load of Na⁺ (67%) is reabsorbed by the proximal tubule. An additional 25% is reabsorbed by the thick ascending limb of Henle's loop, and the remainder by the distal tubule and collecting duct.

The following discussion considers only the renal handling of Na⁺. Although not specifically addressed, Cl⁻ reabsorption is regulated in parallel.

In a normal adult, the filtered load of Na⁺ can be calculated as:

$$\text{filtered load of Na}^+ = (\text{GFR})(\text{plasma [Na}^+])$$
$$= (180 \text{ L/day})(140 \text{ mEq/L}) \quad (42\text{-}11)$$
$$= 25,200 \text{ mEq/day}$$

---

*As noted in Chapter 41, urodilatin, a natriuretic peptide produced in the kidney, also acts on the collecting duct to decrease NaCl reabsorption.

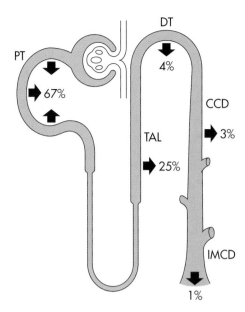

■ Fig. 42-7 Segmental Na⁺ reabsorption. The percentage of the filtered load of Na⁺ reabsorbed by each nephron segment is indicated. *PT,* Proximal tubule; *TAL,* thick ascending limb; *DT,* distal tubule; *CCD,* cortical collecting duct; *IMCD,* inner medullary collecting duct.

With a typical diet, less than 1% of this filtered load is excreted in the urine (approximately 140 mEq/day). Because of the large filtered load of Na⁺, it is important to recognize that small changes in Na⁺ reabsorption by the nephron can profoundly affect Na⁺ balance and thus the volume of ECF. For example, an increase in Na⁺ excretion from 1% to 3% of the filtered load represents an additional loss of approximately 500 mEq/day. Because ECF [Na⁺] is 140 mEq/L, Na⁺ loss of this magnitude would decrease ECF volume by more than 3 L (water excretion would parallel the loss of Na⁺ to maintain body fluid osmolality constant; 500 mEq/day ÷ 140 mEq/L = 3.6 L/day of fluid loss).

In euvolemic subjects the collecting duct is the main nephron segment where Na⁺ reabsorption is adjusted to maintain excretion at a level appropriate for dietary intake. However, other portions of the nephron also play a role in this process. Because the reabsorptive capacity of the collecting duct is limited, these other portions of the nephron must reabsorb the bulk of the filtered load of Na⁺. Thus, during euvolemia, Na⁺ handling by the nephron can be explained by two general processes:

1. Na⁺ reabsorption by the proximal tubule, Henle's loop, and the distal tubule is regulated so that a relatively constant portion of the filtered load of Na⁺ is delivered to the collecting duct. As indicated in Fig. 42-7, the combined action of these nephron segments reabsorbs 96% of the filtered load of Na⁺. The remaining 4% of the filtered load is delivered to the beginning of the collecting duct.

2. Reabsorption of this remaining portion of the filtered load of Na⁺ by the collecting duct is regulated so that the amount of Na⁺ excreted in the urine matches the amount ingested in the diet. Thus, the collecting duct makes final adjustments in Na⁺ excretion to maintain the euvolemic state.

Mechanisms for maintaining constant Na⁺ delivery to the collecting duct. A number of mechanisms maintain delivery of a constant fraction of the filtered load of Na⁺ to the beginning of the collecting duct. These mechanisms are autoregulation of GFR, and thus the filtered load of Na⁺; glomerulotubular balance; and load dependency of Na⁺ reabsorption by Henle's loop and the distal tubule.

Autoregulation of GFR (see Chapter 40) allows for the maintenance of a relatively constant filtration rate over a wide range of perfusion pressures. Because the filtration rate is constant, the amount of the filtered load of Na⁺ delivered to the nephrons is also constant.

Despite the autoregulatory control of GFR, small variations do occur. If these changes were not compensated for by an appropriate adjustment in Na⁺ reabsorption by the nephron, marked changes in Na⁺ excretion would result. However, Na⁺ reabsorption in the euvolemic state, especially by the proximal tubule, does change parallel to changes in GFR. This phenomenon is called **glomerulotubular (G-T) balance.** By this process, reabsorption of Na⁺, primarily by the proximal tubule, is adjusted to match the GFR. Thus, if GFR increases, the amount of Na⁺ reabsorbed by the proximal tubule also increases. The opposite occurs if GFR decreases. (G-T balance is further described in Chapter 41).

The final mechanism that helps maintain the constant delivery of Na⁺ to the beginning of the collecting duct involves the ability of Henle's loop and the distal tubule to increase their Na⁺ reabsorptive rates in response to increased delivery. Of these two segments, Henle's loop, particularly the thick ascending limb, has the greater capacity to increase Na⁺ reabsorption in response to increased delivery. The mechanism by which the thick ascending limb increases its Na⁺ reabsorptive rate in response to an increased delivered load is not completely understood.

Regulation of collecting duct Na⁺ reabsorption. When the delivery rate of Na⁺ is constant, small adjustments in collecting duct reabsorption are sufficient to balance excretion with intake. (Recall that a 2% change in the fractional excretion of Na⁺ would produce more than a 3 L change in the volume of ECF.) Aldosterone is the primary regulator of collecting duct reabsorption, and thus of Na⁺ excretion, under this condition. When aldosterone levels are elevated, Na⁺ reabsorption by the principal cells of the collecting duct is increased (excretion decreased). When aldosterone levels are suppressed, Na⁺ reabsorption is decreased (excretion increased).

In addition to aldosterone, a number of other factors alter collecting duct Na⁺ reabsorption, including ANP, urodilatin, and sympathetic nerves. However, at present, the relative roles of these other factors in the regulation of collecting duct Na$^+$ reabsorption during euvolemia are not clear.

As long as variations in the dietary intake of NaCl are minor, the mechanisms described above can regulate renal Na$^+$ excretion appropriately, thereby maintaining euvolemia. However, these mechanisms cannot effectively handle significant changes in NaCl intake. When NaCl intake significantly increases, volume expansion or contraction occurs. In such cases, additional factors are called into play that act on the kidneys to adjust Na$^+$ reabsorption to reestablish the euvolemic state.

■ Control of Na$^+$ Excretion with Volume Expansion

During volume expansion, the volume sensors send signals to the kidneys, resulting in an increase in the excretion of NaCl and water. The signals acting on the kidneys include

1. Decreased activity of the renal sympathetic nerves.
2. Release of ANP from atrial myocytes and of urodilatin from distal tubule cells.
3. Inhibition of ADH secretion from the posterior pituitary.

4. Decreased renin secretion, and thus decreased production of angiotensin II.
5. Decreased secretion of aldosterone, due to reduced angiotensin II levels, and elevated ANP levels.

The integrated response of the nephron to these signals is illustrated in Fig. 42-8. The important difference between a situation involving an increase in ECV and that involving the euvolemic state is that the renal response is not limited to the collecting duct; rather, it involves the entire nephron.

Three general responses to an increase in ECV occur (Fig. 42-8). The numbers correlate to those encircled in the figure.

1. *GFR increases.* GFR increases primarily as a result of the decrease in sympathetic nerve activity. Sympathetic fibers innervate the afferent and efferent arterioles of the glomerulus and control their diameter. Decreased sympathetic nerve activity leads to their dilation. Because this effect appears to be greater on the afferent arteriole, the hydrostatic pressure within the glomerular capillary is increased, and GFR increases. ANP has also been shown to increase GFR by dilating the afferent and constricting the efferent arterioles. Thus, the increased ANP levels found with this condition are also likely to contribute to this response. With the increase in GFR, the filtered load of Na$^+$ increases.

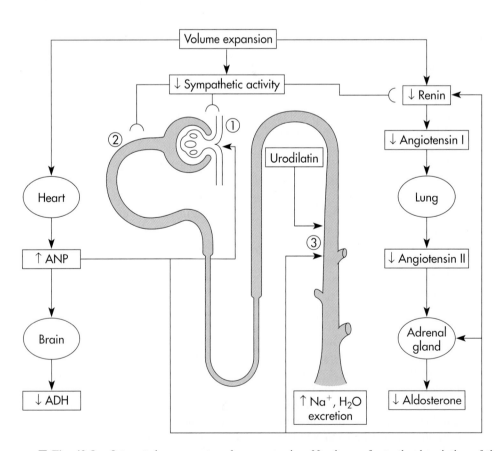

■ Fig. 42-8   Integrated response to volume expansion. Numbers refer to the description of the response in the text. *ANP,* Atrial natriuretic peptide.

2. *Reabsorption of Na+ decreases in the proximal tubule.* Several mechanisms appear to be involved in reducing Na+ reabsorption by the proximal tubule, but the precise role of each of these mechanisms remains controversial. Because activation of the sympathetic nerve fibers innervating this nephron segment stimulates Na+ reabsorption, the decreased sympathetic nerve activity resulting from volume expansion may contribute to the decreased Na+ reabsorption that occurs. In addition, angiotensin II directly stimulates Na+ reabsorption by the proximal tubule. Because angiotensin II levels are also reduced under this condition, it is possible that proximal tubule Na+ reabsorption is decreased as a result. The increased hydrostatic pressure within the glomerular capillaries also leads to an increase in the hydrostatic pressure within the peritubular capillaries. This alteration in the capillary Starling forces reduces the absorption of solute (e.g., NaCl) and water from the lateral intercellular space, thus reducing tubular reabsorption (see Chapter 41 for the mechanism).

3. *Na+ reabsorption decreases in the collecting duct.* Both the increase in the filtered load and the decrease in proximal tubule NaCl reabsorption result in the delivery of large amounts of NaCl to Henle's loop and the distal tubule. Because increased activity of both sympathetic nerves and aldosterone stimulates NaCl reabsorption by

Henle's loop, the reduced nerve activity and low aldosterone levels seen with volume expansion could in theory reduce NaCl reabsorption by this nephron segment. However, because reabsorption by the thick ascending limb is load dependent, these effects are offset, and the fraction of the filtered load of Na+ reabsorbed by Henle's loop is actually increased. Nevertheless, the amount of Na+ delivered to the beginning of the collecting duct is increased compared with the euvolemic state (Fig. 42-9).

The amount of Na+ delivered to the beginning of the collecting duct varies in proportion to the degree of volume expansion. This increased load of Na+ overwhelms the reabsorptive capacity of the collecting duct, which is even further reduced by the actions of ANP of urodilatin and by the decrease in the circulating levels of aldosterone.

The final component in the response to volume expansion is the excretion of water. As Na+ excretion increases, plasma osmolality begins to fall. This results in decreased secretion of ADH. ADH secretion is also decreased in response to the elevated levels of ANP. In addition, ANP and urodilatin inhibit the action of ADH on the collecting duct. Together, these effects decrease water reabsorption by the collecting duct, thereby increasing water excretion by the kidneys. Thus, the excretion of Na+ and water occurs in concert; euvolemia is restored, and body fluid osmolality remains constant. As already noted, the time

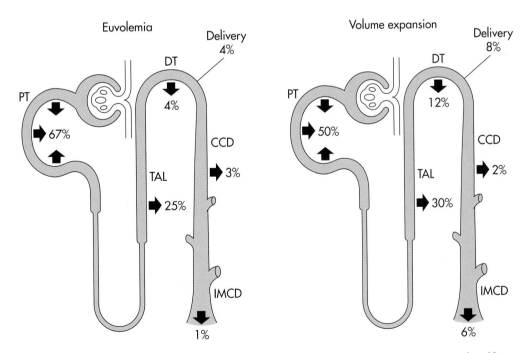

■ **Fig. 42-9**   Segmental Na+ reabsorption during euvolemia and during volume expansion. Note that with volume expansion, delivery of Na+ to the collecting duct is increased from 4% to 8%. With inhibition of Na+ reabsorption by the collecting duct, Na+ excretion is increased from 1% to 6%. *PT,* Proximal tubule; *TAL,* thick ascending limb; *DT,* distal tubule; *CCD,* cortical collecting duct; *IMCD,* inner medullary collecting duct.

course of this response (hours to days) depends on the magnitude of the increase in ECF. Thus, if the degree of volume expansion is small, the mechanisms just described will generally return ECF to its normal level within 24 hours. However, with large degrees of volume expansion, the response can take several days.

In summary, the nephron's response to volume expansion involves the integrated action of all its parts. The filtered load is increased, proximal tubule reabsorption is reduced (GFR is increased, while proximal reabsorption is decreased; thus, G-T balance does not occur under this condition), and the delivery of NaCl to the beginning of the collecting duct is increased. This increased delivery, along with inhibition of collecting duct reabsorption, results in the excretion of a larger fraction of the filtered load of Na^+, thus restoring euvolemia.

■ *Control of Na^+ Excretion with Volume Contraction*

During volume contraction, the sensors send signals to the kidneys, which reduce Na^+ and water excretion. The signals acting on the kidneys include

1. Increased renal sympathetic nerve activity.
2. Increased secretion of renin, which results in ele-

vated angiotensin II levels and thus increased secretion of aldosterone by the adrenal cortex.
3. Inhibition of ANP secretion by the atrial myocytes and urodilatin secretion by the distal tubule.
4. Stimulation of ADH secretion by the posterior pituitary.

The integrated response of the nephron to these signals is illustrated in Fig. 42-10.

The nephron's response to ECV contraction involves all nephron segments. The general response is as follows. The numbers correlate to those encircled in Fig. 42-10.

1. *GFR decreases.* Afferent and efferent arteriolar constriction occurs as a result of increased renal sympathetic nerve activity. The effect appears to be greater on the afferent arteriole, causing the hydrostatic pressure in the glomerular capillary to fall, and thereby decreasing the GFR. This decrease in GFR in turn reduces the filtered load of Na^+.
2. *Na^+ reabsorption by the proximal tubule is increased.* Several mechanisms appear to be involved in augmenting Na^+ reabsorption in this segment. For example, increased sympathetic nerve activity and angiotensin II directly stimulate proximal tubule Na^+ reabsorption. The decreased hydrostatic pressure within the glomerular capillaries also leads to a decrease in the hydrostatic pressure

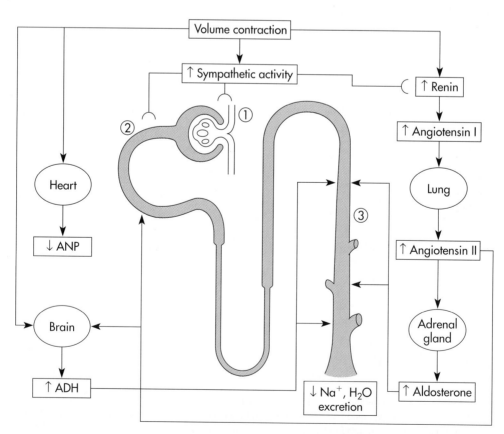

■ **Fig. 42-10**   Integrated response to volume contraction. The circled numbers correlate with the description in the text. Urodilatin levels are also decreased but are not depicted. *ANP,* Atrial natriuretic peptide.

within the peritubular capillaries. This alteration in the capillary Starling forces facilitates the movement of fluid from the lateral intercellular space into the capillary, thereby stimulating proximal tubule reabsorption of solute and water (see Chapter 41 for a complete description of this mechanism).

3. *Na⁺ reabsorption by the collecting duct is enhanced.* The reduction in filtered load and enhanced proximal tubule reabsorption result in decreased delivery of Na⁺ to Henle's loop and the distal tubule. Increased sympathetic nerve activity and aldosterone stimulate Na⁺ reabsorption by the thick ascending limb and distal tubule. Because sympathetic nerve activity is increased and aldosterone levels are elevated during volume contraction, the potential for increased Na⁺ reabsorption by these segments exists. However, because Na⁺ transport by the thick ascending limb and distal tubule is load dependent, the stimulatory effects of increased sympathetic nerve activity and aldosterone are offset. Therefore, the fraction of the filtered load of Na⁺ reabsorbed by these segments is actually less than that seen in the euvolemic state. Nevertheless, the net result is that less Na⁺ is delivered to the beginning of the collecting duct. This process is illustrated in Fig. 42-11.

The small amount of Na⁺ delivered to the collecting duct is almost completely reabsorbed, because transport

in this segment is enhanced. This stimulation of collecting duct Na⁺ reabsorption is primarily due to increased aldosterone levels. Additionally, ANP and urodilatin, which inhibit collecting duct reabsorption, are not present.

Finally, water reabsorption by the collecting duct is enhanced by ADH, the levels of which are elevated owing to activation of the low- and high-pressure vascular baroreceptors, as well as by the elevated levels of angiotensin II. As a result, water excretion is reduced and, together with the Na⁺ retained by the kidneys, euvolemia is reestablished and body fluid osmolality remains constant. The time course of this reexpansion (hours to days), and the degree to which euvolemia is attained, depend on the magnitude of the volume contraction as well as the dietary intake of Na⁺. Thus, the kidneys can reduce Na⁺ excretion, and euvolemia will be restored to its normal level as NaCl is ingested (i.e., increasing NaCl intake will allow euvolemia to be reestablished more quickly).

In summary, the nephron's response to volume contraction involves the integrated action of all its segments. The filtered load of Na⁺ is decreased, proximal tubule reabsorption is enhanced (GFR is decreased, while proximal reabsorption is increased; thus, G-T balance does not occur under this condition), and the delivery of Na⁺ to the beginning of the collecting duct is reduced. This decreased delivery, together with enhanced Na⁺ reabsorption by the collecting duct, virtually eliminates Na⁺ from the urine.

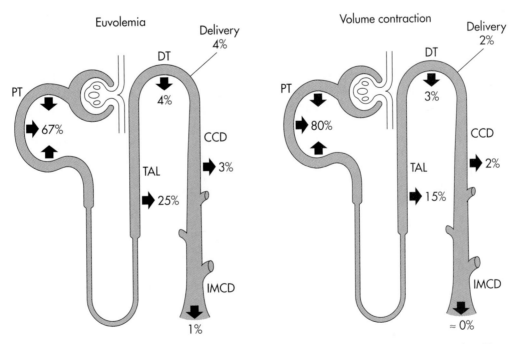

■ **Fig. 42-11** Segmental Na⁺ reabsorption during euvolemia and during volume contraction. Note that with volume contraction, delivery of Na⁺ to the collecting duct is reduced from 4% to 2%. The collecting duct reabsorbs virtually all the Na⁺ it receives, and Na⁺ excretion is reduced to near zero. *PT,* Proximal tubule; *TAL,* thick ascending limb; *DT,* distal tubule; *CCD,* collecting duct; *IMCD,* inner medullary collecting duct.

■ *Edema and the Role of the Kidney*

Edema is the accumulation of excess fluid within the interstitial space. The Starling forces across the capillaries determine the movement of fluid into and out of the vascular compartment and the interstitial space (see Chapter 27). Alterations of these forces under pathological conditions can lead to increased movement of fluid from the vascular space into the interstitium, resulting in edema. However, for edema to be detected clinically (e.g., swelling of ankles), NaCl and water must be retained by the kidneys.

The role of the kidneys in edema can be appreciated by recognizing that the interstitial compartment must contain 2 to 3 L of excess fluid before edema is detectable. The source of this fluid is the vascular compartment (i.e., plasma), which normally has a volume of 3 to 4 L. Thus, the movement of 2 to 3 L out of the plasma compartment into the interstitial compartment would result in a marked decrease in blood pressure. As described below, a marked decrease in blood pressure would prevent further movement of fluid from the vascular compartment into the interstitial compartment. However, retention of NaCl and water by the kidneys replenishes the plasma volume, thereby maintaining the blood pressure. As a result, accumulation of fluid in the interstitial compartment continues, and edema develops.

The Starling forces and their role in determining fluid movement across the capillary wall are explained in Chapter 27. Edema results from a change in the Starling forces that alter these fluid dynamics. Recall that fluid movement across the capillary wall is driven by hydrostatic and oncotic pressure gradients:

$$\text{fluid flow} = K_f [(P_c - P_i) - \sigma(\pi_c - \pi_i)] \quad (42\text{-}12)$$

where K_f is the filtration coefficient of the capillary wall (a measure of the intrinsic permeability and the surface area available for fluid flow); P_c and P_i are the hydrostatic pressures within the lumen of the capillary and the interstitium, respectively; σ is the reflection coefficient for protein across the capillary wall (approximately 0.9 for skeletal muscle); and π_c and π_i are the oncotic pressures generated by protein within the capillary lumen and the interstitium, respectively.

Alterations in capillary hydrostatic pressure (P_c) and plasma oncotic pressure (π_c) are the most common changes in Starling forces associated with the formation of generalized edema. An increase in capillary hydrostatic pressure, usually as a result of elevated venous pressure, causes fluid to move out of the capillary and accumulate in the interstitial space. A decrease in the oncotic pressure of plasma will also cause increased movement of fluid out of the capillary and into the interstitial space.

With renal diseases that produce the **nephrotic syndrome,** the permeability of the glomerular capillary is abnormally high and causes large quantities of albu-

min to be filtered and lost in the urine (proteinuria). If the rate of loss exceeds the rate at which albumin is synthesized by the liver, plasma albumin concentration will fall. The resultant change in π_c contributes to the formation of edema in this condition.

Because the liver synthesizes many of the plasma proteins, including albumin, **hypoalbuminemia** often occurs in individuals with liver failure. The reduced plasma protein concentration contributes to the formation of edema and ascites (accumulation of fluid in the peritoneal cavity) in these individuals.

Any alteration in Starling forces that results in the accumulation of excess fluid in the interstitial space will simultaneously decrease plasma volume. If the plasma volume is not maintained at a near-normal level, this fluid accumulation is self-limiting. Consider the situation that exists with heart failure. Because of decreased cardiac performance, venous pressure is elevated. This raises capillary hydrostatic pressure, and fluid accumulates in the interstitium. Because the source of this fluid is the plasma, and if we assume that plasma volume is not maintained by some mechanism (see below), plasma volume would decrease. Falling plasma volume would in turn decrease venous pressure and capillary hydrostatic pressure, and movement of fluid into the interstitium would cease.

Fig. 42-12 illustrates what occurs when an alteration in the capillary Starling forces causes fluid accumulation in the interstitium. As fluid moves from the vascular compartment into the interstitium, vascular volume is decreased. The volume sensors detect this as volume contraction and send signals to the kidneys that decrease the excretion of NaCl and water by the kidneys. This retention of NaCl water serves to restore the vascular volume (i.e., plasma volume). With restoration of plasma volume, and assuming the condition altering the Starling forces still exists (e.g., untreated heart failure), additional fluid will move into the interstitium, and edema will result. This cycle will continue until a new steady state is reached at the capillary level, such that the amount of fluid moving out of the capillary lumen into the interstitium is again balanced by the amount moving in the opposite direction. This steady state can be attained even when the underlying cause is uncorrected. As edema fluid accumulates in the interstitial compartment, the hydrostatic pressure in this compartment increases. This pressure increase occurs as a result of the limited compliance of the surrounding tissue (e.g., skin.) Eventually, the hydrostatic pressure within the interstitium will rise to a level at which net accumulation in the interstitial compartment ceases.

The importance of NaCl retention by the kidneys in edema provides two approaches for treatment. The first involves dietary manipulation. The ultimate source of NaCl is the diet. Thus, if dietary intake of NaCl is restricted, the amount that can be retained by the kidneys

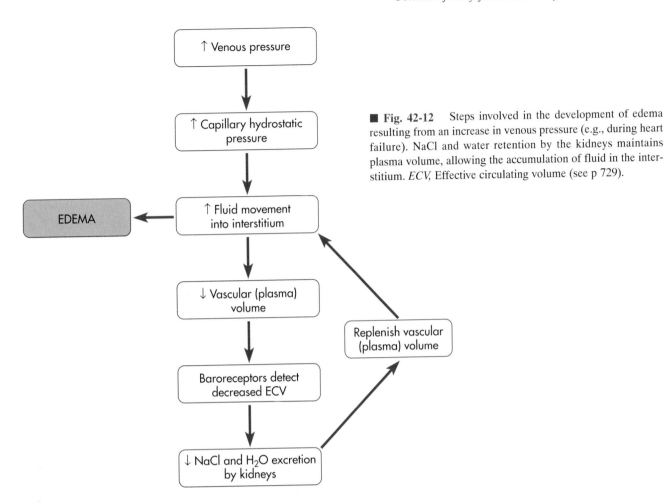

■ **Fig. 42-12** Steps involved in the development of edema resulting from an increase in venous pressure (e.g., during heart failure). NaCl and water retention by the kidneys maintains plasma volume, allowing the accumulation of fluid in the interstitium. *ECV,* Effective circulating volume (see p 729).

is reduced, and edema is limited. The second approach is to inhibit the kidneys' ability to retain NaCl. This inhibition is accomplished by the use of diuretics, which inhibit Na^+ transport mechanisms in the nephron. Thus, NaCl excretion is increased and NaCl retention blunted.

■ *Summary*

1. The osmolality and volume of the body fluids are maintained within a narrow range, despite wide variation in water and solute intake. The kidneys play the central role in this regulatory process by virtue of their ability to vary the excretion of water and solutes.

2. Regulation of body fluid osmolality requires that water intake matches water loss from the body. Regulation of body fluid osmolality involves the integrated interaction of the ADH secretory and thirst centers of the hypothalamus, and the ability of the kidneys to excrete urine that is either hypo-osmotic or hyperosmotic with respect to the body fluids. When body fluid osmolality increases, ADH secretion and thirst are stimulated. ADH acts on the kidneys to increase the permeability of the collecting duct to water. Hence, water is reabsorbed

from the lumen of the collecting duct, and a small volume of hyperosmotic urine is excreted. This renal conservation of water, together with increased water intake, restores body fluid osmolality to normal. When body fluid osmolality decreases, ADH secretion and thirst are suppressed. In the absence of ADH, the collecting duct is impermeable to water, and a large volume of hypo-osmotic urine is excreted. With this increased excretion of water, and with a decreased intake of water caused by suppression of thirst, the osmolality of the body fluids is restored to normal.

3. Central to the process of concentrating and diluting the urine is Henle's loop. The reabsorption of NaCl by Henle's loop allows the separation of solute and water, which is essential for the formation of hypo-osmotic urine. By this same mechanism, the interstitial fluid in the medullary portion of the kidney is rendered hyperosmotic. This hyperosmotic medullary interstitial fluid in turn provides the osmotic driving force for the reabsorption of water from the lumen of the collecting duct when ADH is present.

4. Disorders of water balance alter body fluid osmolality. Changes in body fluid osmolality are manifest by a change in plasma $[Na^+]$. Positive water balance (intake >

excretion) results in a decrease in body fluid osmolality and hyponatremia. Negative water balance (intake < excretion) results in an increase in body fluid osmolality and hypernatremia.

5. Maximal excretion of solute-free water by the kidneys requires normal nephron function (especially the thick ascending limb of Henle's loop), adequate delivery of tubular fluid to the nephrons, and the absence of ADH. Maximal reabsorption of solute-free water by the kidneys requires normal nephron function (especially the thick ascending limb of Henle's loop), adequate delivery of tubular fluid to the nephrons, a hyperosmotic medullary interstitium, the presence of ADH, and responsiveness of the collecting duct to ADH.

6. The volume of ECF is determined by Na^+ balance. When intake of Na^+ exceeds excretion, positive Na^+ balance exists and volume expansion occurs. Conversely, when excretion of Na^+ exceeds intake, negative Na^+ balance exists and volume depletion occurs. The kidneys are the primary route for Na^+ excretion from the body.

7. The coordination of Na^+ intake and excretion, and thus the maintenance of euvolemia, requires the integrated action of the kidneys, the cardiovascular system, and the sympathetic nervous systems. Sensors throughout the body (most importantly the low- and high-pressure vascular volume sensors) monitor the effective circulating volume. Neural and hormonal signals then modulate renal NaCl excretion to match it to intake.

8. During euvolemia, Na^+ excretion by the kidneys is matched to the amount of Na^+ ingested in the diet. The kidneys accomplish this matching by reabsorbing virtually all the filtered load of Na^+ (typically less than 1% of the filtered load is excreted). During euvolemia, the collecting duct adjusts urinary NaCl excretion to effect Na^+ balance. The major factor that regulates collecting duct Na^+ reabsorption is aldosterone, which acts to stimulate Na^+ reabsorption.

9. With volume expansion, low- and high-pressure volume sensors initiate a response that ultimately leads to increased excretion of Na^+ by the kidneys and the reestablishment of euvolemia. The components of this response include a decrease in sympathetic neural outflow to the kidney, a suppression of the renin-angiotensin-aldosterone system, and release of atrial natriuretic peptide from the cardiac atria. At the level of the kidneys, the GFR is enhanced, thereby increasing the filtered load of Na^+. Na^+ reabsorption by the proximal tubule and collecting duct is reduced. Together, these changes in renal Na^+ handling enhance Na^+ excretion. With volume contraction, the above sequence of events is reversed.

10. The development of generalized edema requires that the Starling forces across capillary walls favor the accumulation of fluid in the interstitium, and that NaCl and water are retained by the kidneys.

■ Self-Study Problems

1. An individual's blood is drawn, and the following values are obtained.

Plasma $[Na^+]$	135 mEq/L	(n*: 135-147 mEq/L)
Serum [glucose]	100 mg/dl	(n*: 70-110 mg/dl)
Serum [urea]	100 mg/dl	(n*: 7-18 mg/dl)
P_{osm}	310 mOsm/kg H_2O	(n*: 280-295 mOsm/kg H_2O)

Would plasma ADH levels in this individual be elevated or suppressed?

2. In the table below, indicate the expected osmolality of tubular fluid in the absence and presence of ADH (assume that the plasma osmolality is 300 mOsm/kg H_2O and that the osmolality of the medullary interstitium is 1200 mOsm/kg H_2O at the papilla).

Nephron site	0-ADH	Max. ADH
Proximal tubule	_____	_____
Beginning of descending thin limb	_____	_____
Beginning of ascending thin limb	_____	_____
End of thick ascending limb	_____	_____
End of cortical collecting duct	_____	_____
Urine	_____	_____

3. The ability of the kidneys to maximally concentrate the urine is impaired under each of the following conditions:

a. Administration of a diuretic that inhibits active NaCl transport by the thick ascending limb of Henle's loop.
b. Nephrogenic diabetes insipidus.

What are the mechanisms responsible for the observed impairment in the kidneys' concentrating ability during each of these conditions?

4. An individual must excrete 800 mOsm of solute in a 24-hour period. What volume of urine is required if the individual can concentrate the urine to only 400 mOsm/kg H_2O? What volume of urine is required if this individual can concentrate the urine to 1200 mOsm/kg H_2O?

5. An individual develops an acute episode of vomiting and diarrhea and loses 3 kg in body weight over a 24-hour period. A blood sample shows that plasma $[Na^+]$ is normal at 145 mEq/L. Indicate whether the following parameters would be increased, decreased, or unchanged from what they were before this illness (i.e., normal values).

Plasma osmolality	_____
ECF volume	_____
Plasma ADH levels	_____
Urine osmolality	_____
Sensation of thirst	_____

n, Normal.

6. An individual is euvolemic and ingests a diet that contains 200 mEq/day of Na^+ on average. What would the Na^+ excretion rate of this individual be over a 24-hour period?

7. Indicate on the following table whether the signals listed are increased or decreased by the indicated change in effective circulating volume.

Regulatory signals	Volume expansion	Volume contraction
Renal sympathetic nerves	_____	_____
ANP	_____	_____
Renin-angiotensin	_____	_____
Aldosterone	_____	_____
Vasopressin	_____	_____

8. A patient with heart failure has developed edema with swelling of the ankles and fluid in the lungs. During the past 2 weeks, the individual's weight has increased by 4 kg. Assuming that the entire weight gain is the result of the accumulation of fluid, calculate the following:

Volume of accumulated fluid: _____ L
Amount of Na^+ retained by the kidneys: _____ mEq

■ *Bibliography*

Journal articles

Bichet DG: Vasopressin receptors in health and disease, *Kidney Int* 49:1706, 1996.

Brenner BM, et al: Diverse biological actions of atrial natriuretic peptide, *Physiol Rev* 70:665, 1990.

Hays RM: Cellular and molecular events in the action of antidiuretic hormone, *Kidney Int* 49:1700, 1996.

Hediger MA, et al: Structure, regulation and physiological role of urea transporters, *Kidney Int* 49:1615, 1996.

Knepper MA, et al: Renal aquaporins, *Kidney Int* 49:1712, 1996.

Books and monographs

Fitzsimmons JT: *Physiology and pathophysiology of thirst and sodium appetite.* In Seldin DW, Giebisch G, editors: *The kidney: physiology and pathophysiology,* ed 2, New York, 1992, Raven Press.

Gonzalez-Campoy JM, Knox FG: *Integrated responses of the kidney to alterations in extracellular fluid volume.* In Seldin DW, Giebisch G, editors: *The kidney: physiology and pathophysiology,* ed 2, New York, 1992, Raven Press.

Gunning ME, Ingelfinger JR, King AJ, Brenner BM: *Vasoactive peptides and the kidney.* In Brenner BM, editor: *The kidney,* ed 5, Philadelphia, 1996, WB Saunders.

Hall JE, Brands MW: *The renin-angiotensin-aldosterone systems: renal mechanisms and circulatory homeostasis.* In Seldin DW, Giebisch G, editors: *The kidney: physiology and pathophysiology,* ed 2, New York, 1992, Raven Press.

Harris HW Jr, Zeidel ML: *Cell biology of vasopressin.* In Brenner BM, editor: *The kidney,* ed 5, Philadelphia, 1996, WB Saunders.

Knepper MA, Rector FC Jr: *Urine concentration and dilution.* In Brenner BM, editor: *The kidney,* ed 5, Philadelphia, 1996, WB Saunders.

Lassiter WE, Gottschalk CW: *Regulation of water balance: urine concentration and dilution.* In Schrier RW, Gottschalk CW, editors: *Diseases of the kidney,* ed 5, Boston, 1992, Little, Brown.

Miller JA, Tobe SW, Skorecki KL: *Control of extracellular fluid volume and the pathophysiology of edema.* In Brenner BM, editor: *The kidney,* ed 5, Philadelphia, 1996, WB Saunders.

Palmer BF, Alpern RJ, Seldin DW: *Pathophysiology of edema formation.* In Seldin DW, Giebisch G, editors: *The kidney: physiology and pathophysiology,* ed 2, New York, 1992, Raven Press.

Robertson GL: *Regulation of vasopressin secretion.* In Seldin DW, Giebisch G, editors: *The kidney: physiology and pathophysiology,* ed 2, New York, 1992, Raven Press.

Robertson GL, Berl T: *Pathophysiology of water metabolism.* In Brenner BM, editor: *The kidney,* ed 5, Philadelphia, 1996, WB Saunders.

Rose BD, Rennke HG: *Regulation of salt and water balance.* In Rose BD, Rennke HG, editors: *Renal pathophysiology—the essentials,* Baltimore, 1994, Williams & Wilkins.

Roy DR, Layton HE, Jamison RL: *Countercurrent mechanism and its regulation.* In Seldin DW, Giebisch G, editors: *The kidney: physiology and pathophysiology,* ed 2, New York, 1992, Raven Press.

Teitelbaum I, Kelleher SP, Berl T: *Diabetes insipidus and the syndrome of inappropriate antidiuretic hormone secretion.* In Brenner BM, editor: *The kidney,* ed 5, Philadelphia, 1996, WB Saunders.

CHAPTER
43

Potassium, Calcium, and Phosphate Homeostasis

■ K+ Homeostasis

Potassium (K+) is one of the most abundant cations in the body and is critical for many cell functions. Despite wide fluctuations in dietary K+ intake, its concentration in cells and extracellular fluid (ECF) remains constant. Two sets of regulatory mechanisms safeguard K+ homeostasis. First, certain mechanisms regulate the potassium [K+] in the ECF.* Second, other mechanisms keep the amount of K+ in the body constant by adjusting renal K+ excretion to match dietary K+ intake. It is the kidneys that regulate K+ excretion. In this chapter we focus on the hormones and the factors that influence the [K+] in the ECF compartment and those that regulate the amount of K+ excreted in the urine.

Total body K+ constitutes 50 mEq/kg of body weight, or 3500 mEq for a 70-kg individual. Ninety-eight percent of the K+ in the body is located within cells, where its average concentration is 150 mEq/L. A high intracellular concentration of K+ is required for many cell functions, including cell growth and division and volume regulation. Only 2% of total body K+ is located in the ECF, where its normal concentration is approximately 4 mEq/L. When the [K+] of the ECF exceeds 5.0 mEq/L, **hyperkalemia** exists. Conversely, **hypokalemia** exists when the [K+] of the ECF is less than 3.5 mEq/L.

The large concentration difference of K+ across cell membranes ($\approx$ 146 mEq/L) is maintained by the operation of Na+, K+-ATPase. This K+ gradient is important in maintaining the potential difference across cell membranes (see also Chapters 2 and 22). Thus, K+ is critical for the excitability of nerve and muscle cells, as well as for the contractility of cardiac, skeletal, and smooth muscle cells (Fig. 43-1).

---

*The [K+] in the ECF is monitored in the clinical setting by measuring the plasma [K+]. For simplicity, in this book we use plasma [K+] interchangeable with ECF [K+].

Cardiac arrhythmias are produced by both hypokalemia and hyperkalemia. Fig. 43-2 illustrates several electrocardiograms (ECGs) from patients with various levels of plasma [K+]. The first sign of hyperkalemia is the appearance of tall, thin T waves. Further increases in plasma [K+] prolong the PR interval, depress the ST segment, and lengthen the QRS interval. Finally, as plasma [K+] approaches 10 mEq/L, the P wave disappears, the QRS interval broadens, the ECG appears as a sine wave, and the ventricles fibrillate (i.e., manifest rapid, uncoordinated contractions of muscle fibers). Hypokalemia prolongs the QT interval, inverts the T wave, and lowers the ST segment. The ECG is a fast and easy way to determine whether changes in plasma [K+] are influencing the heart and other excitable cells. In contrast, measurements of plasma [K+] by the clinical laboratory require a blood sample, and values are often not immediately available.

■ Internal K+ Distribution

After a meal, the K+ absorbed by the gastrointestinal tract enters the ECF within minutes (Fig. 43-3). If the K+ ingested during a normal meal (~133 mEq) were to remain in the ECF compartment, plasma [K+] would increase by a potentially lethal 2.4 mEq/L (33 mEq added to 14 L of ECF = Δ2.4 mEq/L). This rise in plasma [K+] is prevented by the rapid uptake of K+ into cells. *Because the excretion of K+ by the kidneys after a meal is relatively slow (hours), the buffering of K+ by cells is essential to prevent life-threatening hyperkalemia.* To maintain total body K+ constant, all the K+ absorbed by the gastrointestinal tract must eventually be excreted by the kidneys. K+ excretion is slow; after 6 hours it is completely eliminated from the body.

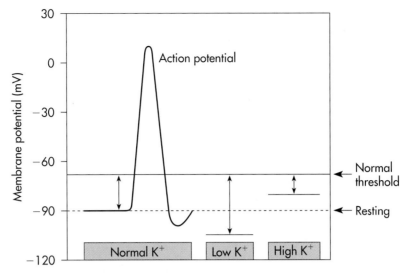

■ **Fig. 43-1**   Effects of variations in plasma [K⁺] on the resting membrane potential of skeletal muscle. Hyperkalemia causes the membrane potential to become less negative, which decreases the excitability by inactivating fast Na⁺ channels. Hypokalemia hyperpolarizes the membrane potential, thereby reducing excitability.

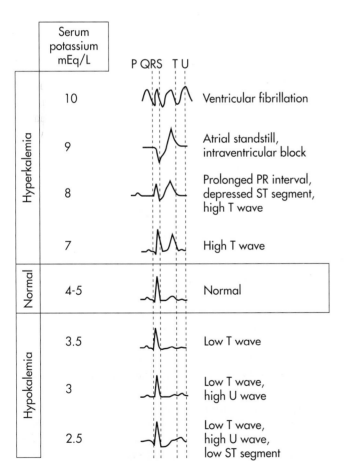

■ **Fig. 43-2**   Electrocardiograms from individuals with varying plasma [K⁺]. Hyperkalemia increases the height of the T wave; hypokalemia inverts the T wave. See text for details. (Modified from Barker L, Burton J, Zieve P: *Principles of ambulatory medicine,* Baltimore, 1982, Williams & Wilkins.)

Several hormones promote the uptake of K⁺ into cells after a rise in plasma [K⁺], and this increased uptake prevents dangerous hyperkalemia. As illustrated in Fig. 43-3 and summarized in Table 43-1, these hormones include epinephrine, insulin, and aldosterone. All these hormones increase K⁺ uptake into skeletal muscle, liver, bone, and red blood cells by stimulating the Na⁺, K⁺-ATPase pump. Acute stimulation of K⁺ uptake (i.e., within minutes) is mediated by increased turnover rate of existing Na⁺, K⁺-ATPase, whereas the chronic increase in K⁺ uptake (i.e., within hours to days) is mediated by an increase in Na⁺, K⁺-ATPase. A rise in plasma [K⁺] that follows K⁺ absorption by the gastrointestinal tract stimulates insulin secretion from the pancreas, aldosterone release from the adrenal cortex, and epinephrine secretion from the adrenal medulla. In contrast, a decrease in plasma [K⁺] inhibits release of these hormones. Whereas insulin and epinephrine act within a few minutes, aldosterone requires about 1 hour to stimulate K⁺ uptake into cells.

Epinephrine. Catecholamines affect the distribution of K⁺ across cell membranes by activating α- and β_2-adrenergic receptors. Stimulation of α receptors releases K⁺ from cells, especially in the liver, whereas stimulation of β_2 receptors causes K⁺ uptake by cells.

α-Receptor activation post exercise is important in preventing hypokalemia. The rise in plasma [K⁺] after a K⁺-rich meal is greater if the subject has been pretreated with **propranolol,** a β-adrenergic blocker. Furthermore, the release of epinephrine during stress (e.g., myocardial ischemia) can rapidly lower plasma [K⁺].

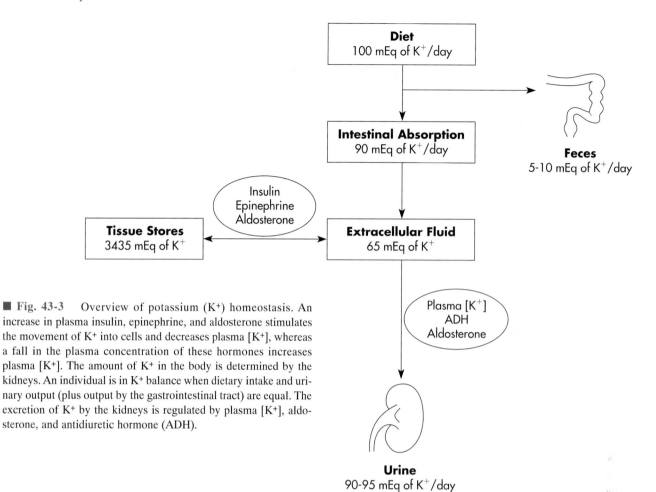

■ Fig. 43-3 Overview of potassium (K⁺) homeostasis. An increase in plasma insulin, epinephrine, and aldosterone stimulates the movement of K⁺ into cells and decreases plasma [K⁺], whereas a fall in the plasma concentration of these hormones increases plasma [K⁺]. The amount of K⁺ in the body is determined by the kidneys. An individual is in K⁺ balance when dietary intake and urinary output (plus output by the gastrointestinal tract) are equal. The excretion of K⁺ by the kidneys is regulated by plasma [K⁺], aldosterone, and antidiuretic hormone (ADH).

■ Table 43-1 Major factors and hormones influencing the distribution of K⁺ between the intracellular and extracellular fluid compartments

Physiological: keep plasma [K⁺] constant

Epinephrine
Insulin
Aldosterone

Pathophysiological: displace plasma [K⁺] from normal

Acid-base balance
Plasma osmolality
Cell lysis
Exercise

Insulin. Insulin also stimulates K⁺ uptake into cells. The importance of insulin in stimulating K⁺ uptake is illustrated by two observations. First, the rise in plasma [K⁺] after a K⁺-rich meal is greater in individuals with diabetes mellitus (i.e., insulin deficiency) than in normal people. Second, infusion of insulin (and glucose to prevent insulin-induced hypoglycemia) can be used to correct hyperkalemia. *Insulin is the most important hormone that shifts K⁺ into cells after ingestion of K⁺ in a meal.*

Aldosterone. Aldosterone, like catecholamines and insulin, also promotes K⁺ uptake into cells. A rise in

aldosterone levels (e.g., **primary aldosteronism**) causes hypokalemia, while a fall in aldosterone levels (e.g., **Addison's disease**) causes hyperkalemia. As discussed below, aldosterone also stimulates urinary K⁺ excretion. Thus, aldosterone alters plasma [K⁺] by acting on K⁺ uptake into cells and by altering urinary K⁺ excretion.

Thus far, our discussion has focused on hormones that keep the distribution of K⁺ across cell membranes constant. Other factors are not homeostatic mechanisms, because they displace normal plasma [K⁺] levels. Table 43-1 summarizes these factors.

Acid-base balance. In general, metabolic acidosis increases plasma [K⁺], whereas metabolic alkalosis decreases plasma [K⁺]. In contrast, respiratory acid-base disorders have little or no effect on plasma [K⁺]. A metabolic acidosis produced by the addition of inorganic acids (e.g., HCl, H_2SO_4) increases plasma [K⁺] to a much greater extent than does a similar acidosis produced by the accumulation of organic acids (e.g., lactic acid, acetic acid, keto acids). The reduced pH promotes movement of H⁺ into cells and the reciprocal movement of K⁺ out of cells. Metabolic alkalosis has the opposite effect; plasma [K⁺] decreases as K⁺ moves into cells and H⁺ exits cells. The mechanism responsible for this shift is not fully understood. It has been proposed that the movement of H+ occurs as the cells buffer changes in the [H+] of the ECF. As H+ moves across the cell membranes, K+ moves in the opposite direction, and thus cations are neither gained nor lost across the cell membranes. Although organic acids produce a metabolic acidosis, they do not cause significant hyperkalemia. Two possible explanations have been suggested for the reduced effect of organic acids in causing hyperkalemia. First, the organic anion may enter the cell with H+, thereby eliminating the need for K+/H+ exchange across the membrane. Second, organic anions may stimulate insulin secretion, which moves K+ into cells. This movement may counteract the direct effect of the acidosis, which moves K+ out of cells.

Plasma osmolality. The osmolality of the plasma also influences the distribution of K+ across cell membranes. An increase in the osmolality of the ECF enhances K+ release by cells and thus increases extracellular [K+]. The plasma K+ level may increase by 0.4 to 0.8 mEq/L for a 10 mOsm/kg H_2O elevation in plasma osmolality. Hypoosmolality has the opposite action. The alterations in plasma [K+] associated with changes in osmolality are related to changes in cell volume. For example, as plasma osmolality increases, water will leave cells because of the osmotic gradient across the plasma membrane. Water leaves cells until the intracellular osmolality equals that of the ECF. This loss of water shrinks cells and causes the [K+] to rise. The rise in intracellular [K+] provides a driving force for the exit of K+ from the cells. This sequence increases plasma [K+]. A fall in plasma osmolality has the opposite effect.

Cell lysis. Cell lysis causes hyperkalemia. The hyperkalemia results from the addition of intracellular K+ to the ECF.

Severe trauma (e.g., burns), and some diseases such as **tumor lysis syndrome** and **rhabdomyolysis** (i.e., destruction of skeletal muscle), cause cell destruction and release of K+ (and other cell solutes) into the ECF. In addition, **gastric ulcers** may cause seepage of red blood cells into the gastrointestinal tract. The blood cells are digested, and the K+ released from the cells is absorbed and can cause hyperkalemia.

Exercise. During exercise, more K+ is released from skeletal muscle cells than during rest. Release of K+ during the recovery phase of the action potential and the ensuing hyperkalemia depends on the degree of exercise. In subjects walking slowly the plasma [K+] increases by 0.3 mEq/L, and levels may increase by up to 2.0 mEq/L or more above normal with more vigorous exercise.

Exercise-induced changes in plasma [K+] usually do not produce symptoms and are reversed after several minutes of rest. However, in individuals (1) with certain endocrine disorders that affect the release of insulin, epinephrine, or aldosterone; (2) whose ability to excrete K+ is impaired (e.g., in renal failure); or (3) who take certain medications, such as β-adrenergic blockers, exercise can lead to potentially life-threatening hyperkalemia. For example, during exercise, plasma [K+] may increase by 2 to 4 mEq/L or more in individuals taking β-adrenergic blockers for hypertension.

Because acid-base balance, plasma osmolality, cell lysis, and exercise do not maintain plasma [K+] at a normal value, they therefore do not contribute to K+ homeostasis. The extent to which these pathophysiological states alter plasma [K+] depends on the integrity of the homeostatic mechanisms that regulate plasma [K+] (e.g., secretion of epinephrine, insulin, and aldosterone).

■ K+ Excretion by the Kidneys

The kidneys play the major role in maintaining K+ balance. As illustrated in Fig. 43-3, the kidneys excrete 90% to 95% of the K+ ingested in the diet. Excretion equals intake even when intake increases by as much as tenfold. This balance of urinary excretion and dietary intake underscores the importance of the kidneys in maintaining K+ homeostasis. Although small amounts of K+ are lost each day in the stool and sweat ($\approx$ 5% to 10% of the K+ ingested in the diet), this amount is essentially constant, is not regulated, and therefore is relatively much less important than is the K+ excreted by the kidneys.* *The main event in determining urinary K+ excretion is K+ secretion from the blood into the tubular fluid by the cells of the distal tubule and collecting duct system.* The transport pattern of K+ by the major nephron segments is illustrated in Fig. 43-4.

Because K+ is not bound to plasma proteins, it is freely filtered by the glomerulus. When normal individuals ingest an average diet, urinary K+ excretion is 15% of the amount filtered. Accordingly, K+ must be reabsorbed along the nephron. When dietary K+ intake increases, however, K+ excretion can exceed the amount filtered. Thus, K+ can also be secreted.

The proximal tubule reabsorbs 67% of the filtered K+ under most conditions. Approximately 20% of the filtered K+ is reabsorbed by Henle's loop and, as with the proximal tubule, the amount reabsorbed is a constant fraction of the amount filtered. In contrast to these segments, which are capable of only reabsorbing K+, the distal tubule and the collecting duct are able to either reabsorb or secrete K+. The rate of K+ reabsorption or secretion by the distal tubule and the collecting duct depends on a variety of hormones and factors. When K+ intake is normal (100 mEq/day), K+ is secreted. A rise in dietary

---

*Loss of K+ in the feces can become significant during periods of diarrhea.

K⁺ intake increases K⁺ secretion. K⁺ secretion can increase the amount of K⁺ appearing in the urine so that it approaches 80% of the amount filtered (Fig. 43-4). In contrast, a low-potassium diet activates K⁺ reabsorption along the distal tubule and collecting duct, so that urinary excretion falls to 1% of the K⁺ filtered by the glomerulus (Fig. 43-4). The kidneys are not able to reduce K⁺ excretion to the same low levels as they can for Na⁺ (0.2%). Therefore, hypokalemia can develop in individuals placed on a K⁺-deficient diet.

Because the magnitude and direction of K⁺ transport by the distal tubule and collecting duct are variable, the overall rate of urinary K⁺ excretion is determined by these tubular segments.

In individuals with **advanced renal disease,** the kidneys are unable to eliminate K⁺ from the body. Plasma [K⁺] therefore rises. The resultant hyperkalemia reduces the resting membrane potential (i.e., the voltage becomes less negative), which decreases the excitability of neurons, cardiac cells, and muscle cells by inactivating fast Na⁺ channels in the membrane. Severe, rapid increases in plasma [K⁺] can lead to cardiac arrest and death. In contrast, in patients taking diuretic drugs for hypertension, urinary K⁺ excretion often exceeds dietary K⁺ intake. Accordingly, negative K⁺ balance exists and

hypokalemia develops. This decline in extracellular [K⁺] hyperpolarizes the resting cell membrane potential (i.e., the voltage becomes more negative), which reduces the excitability of neurons, cardiac cells, and muscle cells. Severe hypokalemia can lead to paralysis, cardiac arrhythmia, and death. Hypokalemia can also impair the ability of the kidneys to concentrate the urine and stimulate renal production of NH₄⁺. Therefore, maintenance of a high intracellular [K⁺], a low extracellular [K⁺], and a high K⁺ concentration gradient across cell membranes is essential for a number of cellular functions.

■ Cellular Mechanisms of K⁺ Transport by the Distal Tubule and Collecting Duct

Fig. 43-5 illustrates the cellular mechanism of K⁺ secretion by principal cells in the distal tubule and collecting duct. Secretion from blood into tubular fluid is a two-step process involving (1) K⁺ uptake across the basolateral membrane by Na⁺, K⁺-ATPase and (2) diffusion of K⁺ from the cell into the tubular fluid. The operation of the Na⁺, K⁺-ATPase creates a high intracellular [K⁺], which provides the driving force for K⁺ exit across the apical membrane through K⁺ channels. Although K⁺

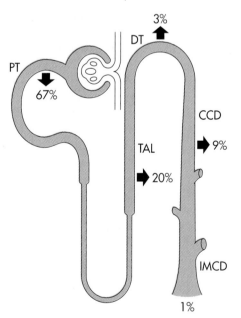
Potassium depletion

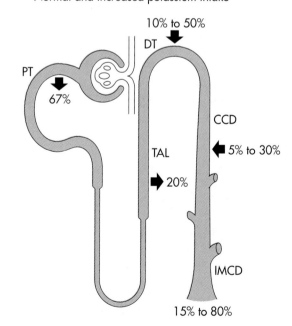
Normal and increased potassium intake

■ **Fig. 43-4**   K⁺ transport along the nephron. K⁺ excretion depends on the rate and direction of K⁺ transport by the distal tubule and the collecting duct. Percentages refer to the amount of filtered K⁺ reabsorbed or secreted by each nephron segment. *Left panel,* Dietary K⁺ depletion. An amount of K⁺ equal to 1% of the filtered load of K⁺ is excreted. *Right panel,* Normal and increased dietary K⁺ intake. An amount of K⁺ equal to 15% to 80% of the filtered load is excreted. *PT,* Proximal tubule; *TAL,* thick ascending limb; *DT,* distal tubule; *CCD,* collecting duct; *IMCD,* inner medullary collecting duct.

channels are also present in the basolateral membrane, K$^+$ preferentially leaves the cell across the apical membrane and enters the tubular fluid. K$^+$ transport follows this route for two reasons. First, the electrochemical gradient of K$^+$ across the apical membrane favors its downhill movement into the tubular fluid. Second, the permeability of the apical membrane to K$^+$ is greater than that of the basolateral membrane. Therefore, K$^+$ preferentially diffuses across the apical membrane into the tubular fluid. The three major factors that control the rate of K$^+$ secretion by the distal tubule and the collecting duct are (Fig. 43-5):

1. The activity of the Na$^+$, K$^+$-ATPase
2. The driving force (electrochemical gradient) for K$^+$ movement across the apical membrane.
3. The permeability of the apical membrane to K$^+$

Any change in K$^+$ secretion results from an alteration in one or more of these factors.

In contrast, the cellular pathways and mechanisms of K$^+$ reabsorption in the distal tubule and collecting duct are not completely understood. Intercalated cells may reabsorb K$^+$ by a H$^+$, K$^+$-ATPase transport mechanism located in the apical membrane. This transporter mediates K$^+$ uptake in exchange for H$^+$. However, the pathway of K$^+$ exit from intercalated cells into the blood is unknown. As we have seen, reabsorption of K$^+$ is activated by a low-K$^+$ diet.

■ Regulation of K$^+$ Secretion by the Distal Tubule and Collecting Duct

Regulation of K$^+$ excretion is achieved mainly by alterations in K$^+$ secretion by principal cells of the distal tubule and collecting duct. *Plasma [K$^+$] and aldosterone are the major physiological regulators of K$^+$ secretion. Antidiuretic hormone (ADH) also stimulates K$^+$ secre-* tion; however, it is less important than plasma [K$^+$] and aldosterone. Other factors, including the flow rate of tubular fluid and acid-base balance, influence K$^+$ secretion by the distal tubule and collecting duct. However, they are not homeostatic mechanisms, because they disturb K$^+$ balance (Table 43-2).

■ Hormones and Factors That Regulate Urinary K$^+$ Excretion

Plasma [K$^+$]. Plasma [K$^+$] is an important determinant of K$^+$ secretion by the distal tubule and collecting duct (Fig. 43-6). Hyperkalemia (e.g., resulting from a high K$^+$ diet or rhabdomyolysis) stimulates secretion within minutes. Several mechanisms are involved. First, hyperkalemia stimulates the Na$^+$, K$^+$-ATPase and thereby increases K$^+$ uptake across the basolateral membrane. This uptake raises intracellular [K$^+$] and increases the electrochemical driving force for K$^+$ exit across the apical membrane. Second, hyperkalemia also increases the permeability of the apical membrane to K$^+$. Third, hyperkalemia stimulates aldosterone secretion by the adrenal cortex, which, as discussed below, acts synergistically with plasma [K$^+$] to stimulate K$^+$ secretion. Fourth, hyperkalemia also increases the flow rate of tubular fluid, which, as discussed below, stimulates K$^+$ secretion by the distal tubule and collecting duct.

Hypokalemia (e.g., caused by a low-K$^+$ diet or diarrhea) decreases K$^+$ secretion by mechanisms opposite to those described for hyperkalemia. Hence, hypokalemia inhibits Na$^+$, K$^+$-ATPase, decreases the electrochemical driving force for K$^+$ efflux across the apical membrane, reduces the permeability of the apical membrane to K$^+$, and causes a reduction in plasma aldosterone levels.

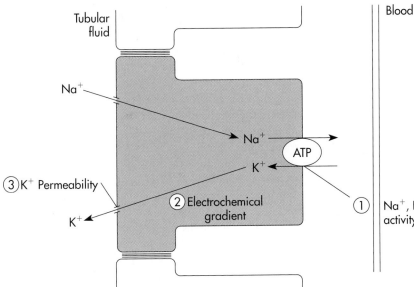

■ **Fig. 43-5** Cellular mechanism of K$^+$ secretion by a principal cell in the distal tubule and collecting duct. The numbers indicate the sites where K$^+$ secretion is regulated: *1,* Na$^+$, K$^+$-ATPase; *2,* electrochemical gradient of K$^+$ across the apical membrane; *3,* K$^+$ permeability of the apical membrane.

■ **Table 43-2**   Major factors and hormones influencing K⁺ excretion

Physiological: keep K⁺ balance constant

Plasma [K⁺]
Aldosterone
Antidiuretic hormone

Pathophysiological: displace K⁺ balance

Flow rate of tubular fluid
Acid-base balance

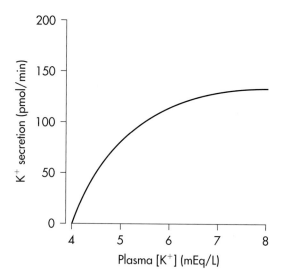

■ **Fig. 43-6**   Relationship between plasma [K⁺] and K⁺ secretion by the distal tubule and cortical collecting duct.

Chronic hypokalemia (plasma [K⁺] <3.5 mEq/L) occurs most often in patients receiving diuretic therapy for hypertension. Hypokalemia also occurs in individuals who vomit, have nasogastric suction, have diarrhea, abuse laxatives, or have **hyperaldosteronism.** Hypokalemia occurs because the excretion of K⁺ by the kidneys exceeds dietary intake of K⁺. Vomiting, nasogastric suction, diuretics, and diarrhea can all cause volume contraction, which in turn stimulates aldosterone secretion (see Chapters 42 and 51). Because aldosterone stimulates K⁺ excretion by the kidneys, its action contributes to the development of hypokalemia.

Chronic hyperkalemia (plasma [K⁺] >5.0 mEq/L) occurs most frequently in individuals with a reduced urinary flow or a low plasma aldosterone level, or in individuals with renal disease whose glomerular filtration rate (GFR) falls to less than 20% of normal. In these individuals, hyperkalemia occurs because the excretion of K⁺ by the kidneys is less than dietary intake of K⁺. Less common causes for hyperkalemia include deficiencies of insulin, epinephrine, or aldosterone secretion, or metabolic acidosis caused by inorganic acids.

Aldosterone. A chronic (i.e., ≥24-hour) elevation in plasma aldosterone concentration enhances K⁺ secretion across the distal tubule and collecting duct by increasing the amount of Na⁺, K⁺-ATPase in principal cells (Fig. 43-7). This uptake elevates cell [K⁺]. Aldosterone also increases the driving force for K⁺ exit across the apical membrane and increases the permeability of the apical membrane to K⁺. Aldosterone secretion is increased by hyperkalemia and by angiotensin II (after activation of the renin-angiotensin system); aldosterone secretion is decreased by hypokalemia and atrial natriuretic peptide (ANP).

Although an acute increase in aldosterone (i.e., within hours) enhances the activity of the Na⁺, K⁺-ATPase, K⁺ excretion does not increase. The reason for this lack of increase relates to the effect of aldosterone on Na⁺ reabsorption and tubular flow. Aldosterone stimulates Na⁺ and thereby water reabsorption and thus decreases tubu-

lar flow. The decrease in flow in turn decreases K⁺ secretion (this process is discussed in more detail later). However, chronic stimulation of Na⁺ reabsorption results in volume expansion, and thereby returns tubular flow to normal. These actions allow the direct stimulatory effect of aldosterone on the distal tubule and collecting duct to increase K⁺ excretion.

Glucocorticoids. Glucocorticoids also stimulate K⁺ excretion. However, this effect is indirect and mediated by an increase in GFR, which increases tubular flow.

Antidiuretic hormone. ADH increases the electrochemical driving force for K⁺ exit across the apical membrane of principal cells by stimulating Na⁺ uptake across the apical membrane. The increased Na⁺ uptake reduces the electrical potential difference across the apical membrane (i.e., the interior of the cell becomes less negatively charged). Despite this effect, ADH does not change K⁺ secretion by these nephron segments. The reason for this relates to the effect of ADH on tubular fluid flow. ADH decreases tubular fluid flow by stimulating water reabsorption. The decrease in tubular flow in turn decreases K⁺ secretion (see below for a discussion). The inhibitory effect of decreased tubular flow offsets the stimulatory effect of ADH on the electrochemical driving force for K⁺ exit across the apical membrane (Fig. 43-8). If ADH did not increase the electrochemical gradient favoring K⁺ secretion, urinary K⁺ excretion would fall as ADH levels increase and urinary flow rates decrease. Hence, K⁺ balance would change in response to alterations in water balance. Thus, these effects of ADH on the electrochemical driving force for K⁺ exit across the apical membrane and tubule flow enable urinary K⁺ excretion to be maintained constant despite wide fluctuations in water excretion.

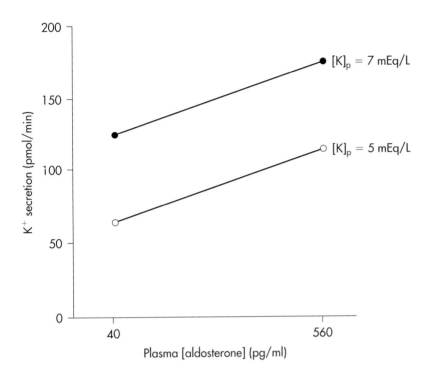

■ **Fig. 43-7** Relationship between plasma aldosterone and K+ secretion by the distal tubule and cortical collecting duct. Note that K+ secretion is further increased when plasma [K+] ([K]$_p$) is increased.

■ *Factors That Perturb K+ Excretion*

Flow of tubular fluid. A rise in the flow of tubular fluid (e.g., with diuretic therapy, ECF volume expansion) rapidly (within minutes) stimulates K+ secretion, whereas a fall in flow (e.g., ECF volume contraction caused by hemorrhage or severe vomiting or diarrhea) reduces K+ secretion by the distal tubule and collecting duct (Fig. 43-9). Increments in tubular fluid flow are more effective in stimulating K+ secretion as dietary K+ intake is increased. Alterations in tubular fluid flow influence K+ secretion by changing the driving force for K+ exit across the apical membrane. As K+ is secreted into the tubular fluid, the [K+] of the fluid increases. The increase in [K+] of the tubular fluid reduces the electrochemical driving force for K+ exit across the apical membrane, thereby reducing the rate of secretion. An increase in tubular fluid flow minimizes the rise in tubular fluid [K+] as the secreted K+ is washed downstream. A second mechanism responsible for flow-dependent stimulation of K+ secretion is related to Na+ reabsorption. A rise in tubular flow increases the amount of Na+ entering the distal tubule and collecting duct, which in turn enhances Na+ reabsorption. The increase in Na+ reabsorption stimulates K+ uptake across the basolateral membrane by increasing the activity of the Na+, K+-ATPase, which promotes K+ secretion. *Because diuretic drugs increase the flow of tubular fluid through the distal tubule and collecting duct, they also enhance urinary K+ excretion.* In contrast, a decline in tubular fluid flow inhibits K+ secretion. This occurs because a decline in tubular fluid flow facilitates the rise in tubular fluid [K+], thereby reducing secretion.

Acid-base balance. Another factor that modulates K+ secretion is the [H+] of the ECF (Fig. 43-10). Acute alterations (over a period of minutes to hours) in the pH of the plasma affect K+ secretion by the distal tubule and collecting duct. **Alkalosis** (a plasma pH above normal) increases H+ secretion, whereas **acidosis** (a plasma pH below normal) decreases K+ secretion. Acute acidosis reduces K+ secretion by two mechanisms: (1) it inhibits Na+, K+-ATPase, thereby reducing cell [K+] and the electrochemical driving force for K+ exit across the apical membrane; and (2) it reduces the permeability of the apical membrane to K+. Alkalosis has the opposite effects.

The effect of metabolic acidosis on K+ excretion is time dependent. When a metabolic acidosis lasts for several days, urinary K+ excretion is stimulated (Fig. 43-11). This occurs because chronic metabolic acidosis decreases water and NaCl reabsorption by the proximal tubule by inhibiting Na+, K+-ATPase in the proximal tubular cells. Hence, the flow of tubular fluid is augmented through the distal tubule and collecting duct. The inhibition of proximal tubular water and NaCl reabsorption also causes a decrease in ECF, thereby stimulating aldosterone secretion. In addition, chronic acidosis caused by inorganic acids increases plasma [K+], which stimulates aldosterone secretion. The rise in tubular fluid flow, plasma [K+], and aldosterone offsets the effects of acidosis on cell [K+] and apical membrane permeability, and K+ secretion rises. Thus, metabolic acidosis may either inhibit or stimulate potassium excretion, depending on the duration of the disturbance.

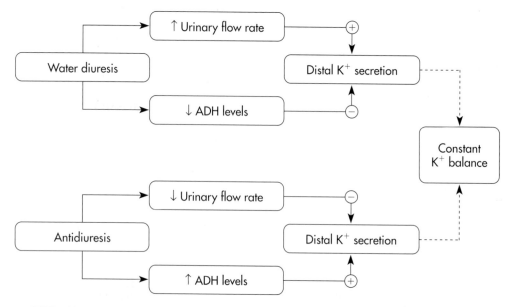

■ **Fig. 43-8**   Opposing effects of ADH on K⁺ secretion by the distal tubule and cortical collecting duct. Secretion is stimulated by an increase in the magnitude of the electrochemical gradient for K⁺ across the apical membrane and perhaps by an increase in the K⁺ permeability of the apical membrane. In contrast, secretion is reduced by a fall in the flow rate of tubular fluid. Because these effects oppose each other, ADH has no net effect on net K⁺ secretion.

■ **Fig. 43-9**   Relationship between tubular flow rate and K⁺ secretion by the distal tubule and cortical collecting duct. A diet high in K⁺ increases the slope of the relationship between flow rate and secretion and increases the maximal rate of secretion. A diet low in K⁺ has the opposite effects. The shaded bar indicates the flow rate under most physiological conditions.

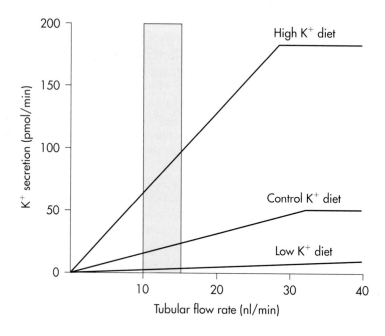

The flow of tubular fluid and acid-base balance do not maintain K⁺ balance at a normal value and therefore do not contribute to K⁺ homeostasis. The extent to which changes in flow and acid-base balance alter K⁺ balance and plasma [K⁺] depends on the integrity of the homeostatic mechanisms that regulate K⁺ balance and plasma [K⁺].

Frequently, as discussed above, the rate of urinary K⁺ excretion is determined by simultaneous changes in hormone levels, acid-base balance, or tubular flow (Table 43-3). The powerful effect of tubular flow often enhances or opposes the response of the distal tubule and collecting duct to hormones and changes in acid-base balance. This interaction can be beneficial, as in the case of hyperkalemia, in which the change in flow enhances K⁺ excretion and thereby restores K⁺ homeostasis. However, this interaction can also be detrimental, as in the case of alkalosis, in which changes in flow and acid-base status perturb K⁺ homeostasis.

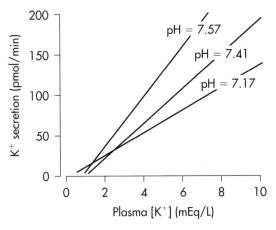

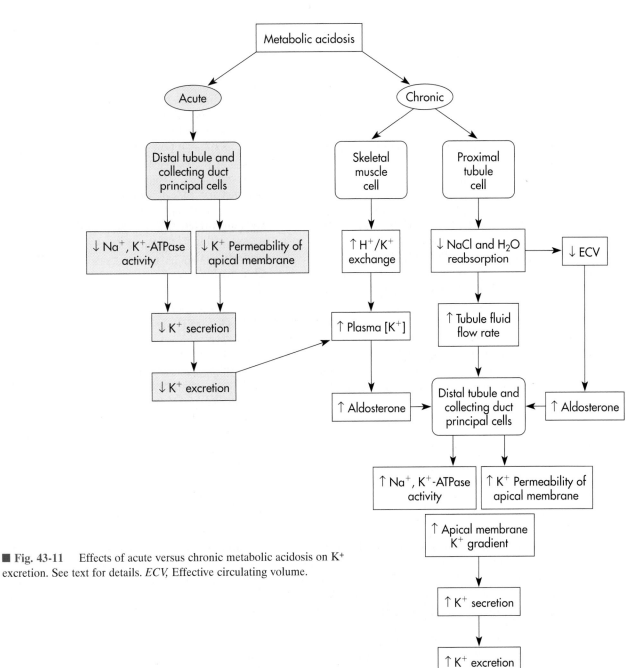

■ **Fig. 43-10**   Effect of plasma pH on the relationship between plasma [K$^+$] and K$^+$ secretion by the distal tubule and collecting duct.

■ **Fig. 43-11**   Effects of acute versus chronic metabolic acidosis on K+ excretion. See text for details. *ECV,* Effective circulating volume.

■ **Table 43-3**   Interaction between the direct/indirect effects of hormones and factors on K⁺ secretion by the distal tubule and collecting duct and flow of tubular fluid

	Direct or indirect	Flow	Urinary excretion
Hyperkalemia	↑	↑	↑↑
Aldosterone			
Acute (<1 hr)	↑	↓	NC
Chronic (>1 hr)	↑	NC	↑
Glucocorticoids	NC	↑	↑
ADH	↑	↓	NC
Acidosis			
Acute	↓	NC	↓
Chronic	↓	↑↑	↑
Alkalosis	↑	↑	↑↑

Modified from Field MJ et al: *Regulation of renal potassium metabolism.* In Narins R, editor: *Textbook of nephrology: clinical disorders of fluid and electrolyte metabolism,* ed 5, New York, 1994, McGraw-Hill. *NC,* No change; *ADH,* antidiuretic hormone.

■ *Overview of Ca⁺⁺ and P_i Homeostasis*

Ca⁺⁺ and inorganic phosphate (P_i)* are multivalent ions that subserve many complex and vital functions. In a normal adult, the renal excretion of these ions is balanced by gastrointestinal absorption. If the plasma concentrations decline substantially, gastrointestinal absorption, bone resorption, and renal tubular reabsorption increase and return plasma concentrations of Ca⁺⁺ and P_i to normal levels. During growth and pregnancy, intestinal absorption exceeds urinary excretion, and these ions accumulate in newly formed fetal tissue and bone. In contrast, bone disease (e.g., **osteoporosis**) or a decline in lean body mass increases urinary multivalent ion loss without a change in intestinal absorption. In these conditions, there is net loss of Ca⁺⁺ and P_i from the body. *The kidneys, in conjunction with the gastrointestinal tract and bone, play a major role in maintaining plasma Ca⁺⁺ and P_i levels.*

■ *Calcium*

Calcium ions play a major role in many processes, including bone formation, cell division and growth, blood coagulation, hormone-response coupling, and electrical stimulus-response coupling (e.g., muscle contraction and neurotransmitter release). Ninety-nine percent of Ca⁺⁺ is stored in bone, 1% is found in the intracellular fluid (ICF) and 0.1% is in the ECF (Table 43-4). The total [Ca⁺⁺] in plasma is 10 mg/dl (2.5 mM or 5 mEq/L), and its concentration is normally maintained within narrow limits. A low ionized plasma [Ca⁺⁺], called

*At physiological pH, inorganic phosphate exists as $HPO_4^=$ and $H_2PO_4^-$ (pK = 6.8). For simplicity, we collectively refer to these ion species as P_i.

■ **Table 43-4**   Body content and distribution of Ca⁺⁺ and P_i

Ion	Body content	Bone	Compartment Intracellular	Compartment Extracellular
Ca⁺⁺	1300 g	99%	1%	0.10%
P_i	700 g	86%	14%	0.03%

hypocalcemia, increases the excitability of nerve and muscle cells and can lead to **hypocalcemic tetany,** which is characterized by skeletal muscle spasms. An elevated ionized plasma [Ca⁺⁺], called **hypercalcemia,** may produce decreased neuromuscular excitability, cardiac arrhythmias, lethargy, disorientation, and even death (see Chapter 48).

Overview of Ca⁺⁺ homeostasis. Ca⁺⁺ homeostasis depends on two factors: (1) the total amount of Ca⁺⁺ in the body and (2) the distribution of Ca⁺⁺ between bone and the ECF compartment. Total body Ca⁺⁺ is determined by the relative amounts of Ca⁺⁺ absorbed by the gastrointestinal tract and excreted by the kidneys (Fig. 43-12). Ca⁺⁺ is absorbed by the gastrointestinal tract through an active, carrier-mediated transport mechanism that is stimulated by **calcitriol,** a metabolite of vitamin D₃ (see also Chapter 48).* Net Ca⁺⁺ absorption is normally 200 mg/day, but it can increase to 600 mg/day when calcitriol levels rise. In adults, Ca⁺⁺ excretion by the kidneys is equal to the amount absorbed by the gastrointestinal tract (200 mg/day), and it changes in parallel with the reabsorption of Ca⁺⁺ by the gastrointestinal tract. Thus, in adults, Ca⁺⁺ balance is maintained because the amount of Ca⁺⁺ ingested in an average diet (1000 mg/day) is equal to the amount lost in the feces (800 mg/day: the amount that escapes absorption by the gastrointestinal tract) plus the amount excreted in the urine (200 mg/day).

The second factor that controls Ca⁺⁺ homeostasis is the distribution of Ca⁺⁺ between bone and the ECF. Three hormones—**parathyroid hormone (PTH),** calcitriol, and **calcitonin**—are the most important hormones that regulate the distribution of Ca⁺⁺ between bone and the ECF and thereby regulate plasma [Ca⁺⁺]. PTH is secreted by the parathyroid glands. Secretion of PTH is stimulated by a decline in plasma [Ca⁺⁺] (i.e., in hypocalcemia). PTH increases plasma [Ca⁺⁺] by

1. Stimulating bone resorption
2. Increasing Ca⁺⁺ reabsorption by the kidneys
3. Stimulating the production of calcitriol, which in turn increases Ca⁺⁺ absorption by the gastrointestinal tract and stimulates bone resorption

The production of calcitriol by the proximal tubule cells of the kidneys is stimulated by hypocalcemia and

*Vitamin D₃ is ingested in the diet and can be synthesized in the skin in the presence of ultraviolet light. Vitamin D₃ is converted in the liver to calcifediol and then in the kidney, primarily in the proximal tubule, to the active metabolite calcitriol (1, 25-(OH)₂-D₃).

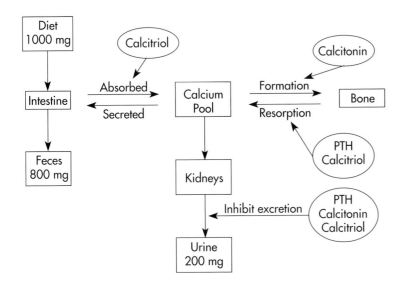

■ **Fig. 43-12** Overview of Ca++ homeostasis. See text for details. *PTH,* Parathyroid hormone.

hypophosphatemia. The effect of hypocalcemia is secondary to increased levels of PTH, which are elevated as a result of the decrease in plasma [Ca++]. The effect of hypophosphatemia is direct, because the decrease in plasma [P_i] stimulates the production of calcitriol by the proximal tubule cells. Calcitriol increases plasma [Ca++] by actions similar to those of PTH (see above).

Calcitonin is also secreted by the parathyroid glands, and its secretion is stimulated by hypercalcemia. Calcitonin decreases plasma [Ca++] mainly by stimulating bone formation (i.e., the deposition of Ca++ in bone). Fig. 43-13 illustrates the relationship between plasma [Ca++] and plasma levels of PTH and calcitonin.

Conditions that lower PTH levels (e.g., vitamin D_3 deficiency or postsurgical hypoparathyroidism after parathyroidectomy due to adenoma) reduce plasma [Ca++] and can cause **hypocalcemic tetany** (intermittent muscular contraction), which is characterized by skeletal muscle spasms. In severe cases, hypocalcemic tetany can cause death by asphyxiation. Hypercalcemia can also cause cardiac arrhythmia and decreased neuromuscular excitability, both of which can be lethal. Clinically, the most common causes of hypercalcemia are **primary hyperparathyroidism** and **malignancy-associated hypercalcemia.** Primary hyperparathyroidism results from the overproduction of PTH caused by a tumor of the parathyroid glands. In contrast, malignancy-associated hypercalcemia occurs in 10% to 20% of all patients with cancer and is caused by secretion of PTH-related peptide (PTHRP), a PTH-like hormone secreted by carcinomas in a variety of organs. Increased levels of PTH and PTHRP cause hypercalcemia and hypercalciuria.

Approximately 50% of the Ca++ in plasma is ionized, 45% is bound to plasma proteins (mainly albumin), and 5% is complexed to several anions, including HCO_3^-, citrate, P_i, and $SO_4^=$ (Table 43-5). The pH of the plasma

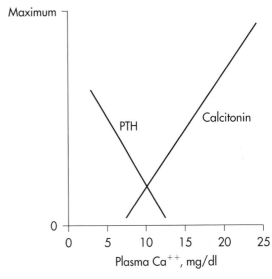

■ **Fig. 43-13** Effect of plasma [Ca++] on plasma levels of PTH and calcitonin. (Modified from Azria M: *The calcitonins: physiology and pharmacology,* Basel, Switzerland, 1989, Karger.)

■ **Table 43-5** Forms of Ca++ and P_i in plasma

Ion	mg/dl	Percentage of total		
		Ionized	*Protein-bound*	*Complexed*
Ca++	10	50%	45%	5%
P_i	4	84%	10%	6%

Ca++ is bound (i.e., complexed) to various anions in the plasma, including HCO_3^-, citrate, P_i, and $SO_4^=$. P_i is complexed to various cations, including Na+ and K+.

influences this distribution. Acidosis increases the percentage of ionized calcium at the expense of Ca++ bound to proteins, whereas alkalosis decreases the percentage of ionized calcium, again by altering Ca++ bound to proteins. Thus, individuals with alkalosis are susceptible to tetany, whereas individuals with acidosis are less susceptible to tetany, even when total plasma Ca++ levels are reduced. The Ca++ available for filtration consists of the ionized fraction and that complexed with anions. Thus, about 55% of the Ca++ in the plasma is available for glomerular filtration.

In patients with **acidosis,** the [H+] of plasma is increased. This increase in [H+] causes more H+ to bind to plasma proteins, HCO_3^-, citrate, P_i, and $SO_4^=$, thereby displacing Ca++. This displacement of Ca++ in turn increases the plasma concentration of ionized Ca++. In contrast, in patients with **alkalosis,** the [H+] of plasma decreases. Some H+ ions dissociate from plasma proteins, HCO_3^-, citrate, P_i, and $SO_4^=$, in exchange for Ca++, thereby decreasing the plasma concentration of ionized Ca++.

Ca++ transport along the nephron. Normally, 99% of filtered Ca++ (i.e., ionized and complexed) is reabsorbed by the nephron. The proximal tubule reabsorbs 70% of filtered Ca++. Another 20% is reabsorbed in Henle's loop (mainly the thick ascending limb), another 9% is reabsorbed in the distal tubule, and <1% is reabsorbed by the collecting duct. About 1% (200 mg/day) is excreted in the urine. This fraction is equal to the net amount absorbed daily by the gastrointestinal tract. Fig. 43-14 summarizes the handling of Ca++ by the different portions of the nephron.

Cellular mechanisms of Ca++ reabsorption. Ca++ reabsorption by the proximal tubule occurs via two pathways: transcellular and paracellular (Fig. 43-15). Ca++ reabsorption across the cellular pathway (i.e., transcellular) accounts for 20% of proximal reabsorption. Ca++ reabsorption through the cell is an active process that occurs in two steps. First, Ca++ diffuses across the apical membrane into the cell down its electrochemical gradient. This gradient is exceptionally steep because the Ca++ concentration in the cell is only 0.4 μM, about 10,000-fold less than that in the tubular fluid (~ 1.5 mM). The cell interior is electrically negative with respect to the luminal side of the apical membrane; this electrical gradient also favors Ca++ entry into the cell, most likely via Ca++ channels. Ca++ leaves the cell across the basolateral membrane against its electrochemical gradient. The mechanism for the exit of Ca++ is thought to occur by a Ca++-ATPase and a 3 Na+-Ca++ antiporter. Eighty percent of Ca++ is reabsorbed between cells across the tight junctions (i.e., paracellular pathway). This passive, paracellular reabsorption of Ca++ occurs by solvent drag along the entire length of the proximal tubule, and is also driven by the positive luminal voltage in the second half of the proximal tubule. Thus, in the proximal tubule, approximately 80% of Ca++ reabsorption is paracellular and 20% is transcellular.

Ca++ reabsorption by Henle's loop is restricted to the thick ascending limb. Ca++ is reabsorbed via a cellular and a paracellular route by mechanisms similar to those

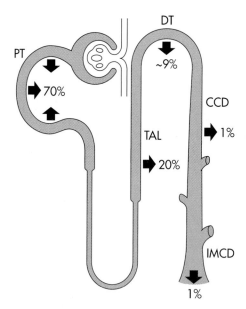

■ **Fig. 43-14**   Transport pattern of Ca++ along the nephron. Percentages refer to the amount of filtered Ca++ reabsorbed by each nephron segment. Approximately 1% of filtered Ca++ is excreted. *PT,* Proximal tubule; *TAL,* thick ascending limb; *DT,* distal tubule; *CCD,* cortical collecting duct; *IMCD,* inner medullary collecting duct.

described for the proximal tubule, with one difference. Ca++ is not reabsorbed by solvent drag in this segment (recall that the thick ascending limb is impermeable to water). In the thick ascending limb, Ca++ and Na+ reabsorption parallel each other because of the significant amount of Ca++ reabsorption that occurs by passive, paracellular mechanisms secondary to Na+ reabsorption and by the generation of the lumen-positive transepithelial voltage. Therefore, *changes in Na+ reabsorption will also cause parallel changes in Ca++ reabsorption by the proximal tubule and the thick ascending limb of Henle's loop.*

In the distal tubule, where the voltage in the tubule lumen is electrically negative with respect to the blood, Ca++ reabsorption is entirely active because Ca++ is reabsorbed against its electrochemical gradient. Ca++ reabsorption by the distal tubule is exclusively transcellular, and the mechanism is similar to that in the proximal tubule and thick ascending limb: uptake across the apical membrane by Ca++-permeable ion channels and exit across the basolateral membrane by Ca++-ATPase and 3 Na+-Ca++ antiporter. *Na+ and Ca++ excretion usually change in parallel. However, this is not always the case because the reabsorption of Ca++ and reabsorption of Na+ by the distal tubule are independent and are differentially regulated. For example, thiazide diuretics inhibit Na+ reabsorption by the distal tubule and stimulate Ca++ reabsorption by this segment. Accordingly, the net effect of thiazide diuretics is to increase urinary Na+ excretion and reduce urinary Ca++ excretion.*

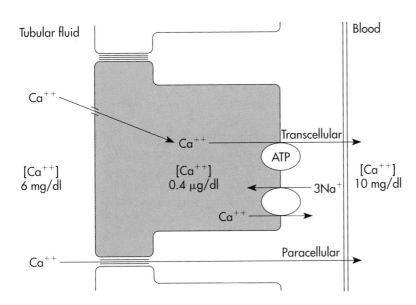

Tubular fluid

Blood

Ca^{++}

Ca^{++}

Transcellular

ATP

$[Ca^{++}]$
6 mg/dl

$[Ca^{++}]$
0.4 µg/dl

$[Ca^{++}]$
10 mg/dl

$3Na^+$

Ca^{++}

Ca^{++}

Paracellular

■ **Fig. 43-15**   Cellular mechanisms of Ca^{++} reabsorption by the proximal tubule. Ca^{++} is reabsorbed by both transcellular and paracellular routes. Although the mechanism of Ca^{++} diffusion into the cell across the apical membrane has not been characterized, it is likely to occur via Ca^{++} channels.

Regulation of urinary Ca^{++} excretion. Urinary Ca^{++} excretion is regulated by PTH, calcitonin, and calcitriol. *PTH exerts the most powerful effect on renal Ca^{++} excretion and is responsible for maintaining Ca^{++} homeostasis.* Overall, this hormone stimulates Ca^{++} reabsorption by the kidneys (i.e., reduces Ca^{++} excretion). Although PTH inhibits the reabsorption of NaCl and fluid, and therefore of Ca^{++}, by the proximal tubule, PTH dramatically stimulates Ca^{++} reabsorption by the thick ascending limb of Henle's loop and the distal tubule. As a result, urinary Ca^{++} excretion declines. Calcitonin and calcitriol also stimulate Ca^{++} reabsorption by the kidneys. Calcitonin stimulates Ca^{++} reabsorption by the thick ascending limb of Henle's loop and the distal tubule, but it is quantitatively less important than PTH. Calcitriol, either directly or indirectly, enhances Ca^{++} reabsorption by the distal tubule. It is also quantitatively less important than PTH.

Several factors disturb Ca^{++} excretion. An increase in plasma $[P_i]$ (e.g., increased dietary intake of P_i) elevates PTH levels, thereby decreasing Ca^{++} excretion. A decline in the plasma $[P_i]$ (e.g., dietary P_i depletion) has the opposite effect. Changes in ECF volume alter Ca^{++} excretion mainly by affecting NaCl and fluid reabsorption in the proximal tubule. Volume contraction increases NaCl and water reabsorption by the proximal tubule, thereby enhancing Ca^{++} reabsorption. Accordingly, urinary Ca^{++} excretion declines. Volume expansion has the opposite effect. Acidosis increases Ca^{++} excretion, whereas alkalosis decreases excretion. The regulation of Ca^{++} reabsorption by pH occurs in the distal tubule by an unknown mechanism.

■ *Phosphate*

P_i is an important component of many organic molecules, including DNA, RNA, ATP, and intermediates of metabolic pathways. It is also a major constituent of bone. Its

concentration in plasma is an important determinant in bone formation and resorption. In addition, urinary P_i is an important buffer (titratable acid) in the maintenance of acid-base balance (see Chapter 44). Eighty-six percent of P_i is located in bone, 14% is in the ICF, and 0.03% is in the ECF (Table 43-4). Normal plasma $[P_i]$ is 4 mg/dl (Table 43-5). Approximately 10% of the P_i in plasma is protein bound and therefore unavailable for ultrafiltration by the glomerulus. According, the $[P_i]$ in the ultrafiltrate is 10% less than in plasma.

Overview of P_i homeostasis. A general scheme of P_i homeostasis is shown in Fig. 43-16. P_i homeostasis depends on two factors: (1) the amount of P_i in the body and (2) the distribution of P_i between the ICF and ECF compartments. Total body P_i is determined by the relative amount of P_i absorbed by the gastrointestinal tract minus the amount excreted by the kidneys. P_i absorption by the gastrointestinal tract occurs by both active and passive mechanisms; P_i absorption increases as dietary P_i rises and it is stimulated by calcitriol. Despite variations in P_i intake of between 800 and 1500 mg/day, the kidneys keep total body P_i constant by excreting an amount of P_i in the urine equal to the amount absorbed by the gastrointestinal tract. Thus, *the kidneys play a vital role in P_i homeostasis.*

The second factor in P_i homeostasis is the distribution of P_i among bone and the ICF and ECF compartments. PTH, calcitriol, and calcitonin regulate the distribution of P_i between bone and ECF. The release of P_i from intracellular stores is stimulated by the same hormones (PTH and calcitriol) that release Ca^{++} from this pool. Thus, the release of P_i is always accompanied by a release of Ca^{++}. In contrast, calcitonin increases bone formation, thereby decreasing plasma $[P_i]$.

The kidneys also play an important role in the regulation of plasma $[P_i]$. A small increase in plasma $[P_i]$ increases the amount of P_i filtered by the glomerulus. Because the kidneys normally reabsorb P_i at a maximal rate, any increase in the amount filtered leads to a rise in urinary P_i excretion. In fact, urinary P_i excretion increases to a value above P_i absorption by the gastrointestinal tract, resulting in a net loss of P_i from the body. This loss of P_i causes plasma $[P_i]$ to fall. In this way, *the kidneys regulate plasma $[P_i]$*. The maximal reabsorptive rate for P_i is variable and is regulated by dietary P_i intake. A high P_i diet decreases the maximal reabsorptive rate of P_i by the kidneys, and a low P_i diet increases the maximal reabsorptive rate. This effect of dietary P_i intake on the maximal P_i transport rate of the kidneys is *independent* of changes in PTH levels.

In patients with **chronic renal failure,** the kidneys cannot excrete P_i and, because of continued P_i absorption by the gastrointestinal tract, P_i accumulates in the body, thereby elevating plasma $[P_i]$. The increased P_i complexes with Ca^{++}, thereby reducing plasma $[Ca^{++}]$. P_i accumulation also decreases the production of calcitriol, which reduces Ca^{++} absorption by the intestine, an effect that further decreases plasma $[Ca^{++}]$. The fall in plasma $[Ca^{++}]$ increases PTH secretion and Ca^{++} release from bone, resulting in **osteitis fibrosa cystica** (i.e., increased bone resorption with replacement fibrous tissue, which makes bone more susceptible to fracture). Chronic **hyperparathyroidism** (i.e., elevated PTH levels) during chronic renal failure can lead to metastatic calcifications in which Ca^{++} and P_i precipitate in arteries, soft tissues, and viscera. Deposition of Ca^{++} and P_i in heart and lung tissue may cause myocardial failure and pulmonary insufficiency, respectively. Prevention and treatment of hyperparathyroidism and P_i retention include a low P_i diet or the administration of a "phosphate binder" (an agent that renders the P_i unavailable for reabsorption by the gastrointestinal tract by forming insoluble P_i salts). Supplemental Ca^{++} and calcitriol are also used.

P_i transport along the nephron. Fig. 43-17 summarizes P_i transport by the various portions of the nephron. The proximal tubule reabsorbs 80% of the P_i filtered by the glomerulus, and the distal tubule reabsorbs 10%. In contrast, Henle's loop and the collecting duct reabsorb only small amounts of P_i. Therefore, 10% of the filtered load of P_i is excreted.

P_i reabsorption by the proximal tubule occurs mainly, if not exclusively, by a transcellular route. As shown in Fig. 43-18, P_i uptake across the apical membrane occurs by a $2Na^+$-P_i symport mechanism. P_i exits across the basolateral membrane, most likely by a P_i-anion antiporter. The cellular mechanism of P_i reabsorption by the distal tubule has not been characterized.

Regulation of urinary P_i excretion. Table 43-6 summarizes the major hormones and factors that regulate urinary P_i excretion. All act on the proximal tubule and either stimulate or inhibit P_i reabsorption. *PTH is the most important hormone that controls P_i excretion.* PTH stimulates cyclic adenosine monophosphate (cAMP) production and inhibits P_i reabsorption by the proximal tubule, thereby increasing P_i excretion. Dietary P_i intake also regulates P_i excretion by mechanisms independent of changes in PTH levels. P_i loading increases excretion, whereas P_i depletion decreases excretion. These changes in dietary P_i intake modulate P_i transport by altering the transport rate of each $2Na^+$-P_i symporter and by increasing the number of transporters.

ECF volume also affects P_i excretion. Volume expansion increases excretion and volume contraction decreases excretion. The effect of the ECF volume of P_i excretion is indirect and may involve changes in hormone levels other than PTH. Acid-base balance also influences P_i excretion: acidosis increases and alkalosis decreases P_i excretion. Glucocorticoids increase the excretion of P_i. Glucocorticoids increase the delivery of P_i to the distal tubule and collecting ducts by inhibit-

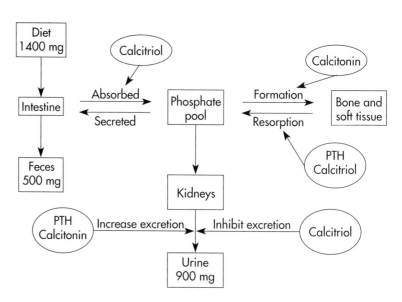

■ **Fig. 43-16**   Overview of P_i homeostasis. See text for details.

ing proximal tubular P_i reabsorption. This inhibition enables the distal tubule and collecting duct to secrete more H^+ and generate more HCO_3^-, because P_i is an important urinary buffer (see Chapter 44 for an explanation). Finally, growth hormone decreases P_i excretion.

In the absence of glucocorticoids (e.g., in **Addison's disease**), P_i excretion is depressed, as is the ability of the kidneys to excrete titratable acid and to generate new HCO_3^-. Growth hormone increases the reabsorption of P_i by the proximal tubule. As a result, growing

children have a plasma $[P_i]$ that is elevated above that found in adults. This higher level of P_i is important for the formation of bone.

■ *Integrated Review of PTH, Calcitriol, and Calcitonin on Ca^{++} and P_i Homeostasis*

Hypocalcemia is the major stimulus of PTH secretion. As summarized in Fig. 43-19, PTH has numerous effects on Ca^{++} and P_i homeostasis. PTH stimulates bone resorption (i.e., release of Ca^{++} and P_i from bone), increases urinary P_i excretion, decreases urinary Ca^{++} excretion, and stimulates the production of calcitriol, which stimulates Ca^{++} and P_i absorption by the intestine. *Because changes in P_i handling in bone, intestine, and the kidneys tend to cancel each other out, PTH increases plasma $[Ca^{++}]$ but has little effect on plasma $[P_i]$. Overall, a rise in plasma PTH levels increases plasma $[Ca^{++}]$ and decreases plasma $[P_i]$. A decline in plasma PTH levels has the opposite effect.*

Calcitriol also plays an important role in Ca^{++} and P_i homeostasis (Fig. 43-20). Calcitriol stimulates Ca^{++} and

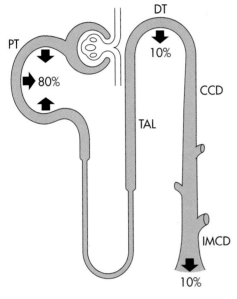

■ **Fig. 43-17** Transport pattern of P_i along the nephron. P_i is reabsorbed primarily by the proximal tubule. Percentages refer to the amount of filtered P_i reabsorbed by each nephron segment. Approximately 10% of filtered P_i is excreted. *PT*, Proximal tubule; *TAL*, thick ascending limb; *DT*, distal tubule; *CCD*, collecting duct; *IMCD*, inner medullary collecting duct.

■ **Table 43-6** Hormones and factors that influence urinary P_i excretion

Increased excretion	Decreased excretion
Increase of PTH	Decrease of PTH
P_i loading	P_i depletion
Volume expansion	Volume contraction
Acidosis	Alkalosis
Glucocorticoids	Growth hormone

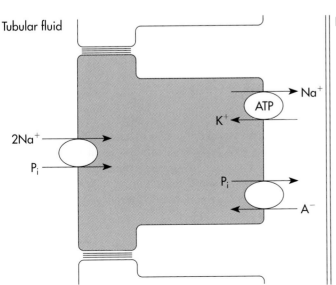

■ **Fig. 43-18** Cellular mechanism of P_i reabsorption by the proximal tubule. The apical transport pathway may operate primarily as a $2Na^+/P_i$ symporter. P_i leaves the cell across the basolateral membrane via a P_i-anion antiporter and possibly via a Na^+/P_i symporter (not shown). A^- indicates an anion.

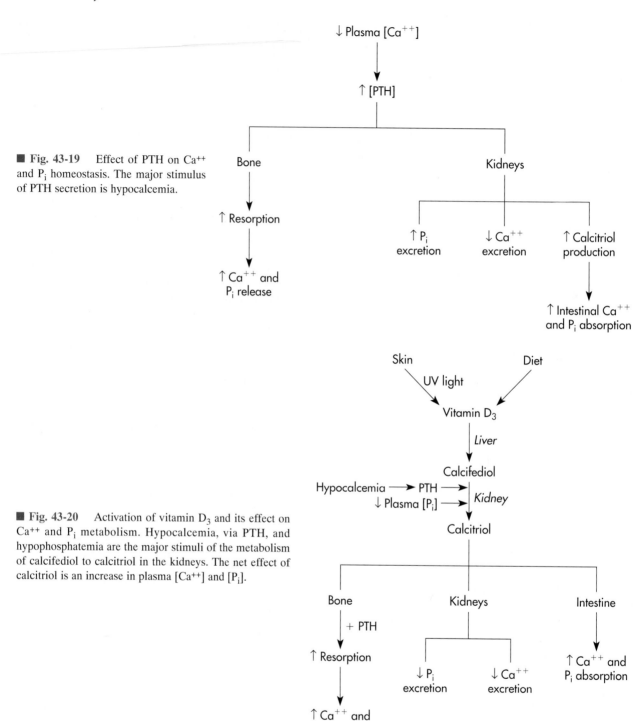

■ Fig. 43-19   Effect of PTH on Ca⁺⁺ and P_i homeostasis. The major stimulus of PTH secretion is hypocalcemia.

■ Fig. 43-20   Activation of vitamin D_3 and its effect on Ca⁺⁺ and P_i metabolism. Hypocalcemia, via PTH, and hypophosphatemia are the major stimuli of the metabolism of calcifediol to calcitriol in the kidneys. The net effect of calcitriol is an increase in plasma [Ca⁺⁺] and [P_i].

P_i absorption by the intestine and Ca⁺⁺ and P_i release from bone, but decreases Ca⁺⁺ and P_i excretion by the kidneys. The net effect of calcitriol is to increase plasma [Ca⁺⁺] and [P_i]. *Thus, the major stimuli of calcitriol production are hypocalcemia via PTH and hypophosphatemia (i.e., a low plasma [P_i]).*

Calcitonin is also an important hormone in Ca⁺⁺ homeostasis because it blocks bone resorption and stimulates Ca⁺⁺ deposition in bone (Fig. 43-21). Calcitonin's modest direct effect on decreasing urinary Ca⁺⁺ excretion

is a relatively minor action of the hormone. The major stimulus of calcitonin secretion is an increase in plasma [Ca⁺⁺]. *Because changes in P_i handling in bone, intestine, and the kidneys tend to cancel each other out, calcitonin decreases plasma [Ca⁺⁺] but has little effect on plasma [P_i].*

Estrogens defend against PTH-mediated resorption of bone. In estrogen-deficient conditions, such as that after menopause, the unabated effect of PTH on bone

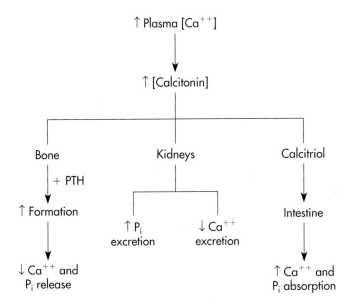

↑ Plasma [Ca^{++}]

↓

↑ [Calcitonin]

Bone   Kidneys   Calcitriol

+ PTH

↑ Formation   ↑ P$_i$ ↓ Ca^{++} Intestine
              excretion   excretion

↓ Ca^{++} and   ↑ Ca^{++} and
P$_i$ release   P$_i$ absorption

■ **Fig. 43-21** Effect of calcitonin on Ca^{++} and P$_i$ homeostasis. The major stimulus of calcitonin secretion is hypercalcemia. The net effect of calcitonin is a reduction in plasma [Ca^{++}]. Quantitatively, therefore, the most important effects of calcitonin are to stimulate bone formation and decrease bone resorption. Although calcitonin reduces urinary Ca^{++} excretion and intestinal Ca^{++} absorption, these effects are relatively minor and have little effect on plasma [Ca^{++}]. The effects of calcitonin on the kidneys and calcitriol production are relatively minor versus its effect on bone.

contributes to the development of **osteoporosis.** Estrogen replacement therapy, which should be accompanied by progesterone, is useful for women at high risk for developing osteoporosis.

■ *Summary*

1. K$^+$ is one of the most abundant cations in the body. It is crucial for many cellular functions, including cell growth and division and the excitability of nerve and muscle.

2. K$^+$ homeostasis is maintained by hormones that regulate plasma [K$^+$] and by the kidneys, which adjust K$^+$ excretion to match dietary K$^+$ intake. Plasma [K$^+$] is maintained by insulin, epinephrine, and aldosterone. In contrast, cell lysis, exercise, and changes in acid-base balance and plasma osmolality disturb plasma [K$^+$].

3. K$^+$ excretion by the kidneys is determined by the rate of K$^+$ secretion by the distal tubule and collecting duct. K$^+$ secretion by these tubular segments is regulated by plasma [K$^+$], aldosterone, and ADH. In contrast, changes in tubular fluid flow and acid-base disturbance disturb K$^+$ excretion by the kidneys.

4. Ca^{++} and inorganic phosphate (P$_i$) are multivalent ions that perform many important functions. The kidneys, in conjunction with the gastrointestinal tract and bone, play a vital role in regulating plasma Ca^{++} and P$_i$ levels.

5. Plasma [Ca^{++}] is regulated by PTH, calcitriol, and calcitonin. Ca^{++} excretion by the kidneys is determined by the net amount of intestinal Ca^{++} absorption, the balance between bone formation and resorption, and the net amount of Ca^{++} reabsorption by the distal tubule and

thick ascending limb of Henle's loop. Ca^{++} reabsorption by the thick ascending limb is regulated by PTH, calcitriol, and calcitonin, which stimulate Ca^{++} reabsorption.

6. Plasma [P$_i$] is regulated by the kidney's maximal reabsorptive capacity of P$_i$. A fall in plasma [P$_i$] stimulates production of calcitriol, which causes the release of P$_i$ from bone into the ECF. Calcitriol also increases P$_i$ absorption by the intestine and decreases urinary P$_i$ excretion.

■ *Self-Study Problems*

1. What would happen to the rise in plasma [K$^+$] after an intravenous K$^+$ load if the subject had a combination of sympathetic blockade and insulin deficiency?

2. What effect would aldosterone deficiency have on urinary K$^+$ excretion? What would happen to plasma [K$^+$] and what effect would this have on K$^+$ excretion?

3. Describe the homeostatic mechanisms involved in maintaining the plasma [K$^+$] after ingestion of a K$^+$-rich meal.

4. If the GFR declined by 50% (i.e., because of loss of one kidney) and the filtered load of K$^+$ also declined by 50%, would the remaining kidney be able to maintain K$^+$ balance? If so, how would this occur? If not, would the subject become hyperkalemic?

5. How is Ca^{++} reabsorption in the proximal tubule dependent on Na$^+$ reabsorption? What would happen to Ca^{++} excretion if a subject was given a diuretic, such as mannitol, that inhibits sodium and water reabsorption by the proximal tubule?

6. What effect would furosemide, an inhibitor of Na^+ reabsorption by the thick ascending limb of Henle's loop, have on urinary Ca^{++} excretion?

7. What would happen to P_i excretion if plasma $[P_i]$ was increased from 4 to 6 mg/dl?

■ *Bibliography*

Journal articles

Friedman PA, Gesek FA: *Cellular calcium transport in renal epithelia: measurement, mechanisms, and regulation, Physiol Rev* 75:429-471, 1995.

Hebert SC: An ATP-regulated, inwardly rectifying potassium channel from rat kidney (ROMK), *Kidney Int* 48:1010-1016, 1995.

Murer H, Biber J: Renal sodium-phosphate cotransport, *Curr Opin Nephrol Hypertens* 3:504-510, 1994.

Books and monographs

Berndt TJ, Knox FG: *Renal regulation of phosphate excretion.* In Seldin DW, Giebisch G, editors: *The kidney: physiology and pathophysiology,* ed 2, New York, 1992, Raven Press.

Giebisch G, Malnic G, Berliner RW: *Control of renal potassium excretion.* In Brenner BM, editor: *The kidney,* ed 5, Philadelphia, 1996, WB Saunders.

Knochel JP, Agarwal R: *Hypophosphatemia and hyperphosphatemia.* In Brenner BM, editor: *The kidney,* ed 5, Philadelphia, 1996, WB Saunders.

Rose BD, Rennke HG: *Disorders of potassium balance.* In Rose BD, Rennke HG: *Renal pathophysiology—the essentials,* Baltimore, 1994, Williams & Wilkins.

Seldin DW, Giebisch G, editors: *The regulation of potassium balance.* New York, 1989, Raven Press.

Stanton BA, Giebisch G: *Renal potassium transport.* In Windhager EE, editor: *Handbook of Physiology:* sect 8, *Renal Physiology,* ed 2, New York, 1992, Oxford University Press.

Suki WN, Rouse D: *Renal transport of calcium, magnesium and phosphate.* In Brenner BM, editor: *The kidney,* ed 5, Philadelphia, 1996, WB Saunders.

Sutton RAL, Dirks JH: *Disturbances of calcium and magnesium metabolism.* In Brenner BM, editor: *The kidney,* ed 5, Philadelphia, 1996, WB Saunders.

Wright FS, Giebisch G: *Regulation of potassium excretion.* In Seldin DW, Giebisch G, editors: *The kidney: physiology and pathophysiology,* ed 2, New York, 1992, Raven Press.

Role of the Kidneys in the Regulation of Acid-Base Balance

The concentration of H^+ in the body fluids is low compared with that of many other ions. For example, Na^+ is present at a concentration some 3 million times greater than that of H^+ ($[Na^+]$ = 140 mEq/L; $[H^+]$ = 40 nEq/L. Because of the low $[H^+]$ of the body fluids, $[H^+]$ is commonly expressed as the negative logarithm, or pH.

Acid-base balance is accomplished through the coordinated functions of the liver, lungs, and kidneys (see also Chapter 36). Acid or base* addition to, or production by, the body must be matched by excretion from the body to maintain acid-base balance. Through metabolism, the liver adds various acid and base equivalents to the extracellular fluid (ECF). Other cells, such as skeletal muscle, can also add acid to the body via metabolism, especially under anaerobic conditions. In a normal adult, acid or base is added to the body fluids by metabolism, and the amount of acid or base added is determined mainly by the diet.

With a normal diet, the body produces approximately 15 to 20 mol of acid per day. Virtually all of this acid is derived from CO_2 ($CO_2 + H_2O \leftrightarrow H_2CO_3$) and is therefore called **volatile acid.** The lungs handle this potential acid load by excreting CO_2 and there is no net effect of this CO_2 on acid-base balance. In addition, the metabolism of food produces acid and base that cannot be excreted by the lungs. In people on a typical meat-containing diet, acid production exceeds base production. This acid, termed **nonvolatile acid,** is produced at a small fraction of the rate of volatile acid production (50 to 100 mmol/day vs. 15 to 20 mol/day). The kidneys, together with various buffers, play an important role in the handling of nonvolatile acid, and thereby minimize the effects of this acid on body fluid pH.

Many of the body's metabolic functions are exquisitely sensitive to pH, and normal function can occur only within a very narrow pH range. The pH range of 6.8 to 7.8 (160 to 16 nEq/L of H^+) in the ECF is generally com-

patible with life. Normally, the pH of the ECF is maintained between 7.35 and 7.45. This chapter examines the mechanisms that maintain the pH of the body fluids within this normal range, with special emphasis on the role of the kidneys.

■ The CO_2/HCO_3^- Buffer System

Bicarbonate (HCO_3^-) is an important buffer of the ECF. Given a plasma $[HCO_3^-]$ of 23 to 25 mEq/L and a plasma volume of 14 L, the bicarbonate within the ECF can potentially buffer 350 mEq of H^+. The CO_2/HCO_3^- buffer system differs from the other buffer systems of the body (e.g., phosphate) because it is regulated by both the lungs and the kidneys. This difference is best appreciated by considering the following reaction:

$$CO_2 + H_2O \overset{CA}{\leftrightarrow} H_2CO_3 \leftrightarrow H^+ + HCO_3^- \qquad (44\text{-}1)$$

The first reaction (hydration/dehydration of CO_2) is the rate-limiting step. This reaction would proceed at a very slow rate without the presence of the enzyme **carbonic anhydrase (CA),** which greatly accelerates the reaction. The second reaction, the ionization of H_2CO_3 to H^+ and HCO_3^-, is virtually instantaneous. To quantitate these reactions, it is convenient and simpler to consider H^+ and HCO_3^- as products, and CO_2 and H_2CO_3 as reactants. Thus:

$$K' = \frac{[H^+][HCO_3^-]}{[CO_2][H_2CO_3]} \qquad (44\text{-}2)$$

Because this simplification combines the dissociation reaction ($H_2CO_3 \leftrightarrow H^+ + HCO_3^-$) with the hydration/dehydration reaction ($CO_2 + H_2O \leftrightarrow H_2CO_3$), K' is not a true dissociation constant. Instead, it is called an **apparent dissociation constant.** The value of K' depends on temperature and solution composition. For plasma at 37° C, K' has a value of $10^{-6.1}$ (pK' = 6.1).

---

*Acids are defined as substances that add H^+ to the body fluids, whereas bases (alkali) remove H^+ from the body fluids.

The terms in the denominator of equation 44-2 represent the total amount of CO_2 dissolved in solution. Most of this CO_2 is in gaseous form, with only 0.3% contained in H_2CO_3. Because the amount of CO_2 in solution depends on its partial pressure (P_{CO_2}) and its solubility (α),* equation 44-2 can be rewritten as:

$$K' = \frac{[H^+][HCO_3^-]}{\alpha P_{CO_2}} \qquad (44\text{-}3)$$

For plasma at 37° C, $\alpha = 0.03$.

Another form of this equation is obtained by solving for $[H^+]$:

$$[H^+] = \frac{K' \alpha P_{CO_2}}{[HCO_3^-]} \qquad (44\text{-}4)$$

Taking the negative logarithm of both sides of the equation yields:

$$-\log[H^+] = \frac{-\log[K'] + -\log\alpha P_{CO_2}}{-\log[HCO_3^-]} \qquad (44\text{-}5)$$

$$pH = \frac{pK' + \log[HCO_3^-]}{\alpha P_{CO_2}} \quad \text{or}$$

$$pH = 6.1 + \log \frac{[HCO_3^-]}{0.03 P_{CO_2}} \qquad (44\text{-}6)$$

Equation 44-6 is the **Henderson-Hasselbalch equation.** This equation shows that the pH of the ECF varies when either $[HCO_3^-]$ or P_{CO_2} is altered. Disturbances of acid-base balance that result from a change in the ECF $[HCO_3^-]$ are called **metabolic acid-base disorders,** whereas those resulting from a change in P_{CO_2} are termed **respiratory acid-base disorders.** These disorders are considered in more detail in a later section of this chapter. The kidneys are primarily responsible for regulating $[HCO_3^-]$, while the lungs control P_{CO_2}.

■ *Metabolic Production of Acid and Alkali*

In the normal individual, the metabolism of dietary foodstuffs produces a number of substances that can impact acid-base status. When insulin is present and tissues are adequately perfused, cellular metabolism of carbohydrates and fats produces large quantities of CO_2 (approximately 15 to 20 mol/day).† As noted, this CO_2 is a potential acid in the body fluids (as H_2CO_3). This volatile acid is excreted from the body by the lungs. The normal diet also contains other substances whose metabolism produces nonvolatile acids.

---

*α is not strictly a gas solubility constant. Rather, it is a constant that relates the P_{CO_2} to the total concentration of H_2CO_3 and the dissolved CO_2 concentration.

†In the absence of insulin, or when tissue hypoxia exists, carbohydrates and fats are incompletely metabolized. Under these conditions, large quantities of nonvolatile acids are produced (e.g., lactic acid and β-hydroxybutyric acid).

Metabolites of amino acids constitute a major portion of nonvolatile acid production. The metabolism of the sulfur-containing amino acids cysteine and methionine yields sulfuric acid. The metabolism of the cationic amino acids lysine, arginine, and histidine yields hydrochloric acid. This acid production is partially offset by the metabolism of the anionic amino acids aspartate and glutamate, which results in the production of HCO_3^-.

In addition to carbohydrates, fats, and amino acids, the diet contains a number of other substances that can impact acid-base balance. For example, ingested phosphate (as $H_2PO_4^-$) constitutes another nonvolatile acid load to the body. A number of organic anions (e.g., citrate) produce HCO_3^- when metabolized. Finally, during the processes of digestion and absorption of gastrointestinal fluid, some HCO_3^- is normally lost in the feces. This HCO_3^- loss is equivalent to the addition of nonvolatile acid to the body. In individuals who eat a typical diet, dietary intake, cellular metabolism, and fecal HCO_3^- loss result in the net addition of approximately 1 mEq/kg body weight of nonvolatile acid to the body each day (50 to 100 mEq/day for most adults). *The production of nonvolatile acids is highly dependent on the diet.* For example, people who eat a vegetarian diet may produce less acid than those who eat meat.

The nonvolatile acids produced during metabolism do not circulate as free acids, but are immediately buffered:

$$H_2SO_4 + 2NaHCO_3 \leftrightarrow Na_2SO_4 + 2CO_2 + 2H_2O \quad (44\text{-}7)$$

$$HCl + NaHCO_3 \leftrightarrow NaCl + CO_2 + H_2O \qquad (44\text{-}8)$$

This buffering process yields Na^+ salts and removes HCO_3^- from the ECF. Buffering of strong acids by HCO_3^- minimizes the tendency for strong acids to lower the pH of the ECF. In order to maintain acid-base balance, the kidneys must excrete these acid salts and replenish the HCO_3^- lost by neutralization of the H^+.

■ *Overview of Renal Acid Excretion*

To maintain acid-base balance, the kidneys must excrete an amount of acid equal to the production of nonvolatile acid. In addition, the kidneys must prevent the loss of HCO_3^- in the urine. This latter task is quantitatively more important, because the filtered load of HCO_3^- is approximately 4320 mEq/day (24 mEq/L × 180 L/day = 4320 mEq/day) compared with only 50 to 100 mEq/day of nonvolatile acid.

Both the reabsorption of filtered HCO_3^- and the excretion of acid are accomplished through the process of H^+ secretion by the nephrons. Thus, in a single day the nephrons secrete approximately 4390 mEq of H^+ into the tubular fluid. Most of this H^+ serves to reabsorb the filtered HCO_3^-, and only 50 to 100 mEq is excreted. As a result of this acid excretion, the urine is normally acidic.

Theoretically, the kidneys could excrete the non-volatile acids and replenish the HCO_3^- lost during titration by reversing the reactions shown in equations 44-7 and 44-8. However, because the pKs of these acids are low, this process would require a urine pH of 1.0, and the minimal urine pH attainable by the kidneys is only 4.0 to 4.5. Consequently, the kidneys cannot excrete the free acids. Instead, they excrete the salts that make up the free acids while excreting H^+ with other anions (i.e., urinary buffers). The primary urinary buffer is phosphate ($HPO_4^=/H_2PO_4^-$). Other constituents of the urine can also serve as buffers (e.g., creatinine), although their roles are less important than that of phosphate. Collectively, the various urinary buffers are called **titratable acid.***

An important mechanism by which the kidneys contribute to the maintenance of acid-base balance is through the synthesis and excretion of **ammonium (NH_4^+).**† The mechanisms involved in this process are discussed in more detail later in this chapter. For now, it is only important to know that for each NH_4^+ excreted in the urine, an HCO_3^- is returned to the systemic circulation, which replenishes the HCO_3^- lost during titration of nonvolatile acid.

In brief, *the kidneys contribute to acid-base homeostasis by reabsorbing the filtered load of HCO_3^- and excreting an amount of acid equivalent to the amount of nonvolatile acid produced through metabolism.* This overall process is termed **net acid excretion (NAE)** and can be quantitated as follows:

$$NAE = [(U_{NH_4^+} \times \dot{V}) + (U_{TA} \times \dot{V})] - (U_{HCO_3^-} \times \dot{V}) \quad (44\text{-}9)$$

where $U_{NH_4^+} \times \dot{V}$ and $U_{TA} \times \dot{V}$ are the rates of excretion (mEq/day) of NH_4^+ and titratable acid (TA); and $U_{HCO_3^-} \times V$ is the amount of HCO_3^- lost in the urine (equivalent to adding H^+ to the body). Again, to maintain acid-base balance, the amount of net acid excretion must equal the amount of nonvolatile acid produced.

■ *HCO_3^- Reabsorption along the Nephron*

Glomerular filtration delivers 4320 mEq/day of HCO_3^- to the nephrons. Fig. 44-1 illustrates the contribution of the various nephron segments to the reabsorption of this HCO_3^-. The reabsorption of HCO_3^- is critically impor-

tant for the prevention of its loss in the urine. Under normal condition, virtually all the filtered HCO_3^- is reabsorbed, and none appears in the urine.

Approximately 80% of the filtered load of HCO_3^- is reabsorbed in the proximal tubule. The cellular mechanisms involved in this reabsorption are illustrated in Fig. 44-2. The apical membrane of the proximal tubule cell contains an Na^+-H^+ antiporter that uses the energy in the lumen-to-cell Na^+ gradient to secrete H^+ into the tubular fluid. Recent evidence indicates that some portion of H^+ is secreted via an H^+-ATPase. Within the cell, H^+ and HCO_3^- are produced in a reaction catalyzed by carbonic anhydrase (see equation 44-1). H^+ is secreted into the tubular fluid, whereas HCO_3^- exits the cell across the basolateral membrane and returns to the peritubular blood.

Although the electrochemical gradient for HCO_3^- favors its passive movement out of the cell across the basolateral membrane, simple diffusion does not appear to occur to a significant degree. Instead, HCO_3^- movement out of the cell across the basolateral membrane is coupled to that of other ions. Most of the HCO_3^- exits via a symporter that couples the exit of 1 Na^+ to 3 HCO_3^-. Additionally, some of the HCO_3^- exits in exchange for Cl^- (via a Cl^--HCO_3^- antiporter).

Within the tubular fluid, the secreted H^+ combines with the filtered HCO_3^- to form H_2CO_3. This H_2CO_3 is rapidly converted to CO_2 and H_2O. Carbonic anhydrase present in the apical membrane and exposed to the tubular fluid contents facilitates the conversion of H_2CO_3 to H_2O and CO_2. Because the tubule is highly permeable to

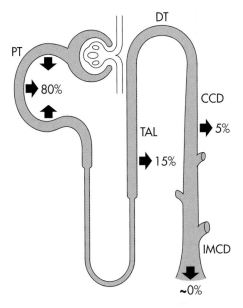

■ **Fig. 44-1** Segmental reabsorption of HCO_3^-. The fraction of the filtered load of HCO_3^- reabsorbed by the various segments of the nephron is shown. Normally, the entire filtered load of HCO_3^- is reabsorbed. *PT,* Proximal tubule; *TAL,* thick ascending limb; *DT,* distal tubule; *CCD,* collecting duct; *IMCD,* inner medullary collecting duct.

---

*The term titratable acid is derived from the method by which these buffers are quantitated in the laboratory. Typically, alkali (OH^-) is added to a urine sample to titrate its pH to that of plasma (i.e., 7.4). The amount of alkali added is equal to the H^+ titrated by these urine buffers, and is thus called titratable acid.

†Traditionally, ammonia (NH_3) was considered a urinary buffer. However, as described later in this chapter, this designation is not consistent with what is currently known about ammonium production and excretion. Consequently, we do not refer to ammonia/ammonium as a urinary buffer.

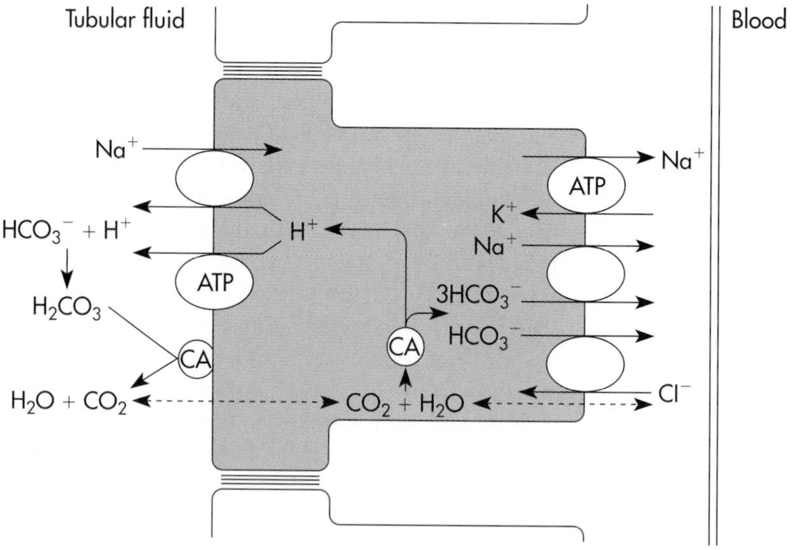

■ **Fig. 44-2** Cellular mechanism for reabsorption of filtered HCO_3^- by cells of the proximal tubule. *CA,* Carbonic anhydrase; *ATP,* adenosine triphosphate. See text for details.

both CO_2 and H_2O, these are rapidly reabsorbed. The net effect of this process is that for each HCO_3^- removed from the tubular fluid, one HCO_3^- appears in the peritubular blood.

An additional 15% of the filtered load of HCO_3^- is reabsorbed by Henle's loop. Most of this HCO_3^- is reabsorbed by the cells of the thick ascending limb. This mechanism for HCO_3^- reabsorption appears to be similar to that described for the proximal tubule. H^+ is secreted into the tubular fluid by an apical membrane Na^+-H^+ antiporter (an H^+-ATPase is not involved in this process). HCO_3^- exits the cell across the basolateral membrane coupled to Na^+ (Na^+-$3HCO_3^-$ symporter) and is returned to the peritubular blood.

The distal tubule and collecting duct reabsorb the small amount of HCO_3^- that escapes reabsorption by the proximal tubule and Henle's loop (5% off the filtered load). This reabsorption does not depend on Na^+ (i.e., apical membrane Na^+-H^+ antiporter), as is the case in the earlier nephron segments. Fig. 44-3 shows the mechanism of HCO_3^- reabsorption by the collecting duct. Here, H^+ secretion occurs via the intercalated cell (see Chapter 40). Within the cell, H^+ and HCO_3^- are produced by the hydration of CO_2; this reaction is catalyzed by carbonic anhydrase. The H^+ is secreted into the tubular fluid by two mechanisms. The first mechanism involves an apical membrane H^+-ATPase. The second mechanism couples the secretion of H^+ to the reabsorption of K^+ via an H^+, K^+-ATPase similar to the mechanism that operates in the stomach (see Chapter 38). The HCO_3^- exits the cell across the basolateral membrane in exchange for Cl^- (via a Cl^--HCO_3^- antiporter) and enters the peritubular capillary blood.

A second population of intercalated cells within the collecting duct secrete HCO_3^- rather than H^+ into the tubular fluid. In contrast to the collecting duct cells described in the above paragraph, these cells appear to have the H^+-ATPase located in the basolateral membrane

and a Cl^--HCO_3^- antiporter in the apical membrane (Fig. 44-3). Their activity can be increased during metabolic alkalosis when the kidneys must excrete excess HCO_3^-. However, under normal conditions, H^+ secretion predominates in the collecting duct.

The apical membrane of the cells of the collecting duct has a low permeability to H^+, and the pH of the tubular fluid can become quite acidic. Indeed, the most acidic tubular fluid along the nephron (pH = 4.0 to 4.5) is produced here. By comparison, the permeability of the proximal tubule to H^+ and HCO_3^- is much higher, and the tubular fluid pH falls to only 6.5 in this segment. As explained below, the ability of the collecting duct to lower the pH of the tubular fluid is critically important for the excretion of urinary buffers as well as ammonium.

■ *Regulation of HCO_3^- Reabsorption*

HCO_3^- reabsorption (i.e., H^+ secretion) is regulated by several factors (Table 44-1). The primary sites for regulation of HCO_3^- reabsorption are the proximal tubule and collecting duct.

Glomerular filtration rate. Because of glomerulotubular balance (see Chapter 41), any change in the filtered load of HCO_3^-, as a result of alterations in the glomerular filtration rate, is matched by an appropriate change in HCO_3^- reabsorption by the proximal tubule. Thus, proximal tubule HCO_3^- reabsorption increases with an increase in filtered load and decreases with a reduced filtered load.

Na^+ balance. Most of the proximal tubule HCO_3^- reabsorption occurs as a result of H^+ secretion by the Na^+-H^+ antiporter located in the apical membrane of the cells. Consequently, factors that regulate Na^+ homeostasis (see Chapter 42) alter HCO_3^- reabsorption secondarily. Thus, volume expansion (i.e., positive Na^+ balance), which inhibits proximal tubule Na^+ reabsorption, also

H$^+$-secreting cell

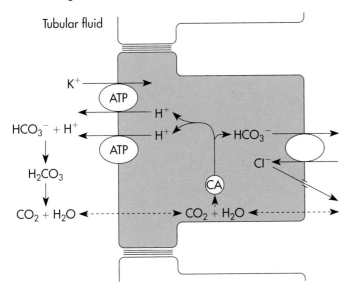

HCO$_3$$^-$-secreting cell

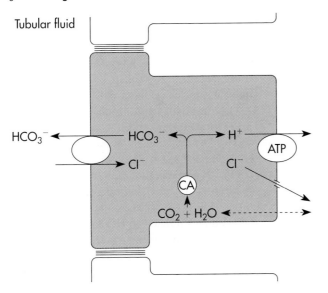

■ **Fig. 44-3**   Cellular mechanisms for reabsorption and secretion of HCO$_3$$^-$ by intercalated cells of the collecting duct. *CA*, Carbonic anhydrase; *ATP*, adenosine triphosphate. See text for details.

decreases the reabsorption of HCO$_3$$^-$. Conversely, HCO$_3$$^-$ reabsorption is enhanced with volume contraction (i.e., negative Na$^+$ balance).

Systemic acid-base balance. As might be expected, changes in systemic acid-base balance also affect HCO$_3$$^-$ reabsorption. Systemic acidosis, whether produced by a decrease in the plasma [HCO$_3$$^-$] (metabolic) or by an increase in the Pco$_2$ (respiratory), stimulates HCO$_3$$^-$ reabsorption all along the nephron (i.e., proximal tubule, Henle's loop, and the collecting duct). This stimulation is believed to occur as a result of acidification of the intracellular fluid (ICF), which in turn steepens the cell-to-lumen H$^+$ gradient and enhances H$^+$ secretion across the apical membrane of the cell.

Acidification of the ICF may also result in the insertion of more transporters into the membranes of the cells. The insertion of H$^+$-ATPase into the apical membrane of collecting duct intercalated cells is an important component of the response to systemic acidosis. Insertion of these acid base–related transporters into the apical, and perhaps also the basolateral, membrane may occur in other nephron segments also. This constitutes an important mechanism for regulating transport in response to systemic acid-base disorders. Metabolic and respiratory alkalosis inhibit HCO$_3$$^-$ reabsorption along the nephron. The mechanisms involved are thought to be the opposite of those for stimulation of HCO$_3$$^-$ reabsorption with acidosis.

■ **Table 44-1**   Factors that regulate HCO_3^- reabsorption (H^+ secretion) by the nephron

Factor	Nephron site of action
Increasing H⁺ secretion	
Increase in filtered load of HCO_3^-	Proximal tubule
Volume contraction	Proximal tubule
Decrease in plasma $[HCO_3^-]$ (↓ pH)	Proximal tubule, thick ascending limb of Henle's loop, and collecting duct
Increase in blood P_{CO_2}	Proximal tubule, thick ascending limb of Henle's loop, and collecting duct
Increase in aldosterone	Collecting duct
Decreasing H⁺ secretion	
Decrease in filtered load of HCO_3^-	Proximal tubule
Volume expansion	Proximal tubule
Increase in plasma $[HCO_3^-]$ (↑ pH)	Proximal tubule, thick ascending limb of Henle's loop, and collecting duct
Decrease in blood P_{CO_2}	Proximal tubule, thick ascending limb of Henle's loop, and collecting duct
Decrease in aldosterone	Collecting duct

Aldosterone. Aldosterone is an important regulatory factor for HCO_3^- reabsorption, especially in the collecting duct. Aldosterone stimulates H^+ secretion by the intercalated cells of the collecting duct. This effect reflects both the direct action of the hormone on the intercalated cell and an indirect effect via aldosterone stimulation of Na^+ reabsorption by the principal cell. With regard to aldosterone's indirect effect (see also Chapters 41 and 42), reabsorption by the principal cells of the collecting duct produces a lumen-negative transepithelial voltage. When Na^+ reabsorption is stimulated by aldosterone, the magnitude of the lumen-negative voltage is increased. This in turn favors intercalated cell H^+ secretion because it reduces the electrochemical gradient against which the apical membrane H^+-ATPase must pump (the H^+-ATPase is affected by a change in voltage).* The cellular mechanism by which aldosterone directly stimulates intercalated cell H^+ secretion probably involves the synthesis of additional transporters and their insertion into the cell membranes. As would be expected, collecting duct H^+ secretion is decreased when aldosterone levels are reduced.

Other factors. Although other factors influence renal H^+/HCO_3^- transport, they are not primarily involved in regulating acid-base balance. For example, parathyroid hormone (PTH) inhibits HCO_3^- reabsorption by the proximal tubule. PTH is primarily involved in the maintenance of Ca^{++} and P_i balance (see Chapters 43 and 48). However, when PTH acts on proximal tubule cells, it also inhibits the Na^+-H^+ antiporter in the apical membrane. Angiotensin II stimulates proximal tubule HCO_3^- reabsorption. This action is related to stimulation of Na^+ reabsorption (see Chapter 42) and is mediated by increased activity of the Na^+-H^+ antiporter. Finally, hypokalemia can stimulate proximal tubule HCO_3^- reabsorption. The mechanism for this stimulation is not completely understood but may reflect hypokalemia-induced acidification of the ICF (see Chapter 43).

■ *Formation of New HCO_3^-: The Role of Ammonia*

As discussed previously, reabsorption of the filtered load of HCO_3^- by the kidneys is important for the maintenance of acid-base balance. HCO_3^- loss in the urine would decrease the plasma $[HCO_3^-]$ and would be equivalent to the addition of H^+ to the body. However, HCO_3^- reabsorption alone does not replenish the HCO_3^- lost during the titration of the nonvolatile acids produced by metabolism. *To maintain acid-base balance, the kidneys must replace this lost HCO_3^- with new HCO_3^-.* A portion of the new HCO_3^- is produced during the titration of urinary buffers such as phosphate and creatinine (Fig. 44-4). In the collecting duct, where tubular fluid contains little or no HCO_3^- owing to HCO_3^- reabsorption in upstream tubular segments, H^+ secreted into tubular fluid combines with a urinary buffer. Thus, H^+ secretion results in excretion of the H^+ with a buffer, and the HCO_3^- produced in the cell from the hydration of CO_2 is added back to the blood.

As noted previously, the primary urinary buffer is phosphate ($HPO_4^=/H_2PO_4^-$). The amount of phosphate excreted each day, and therefore available to serve as a urinary buffer, is derived solely from the diet. Moreover, the amount of P_i excreted is regulated in response to the need to maintain Ca^{++} and P_i balance (see Chapters 43 and 48), and not in response to the need to maintain acid-base balance. However, ammonium is produced by the kidneys, and its synthesis and subsequent excretion are regulated in response to the body's acid-base requirements. Because ammonium excretion is tied to acid-base requirements, it is critically involved in new HCO_3^- formation.

Ammonium is produced in the kidneys by the metabolism of the amino acid glutamine. Glutamine (primarily from the liver) and the Na^+ salts of the nonvolatile acids

*Because the H^+, K^+-ATPase of intercalated cells is electroneutral, indirect stimulation of this transporter by the lumen-negative voltage would not occur.

Tubular fluid

Blood

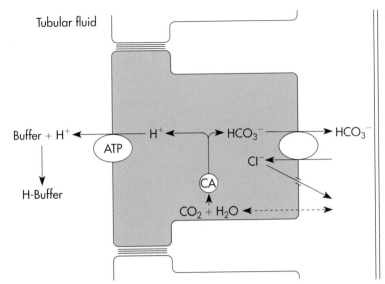

■ **Fig. 44-4**   General scheme for the excretion of H^+ with non-HCO_3^- urinary buffers. The primary urinary buffer is $HPO_4^=$. Other buffers include creatinine. Collectively, the urinary buffers are called titratable acid. For simplicity, only the H^+-ATPase is shown. H^+ secretion by the H^+, K^+-ATPase also titrates luminal buffers. *CA,* Carbonic anhydrase; *ATP,* adenosine triphosphate.

(e.g., Na_2SO_4) are delivered to the kidneys in the renal arterial plasma. The kidneys metabolize the glutamine, excrete NH_4^+ with the acid salts, and return $NaHCO_3$ to the body in the renal vein plasma. An important point to recognize is that the formation of new HCO_3^- by this process depends on the kidney's ability to excrete the NH_4^+ in the urine. If NH_4^+ is not excreted in the urine, but instead enters the systemic circulation, it will titrate plasma HCO_3^-, thus negating the process of generating new HCO_3^-.* The process by which the kidneys excrete NH_4^+ is complex (Fig. 44-5).

Ammonium is produced in proximal tubule cells from glutamine. Each glutamine molecule produces two molecules of NH_4^+ and a divalent anion. Metabolism of this anion ultimately provides two molecules of HCO_3^-:

$$\text{Glutamine} \leftrightarrow 2NH_4^+ + \text{anion}^{-2} \leftrightarrow$$
$$2HCO_3^- + 2NH_4^+ \quad (44\text{-}10)$$

The HCO_3^- exits the proximal tubule cell across the basolateral membrane and enters the peritubular blood as new HCO_3^-. NH_4^+ exits the cell across the apical membrane and enters the tubular fluid. A major mechanism for the secretion of NH_4^+ into the tubular fluid involves the Na^+-H^+ antiporter, with NH_4^+ substituting for H^+. In addition, NH_3 can diffuse out of the cell into the tubular lumen, where it is protonated to NH_4^+. A significant portion of the NH_4^+ secreted by the proximal tubule is reabsorbed by Henle's loop. The thick ascending limb is the primary site of this NH_4^+ reabsorption. NH_4^+ substitutes for K^+ on the 1 Na^+-1 K^+-2 Cl^- symporter. In addition, the lumen-positive transepithelial voltage in this segment drives paracellular reabsorption of NH_4^+.

The reabsorbed NH_4^+ accumulates in the medullary

interstitium, where it exists in chemical equilibrium with NH_3.* NH_4^+ then reenters the tubular fluid of the collecting duct. The mechanism by which NH_4^+ reappears in the collecting duct involves the processes of **nonionic diffusion** and **diffusion trapping.** The collecting duct does not have a specific transport mechanism for the secretion of NH_4^+, nor do the cells have a significant passive permeability to it. However, the cells of the collecting duct are permeable to NH_3, which can diffuse from the medullary interstitium into the lumen of the collecting duct. As described previously, H^+ secretion by the collecting duct intercalated cells results in acidification of the luminal fluid (luminal fluid pH as low as 4.0 to 4.5 can be achieved). Consequently, NH_3 diffusing from the medullary interstitium into the collecting duct lumen (nonionic diffusion) is protonated to NH_4^+ by the acidic tubular fluid. Because the collecting duct is less permeable to NH_4^+ than to NH_3, NH_4^+ is trapped in the tubule lumen (diffusion trapping) and eliminated from the body in the urine.

H^+ secretion by the collecting duct is critical for the excretion of NH_4^+. If collecting duct H^+ secretion is inhibited, the NH_4^+ reabsorbed by the thick ascending limb will not be excreted in the urine. Instead, it will be returned to the systemic circulation, where it will react with HCO_3^- (i.e., be converted to urea by the liver). If this occurs, net acid excretion by the kidneys is reduced, and insufficient quantities of new HCO_3^- are added to the systemic circulation to replenish what was neutralized by the buffering of nonvolatile acids. Whereas new HCO_3^- is produced during the metabolism of glutamine by cells of the proximal tubule, the overall process is not complete until the NH_4^+ is excreted (i.e., the production

---

*The mechanism by which NH_4^+ titrates HCO_3^- is indirect and occurs as a result of the synthesis of urea from NH_4^+ by the liver (i.e., the urea cycle). When urea is synthesized from NH_4^+, H^+ is generated. This H^+ is rapidly buffered by HCO_3^-.

*Ammonia is a weak base that is present as both NH_4^+ and NH_3, with the relative amounts of each species determined by the pKa (pKa = 9.0).

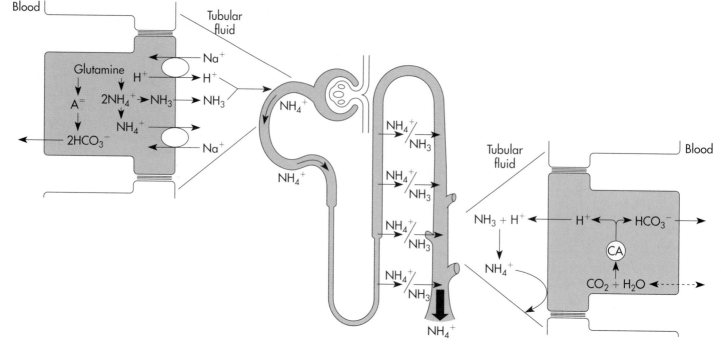

■ Fig. 44-5   Production, transport, and excretion of ammonium by the nephron. Glutamine is metabolized in the proximal tubule to NH_4^+ and HCO_3^-. The NH_4^+ is secreted into the lumen, and the HCO_3^- enters the blood. The secreted NH_4^+ is reabsorbed in Henle's loop primarily by the thick ascending limb, and accumulates in the medullary interstitium, where it exists as both NH_4^+ and NH_3. NH_3 diffuses into the tubular fluid of the collecting duct, and H^+ secretion by the collecting duct leads to accumulation of NH_4^+ in the lumen by the processes of nonionic diffusion and diffusion trapping. For every NH_4^+ excreted in the urine, a "new HCO_3^-" is returned to the systemic circulation. Therefore, the excretion of NH_4^+ can be used as a marker of proximal tubule glutamine metabolism, which in turn determines new HCO_3^- formation.

of urea from NH_4^+ by the liver is prevented). Thus, NH_4^+ excretion can be used as a marker of proximal tubule glutamine metabolism. Because of the stoichiometry of this reaction, one new HCO_3^- is returned to the systemic circulation for each NH_4^+ excreted in the urine.

An important feature of the NH_4^+ system is that it can be regulated. Alterations in ECF pH, presumably by affecting intracellular pH, cause changes in glutamine metabolism (NH_4^+ production) in the proximal tubule cells. During systemic acidosis, the enzymes in the proximal tubule cell, which are responsible for the metabolism of glutamine, are stimulated. This stimulation involves the synthesis of new enzyme and requires several days for complete adaptation. With increased levels of this enzyme, NH_4^+ production is increased, thus allowing enhanced production of new HCO_3^-. Conversely, glutamine metabolism is reduced with alkalosis.

Plasma $[K^+]$ also alters NH_4^+ production. In hyperkalemia, NH_4^+ production is inhibited, whereas hypokalemia stimulates its production. The mechanism by which plasma K^+ alters NH_4^+ production is not fully understood. Alterations in plasma $[K^+]$ may change intracellular $[H^+]$ by exchanging H^+ for K^+ (see Chapter 43), and the change in intracellular pH may then control glutamine metabolism. By this mechanism, exchange of extracellular K^+ for intracellular H^+ during hyperkalemia would

raise intracellular pH, thereby inhibiting glutamine metabolism. The opposite would occur during hypokalemia.

Renal tubule acidosis (RTA) refers to conditions in which urine acidification is impaired. In RTA, the kidneys are unable to excrete a sufficient amount of net acid to balance nonvolatile acid production, and metabolic acidosis results. RTA can occur either by a defect in proximal tubule H^+ secretion/HCO_3^- reabsorption (proximal RTA) or by a defect in distal tubule H^+ secretion (distal RTA).

Proximal RTA can be caused by a variety of hereditary and acquired conditions (e.g., **cystinosis, Fanconi's syndrome,** administration of carbonic anhydrase inhibitors). H^+ secretion by proximal tubule cells is impaired and results in a decrease in the reabsorption of the filtered load of HCO_3^-. Consequently, HCO_3^- is lost in the urine, plasma $[HCO_3^-]$ decreases, and metabolic acidosis ensues.

Distal RTA also occurs in a number of hereditary and acquired conditions (e.g., with **medullary sponge kidney,** with certain drugs such as **amphotericin B,** and secondary to urinary obstruction). Depending on the cause, secretion of H^+ by collecting duct intercalated cells is impaired or the permeability of the collecting duct to H^+ is increased. In either case, the ability to acidify the tubular fluid is impaired. Consequently, nonionic diffusion and diffusion trapping of NH_4^+ is impaired. This impairment in turn decreases net acid excretion, with the subsequent development of metabolic acidosis.

Failure to produce and excrete sufficient quantities of NH_4^+ can also reduce the amount of net acid excreted by the kidneys. In this situation, proximal tubule HCO_3^- reabsorption is normal, as is H^+ secretion by the distal tubule and collecting duct, and the urine pH is maximally acidic. However, because of the lack of sufficient quantities of NH_4^+, net acid excretion is less than net acid production, and metabolic acidosis develops.

If the metabolic acidosis resulting from any of these forms of RTA is severe, individuals must ingest alkali (e.g., $NaHCO_3$) to maintain acid-base balance. In this way, the HCO_3^- lost each day in the titration of nonvolatile acid is replenished by "new HCO_3^-" ingested in the diet.

■ *Response to Acid-Base Disorders*

The pH of the ECF is maintained within a very narrow range (7.35 to 7.45).* Acidosis exists when the blood pH falls below this range, whereas alkalosis exists when the blood pH exceeds this range. When the acid-base disorder results from a primary change in $[HCO_3^-]$, it is called a *metabolic disorder*. When the primary disturbance is an alteration in blood P_{CO_2}, it is called a *respiratory disorder*.

When an acid-base disturbance develops, the body employs a series of mechanisms to defend against the change in the pH of the ECF. *These defense mechanisms do not correct the acid-base disturbance but merely minimize the change in pH imposed by the disturbance.* Restoration of the blood pH to its normal value requires correction of the underlying process or processes that produced the acid-base disorder. For example, metabolism of fats in the absence of insulin leads to the accumulation of keto acids (a nonvolatile acid) in the blood. As a result of this accumulation, metabolic acidosis develops. The acid-base defense mechanisms minimize the fall in pH that occurs in this condition, but normal acid-base balance is not restored until insulin is administered and keto acid production ceases.

The body has three general mechanisms to defend against changes in body fluid pH produced by acid-base disturbances: (1) extracellular and intracellular buffering,

(2) adjustments in blood P_{CO_2} by alterations in the ventilatory rate of the lungs, and (3) adjustments in renal acid excretion.

■ *Extracellular and Intracellular Buffering*

The first line of defense against acid-base disorders is extracellular and intracellular buffering. The response of the extracellular buffers is virtually instantaneous, whereas intracellular buffering is somewhat slower and can take several minutes to complete.

Metabolic disorders that result from the addition of nonvolatile acid or alkali to the body fluids are buffered in both the ECF and ICF. The CO_2/HCO_3^- buffer system is the principal ECF buffer (see equation 44-1). When nonvolatile acid is added to the body fluids or base is lost from the body, HCO_3^- is consumed during the process of neutralizing the acid load, and the plasma $[HCO_3^-]$ is reduced. Conversely, when nonvolatile base is added to the body fluids or acid is lost from the body, H^+ is consumed. This causes more HCO_3^- to be produced from the dissociation of H_2CO_3, and consequently $[HCO_3^-]$ increases.

Although the CO_2/HCO_3^- buffer system is the principal ECF buffer, phosphate and plasma protein provide additional extracellular buffering:

$$H^+ + HPO_4^= \leftrightarrow H_2PO_4^-$$
$$H^+ + \text{protein} \leftrightarrow \text{H-Protein} \qquad (44\text{-}11)$$

The combined action of the CO_2/HCO_3^-, phosphate, and plasma protein buffering processes accounts for approximately 50% of the buffering of a nonvolatile acid load and 70% of a nonvolatile alkali load. The remainder of the buffering under these two conditions occurs intracellularly. Intracellular buffering involves the movement of H^+ into cells (during buffering of nonvolatile acid) or the movement of H^+ out of cells (during buffering of nonvolatile alkali). H^+ is titrated inside the cell by HCO_3^-, phosphate, and the histidine groups on protein.

Bone represents an additional source of extracellular buffer (e.g., $NaHCO_3$, $KHCO_3$, $CaCO_3$, $CaHPO_4$). In chronic acidosis, buffering by bone results in demineralization; in other words Ca^{++} is released from bone as Ca^{++}-containing buffers bind H^+ in exchange for Ca^{++}.

In respiratory acid-base disorders, body fluid pH changes as a result of alterations in $[H_2CO_3]$, which is determined directly by the P_{CO_2} (see equation 44-1). Virtually all buffering in respiratory acid-base disorders occurs intracellularly. When P_{CO_2} rises (respiratory acidosis), CO_2 moves into cells, where it combines with H_2O to form H_2CO_3. H_2CO_3 dissociates to H^+ and HCO_3^-. Some of the H^+ is buffered by cellular proteins, and HCO_3^- exits the cell and raises the plasma $[HCO_3^-]$.

This process is reversed when P_{CO_2} is reduced (respiratory alkalosis). Under this condition, the hydration

---

*For simplicity, the value of 7.40 will be used as normal, and deviations from this single value are deemed abnormal. Similarly, the normal range for P_{CO_2} is 33 to 44 mm Hg. However, a P_{CO_2} of 40 mm Hg is used as the normal reference value. Finally, a value of 24 mEq/L is considered a normal ECF $[HCO_3^-]$, even though the normal range is 22 to 28 mEq/L.

reaction ($H_2O + CO_2 \leftrightarrow H_2CO_3$) is shifted to the left by the decrease in P_{CO_2}. As a result, the dissociation reaction ($H_2CO_3 \leftrightarrow H^+ + HCO_3^-$) also shifts to the left, thereby reducing the plasma $[HCO_3^-]$.

■ *Respiratory Defense*

The lungs are the second line of defense against acid-base disorders. As indicated by the Henderson-Hasselbalch equation (see equation 44-6), changes in P_{CO_2} alter blood pH. An increase in P_{CO_2} decreases pH; a decrease in P_{CO_2} increases pH.

The ventilatory rate determines the P_{CO_2}. Increased ventilation decreases P_{CO_2}, whereas decreased ventilation increases P_{CO_2}. The blood P_{CO_2} and pH are important regulators of the ventilatory rate. Chemoreceptors located in the brain (ventral surface of the medulla) and in the periphery (carotid and aortic bodies) sense changes in P_{CO_2} and $[H^+]$ and alter the ventilatory rate (see Chapter 36). In metabolic acidosis, an increase in $[H^+]$ (decrease in pH) increases the ventilatory rate. Conversely, during metabolic alkalosis, a decrease in $[H^+]$ (increase in pH) leads to a decrease in the ventilatory rate.* The respiratory response to metabolic acid-base disturbances may take effect within several minutes but may require several hours to complete.

> Individuals with insulin-dependent diabetes can develop a metabolic acidosis (secondary to the production of keto acids) if insulin dosages are not adequate. As a compensatory response to this acidosis, the individual develops deep and rapid breathing. This breathing pattern is termed **Kussmaul respiration**. With prolonged Kussmaul respiration, the respiratory muscles can become fatigued. Respiratory compensation can then be impaired and the acidosis can become severe.

■ *Renal Defense*

The third and final line of defense against acid-base disorders is the kidneys. In response to a change in the plasma pH and P_{CO_2}, the kidneys make appropriate adjustments in the excretion of HCO_3^- and net acid. The renal response requires several days to complete because it takes hours to days to increase the synthesis and activity of the enzymes involved in NH_4^+ production.

---

*With maximal hyperventilation, P_{CO_2} can be reduced to approximately 10 mm Hg. Because hypoxia, which is a potent stimulator of ventilation, also develops with hypoventilation, the degree to which P_{CO_2} can be increased is limited. In an otherwise normal individual, hypoventilation cannot raise P_{CO_2} above 60 mm Hg.

In acidosis (increase in $[H^+]$ or P_{CO_2}), secretion of H^+ by the nephron is stimulated, and the entire filtered load of HCO_3^- is reabsorbed. The production and excretion of NH_4^+ are also stimulated, thus increasing net acid excretion by the kidneys (see equation 44-9). The new HCO_3^- generated during the process of net acid excretion is returned to the body, and plasma $[HCO_3^-]$ increases.

In alkalosis (decrease in $[H^+]$ or P_{CO_2}), secretion of H^+ by the nephron is inhibited. As a result, net acid excretion and HCO_3^- reabsorption are reduced. HCO_3^- will appear in the urine, thereby reducing the plasma $[HCO_3^-]$.

> Loss of gastric contents from the body (e.g., during vomiting or nasogastric suction) produces a metabolic alkalosis secondary to the loss of HCl. If the volume of gastric fluid loss is significant, the effective circulating volume (ECV) will also be decreased. Under this condition, the kidneys cannot excrete sufficient quantities of HCO_3^- to compensate for the metabolic alkalosis. HCO_3^- excretion does not occur, because the decreased ECV results in enhanced proximal tubule Na^+ reabsorption and increased levels of aldosterone (see Chapter 42). These responses in turn limit HCO_3^- excretion, because Na^+ reabsorption in the proximal tubule is coupled to H^+ secretion via the Na^+, H^+-ATPase (i.e., HCO_3^- is reabsorbed because of the need to reduce Na^+ excretion). In addition, the elevated aldosterone levels stimulate H^+ secretion by the collecting duct. Thus, individuals who experience significant gastric fluid loss typically have a metabolic alkalosis and a paradoxically acidic urine. Correction of the alkalosis occurs only when the ECV is restored to its normal value. With restoration of ECV, HCO_3^- reabsorption by the proximal tubule will decrease, as will H^+ secretion by the collecting duct. As a result, HCO_3^- excretion will increase and the plasma $[HCO_3^-]$ will return to normal.

■ *Simple Acid-Base Disorders*

Table 44-2 summarizes the primary alterations and the subsequent defense mechanisms for the various simple acid-base disorders. These respiratory and renal defense mechanisms are commonly referred to as **compensatory responses**. Note again that these compensatory mechanisms do not correct the underlying disorder but simply reduce the magnitude of the change in blood pH. Complete recovery from the acid-base disorder requires correction of the underlying cause of the disturbance.

■ *Types of Acid-Base Disorders*

Metabolic acidosis. Metabolic acidosis is characterized by a low plasma $[HCO_3^-]$ and a low plasma pH.

■ **Table 44-2**   Characteristics of simple acid-base disorders

Disorder	Plasma pH	Primary alteration	Defense mechanisms
Metabolic acidosis	↓	↓ plasma $[HCO_3^-]$	ICF and ECF buffers, hyperventilation (↓ Pco_2), ↑ renal NAE excretion
Metabolic alkalosis	↑	↑ plasma $[HCO_3^-]$	ICF and ECF buffers, hypoventilation (↑ Pco_2), ↓ renal NAE excretion
Respiratory acidosis	↓	↑ Pco_2	ICF buffers, ↑ renal NAE excretion
Respiratory alkalosis	↑	↓ Pco_2	ICF buffers, ↓ renal NAE excretion

NAE, Net acid excretion; *ICF,* intracellular fluid; *ECF,* extracellular fluid.

This condition can develop through the addition of non-volatile acid to the body (e.g., in diabetic ketoacidosis), the loss of nonvolatile alkali (e.g., with diarrhea), or the failure of the kidneys to excrete sufficient net acid to replenish the HCO_3^- used to titrate nonvolatile acids (e.g., in renal tubular acidosis or renal failure). As described above, buffering of H^+ occurs in both the ECF and ICF. When pH falls, the respiratory centers are stimulated and the ventilatory rate is increased (respiratory compensation). This increase in respiratory rate reduces Pco_2, which further minimizes the fall in plasma pH. In general, there is a 1.2 mm Hg decrease in Pco_2 for every 1 mEq/L fall in plasma $[HCO_3^-]$. Thus, if plasma $[HCO_3^-]$ were reduced to 14 mEq/L from a normal value of 24 mEq/L, the expected decrease in Pco_2 would be 12 mm Hg, and the measured Pco_2 would be 28 mm Hg (normal Pco_2 = 40 mm Hg).

Finally, renal excretion of net acid is increased. This increased excretion occurs through eliminating all HCO_3^- from the urine (enhanced reabsorption of filtered HCO_3^-) and increasing ammonium excretion (enhanced production of new HCO_3^-). If the process that initiated the acid-base disturbance is corrected, the kidneys' enhanced excretion of acid will ultimately return the pH and $[HCO_3^-]$ to normal. With correction of the pH, the ventilatory rate will also return to normal.

When nonvolatile acid is added to the body fluids, the $[H^+]$ increases (pH decreases) and the $[HCO_3^-]$ decreases. In addition, the concentration of the anion, which is associated with the nonvolatile acid, will increase. This change in the [anion] provides a convenient way to analyze and help determine the cause of a metabolic acidosis, and is known as calculating the anion gap. The **anion gap** represents the difference between the concentration of the major plasma cation (Na^+) and the major plasma anions (Cl^- and HCO_3^-).

$$\text{Anion gap} = [Na^+] - ([Cl^-] + [HCO_3^-]) \quad (44\text{-}12)$$

Under normal conditions, the anion gap is in the range of 8 to 16 mEq/L.* If the anion of the nonvolatile acid is Cl^-, the anion gap will be normal (i.e., the decrease

in $[HCO_3^-]$ is matched by an increase in $[Cl^-]$). The metabolic acidosis associated with diarrhea or renal tubular acidosis has a normal anion gap. In contrast, if the anion of the nonvolatile acid is not Cl^- (e.g., lactate, β-hydroxybutyrate), the anion gap will increase (i.e., the decrease in $[HCO_3^-]$ is not matched by an increase in the $[Cl^-]$, but rather by an increase in the concentration of the unmeasured anion). The anion gap is increased in the metabolic acidosis associated with renal failure, diabetes (ketoacidosis), lactic acidosis, or the ingestion of large quantities of aspirin. Thus, *calculation of the anion gap is a useful way to identify the cause of a metabolic acidosis.*

Metabolic alkalosis. Metabolic alkalosis is characterized by an elevated plasma $[HCO_3^-]$ and an elevated plasma pH. This condition can be caused by the addition of nonvolatile alkali to the body (e.g., ingestion of antacids), as a result of a decreased ECV (e.g., hemorrhage), or more commonly from loss of nonvolatile acid (e.g., loss of gastric HCl with vomiting). Buffering occurs in the ECF and ICF compartments. The increase in pH inhibits the respiratory centers and the ventilatory rate is reduced, thus elevating Pco_2 (respiratory compensation). With appropriate respiratory compensation, Pco_2 increases 0.7 mm Hg for every 1 mEq/L rise in plasma $[HCO_3^-]$.

The renal compensatory response to metabolic alkalosis is to increase the excretion of HCO_3^- by reducing its reabsorption along the nephron. Normally, this response occurs quite rapidly and effectively. However, as already noted, when the alkalosis occurs in the setting of decreased ECV (e.g., vomiting where fluid loss occurs with the H^+ loss), HCO_3^- excretion does not occur. Renal excretion of HCO_3^- will increase, and the alkalosis will be corrected only if volume is restored to normal. Enhanced renal excretion of HCO_3^- will eventually return the pH and $[HCO_3^-]$ to normal, provided that the underlying cause of the initial acid-base disturbance is corrected. With correction of the pH, the ventilatory rate also returns to normal.

Respiratory acidosis. Respiratory acidosis is characterized by elevated Pco_2 and reduced plasma pH. It results from decreased gas exchange across the alveoli, as a result of either inadequate ventilation (e.g., drug-induced depression of the respiratory centers) or impaired gas diffusion (e.g., pulmonary edema, as may occur in cardiovascular disease or lung disease). In contrast to the meta-

---

*An anion gap (i.e., a difference between the concentration of cations and anions) does not actually exist. All cations are balanced by anions. The gap simply reflects the parameters that are measured. In reality:

$[Na^+] + [\text{unmeasured cations}] =$
$\qquad [Cl^-] + [HCO_3^-] + [\text{unmeasured anions}]$

bolic disorders, buffering during respiratory acidosis occurs almost entirely in the intracellular compartment. The increase in P_{CO_2} and decrease in pH stimulate both HCO_3^- reabsorption by the nephron and ammonia excretion (renal compensation). Together, these responses increase net acid excretion and generate new HCO_3^-.

The renal compensatory response takes several days to occur. Consequently, respiratory acid-base disorders are commonly divided into acute and chronic phases. In the acute phase, not enough time has elapsed for the renal compensatory response to occur. And the body relies on intracellular buffering to minimize the change in pH. During this phase, and because of the buffering, plasma $[HCO_3^-]$ increases 1 mEq/L for every 10 mm Hg rise in P_{CO_2}. In the chronic phase, renal compensation occurs, and plasma $[HCO_3^-]$ increases 3.5 mEq/L for each 10 mm Hg rise in P_{CO_2}. Correction of the underlying disorder returns P_{CO_2} to normal, and the renal excretion of acid will decrease to its initial level.

Respiratory alkalosis. Respiratory alkalosis is characterized by reduced P_{CO_2} and elevated plasma pH. It results from increased gas exchange in the lungs, usually due to increased ventilation from stimulation of the respiratory centers (e.g., by drugs or disorders of the central nervous system). Hyperventilation can also occur as a response to anxiety or fear. As noted, buffering is primarily intracellular. In the acute phase of respiratory alkalosis, plasma $[HCO_3^-]$ decreases 2 mEq/L for every 10 mm Hg fall in P_{CO_2}. The elevated pH and reduced P_{CO_2} inhibit HCO_3^- reabsorption by the nephron and reduce ammonia excretion (renal compensation). As a result of these two effects, net acid excretion is reduced. This response takes several days to complete and results in a 5 mEq/L decrease in plasma $[HCO_3^-]$ for every 10 mm Hg reduction in P_{CO_2}. Correction of the underlying disorder will return P_{CO_2} to normal, and renal excretion of acid will increase to its initial level.

■ *Analysis of Acid-Base Disorders*

Analysis of an acid-base disorder is directed at identifying the underlying cause so that appropriate therapy can be initiated. The patient's medical history and associated physical findings often provide valuable clues about the nature and origin of an acid-base disorder. Additionally, analysis of an arterial blood sample is frequently required. Such an analysis is straightforward if approached in a systematic fashion. For example, consider the following data:

$$pH = 7.35$$
$$[HCO_3^-] = 16 \text{ mEq/L}$$
$$P_{CO_2} = 30 \text{ mm Hg}$$

The acid-base disorder represented by these values, or any other set of values, can be determined by the following three-step approach (Fig. 44-6).

1. *Examination of the pH.* By first considering the plasma pH, one can classify the underlying disorder as either an acidosis or an alkalosis. Note that the body's defense mechanisms, by themselves, cannot correct an acid-base disorder. Thus, even if the defense mechanisms are completely operative, the pH still indicates the origin of the initial disorder. In the example shown above, the pH of 7.35 indicates acidosis.

2. *Determination of metabolic vs. respiratory disorder.* Simple acid-base disorders are either metabolic or respiratory. To determine which disorder is present, the $[HCO_3^-]$ and P_{CO_2} must next be examined. As indicated by the Henderson-Hasselbalch equation (see equation 44-6), acidosis could be the result of a decrease in the $[HCO_3^-]$ (metabolic) or an increase in the P_{CO_2} (respiratory). Alternatively, alkalosis could be the result of an increase in the $[HCO_3^-]$ (metabolic) or a decrease in the P_{CO_2} (respiratory). For the above example, the $[HCO_3^-]$ is reduced from normal (normal = 23 to 25 mEq/L), as is the P_{CO_2} (normal = 40 mm Hg). The disorder must therefore be a metabolic acidosis; it cannot be a respiratory acidosis, because the P_{CO_2} is reduced.

3. *Analysis of compensatory response.* Metabolic disorders result in compensatory changes in ventilation and thus in P_{CO_2}, whereas respiratory disorders result in compensatory changes in renal acid excretion and thus in plasma $[HCO_3^-]$. In an appropriately compensated metabolic acidosis, P_{CO_2} will be decreased, whereas it is elevated in a compensated metabolic alkalosis. In respiratory acidosis, complete compensation results in an elevation of $[HCO_3^-]$. Conversely, $[HCO_3^-]$ is reduced in response to respiratory alkalosis. In the above example, P_{CO_2} is reduced from normal, and the magnitude of this reduction (10 mm Hg decrease in P_{CO_2} for an 8 mEq/L increase in $[HCO_3^-]$) is as expected. Therefore, the acid-base disorder is a simple metabolic acidosis with appropriate respiratory compensation.

If the appropriate compensatory response is not present, a mixed disorder should be suspected. A **mixed acid-base disorder** reflects the presence of two or more underlying causes of the acid-base disturbance. A mixed disorder should be suspected when analysis of the arterial blood gas indicates that appropriate compensation has not occurred. For example, consider the following data:

$$pH = 6.96$$
$$[HCO_3^-] = 12 \text{ mEq/L}$$
$$P_{CO_2} = 55 \text{ mm Hg}$$

Following the three-step approach outlined above, it is evident that the disturbance is an acidosis that has both a metabolic component ($[HCO_3^-] < 24$ mEq/L) and a respiratory component ($P_{CO_2} > 40$ mm Hg). Thus, this disorder is mixed. An example of such a disorder is seen in

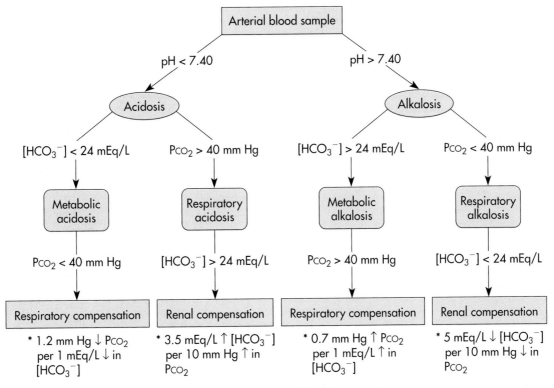

■ Fig. 44-6 An approach to the analysis of simple acid-base disorders.

an individual with a history of chronic pulmonary disease (e.g., emphysema with respiratory acidosis), who develops an acute gastrointestinal illness with diarrhea. Because diarrhea fluid contains HCO_3^-, its loss from the body results in the development of a metabolic acidosis.

A mixed acid-base disorder is also indicated in a patient who has abnormal P_{CO_2} and plasma $[HCO_3^-]$ but in whom the plasma pH is normal. Such a situation can be seen in a patient who has ingested a large quantity of aspirin. The salicylic acid (the active ingredient in aspirin) produces a metabolic acidosis, and at the same time stimulates the respiratory centers, causing hyperventilation and a respiratory alkalosis. Thus, the patient has a reduced plasma $[HCO_3^-]$ and a reduced P_{CO_2}.

■ Summary

1. The pH of the body fluid is maintained within a narrow range by the coordinated function of the lungs, liver, and kidneys. The amount of volatile (CO_2-derived) and nonvolatile acids produced by metabolism, together with any acid or alkali ingested in the diet, must be excreted for acid-base balance to be maintained.

2. The lungs are the excretory route for volatile acids, whereas the kidneys are the route for excretion of nonvolatile acids.

3. The body uses buffer systems to minimize changes in body fluid pH. The CO_2/HCO_3^- buffer system of the ECF is the most important because it is regulated by both the lungs and the kidneys.

4. The kidneys maintain acid-base balance by excreting an amount of acid equal to the amount of nonvolatile acid produced by cellular metabolism and metabolism of food. The kidneys also prevent the loss of HCO_3^- in the urine by reabsorbing virtually all the HCO_3^- that is filtered at the glomerulus. Both the reabsorption of filtered HCO_3^- and the excretion of acid are accomplished by secretion of H^+ by the nephrons.

5. Urinary buffers are necessary for effective excretion of acid, because the minimum pH of the urine is only 4.0 to 4.5. Phosphate is the primary urinary buffer. The production (glutamine metabolism) and excretion of ammonium are critical to the generation of new HCO_3^- by the kidneys. Ammonium production by the kidneys and its subsequent excretion are regulated in response to acid-base disturbances.

6. Respiratory acid-base disorders result from primary alterations in the blood P_{CO_2}. Elevation of P_{CO_2} produces acidosis, and the kidneys respond by increasing excretion of acid. Conversely, reduction of P_{CO_2} produces alkalosis, and renal acid excretion is reduced. The kidneys respond to respiratory acid-base disorders over several hours to days.

7. Metabolic acid-base disorders result from primary alterations in the plasma $[HCO_3^-]$, which in turn result from addition of acid to, or loss of alkali from, the body. In response to metabolic acidosis, pulmonary ventilation is increased, which decreases the P_{CO_2}. An increase in the $[HCO_3^-]$ causes alkalosis. Alkalosis decreases pulmonary ventilation, which elevates the P_{CO_2}. The pulmonary response to metabolic acid-base disorders occurs in a matter of minutes.

■ Self-Study Problems

1. If there were no urinary buffers, how much urine (L/day) would the kidneys have to produce to excrete net acid equal to the amount of nonvolatile acid produced from metabolism? Assume that nonvolatile acid production is 70 mEq/day and the minimum urine pH is 4.0.

2. In the following table, indicate the simple acid-base disorder that exists for the laboratory data given. Use as normal values: pH = 7.40; $[HCO_3^-]$ = 24 mEq/L; and P_{CO_2} = 40 mm Hg.

pH	[HCO_3^-] mEq/L	Pco_2 mm Hg	Disorder
7.34	15	29	_____
7.49	35	48	_____
7.47	14	20	_____
7.34	31	60	_____
7.26	26	60	_____
7.62	20	20	_____
7.09	15	50	_____
7.40	15	25	_____

3. What effect would administration of a drug that inhibits carbonic anhydrase be expected to have on urinary HCO_3^- excretion, and by what mechanism? What type of acid-base disorder could result from the use of this drug?

4. A previously healthy individual develops a gastrointestinal illness with nausea and vomiting. After 12 hours of this illness, the following laboratory data are obtained:

Body weight:	70 kg
Blood pressure:	120/80 mm Hg
Plasma pH:	7.48
Pco_2:	44 mm Hg
Plasma [HCO_3^-]:	32 mEq/L
Urine pH:	7.5

What is the acid-base disorder of this individual? What was its origin?

The illness continues, and 48 hours later the following laboratory data are obtained:

Body weight:	68 kg
Blood pressure:	80/40 mm Hg

Plasma pH:	7.50
Pco_2:	48 mm Hg
Plasma [HCO_3^-]:	36 mEq/L
Urine pH:	6.0

Has the acid-base disturbance changed? How do you explain the paradoxical decrease in urine pH?

■ Bibliography

Journal articles

Alpern R et al: Renal proximal tubule response to acid, *News Physiol Sci* 10:77, 1995.

Capasso G et al: Acidification in mammalian cortical distal tubule, *Kidney Int* 45:1543, 1994.

Gluck S et al: Physiology and biochemistry of the kidney vacuolar H+-ATPase, *Annu Rev Physiol* 58:427, 1996.

Hamm LL, Hering-Smith KS: Acid-base transport in the collecting duct, *Semin Nephrol* 13:246, 1993.

Lemann J, Lennon EJ: Role of diet, gastrointestinal tract and bone in acid-base homeostasis, *Kidney Int* 1:275, 1994.

Smulder YM et al: Renal tubular acidosis, pathophysiology and diagnosis, *Arch Intern Med* 156:1629, 1996.

Wingo C et al: Function and structure of H-K-ATPase in the kidney, *Am J Physiol* 269:F1, 1995.

Books and monographs

Alpern RJ, Emmett M, Seldin DW: *Metabolic alkalosis*. In Seldin DW, Giebisch G, editors: *The kidney: physiology and pathophysiology*, ed 2, New York, 1992, Raven Press.

Alpern RJ, Rector FC Jr: *Renal acidification mechanisms*. In Brenner BM, editor: *The kidney*, ed 5, Philadelphia, 1996, WB Saunders.

DuBose TD Jr, Cogan MG, Rector FC Jr: *Acid-base disorders*. In Brenner BM, editor: *The kidney*, ed 5, Philadelphia, 1996, WB Saunders.

Emmett M, Alpern RJ, Seldin DW: *Metabolic acidosis*. In Seldin DW, Giebisch G, editors: *The kidney: physiology and pathophysiology*, ed 2, New York, 1992, Raven Press.

Flessner MF, Knepper MA: *Renal acid-base transport*. In Seldin DW, Giebisch G, editors: *The kidney: physiology and pathophysiology*, ed 2, New York, 1992, Raven Press.

Halperin ML et al: *Biochemistry and physiology of ammonium excretion*. In Seldin DW, Giebisch G, editors: *The kidney: physiology and pathophysiology*, ed 2, New York, 1992, Raven Press.

Hamm LL, Alpern RJ: *Cellular mechanisms of renal tubular acidification*. In Seldin DW, Giebisch G, editors: *The kidney: physiology and pathophysiology*, ed 2, New York, 1992, Raven Press.

Madias NE, Cohen JJ: *Respiratory alkalosis and acidosis*. In Seldin DW, Giebisch G, editors: *The kidney: physiology and pathophysiology*, ed 2, New York, 1992, Raven Press.

Rose BD, Rennke HG: *Acid-base physiology and metabolic alkalosis*. In Rose BD, Rennke HG: *Renal pathophysiology—the essentials*, Baltimore, 1994, Williams & Wilkins.

Rose BD, Rennke HG: *Metabolic acidosis*. In Rose BD, Rennke HG: *Renal pathophysiology—the essentials*, Baltimore, 1994, Williams & Wilkins.

Seldin DW, Giebisch G, editors: *The regulation of acid-base balance*, New York, 1990, Raven Press.

THE ENDOCRINE SYSTEM

Saul M. Genuth

General Principles of Endocrine Physiology

Endocrinology was once classically defined as a discipline concerned with the "internal secretions of the body." The original concept of the endocrine system held that hormones, which are chemical substances liberated by specific types of cells, are carried by the bloodstream to act on distant target cells. This concept represented a major advance in physiological understanding. It suggested a basic mechanism for maintaining the stability of the internal milieu of the cells in the face of irregular nutrient, mineral, and water fluxes and of physical alterations in the body's environment. It also suggested that secretion of a hormone was evoked by a specific change in that milieu. As a result of the hormone's subsequent action on its target cells, the change was counteracted, and chemical or physical **homeostasis** (the desired status quo) was restored. However, from this basic homeostatic notion has grown an increasingly complex picture of the mission and concept of the endocrine system. The mission includes regulation of cellular proliferation and differentiation, growth and body maturation, body mass and its components, reproduction, senescence, and behavior.

A diversity of "classic" endocrine cell types (pituitary, thyroid, adrenal, gonadal, parathyroid, pancreatic islet) have been found and their locations, glandular organization, and molecular species of hormones have been identified. Originally, nonendocrine cell types have also been discovered to produce and secrete substances that act upon other cells. These cells include renal cells (erythropoietin); cardiac atrial and ventricular cells (atrial natriuretic hormones); endothelial cells (endothelin, nitric oxide); various lymphocytes, monocytes, and macrophages (interleukins, interferons); platelets and mesenchymal cells (growth factors, annexins, integrins); adipose cells (leptin); and placental cells (practically all known hormones). Thus, the number and molecular variety of hormones have multiplied, and the basic premise of endocrinology has been adapted to many other disciplines.

Target cells of hormone action are also diverse and include other hormone-producing cells. Some hormones require chemical modification at intermediate sites between the gland or cell of origin and the target cells before their mission can be accomplished. A complementary group of target cell substances—hormone receptors—also play an essential role in mediating hormone action. In addition, the activation of these receptors evokes responses that involve multiple intracellular mechanisms.

Much of the control of hormone secretion depends on the feedback principle described below. Moreover, important functional interrelationships among the endocrine, neural, and immune systems have been identified. Because of the complexity and diversity of the components of the endocrine system, students may be overwhelmed unless they can relate the functional characteristics of each component to a set of unifying principles. The major purpose of this chapter is to provide such a framework for the subsequent chapters of this book.

■ *Relationship between Endocrine and Neural Physiology*

In a conceptual sense, the nervous system and the endocrine system have important functional similarities. Each is basically a system for signaling. Each operates in a stimulus-response manner. Each transmits signals that in some cases are highly localized, narrow, and unitary in purpose and in other cases are widespread, broad, and diverse in purpose. Each system is crucial to the cooperative physiological functioning of the highly differentiated cells, tissues, and organs that make up the human organism. Therefore, *the nervous system and the endocrine system together integrate incoming stimuli in order to integrate the organism's response to changes in its external and internal environment*. Recent advances in immunohistochemistry, cellular physiology, and molecular biology reveal increasingly intimate relationships between neural function and hormone secretion. As a result of this research, the very distinction between a hormone and a neurotransmitter has become blurred. Indeed, a circulating hormone might be characterized as a signal molecule freed from the confines of an axon to reach all responsive cells, or a neurotransmitter might be characterized as a signal molecule captured from the circulation to provide a restricted chemical connection between two distant cells.

This close relationship between the nervous and endocrine systems is illustrated by several common characteristics:

1. Neurons and endocrine cells can secrete into the bloodstream.
2. Endocrine cells and neurons generate electrical potentials and can be depolarized.
3. Peptides originally discovered as products of endocrine cells have neurotransmitter functions also. Likewise, molecules nominally considered to be neurotransmitters can act as hormones.
4. A single cell can produce both biogenic amine neurotransmitters and peptide hormone molecules.
5. A single gene can be transcribed and translated to yield either a peptide neurotransmitter or a peptide hormone, or both.

Two examples illustrate the coordinated function of the endocrine and nervous systems. The first example concerns regulation of plasma glucose levels. A fall in the plasma glucose to a dangerously low level is sensed in the brain and liver. The sympathetic nervous system; neurohormones from the hypothalamus; and hormones from the anterior pituitary gland, adrenal cortex, adrenal medulla, and pancreatic islets all act on target cells in liver, muscle, and adipose tissue to restore plasma glucose to normal. The second example concerns regulation of blood volume. A significant decrease in the circulating blood volume is sensed by baroreceptors, the cardiac atria, the kidney, and the brain. The sympathetic nervous system; a neurohormone from the posterior pituitary gland; and hormones from the cardiac atria, adrenal medulla, adrenal cortex, and kidney act on target cells in blood vessels and kidney to restore blood volume.

Confirmation of a close relationship between the endocrine and immune systems is also emerging. Immune cells secrete **cytokines,** and these molecules act on target cells through mechanisms analogous to those of hormones. Endocrine cells may themselves be targets of these cytokines; these interactions are used to coordinate immune responses and endocrine responses to a stimulus or to reinforce hormonal actions. In addition, a number of classic hormones are present in, and are likely synthesized by, immune cells. Hormones from this source may act in a local fashion, even on their cells of origin.

The spectrum of hormonal signaling encompasses endocrine, neurocrine, paracrine, and autocrine effects (Fig. 45-1). **Endocrine** function is transmission of a molecular signal from a classic endocrine cell through the bloodstream to a distant target cell. **Neurocrine** function is

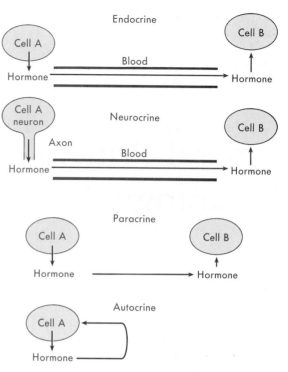

■ **Fig. 45-1** Schematic representation of mechanisms for cell-to-cell signaling via hormone molecules. In *endocrine function,* the signal is carried to a distant target via the bloodstream. In *neurocrine function,* the hormone signal originates in a neuron, and after axonal transport to the bloodstream it is carried to a distant target cell. In *paracrine function,* the hormone signal is carried to an adjacent target cell over short distances via the interstitial fluid. In *autocrine function,* the hormone signal acts back on the cell of origin or adjacent identical cells.

transmission of a molecular signal from a neuron down its axon and then into the bloodstream to a distant target cell. **Paracrine** function is transmission of a molecular signal from one cell type to a neighboring different cell type by diffusion through intercellular fluid channels or gap junctions. **Autocrine** function is transmission of a molecular signal through the intercellular fluid or gap junctions to neighboring identical cells or back to the cell of origin.

According to the route by which it is transmitted, the same messenger molecule may function as an endocrine hormone (bloodstream conveyance), as a neurotransmitter (axonal conveyance), as a neurohormone (combined axonal and bloodstream conveyance), or as a paracrine or autocrine hormone (local conveyance). The effect produced by the signaling molecule then depends on the target cell and the intracellular mechanisms that are activated. For example, a hypothalamic cell (see Chapter 49) may secrete the neurohormone **somatostatin** into blood, which reaches the pituitary gland and inhibits the release of growth hormone from that gland. A brain cell may transmit somatostatin to a second brain cell in order to alter behavior. Finally, a cell in the pancreatic islets may release somatostatin into the fluid bathing adjacent cells and inhibit their release of insulin (see Chapter 47).

The close relationship between the neural and endocrine systems is well illustrated by some endocrine diseases. For example, in families with the **multiple endocrine adenoma syndrome type 2,** neoplasms of the parathyroid glands that secrete parathyroid hormone and cause hypercalcemia, and neoplasms of the adrenal medulla (a sympathetic nervous system component) that secrete norepinephrine and cause hypertension, coexist in the same individual. In other instances, a single bronchial neoplasm may secrete the neurotransmitter serotonin and the pituitary hormone adrenocorticotropin. These substances cause vascular flushes and a syndrome of cortisol excess, respectively, in affected individuals.

■ *Types of Hormones*

Hormone molecules fall into three general chemical classes. The **amines**—thyroid hormones and catecholamines—originate from the amino acid tyrosine and retain the aliphatic α-amino group. Introduction of a second hydroxyl group in the benzene ring is characteristic of the catecholamines, whereas iodination of the benzene ring distinguishes thyroid hormone. The second group of hormones is composed of **proteins** and **peptides.** In some instances, protein hormones with similar structures but different missions have originated from a common ancestral gene during evolution. In other instances, a single progenitor protein gives rise to several hormone "offspring" of different sizes, some with differing and some with overlapping actions. The third chemical group of hormones consists of the **steroids,** which include adrenocortical and reproductive gland hormones and the active metabolites of vitamin D. Cholesterol is the common precursor in this class. Modification of side chains, hydroxylation at various sites, and ring aromatization confer individual biological activities on various members of this group.

■ *Hormone Synthesis*

■ *Protein or Peptide Hormone Synthesis*

Protein or peptide hormones are synthesized on the rough endoplasmic reticulum in the same way as other proteins. The appropriate amino acid sequence is dictated by a specific messenger RNA that results from transcription of the hormone gene. In general, a single gene determines the structure and synthesis of a single protein or peptide hormone. However, multiple genes containing the same sequence or slightly different sequences that direct synthesis of a single peptide hormone in different cells have also been described. Alternatively, a single gene may give rise to more than one primary RNA message by inclusion or exclusion of particular exons during gene processing.

Thus, one gene may direct the synthesis of different peptides in various cells.

The DNA molecules for protein hormones are now readily cloned and structured, allowing the structure of the primary gene product to be deduced. This research has led, in some cases, to the discovery of previously unknown additional peptide products whose function remains to be ascertained. Recombinant DNA technology also facilitates synthesis of authentic human protein hormones such as insulin and growth hormone for therapeutic purposes.

The process of peptide hormone synthesis is illustrated in Fig. 45-2. Translation of messenger RNA begins with an N-terminal signal peptide sequence. Translation then temporarily ceases while this signal peptide attaches the messenger RNA to the endoplasmic reticulum receptors via "docking proteins." Translation then resumes until the entire encoded peptide sequence, known at this stage as a **preprohormone,** is formed. The signal peptide is then cleaved, resulting in a **prohormone,** which is simultaneously directed into the cisternal space for transport to the Golgi apparatus. Along with the hormone, the prohormone contains other peptide sequences, some of which may function to ensure proper folding of the hormone peptide chain that permits it to form intramolecular linkages. Other peptide sequences within the prohormone may have related or independent functions and may be cosecreted with the hormone. Within the Golgi apparatus, the prohormone is packaged for storage in **secretory granules.** These granules may contain proteolytic enzymes necessary for subsequent conversion of the prohormone to the hormone or for elimination of copeptides. Golgi processing of prohormones to hormones may also involve glycosylation and phosphorylation. In addition, many secretory granules of peptide hormones contain a soluble acidic protein of unknown function called **chromogranin.**

■ *Amino and Steroid Hormone Synthesis*

The amine hormones are synthesized from tyrosine, whereas the steroid hormones and vitamin D are synthesized from cholesterol. Each type requires a sequential series of discrete enzymatic reactions. Further alterations that increase or modify the biological activity of these hormones may occur outside the gland of origin. This multiplicity of distinctive steps means that a variety of defects in hormone generation can and do arise. These defects can result from single gene–single enzyme mutations or from selective drug-induced enzyme inhibition.

Genetic diseases involving deficient or abnormal synthesis of peptide or protein hormones (e.g., insulin) usually involve the hormone gene itself. Single amino acid substitutions or deletions can give rise to a mutant gene, which may express a product that cannot be

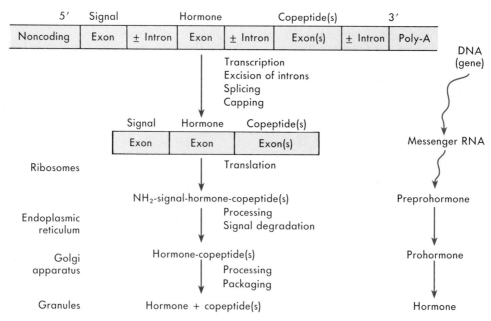

■ Fig. 45-2 Schematic representation of peptide hormone synthesis. In the nucleus, the primary gene transcript undergoes excision of introns, splicing of the exons, capping of the 5′ end, and addition of poly-A at the 3′ end. The resultant mature messenger RNA enters the cytoplasm, where it directs the synthesis of a preprohormone peptide sequence on ribosomes. In this process the N-terminal signal is removed, and the resultant prohormone is transferred vectorially into the endoplasmic reticulum. The prohormone undergoes further processing and packaging in the Golgi apparatus. After final cleavage of the prohormone within the granules, they contain the hormone and copeptides ready for secretion by exocytosis.

processed or secreted normally or that has reduced biological activity. In the case of thyroid or steroid hormones or vitamin D, the product of the mutant gene is usually an enzyme that catalyzes one of the reactions in the biosynthetic sequence for the affected hormone. The resultant clinical state may reflect both the deficiency of the hormone product (e.g., cortisol) and excess accumulation of a precursor that leads to overproduction of another product (e.g., an androgen).

■ *Hormone Release*

■ *Release of Protein and Catecholamine Hormones*

Both protein and catecholamine hormones are stored in secretory granules. These hormones are released from the granules by **exocytosis** (Fig. 45-3). The extracellular stimulus to secretion is usually followed by an immediate rise in the concentration of cytosolic calcium, which is first mobilized from intracellular bound stores and then taken up from extracellular fluid through plasma membrane channels. This increase in the intracellular Ca^{++} concentration initiates movement of secretory vesicle organelles to appropriate sites in the plasma membrane, a process facilitated by specific vesicle-associated proteins, a **guanosine triphosphate (GTP)**–binding protein, and microtubule and microfilament elements. A sec-

ondary rise in **cyclic adenosine monophosphate (cAMP)** often follows. After fusion of the granule and plasma membranes, gap junctions and small pores form, and the hormone is released into the extracellular fluid along with copeptides, cleavage enzymes, chromogranin, and any other granule contents. The membrane material from the empty core may then be reprocessed. In addition to this stimulated release of protein hormones from storage granules by exocytosis, a low, direct, basal rate of *constitutive* secretion of newly synthesized prohormones, partially processed prohormones, or the hormones themselves can also occur.

■ *Release of Thyroid and Steroid Hormones*

Thyroid and steroid hormones are not stored within discrete granules, although the hormones may be compartmentalized in the cell. Once the hormones have appeared in free form within the cytoplasm, they apparently leave the cell by simple transfer through the plasma membrane.

■ *Other Forms of Hormone Release*

These modes of hormone synthesis and release are essentially unicellular. However, more complicated patterns of hormone production also occur. Two adjacent cell types in a single gland may interact so that hormone A from

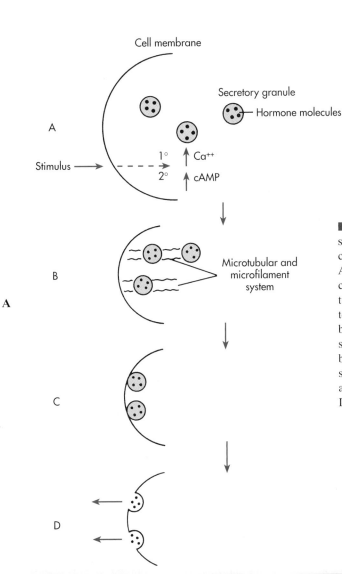

Cell membrane

Secretory granule

Hormone molecules

A

Stimulus →

1° ↑ Ca⁺⁺
2° ↑ cAMP

B — Microtubular and microfilament system

C

D

A

■ **Fig. 45-3** **A,** Secretion of peptide hormones via exocytosis is initiated *(A)* by application of a stimulus that raises intracellular Ca⁺⁺ levels and also usually raises cytosolic cyclic AMP (cAMP). The secretory granules are lined up and translocated to the plasma membrane *(B)* via activation of a microtubular and microfilament system. The membrane of the secretory granule fuses with that of the cell *(C)*. The common membrane is lysed *(D)*, releasing the hormone into the interstitial space. **B,** Insulin secretory granules in a β cell being stimulated by glucose. The arrow indicates a granule undergoing exocytosis. (From Lacy PE: Beta cell secretion—from the standpoint of a pathobiologist, *Diabetes* 19:895, 1970. From the American Diabetes Association.)

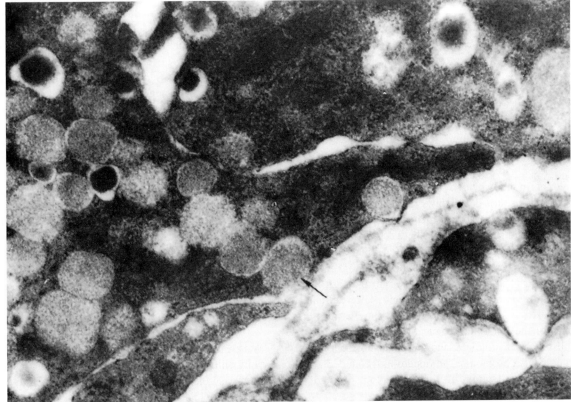

B

cell A is modified in cell B to produce hormone B, a hormone with an entirely different spectrum of biological effects. For example, estrogens (hormone B) are produced from androgens (hormone A) in the ovaries. Peripheral tissues, such as adipose tissue, that are ordinarily considered to be nonendocrine may also carry out similar conversions.

A second mode of hormone production involves modification of a precursor molecule of low activity to one of higher activity by successive steps that take place in several different tissues. For example, a sterol synthesized in the skin requires actions by the liver and kidney to produce the most potent vitamin D hormone.

In yet a third mode of hormone production, peptide hormones can even be produced in the circulation itself from a protein precursor. A prototype for this pattern is the synthesis of angiotensin—a peptide hormone—from a protein secreted by the liver and acted on sequentially by enzymes released from the kidney and the lung.

■ *Regulation of Hormone Secretion*

Some of the general mechanisms that govern the secretion of hormones are summarized as follows:

Feedback control

Hormone-hormone
Substrate-hormone
Mineral-hormone

Neural control	*Chronotropic control*
Adrenergic	Oscillating
Cholinergic	Pulsatile
Dopaminergic	Diurnal rhythm
Serotoninergic	Sleep-wake cycle
Endorphinergic-	Menstrual rhythm
enkephalinergic	Seasonal rhythm
Gabaergic	Developmental rhythm

The feedback principle is universally operative in the control of hormone secretion. *Negative feedback, which is most common, acts to limit the excursions in output of each partner in the pair* (Fig. 45-4). In the simplest example, hormone A, which stimulates secretion of hormone B, will in turn be inhibited by an excess of hormone B. This straightforward mechanism characterizes the usual relationship that exists between hormones of the pituitary gland and their target glands. Secretion of a hormone that either accelerates the production or retards the utilization of a particular substrate will increase the concentration of the substrate in plasma. The resultant circulating excess of that substrate will inhibit further secretion of the hormone, while a circulating deficit of that substrate will stimulate secretion of the hormone. On the other hand, a hormone that impedes the production or accelerates the utilization of a particular substrate will decrease the plasma concentration of the substrate. Secretion of such a hormone will be stimulated by a circulating excess but inhibited by a circulating deficit of the substrate.

Positive feedback, which is less common, *acts to amplify the initial biological effect of the hormone.* Thus, hormone A, which stimulates secretion of hormone B, may in turn be initially stimulated to greater secretion rates by hormone B, but only through a limited dose-response range. Once sufficient biological momentum for secretion of hormone B is reached, other influences, including negative feedback, will reduce the response of hormone A to fit the final biological purpose.

Neural control acts to evoke or suppress hormone secretion in response to both external and internal stimuli. Hormone secretion may arise from visual, auditory, olfactory, gustatory, tactile, or pressure stimuli and may be perceived consciously or unconsciously. Pain, emotion, sexual excitement, fright, injury, stress, and changes in blood volume can all modulate hormone secretion through neural mechanisms. Examples include the release of **oxytocin,** which fills the milk ducts in response to the stimulus of suckling, or the release of **aldosterone,** which augments the circulatory volume in response to upright posture.

Many hormones are secreted in distinct pulses. Furthermore, certain patterns of hormone secretion are dictated by rhythms that may be genetically encoded or acquired. Circadian or daily rhythms can be demonstrated even within certain individual cells in culture. For example, pineal gland cells show regular and coordinated 24-hour variation in synthesis of the hormone **melatonin,** in the enzyme *N*-acetyltransferase necessary for melatonin synthesis, and in the stimulatory molecule cAMP. A similar intrinsic 24-hour cycle can be demonstrated for a number of whole organism endocrine and neural physiological processes, even in a timeless environment lacking day or night. The suprachiasmatic nucleus of the hypothalamus is the center for intrinsic oscillations or cycles; that is, it is the circadian clock. This clock coordinates endocrine rhythms with metabolic and behavioral rhythms (e.g., food seeking). The intrinsic 24-hour cycle is entrained with the light-dark, day-night cycle of the physical environment by direct and indirect input from the retina (Fig. 45-5). Modifications of the intrinsic cycle occur via light signals from the retina as well as signals from the thalamus, midbrain, hippocampus, and pineal gland. Endocrine and related rhythms are also affected by the sleep-wake cycle via the circadian clock. In addition, input from the reticular activating substance and sleep centers to hypothalamic neurons that govern specific pituitary hormones (see Chapter 49) mediates sleep-wake effects independently from the circadian clock.

When the circadian clock is altered, the secretion of various hormones is also altered. For example, in jet lag, a sudden artificial shift in clock time abruptly

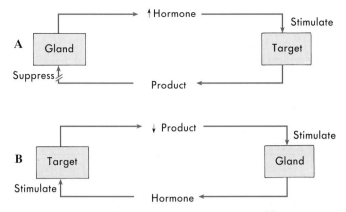

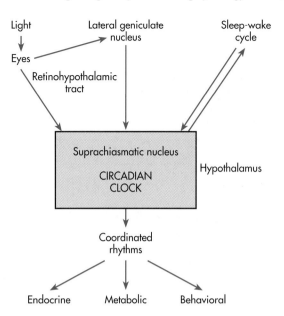

■ **Fig. 45-4** Negative feedback principle. **A,** A primary increase in hormone secretion stimulates a greater output of product from the target cell. The product then feeds back on the gland to suppress further hormone secretion. In this fashion, hormone excess is limited or prevented. **B,** A primary decrease in output of product from the target cell stimulates the gland to secrete hormone. The hormone then stimulates a greater output of product from the target cell. In this fashion, the product deficiency is limited or corrected.

alters day-night and sleep-wake entrained cycles of secretion of a variety of hormones, including melatonin and cortisol. Re-establishment of normal cycles cued by the new clock time reflects entrainment of the circadian clock to an altered environment and often requires several days. An important clinical example occurs when major medical or surgical stress overrides the circadian clock and causes a pattern of hormonal release and metabolism that stimulates mobilization of endogenous fuels, such as glucose or free fatty acids, and augments their delivery to critical organs. In contrast, growth and reproductive processes are suppressed (see Chapter 51).

Seasonal variation in hormone secretion also occurs, which may reflect the influence of temperature, tides, and variations in the length of daylight on the rhythm of the circadian clock. Some of these rhythms appear atavistic in humans and have probably served to fulfill biological needs of evolutionary ancestors. Perhaps the most intriguing of all are those patterns of hormone secretion that coincide with and are unique to developmental stages, such as the onset of puberty. A diverse and still growing number of neurotransmitter molecules carries these signals to the endocrine cells.

■ *Hormone Action*

Three major sequential steps are involved in eliciting the response of a target cell to a hormonal stimulus:

1. The hormone must be recognized and bound by a specific receptor on the surface or within the target cell.

■ **Fig. 45-5** The origin of circadian rhythms in endocrine gland secretion, metabolic processes, and behavioral activity. A clock with an intrinsic 24- to 25-hour cycle is located in the suprachiasmatic nucleus of the hypothalamus. This free-running clock is entrained by environmental light signals to the external 24-hour day. It is also influenced by, and in turn can influence, the sleep-wake cycle, which also has independent effects on hormone secretion. (Modified from Turek FW: Circadian rhythms, *Recent Prog Horm Res* 49:43-90, 1994, with permission of Academic Press.)

2. The hormone receptor complex must then be coupled to a signal-generating mechanism in the target cell or act as one itself.
3. The generated signal (second messenger) then changes intracellular processes quantitatively by altering the activity or concentration of enzymes, other functional proteins, and structural proteins (Fig. 45-6).

There are two basic schemes for accomplishing these steps. The first is mainly employed by peptide/protein and catecholamine hormones. The receptor for the hormone and the signal-generating system is located within or immediately adjacent to the plasma membrane of the cell. In this case, the essential information for triggering the response actually lies in the receptor molecule. By occupying the receptor, the hormone changes the receptor's conformation and allows transmission of the information that the receptor contains. Thus, the hormone in this scheme is primarily only an extracellular signal. This type of hormone response is elicited within seconds to minutes. In the second scheme, which is employed mainly by steroid and thyroid hormones, the hormone must enter the cell, occupy the receptor, and in combination with the receptor, interact with DNA molecules in the nucleus to generate a message. In this situation, the DNA molecules act as second messengers, and the essential information for triggering a response lies in the hor-

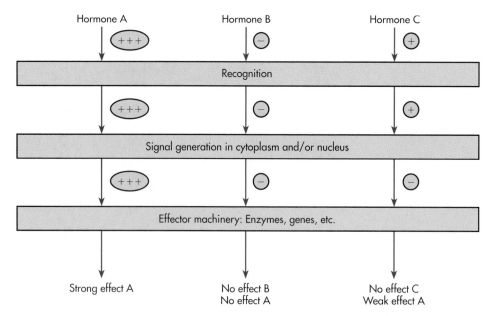

■ **Fig. 45-6**   Hormone-cell interaction. Hormone A is recognized by this cell through binding with its specific receptor. An intracellular signal is generated that stimulates the appropriate enzymatic machinery, and effect A is produced. Hormone B is not recognized because the cell lacks a receptor for it. Thus, hormone B cannot produce effect A in this cell even though it might operate through an identical enzymatic machinery in its own target cell. Hormone C may be slightly recognized by this cell through individual overlap with the receptor to hormone A. Although a weak intracellular signal may be generated, no effect of C results because the cell lacks the appropriate enzymatic machinery. To a minor extent, however, hormone C may produce effect A.

mone and the receptor, coupled together. Thus, the hormone is a true intracellular signal. This type of hormonal action requires minutes to hours, or even days, for its full expression.

■ *Receptor Kinetics*

A given hormone may act through somewhat different receptor molecules in different target cells. However, multiple actions of a given hormone in the same target cell are usually initiated by binding to a sole receptor molecule. The large number of receptor molecules per cell often guarantees that receptor availability will not be rate limiting for hormone action.

Receptors are protein molecules that associate with their cognate hormones in reversible reactions that appear to obey the following molecular chemical kinetics:

$$H + R = HR \qquad (45\text{-}1)$$

$$K_{assoc} = \frac{HR}{[H]\,[R]} \qquad (45\text{-}2)$$

$$\frac{[HR]}{[H]} = K_{assoc} \times [R] \qquad (45\text{-}3)$$

where

H = free hormone in solution
R = unoccupied receptor

HR = bound hormone = occupied receptor
R_0 = initial receptor capacity = [R] + [HR]
K_{assoc} = affinity constant

If a constant amount of receptor is incubated in vitro with increasing concentrations of hormone, the amount of bound hormone increases until receptor occupancy reaches 100%. At this point, the number of bound hormone molecules equals the total number of originally available receptor molecules, that is, the initial receptor capacity (R_0). At the same time, as the free hormone concentration approaches infinity and the receptor occupancy approaches 100%, the ratio of bound hormone to free hormone progressively decreases and approaches zero. That is, as

$$[H] \rightarrow \text{Infinity}$$

$$[HR] \rightarrow R_0 \qquad (45\text{-}4)$$

$$\frac{[HR]}{[H]} \rightarrow 0$$

The data obtained by incubating receptors with increasing amounts of hormone can be plotted in a meaningful way by simple substitution in equation 45-3. Since

$$[R] = R_0 - [HR]$$

$$\frac{[HR]}{[H]} = K_{assoc} \times (R_0 - [HR]) \qquad (45\text{-}5)$$

$$\frac{[HR]}{[H]} = K_{assoc} \, [HR] + K_{assoc} \, R_0 \qquad (45\text{-}6)$$

$$\frac{\text{Bound hormone}}{\text{Free hormone}} = K_{assoc} \times \text{Bound hormone} + K_{assoc} \times \text{Receptor capacity}$$

Plotting the ratio of bound hormone to free hormone as a function of bound hormone theoretically yields a straight line (Fig. 45-7, *B*). This is called a **Scatchard plot.** The slope of the line equals the negative of the association constant (K_{assoc}), and the x intercept equals R_0 (the receptor capacity).

In reality, many Scatchard plots of hormone binding to receptor yield exponential curves (Fig. 45-7, *B*). Such a curve suggests that hormone occupancy of a relatively small number of receptors decreases the affinity of nearby unoccupied receptor molecules for the hormone. However, in many instances, occupancy of only 5% to 10% of the total available receptor molecules is enough to yield full (i.e., maximal) biological action of the hormone. In these cases, therefore, the declining affinity of receptor for hormone does not impede hormone action quantitatively, but it may reduce the duration of hormone effect or protect the cell from a sudden massive excess of hormone.

Regulation of its hormone receptor provides another mechanism for regulating hormone action. Rearrangement of equation 45-5 to provide an expression for HR yields

$$[HR] = R_0 \times \frac{K_{assoc} \, [H]}{K_{assoc} \, [H] + I} \qquad (45\text{-}7)$$

Thus, HR is directly proportional to R_0, the initial receptor number. An increase in receptor number (R_0) raises the maximal [HR] obtainable at saturating concentrations of hormone. Thus, increasing the number of receptors would raise the maximal responsiveness of the cell for those hormone effects in which receptor binding, rather than a later step in hormone action, is rate limiting. This is generally the case for steroid and thyroid hormones. At submaximal hormone concentrations, the increase in [HR] produced by an increase in R_0 would enhance the sensitivity of the cell. This is commonly seen with peptide hormones.

Receptor capacity is often regulated by the level of its specific hormone. In many instances, the regulation is inverse; that is, a sustained excess of hormone decreases the number of its receptors per cell. This process, which is called **down-regulation,** acts to lessen the effect of chronic exposure to excess hormone. However, in some instances, intermittent exposure of the target cells to low concentrations of the hormone creates a direct relationship; that is, the hormone appears to recruit its own receptors. This process, which is called **up-regulation,** amplifies the cell's response to the hormone. An increase in receptor affinity (K_{assoc}) will also increase [HR] and the sensitivity of the cell to hormone stimulation. Affinity can be altered by phosphorylation of the receptor and by

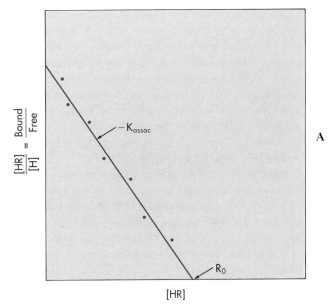

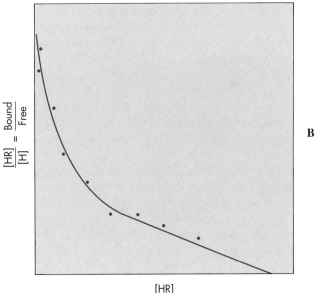

■ **Fig. 45-7** Scatchard plot. **A,** A linear plot results when the hormone reacts with a single receptor class and no cooperativity is present. The negative of the association constant, K_{assoc}, equals the slope of the line. The receptor number, R_0, equals the intercept with the x axis. **B,** An exponential plot results when hormone occupancy of one receptor molecule alters the local affinity of a second nearby molecule for the hormone. This phenomenon is called *negative cooperativity.*

factors such as ambient pH, osmolality, ion concentrations, and substrate levels.

■ *Plasma Membrane Receptor Systems*

Peptide and catecholamine hormone receptors are large glycoproteins, often composed of subunits, of molecular weight 50,000 to 200,000. Each molecule extends completely through the plasma membrane (see Fig. 5-5). A specific extracellular site or sites in the N-terminus portion of the receptor binds the hormone. The intramembranous portion may simply span the plasma membrane once, or wind in and out of it a number of times, typically seven times. The latter configuration anchors the receptor and also allows interaction with more than one signal-generating mechanism within the plasma membrane. The intracellular C-terminus tail of the receptor may contain a separate signal-generating mechanism.

Receptors tend to be concentrated in cellular microvilli. Hormone binding to these receptors may change their conformation and their distribution within the plasma membrane, and causes clustering of the hormone-receptor complexes. After receptor activation is completed, the complexes are internalized at these sites by **endocytosis.** Within the cell, lysosomes degrade the complex. Either the individual hormone and receptor molecules are destroyed or the receptor molecules are recycled back into the plasma membrane. It is possible that some internalized hormone-receptor complexes can also mediate intracellular actions of the hormone before being disrupted.

Some plasma membrane receptors resemble immunoglobulins in structure. Certain individuals susceptible to **autoimmune diseases** develop antibodies to their own hormone receptors. When such antibodies react with the receptor molecules, they may block access of the hormone to the receptor and cause hypofunction of the target cells (e.g., the **"resistant ovary" syndrome**). Alternatively, the antibody receptor combination mimics the hormone receptor interaction and causes hyperfunction of the target cells (e.g., hyperthyroidism caused by **Graves' disease;** see Chapter 50).

■ *Coupling by G Proteins*

For many hormones, occupancy of the plasma membrane receptor initiates a sequence of reactions within the membrane bilayer. *Several families of coupling molecules known as G proteins (see Chapter 5) functionally link various receptors to nearby effector molecules. The latter in turn generate second messengers that mediate the hormones' intracellular actions* (Fig. 45-8). G proteins are trimers; each has a unique α subunit and β-dimer subunit that is similar among family members. The α subunits bind to receptors, to effector molecules, and to guanosine diphosphate (GDP) and guanosine triphosphate (GTP). The β-dimeric subunit may serve to attach the G protein to the plasma membrane.

In its inactive state, the G protein is bound to GDP. When a hormone binds to a receptor, the appropriate adjacent G protein α subunit binds to the occupied receptor. The G protein then releases its bound GDP and binds instead to GTP. The displacement of GDP by GTP causes the α subunit of the G protein to dissociate from both the hormone receptor and from its own β-γ subunit. At this point, the G protein—which consists of the α subunit and GTP—is activated. The α subunit–GTP then moves to and binds to a nearby membrane effector molecule, such as the enzyme **adenylyl cyclase,** an ion channel carrier protein, or the enzyme **phospholipase C.** The activity of the effector molecule is either stimulated or inhibited by the binding of the α subunit–GTP complex. In binding to an effector molecule, the α subunit then catalyzes the hydrolysis of its bound GTP to GDP and inorganic phosphate. The α subunit–GDP then reassociates with its β-γ dimer, thereby reconstituting the original inactive G protein. The G protein is now free to interact with another hormone-occupied receptor molecule and start another cycle. This coupling cycle is repeated with the G protein α subunit shuttling between receptor and effector molecules until the hormone dissociates from its receptor or is internalized and degraded. Mg^{++} is required for the G-protein cycle, which is driven by the energy derived from the hydrolysis of GTP to GDP. Because the effector generates many intracellular second messenger molecules, the G-protein mechanism of signal transduction greatly amplifies the original extracellular hormone signal (see also Chapter 5).

■ *Second Messengers*

G proteins couple hormone-receptor complexes to at least three main effector systems: the adenylyl cyclase–cAMP system, the calcium-calmodulin system, and the membrane phospholipase–phospholipid system (see Chapter 5).

The **adenylyl cyclase–cAMP** system was the first to be described and initiated the concept of a second messenger. The plasma membrane enzyme adenylyl cyclase catalyzes formation of cAMP from adenosine triphosphate (ATP), with Mg^{++} as cofactor. A stimulatory G protein (G$_s$) therefore increases intracellular cAMP levels, whereas an inhibitory G protein (G$_i$) decreases cAMP levels.

An increase in cAMP stimulates the activation of **protein kinase A** (Fig. 45-9). Activation of protein kinase A in turn allows it to activate a number of enzymes in numerous metabolic pathways by phosphorylating their kinases. Alternatively, cAMP-stimulated phosphorylation may deactivate other enzymes. Thus, after a hormone binds to its receptor, this system generates a cascade of effects that ultimately changes the flux of metabolites in the cell. In the end, either the storage or the release of an important metabolite may be facilitated. Activation or deactivation of reciprocal pathways by the same hormone can augment the result, for example, by simultaneously inhibiting the release pathway while stimulating the storage pathway. Adenylyl cyclase and

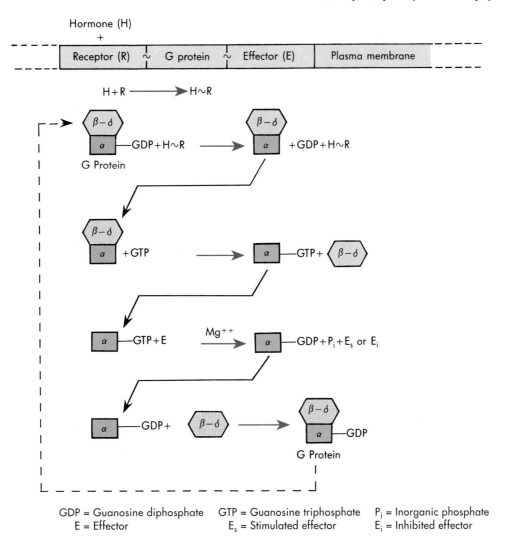

$$\text{Hormone (H)}$$
$$+$$

| Receptor (R) | ∼ | G protein | ∼ | Effector (E) | Plasma membrane |

$$H + R \longrightarrow H{\sim}R$$

GDP = Guanosine diphosphate   GTP = Guanosine triphosphate P_i = Inorganic phosphate
E = Effector E_s = Stimulated effector E_i = Inhibited effector

■ **Fig. 45-8**   Mechanism of G protein–mediated hormone actions. G protein transduces the hormone-receptor complex message to either stimulate or inhibit the effector in the plasma membrane. A GDP-GTP cycle fuels the sequence. See text for detailed description.

cAMP are ubiquitously distributed. Therefore, the specificity of enzyme responses to a particular hormone may also depend on the compartmentalization of increase in cAMP within the cell or on the proximity of the activated adenylyl cyclase to target enzyme(s).

cAMP may also act as a hormone second messenger by altering gene expression. Target DNA molecules have a **cAMP regulatory element (CRE)** that binds a protein transcription factor known as **cAMP response element binding protein (CREB).** cAMP activates protein kinase A; the catalytic subunit of the enzyme is then free to be translocated into the nucleus, where it phosphorylates CREB. The phosphorylated CREB is then capable of binding to CRE in a complex with another transcription protein, such as activated transcription factor-1. The final result of these reactions is the stimulation or inhibition of RNA polymerase and transcription of the target gene, and hence the stimulation or inhibition of synthesis of a specific protein.

The actions of cAMP are terminated when it is hydrolyzed. This reaction is catalyzed by the enzyme **phosphodiesterase.** Because the activity of phosphodiesterase is also modulated by hormones via a G protein, the level of cAMP is under dual regulation. Two hormones can function antagonistically if one stimulates adenylyl cyclase and the other stimulates phosphodiesterase.

A second system for transduction of the hormone signal is the **calcium-calmodulin system** (Fig. 45-10). As a result of hormone occupancy of its receptor, a specific G protein activates channels in the plasma membrane through which extracellular calcium can enter the cytoplasm. Calcium may also be mobilized from intracellular reservoirs in the endoplasmic reticulum and possibly the mitochondria. Ca^{++} can function as a second messenger, by transiently interacting with hundreds of binding proteins and target effector molecules. The overall results are influenced by several factors, including the

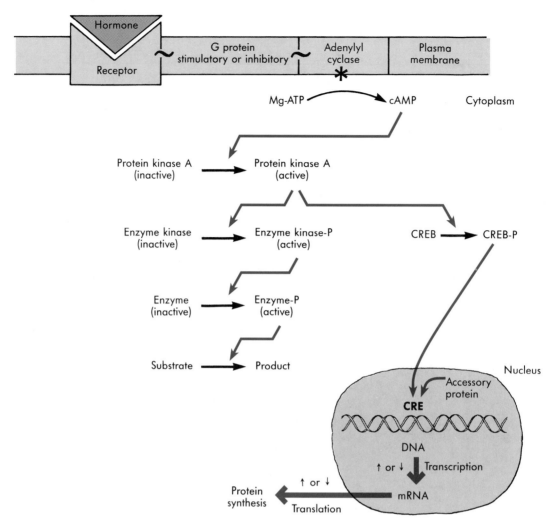

■ Fig. 45-9   Mechanism of hormone action via cAMP as second messenger. The hormone-receptor complex, via a G protein, either stimulates or inhibits adenylyl cyclase. If stimulated, cAMP is synthesized from ATP. cAMP activates protein kinase A, leading to a cascade of phosphorylations that ultimately activates or inactivates target enzymes. The latter regulate metabolic pathways. In addition, activated protein kinase A phosphorylates a cAMP response element binding *(CREB)* protein, which acts as a transcription factor by interacting with a cAMP regulatory element *(CRE)* on target DNA molecules.

restriction of calcium diffusion in the cytosol, spatial localization of target molecules, the broad spectrum of protein affinities for Ca⁺⁺ (which range from 10 nM to 1000 nM), and the duration of hormone-receptor interaction. Cytosolic calcium particularly combines with a ubiquitous and specific binding protein, **calmodulin,** in various proportions. The different calcium-calmodulin complexes activate or deactivate a variety of calcium-dependent enzymes. In this fashion, metabolite levels within the cell can be altered.

A third system for transduction of the initial hormone receptor signal is through intermediates generated from specific **plasma membrane phospholipids** (Fig. 45-11). The key phospholipid in this system is **phosphatidylinositol,** which undergoes further phosphorylation to phosphatidylinositol-4,5-bisphosphate. Hormone occu-

pancy of its receptor initiates a G-protein activation of the membrane-bound enzyme **phospholipase C.** Activated phospholipase C splits phosphatidyl-4,5-bisphosphate into a **diacylglycerol** and **inositol-1,4,5-trisphosphate.** The diacylglycerols are potent activators of the enzyme **protein kinase C,** which is calcium dependent. Diacylglycerol markedly increases the enzyme's affinity for calcium. Inositol trisphosphate (IP$_3$), released simultaneously with diacylglycerol, binds to a specific IP$_3$ receptor on the endoplasmic reticulum. This binding leads to formation of a channel through which calcium sequestered in the endoplasmic reticulum flows into the cytosol. Therefore, the combined products of phospholipase C action on phosphatidylinositol bisphosphate greatly amplify protein kinase C activity. In turn, protein kinase C phosphorylates and thereby activates or deacti-

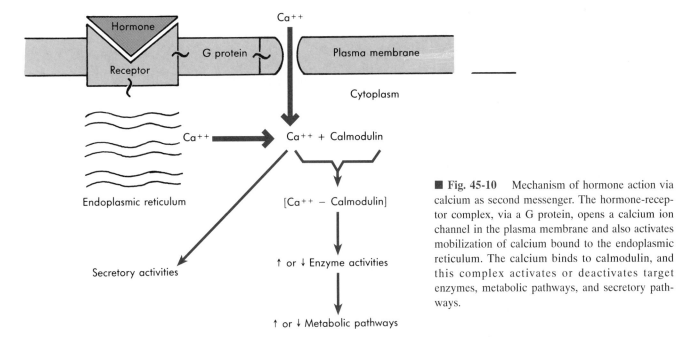

■ **Fig. 45-10** Mechanism of hormone action via calcium as second messenger. The hormone-receptor complex, via a G protein, opens a calcium ion channel in the plasma membrane and also activates mobilization of calcium bound to the endoplasmic reticulum. The calcium binds to calmodulin, and this complex activates or deactivates target enzymes, metabolic pathways, and secretory pathways.

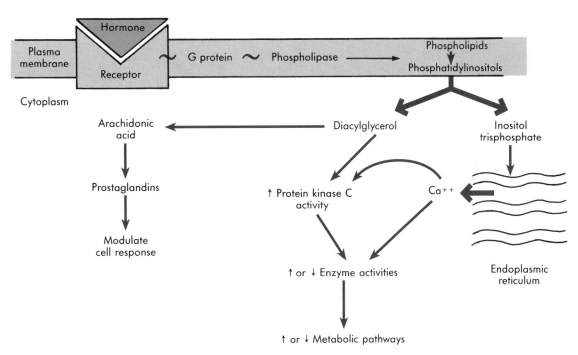

■ **Fig. 45-11** Mechanism of hormone action via membrane phospholipids. The hormone-receptor complex, via a G protein, activates phospholipase C, which then releases diacylglycerol and inositol trisphosphate from membrane-bound phosphoinositides. Inositol trisphosphate mobilizes calcium from the endoplasmic reticulum. Calcium with diacylglycerol activates protein kinase C, which phosphorylates target enzymes, increasing or decreasing metabolic pathways. Diacylglycerol also yields arachidonic acid for synthesis of modulating prostaglandins.

vates numerous enzymes involved in hormone actions. Finally, arachidonic acid, which is derived from subsequent hydrolysis of the diacylglycerol, serves as a substrate for the rapid synthesis of **prostaglandins.** The prostaglandins are also modulators of hormonal responses.

Although rare, diseases caused by mutant genes for receptors or G proteins have provided much insight into mechanisms of hormone action. For example, the reduced activity of a mutant α subunit of a stimulatory G protein leads to diminished cAMP levels and consequently deficient action of parathyroid hormone and resultant **hypocalcemia** (see Chapter 48). Another mutant G protein is constitutively overactive and is associated with continuous hypersecretion of growth hormone causing the disease **acromegaly** (see Chapter 49). Mutant nuclear receptors for thyroid hormone lead to **hypothyroidism** because thyroid hormone target cells cannot respond normally to this hormone (see Chapter 50).

Two other mechanisms of signal generation from plasma membrane receptors that do not require G-protein intermediaries are known. In each, the transducers lie in the intracytoplasmic tail of the receptor (Fig. 45-12). In one of these mechanisms, binding of the protein hormone changes the conformation of the receptor and exposes sites on its intracellular portion that are capable of receptor autophosphorylation. As a result, the receptor itself becomes a **tyrosine kinase** that phosphorylates tyrosine residues on intracellular protein substrates. This phosphorylation of tyrosine residues initiates a cascade of serine and threonine phosphorylations of enzyme kinases and phosphatases, which causes multiple intracellular events. These effects include alterations in cellular metabolism as well as cellular proliferation and differen-

tiation. **Insulin** is an example of a hormone that acts in this manner. In the second analogous mechanism, hormone binding initiates a conformational change in the intracytoplasmic tail of the receptor that exposes sites to which a class of cytoplasmic tyrosine kinases bind and are then activated. The sequence of events that follows is similar to those in the example just described, in which the receptor itself becomes a tyrosine kinase. Growth hormone is an example of this type of hormone action.

Another second messenger that results from hormone interaction with plasma membrane receptors is **cyclic guanosine monophosphate** (cGMP) arising from the action of **guanylyl cyclase** on GTP. Furthermore, a G protein that modulates cGMP phosphodiesterase activity also regulates cGMP levels. cGMP then activates **protein kinase G** and initiates a cascade of subsequent enzyme activations characteristic of this signaling system. Finally, peptide and protein hormones also cause increases or decreases in the concentration, as opposed to the activity, of enzymes and their messenger RNAs. These changes in concentration involve modification of gene expression and/or stabilization of mRNA levels. Because the cAMP mechanism described earlier cannot explain all these effects, there must be other mecha-

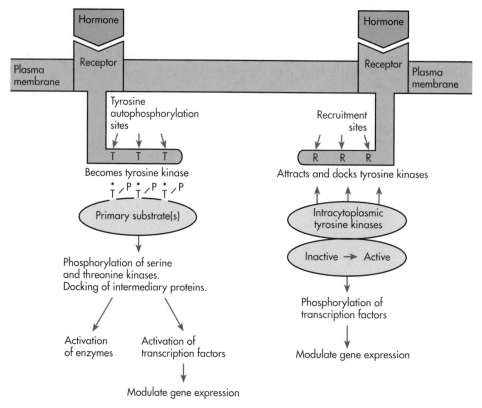

■ **Fig. 45-12** Mechanism of hormone action via tyrosine kinase activation. In one case shown on the left, occupancy of a site on the extracellular portion of the receptor activates autophosphorylation of tyrosine residues in the intracellular tail of the receptor. This creates tyrosine kinase activity of the receptor itself. The receptor then phosphorylates multiple sites in an intracellular protein substrate, setting into motion a cascade of events leading to enzyme activations and gene transcriptions. In the case shown on the right, the intracellular tail of the receptor attracts and docks other nearby tyrosine kinases, which then phosphorylate cytoplasmic substrates such as transcription factor proteins, ultimately modulating gene expression.

nisms for transmitting signals from the hormone-occupied plasma membrane receptor to specific target DNA molecules.

As complex as each of these systems seems individually, it must also be appreciated that a single hormone may operate through one or more of them simultaneously or in sequence. Thus, each messenger may subserve a different function of a single hormone. Moreover, the systems can interact with each other in important ways. For example, calcium-calmodulin can stimulate not only adenylyl cyclase activity itself, but also the activity of phosphodiesterase, the enzyme that hydrolyzes cAMP. Thus, cAMP levels, initially increased by a rapid hormone activation of adenylyl cyclase, may be subsequently dampened by a later response to the same hormone that activates phosphodiesterase. Likewise, in some situations, cAMP and protein kinase A products can inhibit the activity of the phospholipid messenger system by decreasing the generation of diacylglycerols. Thus, an early stimulation of cell processes by hormone action through protein kinase C may be later dampened by hormone action through protein kinase A. Finally, cAMP-activated phosphorylation of plasma membrane receptors themselves may decrease their affinity for hormones. This decrease in hormone affinity constitutes still another negative feedback mechanism for limiting hormone action or duration.

■ *Intracellular Receptor Systems*

An entirely different mechanism of signal transduction is characteristic of thyroid hormones, adrenal and gonadal steroid hormones, and vitamin D. In contrast to peptide and catecholamine hormones, these hormones enter the cell and bind within minutes to receptors located in the nucleus. Alternatively, the hormones first bind to receptors in the cytoplasm, and the resultant complexes are then transferred to the nucleus (Fig. 45-13). These receptors are large oligomeric and usually phosphorylated pro-

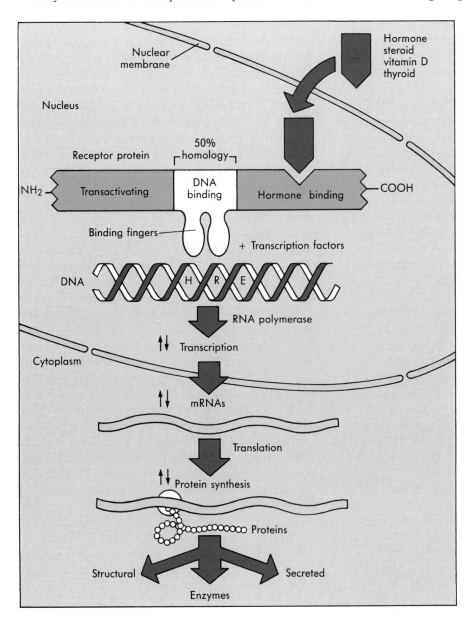

■ **Fig. 45-13**   Mechanism of action of vitamin D, steroid, and thyroid hormones. The hormone combines with the C-terminus of a specific intracellular receptor protein. The DNA-binding midportion of the receptor protein changes conformation, permitting it to interact with a hormone regulatory element in target DNA molecules. Gene transcription and synthesis of protein products are thereby stimulated or repressed.

teins. They are all coded for by a superfamily of genes related to the *cis*-oncogenes, and they contain three functional domains. The variable C-terminus domain binds the ligand hormone and is unique to each of these receptors. The middle domain of approximately 70 amino acids exhibits up to 50% homology with the middle domains of the other receptors in this class. The middle domain contains a DNA-binding site formed by two helical zinc fingers (Fig. 45-13). These receptor fingers attach to DNA molecules and are responsible for the specificity of DNA binding. The remaining N-terminus domain, which is highly variable in length and constituent amino acids, has transactivating functions.

In general, hormone receptors located in the target cell cytoplasm are inactive by themselves. Thus, they must be activated in some way in order to initiate intracellular events. In one model of activation, which is characteristic of adrenal steroid hormones, the unoccupied receptor may be complexed via its C-terminus domain to a blocking molecule, such as a **heat shock protein.** The hormone displaces the blocking protein when it binds to the receptor. This unblocking of the receptor permits it to be translocated into the nucleus, undergo dimerization (usually into homodimers), and bind to a specific site on a target DNA molecule, sometimes with the help of another acceptor protein. This DNA site, usually only 8 to 15 base pairs long, is known as a *hormone regulatory unit (HRE)*. Each half of an HRE site, which are oriented as palindromes, binds one of the two hormone-receptor monomers in the dimeric complex. The HRE is usually upstream from the basal promoter site at the 5′ end of the gene. With the gene now also fixed to the nuclear matrix, transactivating elements in both the N-terminus and C-terminus domains of the receptor stimulate RNA polymerase activity, and the gene is transcribed. Negative regulatory elements also exist in DNA molecules. Occupancy of a negative regulatory HRE by the hormone-receptor complex suppresses basal rates of transcription.

In another general model of activation, which is characteristic of thyroid hormones and vitamin D, the unoccupied receptor molecule is already attached to DNA binding sites and prevents gene transcription. The hormone enters the nucleus, binds to its receptor, and relieves the suppressive effect of the unliganded receptor. In a variant of this model, hormone binding causes dissociation of the two identical receptor monomers constituting the homodimer; this dissociation permits formation of heterodimers. For example, the thyroid receptor reassociates into a heterodimer consisting of an original thyroid hormone monomer and a retinoid receptor monomer. This heterodimer can then activate transcription of the DNA molecule.

In addition to these direct effects of hormone receptors of the steroid, thyroid, and vitamin D classes on specific target genes, another important mechanism involves the proto-oncogenes **cJun** and **cFos.** These two peptides form a heterodimer known as *AP-1* (activating protein-1),

which has its own cognate site on numerous DNA molecules. Hormone-receptor complexes can interact with AP-1 bound to genes and thereby stimulate or repress their transcription. The unoccupied or hormone-complexed receptor may also interact with cJun or cFos molecules individually. In this manner, the proliferation of target cells can be turned on or off by this class of hormones. Finally, steroid and similar hormones can also produce cascade effects within the cell. The gene expressing a regulatory protein or a transcription factor, such as cJun or cFos, can itself be rapidly activated by the hormone-receptor complex. This early product of hormone action can then facilitate later activation of more specific target genes as described above.

Once transactivated by hormone receptors, promoter nucleotide sequences in the DNA molecule initiate transcription at the start site of the specific gene message by RNA polymerase II. The resultant "immature" RNA then undergoes maturation to messenger RNA by capping, excision of untranslated nucleotide sequences, and splicing. Translation of the RNA message in the cytoplasm results in synthesis of specific target proteins of the hormone.

The magnitude of gene transcriptional effects of these hormones depends on several factors, including (1) the intracellular concentration of active hormone molecules, which may require conversion of a hormone precursor to the active molecule in situ; (2) the concentration and affinity of hormone receptor molecules and transcription factors; (3) the concentrations of nonspecific factors, such as RNA polymerase, the enzymes of protein synthesis or of processing of transfer RNA, and of amino acid substrates; and (4) the stage of the cell cycle.

The specificity of these hormone effects on target cells depends on (1) the presence of target genes that have not been "closed" during differentiation of the cell; (2) hormone receptors, some of which exist as isoforms specific to certain cells; and (3) transcription factors or other hormone-receptor acceptor proteins in the nucleus that are cell specific. Although each hormone has its own subset of target genes, the nuclear actions of two different hormones can overlap.

The importance of steroid and thyroid hormone nuclear effects is illustrated by the fact that each regulates about 1% of all the genes expressed by some cells. The proteins whose synthesis is regulated up or down by these hormones may be enzymes, structural proteins, receptor proteins, transcriptional proteins that regulate the expression of other genes, or proteins that are exported by the cell. By this hormone mechanism, enzymes are either induced or repressed rather than rapidly activated or inactivated. Response of metabolic pathways can be either accelerated or retarded. Other consequences of hormone action include alterations in the processing of the primary RNA product, in the turnover of messenger RNA molecules, or in post-translational modification of proteins. The transcription mechanism of steroid and thyroid hormones explains why hours are usually required for many of their biological effects to become evident or to disappear.

■ *Responsivity to Hormones*

The final outcome of the interaction of any hormone with its target cells depends on a number of factors. These factors include hormone concentration; receptor number; duration of exposure; intervals between consecutive exposures; intracellular conditions, such as concentrations of rate-limiting enzymes, cofactors or substrates; and the concurrent effects of antagonistic or synergistic hormones.

Hormonal effects are not "all-or-none" phenomena. The dose-response curve for the action of a hormone is generally complex and often exhibits a sigmoidal shape (Fig. 45-1, *A*). An intrinsic basal level of activity may be observed independent of added hormone and long after any previous exposure. A certain minimal threshold concentration of hormone is then required to elicit a measurable response. *The effect obtained at saturating doses of hormone defines the maximal responsiveness of the target cell. The concentration of hormone required to elicit a half-maximal response is an index of the sensitivity of the target cell.* Alterations in the dose-response curve in vivo can take two general forms (Fig. 45-14, *B*). First, a decrease in maximal responsiveness could be caused by

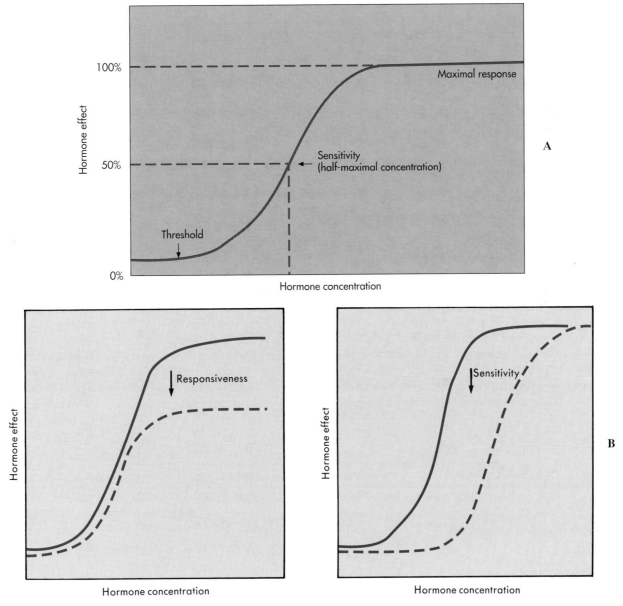

■ **Fig. 45-14**   **A,** The general shape of a hormone dose-response curve. Sensitivity is most often expressed as the concentration of the hormone that produces a half-maximal response. **B,** Alterations in the dose-response curve can take the form of a change in maximal responsiveness *(left panel),* a change in sensitivity *(right panel),* or both.

a decrease in the number of functional target cells, the total number of receptors per cell, the concentration of an enzyme being activated by the hormone, or the concentration of a precursor essential to the final product of hormone action; it could also be caused by an increase in the concentration of a noncompetitive inhibitor. Second, a decrease in hormone sensitivity could be caused by a decrease in the number or affinity of hormone receptors, alterations in the concentration of modulating cofactors, an increase in the rate of hormone degradation, or increases in antagonistic hormones.

The normal range of responsiveness to a hormone is usually rather broad and is in part a result of the physiological variability created by the aforementioned factors within and among normal individuals. However, the exquisiteness and precision with which hormonal effects can be modulated are important components in achieving one major objective of hormonal regulation: metabolic stability.

Obesity is a good example of a condition in which sensitivity to a hormone, insulin, is considerably diminished. Moreover, in **type 2 diabetes** (non–insulin-dependent diabetes), both sensitivity and maximal responsiveness to insulin are reduced, causing high plasma glucose levels.

■ *Hormone Transport*

After secretion, hormones enter pools characterized by widely varying size, volume of distribution, degree of compartmentalization, and fractional turnover rates. Initially, all hormones enter the plasma pool, where they may circulate either as free molecules or bound to specific carrier proteins. Catecholamine and the majority of peptide and protein hormones circulate unbound. In contrast, steroid and thyroid hormones and vitamin D circulate bound to specific globulins that are synthesized in the liver. The extent of protein binding markedly influences the exit rates of hormones from plasma into interstitial fluid and hence to target cells. As noted in Table 45-1, the plasma half-life of a hormone is directly correlated with the percentage of protein binding. For example, thyroxine is 99.95% protein bound and has a plasma half-life of 6 days, whereas aldosterone is only 15% bound and has a plasma half-life of 25 minutes. Larger and more complex protein hormones tend to have longer half-lives than do smaller proteins and peptides. In addition, hormone exit from plasma is not necessarily irreversible. In some instances, hormone molecules may return to plasma from other compartments, possibly after dissociation from cell membrane receptors. The return to plasma can occur by way of the lymphatic channels.

■ *Hormone Disposal*

Irreversible removal of hormone is a result of target cell uptake, metabolic degradation, and urinary or biliary excretion. The sum of all removal processes is expressed by the metabolic clearance rate (MCR). In a steady state, MCR is defined as volume of plasma cleared/unit time, which equals mass removed/unit time divided by circulating mass/unit volume, that is,

$$\text{MCR} = \frac{\text{mg/minute removed}}{\text{mg/ml of plasma}} = \frac{\text{ml cleared}}{\text{minute}} \quad (45\text{-}8)$$

MCR is one expression of the efficiency with which a hormone is removed from plasma. The ratio of MCR to the volume of distribution of a hormone is a measure of its fractional turnover rate (K). The plasma half-life, which is inversely related to K, is a cruder but more conveniently determined index of hormone removal. As shown in Table 45-1, MCR is inversely correlated with plasma half-life.

The kidney and liver are the major sites of hormone extraction and degradation. Renal clearance of hormone is reduced greatly by protein binding to globulins in the plasma; for example, less than 1% of secreted cortisol

■ **Table 45-1**   Correlation of plasma half-life and metabolic clearance of hormones with their structure and degree of protein binding

Hormone	Protein binding (%)	Plasma half-life (days)	Metabolic clearance (ml/min)
Thyroid			
Thyroxine	99.97	6	0.7
Triiodothyronine	99.7	1	18
Steroids			
Cortisol	94	0.07	140
Testosterone	89	0.04	860
Aldosterone	15	0.016	1100
Proteins			
Thyrotropin (molecular weight 28,000)	Nil	0.034	50
Insulin (molecular weight 6000)	Nil	0.006	800

appears unchanged in the urine, because only the small, free fraction of plasma cortisol is filtered by the glomerulus. On the other hand, about 30% of cortisol metabolites are excreted in the urine, because they are generally unbound or only loosely bound to protein. Peptide and smaller protein hormones are filtered to some degree by the glomerulus. Usually, however, they subsequently undergo tubular reabsorption and degradation within the kidney, so that only a small fraction finally appears in the urine.

Metabolic degradation occurs by enzymatic processes that include proteolysis, oxidation, reduction, hydroxylation, decarboxylation, and methylation. Virtually all hormones are extracted from the plasma and degraded to some extent by the liver. In addition, glucuronidation and sulfation of hormones or their metabolites may be carried out, and the conjugates are subsequently excreted in the bile or the urine. Some hormonal degradation appears to take place during interaction with target tissues. As noted previously, a portion of the hormone–plasma membrane receptor complex is internalized within the target cell, and hormone may be degraded within the cell. Hormone action and hormone degradation may be quantitatively linked in these situations.

■ *Hormone Measurement*

The most common and useful method for measuring hormones is immunoassay. Monoclonal antibodies can be produced that react with protein and peptide hormones as well as to steroid, thyroid, and vitamin D molecules after they are chemically conjugated to a protein such as albumin. These antibodies react with the respective hormones at concentrations in the picomolar range, and a variety of indicator techniques, including radioactivity, enzyme activity, and chemiluminescence, can then be used to quantitate the results. Immunoassays can usually be made sensitive enough to distinguish low plasma hormone levels from normal, and specific enough to distinguish plasma hormones from circulating precursor molecules and products of hormone metabolism. However, sensitive biological assays can also be required to obtain correct physiological or diagnostic information. For example, the bioactivity of protein hormones may vary with their degree of glycosylation and at different times. Certain pituitary hormones show such variation during the menstrual cycle. An immunoassay may show little change in molecular concentration at some point because glycosylation does not alter the hormone epitope with which the immunoassay antibody is reacting. Nevertheless, concentrations of hormone capable of exerting biological effects are, in fact, different at that point. Another example is seen in diseases in which a mutant hormone is secreted—one that has low biological activity but retains the critical antigenic sequence. An immunoassay would show normal or even high plasma

levels (from negative feedback) of the hormone when there is actually a deficiency of hormone actions on target tissues.

■ *Estimates of Hormone Secretion*

■ *Secretion Rate*

Absolute quantitation of the output of a single hormone by an individual gland can be accomplished in vivo only by catheterization of the blood supply to the gland. The arterial (A) and venous (V) concentrations of hormone, in mass per unit volume, and the blood flow (BF) across the gland, in volume per unit time, must be measured. The rate of secretion in mass per unit time is then $(V - A) \times BF$. This method for assessing secretion rate is suitable for animal studies but is not applicable to clinical circumstances.

Sampling of veins that drain glands can be used diagnostically to localize the source of excess hormone production. This kind of sampling can be used for multiple glands, such as the parathyroid glands, or for hormones, such as steroids, that may be secreted from either the adrenal glands or the gonads. A microtumor that secretes excess amounts of a hormone may exist within the already small pituitary gland. Its presence can be identified, and it can be localized to the correct side of the gland by sampling blood from veins draining the right and left sides, respectively. This procedure is helpful in cases in which radiologic methods cannot detect such a small tumor.

■ *Production Rate*

A less direct but frequently satisfactory method of estimating hormone secretion in physiological investigations is the measurement of the production rate (PR) in mass per unit time. PR is the total amount of the hormone entering the peripheral circulation per unit time; in a steady state, it will equal the total amount of hormone leaving the circulation. Therefore, production rate is determined by measuring plasma concentration (P) and the MCR (see p 796):

$$PR = P \times MCR \qquad (45\text{-}9)$$

■ *Plasma Levels*

A simple plasma concentration provides a valid index of hormone production rate when the metabolic clearance of the hormone is within normal limits and can be taken as a constant; since $PR = P \times MCR$, PR is proportional to P if MCR is a constant. This equation is the theoretical basis for employing plasma hormone measurements alone as an index of activity of the gland of origin. However, the release of many hormones is characterized by episodic spurts and diurnal variation. In such cases, it may be hazardous to draw conclusions from a single plasma value, and multiple measurements taken at different times of the day may be needed.

■ *Urinary Excretion*

Measurement of urinary hormone excretion is cumbersome because it requires accurately timed collections. However, it offers the advantage of, in effect, averaging plasma fluctuations over the collection period. Furthermore, in some instances, the quantity of a hormone metabolite in the urine far exceeds the plasma or urinary level of the hormone itself, and is therefore more easily measurable.

Urinary excretion of a hormone or a metabolite is a valid index of production rate (and hence secretion rate) when the following two conditions are fulfilled: (1) the kidney must be contributing its usual fraction of the total metabolic clearance; and (2) within the kidney itself, the usual proportioning of hormone between intrarenal degradation and urinary excretion must be maintained. The chief sources of error in employing urinary excretion as a reflection of hormone secretion are general impairment in renal function, a change in the pattern of degradation to a metabolic product excreted differently by the kidney, and incomplete collections of urine. When diurnal variation in hormone secretion or metabolism is not a factor, incomplete or untimed collections can be compensated for by indexing urinary hormone concentration to the urinary creatinine concentration in the sample.

■ *Summary*

1. The function of the endocrine system is to regulate metabolism, fluid status, growth, maturation and sexual development, senescence, and behavior. The endocrine and nervous systems work conjointly to maintain homeostasis.

2. Hormones are signaling molecules that are conveyed by the bloodstream (endocrine), by neural axons and the bloodstream (neurocrine), or by local diffusion (paracrine, autocrine).

3. Hormone molecules may be proteins, peptides, catecholamines, steroids, or iodinated tyrosine derivatives.

4. Protein and peptide hormone synthesis involves processing of a primary gene transcript called a prohormone. Such processing includes proteolytic cleavage, glycosylation, and phosphorylation. Thyroid hormone and cate-

cholamines are synthesized from tyrosine, whereas steroid hormones and vitamin D arise from cholesterol by multiple enzyme reactions.

5. Peptide and protein hormones and catecholamines are stored in granules and secreted by exocytosis. Thyroid hormone is stored within protein molecules in large quantities; steroid hormones are not stored at all. Both are released by diffusion.

6. Protein and peptide and catecholamine hormones act on target cells via specific protein receptors located in the plasma membranes; the hormone-receptor complexes transduce signals through second messengers. Stimulatory or inhibitory G proteins link the receptor to membrane mechanisms that generate cAMP, Ca^{++}, diacylglycerols, and inositol trisphosphate. These molecules act intracellularly to increase or decrease enzyme activities. Other receptors activate tyrosine kinase sites, which leads to similar effects on enzymes. All of these effects are rapid.

7. Thyroid and steroid hormones act by means of specific protein receptors located in the nucleus. The hormone-receptor complex interacts with promoter elements or negative elements in DNA molecules and with transcription factors to induce or repress expression of target genes. In turn, these changes in gene activity lead to increases or decreases in the concentration of enzymes and other cell proteins. These effects are slower.

8. The sensitivity of an organism to hormone action is expressed as the hormone concentration that produces half-maximal activity. The sensitivity can be influenced by changes in receptor number, affinity, hormone degradation rate, or competitive antagonists. The maximal effect produced by saturating concentrations of hormone can be influenced by the number of target cells, receptor number, concentration of target enzymes, or noncompetitive antagonists.

9. Hormone secretion is measured directly by arteriovenous concentration gradients and flow rates across the gland. Clinically, plasma levels and urinary excretion rates are used as indirect indices of hormonal secretion rates. These results are valid as long as metabolic or renal clearance of the hormone is normal.

■ *Self-Study Problems*

1. How do the mechanisms of action of peptide hormones differ from those of steroid or thyroid hormones?

2. How does negative feedback regulate hormone secretion?

■ *Bibliography*

Journal articles

Alford FP et al: Temporal patterns of circulating hormones as assessed by continuous blood sampling, *J Clin Endocrinol Metab* 36:108, 1973.

Birnbaumer L et al: Molecular basis of regulation of ionic channels by G proteins, *Recent Prog Horm Res* 45:121, 1989.

Bost KL et al: Similarity between the corticotrophin ACTH receptor and a peptide encoded by an RNA that is complementary to ACTH mRNA, *Proc Natl Acad Sci* 82:1372, 1985.

Carson-Jurica MA et al: Steroid receptor family: structure and function, *Endocr Rev* 11:201, 1990.

Chambon P et al: Promoter elements of genes coding for proteins and modulation of transcription by estrogens and progesterone, *Recent Prog Horm Res* 40:1, 1984.

Combarnous Y: Molecular basis of the specificity of binding of glycoprotein hormones to their receptors, *Endocr Rev* 13:670, 1992.

Fradkin JE et al: Specificity spillover at the hormone receptor: exploring its role in human disease, *N Engl J Med* 320:640, 1989.

Freedman LP: Anatomy of the steroid receptor zinc finger region, *Endocr Rev* 13:129, 1992.

Glass CK: Differential recognition of target genes by nuclear receptor monomers, dimers, and heterodimers, *Endocr Rev* 15:391, 1994.

Gordon P et al: Internalization of polypeptide hormones; mechanism, intracellular localization and significance, *Diabetologia* 18:263, 1980.

Inagami T, Naruse M, Hoover R: Endothelium as an endocrine organ, *Annu Rev Physiol* 57:171, 1995.

Lacy PE: Beta cell secretion—from the standpoint of a pathobiologist, *Diabetes* 19:895, 1970.

Lefkowitz R et al: Mechanisms of membrane-receptor regulation: biochemical, physiological, and clinical insights derived from studies of the adrenergic receptors, *N Engl J Med* 310:1570, 1984.

Reiter RJ: Pineal melatonin: cell biology of its synthesis and of its physiological interactions, *Endocr Rev* 12:151, 1991.

Ralff CJ, Kushner PJ, Baxter JD: The nuclear hormone receptor gene superfamily, *Annu Rev Med* 46:443, 1995.

Sherwin RS et al: A model of the kinetics of insulin in man, *J Clin Invest* 53:1481, 1974.

Spiegel AM: Guanine nucleotide binding protein and signal transduction, *Vitam Horm* 44:47, 1988.

Spiegel AM, Shenker A, Weinstein LS: Receptor-effector coupling by G proteins: implications for normal and abnormal signal transduction, *Endocr Rev* 13:536, 1992.

Tait JF: The use of isotopic steroids for the measurement of production rates in vivo, *J Clin Endocrinol* 23:1285, 1963.

Turek FW: Circadian rhythms, *Recent Prog Horm Res* 4:43, 1994.

Wilkin TJ: Mechanisms of disease: receptor autoimmunity in endocrine disorders, *N Engl J Med* 323:1318, 1990.

Zor U: Role of cytoskeletal organization in the regulation of adenylate cyclase–cyclic adenosine monophosphate by hormones, *Endocr Rev* 4:1, 1984.

Books and monographs

Arendt J: *The pineal gland: basic physiology and clinical implications.* In DeGroot LJ, editor: *Endocrinology,* ed 3, Philadelphia, 1995, WB Saunders.

Chin WW: *Hormonal regulation of gene expression.* In DeGroot LJ, editor: *Endocrinology,* ed 3, Philadelphia, 1995, WB Saunders.

Exton JH, Blackmore PF: *Calcium-mediated hormonal responses.* In DeGroot LJ, editor: *Endocrinology,* ed 2, Philadelphia, 1989, WB Saunders.

Gammeltoft S, Kahn CR: *Hormone signaling via membrane receptors.* In DeGroot LJ, editor: *Endocrinology,* ed 3, Philadelphia, 1995, WB Saunders.

Gershengorn MC, Perlman JH: *Second messenger signaling pathways: phosphatidylinositol and calcium.* In DeGroot LJ, editor: *Endocrinology,* ed 3, Philadelphia, 1995, WB Saunders.

Habener JF: *Genetic control of hormone formation.* In Wilson FJ, Foster DF, editors: *Textbook of endocrinology,* ed 8, Philadelphia, 1992, WB Saunders.

Habener JF: *Cyclic AMP second messenger signaling pathway.* In DeGroot LJ, editor: *Endocrinology,* ed 3, Philadelphia, 1995, WB Saunders.

Kahn CR, Smith RJ, Chin WW: *Mechanism of action of hormones that act at the cell surface.* In Wilson JD, Foster DF, editors: *Textbook of endocrinology,* ed 8, Philadelphia, 1992, WB Saunders.

Mester J, Baulieu E-E: *Nuclear receptor superfamily.* In DeGroot LJ, editor: *Endocrinology,* ed 3, Philadelphia, 1995, WB Saunders.

Nishizuka Y: *Membrane phospholipids and the mechanism of action of hormones.* In LaBrie F, Proulx L, editors: *Endocrinology,* Proceedings of the 7th International Congress of Endocrinology, Quebec City, 1984, Amsterdam, 1984, Elsevier.

Yalow RS, Berson SA: *Introduction and general considerations.* In Odell WD, Daughaday WH, editors: *Principles of competitive protein-binding assays,* Philadelphia, 1971, JB Lippincott.

Whole Body Metabolism

Metabolism can be broadly defined as the sum of all the chemical (and physical) processes involved in (1) producing energy from exogenous and endogenous sources, (2) synthesizing and degrading structural and functional tissue components, and (3) disposing of the resultant waste products of these reactions. Regulating the rate and direction of many aspects of metabolism is one of the major functions of the endocrine system. Therefore, a firm grasp of the fundamentals of metabolism is essential to an understanding of the important influence of hormones on body functions.

■ *Energy Metabolism*

■ *Balance*

The laws of thermodynamics require that overall energy balance be constantly maintained in living organisms during periods of stable weight. However, energy may be acquired in various forms, stored in other forms, and expended in many different ways. Therefore, numerous interconversions of chemical, mechanical, and thermal energy are possible within the basic requirement that *in the steady state, energy input must always equal energy output.* Fig. 46-1 illustrates this overall flow of energy through the human organism.

■ *Energy Input*

Energy input consists of foodstuffs, which are classified into three major chemical categories: carbohydrate, fat, and protein. The complete combustion of each chemical type yields characteristic amounts of energy, expressed as joules or kilocalories per gram (1 kcal = 4184 joules). Combustion of each class of foodstuff requires characteristic amounts of oxygen, depending on the proportions of carbon, hydrogen, and oxygen in the substance. However, the energy yield from each class of foodstuff per liter of oxygen used is similar because the ratio of carbon to

hydrogen atoms is also similar in each class (Table 46-1). Within the body, the carbon skeletons of both carbohydrate and protein can be converted to fat and their potential energy is stored more efficiently in this manner. The carbon skeletons of protein can also be converted to carbohydrate when that energy source is specifically needed. However, no significant conversion of carbon skeletons of fat to carbohydrate takes place in the body.

■ *Energy Output*

Energy output can be divided into several distinct and measurable components:

1. At rest, energy is expended in a myriad of synthetic and degradative chemical reactions; in generating and maintaining gradients of ions and other molecules across cell and organelle membranes; in the creation and conduction of signals, particularly in the nervous system; in the mechanical work of respiration and circulation of the blood; and in obligate heat loss to the environment. The absolute minimal energy expenditure of the body is called the **basal** or **resting metabolic rate (BMR** or **RMR)**. In the adult human, BMR amounts to an average daily expenditure of 20 to 25 kcal (84 to 105 kjoules)/kg body weight (or 1.0 to 1.2 kcal/min) and requires the use of approximately 200 to 250 ml oxygen/min. About 40% of the BMR is accounted for by the central nervous system and 20% to 30% by the skeletal muscle mass. Eighty percent of the interindividual variance in BMR is accounted for by fat-free mass, fat mass, age, and gender. The BMR is linearly related to lean body mass and to body surface area. It declines in the elderly, partly because lean body mass declines with age. Women have slightly lower BMRs than men. Studies of identical twins and families suggest that some of the remaining variation in BMR is genetically determined. During sleep, BMR falls 10% to 15%. BMR is increased by raising environmental temperature.

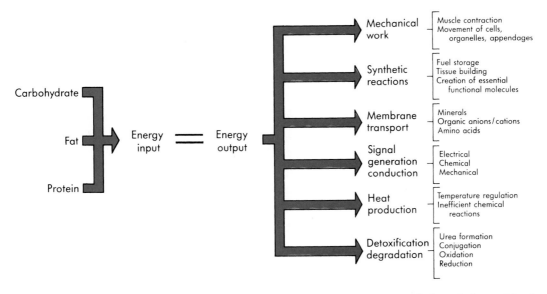

■ **Fig. 46-1** Overview of energy balance. In a steady state, input as caloric equivalents of food equals output as caloric equivalents of various forms of mechanical and chemical work and heat.

■ **Table 46-1** Energy equivalents of foodstuffs

	Kilocalories produced per gram	O_2 used (L/g)	Kilocalories produced per liter of O_2	Respiratory quotient
Carbohydrate	4.2	0.84	5.0	1.00
Fat	9.4	2.00	4.7	0.70
Protein	4.3*	0.96*	4.5	0.80
Typical fuel mix	—	—	4.8	0.85

*Each gram of protein oxidized yields 0.16 g of urinary nitrogen. Thus, these values should be multiplied by 6.25 to express them per gram of urinary nitrogen.

During fever, BMR also increases because a high body temperature accelerates enzyme-catalyzed reactions. The increase in BMR requires an increase in respiratory rate to supply the needed oxygen and dispose of extra carbon dioxide (CO_2). An increase in caloric intake is also required to prevent weight loss if the illness is prolonged.

2. Ingestion of food causes a small obligate increase in energy expenditure, referred to as **diet-induced thermogenesis.** This expenditure is partly explained by the cost of digestion and the increased rate of reactions involved in the disposition of the ingested calories, such as storage of glucose in the large molecule, glycogen, or degradation of amino acids to urea.

3. **Nonshivering thermogenesis** refers to energy expended for the purpose of producing heat, either in an *obligatory* manner to maintain a constant thermoneutral state, or in a *facultative* manner when an individual is acutely exposed to cold. All tissues contribute to the obligatory thermogenic process. This kind of energy expenditure may also be evoked and may compensate for a prolonged intake of excess calories as a means of limiting weight gain.

4. Energy is also expended by sedentary individuals in spontaneous physical activity such as "fidgeting," at least some of which is unconscious and seemingly purposeless.

5. The additional energy expended in occupational labor and purposeful exercise (Table 46-2) varies greatly among individuals, as well as from day to day and from season to season. This component generates the greatest need for variation in daily caloric intake and underscores the importance of energy stores to buffer temporary discrepancies between energy output and intake.

Of a total average daily expenditure of 2300 kcal (9700 kjoules) in a sedentary adult, basal metabolism accounts for 60% to 70%, dietary and obligatory thermogenesis for 5% to 15%, and spontaneous physical activity for 20% to 30%. Up to an additional 4000 kcal may be used in daily physical work. During short periods of occupational or recreational exercise, energy expenditure can increase more than tenfold over basal levels.

■ **Table 46-2** Estimates of energy expenditure in adults

Activity	Calorie expenditure (kcal/min)
Basal	1.1
Sitting	1.8
Walking, 2.5 miles/hr	4.3
Walking, 4.0 miles/hr	8.2
Climbing stairs	9.0
Swimming	10.9
Bicycling, 13 miles/hr	11.1
Household domestic work	2-4.5
Factory work	2-6
Farming	4-6
Building trades	4-9

Data from Kottke FJ: *Animal energy exchange.* In Altman PL, editor: *Metabolism,* Bethesda, Md, 1968, Federation of American Society for Experimental Biology.

■ *Energy Generation*

■ *Generation of Adenosine Triphosphate from Foodstuffs*

The basic chemical currency of energy in all living cells are the two high-energy phosphate bonds contained in **adenosine triphosphate (ATP).** To a lesser extent, other purine and pyrimidine nucleotides (guanosine triphosphate, cytosine triphosphate, uridine triphosphate, inosine triphosphate) also serve as energy sources after the energy from ATP is transferred to them. In muscle, creatine phosphate is a particularly important high-energy molecule.

The two terminal P-O bonds of ATP each contain about 12 kcal of potential energy per mole under physiological conditions. These bonds are in constant flux. They are generated by oxidative reactions and are broken as the energy is either (1) transferred into other high-energy bonds involved in synthetic reactions (e.g., amino acid + ATP → amino acyl AMP), (2) expended in creating lower-energy phosphorylated metabolic intermediates (e.g., glucose + ATP → glucose-6-phosphate), or (3) converted to mechanical work (e.g., propulsion of spermatozoa). Because the production and transfer of energy is only 65% efficient, about 18 kcal of substrate are required to generate each terminal P-O bond of ATP. At any particular moment, the total body content of ATP would suffice for little more than 1 minute of energy use. In a normal day when 2300 kcal are turned over, about 128 moles, or 63 kg, of ATP (a mass approximating body weight) are generated and expended. An overview of energy production with generation of ATP from the major substrates is shown in Fig. 46-2.

Combustion of carbohydrate. The combustion of carbohydrates, chiefly glucose with lesser amounts of fructose and galactose, involves two major phases:

1. During the cytoplasmic anaerobic phase known as **glycolysis** (Embden-Meyerhof pathway), each partially oxidized glucose molecule yields two molecules of pyruvate but only 8% of its energy content.

Glycolysis can serve only briefly as a sole source of energy because (1) the body supply of glucose is limited and (2) the accumulated pyruvate must be siphoned off by reduction to lactate, a metabolite that in excess amounts is noxious.

2. During the mitochondrial aerobic phase, the two pyruvate molecules are oxidized to CO_2 by the **citric acid cycle (Krebs) cycle,** and the remaining energy is liberated. In this pathway, acetyl coenzyme A (acetyl CoA), initially formed by oxidative decarboxylation of pyruvate, is condensed with oxaloacetate to form citrate. Through a cyclic series of reactions, the carbons of acetyl CoA appear as CO_2, and oxaloacetate is regenerated.

Combustion of fatty acids. The combustion of fatty acids, the major energy component of fats, takes place in the mitochondria through a repetitive biochemical sequence known as beta oxidation. In this process, two carbons in the form of acetyl CoA are released at a time until the entire fatty acid molecule is broken down. The acetyl CoA enters the citric acid cycle and is disposed of (as already described). In the liver, a variable portion of fatty acid oxidation stops at the last four carbons and yields acetoacetic and β-hydroxybutyric acids. The production of these ketoacids results from an imbalance between the flow of fatty acids into the liver mitochondria and the capacity of the citric acid cycle to dispose of acetyl CoA. The water-soluble ketoacids are released by the liver to be oxidized in other tissues as additional energy substrates.

Accelerated production of ketoacids occurs when carbohydrate intake is low or when fasting is prolonged beyond the usual overnight period. **Ketosis** can produce severe metabolic acidosis in humans deprived of the key hormone *insulin*, as in insulin-dependent or type 1 diabetes mellitus.

Combustion of protein. The combustion of protein first requires hydrolysis to its component amino acids. Each of these amino acids then undergoes degradation by individual pathways, which ultimately lead to intermediate compounds of the citric acid cycle and then to acetyl CoA and CO_2.

The combustion of all foodstuffs yields large numbers of hydrogen atoms. These hydrogens are oxidized to H_2O in the mitochondria in linkage with the phosphorylation of adenosine diphosphate (ADP) to ATP (Fig. 46-2). In these reactions, three high-energy P-O bonds are formed for each atom of oxygen used. This process yields 60% to 65% of the usable chemical energy in foodstuffs.

■ *Respiratory Quotient*

In the process of oxidizing substrates to meet basal energy needs, the proportion of carbon dioxide produced (Vco_2) to oxygen used (Vo_2) varies according to the fuel

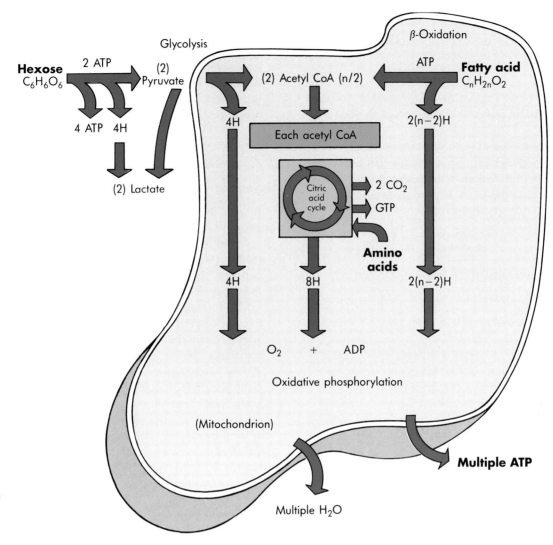

■ **Fig. 46-2** Overview of energy production. Glycolysis and each turn of the citric acid cycle supply only 2 adenosine triphosphate (ATP) equivalents apiece. ATP is generated mainly when hydrogens removed from carbohydrate, fat, or protein substrates are oxidized in the mitochondria. *ADP*, Adenosine diphosphate; *GTP*, guanosine triphosphate.

mix. The ratio of V_{CO_2} to V_{O_2} is known as the **respiratory quotient (RQ).** As indicated by the following equations, RQ equals 1.0 for oxidation of carbohydrate (e.g., glucose), whereas RQ equals 0.70 for oxidation of fat (e.g., palmitic acid).

For carbohydrates:

$$C_6H_{12}O_6 + 6\ O_2 \rightarrow 6\ CO_2 + 6\ H_2O$$
Glucose

$$RQ = \frac{6\ CO_2}{6\ O_2} = 1.0 \qquad (46\text{-}1)$$

For fats:

$$C_{15}H_{31}COOH + 23\ O_2 \rightarrow 16\ CO_2 + 16\ H_2O$$
Palmitic acid

$$RQ = \frac{16\ CO_2}{23\ O_2} = 0.70 \qquad (46\text{-}2)$$

The RQ for protein reflects the individual RQs of the amino acids, and it averages 0.80. Ordinarily, protein is only a minor energy source. The small contribution of protein oxidation to the overall RQ can be corrected for by measuring the urinary excretion of the nitrogen that results from the metabolism of amino acids.

By determining the RQ, corrected for protein, one can calculate the proportion of carbohydrate and fat in the fuel mix being oxidized.

For example, when the O_2 consumed = 210 ml/min and the CO_2 produced = 174 ml/min:

$$RQ = \frac{174}{210} = 0.83$$

If C is the proportion of energy produced by carbohydrate oxidation and F is the remaining proportion of energy produced by fat oxidation, then:

$$1 \times C + 0.7 \times F = 0.83$$

Since C + F = 1:

$$1 \times C + 0.7 \times (1 - C) = 0.83$$
$$C = 0.43$$
$$F = 0.57$$

That is, 43% of the calories are being provided by carbohydrate oxidation and 57% of the calories by fat oxidation.

With a knowledge of the actual rate of energy expenditure in kilocalories per minute and the standard values of 4 kcal/g of carbohydrate and 9 kcal/g of fat, it is possible to calculate the actual rates of oxidation of carbohydrate and fat, respectively, in grams per minute:

$$210 \text{ ml of } O_2 \text{ consumed per minute} = 1.05 \text{ kcal/min}$$
$$4 \times \text{a gram of carbohydrate} = 0.43 \times 1.05$$

Therefore, a gram of carbohydrate = 0.113/min.

$$9 \times \text{a gram of fat} = 0.57 \times 1.05$$

Therefore, a gram of fat = 0.067/min.

From the above calculations, it is possible to alter the fuel mix to compensate for clinically impaired respiratory function. By increasing the proportion of fat, a lesser amount of CO_2 is produced for the same quantity of O_2 expended; that is, the demand on the individual's ventilation is reduced (see Chapter 36).

In the resting adult, the rate of glucose oxidation is approximately 120 mg/min (170 g/day), whereas that of fat oxidation is approximately 60 mg/min (90 g/day). Thus, in caloric equivalents, glucose supplies about 45% of the energy required for basal metabolism. The central nervous system is an obligate glucose consumer and uses the major portion of this fuel. Estimates of cerebral glucose use are 125 to 150 g/day. In contrast, the large muscle mass oxidizes primarily fatty acids in resting individuals. However, like all tissues, the muscle mass uses at least some glucose in order to maintain sufficient concentrations of citric acid cycle intermediates for efficient disposal of acetyl CoA and completion of fatty acid oxidation.

■ *Energy Storage and Transfers*

■ *Storage*

In humans, the intake of energy in the form of food is periodic. The time course of energy intake does not match either the constant rate of energy expenditure in the basal state or that expended during intermittent muscle work. Therefore, the organism must have mechanisms for storing ingested energy for future use.

Fat stores. The greatest part of energy reserves (75%) is in the form of fat as triglycerides, which are stored in adipose tissue (Fig. 46-3). In normal-weight humans, fat constitutes 10% to 30% of body weight, but it can reach 80% in very obese individuals. Fat is a particularly efficient storage fuel because of its high caloric density (9 kcal/g) and because it obligates little additional weight as intracellular water. Fat stores can supply energy needs for up to 2 months in totally fasted individuals of normal weight. Triglycerides are formed by esterification of free fatty acids (FFAs) (largely derived from the diet) with α-glycerol phosphate. However, FFAs can also be synthesized from acetyl CoA derived from oxidation of glucose. In this way, carbohydrate can be converted to fat in liver and adipose tissue and its energy stored in this more efficient form (Fig. 46-4). In humans, however, this process accounts for relatively little glucose use.

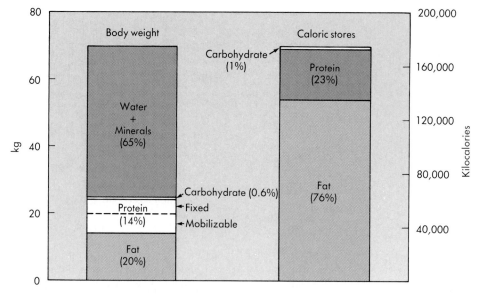

■ **Fig. 46-3** The composition of an average 70-kg human shown in terms of weight *(left)* and caloric stores *(right)*. Note the trivial proportion of carbohydrate stores relative to fat stores.

Protein stores. Protein (4 kcal/g) constitutes almost 25% of the potential energy reserves (Fig. 46-3), and the component amino acids can contribute to the supply of essential glucose. However, virtually all proteins serve some vital structural or functional role. Therefore, their use as a major source of energy is deleterious and arises only as a last resort before death from fasting.

Glycogen. Carbohydrate (4 kcal/g) in the form of a glucose polymer, **glycogen,** forms less than 1% of total energy reserves (Fig. 46-3). However, this portion is critical for support of central nervous system metabolism and for short bursts of intense muscle work. Approximately one fourth of the glycogen stores (75 to 100 g) is in the liver, and about three fourths (300 to 400 g) is in muscle mass. Liver glycogen can be made available to other tis-

sues by the process of **glycogenolysis** and glucose release. Muscle glycogen can be used only by muscle, because this tissue lacks the enzyme glucose-6-phosphatase, which is required for release of glucose into the bloodstream.

Glycogen can be formed from all three major dietary sugars. In addition, in the liver (and to a much lesser extent, in the kidney), glucose itself can be synthesized de novo from the three carbon precursors pyruvate, lactate, and glycerol, and from parts of the carbon skeleton of all 20 amino acids in protein (except leucine and lysine). This process, known as **gluconeogenesis,** converts two pyruvate molecules to glucose. However, gluconeogenesis is not a simple reversal of the reactions of glycolysis (Fig. 46-4). The chemical free energy change

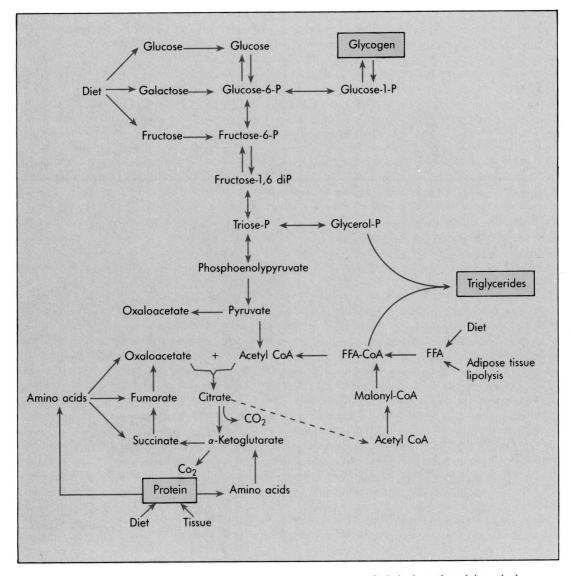

■ **Fig. 46-4** Chemical pathways of energy transfer and storage. Carbohydrates funnel through glucose-6-phosphate to be stored as glycogen or to undergo glycolysis to pyruvate and be used for synthesis of fatty acids. The latter are esterified with glycerol-phosphate and stored as triglycerides. Amino acids arising from protein are converted to glucose via citric acid cycle intermediates and pyruvate in the process known as gluconeogenesis.

is too large to permit efficient backward flow of the glycolytic reactions at three steps: (1) pyruvate to phosphoenolpyruvate, (2) fructose-1,6-biphosphate to fructose-6-phosphate, and (3) glucose-6-phosphate to glucose. Substitution of simple phosphatase reactions reverses the last two steps. However, the first step requires energy input in the form of ATP and guanosine triphosphate. It is also important to realize that *net glucose synthesis cannot occur from acetyl CoA,* even though carbon atoms from acetyl CoA can become part of oxaloacetate and then part of glucose molecules by means of the citric acid cycle. Thus, fat can contribute to carbohydrate stores only by way of the 3-carbon glycerol moiety of triglycerides.

■ *The Cost of Energy Storage Transfer*

The processes of energy storage and transfer themselves expend energy. This energy requirement partly accounts for the stimulation of oxygen use after a meal (diet-induced thermogenesis). The cost of storing dietary fatty acids as triglycerides in adipose tissue is only 3% of the original calories, and the cost of storing glucose as glycogen is only 7% of the original calories. In contrast, conversion of carbohydrate to fat uses up 23% of the original calories, and a similar amount is expended in storing dietary amino acids as protein or in converting them to glycogen.

■ *Relationships between Substrate Use and Synthesis*

Because glucose and fatty acids are alternative and in effect competing energy substrates, some relationship between their use and their synthesis and storage within cells is expected. Under circumstances in which fatty acid supply and plasma FFA levels are increased, glucose uptake by cells is decreased (Randle fatty acid–glucose cycle). Furthermore, intermediates produced during fatty acid oxidation slow down glycolysis and promote gluconeogenesis. Thus, increased use of fatty acids as fuel shifts glucose metabolism away from oxidation in liver and muscle. In addition, in the liver, increased fatty acid use shifts glucose metabolism from storage as glycogen to release into the bloodstream.

Conversely, when dietary glucose is plentiful, glycolysis is augmented, more acetyl CoA is generated from pyruvate, and more citrate is formed in the mitochondria (Fig. 46-3). The citrate diffuses back into the cytoplasm, where it is a potent activator of the first step in the synthesis of fatty acids (acetyl CoA → malonyl CoA). Citrate is also split into acetyl CoA and oxaloacetate; the acetyl CoA provides substrate for fatty acid synthesis. Furthermore, other glucose molecules are oxidized via the pentose shunt pathway, which generates NADPH, also needed for fatty acid synthesis. Thus, when the sup-

ply of glucose is plentiful, some net conversion of glucose carbon to fatty acid carbon occurs with the following stoichiometry:

$$4^{1}/_{2} \text{ glucose} + 4 \text{ O}_2 \rightarrow \text{Palmitic acid} + 11 \text{ CO}_2$$

The resultant RQ is $11 \div 4 = 2.75$. Therefore, whenever the RQ in a human is greater than 1.0, **lipogenesis** from glucose is likely to be occurring. In addition, glycolysis will produce more glycerol phosphate from triose phosphates. The combination of increased fatty acid synthesis and glycerol phosphate availability results in accentuated synthesis of triglycerides and reduced oxidation of fat. Thus, increased carbohydrate utilization shifts fat metabolism from oxidation to storage. *Many of these intrinsic chemical checks and balances are also reinforced by hormonal effects, particularly those of insulin and glucagon.*

■ *Energy Transfer between Organs*

In addition to these intracellular relationships, transfer of energy between organs is another important aspect of metabolism. The stored energy contained within adipose tissue triglycerides is transported in the form of FFAs to the liver. There, part of their energy (but not their carbon atoms) is effectively transferred to glucose molecules, because as fatty acids are oxidized, gluconeogenesis is stimulated concurrently, as previously described. The newly synthesized glucose molecules can then be transported to muscle tissue, where their energy is released during glycolysis and applied to muscle contraction. Furthermore, if the rate at which lactate is produced in the muscle during glycolysis exceeds the ability of the muscle to oxidize it in the citric acid cycle, the lactate can be returned to the liver, where it may again be built back up into glucose molecules. *From this standpoint, the liver is a flexible and versatile organ that can transmute and transfer energy from fuel depots to working tissues.*

■ *Carbohydrate Metabolism*

Dietary carbohydrates are broken down into various sugars (hexoses), the most important of which are glucose, fructose, and galactose. In addition to serving as energy sources, sugars are components of glycoproteins, glycopeptides, and glycolipids. These substances have structural and functional roles in basement membrane collagen, mucopolysaccharides, nerve cell myelin, hormones, and hormone receptors.

Glucose is the central molecule in carbohydrate metabolism. Other sugars are metabolized through the glucose pathways. The initial step in glucose metabolism is transport of the hexose across the cell membrane down a normally large concentration gradient from extracellular fluid to cytoplasm. This process, called *facilitated dif-*

fusion, is different from active transport against a concentration gradient (see Chapter 1). Facilitated diffusion is carried out by a family of glucose transport proteins (referred to as Glut-1, Glut-2, Glut-3, etc.) that are coded for by closely related genes. Each transport protein spans the plasma membrane 12 times, and both its amino and carboxy termini are located within the cytoplasm. The Glut-1 transporter is expressed constitutively and is responsible for the low level of basal glucose uptake required to sustain the energy generation process carried out by all cells. The number of these transporters is increased by fasting and decreased by an excess of glucose. The Glut-4 transporter is expressed exclusively in cardiac and skeletal muscle and adipose tissue and is specifically responsible for the glucose utilization that is stimulated by the hormone insulin (see Chapter 47). Glut-2 is expressed by hepatic and renal tubular cells that transfer glucose out of the cell and into the extracellular fluid and plasma. Glut-2 is also present in insulin-secreting cells of the pancreatic islets, where it maintains virtual equilibrium between the glucose concentrations in the extracellular fluid and cytoplasm.

Basal plasma glucose levels are closely regulated around an average concentration of 80 mg/dl^{-1} (4.5 μmol/L^{-1}), with a range of 60 to 110 mg/dl^{-1}.

> When the plasma glucose level falls progressively below 60 mg/dl^{-1}, brain uptake of glucose and utilization of oxygen decrease in parallel. If the homeostatic mechanisms described in Chapter 45 fail, central nervous system function becomes progressively impaired. Convulsions, coma, and death may ensue.

The major products of glycolysis, lactate and pyruvate, circulate at average concentrations of 0.7 and 0.07 mM, respectively. This 10:1 ratio of lactate to pyruvate ordinarily prevails, even when the glycolytic rate changes, as long as oxygen is plentiful.

> When tissues are deprived of oxygen because of impaired circulation or respiration, the equilibrium between lactate and pyruvate shifts greatly toward lactate, the reduced molecule. Plasma concentrations of lactate as high as 30 mM may develop and produce severe metabolic acidosis (blood pH as low as 6.8). Gastrointestinal symptoms may be followed by progressive loss of consciousness and total system failure, often ending in death.

In the basal state, glucose turnover is about 2 mg/kg^{-1}/min^{-1} (11 μmol/kg^{-1}/min^{-1}), which is equivalent to about 9 g/hr^{-1} or 225 g/day^{-1} in adults. Approximately 55% of glucose use results from terminal oxidation, of which the brain accounts for the greatest part (Fig. 46-5). Another 20% results from glycolysis; the resultant lactate then returns to the liver for resynthesis into glucose (Cori cycle). Reuptake by the liver and other

splanchnic tissues accounts for the remaining 25% of glucose use. Most glucose use (about 70%) in the basal state is independent of insulin, a hormone with otherwise important regulatory effects on glucose metabolism.

The circulating pool of glucose is only slightly larger than the liver's glucose output in 1 hour. This pool is sufficient to maintain brain oxidation only for several hours, even if all other glucose use ceases. The limitations of the circulating glucose supply emphasize the crucial importance of continuous hepatic production of glucose in the fasting state. About 75% of this production results from glycogenolysis and 25% from gluconeogenesis. Hepatic uptake and subsequent use of circulating lactate account for more than half the glucose supplied by gluconeogenesis. The remainder is largely accounted for by amino acids, especially alanine. The supply of lactate comes from glycolysis in muscle, red blood cells, white blood cells, and a few other tissues. The amino acid precursors come from proteolysis of muscle. Despite the importance of precursors, however, simply increasing their supply does not increase the rate of gluconeogenesis. The necessary enzymes (Fig. 46-4) must also be up-regulated by hormonal modulation or by hepatic autoregulatory responses to the falling glucose concentrations.

When an individual ingests glucose after overnight fasting, approximately 70% of the load is assimilated by peripheral tissues, mainly muscle, and about 30% by splanchnic tissues, mainly the liver. Only 20% to 30% of a glucose load is oxidized during the 3 to 5 hours required for its absorption from the gastrointestinal tract. The remainder is stored as glycogen, partly in muscle and partly in liver. Glucose initially stored as muscle glyco-

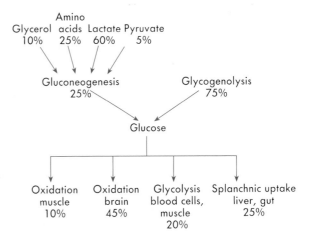

■ **Fig. 46-5** Quantitative overview of glucose turnover in overnight fasted humans. The disposal of circulating glucose *(lower portion)* is largely by oxidation and glycolysis, with the brain acting as the single largest consumer. The production of glucose in the circulation *(upper portion)* is largely from glycogenolysis. The proportionate contribution of glucose precursors to gluconeogenesis, with lactate predominating, is also shown. The average overall rate of glucose turnover is 2.0 mg/kg/min or 11 μmol/kg/min.

gen can later be transferred to the liver by undergoing glycolysis to lactate, which is released into the circulation; the lactate is then taken up by the liver, rebuilt into glucose, and stored as glycogen in that organ. During the period of peak absorption of exogenous glucose, hepatic output of the sugar is largely unnecessary and is greatly reduced from basal levels. These metabolic adaptations are facilitated by coordinated secretion of the pancreatic islet hormones insulin and glucagon.

■ *Protein Metabolism*

The average adult body contains 10 kg of protein, of which about 6 kg is metabolically active. This pool turns over continuously at a rate of 3 to 5 g/kg body weight/day; the degradative and synthetic reactions involved are estimated to account for 20% of the BMR. Of the amino acids released daily by proteolysis from muscle, the main endogenous repository for protein, a large part cycles back into protein synthesis. However, as much as 50 g is degraded. Therefore, daily dietary intake of 50 g of protein or 0.8 g/kg is ordinarily sufficient to replace what is lost by degradation. When accretion of lean body mass takes place (e.g., in growing children, pregnant women, or persons recovering from previous weight loss), daily protein requirements increase to 1.5 to 2.0 g/kg^{-1}.

All proteins are composed of the same 20 amino acids. Ten are **essential amino acids** because their carbon skeletons, the corresponding α-ketoacids, cannot be synthesized by humans. (The essential amino acids are threonine, methionine, valine, leucine, isoleucine, phenylalanine, tyrosine, tryptophane, lysine, and [in infants] histidine.) Once present in the body, however, the carbon skeletons can be converted to the essential amino acids by transamination. The other 10 amino acids are the **nonessential amino acids.** These amino acids can be synthesized endogenously because the appropriate carbon skeletons can be built from glucose metabolites in the citric acid cycle. The essential amino acids must be supplied in the diet, with individual minimal requirements ranging from 0.5 to 1.5 g/day^{-1}. All 20 amino acids are required for normal protein synthesis; therefore, a deficiency of even one essential amino acid disrupts this process.

Protein sources vary greatly in their biological effectiveness, depending in part on the ratio of essential to nonessential amino acids. Milk and egg proteins are of the highest quality in this regard. During infancy and childhood, about 40% of the protein intake should consist of essential amino acids in order to support growth. In adults, this requirement falls to 20%. In addition to their incorporation into proteins, many of the amino acids, including some essential ones, are precursors for important molecules, such as purines, pyrimidines, polyamines, phospholipids, creatine, carnitine, methyl

donors, thyroid and catecholamine hormones, and neurotransmitters.

The plasma concentrations of the individual amino acids range widely from 20 to 500 μmol/L^{-1}. All 20 amino acids can be completely oxidized to CO_2 and H_2O after removal of the amino group. Each traverses a specific degradative pathway. However, all these pathways converge into three general metabolic processes: **gluconeogenesis, ketogenesis,** and **ureagenesis.** Except for leucine and lysine, all the amino acids can contribute carbon atoms for the synthesis of glucose. Five ketogenic amino acids give rise either to acetoacetate or its CoA precursors. In the degradation of all amino acids, ammonia is released. Ammonia, incorporated mainly into glutamine and alanine molecules, is then transported to the liver. In the liver, ammonia is "detoxified" by incorporation into urea, a metabolically inert molecule. The synthesis of urea by the Krebs-Henseleit cycle is depicted in Fig. 46-6. The urea resulting from protein degradation is excreted by the kidney (see Chapter 42).

In the healthy adult under steady-state conditions, the total daily nitrogen excreted in the urine as urea plus ammonia, along with minor losses of nitrogen in the feces (0.4 g/day^{-1}) and skin (0.3 g/day^{-1}), is equal to the nitrogen released during metabolism of exogenous and endogenous protein. Such an individual is said to be in **nitrogen balance.** In the absence of dietary protein intake, the sum of urea plus ammonia nitrogen in the urine reflects almost quantitatively the rate of endogenous protein degradation. Because the nitrogen from the degraded protein is not being replaced, such an individual is said to be in **negative nitrogen balance.** *When protein breakdown is greatly accelerated by tissue trauma or disease, urinary urea plus ammonia nitrogen may exceed protein nitrogen intake.* Again, the individual is said to be in **negative nitrogen balance.** Conversely, in a growing child or in a previously malnourished individual undergoing protein repletion with gain in body mass, urinary

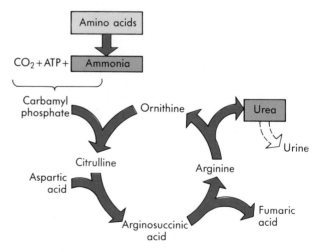

■ **Fig. 46-6** The Krebs-Henseleit urea cycle for disposal of ammonia generated by the metabolism of amino acids.

urea plus ammonia nitrogen excretion is less than the intake of protein nitrogen. This individual is said to be in **positive nitrogen balance.**

Protein deficiency can occur in various settings, ranging from poor third world countries to hospitals and nursing homes in the United States. In the former, the available protein supply is either too low or expensive. In the latter, protein deficiency results from nutritional miscalculations during assisted or artificial feeding. Selective protein deficiency with sufficient caloric intake leads to **kwashiorkor.** Signs and symptoms of this condition include low plasma albumin levels, edema (fluid retention), fragile hair and skin, reduced healing of wounds, and depressed cellular immune function with increased infections.

Measurements of external nitrogen balance do not themselves quantitate the dynamic internal equilibrium between protein synthesis and protein degradation. Protein degradation must be estimated by labeling body protein with an isotopic amino acid tracer, such as ^{15}N-glycine, and determining the flux of protein from measurements of ^{15}N-specific activity. Such studies show that healthy adults receiving isocaloric diets containing adequate protein degrade and synthesize protein at a rate of 3 to 4 g/kg/day. Individual synthesis rates for most proteins are not known, but the hepatic synthesis of albumin accounts for about 5% of the total. The rate of total body

protein synthesis is diminished when the diet is severely deficient in energy, in total protein, or in one of the essential amino acids. In such situations, the rate of protein degradation usually also diminishes, but not to the same extent as synthesis, so that net loss of body protein results.

In addition to the flux of total body protein, each individual amino acid undergoes its own unique turnover. It is instructive to contrast the turnover of two amino acids: leucine, an essential amino acid, and alanine, a nonessential amino acid.

The only source of leucine in the postabsorptive state is endogenous protein degradation (Fig. 46-7, *A*). Oxidation accounts for 20% of leucine disappearance from plasma, whereas 80% is reincorporated into new protein molecules. From a knowledge of the rate of leucine production (0.2 mg/kg/min) and the average leucine content of protein (8%), the rate of proteolysis can be estimated at 2.5 mg/kg/min. Hormonal effects on protein breakdown can then be assessed in this way. After ingestion of food, leucine oxidation diminishes and more leucine is used for protein synthesis. *However, because leucine oxidation is continuous and irreversible, a daily dietary intake of approximately 1 g of leucine must be provided.* During prolonged fasting, oxidation of leucine contributes slightly to energy needs. More important, leucine produced by catabolism of dispensable proteins helps maintain the synthesis of other more critical proteins.

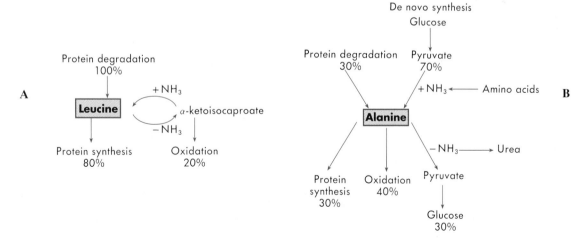

■ **Fig. 46-7** **A,** Quantitative turnover of leucine, *an essential amino acid,* in overnight fasted humans. Protein degradation is the only source for this amino acid whose carbon skeleton (*α*-ketoisocaproate) cannot be synthesized. Most leucine disposal is effected via reincorporation into protein synthesis. The leucine that is lost daily by oxidation must be replaced by dietary intake. **B,** Quantitative turnover of alanine, *a nonessential amino acid,* in overnight fasted humans. Alanine production is mostly by de novo synthesis from pyruvate, with a lesser contribution from protein degradation. Alanine disposal takes place via reincorporation into protein, oxidation, and gluconeogenesis. Alanine molecules, which arise from pyruvate and are reconverted to pyruvate, act as carriers for ammonia transferred from other amino acids. (Data in **A** from Matthews D et al: *Am J Physiol* 238:473, 1980; data in **B** from Chochinov R et al: *Diabetes* 27:287, 1978.)

The turnover of alanine in the postabsorptive state is more complex (Fig. 46-7, *B*). About 30% of alanine is produced from protein degradation. The other 70% of alanine arises from de novo synthesis: the carbon skeleton of alanine comes from glucose by way of pyruvate, and the amino group of alanine by transamination from other amino acids. The disposal of plasma alanine reflects three major routes and processes: about 40% is oxidized via the citric acid cycle after reconversion to pyruvate, about 30% reappears as glucose via gluconeogenesis from pyruvate, and the remaining 30% is reused for protein synthesis. Fig. 46-7, *B* shows that a glucose-alanine cycle, analogous to the glucose-lactate (Cori) cycle, can be envisioned. In this cycle, alanine functions as a carrier of amino groups from muscle to liver. Except for glutamine, alanine is the predominant amino acid released by muscle. It is formed there from pyruvate by transamination from other amino acids released during muscle proteolysis. Alanine is then extracted by the liver, where the amino group is removed for urea synthesis and thereby regenerates pyruvate for gluconeogenesis. Fig. 46-7, *B* also shows that although alanine is a gluconeogenic amino acid, no *net* synthesis of glucose from protein results from this particular pathway. Carbon atoms merely shuttle from one glucose molecule to another via pyruvate and alanine.

■ Fat Metabolism

Fat usually represents almost half the total daily substrate for oxidation (about 100 g, or 900 kcal). The usual daily intake in the United States is also approximately 100 g, or 40% of total calories. The major component of both dietary and storage fat consists of triglycerides. Exogenous triglycerides from the diet are absorbed as chylomicrons, whereas endogenous triglycerides are synthesized largely in the liver. Both consist of long-chain saturated (palmitic and stearic) and monounsaturated (oleic) fatty acids esterified to glycerol. Because these fatty acids can also be synthesized in the liver and adipose tissue, in an overall sense, no strict dietary requirement exists for fat. De novo synthesis of FFA from carbohydrate ordinarily occurs at a low rate, however.

About 3% to 5% of fatty acids are polyunsaturated and cannot be synthesized in the body. These fatty acids are termed **essential dietary fatty acids** (linoleic, linolenic, and arachidonic) because they are required as precursors for certain membrane phospholipid and glycolipid substances, as well as for important intracellular mediators known as prostaglandins. Another component of fat, the steroid molecule cholesterol, serves a variety of specific functions in membranes and is the precursor for bile acids and steroid hormones. Cholesterol is both ingested and synthesized by most cells.

■ Concentrations of Important Plasma Lipids

Table 46-3 presents the average basal concentrations of the most important plasma lipids. Although FFAs circulate at the lowest concentration, their plasma half-life is by far the shortest (2 minutes) and their rate of turnover is the greatest (up to 200 g/day). From 30% to 40% of plasma FFA molecules are oxidized, largely by muscle, where they are the major fuel; 50% to 70% are re-esterified, cycling back to triglycerides. The rate of oxidation is largely proportional to the plasma FFA concentration. Plasma FFA derived from dietary fat or adipose tissue stores contributes 50% of total lipid oxidation; the remainder mainly comes from oxidation of intracellular lipids prestored in heart, muscle, and liver. Plasma ketoacids, derived from beta oxidation, can also be oxidized by muscle, but they become an important fuel only in muscle and in the central nervous system during prolonged fasting.

■ Production, Transport, and Fate of Plasma Lipoproteins

The production, transport, and fate of plasma lipoproteins are very complex. Triglycerides and cholesterol, which form the major components of plasma lipids (Table 46-3), circulate as complex lipoprotein particles ranging in size from 75 to 1500 μm. The nonpolar, hydrophobic core of these particles contains triglyceride and cholesterol esters, whereas their polar, hydrophilic surfaces consist of phospholipid, cholesterol, and apoproteins. The plasma lipoproteins are classified according to their physical densities (Table 46-4). As would be expected, the lowest density particles contain primarily triglycerides. As the particles increase in density, the triglyceride proportion decreases while that of phospholipid and protein increases. Numerous apoproteins, varying in size and charge, are found among the lipoprotein classes. *The varied functions of apoproteins include facilitation of triglyceride transport out of the intestine and liver, activation of enzymes of lipoprotein metabolism, and attachment of the lipoprotein particles to specific cell surface receptors.* Apoproteins can also be

■ **Table 46-3** Average lipid concentrations in postabsorptive plasma

	mg/dl	*μmole/L*
Ketoacids	10	0.1
Free fatty acids	10	0.4
Triglycerides	100	1.2
Cholesterol (total)	185	4.8
Low density	120	
High density	50	
Very low density	15	

exchanged by lipoprotein particles, a process that facilitates the normal traffic of lipids through the blood.

Chylomicrons are formed from dietary fat and circulate only after a meal. These chylomicrons are transported across the intestinal wall into the blood, as detailed in Chapter 39. They are rapidly cleared from plasma, their half-life being 5 minutes. On the capillary endothelial surfaces of adipose tissue, muscle, and heart, chylomicron triglyceride is partly hydrolyzed by the enzyme **lipoprotein lipase** (Fig. 46-8). This enzyme is activated by apoprotein CII. The liberated FFAs are transported across the endothelial cells and taken up for resynthesis and storage as intracellular triglycerides. The remaining particles, known as **chylomicron remnants,** now contain less triglyceride and are enriched with cholesterol esters by interaction with **high-density lipoprotein (HDL) particles.** These remnants have also acquired apoprotein E, which, with apoprotein B48, directs their uptake by the liver. In the liver, the remnants are degraded to FFAs, glycerol, and free cholesterol; their portion becomes part of amino acids. Thus, the net result of chylomicron metabolism is to transfer most of the dietary triglycerides to adipose tissue and the dietary cholesterol to the liver.

Very-low-density lipoprotein (VLDL) particles are the major source of plasma triglycerides in the postabsorptive state. VLDL particles are synthesized and secreted largely by the liver, with a smaller contribution from the intestine. Under normal dietary circumstances, about 15 g of VLDL are produced per day. However, this amount can increase threefold to sixfold to accommodate high-calorie or high-carbohydrate diets. VLDL particles have a plasma half-life of about 2 hours. The initial phase of VLDL metabolism follows the same route as chylomicrons (Fig. 46-8). After lipolysis by lipoprotein lipase and interaction with HDL particles, the partially triglyceride-depleted and cholesterol-enriched particle is called **intermediate-density lipoprotein (IDL)** (Table 46-4). About half of the IDL particles are taken up by the liver, directed by apoprotein E and apoprotein B100. However, the other 50% is converted to **low-density lipoprotein (LDL)** particles in the blood and liver. These particles transfer exogenous and endogenous cholesterol to other tissues.

LDL is the major cholesterol-containing compound in plasma (Table 46-3) and it turns over with a half-life of 24 hours. The average daily amount of cholesterol absorbed from the diet (300 mg) plus the average amount synthesized (600 mg) is balanced by daily excretion of cholesterol in the form of bile salts and neutral steroids. Hepatic synthesis of cholesterol varies inversely with the dietary intake, thereby maintaining a constant input.

The cholesterol esters in LDL particles, generated as described earlier, are taken up by numerous cells that have specific LDL receptors that recognize the LDL particles, apoprotein E and apoprotein B100 (Fig. 46-8). Once internalized in a cell, cholesterol esters are hydrolyzed in lysosomes to free cholesterol, which is then used by different cells for various purposes. Cholesterol may also be re-esterified (a reaction catalyzed by acyl-CoA-cholesterol acyltransferase) and then stored.

The free cholesterol level within the cell regulates itself. Cholesterol diminishes its own further uptake into the cell by down-regulating the LDL receptor. Cholesterol also reduces its own intracellular de novo synthesis by suppressing the rate-limiting enzyme hydroxymethylglutaryl-CoA (HMG-CoA) reductase.

HDL particles (Table 46-4) perform crucial functions in transferring lipid components between other lipoprotein particles and ultimately between organs. They also facilitate enzyme activities in the metabolism of lipoproteins. HDL particles synthesized in the liver contain primarily apoprotein C and apoprotein E; those that are synthesized in the intestine contain primarily apoprotein A. Nascent HDL is released as small, relatively dense spherical particles. Shortly after entering the circulation, they acquire phospholipids and a bilayer, discoid shape and equilibrate their apoprotein contents. The plasma half-life of HDL is 5 to 6 days.

HDL assists in the previously described hydrolysis of chylomicron and VLDL triglycerides to FFA (Fig. 46-8) by providing apoprotein C for the activation of lipoprotein lipase. HDL also facilitates the flow of excess plasma triglycerides back to the liver, the flow of cholesterol to peripheral cells, and reverse transport of cholesterol back to the liver (Figs. 46-8 and 46-9). In this process, the smaller and denser subfraction HDL_3 accepts free cholesterol from peripheral cells and from remnant and IDL particles. This free cholesterol is then esterified by the plasma enzyme **lecithin-cholesterol acyltransferase (LCAT);** this esterification is activated

■ **Table 46-4**   Major lipoprotein classes

			Cholesterol			
	Density	*Triglyceride (%)*	*Free (%)*	*Esters (%)*	*Phospholipid (%)*	*Protein (%)*
Chylomicrons	<0.94	85	2	4	8	2
VLDL	0.94-1.006	60	6	16	18	10
IDL	1.006-1.019	30	8	22	22	18
LDL	1.019-1.063	7	10	40	20	25
HDL	1.063-1.21	5	4	15	30	50

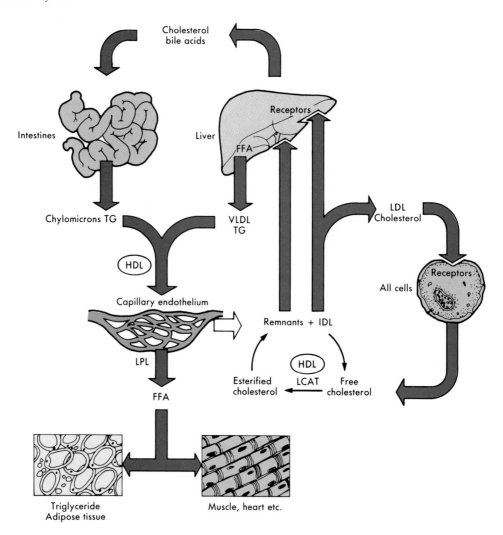

■ **Fig. 46-8**   Schematic overview of lipoprotein metabolism and major aspects of lipid turnover in humans. Exogenous triglycerides (*TG,* chylomicrons absorbed from the intestine) and endogenous triglycerides (very-low-density lipoproteins, *VLDL,* produced in the liver) both give rise to free fatty acids (*FFA*) for storage in adipose tissue and oxidation in muscle. High-density lipoprotein (*HDL*) particles facilitate, and the enzyme lipoprotein lipase *(LPL)* directly catalyzes, liberation of the FFA from TG. The resultant particles, called remnants from chylomicrons and intermediate-density lipoproteins *(IDL)* from VLDL, undergo further change in the circulation, which is also facilitated by HDL. The ratio of esterified cholesterol to free cholesterol is increased in the remnant and IDL particles by the enzyme lecithin-cholesterol acyltransferase *(LCAT).* The remnant particles are then taken up by the liver for further metabolism. The IDL particles are partly taken up by the liver and partly converted to cholesterol-rich low-density lipoprotein *(LDL)* particles. The latter are then taken up by virtually all cells after interaction with specific LDL receptors. Cholesterol, either synthesized in the liver or extracted from remnant and IDL particles, is also excreted into the intestine, partly as bile acids.

by HDL apoprotein A_1. The cholesterol ester is then exchanged for triglycerides in other particles by the cholesterol-ester transfer protein; in this exchange process, the HDL changes to the larger and less dense HDL_2 subfraction. The exchanged cholesterol esters can either be delivered to the peripheral cells as LDL particles or be delivered to the liver, where they are taken up as part of remnant, IDL, and LDL particles. This latter process is called *reverse cholesterol transport.* The HDL_2 can itself

cycle back to HDL_3, as the triglycerides acquired in these exchanges are hydrolyzed by hepatic lipase (Fig. 46-9). The process of reverse cholesterol transport contributes significantly to the maintenance of physiologically appropriate and "healthy" lipoprotein levels.

The factors that influence the relative proportions of LDL and HDL particles are of great public health importance because cholesterol taken up from plasma

Reverse Cholesterol Transport

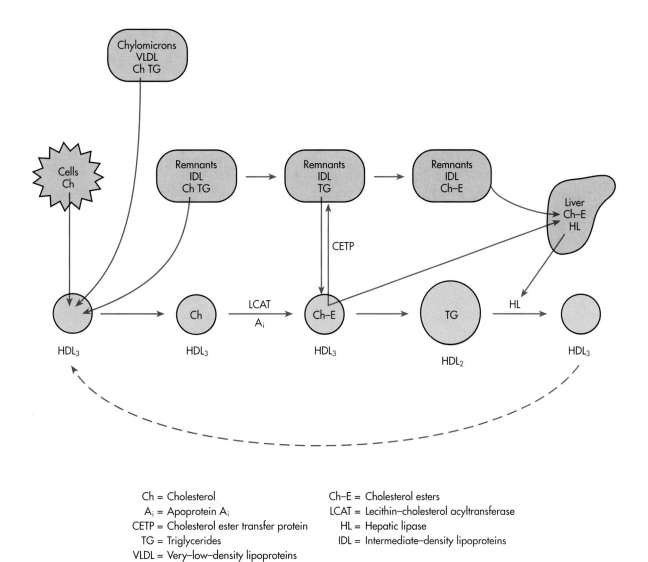

Ch = Cholesterol
A_i = Apoprotein A_i
CETP = Cholesterol ester transfer protein
TG = Triglycerides
VLDL = Very–low–density lipoproteins

Ch–E = Cholesterol esters
LCAT = Lecithin–cholesterol acyltransferase
HL = Hepatic lipase
IDL = Intermediate–density lipoproteins

■ **Fig. 46-9** Functioning of high-density lipoprotein *(HDL)*. HDL_3 particles accept and esterify cholesterol from cells and other lipoprotein particles. Apoprotein A_1 activates the key enzyme LCAT. The resultant particle exchanges cholesterol esters for triglycerides with chylomicrons and VLDL, becoming more buoyant HDL_2 particles. These in turn are relieved of the triglycerides by the action of hepatic lipase and cycle back to HDL_3 particles.

by macrophages as LDL particles is an essential component of atherosclerotic plaques in major blood vessels. *HDL particles help prevent this plaque formation by facilitating cellular LDL uptake.* LDL levels are higher in men than in women and are increased by androgens, smoking, obesity, a sedentary life style, a high saturated fat intake, and certain drugs. HDL levels are lower in men than in women and are decreased by androgens, smoking, obesity, a high polyunsaturated fat diet, and non–insulin-dependent type 2 diabetes. HDL levels are increased by estrogens, exercise conditioning, and moderate alcohol intake. *These effects partly explain the fact that male gender, a lack of physical fitness, obesity, and smoking are strong risk factors for atherosclerotic premature cardiovascular disease and death.* After menopause, the relative protection enjoyed by women disappears. Strenuous public health efforts are under way to screen individuals for a high LDL/HDL ratio (>4.0) and to lower the ratio by decreased intake of saturated fat to less than 30% of total calories, weight reduction, cessation of smoking, and increased exercise.

Major abnormalities in lipoprotein levels are also caused by genetic defects in the pathways of lipid metabolism. A deficiency in lipoprotein lipase activity leads to excessive and prolonged chylomicron and triglyceride levels after ingestion of fat-containing meals; these high levels can cause severe inflammation of the pancreas. Mutations that cause deficient or low-affinity cell surface LDL receptors lead to extremely high plasma LDL cholesterol levels, visible deposits of cholesterol in skin and tendons, and premature coronary artery disease **(familial hypercholesterolemia).** Synthesis of an abnormal apoprotein E, which cannot efficiently direct lipoprotein particles to interact with cell receptors, leads to accumulation of chylomicron remnants and IDL in plasma. In this situation, both triglyceride and cholesterol levels are elevated, a condition that increases the risk of coronary artery disease. Another cause of this dual abnormality is excessive production of apoprotein B100 **(familial-combined hyperlipidemia).** Conversely, a deficiency of apoprotein B leads to very low levels of chylomicrons, VLDL, and LDL in plasma, but with pathological accumulation of triglycerides in the intestines and the liver.

■ *Metabolic Adaptations*

■ *Fasting*

In the fasting state, the individual totally depends on endogenous substrates for energy (Fig. 46-10). Mobilization of glucose provides essential fuel for the central nervous system; release of FFAs provides for the oxidative needs of the other tissues. An increase in protein degradation to amino acids is also a fundamental feature of this response. The fasting individual is said to be in a state of **catabolism,** because carbohydrate, fat, and protein stores all decrease.

During fasting, the liver initially supplies glucose to the circulation by augmenting glycogenolysis. After 12 to 15 hours of fasting, however, hepatic glycogen stores are greatly depleted, and a rapid enhancement of gluconeogenesis fills the void. To supply glucose precursors, 75 to 100 g of muscle protein are broken down daily during the first few days of a fast. This muscle breakdown is reflected in a rising excretion of urea in the urine. Gluconeogenesis is also enhanced by the provision of 15 to 20 g of glycerol daily, which is released during the accelerated lipolysis of triglycerides in adipose tissue.

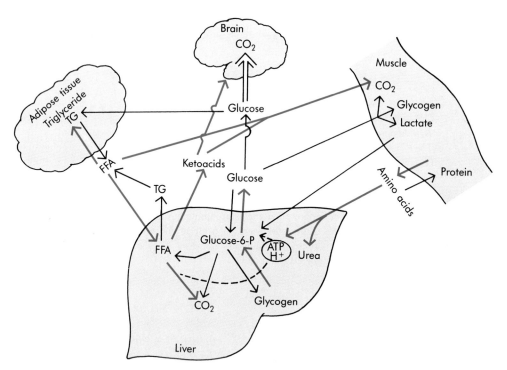

■ **Fig. 46-10**   Pattern of substrate flow in the fasting state. Adipose tissue increases free fatty acid (FFA) supply to the liver, where FFA is used for energy, for ketogenesis, and to generate ATP and reducing equivalents for gluconeogenesis. In muscle, FFA oxidation spares glucose use. Muscle increases amino acid flow to the liver for use in gluconeogenesis. The ammonia released from the amino acids is detoxified by incorporation into urea. Hepatic glucose production from glycogenolysis and gluconeogenesis is augmented. Glucose uptake by the liver, adipose tissue, and muscle is diminished, but uptake by the brain is sustained. Ketoacid production by the liver and eventually ketoacid use by peripheral tissues are increased. *TG,* Triglycerides; Glucose-6-P, glucose-6-phosphate; *colored arrows,* increased flow of fuel; *black arrows,* decreased flow of fuel.

Glucose oxidation in muscle and liver is spared as increasing quantities of FFAs become available. Muscle lipoprotein lipase activity increases to facilitate uptake of triglycerides for oxidation; adipose lipoprotein lipase activity decreases to dampen uptake of triglyceride for storage.

A portion of fatty acid oxidation in liver yields the ketoacids β-hydroxybutyrate and acetoacetate, which spare the use of glucose by muscle cells. The shift away from glucose and toward fatty acid oxidation lowers the respiratory quotient. These adaptations are reflected in changing plasma concentrations of substrates (Fig. 46-11). Levels of glucose and the major gluconeogenic amino acid, alanine, decrease, whereas levels of FFAs, glycerol, and branched-chain amino acids, such as leucine, increase. High levels of the strong ketoacids produce a tendency to metabolic acidosis with a slight reduction in blood pH. Much of this pattern of adaptation is mediated by hormonal modification, particularly decreasing insulin production and increasing glucagon production (Fig. 46-11).

After a few days, other important adaptations occur. Total energy expenditure, reflected in the BMR, decreases 10% to 20% and limits the drain on energy stores. The central nervous system no longer depends entirely on glucose as an energy source, and two thirds of its needs are eventually met by the ketoacids. As less glucose is needed for oxidation, gluconeogenesis diminishes and protein breakdown declines to 25 to 30 g/day^{-1}. Protein synthesis also decreases. In long-term fasting, body weight diminishes by an average of 300 g/day^{-1}, of which two thirds is accounted for by fat and one third by lean tissue. As long as sufficient fluid is ingested, an individual of normal weight can survive a fast of up to 60 days. At this time, fat stores are almost exhausted, protein degradation rapidly accelerates, and death follows. This flow of substrates, shown in Fig. 46-10, is reversed after feeding. Glucose enters the plasma from dietary carbohydrate, FFAs from dietary triglycerides, and amino acids from protein. Each substrate is stored as described, and the individual is said to be in a state of **anabolism.**

■ *Exercise*

The metabolic response to exercise resembles the response to fasting, in that the mobilization and generation of fuels for oxidation are dominant factors. The type and amounts of expended substrate vary with the intensity and duration of the exercise (Fig. 46-12). During very intense, short-term exercise (e.g., a 10- to 15-second sprint), stored creatine phosphate and ATP provide the energy at a rate of approximately 50 kcal/min^{-1}. When these stores are depleted, additional intense exercise for up to 2 minutes can be sustained by breakdown of muscle glycogen to glucose-6-phosphate, with glycolysis

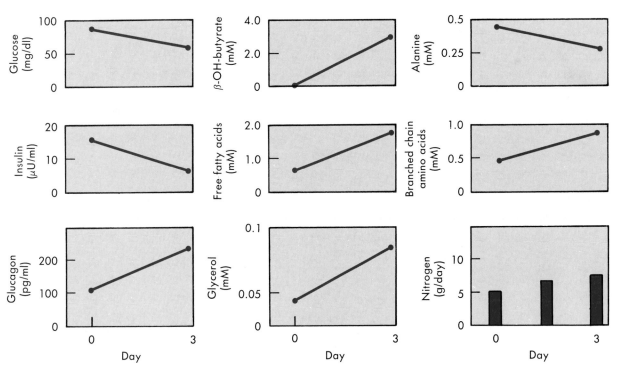

■ Fig. 46-11 Changes in plasma substrate levels, urine nitrogen excretion, and plasma insulin and glucagon during 3 days of fasting in humans. Note the rise in lipid-derived fuels and products of proteolysis. These changes are mediated in part by a fall in insulin and a rise in glucagon (hormones from the pancreatic islets). (Redrawn from Felig P et al: *J Clin Invest* 48:584, 1969. From the American Society for Clinical Investigation.)

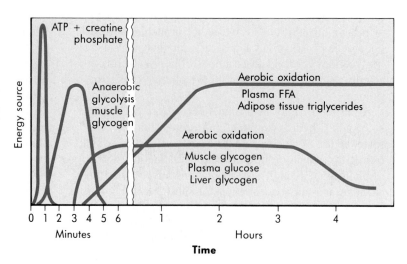

■ **Fig. 46-12**   Energy sources during exercise. Note the sequential use of stored high-energy phosphate bonds, glycogen, circulating glucose, and circulating free fatty acids *(FFA)*. The latter dominate in sustained exercise.

yielding the necessary energy (at a rate of 30 kcal/min^{-1}). This **anaerobic** phase is not limited by depletion of muscle glycogen at this point, but rather by the rapid accumulation of lactic acid in the exercising muscles and the circulation.

After several minutes of exhaustive anaerobic exercise, an oxygen debt of 10 to 12 L can be built up. This debt must be repaid before the exercise can be repeated. From 6 to 8 L of oxygen are required either to rebuild the accumulated lactic acid back into glucose in the liver or to oxidize it to CO_2. About 2 L of oxygen are required to replenish normal muscle ATP and creatine phosphate content. An additional 2 L of oxygen will replenish the oxygen normally present in the lungs and body fluids and oxygen bound to myoglobin and hemoglobin.

For less intense but longer periods of exercise, **aerobic** oxidation of substrates is required to produce the necessary energy (at a maximum of about 12 kcal/min^{-1}). Substrates from the circulation are added to muscle glycogen (Fig. 46-12). After a few minutes, glucose uptake from the plasma increases dramatically, up to thirtyfold in some muscle groups. Resting glucose uptake by muscle is regulated by the hormone insulin, and this effect increases somewhat with exercise. However, an entirely separate insulin-independent factor comes into play during exercise, one that markedly enhances glucose transfer into muscle cells. To offset the drain of glucose by muscle and maintain a normal plasma glucose level, hepatic glucose production must increase up to fivefold. Initially, the glucose produced is largely from glycogenolysis. Indeed, endurance can be improved by high-carbohydrate feedings for several days before prolonged exercise (e.g., a marathon run), because this carbohydrate "loading" increases both liver and muscle glycogen stores. With exercise of longer duration, however, gluconeogenesis becomes increasingly important as liver glycogen stores become depleted. To support gluconeogenesis, amino acids are increasingly released by muscle proteolysis, and their fractional uptake by the

liver is enhanced. The activities of key gluconeogenic enzymes such as **phosphoenolpyruvate carboxykinase (PEPCK)** are increased, and even transcription of their genes is induced. These events are coordinated by increased sympathetic neural activity and the relative effects of the hormones glucagon and insulin (see Chapter 47).

Eventually, fatty acids liberated from adipose tissue triglycerides become the predominant substrate and supply two thirds of the energy needs during sustained exercise. Except for increases in circulating pyruvate and lactate levels resulting from greatly enhanced glycolysis, the pattern of change in the other plasma substrates is similar to that of fasting (Fig. 46-11), but it occurs over a much shorter time frame.

During recovery from exercise, muscle and liver glycogen stores must be rebuilt, and these processes require energy input. Some energy is also needed during this period to recycle unexpended FFAs back into triglycerides.

Several diseases that affect muscle function and exercise capacity result from genetic defects in energy-generating steps. First, in **McArdle's disease** or **muscle phosphorylase deficiency,** glycogen cannot be rapidly broken down to glucose-6- phosphate (Fig. 46-4), and hence pain and weakness occur during even brief exercise. The impairment in glycolysis from lack of substrate is demonstrated by a failure of lactate levels to rise in a draining vein after anaerobic forearm muscle exercise when the arterial inflow is occluded. Second, in **von Gierke's disease** or **glucose-6-phosphatase deficiency,** hepatic glucose release is impaired, which limits the supply of glucose during the early phase of exercise. Third, deficiencies of beta-oxidation enzymes (Fig. 46-2) or of **carnitine** or **carnitine palmitoyl transferase** (required to transfer FFAs into the mitochondria) prevent efficient use of FFAs. As a result, exercise capacity is reduced and exercise produces muscle weakness and pain. The second and third conditions also lead to hypoglycemia during fasting, because hepatic glucose production is decreased.

■ Regulation of Energy Stores

The preponderance of stored energy consists of fat, and individuals vary greatly in the amounts and percentages of body weight accounted for by adipose tissue. What determines the physiologically proper quantity of this energy reserve, and what regulates it? Does an ideal relationship exist between total fat mass and either total body weight or total lean body mass? Do all adipose tissue sites function in the same way as storage depots?

It is estimated that about 25% of the variance in total body fat and 30% to 35% of the variance in subcutaneous truncal and abdominal fat is accounted for by genetic factors. A genetic influence on fat mass is supported by (1) the tendency for body mass of adopted children to correlate better with that of their biological parents than with that of their adoptive parents; (2) the much greater similarity of adipose stores in identical (monozygotic) twins, whether reared together or apart, than in fraternal (dizygotic) twins; (3) the greater correlation between the total weight gains and increases in abdominal fat of identical twins than in fraternal twins when fed a caloric excess; (4) the identification of genes that inexorably cause obesity in animal models that exhibit autosomal recessive inheritance of the trait; and (5) the isolation of one such mouse gene from the analogous human chromosome and the demonstration of its product (a peptide named **leptin**) in human adipose tissue and plasma.

Environmental and cultural influences on energy stores, specifically the quality and quantity of the food available, are suggested by the excessive weight gain of certain laboratory animals in response to presentation of high-fat or "junk food" diets, as well as by the much greater prevalence of obesity in affluent and relatively sedentary westernized societies than in other populations. Also, the human species has more energy-storage adipose cells per unit body mass than any other species except whales; this high adipose cell content may contribute to a propensity for larger fat masses.

Some data suggest the existence of a particular set point for energy stores in each individual. Once adult weight is reached, it tends to be constant, at least until middle age, at which point most humans incur at least a modest weight gain that leads to a higher proportion of body fat. Abdominal fat particularly increases with age, and more so in men. Normal and genetically obese laboratory rodents subjected to forced overfeeding or underfeeding experiments return to their normal weight and degree of fatness when again allowed free access to food. In rodents, this compensatory control of appetite (caloric

Box 46-1   *Modulators of feeding behavior*

Stimulate	Inhibit
Neuropeptide Y	Leptin
Endorphins	Epinephrine/norepinephrine
Galanin	Serotonin
Norepinephrine	Urocortin
γ-Amino butyric acid	Corticotropin-releasing hormone
Cortisol	Glucagon-like peptide-1
	Cholecystokinin
	Calcitonin
	Bombesin
	Enterostatin
	Insulin

and nutrient intake) appears to reside in the lateral hypothalamus (a hunger center) and in the ventromedial hypothalamus (a satiety center).

Humans who suffer damage to the hypothalamus from neoplasms or infiltrative disorders, such as **sarcoidosis,** sometimes gain large amounts of weight to new plateaus of obesity. Conversely, in the hypothalamic dysfunction of **anorexia nervosa,** weight is maintained at low, even life-threatening levels.

A variety of afferent signals to the hypothalamus contribute to the stimulation of appetite. These signals include the sight, smell, taste, sweetness, and palatability of food; a 15% reduction in plasma glucose; and a decrease in FFA oxidation in the liver. Eating is inhibited by glucose in the duodenum or portal vein. A variety of neuropeptides in the brain, some also with gastrointestinal location and function, and a variety of neurotransmitters carry appetite regulatory signals to and within the central nervous system (Box 46-1). Some appear to be nutrient specific, such as serotonin (glucose) and enterostatin (fat). Some are under hormonal regulation, and some also interact. For example, insulin strongly inhibits the synthesis of neuropeptide Y, a potent stimulator of food intake; cortisol inhibits synthesis of corticotropin-releasing hormone, an appetite suppressor.

Homeostatic setting of energy stores also occurs by regulation of energy expenditure. In the animal experiments described above, spontaneous return to normal weight from an excess or a deficit of fat mass was accomplished by decreases or increases in daily energy expenditure, respectively. The same phenomenon has been documented both indirectly and directly in human investigations involving normal-weight and obese individuals. Such compensation may occur via obligatory non-shivering thermogenic processes, such as "futile cycles" that are wasteful of ATP (e.g., glucose → glucose-6-phosphate → glucose), ion pumping via the membrane enzyme Na^+, K^+-ATPase, or uncoupling of ATP formation from mitochondrial oxidation. In animals,

brown adipose tissue (BAT) seems specifically designed for such purposes. Its large mitochondria are stimulated by an uncoupling **protein,** also called **thermogenin,** that disassociates ATP production from oxygen utilization, and thereby generates heat without producing useful chemical or mechanical work. Thermogenin production is regulated by sympathetic nervous system signals, that is, norepinephrine interacting with B₃ receptors. Although BAT is clearly present and probably functional in human newborns who must suddenly adapt to a lowering of environmental temperature, this type of adipose tissue is also present but difficult to detect and even harder to quantitate in adult humans. A new and related **uncoupling protein** has recently been discovered in white adipose tissue of humans.

If there is a hypothalamic set point for energy stores in each individual, how does the hypothalamus sense and quantitate peripheral fat mass? One answer is now clear. Leptin, the obesity gene product discovered in obese mice and produced by adipose tissue, serves such a role.

In one mouse model, leptin is deficient because of a mutant leptin gene, and the animal is obese. This animal overeats, has a low BMR and low body temperature, and is inactive physically. Replacement therapy with leptin corrects all of these abnormalities and causes weight loss. In another mouse model, the obese animal has elevated levels of leptin, but the leptin receptor in the hypothalamus is defective because of a mutant gene. Treatment with leptin has no effect.

Discovery of leptin and its receptor now suggests at least one reasonable scheme for the regulation of energy stores (Fig. 46-13). When adipose tissue mass expands beyond a designated set point (because of an increased number of cells with normal triglyceride content, or a normal number of cells with increased triglyceride content, or both), leptin synthesis and secretion increase. The resultant elevated plasma leptin concentration leads to greater occupancy of leptin plasma membrane receptors in the hypothalamus and other areas of the brain. Leptin stimulation sets into motion multiple response mecha-

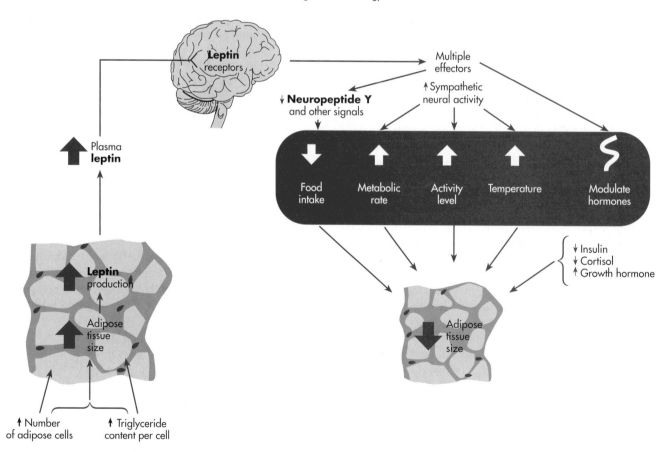

Feedback Regulation of Energy Stores

■ **Fig. 46-13** Overview of a current concept of regulation of energy stores. Leptin production and release and plasma levels are proportional to adipose mass and "report" the size of the latter to the hypothalamus and other brain areas. The occupied leptin receptor initiates a series of effector mechanisms that adjust the adipose mass downward when it increases beyond a set point that is physiologically optimal. Effector mechanisms decrease food intake, increase energy expenditure, and modulate secretion of hormones in order to decrease lipogenic activity and increase lipolytic activity of adipose tissue.

nisms that decrease adipose tissue mass. These endocrine, neural, and neurocrine mechanisms include decreasing food intake by decreasing production of appetite stimulators, such as neuropeptide Y; increasing energy expenditure by increasing BMR, body temperature, and physical activity; and changing the hormonal set in order to reduce lipogenesis in adipose tissue cells.

Plasma leptin levels do not increase acutely after food intake; thus, leptin probably does not act as an immediate regulator of energy turnover. Fasting for several days decreases leptin, while continuous hyperinsulinemia increases leptin. These responses may be the result of subtle decreases and increases in adipose mass, respectively, as well as a direct effect of insulin on leptin production.

Pathological accumulation of energy stores as fat (i.e., obesity) is a major health problem in many countries. A body weight 20% above desirable or ideal increases the risk of such disorders as diabetes, hypertension, and cardiovascular disease; a body weight 40% to 50% above desirable greatly increases the risk of death. Accumulation of fat in abdominal and particularly visceral depots confers especially high risk. The exact cause or causes of human obesity are not known. Some obese individuals overeat and recognize an inability to control it; most, however, report lower caloric intakes than they are actually ingesting. Because there are tight physiological controls on how many calories can be stored as carbohydrate or as protein, an excessive intake of fat is easier to envision as the source of calories if obesity results from an abnormality on the input side of the energy equation. Fatty acid oxidation is independent of fat intake, whereas oxidation of carbohydrate and protein is stimulated by their respective intakes.

Many obese individuals also behave as if they have an elevated set point for energy stores. These individuals appear to "defend" this set point tenaciously by decreasing energy expenditure when caloric intake is reduced by dieting and significant amounts (e.g., 19%) of weight are lost. In some studies, nonobese infants or adults with lower BMRs are at greater risk for future weight gain. However, once obesity is present and static, BMR, diet-induced thermogenesis, and the energy cost of exercise are generally equal to or greater than those of normal weight individuals. Thus, a continuous deficit in energy expenditure is an unlikely single explanation for obesity.

In obese humans the profile of certain hormones involved in regulation of fat metabolism (increased insulin and cortisol, decreased growth hormone) generally favors deposition rather than mobilization of fat. Endorphin levels are elevated, which suggests involvement of that neuropeptide in central appetite stimulation. In addition, adipose tissue of obese humans contains elevated levels of lipoprotein lipase, the key enzyme that transfers circulating triglycerides into cells. None of these abnormalities has been proved to be the primary cause of human obesity.

The initial studies of leptin in obese humans suggest that absolute leptin deficiency is an extremely rare cause of their obesity. Their plasma leptin levels are elevated and correlate with their increased fat mass. Messenger RNA levels for leptin are increased in their adipose cells and also correlate with their fat mass. Hence, it appears that the peripheral signal indicating that energy stores are too large is being generated, but it is not being received or acted upon normally in the hypothalamus. Thus, human obesity is likely to result from defects in the leptin receptor, in generation of its second messenger or effector mechanism within the leptin target cell(s) or in other effector cells further downstream (Fig. 46-13). Whether partial resistance to leptin can be overcome by sufficient exogenous leptin therapy is not known. Until this point is elucidated, treatment of obesity by dieting, disciplined exercise, behavior modification, and drugs that may act favorably at some point in the complex system that sets energy stores is palliative but not a cure.

■ *Summary*

1. Energy input as carbohydrate, fat, and protein calories must equal energy expenditure if body weight is to remain constant. Energy expenditure is composed of basal, diet-induced thermogenesis and sedentary activity components plus exercise and heavy labor needs. Basal metabolic rate (60% to 70% of total) is proportional to body mass, is in part genetically determined, and declines with aging.

2. Fatty acids are the major fuel in most tissues except for the central nervous system and red blood cells, where glucose is ordinarily the obligatory oxidative substrate. Depending on availability, fatty acids and glucose are competitive substrates in muscle mass and liver. Use of one spares use of, and may increase production of, the other.

3. Anaerobic glycolysis, beta oxidation of fatty acids, and disposal of acetyl CoA by the Krebs cycle are the biochemical mechanisms that generate ATP by oxidative phosphorylation. The overall efficiency of energy yield is 65%.

4. Energy is primarily stored as adipose tissue triglycerides. Lesser and less readily mobilizable amounts of energy are stored as protein. Carbohydrate stores are trivial; hence, the need for efficient glucose production by the liver (gluconeogenesis) to maintain a supply for the brain.

5. During long-term fasting, gluconeogenesis from amino acids, glycerol, and lactate is required to sustain central nervous system metabolism and other critical functions dependent on glucose. The pathway of gluconeogenesis is partly a reversal of glycolysis, but it requires special steps from pyruvate. Increased use of fatty acids during fasting greatly increases production of the ketoacids β-hydroxybutyrate and acetoacetate.

6. Endogenous protein turnover obligates a daily ingestion of protein, in particular, essential amino acids such as leucine. Essential amino acids are irreversibly degraded, and their carbon skeletons cannot be synthesized. The carbon skeletons of nonessential amino acids, such as alanine, are degraded and resynthesized daily. Protein synthesis requires the availability of all 20 amino acids.

7. Fat metabolism involves a variety of circulating lipoprotein particles that transfer triglycerides and cholesterol, either originating in the diet or from hepatic synthesis, to and from peripheral tissues and the liver. Low-density lipoprotein particles, rich in cholesterol, play a role in the development of atherosclerosis, whereas high-density lipoprotein particles have a protective effect.

8. Energy needs during exercise are met in sequence by stored muscle creatine phosphate plus ATP, stored muscle glycogen, anaerobic glycolysis, and (finally) aerobic oxidation of glucose and then fatty acids taken up from the plasma. These substrates are supplied by hepatic glycogenolysis and gluconeogenesis and adipose tissue lipolysis, respectively.

9. Correlation of energy intake and expenditure with energy stores is a complex process, controlled in the hypothalamus and involving numerous amine and peptide neurotransmitters and neuromodulators. The hypothalamus senses adipose tissue mass (energy stores) by reception of leptin, a circulating signal generated in adipose cells. Obesity can result from an altered set point of energy stores, from unregulated caloric intake, or from decreased energy use. Resistance to the action of leptin could be one cause of obesity.

■ *Self-Study Problems*

1. What are the elements of the system that regulates energy intake, storage, and expenditure?

2. What metabolic adjustments permit a normal human to survive up to 60 days of total fasting?

■ *Bibliography*

Journal articles

Bogardus C et al: Familial dependence of the resting metabolic rate, *N Engl J Med* 315:96, 1986.

Bouchard C, Després J-P, Mauriège P: Genetic and nongenetic determinants of regional fat dstribution, *Endocr Rev* 14:72, 1993.

Bray GA, York DA, Fisler JS: Experimental obesity, *Vitam Horm* 45:1, 1988.

Cahill GF: Starvation in man, *N Engl J Med* 282:668, 1970.

Caro JF et al: Leptin: the tale of an obesity gene, *Diabetes* 45:1455, 1996.

Dallman MF et al: The neural network that regulates energy balance is responsive to glucocorticoids and insulin and also regulates HPA axis responsivity at a site proximal to CRF neurons, *Ann NY Acad Sci* 771:730, 1995.

Eckel RH: Lipoprotein lipase: a multifunctional enzyme relevant to metabolic diseases, *N Engl J Med* 320:1060, 1989.

Exton JH: Gluconeogenesis, *Metabolism* 21:945, 1972.

Felig P et al: Amino acid metabolism during prolonged starvation, *J Clin Invest* 48:584, 1969.

Ferrannini E et al: The disposal of an oral glucose load in healthy subjects: a quantitative study, *Diabetes* 34:580, 1985.

Foster D: From glycogen to ketones—and back (Banting Lecture 1984), *Diabetes* 33:1188, 1984.

Giesecke K et al: Protein and amino acid metabolism during early starvation as reflected by excretion of urea and methylhistidines, *Metabolism* 38:1196, 1989.

Groop LC et al: Role of free fatty acids and insulin in determining free fatty acid and lipid oxidation in man, *J Clin Invest* 87:83, 1991.

Harris RBS: Role of set-point theory in regulation of body weight, *FASEB J* 4:3310, 1990.

Haymond M, Miles J: Branched chain amino acids as a major source of alanine nitrogen in man, *Diabetes* 31:86, 1982.

Jansky L: Humoral thermogenesis and its role in maintaining energy balance, *Physiol Rev* 75:237, 1995.

Katz L et al: Splanchnic and peripheral disposal of oral glucose in man, *Diabetes* 32:675, 1983.

Klein S, Coppack SW, Mohamed-Ali V, Landt M: Adipose tissue leptin production and plasma leptin kinetics in humans, *Diabetes* 45:984, 1996.

Klein S, Goran M: Energy metabolism in response to overfeeding in young adult men, *Metabolism* 42:1201, 1993.

Morley JE, Levine AS: Nutrition: the changing scene—the central control of appetite, *Lancet* 1:398, 1983.

Ravussin E et al: Determinants of 24-hour energy expenditure in man: methods and results using a respiratory chamber, *J Clin Invest* 78:1568, 1986.

Ravussin E, Swinburn BA: Energy expenditure and obesity, *Diabetes Rev* 4:403, 1996.

Reeds P, James W: Nutrition: the changing scene—protein turnover, *Lancet* 1:571, 1983.

Roberts SB et al: Dietary energy requirements of young adult men, determined by using the doubly labeled water method, *Am J Clin Nutr* 54:499, 1991.

Schaefer E et al: Pathogenesis and management of lipoprotein disorders, *N Engl J Med* 312:1300, 1985.

Segal KR, Landt M, Klein S: Relationship between insulin sensitivity and plasma leptin concentration in lean and obese men, *Diabetes* 45:988, 1996.

Sims EAH: Energy balance in human beings: the problems of plentitude, *Vitam Horm* 43:1, 1986.

Sims EAH, Danforth E Jr: Expenditure and storage of energy in man, *J Clin Invest* 79:1019, 1987.

Tall AR: Plasma high density lipoproteins, *J Clin Invest* 86:379, 1990.

Wasserman DH: Regulation of glucose fluxes during exercise in the postabsorptive state, *Annu Rev Physiol* 57:191, 1995.

Wasserman DH, Cherrington AD: Hepatic fuel metabolism during muscular work: role and regulation, *Am J Physiol* 260:E811, 1991.

Wolfe BM et al: Effect of elevated free fatty acids on glucose oxidation in normal humans, *Metabolism* 37:323, 1988.

Books and monographs

Flatt JP: *The biochemistry of energy expenditure.* In Bray G, editor: *Recent advances in obesity research, II.* Proceedings of the 2nd International Congress on Obesity, Los Angeles, 1978, Newman Publishing.

Kimball SR, Flaim KE, Peavy DE, Jefferson LS: *Protein metabolism.* In Rifkin H, Porte D Jr, editors: *Diabetes mellitus,* ed 4, New York, 1990, Elsevier Scientific Publishing.

Leibowitz SF: *Brain neurotransmitters and hormones in relation to eating behavior and its disorders.* In Bjorntorp P, Brodoff BN, editors: *Obesity,* Philadelphia, 1992, JB Lippincott.

McGarry JD, Foster DW: *Ketogenesis.* In Porte D Jr, Sherwin RS, editors: *Ellenberg & Rifkin's diabetes mellitus,* ed 5, Stamford, Conn, 1996, Appleton & Lange.

Seifter S, Englard S: *Carbohydrate metabolism.* In Rifkin H, Porte D Jr, editors: *Diabetes mellitus,* ed 4, New York, 1990, Elsevier Scientific Publishing.

Shulman GI, Barrett EJ, Sherwin RS: *Integrated fuel metabolism.* In Porte D Jr, Sherwin RS, editors: *Ellenberg & Rifkin's diabetes mellitus,* ed 5, Stamford, Conn, 1996, Appleton & Lange.

Woods SC, Kaiyala K, Porte D Jr, Schwartz MW: *Food intake and energy balance.* In Porte D Jr, Sherwin RS, editors: *Ellenberg & Rifkin's diabetes mellitus,* ed 5, Stamford, Conn, 1996, Appleton & Lange.

Hormones of the Pancreatic Islets

■ *Anatomy of the Pancreatic Islets*

The islets of the pancreas secrete two major hormones, **insulin** and **glucagon.** These hormones are rapid and powerful regulators of metabolism. *Together they coordinate the flow and metabolic fate of endogenous glucose, free fatty acids (FFAs), amino acids, and other substrates to ensure that energy needs are met in the basal state and during exercise. In addition, they coordinate the efficient disposition of the nutrient input from meals.* They accomplish these functions primarily by actions on the liver, muscle mass, and adipose tissue. Other secretory peptide products of islet cells (including amylin, pancreastatin, somatostatin, and pancreatic polypeptide) play subsidiary, if any, roles in the regulation of metabolism outside the gastrointestinal tract.

The strategic location of the pancreatic islets reflects these functions. Insulin and glucagon are released in response to nutrient inflow from the gut and to gastrointestinal secretagogues. The products of the exocrine pancreas are also released in response to such stimuli. The proximity of the islets to the pancreatic acini may also permit them to have local effects on exocrine pancreatic function. Islet hormones are secreted into the pancreatic vein and then into the portal vein, where they join the nutrient stream after meals. This arrangement preferentially exposes the liver, which is the central organ in substrate traffic, to higher islet hormone concentrations than those the peripheral tissues receive. In addition, the liver can extract variable amounts of insulin and glucagon on their first pass through this organ. In this manner, the liver can modulate the hormones' availability to other tissues. *Insulin and glucagon are often secreted and act in reciprocal fashion—when one is needed, the other usually is not. Therefore, the ratio of their concentrations may be more critical than their actual concentrations.*

There are approximately 1 million islets in the pancreas, and they constitute 1% to 1.5% of the human pancreatic mass. Each islet contains, on average, 2500 cells composed of four types. β cells, the unique source of insulin, make up 60% to 70%; α cells, the source of glucagon, 20% to 25%; and δ cells, the source of somato-statin, 10%. The remainder are mostly PP cells, the source of pancreatic polypeptide.

The microscopic structure, vascular supply, and distribution of the islets are important to islet function. Each islet consists of a core of β cells (Fig. 47-1, *A*) with either a mantle of α and/or δ cells or a mantle of δ and PP cells. If islets are disaggregated experimentally and the individual cells dispersed, these cells spontaneously reaggregate into islets if the cells are brought back together again in culture. Gap junctions exist between neighboring islet cells (Fig. 47-1, *B*) and permit the flow of molecules (that exert possible paracrine effects) and electrical currents between them.

The endocrine cells of the islets arise from common endodermal ancestors in the pancreatic ducts. A transcription factor called insulin-promoter-factor-1 is required for the specific differentiation of β cells and for the induction of insulin synthesis. Islet cells also display features characteristic of neuroectodermal cells, such as membrane polarization/depolarization and synthesis of neurotransmitter amines (e.g., gamma-aminobutyric acid [GABA]). Developmental factors lead to the selective expression of different hormone genes in these cells. The islets are identifiable by the fourth week of human gestation and are able to secrete insulin by the tenth week.

The islets are exceedingly well vascularized; they receive 10% of the pancreatic blood supply. Small arterioles enter the core of the islet and break up into a network of capillaries with fenestrated endothelium. These capillaries then converge into venules, which carry the blood to the mantle of the islet. This portal arrangement allows high concentrations of insulin from the β cell core to bathe the α, δ, and PP cells of the respective mantles. This type of vascular pattern also suggests paracrine effects of insulin on the other islet cells. Each β and α cell has a basal (arterial) and an apical (venous) face. Between the lateral surfaces of neighboring β cells run canaliculi that span the distance between the arteriolar and venous ends of the cell. These canaliculi carry interstitial fluid in a venous direction and permit selective exposure of the lateral cell surfaces to regulatory molecules, such as glucose (Fig. 47-2).

The islets are innervated by parasympathetic, sympathetic, and peptidergic nerves. The δ cells in the mantle are dendritic in shape and send granule-containing processes into the β-cell core; these features suggest a neurocrine pathway of intra-islet regulation.

Within the islet cells, hormones are stored in secretory granules with smooth membranes. These secretory granules are more heavily distributed in the apical venous (secretory) side of the cell (Fig. 47-2). Islet cells also contain a system of microtubules that are often arranged in parallel bundles that separate linear rows of secretory granules. In addition, microfilaments containing myosin and actin form a web adjacent to the plasma membrane and in association with the microtubules. These structures probably facilitate active movement of the secretory granules to the plasma membrane.

■ *Insulin*

■ *Structure and Synthesis*

The structure of insulin and the process by which insulin is synthesized are presented in some detail as an example of how a complex protein/peptide is made.

Structure. Insulin consists of two straight peptide chains (called the A and B chains) that are linked together (Fig. 47-3). Its molecular weight is 6000. The A chain, containing 21 amino acids, and the B chain, containing 30 amino acids, are connected by two disulfide bridges. In addition, the A chain contains an intrachain disulfide ring (Fig. 47-3). The tertiary structure of insulin is determined by the N-terminal and C-terminal amino acids of the A chain and the hydrophobic character of the amino acids at the C terminal of the B chain. This tertiary structure is critical to the biological activity of insulin, which resides within the B chain. Insulin monomers readily form a crystalline hexameric unit with two zinc atoms.

Crystalline zinc insulin (CZI) is the most important pharmaceutical preparation used in the management of **diabetes mellitus.** It is a "fast-acting" insulin that is injected subcutaneously to obtain the prompt effect needed in diabetic emergencies or to prevent excessive hyperglycemia after meals. Slower-acting insulins are made by altering buffers, pH, and/or zinc concentrations or adding other substances to CZI. These pharmaceutical insulin preparations are absorbed more slowly from the skin and provide a long-acting supply of insulin that mimics basal insulin delivery. Knowledge of the amino acid sequences and three-dimensional structure of insulin (and related insulin growth factors) has now permitted the design of insulin analogs that are made by substituting, deleting, or changing the sequence of amino acids at strategic sites in the molecule. Such new insulin analogs provide pharmacologic therapy

that more closely mimics normal insulin secretion patterns (see below).

Synthesis. The process of insulin synthesis is diagrammed in Fig. 47-4. The insulin gene is the ancestral member of a superfamily of genes that encode a variety of insulin-like growth factor molecules. It is composed of four exons and two introns. The gene directs the synthesis of preproinsulin, an insulin precursor with a molecular weight of 11,500. Preproinsulin contains four sequential peptides: an N-terminal signal peptide, the B chain of insulin, a connecting peptide, and the A chain of insulin (Fig. 47-3). The N-terminal signal peptide is rapidly cleaved from the molecule at the site of synthesis while the proinsulin chain is being completed. As proinsulin is guided to the Golgi apparatus, disulfide linkages are established that yield the "folded" proinsulin molecule with a molecular weight of 9000. The disulfide bonded A and B chains of insulin are linked by a connecting peptide (C peptide) through two basic residues each of which are located at the C terminal of the B chain and the N terminal of the A chain (Fig. 47-3). During its packaging into granules by the Golgi apparatus, proinsulin is slowly cleaved by specific trypsin-like and carboxypeptidase-like enzymes that split off the arg-arg and lys-arg residues, respectively. The resultant insulin molecule, along with the C-peptide molecule, is retained in the granules and released by exocytosis in equimolar amounts. Insulin becomes associated with zinc as the secretory granules mature. The zinc insulin crystals form the dense central core of the granule, whereas C peptide is present in the clear space between the granule membrane and the core.

In the trans-Golgi region, 99% of proinsulin is processed in a manner that results in storage granules for regulated insulin release. The remaining 1% of proinsulin escapes storage in granules; this "free" proinsulin maintains a low rate of constitutive insulin secretion. *Insulin synthesis is stimulated by glucose or feeding and is decreased by fasting.* Glucose rapidly increases translation of the insulin mRNA and more slowly increases transcription of the insulin gene. A cyclic AMP (cAMP) regulatory element and a separate glucose regulatory element have been identified in the insulin gene. *In general, synthesis and secretion of insulin are closely linked.*

■ *Insulin Secretion*

A large number of factors stimulate or inhibit insulin release (Table 47-1). Because of the preeminent importance of glucose in metabolism, the mechanism whereby this substrate acutely stimulates insulin secretion has been intensively investigated. The following sequence occurs during this stimulation (Fig. 47-5):

1. A specific transporter **(Glut-2),** concentrated in the microvilli of the canaliculi between β cells (Fig.

A

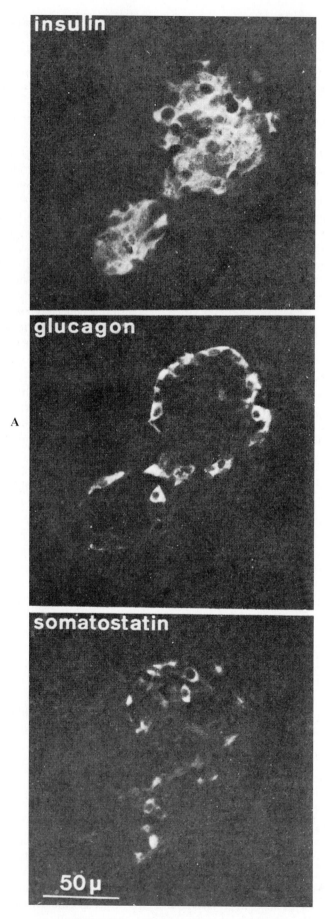

■ **Fig. 47-1**   For legend see opposite page.

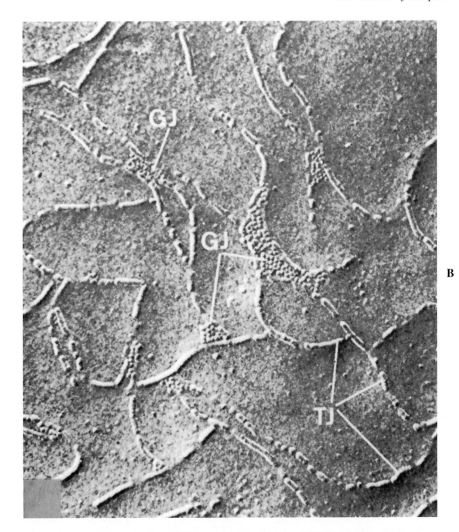

B

■ **Fig. 47-1, cont'd** **A,** Human islet stained by immunohistochemical methods shows the predominance and central core location of β cells and the peripheral distribution of α cells and δ cells. (From Unger RH et al: Insulin, glucagon, and somatostatin secretion in the regulation of metabolism, *Annu Rev Physiol* 40:307, 1978.) **B,** Electron micrograph of adjacent β and α cells in an islet showing the presence of gap junctions *(GJ)* and tight junctions *(TJ)* between them. (From Orci L et al: Cell contacts in human islets of Langerhans, *J Clin Endocrinol Metab* 41:841, 1975.)

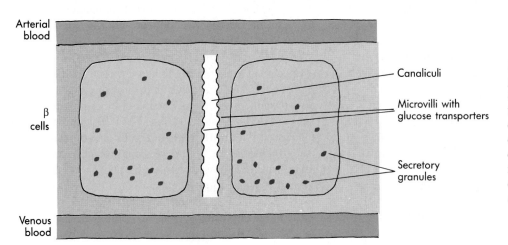

■ **Fig. 47-2** Orientation of islet β cells to their circulatory supply. Secretory granules are concentrated on the venous face of the cell. Glucose transporters are concentrated in microvilli on the lateral surfaces in contact with channels (canaliculi) that contain intercellular fluid and connect arterial and venous vessels.

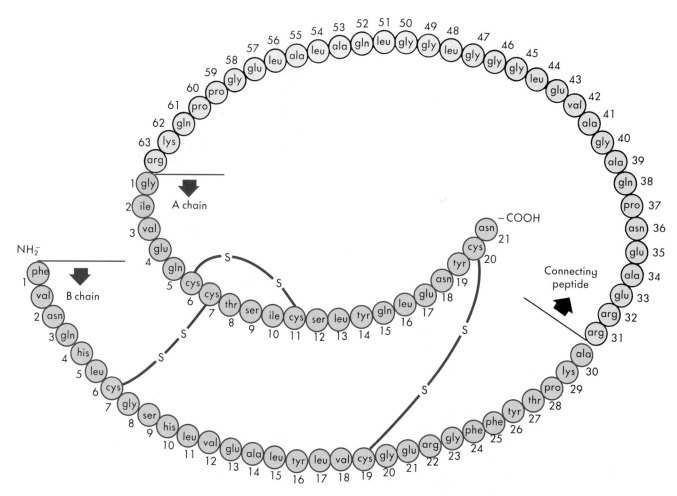

■ **Fig. 47-3**   The structure of porcine proinsulin. The solid area is the insulin molecule released by cleavage of the connecting peptide. (Redrawn from Shaw WN, Chance RE: Effect of porcine proinsulin in vitro on adipose tissue and diaphragm of the normal rat, *Diabetes* 17:737, 1968. From the American Diabetes Association.)

47-2), facilitates diffusion of glucose into the β cell. This helps maintain the glucose concentration in the β cell at a level that is essentially equal to that of the interstitial fluid.

2. *The enzyme glucokinase appears to function as the fundamental glucose sensor that controls the subsequent β-cell response.* The enzyme has a K_m for glucose of 5 to 8 mM, which is in the physiological range. Phosphorylation of glucose by glucokinase is the first and rate-limiting step in islet glucose use. An insulin-releasing signal is generated downstream from glucose-6-phosphate, and the subsequent rate of insulin secretion parallels that of glucose oxidation.

3. At the same time that glucose is being oxidized, rapid increases occur in intracellular ATP concentration; the ATP/ADP ratio; and concentrations of NADH, NADPH, and H^+.

4. An ATP-sensitive K^+ channel closes, K^+ efflux from the β cell is suppressed, and the cell depolarizes. Depolarization opens a voltage-regulated Ca^{++} channel, and the concentration of intracellular Ca^{++}

rapidly increases. The elevated Ca^{++} concentration activates the mechanism for secretory granule movement along the microtubules (see Fig. 45-3), perhaps via a myosin light chain kinase. A monomeric G protein (GTPase) attached to the secretory vesicle interacts with special plasma membrane proteins (fusins). This interaction leads to the fusion of the granule with the membrane. Exocytosis of insulin follows.

All the above processes occur within 1 minute of exposure to glucose. A similar sequence with specific transporters and enzymatic steps probably underlies the less prominent stimulatory action of other fuels, such as amino acids and ketoacids (Fig. 47-5). In addition, a secondary rise in cAMP levels in β cells also follows exposure to glucose; a cAMP-dependent protein kinase stimulates insulin release, possibly by phosphorylating the proteins involved in exocytosis (Fig. 47-5). Stimulatory G proteins mediate the insulin-releasing effects of peptides such as glucagon, whereas inhibitory G proteins mediate the insulin-suppressive effects of peptides such

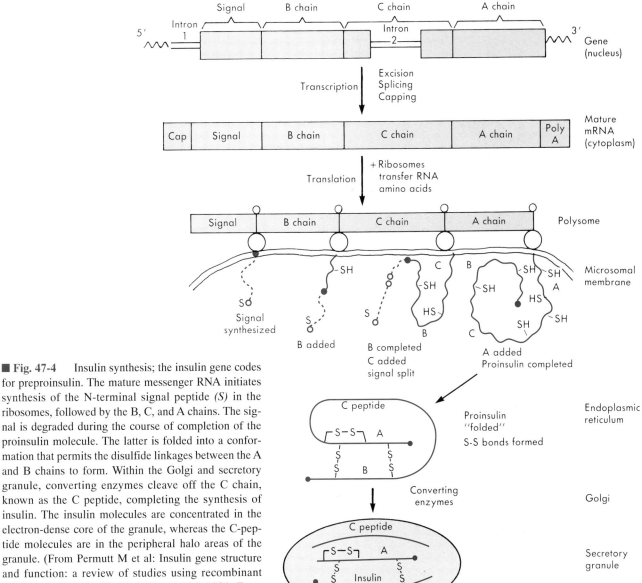

■ Fig. 47-4 Insulin synthesis; the insulin gene codes for preproinsulin. The mature messenger RNA initiates synthesis of the N-terminal signal peptide *(S)* in the ribosomes, followed by the B, C, and A chains. The signal is degraded during the course of completion of the proinsulin molecule. The latter is folded into a conformation that permits the disulfide linkages between the A and B chains to form. Within the Golgi and secretory granule, converting enzymes cleave off the C chain, known as the C peptide, completing the synthesis of insulin. The insulin molecules are concentrated in the electron-dense core of the granule, whereas the C-peptide molecules are in the peripheral halo areas of the granule. (From Permutt M et al: Insulin gene structure and function: a review of studies using recombinant DNA methodology, *Diabetes Care* 7:386, 1984. From the American Diabetes Association; and from Steiner DF et al. In Degroot LJ et al: *Endocrinology,* vol 2, New York, 1979, Grune & Stratton.)

■ Table 47-1   Insulin secretion

Increased by		Decreased by
D-Glucose	Glucagon	Fasting
Galactose	Glucagon-like	Exercise
Mannose	peptide 1	Endurance training
Glyceraldehyde	Gastric inhibitory	Somatostatin
Protein	polypeptide	Galanin
Arginine	Secretin	Pancreastatin
Lysine	Cholecystokinin	Leptin
Leucine	Vagal activity	Interleukin-1
Alanine	Acetylcholine	α-Adrenergic activity
Ketoacids	β-Adrenergic	Prostaglandin E$_2$
Free fatty acids	activity	Diazoxide
Potassium	Sulfonylurea	
Calcium	drugs	

as somatostatin (Fig. 47-5). A stimulatory G protein linked to phospholipase C mediates the ability of acetylcholine to stimulate insulin release via generation of phosphatidylinositol second messengers and increased protein kinase C activity.

A class of **sulfonylurea drugs** stimulates insulin release by binding to one component of the K$^+$ channel and directly closing it. These drugs are used in the treatment of **type 2 non–insulin-dependent diabetes** to increase insulin secretion. In contrast, the drug **diazoxide** opens the K$^+$ channel and thereby inhibits insulin release. Diazoxide is useful in the treatment of hyperinsulinism.

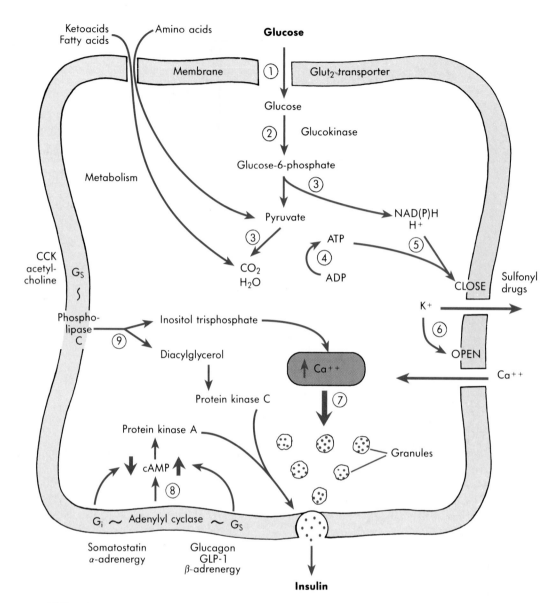

■ **Fig. 47-5**   Current concepts of regulation of insulin secretion by the β cell. Glucose transport *(1)* and *glucokinase*-catalyzed phosphorylation *(2)* raise glucose-6-phosphate levels. Metabolism *(3)* subsequently leads to increased adenosine triphosphate (ATP) levels *(4)* and NAD(P)H levels *(5)* that inhibit or close a potassium channel *(6)* and open a calcium channel *(6)*. Increased calcium levels then trigger exocytosis of insulin granules *(7)*. Other modulators of secretion act via the adenylyl cyclase–cAMP–protein kinase pathway *(8)* and the phospholipase-phosphoinositide pathway *(9)*. *SU,* Sulfonylurea; *GLP-1,* glucagon-like-peptide-1; *CCK,* cholecystokinin; *NAD(P)H,* reduced nicotine adenine dinucleotide phosphate; *ADP,* adenosine diphosphate.

Many nuances exist in glucose-stimulated insulin release. For example, newly synthesized insulin molecules are preferentially secreted. In addition, individual β cells differ in their sensitivity to glucose, and only some of them respond at any one time. Those at the center of the islet show greater and faster responsiveness. If β cells are dispersed or their gap junctions are functionally blocked, insulin secretion is markedly reduced; these observations demonstrate the importance of cell-to-cell signaling in insulin secretion. Finally, an intrinsic, non-neural oscillation of membrane potential, cytoplasmic Ca++ concentration, and insulin release exists,

with a cycle of 13 to 15 minutes. Because plasma insulin levels follow a similar cycle, a pacemaker (which has not been identified) must coordinate islet function throughout the pancreas.

In rare instances, mild diabetes mellitus is caused by genetic abnormalities in proinsulin structure, insulin structure, or the structure of molecules involved in insulin release. Some mutant genes express insulin molecules with reduced biological activity or proinsulin molecules that cannot be processed correctly. Other mutant genes express Glut-2 transporters or glu-

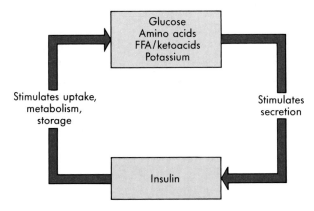

■ **Fig. 47-6** Feedback relationship between insulin and nutrients. Those nutrients that stimulate insulin secretion are the same nutrients whose disposal is facilitated by insulin. *FFA,* Free fatty acids.

cokinases with reduced affinity for glucose, and thus impair glucose sensing by β cells.

■ *Regulation of Insulin Secretion*

In the broadest sense, insulin secretion is governed by a feedback relationship with exogenous nutrient supply (Fig. 47-6). When substrate supply is abundant, insulin is secreted in response. Insulin then stimulates use of these incoming nutrients and simultaneously inhibits the mobilization of analogous endogenous substrates. When nutrient supply is low or absent, insulin secretion is dampened and mobilization of endogenous fuels is enhanced.

Glucose is the insulin stimulant of greatest importance in humans. Because insulin in turn stimulates the use of glucose, this substrate-hormone pair forms a feedback system for close regulation of plasma glucose levels. The relationship between plasma insulin and plasma glucose is sigmoidal (Fig. 47-7). Virtually no insulin is secreted below a plasma glucose threshold of about 50 mg/dl. A half-maximal insulin secretory response occurs at a plasma glucose level of about 150 mg/dl; a maximal insulin response occurs at levels of 300 mg/dl.

Both in vitro and in vivo, insulin secretion exhibits a biphasic response to a continuous glucose stimulus (Fig. 47-8). Within seconds of exposure to glucose, an immediate pulse of insulin is released that peaks at 1 minute and then returns toward baseline. After 10 minutes of continuous stimulation, a second phase of secretion begins. During this phase, insulin plasma levels rise more slowly and reach a second plateau, which can be maintained for many hours in normal individuals. This biphasic response may result from (1) rapid insulin generation followed by the slow removal of a substance that is formed after glucose stimulation and acts as a feedback inhibitor of insulin release, (2) granules with different sensitivities to glucose, and (3) glucose stimulation of insulin synthesis that sustains the later secretory phase.

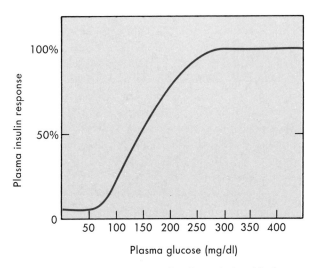

■ **Fig. 47-7** Approximate in vivo relationship between plasma glucose and insulin secretion, the latter being assessed by the plasma insulin response to stepwise infusion of glucose in humans. No insulin is secreted below a plasma glucose level of 50 mg/dl. Half-maximal secretion occurs at 125 to 150 mg/dl. (Redrawn from Karam JH et al: "Staircase" glucose stimulation of insulin secretion in obesity; measurement of beta cell sensitivity and capacity, *Diabetes* 23:763, 1974. From the American Diabetes Association.)

When glucose is given orally, a greater insulin response is elicited than when plasma glucose is comparably elevated by intravenous administration. This augmented insulin response to oral glucose is accounted for by one or more gastrointestinal hormones that are released in response to meals and are capable of potentiating glucose-stimulated insulin secretion (Table 47-1). Glucagon-like peptide 1 and gastric inhibitory polypeptide are the most important of these insulinogogues. This prompt gastrointestinal mechanism of insulinogenesis moderates the early rise in plasma glucose that follows the ingestion and absorption of a carbohydrate meal. In contrast, somatostatin released within pancreatic islets *(paracrine* or *neurocrine)* and from intestinal cells *(endocrine)* may dampen insulin responses to meals.

Insulin secretion is also stimulated by amino acids that result from digestion of protein in a meal. The basic amino acids, arginine and lysine, are the most potent stimulants; leucine, alanine, and others contribute modestly to this effect. Glucose and amino acids are synergistic stimulators of insulin release, so that the plasma insulin rise that follows a meal represents more than the additive effect of its carbohydrate and protein content. Triglycerides and fatty acids exert only a small stimulatory effect on insulin release in humans. In fact, these small effects may be mostly indirect and exerted by means of gastric inhibitory polypeptide. Ketoacids at concentrations that prevail during prolonged fasting (see Fig. 46-11) modestly stimulate insulin secretion; this effect may help sustain a critical low level of insulin when β-cell stimulation by ingested nutrients is absent.

Both potassium and calcium are essential for normal insulin responses to glucose. Thus, relative insulin deficiency occurs in subjects depleted of potassium, calcium, or the calcitropic hormone, vitamin D. Magnesium exerts at least a modulatory effect. Sympathetic nerves and epinephrine stimulate insulin secretion via β-adrenergic receptors but inhibit insulin secretion via α-adrenergic receptors. Parasympathetic activity via the vagus nerve increases insulin release. In addition, a cephalic phase of insulin secretion precedes the entrance of food into the gastrointestinal tract.

An increase in the number of β cells (hyperplasia) can also lead to an increase in insulin secretion. A variety of other hormones directly or indirectly cause hyperplasia of the β cells and a subsequent increase in insulin secretion, largely by antagonizing insulin action and increasing insulin need by peripheral tissues. These hormones include cortisol, growth hormone, estrogen-progesterone, human placental lactogen, and thyroid hormones. Insulin has a negative feedback effect on its own secretion, and this effect is independent of any effect on plasma glucose. Leptin can also inhibit insulin release, an action which closes a negative feedback loop between the two hormones (see Chapter 46).

The net result of these many influences on insulin secretion is to maintain an average basal peripheral

plasma insulin level of 10 μU/ml (6×10^{-11} M) in humans. After several days of fasting, this value declines over 50%. A similar decrease occurs during prolonged exercise. Plasma insulin levels increase threefold to tenfold after a typical meal and usually peak 30 to 60 minutes after eating is initiated (Fig. 47-9). Plasma C peptide, coreleased with insulin, fluctuates similarly (Fig. 47-9). In addition to the intrinsic low-level 15-minute cycles and the bursts of insulin secretion stimulated by meals, a higher amplitude insulin cycle exists. This cycle has a 2-hour frequency entrained by glucose and represents feedback regulation. The liver is regularly exposed to insulin concentrations two or three times higher than those of other organs in the basal state, and transiently five to ten times higher after β-cell stimulation.

Obesity markedly increases insulin secretion (Fig. 47-9), whereas physical conditioning produced by habitual exercise decreases it. These alterations at least partly reflect decreases and increases, respectively, in responsiveness to insulin action. The hyperinsulinemia that accompanies excess weight gain and a sedentary life style is a risk factor (though not necessarily a causative agent) for the later development of **type 2 non–insulin-dependent diabetes mellitus,** as well as for cardiovascular disease and mortality.

In addition to resistance to insulin action and compensatory hyperinsulinemia, more subtle abnormalities in insulin secretion occur in the early phase of type 2 diabetes. These abnormalities, which include altered cyclicity, diminished pulse frequency, and a delayed response to rising glucose levels, evolve later into a complete loss of recognition of glucose as a stimulus for insulin secretion. Finally, other nutrient and pharmacologic stimuli also become ineffective, and therapy with insulin is required.

Insulin circulates unbound to any carrier protein. Its half-life in plasma is 5 to 8 minutes and its metabolic clearance rate is 800 ml/min. Estimates of basal insulin delivery rate to the peripheral circulation in humans are about 0.5 to 1 unit/hr (20 to 40 μg/hr). During meals, the delivery rate increases up to tenfold, and the total daily peripheral delivery of insulin is about 30 units. If the amount of insulin removed during its first pass through the liver is accounted for (approximately 50% of portal vein insulin), the actual β-cell secretory rate becomes approximately 60 units/day. The liver decreases its extraction of insulin in response to glucose and meals. As a result, a greater amount of insulin is allowed to escape to the periphery for stimulation of nutrient uptake.

Insulin is metabolized largely in the kidney and liver by specific enzymes that split the disulfide bonds and separate the A and B chains. Very little insulin is excreted unchanged in the urine. Degradation of insulin also occurs in association with its plasma membrane receptor after internalization by target cells.

Glucose infusion

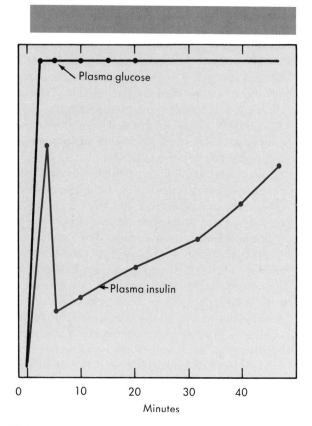

■ Fig. 47-8   Insulin response to glucose infusion shows a rapid first phase of release followed by a fall and a later, slower second phase.

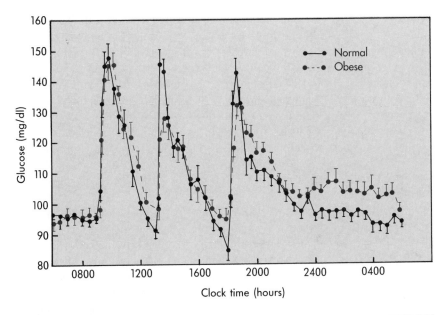

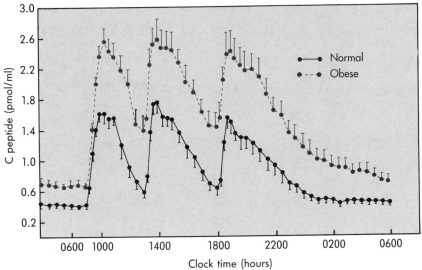

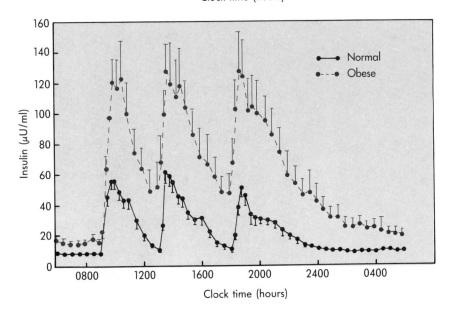

■ **Fig. 47-9** Twenty-four-hour profiles of plasma glucose, C peptide, and insulin in normal weight *(solid lines)* and obese *(dotted lines)* humans. Note the parallel increases with each meal, the rapid return toward baseline, and the exaggerated β cell responses in obesity. (Redrawn from Polonsky K et al: *J Clin Invest* 81:442, 1988. From the American Society for Clinical Investigation.)

Although C peptide is secreted in amounts that are equimolar to insulin, its basal peripheral plasma levels are approximately fivefold higher, averaging 1 ng/ml (3×10^{-10} M). This difference is caused by a lower rate of metabolic clearance for C peptide. In contrast to insulin, C peptide is not extracted by the liver to any significant degree. Therefore, plasma (and even urine) C-peptide measurements can actually provide more accurate information about β-cell function than do insulin measurements in some circumstances. Proinsulin is also constitutively released by the β cell in the basal state; during glucose stimulation, proinsulin levels increase more slowly and to a lesser degree than insulin. Although proinsulin exhibits some biological insulin activity (about 5% to 10% that of insulin), at present no function can be ascribed to it or to C peptide.

Hypersecretion of insulin is usually caused by a tumor of the β cells. The cardinal manifestation is a low plasma glucose level (<50 mg/dl) in the fasting state. Because the sympathetic nervous system is quickly activated by abrupt hypoglycemia, bursts of insulin hypersecretion produce episodes of rapid heart rate, nervousness, sweating, and hunger. With sustained insulin excess and persistent hypoglycemia, disturbed central nervous system function is manifested by bizarre behavior, defects in cerebration, loss of consciousness, or convulsions. The need to ingest large amounts of carbohydrate combined with the stimulating effect of insulin on fat storage produces weight gain. The diagnosis of a β-cell tumor is established by demonstrating fasting plasma insulin and C-peptide levels that are inappropriately high for the prevailing glucose levels. Removal of the tumor cures the condition. Failing that, drugs that inhibit insulin secretion palliate the hypoglycemia.

■ *Insulin Actions*

The effects of insulin are broad in scope, involve many organs and intracellular pathways, and are metabolically critical. In the following discussion, the cellular mechanisms of insulin action are presented first. Tissue and inter-organ effects are then discussed. Finally, the total body effects of insulin are correlated with its secretion.

Insulin action on cells. The first and overall rate-limiting step in insulin action is the transport of insulin through the capillary wall. Once it arrives at the target cell, insulin combines with a plasma membrane glycoprotein receptor of the type shown in Fig. 45-12. This tetramer contains an extracellular α subunit that is disulfide-bonded to a β subunit; this β subunit transverses the plasma membrane and largely resides within the cytoplasm. Two such identical α-β dimers are joined extra-

cellularly by another disulfide (Fig. 47-10). The β subunit has 194 extracellular residues, a 23-*N*-amino acid transmembrane anchor, and an intracytoplasmic component with 403 residues.

The insulin receptor gene is a member of a superfamily that codes for other growth factor receptors. Its structure is shown in Fig. 47-11. The insulin receptor gene illustrates how the many functions of a receptor can be packaged in a DNA molecule. The gene, which contains 22 exons (Fig. 47-11), codes for a proreceptor molecule. This proreceptor contains, in sequence, a signal peptide, the α subunit, a proreceptor processing site, and the β subunit. After translation and removal of the signal peptide, two proreceptor molecules associate into a disulfide dimer. After this disulfide dimer is formed, a basic amino acid cleavage site on each dimer is removed. This cleavage yields the discrete α and β subunits of the insulin receptor linked by disulfide bonds. Of great importance to receptor function are exons 17 to 21, which code for its tyrosine kinase activity.

After insulin binds to the insulin receptor on a target cell, a conformational change occurs that leads to aggregation of receptors. The hormone-receptor complex is subsequently internalized by endocytosis; the hormone is degraded; and the receptor is either degraded, stored, or recycled back to the plasma membrane. Insulin downregulates the insulin receptor by increasing its rate of degradation and suppressing its synthesis. This phenomenon is one reason why obese subjects have a decreased sensitivity to insulin (Fig. 47-9). For some actions, full biological activity of insulin is expressed when only 5% of its receptor sites are occupied.

Insulin binding to its receptor causes multiple events to occur at several locations, including the plasma membrane itself, the cytoplasm, and the nucleus. These events include the following:

1. Initial signal transduction occurs via the receptor **tyrosine kinase** activity that resides in the intracytoplasmic portion of the β subunit. This kinase is inactive when the extracellular α subunit of the receptor is unoccupied by insulin. When a single molecule of insulin binds to its α-subunit site, this kinase is activated. The process of activation possibly takes place via a conformational change transmitted through the receptor molecule. Once the receptor kinase activity is stimulated, it autophosphorylates its β subunit at three key tyrosines, with ATP as substrate.

2. The now fully active tyrosine kinase phosphorylates tyrosines on one or two specific **insulin receptor substrates** (IRS-1 and IRS-2). Each of these IRS phosphotyrosines serves as a docking site and possibly an activating site for other protein kinases, protein phosphatases, and facilitatory proteins that link to membrane G proteins, phospholipases, and ion channels. Many of these subsidiary steps involve serine and threonine phosphorylation.

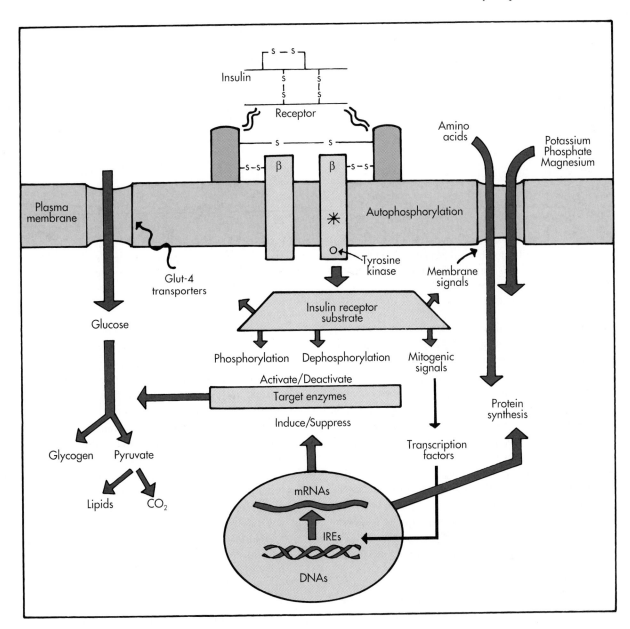

■ **Fig. 47-10**   Mechanisms of insulin action on cells. Binding of insulin to the subunit of its receptor causes autophosphorylation by ATP of an intracellular β-subunit receptor site that generates tyrosine kinase activity. The receptor tyrosine kinase then phosphorylates an insulin receptor substrate or substrates. The latter begins a cascade of serine and threonine phosphorylations, which activate or deactivate target enzymes of glucose metabolism. Docking of other regulatory proteins to the insulin receptor substrate initiates other cascades that stimulate or repress gene transcription via insulin response elements *(IREs)* in DNA molecules. Glucose transporters are moved to the plasma membrane and facilitate glucose entry. Also independently, amino acid, potassium, magnesium, and phosphate entries into the cell are facilitated. Mitogenic proteins are activated that increase transcription factors required to stimulate gene expression concerned with cell growth.

3. IRS phosphorylation is followed by several different cascades of events that ultimately activate or deactivate numerous enzymes, translocate glucose transport proteins to the plasma membrane, and repress or transcribe genes in the nucleus of the target cell. Although knowledge about the detailed mechanisms of these cascades is still evolving, several mechanisms have been delineated. One is activation of **phosphatidylinositol-3-kinase** (PI-3-kinase), an enzyme that generates phosphatidylinositol-3-4 and -3,4,5 phosphates. (These molecules are distinct from the second messenger, inositol-1,4,5 trisphosphate.) The PI-3 phosphates may stimulate translocation of glucose transport proteins to the plasma membrane. Other downstream products of PI-3 kinase are S6 kinases that phosphorylate nuclear accessory proteins involved in gene transcription.

Insulin receptor gene

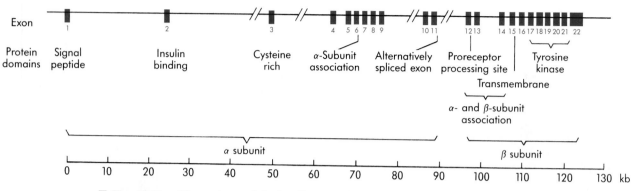

■ **Fig. 47-11** The anatomy of the insulin receptor gene. The final gene product contains two sulfhydryl-bonded subunits. Two of these monomers associate to form the receptor molecule (see Fig. 47-10). (Modified from Seino S, Seino M, Bell GI: *Diabetes* 39:129, 1990. From the American Diabetes Association.)

4. Another IRS-1–initiated step involves **growth receptor binding protein-2 (GRB-2).** This intermediary facilitates the binding of GTP to **ras,** a proto-oncogene that resides in the plasma membrane. When thus activated, ras starts another series of reactions that stimulate cell growth and differentiation. Other ras products participate in insulin activation of the enzyme **glycogen synthase.** Yet another key modulator of growth and metabolic events included in this web of IRS-1 signaling is **mitogen-activated protein kinase (MAP kinase).** The proto-oncogene **cJun** is a factor in this pathway.

5. For certain insulin actions, phospholipase C–generated second messengers (i.e., inositol-1,4,5 trisphosphate and diacyl glycerol) are needed to produce the full hormone effect.

6. Finally, in some target cells, insulin action lowers cAMP levels by activating phosphodiesterase (see Chapter 45) and reduces cAMP effectiveness by inhibiting its binding to protein kinase A.

The cellular physiological result of many of the above effects is a rapid shift of metabolic directions in the cytoplasm and mitochondria. This shift is brought about by activating or deactivating critical enzymes through either their phosphorylation or their dephosphorylation. Such shifts are reinforced and prolonged, however, by the nuclear effects emanating from the initial receptor and plasma membrane steps. Although no single consensus DNA sequence acts as an insulin regulatory element (IRE) that accounts for all insulin effects on gene transcription, numerous target DNA molecules exist. Both induction (e.g., glucokinase) and repression (e.g., phosphoenolpyruvate carboxykinase) of gene expression occur. These effects are likely mediated by various insulin-activated transcriptional proteins that bind to one or more DNA molecules.

The insulin signal rapidly stimulates a number of processes (Fig. 47-10). Within 1 minute, glucose transport into muscle and adipose cells is increased up to twentyfold by activation of a glucose carrier system in the plasma membrane. Insulin rapidly recruits the glucose transporter **Glut-4,** that is specifically expressed in muscle and adipose tissue, from a cytoplasmic pool of vesicles to the plasma membrane. Insulin also increases the activity of the transporter. Transcription of the Glut-4 gene is stimulated more slowly. Glut-4 then facilitates diffusion of glucose down its concentration gradient. This process does not require energy. The importance of this insulin action is underscored by the fact that at low physiological insulin concentrations, glucose transport is the rate-limiting step in glucose use. At high physiological insulin concentrations, such as after a meal, the rate-limiting step shifts to an unknown point in intracellular glucose metabolism. In an independent manner, insulin also facilitates the cellular uptake of the amino acids that utilize transporter system A (see Chapter 1), as well as uptake of potassium, magnesium, and phosphate (Fig. 47-10).

After glucose and amino acids are transported into the cytoplasm, insulin then directs the disposition of these substances. Conversion of glucose to glycogen, to pyruvate and lactate, and to fatty acids is all stimulated to varying degrees. Synthesis of specific proteins, such as albumin, casein, and a number of enzymes from the amino acids, is selectively enhanced. Inhibition of proteolytic and lipolytic enzymes protects protein and triglyceride stores. Another insulin-stimulated action of metabolic importance is the translocation of Na$^+$, K$^+$-ATPase to the plasma membrane, thus increasing energy expenditure. Finally, insulin inhibits the translocation of its own receptor to the plasma membrane, thereby limiting the extent of the hormone's actions.

An estimated 14 million people in the United States. have **type 2 non–insulin-dependent diabetes mellitus,** and the incidence is increasing worldwide.

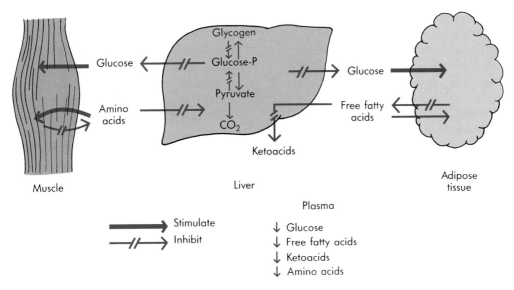

Because a major cause of this form of diabetes is
resistance to insulin, much research into mechanisms
of insulin action is motivated by the need to pinpoint
the defects and find specific remedies. With uncommon individual or family exceptions, mutations in the
insulin receptor, its kinase activity, Glut-4, IRS-1,
glycogen synthase, and several other enzymes and
receptors involved in glucose metabolism have thus
far been eliminated as the primary cause of hyperglycemia in the usual patient. In patients with various
mutant insulin receptors, diabetes ranges from mild, in
which the defect merely decreases somewhat the
receptor affinity for insulin, to lethal in infancy, in
which the defect completely prevents the receptor
from being properly processed or translocated to the
plasma membrane.

Actions on flow of fuels. *Insulin is the hormone of
abundance. When the influx of nutrients exceeds concurrent energy needs and rates of anabolism, insulin
induces efficient storage of the excess nutrients while
suppressing mobilization of endogenous substrates.* The
stored nutrients can then be made available during subsequent fasting periods to maintain glucose delivery to
the central nervous system and free fatty acid delivery to
the muscle mass and viscera. *The major targets for
insulin action are the liver, the adipose tissue, and the
muscle mass.* Fig. 47-12 displays the general flow of
substrates produced by insulin; Fig. 47-13 shows the
important metabolic control points at which insulin acts
directly or indirectly in the liver.

Carbohydrates. Insulin stimulates glucose oxidation
and storage while simultaneously inhibiting glucose
production. Therefore, insulin either lowers the basal
circulating glucose concentration or limits the rise in
plasma glucose that results from a dietary carbohydrate

load. These actions are accomplished by a number of
insulin effects.

LIVER. In the liver, extracellular glucose levels equilibrate rapidly with intracellular levels by means of the
Glut-2 transporter. Insulin enhances inward movement of
glucose by inducing hepatic glucokinase, which catalyzes phosphorylation of the incoming glucose to glu-
cose-6-phosphate. Insulin then promotes storage of glucose as glycogen by activating the glycogen synthase
enzyme complex. At the same time, insulin stimulates
glycolysis, which converts glucose to pyruvate and lactate, by increasing the activities of the committed
enzymes phosphofructokinase and pyruvate kinase.
Oxidation of the pyruvate and lactate is stimulated by
increased pyruvate dehydrogenase activity. Insulin also
rapidly inhibits hepatic glycogenolysis and therefore
hepatic glucose output by decreasing glycogen phosphorylase activity and also by decreasing glucose-6-phos-
phatase levels (Fig. 47-13).

In addition, insulin inhibits gluconeogenesis. This
inhibition is accomplished by decreasing the hepatic
uptake of precursor amino acids and their availability
from muscle (Fig. 47-12). Insulin also decreases the levels or activities of the committed gluconeogenic enzymes
pyruvate carboxylase, phosphoenolpyruvate carboxykinase, and fructose-1,6-biphosphatase. Thus, pyruvate is
shunted toward acetyl CoA in the mitochondria; the
acetyl CoA can be returned to the cytoplasm via citrate,
regenerated as acetyl CoA, and directed into fatty acid
synthesis.

Many hepatic effects of insulin require concurrent
administration of glucose and represent amplification of
biochemical events that are induced by glucose itself.
Some of these effects are also augmented because insulin
inhibits the secretion of glucagon, a hormone with effects
that are antagonistic to those of insulin.

If plasma insulin is raised by continuously infusing insulin in the basal state, the plasma glucose level declines as hepatic glucose output falls. However, hepatic glucose production quickly recovers from its low point after a short time. This recovery reflects three counter-regulatory processes: (1) an autoregulatory response of the liver to a lowered plasma glucose concentration, probably mediated by the direct effects of glucose on phosphorylase and other enzymes; (2) a sensing of hypoglycemia by the hypothalamus, leading to stimulation of glucose output via activation of the sympathetic nervous system; and (3) a sensing of hypoglycemia by the α cells of the pancreatic islets, which then secrete the insulin antagonist glucagon. These mechanisms protect the central nervous system from glucose deprivation caused by the unchecked action of insulin.

MUSCLE. Insulin stimulates the transport of glucose into muscle cells. Depending on the insulin concentration, 20% to 50% of the glucose that enters undergoes oxidation, mainly caused by activation of pyruvate dehydrogenase. The remainder is specifically directed into storage as glycogen by insulin activation of glycogen synthase. Muscle blood flow also increases as a consequence of insulin action. Slow twitch "high oxidative" type I fibers, which depend more on fatty acid fuel, are actually more sensitive to insulin action on glucose uptake than are the fast twitch "glycolytic" and more glucose-dependent type II muscle fibers.

ADIPOSE TISSUES. In adipose tissue also, insulin stimulates the transport of glucose into the cells. Much of this glucose is then converted to α-glycerophosphate, which is used in the esterification of fatty acids and permits

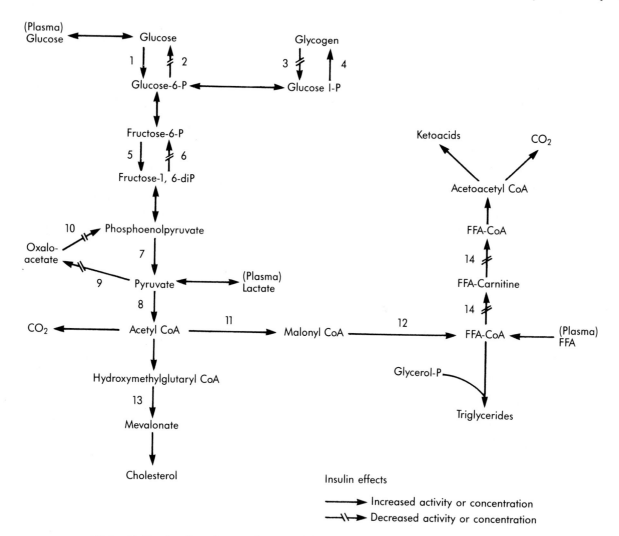

■ **Fig. 47-13**   Insulin actions on glucose and fatty acid metabolism in the liver. The pathway from pyruvate to glucose via oxaloacetate constitutes gluconeogenesis. Acetyl CoA generated from pyruvate can be converted to fatty acids via malonyl CoA. The key enzymes involved that are influenced by insulin are as follows: *1,* glucokinase; *2,* glucose-6-phosphatase; *3,* phosphorylase; *4,* glycogen synthase; *5,* phosphofructokinase; *6,* fructose-1,6-biphosphatase; *7,* pyruvate kinase; *8,* pyruvate dehydrogenase; *9,* pyruvate carboxylase; *10,* phosphoenolpyruvate carboxykinase; *11,* acetyl-CoA carboxylase; *12,* fatty acid synthase; *13,* hydroxy-methylglutaryl-CoA reductase; and *14,* carnitine acyltransferase.

their storage as triglycerides. To a minor extent, glucose can also be converted to fatty acids (Fig. 47-13).

Fat metabolism. The metabolism of both endogenous and exogenous fat is profoundly influenced by insulin. *The net overall effect of insulin is to enhance storage and to block mobilization and oxidation of fatty acids* (Fig. 47-12). Insulin rapidly lowers the circulating levels of FFAs and ketoacids and may eventually reduce the level of triglycerides.

ADIPOSE TISSUES. *In adipose tissue, the storage of fat is stimulated by insulin in several ways.* Most important, insulin profoundly inhibits **hormone-sensitive adipose tissue lipase** activity. It accomplishes this inhibition by decreasing the levels of cAMP and inhibiting protein kinase A. By suppressing lipolysis and the release of stored fatty acids, insulin lowers their rate of delivery to the liver and peripheral tissues. A major consequence is a marked reduction in the generation of ketoacids. In addition, insulin stimulates the use of ketoacids by the peripheral tissues. *Thus, insulin is the major and perhaps the sole antiketogenic hormone.*

Insulin also actively promotes deposition of circulating fat into adipose tissue by activating key enzymes necessary for this process. The enzyme adipose tissue lipoprotein lipase, which catalyzes hydrolysis of very-low-density lipoprotein (VLDL) and chylomicron triglycerides to FFA (see Chapter 46), is induced by insulin. The action of this enzyme makes FFAs available for transfer into adipose cells (Fig. 47-12). α-Glycerophosphate, needed for esterification of the FFAs, is generated from glyceraldehyde phosphate; the necessary enzyme, glyceraldehyde phosphate dehydrogenase, is also induced by insulin.

MUSCLE. Within muscle, insulin suppresses the enzyme lipoprotein lipase in inverse proportion to its stimulation of glucose uptake. Thus in muscle, FFA uptake and oxidation are inhibited by insulin, especially in the type I oxidative fibers that depend most on FFAs. These overall actions of insulin within muscle reinforce the principle that glucose and FFAs are competitive energy substrates.

LIVER. *Within the liver, insulin is also antiketogenic and lipogenic.* Under the influence of insulin, FFAs entering from the circulation are shunted away from β oxidation and ketogenesis (Figs. 47-12 and 47-13). They are instead re-esterified with D-glycerophosphate, derived either from insulin-stimulated glycolysis or from glycerol via the enzyme glycerophosphate kinase. Fatty acids are also synthesized from glucose under the influence of insulin. Mitochondrial acetyl CoA generated from pyruvate by the action of pyruvate dehydrogenase is transferred to the cytoplasm, where it is converted to malonyl CoA by the action of acetyl-CoA carboxylase. This rate-limiting step in fatty acid synthesis is activated by insulin, which also induces the final enzyme involved, fatty acid synthase. Moreover, insulin increases the activity of the hexose monophosphate shunt by inducing the enzyme glucose-6-phosphate dehydrogenase. This shunt generates the supply of reduced triphosphopyridine nucleotide, which is also needed for fatty acid synthesis.

The antiketogenic action of insulin in the liver may also be mediated by stimulation of malonyl-CoA formation, because malonyl CoA inhibits the enzyme carnitine acyltransferase (Fig. 47-13). The latter enzyme is responsible for transferring FFAs from the cytoplasm into the mitochondria for oxidation and conversion to ketoacids.

Insulin also favors hepatic synthesis of cholesterol from acetyl CoA by activating the rate-limiting enzyme hydroxymethylglutaryl-CoA reductase. In parallel with increasing hepatic triglyceride storage, insulin decreases apolipoprotein B synthesis; the net result is an acute suppression of VLDL release. However, under conditions of continuous, long-term hyperinsulinemia, the high rate of VLDL synthesis ultimately elevates circulating triglyceride levels.

Protein metabolism. Insulin enhances protein and amino acid sequestration in all target tissues (Fig. 47-12). *Thus, insulin is an anabolic hormone.* If administered in the basal state, insulin lowers the plasma levels of many amino acids. During the assimilation of a protein meal, the increase in insulin secretion limits the rise of plasma amino acid levels, especially of the essential branched-chain amino acids leucine, valine, and isoleucine. In muscle, insulin stimulates the sodium-dependent transport of amino acids across the muscle cell membrane. Although insulin stimulates the general rate of protein synthesis in vitro, this stimulation is evident in vivo mostly when amino acids are in abundance after a meal. (In the basal state, insulin limits the availability of endogenous amino acids for new protein synthesis.) The mechanisms include increases in gene transcription for numerous proteins (e.g., albumin), in rates of mRNA translation, in general RNA synthesis, and in ribosome synthesis. RNA degradation is decreased by insulin.

Even more dramatically, *insulin inhibits proteolysis.* This action is manifested by suppression of release of branched-chain and aromatic amino acids from muscle and inhibition of their oxidation. In contrast, insulin has little effect on the flux of alanine.

As noted, the genes for insulin and its receptor are related to genes that encode a variety of tissue growth factors. These growth factors include somatomedins (insulin-like growth factors 1 and 2 [IGF-1 and IGF-2]), epidermal growth factor, nerve growth factor, and relaxin. Insulin is not only a general anabolic hormone, but it also stimulates the synthesis of macromolecules in tissues such as cartilage and bone and thereby directly contributes to body growth. It also indirectly contributes to growth by stimulating the transcription of other related gene growth factors such as IGF-1 and by suppressing the gene for one of the IGF-1–binding proteins. The insulin-deprived young animal or human has a reduced lean body mass and may be profoundly retarded in height and maturation.

Other actions. Both protein anabolism and the storage of glucose as glycogen require the concurrent cellular uptake of potassium, phosphate, and magnesium. Insulin stimulates translocation of all three minerals into muscle cells and of potassium and phosphate into the liver. Therefore, insulin, secreted in response to a carbohydrate load, lowers serum potassium, phosphate, and magnesium levels, and is considered to be one of the normal regulators of potassium balance. Another effect of insulin on electrolyte balance is to increase reabsorption of potassium, phosphate, and sodium by the tubules of the kidney. These renal effects contribute to anabolism by conserving vital intracellular electrolytes. Sodium is necessary for formation of the additional extracellular fluid required when lean body mass is undergoing expansion.

The overall consumption of glucose by the central nervous system is independent of insulin. However, selected areas of the brain, particularly the hypothalamus and its adjacent capillary endothelium, contain insulin receptors and are insulin responsive. Insulin also reaches the cerebrospinal fluid from plasma and, when injected into the cerebral ventricles of primates, decreases food intake. This action is partly mediated by a direct suppressive effect on neuropeptide Y release (see Chapter 46). In addition, continuous insulin excess increases body weight and adipose mass, and with the latter, leptin levels increase to induce satiety. If endogenous or exogenous insulin causes hypoglycemia, food intake will be stimulated by other pathways and contribute to weight gain.

Correlation of insulin secretion and action. The insulin sensitivity of tissues relates well to prevailing plasma insulin levels in various physiological states (Fig. 47-14). Suppression of lipolysis and FFA mobilization and consequent ketogenesis are the most sensitive insulin actions. Slightly less sensitive insulin actions are inhibition of hepatic glucose production and of muscle proteolysis, as exemplified by release of branched-chain amino acids (Fig. 47-14). Stimulation of muscle glucose uptake requires considerably higher insulin concentrations.

The normal postabsorptive plasma insulin concentration of about 10 μU/ml permits a finely regulated flow of FFA substrates for energy, with minimal ketogenesis during the daily nocturnal fasting period. In addition, sufficient glycogenolysis is permitted to sustain the plasma glucose level. Shortly after a person eats, insulin concentrations rise to 30 μU/ml and hepatic glucose output becomes greatly suppressed. With a further increase to postprandial levels of 50 to 100 μU/ml, muscle proteolysis is inhibited and glucose uptake (and amino acid uptake) by peripheral tissues is strongly stimulated. These processes facilitate the use of substrate at a time of abundance. Under maximal insulin stimulation at approximately 200 μU/ml, peripheral glucose use increases from 2 to 12 mg/kg/min. Of this total increase, two thirds is accounted for by storage as glycogen. *Thus, the β cell responds to the physiological need of the moment by delivering insulin at rates that provide appropriate hormone concentrations for regulating substrate fluxes.*

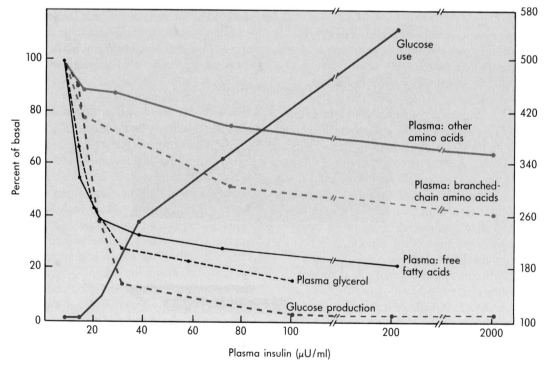

Dose-response curves for insulin action in humans

■ **Fig. 47-14**   Plasma dose-response curves for insulin actions in humans. Note the marked sensitivity of inhibition of lipolysis and glucose production by insulin, with lesser sensitivity for stimulation of glucose production. The effects on amino acid metabolism are intermediate.

A further subtlety is appreciated when the response of each individual's β cells to glucose is compared with the person's peripheral glucose uptake in response to insulin (Fig. 47-15): the least insulin-sensitive individuals secrete the greatest amount of insulin, and vice versa. This fine coordination between insulin availability (β-cell function) and insulin need (tissue responsiveness) maintains the plasma glucose concentration in a narrow range. The feedback operates in obese and in elderly individuals, in whom insulin secretion rates rise to accommodate decreased tissue sensitivity. The feedback also occurs in physically trained individuals, in whom insulin secretion falls as tissue sensitivity to the hormone increases. During puberty, a selective resistance to insulin action on glucose metabolism leads to an increase in insulin secretion that facilitates cellular amino acid uptake for tissue growth.

It should be apparent by now that complete lack of insulin actions would cause a major and life-threatening metabolic disturbance. Primary deficiency of insulin as a consequence of selective β-cell destruction is known as **type 1** or **insulin-dependent diabetes mellitus.** The disease usually results from a genetically conferred vulnerability to an environmental insult that initiates a destructive autoimmune process. As a consequence of the lack of insulin, hepatic glucose production is uninhibited and the efficiency of peripheral glucose use is reduced. A new equilibrium between these processes is reached at a very high plasma glucose level of 300 to 1000 mg/dl. An increased rate of gluconeogenesis is supported by uninhibited proteolysis. Uninhibited lipolysis and ketogenesis elevate the plasma levels of FFAs and of the strong carboxylic acids, acetoacetic and β-OH-butyric. As they are neutralized by sodium bicarbonate, carbonic acid is formed, which dissociates to carbon dioxide and water. Compensatory pulmonary hyperventilation lowers P_{CO_2}, but despite this compensation, the blood pH may finally fall to less than 6.8, and death from diabetic ketoacidosis ensues.

Before this terminal point is reached in type 1 diabetes mellitus, a classic constellation of symptoms is observed. Because of the high plasma glucose levels, the filtered load exceeds the renal tubular capacity for reabsorption of glucose. Glucose is therefore excreted in the urine in large quantities, causing, by its osmotic effect, increased excretion of water and salts and frequent urination. Thirst is stimulated by the hyperosmolality of the plasma and by the hypovolemia. The loss of glucose is also a caloric drain, which the patient attempts to recoup by eating more. This response adds to hyperglycemia, as the insulin-deficient individual is unable to store carbohydrate efficiently. Exercise capacity may be impaired because of the reduction in muscle and liver glycogen stores. The end result is a catabolic state manifested by loss of lean body mass, adipose tissue, and body fluids.

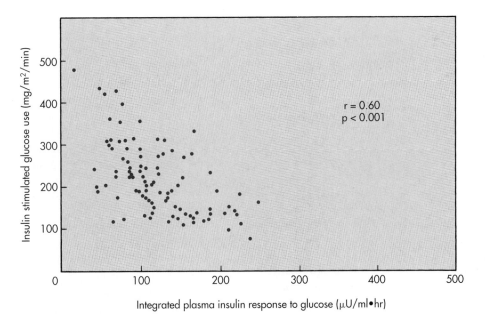

■ **Fig. 47-15** Relationship between responsiveness of peripheral tissue glucose uptake to insulin and responsiveness of β cells to glucose. Note that the less responsive tissues are to insulin, the greater is the amount of insulin secreted when glucose is provided orally to humans. This feedback system helps to maintain plasma glucose in the physiological range. (Modified from Hollenbeck C, Reaven GM: Variations in insulin-stimulated glucose uptake in healthy individuals with normal glucose tolerance, *J Clin Endocrinol Metab* 64:1169, 1987. From the Endocrine Society.)

Negative balances of nitrogen, potassium, phosphate, magnesium, and other intracellular components develop as these substances are excreted in the urine.

Osmotic fluid shifts secondary to the high plasma glucose level, and its conversion to other sugars, such as sorbitol, may cause swelling of the lens of the eye, blurred vision, and even formation of cataracts. Numerous proteins, including hemoglobin, albumin, and collagen, are nonenzymatically glucosylated by formation of an adduct between the aldehyde group of glucose and the N terminus or other free amino groups in these proteins. End products of protein glycosylation contribute to long-term tissue damage in the retina, kidneys, nerves, and cardiovascular system.

Insulin therapy systematically lowers plasma levels of glucose, FFAs, and ketoacids to normal and reduces urine nitrogen losses (Fig. 47-16). This result is achieved by the direct actions of insulin, as well as by normalizing the unrestrained secretion of glucagon that results from insulin deficiency and contributes to the hyperglycemia and ketoacidemia (Fig. 47-16). In diabetic ketoacidosis, fluid volume replacement along with potassium (to prevent hypokalemia from insulin action) is also essential to recovery.

Other β-cell products. In addition to insulin, the β-cell granule also contains peptides that are structurally unrelated to insulin. Although these peptides are synthesized by direction of other genes, they are packaged with insulin and coreleased during exocytosis. **Amylin** is a 37-amino acid peptide synthesized from a precursor that is expressed by a calcitonin-related gene (see Chapter 48). The granule content and the plasma levels of amylin, both in the basal state and after stimulation, are approximately 1% to 2% of those of insulin. Amylin is a noncompetitive antagonist to insulin, especially by decreasing glucose uptake and metabolism in muscle. Amylin also tends to polymerize, and fibrils containing this peptide accumulate extracellularly within the islets of individuals with type 2 non–insulin-dependent diabetes mellitus. The physiological and pathophysiological roles of amylin remain to be determined.

Pancreastatin is a 49-amino acid peptide that is structurally related to and may be a product of the processing of chromogranin A (see Chapter 45). This peptide inhibits insulin secretion. Because it is coreleased with insulin from the β-cell granule, pancreastatin may participate in an autofeedback regulation of insulin secretion.

■ Glucagon

■ Structure and Synthesis

Glucagon is a single, straight-chain peptide hormone of 29 amino acids and molecular weight of 3500. The N-terminal residues 1 to 6 are essential for receptor binding and for biological activity.

Glucagon is synthesized from a preproglucagon precursor by islet α cells (Fig. 47-17). The gene that encodes glucagon is a member of a superfamily that codes for vasoactive intestinal peptide, gastric inhibitory peptide, secretin, and growth hormone–releasing hormone (see Chapters 38 and 49). The functions of the copeptides produced by the α cells (Fig. 47-17) are unknown. In specific intestinal cells, processing of preproglucagon yields glucagon-like peptides of several types, instead of glucagon (Fig. 47-17). Both glucose and insulin decrease α-cell glucagon synthesis by repressing transcription of the glucagon gene. Both a cAMP-responsive element and an insulin-responsive element are present in the gene. The directional blood flow in the islets promotes the bathing of mantle α cells with high concentrations of inhibitory insulin from the core β cells. Glucagon is stored in dense granules and is released by exocytosis. This process is inhibited if α-cell Ca^{++} levels are decreased.

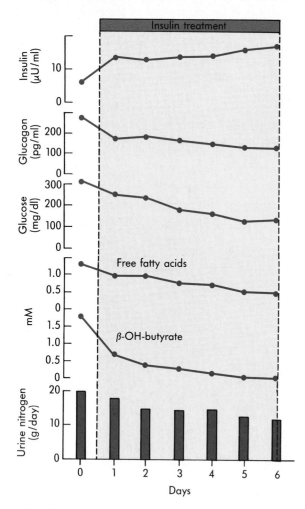

■ **Fig. 47-16** The effects of insulin replacement on plasma hormone and substrate levels and on urine losses of glucose and nitrogen in insulin-deficient diabetic humans. Note that this is a mirror image of the changes in substrates that characterize the adaptation to fasting shown in Fig. 46-11.

■ *Regulation of Secretion*

The most important principle governing glucagon secretion is the maintenance of normoglycemia in the face of increased tissue glucose demand. Exactly opposite to insulin secretion, glucagon is secreted in response to glucose deficiency and acts to increase circulating glucose levels (Fig. 47-18). Hypoglycemia causes a twofold to fourfold increase in plasma glucagon levels, whereas hyperglycemia lowers them approximately 50%. Although glucose directly regulates glucagon secretion in vitro, its effect is strongly modulated by insulin. Glucagon secretion is stimulated much more by low glucose levels if insulin is absent. Conversely, the presence of insulin greatly potentiates the suppressive effect of high glucose levels on the α cell.

Glucagon secretion is also stimulated by a protein meal and, most effectively, by amino acids such as arginine and alanine. However, this α-cell response to protein is greatly dampened if glucose is administered concurrently. This interaction partly occurs via insulin; positive glucagon responses to amino acids are restrained by insulin excess and augmented by insulin deficiency. FFAs and glucose exert a suppressive effect on the glucagon response. Glucagon responses to orally ingested nutrients (as opposed to the responses to intravenous delivery) may also be reinforced by the release of gastrointestinal secretagogues that augment insulin secretion. Important exceptions are GLP-1 (a proglucagon product of the intestine) (Fig. 47-17) and secretin, both of which inhibit α-cell glucagon release.

The sum of all these individual influences is that the ingestion of ordinary meals produces much less variation in plasma glucagon levels than in plasma insulin levels. These differences are partly explained by the offsetting effects of the carbohydrate and protein portions of the meal on the α cell, compared with the synergistic effects of these nutrients on the β cell.

Fasting for several days increases plasma glucagon levels twofold. Exercise of sufficient intensity and duration also increases plasma glucagon levels. Neural mechanisms may mediate some of these responses. In particular, vagal stimulation and acetylcholine acutely increase glucagon secretion. The neurohormone somatostatin inhibits the secretion of glucagon, probably by paracrine or neurocrine effects made possible by the islet microarchitecture (Fig. 47-1).

A variety of stresses, including infection, burns, tissue infarction, and major surgery, rapidly increase glucagon secretion. This increased secretion is probably mediated by the sympathetic nervous system via outflow from the ventromedial hypothalamus to α-adrenergic receptors in the α cells. The excess glucagon often leads to clinically significant hyperglycemia, particularly in individuals who have diabetes mellitus.

Monomeric α-cell glucagon circulates unbound in plasma at a basal concentration of 50 to 100 pg/ml (2×10^{-11} M). It has a half-life of 6 minutes. The daily secretion rate of glucagon is estimated to be 100 to 150 μg.

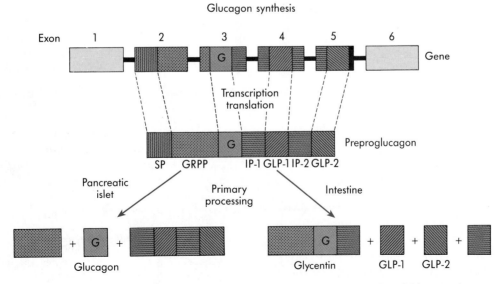

■ **Fig. 47-17** Glucagon synthesis. The gene is composed of six exons that yield preproglucagon. After elimination of the signal peptide *(SP)*, the α cells of the pancreas process proglucagon to glucagon, a glucagon-related polypeptide *(GRPP)*, and a C-terminal peptide. In the intestinal L cells, glucagon itself is not produced, but glucagon-like peptides 1 and 2 *(GLP-1 and GLP-2)* are secreted along with a larger glucagon-containing peptide called glycentin. *IP-1,* Intervening peptide-1; *IP-2,* intervening peptide-2. (Modified from Phillipe J: Structure and pancreatic expression of the insulin and glucagon gene, *Endocr Rev* 12:252, 1991. From the Endocrine Society.)

The ratio of portal vein to peripheral vein glucagon concentrations is about 1.5 in the basal state, and about 50% of glucagon is extracted by the liver during a single passage. The kidney is the other major site of glucagon degradation. Less than 1% of the glucagon filtered by the glomerulus is excreted in the urine.

■ *Hormone Actions*

In almost all respects, the actions of glucagon are exactly opposite to those of insulin. Glucagon promotes mobilization rather than storage of fuels, especially glucose (Fig. 47-19). Both hormones act at similar control points in the liver (Table 47-2, Fig. 47-13). Glucagon may even be viewed as the primary hormone that regulates hepatic glucose production and ketogenesis, insulin's role being that of glucagon antagonist.

Glucagon binds to a hepatic plasma membrane glycoprotein receptor; the resultant signal is transduced via a stimulatory G protein, adenylyl cyclase, and cAMP as second messenger (see Figs. 45-8 and 45-9). cAMP-activated protein kinase A initiates a cascade of phosphorylations that activate or deactivate a number of enzyme kinases or phosphatases by covalent modification of the enzyme structures. The first and best-studied example is phosphorylase, the enzyme that degrades glycogen. Activated protein kinase A converts inactive phosphorylase kinase to active phosphorylase kinase. The latter then converts inactive phosphorylase to active phosphorylase, and the rate of glycogenolysis increases. In contrast, phosphorylation of the enzymes phosphofructokinase and pyruvate kinase decreases their activity so that the rate of glycolysis is decreased.

The dominant effect of glucagon is on the liver. (Its actions on adipose tissue and muscle are minor unless insulin is virtually absent.) In the liver, glucagon exerts an immediate and profound glycogenolytic effect through activation of glycogen phosphorylase. The glucose-1-phosphate released as a result of glycogen phos-

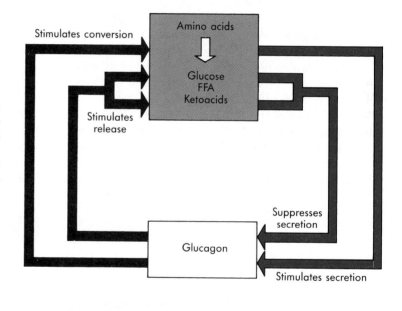

■ Fig. 47-18 Feedback relationship between glucagon and nutrients. Glucagon stimulates production and release of glucose, free fatty acids *(FFA)*, and ketoacids, which in turn suppress glucagon secretion. Amino acids stimulate glucagon secretion, and glucagon in turn stimulates the conversion of amino acids to glucose.

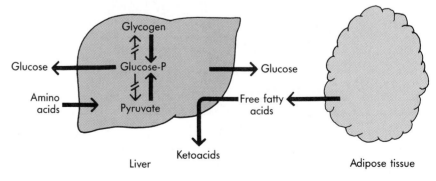

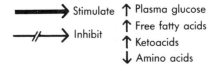

■ Fig. 47-19 The effect of glucagon on the overall flow of fuels results in tissue release of glucose, fatty acids, and ketoacids into the circulation and hepatic uptake of amino acids for gluconeogenesis.

phorylase activation is prevented from undergoing resynthesis to glycogen by a simultaneous inhibition of glycogen synthase. Glucagon also stimulates gluconeogenesis by several mechanisms. The hepatic extraction of amino acids, especially alanine, is increased. The activities and concentrations of gluconeogenic enzymes are increased, whereas those of glycolysis are decreased.

The enzyme pair phosphofructokinase and fructose-1,6-biphosphatase determine the direction and magnitude of the flow between fructose-6-phosphate and fructose-1,6-biphosphate, and therefore the relative rates of glycolysis and gluconeogenesis (Fig. 47-13). The activities of these two enzymes in turn are reciprocally related to the level of fructose-2,6-biphosphate. The concentration of this important metabolite is regulated by the unique bidirectional enzyme 6-phosphofructo-2-kinase/fructose-2,6-biphosphatase, which is very sensitive to the islet hormones (Fig. 47-20).

When phosphorylated, this bidirectional enzyme is a phosphatase that decreases fructose-2,6-biphosphate levels; when dephosphorylated, the enzyme is a kinase that increases fructose-2,6-biphosphate levels. Glucagon action phosphorylates the enzyme and lowers fructose-2,6-biphosphate levels; this in turn decreases phosphofructokinase and increases fructose-1,6-biphosphatase activities (Fig. 47-20). The result is an increase in gluconeogenesis and a decrease in glycolysis. Insulin action dephosphorylates the bidirectional enzyme and has exactly the opposite effects on fructose-2,6-biphosphate levels (Fig. 47-20). The result is a decrease in gluconeogenesis and an increase in glycolysis.

The crucial importance of glucagon to the maintenance of basal hepatic glucose output is shown by the marked decline that follows the selective inhibition of glucagon secretion. The powerful glycogenolytic and hyperglycemic action of glucagon is exhibited at plasma hormone concentrations of 150 to 500 pg/ml, and occurs even in the presence of insulin somewhat above basal levels (20 to 30 μU/ml). However, this action is transient; the acute stimulation of hepatic glucose output, which occurs during continuous glucagon administration,

wanes after about 30 minutes because of hepatic autoregulation by hyperglycemia and stimulation of insulin release. However, if glucagon is given in a more physiological, fluctuating pattern, each increase in the hormone causes a pulse of glucose output.

Glucagon has little or no influence on glucose use by peripheral tissues. Thus, hyperglucagonemia has no effect on the plasma glucose levels that are generated by an exogenous glucose load, as long as the insulin response to the glucose stimulus is normal. The gluconeogenic action of glucagon is also reflected in the ability of the hormone to increase the rate of disposal of amino acids and their degradation to urea. However, glucagon has no particular influence on branched-chain amino acid levels, which suggests that it has little or no effect on muscle proteolysis.

Another important intrahepatic action of glucagon is to direct incoming FFAs away from triglyceride synthesis and toward β-oxidation. Thus, glucagon is a ketogenic as well as a hyperglycemic hormone. Glucagon inactivates acetyl-CoA carboxylase, which catalyzes the rate-limiting step in FFA synthesis from cytoplasmic acetyl CoA (Fig. 47-13). This inactivation results in lower levels of malonyl CoA, an allosteric inhibitor of carnitine acyltransferase. In turn, lower levels of malonyl CoA allow a faster rate of influx of fatty acyl CoA into the mitochondrion for conversion to ketoacids. Glucagon also activates adipose tissue lipase, and thereby increases lipolysis and the delivery of FFAs to the liver. Although the ketogenic actions of glucagon are physiologically very relevant, they are easily nullified by rather small amounts of insulin, particularly at the adipose tissue locus. Finally, hepatic hydroxy-methylglutaryl-CoA reductase activity is inhibited by glucagon, thereby decreasing hepatic cholesterol synthesis.

Other actions of glucagon include inhibition of renal tubular sodium resorption; thus, it causes natriuresis. Activation of myocardial adenylyl cyclase causes a modest increase in cardiac output. Glucagon may also be synthesized in the central nervous system and may act locally in the regulation of appetite.

■ **Table 47-2**   Contrasting effects of insulin and glucagon on key enzymes in hepatic glucose metabolism

Enzyme	Activity		Gene expression	
	Insulin	*Glucagon*	*Insulin*	*Glucagon*
Gluconeogenesis and glucose export				
Glucose-6-phosphatase Fructose-1,6-biphosphatase Phosphoenolpyruvate carboxykinase	↓	↑	↓	↑
Pyruvate				
Glucokinase 6-Phosphofructo-1-kinase Pyruvate kinase	↑	↓	↑	↓
Glycolysis and glucose oxidation				

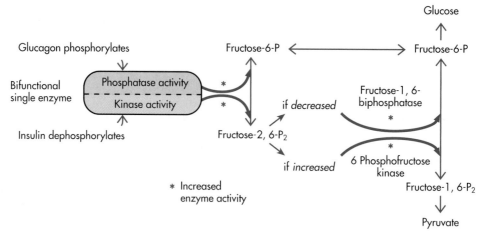

■ **Fig. 47-20** Regulation of the relative rates of gluconeogenesis and glycolysis by the actions of islet hormones on a single bifunctional enzyme. Insulin causes dephosphorylation of the enzyme, making it a kinase, which raises the level of fructose-2,6-biphosphate. This intermediate stimulates the activity of 6-phosphofructose kinase and shifts metabolism toward pyruvate (glycolysis). Glucagon phosphorylates the bifunctional enzyme, making it a phosphatase, which lowers the level of fructose-2,6-biphosphate, thereby increasing the activity of fructose-1,6-biphosphatase and shifting metabolism toward glucose (gluconeogenesis).

■ *Insulin:Glucagon Ratio*

It should now be apparent that the direction of substrate fluxes is very sensitive to the relative availability of insulin and glucagon (compare Figs. 47-12 and 47-19). The usual molar ratio of insulin to glucagon in plasma is about 2.0. Under circumstances that require mobilization and increased use of endogenous substrates, the insulin:glucagon ratio drops to 0.5 or less. This decreased ratio is seen in fasting and in prolonged exercise, and is caused by both decreased insulin secretion and increased glucagon secretion. A low insulin:glucagon ratio facilitates increased glycogenolysis, amino acid mobilization, and gluconeogenesis to maintain glucose supply to the central nervous system. Lipolysis is also enhanced, which increases FFA flow to muscle and liver for oxidation. During exercise, the low insulin:glucagon ratio still permits muscle glucose uptake, which is stimulated by an exercise-specific mechanism that is independent of insulin.

Maintenance of a low insulin:glucagon ratio is critical in the neonatal period when the infant is abruptly cut off from maternal fuel supplies but is not yet able to efficiently assimilate exogenous fuel from its gastrointestinal tract. When this ratio is excessive—as may occur in infants born of diabetic mothers—hypoglycemia may result.

Conversely, under circumstances in which substrate storage is advantageous, such as after a pure carbohydrate load or a mixed meal, the insulin:glucagon ratio rises to 10 or more, mainly because of increased insulin secretion. The high ratio enhances glucose uptake, oxidation, and conversion to liver and muscle glycogen, while it suppresses unneeded proteolysis and lipolysis. An interesting example of only a small and insignificant change in the insulin:glucagon ratio occurs after a subject ingests a pure protein meal. In this situation, insulin secretion increases, preventing unneeded proteolysis and facilitating muscle uptake of some amino acids and their incorporation into proteins. At the same time, glucagon secretion also increases. This increase in glucagon prevents the decrease in hepatic glucose output and hypoglycemia that would ensue if the extra insulin action were completely unopposed. Ingestion of pure fat has little influence on the insulin:glucagon ratio. After a mixed meal, however, the increase in the ratio facilitates clearance of chylomicrons by activation of adipose tissue lipoprotein lipase.

Primary glucagon excess is produced by α-cell tumors. Plasma levels of glucose and of ketoacids are only modestly elevated. The marked increase in gluconeogenesis causes a generalized reduction of plasma amino acids and an increase in urinary nitrogen. The catabolic action of the hormone is exhibited by loss of weight and by a peculiar, destructive skin lesion. Severe diabetes mellitus is uncommon because of the compensatory increase in insulin secretion.

The predictable consequence of glucagon deficiency would be fasting hypoglycemia. In fact, cases of fasting hypoglycemia caused by glucagon deficiency have rarely been documented. Other hormonal adjustments likely sustain plasma glucose when glucagon is deficient. However, glucagon secretion in

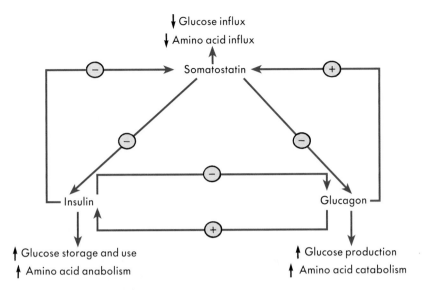

↓ Glucose influx
↓ Amino acid influx

Somatostatin

− Insulin

Glucagon

↑ Glucose storage and use
↑ Amino acid anabolism

↑ Glucose production
↑ Amino acid catabolism

■ **Fig. 47-21** Schema interrelating the effects of somatostatin, insulin, and glucagon on each other's secretion with their effects on glucose and amino acid metabolism. (Modified from Unger RH et al: Insulin, glucagon, and somatostatin secretion in the regulation of metabolism, *Annu Rev Physiol* 40:307, 1978.)

response to insulin-induced hypoglycemia can become greatly impaired in type 1 diabetes. The lack of glucagon markedly increases the risk of severe "insulin reactions" if such a patient injects too much insulin, misses a meal, or exercises heavily.

■ *Somatostatin Secretion and Action*

Somatostatin functions primarily as an inhibitor of growth hormone secretion (see Chapter 49), but it is also synthesized by the δ cells of the pancreatic islets and by intestinal cells. In the δ cells, the processing of the primary somatostatin gene product, prosomatostatin, yields mostly a 14-amino acid peptide (SS-14). In intestinal cells, a 28-amino acid peptide with an N-terminal extension is probably the major product (SS-28). Many of the biological actions of these products are similar. Somatostatin secretion is stimulated by glucose, amino acids, FFAs, a variety of gastrointestinal hormones, glucagon, and β-adrenergic and cholinergic neurotransmitters. It is inhibited by insulin and α-adrenergic neurotransmitters. Exocytosis of somatostatin granules is stimulated by cAMP. Plasma levels of SS-28, but not of SS-14, increase with mixed meals.

Somatostatin is a profound inhibitor of both insulin and glucagon secretion. The administration of somatostatin also decreases the assimilation rate of all nutrients from the gastrointestinal tract. This effect is accomplished by inhibitory actions on gastric, duodenal, and gallbladder motility; on the secretion of hydrochloric acid, pepsin, gastrin, secretin, and intestinal juices; and on pancreatic exocrine function. Somatostatin also inhibits the absorption of glucose, xylose, and triglycerides across the mucosal membrane. SS-14 and SS-28 may participate in a feedback arrangement, whereby entrance of food into the gut stimulates their release in order to prevent rapid nutrient overload. SS-14 may be released locally and may act in neurocrine and paracrine fashion to limit insulin and

glucagon responses to meals. SS-28, which is released in particular after ingestion of fat, may function as a true hormone: that is, it may reach the pancreatic islets via the bloodstream. The interaction among the α cells, β cells, δ cells, and intestinal cell products may coordinate the rates of bulk movement, digestion, and absorption of nutrients with the rates of nutrient uptake by the liver and peripheral tissues (Fig. 47-21).

Somatostatin analogs are now used therapeutically to alleviate diarrhea caused by unregulated gastrointestinal hormone secretion. They are also employed to inhibit unregulated release of various peptide and protein hormones by neoplasms. Tumors of the δ cells produce somatostatin excess. Signs and symptoms of somatostatin excess include inhibition of nutrient absorption, excess stool fat, and weight loss. Plasma insulin and glucagon levels are low, and the low insulin level may lead to modest hyperglycemia.

■ *Pancreatic Polypeptide*

Pancreatic polypeptide is a specific product of the PP cells. It has 36 amino acids and a distinctive C-terminal tyrosine-amide residue. It belongs to a family of similar molecules, including neuropeptide Y in the hypothalamus. PP is secreted in response to food ingestion via gastrointestinal secretagogues and cholinergic stimulation. PP is also stimulated by hypoglycemia and inhibited by glucose administration. Its best-defined action is to inhibit exocrine pancreatic secretion, partly by inhibiting the uptake of precursor amino acids by the acinar cells. Its true physiological importance is unclear, but elevated plasma levels of PP serve as markers for the presence of islet cell tumors and their response to treatment. A failure of plasma PP to increase when plasma glucose is sharply reduced suggests loss of cholinergic pancreatic islet innervation.

■ *Summary*

1. The pancreatic islets are composed of insulin-secreting β cells (the majority), glucagon-secreting α cells, somatostatin-secreting δ cells, and pancreatic polypeptide(PP)–secreting cells. The microarchitecture and blood flow arrangements permit paracrine and neurocrine functioning, as well as direct cell-to-cell communication through gap junctions.

2. Insulin is a major glucoregulatory, antilipolytic, antiketogenic, and anabolic hormone. It consists of two straight-chain peptides held together by disulfide bonds and synthesized from a single-chain precursor (proinsulin).

3. Insulin secretion is stimulated primarily by glucose and food intake, but also by other fuels, gastrointestinal peptides, and cholinergic and β-adrenergic stimuli. Release is inhibited by fasting and by exercise, both circumstances in which fuel mobilization is required.

4. Insulin promotes fuel storage. Its effects in order of increasing insulin doses required are inhibition of adipose tissue lipolysis and of ketogenesis; inhibition of hepatic glycogenolysis, gluconeogenesis, and glucose release; inhibition of muscle proteolysis; and stimulation of muscle glucose uptake and storage as glycogen. Insulin also stimulates cellular uptake of amino acids, phosphate, and magnesium, as well as synthesis of numerous proteins.

5. Insulin acts through a plasma membrane receptor that phosphorylates itself after binding insulin, and thereby acquires tyrosine kinase activity. The activated receptor phosphorylates an insulin receptor substrate or substrates. From this phosphorylation flows a cascade of modulation of the activities of numerous enzymes involved in glucose and fatty acid metabolism. In addition, gene transcription of numerous enzymes and proteins essential to cell growth is induced or repressed.

6. Insulin decreases plasma levels of glucose, free fatty acids (FFAs), ketoacids, glycerol, and branched-chain and other amino acids. Insulin deficiency leads to hyperglycemia, loss of lean body and adipose tissue mass, growth retardation, and ultimately metabolic ketoacidosis.

7. Glucagon is a straight-chain peptide released in response to hypoglycemia and to amino acids. Its secretion is suppressed by glucose, FFAs, and insulin. Glucagon secretion increases during prolonged fasting and exercise.

8. Glucagon is an insulin antagonist that promotes mobilization of glucose. It acts primarily on the liver to stimulate glycogenolysis and gluconeogenesis, as well as fatty acid oxidation and ketogenesis. cAMP is its second messenger, and covalent modification of enzyme activities by phosphorylation is the main mechanism of action.

Glucagon increases the plasma levels of glucose, FFAs, and ketoacids, but it decreases amino acid levels.

9. The insulin:glucagon ratio controls the relative rates of glycolysis and gluconeogenesis by altering hepatic fructose-2,6-biphosphate levels. This metabolite in turn regulates the rate and direction of flow between fructose-1-phosphate and fructose-1,6-biphosphate. The two hormones have antagonistic effects at numerous other liver enzyme steps in glucose and fatty acid metabolism.

10. Somatostatin is a neuropeptide of islet and intestinal cell origin. It decreases the motility of the gastrointestinal tract, gastrointestinal secretions, digestion and absorption of nutrients, and secretion of both insulin and glucagon. Somatostatin is secreted in response to meals; its actions, along with those of insulin and glucagon, probably coordinate nutrient input with substrate disposal.

■ *Self-Study Problems*

1. Describe the pathophysiological sequence that follows acute insulin deficiency.

2. Describe the islet hormonal responses to a mixed meal.

■ *Bibliography*

Journal articles

Amiel SA et al: Insulin resistance of puberty: a defect restricted to peripheral glucose metabolism, *J Clin Endocrinol Metab* 72:277, 1991.

Boden G et al: Role of glucagon in disposal of an amino acid load, *Am J Physiol* 259:E225, 1990.

Bonadonna RC et al: Dose-dependent effect of insulin on plasma free fatty acid turnover and oxidation in humans, *Am J Physiol* 259:E726, 1990.

Cahill GF: Starvation in man, *N Engl J Med* 282:668, 1970.

Cheatham B, Kahn CR: Insulin action and the insulin signaling network, *Endocr Rev* 16:117, 1995.

Dupre J, Behme MT, Hramiak IM, Longo CJ: Hepatic extraction of insulin after stimulation of secretion with oral glucose or parenteral nutrients, *Metabolism* 42:921, 1993.

Exton JH: Some thoughts on the mechanism of action of insulin, *Diabetes* 40:521, 1991.

Fehmann H-C, Göke R, Göke B: Cell and molecular biology of the incretin hormones glucagon-like peptide-I and glucose-dependent insulin releasing polypeptide, *Endocr Rev* 16:390, 1995.

Frank HJL et al: A direct in vitro demonstration of insulin binding to isolated brain microvessels, *Diabetes* 30:757, 1981.

Fukagawa NK et al: Insulin dose-dependent reductions in plasma amino acids in man, *Am J Physiol* 250:E13, 1986.

Gottesman I et al: Insulin increases the maximum velocity for glucose uptake without altering the Michaelis constant in man: evidence that insulin increases glucose uptake merely by providing additional transport sites, *J Clin Invest* 70:1310, 1982.

Granner DK, Andreone TL: Insulin modulation of gene expression, *Diabetes Metab Rev* 1:139, 1985.

Hollenbeck C, Reaven GM: Variations in insulin-stimulated glucose uptake in healthy individuals with normal glucose tolerance, *J Clin Endocrinol Metab* 64:1169, 1987.

Inoue H, et al: Isolation, characterization, and chromosomal mapping of the human insulin promoter factor 1 (IPF-1) gene, *Diabetes* 45:789, 1996.

Itoh M et al: Antisomatostatin gamma globulin augments secretion of both insulin and glucagon in vitro: evidence for a physiologic role for endogenous somatostatin in the regulation of pancreatic alpha and beta cell function, *Diabetes* 29:693, 1980.

Jackson RA et al: Influence of aging on glucose homeostasis, *J Clin Endocrinol Metab* 55:840, 1982.

Jefferson LS: Role of insulin in the regulation of protein synthesis, *Diabetes* 29:487, 1980.

Kahn CR: Insulin action, diabetogenes, and the cause of type II diabetes, *Diabetes* 43:1066, 1994.

Kahn SE: Regulation of β-cell function in vivo, *Diabetes Metab Rev* 4:372, 1996.

Kahn SE et al: Evidence of cosecretion of islet amyloid polypeptide and insulin by beta cells, *Diabetes* 39:634, 1990.

Katz L et al: Splanchnic and peripheral disposal of oral glucose in man, *Diabetes* 32:675, 1983.

Kimball SR, Vary TC, Jefferson LS: Regulation of protein synthesis by insulin, *Annu Rev Physiol* 56:321, 1994.

King DS et al: Insulin secretory capacity in endurance-trained and untrained young men, *Am J Physiol* 259:E155, 1990.

Krasinski SD et al: Pancreatic polypeptide and peptide YY gene expression, *Ann NY Acad Sci* 611:73, 1990.

Liljenquist JE et al: Evidence for an important role of glucagon in the regulation of hepatic glucose production in normal man, *J Clin Invest* 59:369, 1977.

Magnuson MA: Glucokinase gene structure: functional implications of molecular genetic studies, *Diabetes* 39:523, 1990.

Marchetti P et al: Pulsatile insulin secretion from isolated human pancreatic islets, *Diabetes* 43:827, 1994.

Matschinsky FM: Glucokinase as glucose sensor and metabolic signal generator in pancreatic beta cells and hepatocytes, *Diabetes* 39:647, 1990.

Matschinsky FM, Sweet IR: Annotated questions and answers about glucose metabolism and insulin secretion of β-cells, *Diabetes Metab Rev* 4:130-144, 1996.

Meda P et al: Rapid and reversible secretion change during uncoupling of rat insulin-producing cells, *J Clin Invest* 86:759, 1990.

Mueckler M: Family of glucose-transporter genes: implications for glucose homeostasis and diabetes, *Diabetes* 39:6, 1990.

Nair S et al: Effect of intravenous insulin treatment on in vivo whole body leucine kinetics and oxygen consumption in insulin deprived type I diabetic patients, *Metabolism* 36:491, 1987.

Nurjhan N et al: Insulin dose-response characteristics for suppression of glycerol release and conversion to glucose in humans, *Diabetes* 35:1326, 1986.

Olefsky JM: The insulin receptor: a multifunctional protein, *Diabetes* 39:1009, 1991.

Orskov C et al: Proglucagon products in plasma of noninsulin-dependent diabetics and nondiabetic controls in the fasting state and after oral glucose and intravenous arginine, *J Clin Invest* 87:415, 1991.

Philippe J: Structure and pancreatic expression of the insulin and glucagon genes, *Endocr Rev* 12:252, 1991.

Polonsky KS, Given BD, Van Cauter E: Twenty-four-hour profiles and pulsatile patterns of insulin secretion in normal and obese subjects, *J Clin Invest* 81:442, 1988.

Reichlin S: Somatostatin, *N Engl J Med* 309:1495, 1983

Robertson RP, Seaquist ER, Walseth TF: G proteins and modulation of insulin secretion, *Diabetes* 40:1, 1991.

Saltiel AR: Second messengers of insulin action, *Diabetes Care* 13:244, 1990.

Schwartz MW et al: Insulin in the brain: a hormonal regulator of energy balance, *Endocr Rev* 13:387, 1992.

Schwartz TW: Pancreatic polypeptide: a hormone under vagal control, *Gastroenterology* 85:1411, 1983.

Seino S, Seino M, Bell GI: Human insulin receptor gene, *Diabetes* 39:129, 1990.

Stephens JM, Pilch PF: The metabolic regulation and vesicular transport of GLUT4, the major insulin-responsive glucose transporter, *Endocr Rev* 4:529, 1995.

Sturis J et al: Entrainment of pulsatile insulin secretion by oscillatory glucose infusion, *J Clin Invest* 87:439, 1991.

Thiebaud D et al: The effect of graded doses of insulin on total glucose uptake, glucose oxidation, and glucose storage in man, *Diabetes* 31:957, 1982.

Unger RH et al: Insulin, glucagon, and somatostatin secretion in the regulation of metabolism, *Annu Rev Physiol* 40:307, 1978.

Weigle DS: Pulsatile secretion of fuel regulatory hormones, *Diabetes* 36:764, 1987.

Weir GC, Bonner-Weir S: Islets of Langerhans: the puzzle of intraislet interactions and their relevance to diabetes, *J Clin Invest* 85:983, 1990.

Wollheim CB, Lang J, Regazzi R: The exocytotic process of insulin secretion and its regulation by Ca++ and G-proteins, *Diabetes Metab Rev* 4:276, 1996.

Books and monographs

Cheatham B, Kahn CR: *The biochemistry of insulin action.* In LeRoith D, Taylor SI, Olefsky JM, editors: *Diabetes mellitus,* Philadelphia, 1996, Lippincott-Raven.

Cook DL, Taborsky GJ: *β-cell function and insulin secretion.* In Rifkin H, Porte D, editors: *Diabetes mellitus,* New York, 1990, Elsevier Scientific.

Czech MP, Erwin JL, Sleeman MW: *Insulin action on glucose transport.* In LeRoith D, Taylor SI, Olefsky JM, editors: *Diabetes mellitus,* Philadelphia, 1996, Lippincott-Raven.

Flakoll P, Carlson MG, Cherrington A: *Physiologic action of insulin.* In LeRoith D, Taylor SI, Olefsky JM, editors: *Diabetes mellitus,* Philadelphia, 1996, Lippincott-Raven.

Malaisse WJ: *Insulin secretion and beta cell metabolism.* In DeGroot LJ, editor: *Endocrinology,* Philadelphia, 1994, WB Saunders.

O'Brien RM, Granner DK: *Insulin action: gene regulation.* In LeRoith D, Taylor SI, Olefsky JM, editors: *Diabetes mellitus,* Philadelphia, 1996, Lippincott-Raven.

Polonsky KS, O'Meara NM: *Secretion and metabolism of insulin, proinsulin and C-peptide.* In DeGroot LJ, editor: *Endocrinology,* Philadelphia, 1994, WB Saunders.

Steiner DF et al: *Chemistry and biosynthesis of the islet hormones: insulin, islet amyloid polypeptide (amylin), glucagon, somatostatin and pancreatic polypeptide.* In DeGroot LJ, editor: *Endocrinology,* Philadelphia, 1994, WB Saunders.

Unger RH, Orci L: *Glucagon.* In Rifkin H, Porte D, editors: *Diabetes mellitus,* New York, 1990, Elsevier Scientific.

Endocrine Regulation of Calcium and Phosphate Metabolism

A complex regulatory system maintains the normal amounts of calcium, phosphate, and the related mineral magnesium in the body. The key hormones that regulate the amounts of calcium and phosphate are **parathyroid hormone (PTH),** a peptide, and **vitamin D,** a sterol. *These hormones act on three organ systems—the intestinal tract, the bone, and the kidneys—to maintain calcium and phosphate levels in the face of environmental changes (e.g., diet) and internal demands (e.g., pregnancy).* Before detailing these hormonal mechanisms of regulation, an overview of calcium and phosphate metabolism, as well as related structural and functional aspects of bone mass, is presented. Without this introduction, it is difficult to understand how the individual endocrine components of the system work together.

■ *Overview of Calcium and Phosphate Metabolism*

■ *Calcium*

The calcium ion is fundamentally important to all biological systems. Because of its importance, the concentration of calcium is maintained within specific limits of physiological tolerance in several compartments. The resting intracellular cytosolic concentration of free calcium is only 10^{-7} M. This value can increase transiently 10- to 100-fold when the calcium ions are involved in creation or maintenance of action potentials, contraction and motility, cytoskeletal rearrangements, cell division, secretion, and modulation of enzyme activities. In absolute terms, however, this transient increase represents movement of exquisitely small amounts of calcium into the cell cytoplasm from either extracellular fluid or intracellular reservoirs. Both the initial entry and subsequent extrusion of calcium into and out of these reservoirs take place very rapidly, and the amounts exchanged are balanced. Despite the small amount of calcium

involved in these processes, calcium ions constitute a cellular ionic signal of unusual speed and a large dynamic range of amplitude and sensitivity.

The total pool of intracellular free calcium is estimated to be only 0.2 mg. An additional 9 g of intracellular calcium is present in a bound form in the endoplasmic reticulum, the mitochondria, and the plasma membrane. This intracellular calcium constitutes an immediately accessible storage pool and also contributes to the structural integrity of the cell.

The extracellular concentration of free calcium is approximately 10^{-3} M, or four orders of magnitude higher than the intracellular concentration. This large gradient is maintained by specialized membranes and calcium pumps (see Chapter 1). Maintenance of the proper extracellular concentration is essential for generation of normal membrane potentials and neurotransmission, for calcium uptake into the cells in the course of contraction and exocytosis, for normal blood clotting, and for modulation of plasma enzyme activities. The total extracellular pool of calcium weighs about 1 g. The skeleton and teeth contain 1 to 2 kg of calcium, depending on body size, or 99% of the total amount. This pool of bound calcium functions in skeletal structure, protection of internal organs, and locomotion.

The level of total calcium (free and bound) in the plasma ranges from 8.6 to 10.6 mg/dl (2.15 to 2.65 mmol/L = 4.3 to 5.3 mEq/L).* For any individual, however, the variation from day to day is generally less than 10%. Approximately 50% of plasma calcium is in the ionized, biologically active form. Ten percent is complexed in nonionic but ultrafilterable forms, such as calcium bicarbonate; much of the plasma calcium is bound to albumin; and 40% is bound to proteins, mainly albumin. Because of this binding, total plasma calcium rises

---

*The normal limits vary by as much as 0.5 mg/dl from laboratory to laboratory, depending on the method employed.

and falls with the albumin concentration, even into abnormal ranges. These fluctuations have no adverse biological consequences as long as the ionized calcium concentration remains normal. As the pH of the blood increases, however, the equilibrium between ionized and protein-bound calcium shifts toward the latter state. *Thus, alkalosis decreases and acidosis increases the plasma ionized calcium concentration.*

The plasma ionized calcium concentration can drop below normal: when (1) there is a total body calcium deficit, (2) a sudden shift in internal balance causes calcium to be taken up into bone faster than the extracellular calcium pool can be replenished, or (3) plasma protein binding to calcium increases, for example, in response to respiratory alkalosis secondary to hyperventilation. A decreased concentration of ionized calcium in the plasma causes neuromuscular irritability, manifested by numbness and tingling sensations, tetanic muscle contractions in the hands and feet, and, most dangerously, spasm of muscles in the larynx and consequent airway obstruction. Central nervous system irritability can cause seizures. When plasma ionized calcium is high, reduced neurotransmission causes muscle weakness, decreased intestinal motility, impaired mentation, and even coma.

Fig. 48-1 details the normal turnover of calcium in the body. Although daily dietary calcium can range from 200 to 2000 mg, the intake of many adults is below the recommended minimum of 800 mg. The percentage of dietary calcium absorbed from the intestine is inversely related to intake, but the relationship is curvilinear. An adaptive increase in fractional absorption is one important mechanism for maintaining normal body calcium stores when the diet does not contain adequate calcium. Conversely, an adaptive decrease in absorption prevents overload when the diet supplies too much calcium. At a daily intake of 1000 mg of calcium, about 35% is absorbed. The same amount of calcium, 350 mg, must ultimately be excreted to maintain balance. About 150 mg is secreted back into the intestine and excreted in the stools, along with the unabsorbed fraction from the diet. The remaining 200 mg is excreted in the urine. The kidneys filter about 10,000 mg of calcium per day (non–protein-bound calcium concentration × glomerular filtration rate = 60 mg/L × 170 L/day). However, approximately 98% is reabsorbed in the tubules. Adjustment of the small fraction of filtered calcium that is finally excreted provides a sensitive means of maintaining calcium balance. *Both dietary calcium intake and absorption from the intestine are diminished in elderly individuals. This decreased calcium input contributes to declining bone mass and the increased risk of fracture in the aged (osteoporosis).*

Calcium enters and exits from an extracellular pool of 1000 mg, which is in equilibrium with a rapidly exchanging pool of several times that size. This pool probably represents the surface of recently or partially mineralized bone. Approximately 500 mg of calcium is "irreversibly" removed from the extracellular space by bone formation, and the same amount is returned to it by bone resorption in the steady-state process that constitutes normal **bone remodeling.**

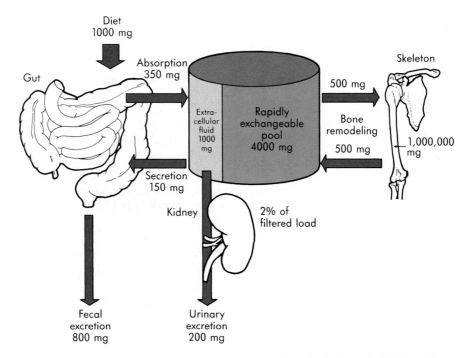

■ **Fig. 48-1**   Average daily calcium turnover in humans. Note both the external balance between intake and excretion and the internal balance between entry into and exit from bone.

■ *Phosphate*

The phosphate ion is also critically important to all biological systems. Phosphate is an integral component of numerous intermediates in the metabolism of carbohydrates, lipids, and proteins. It forms part of the structure of high-energy transfer and storage compounds, such as adenosine triphosphate (ATP) and creatine phosphate; of cofactors such as NAD, NADP, and thiamine pyrophosphate; of second messengers such as cAMP and inositol trisphosphate; and of DNA and RNA. Phosphate functions as a covalent modifier of many enzymes. Inside cells, it is an important anion that balances the cations K^+ and Mg^{++}, and a major constituent of the crystalline structure of bone and teeth. Of the total body phosphate content, 85% is contained in the skeleton and 6% in muscle.

The normal concentration of phosphate in the plasma is 2.5 to 4.5 mg/dl (0.81 to 1.45 mmol/L). Because the valence of phosphate changes with pH, it is less convenient to express phosphate concentration in milliequivalents per liter, as was done for calcium. The turnover of phosphate is shown in Fig. 48-2. About 70% of the phosphate ingested is absorbed by the intestine. In contrast to calcium, this absorbed amount remains relatively constant. Thus, the relationship between intake and absorption of phosphate from the intestine is more linear than that for calcium, Also, although adaptive regulation of phosphate absorption exists, it is less important than that of calcium. Therefore, urinary excretion provides the major mechanism for preserving phosphate balance. Of the daily filtered load of approximately 6000 mg (plasma concentration × glomerular filtration rate = 35 mg/L ×

170 L/day), the renal tubules can reabsorb from 70% to 100%, with an average of 90%. Regulation of phosphate absorption by the renal tubules provides the flexibility necessary to compensate for large swings in dietary intake.

Soft tissue stores of phosphate, such as those in the muscle mass, undergo rapid transfer with the extracellular fluid pool of phosphate. This transfer process is an important factor in the minute-to-minute regulation of plasma phosphate concentration. About 250 mg, or half the total extracellular fluid pool of 500 mg, enters and leaves the bone mass daily in the process of bone remodeling.

> Severe phosphate depletion can lead to skeletal muscle weakness, cardiac and respiratory muscle dysfunction, loss of red blood cell membrane integrity, and abnormal formation of bone.

The divalent cation magnesium (Mg^{++}) is related in some metabolic respects to calcium and phosphate. Magnesium is essential in neuromuscular transmission and serves as a cofactor in numerous enzyme reactions, most notably those involving energy transfers via ATP and those involved in protein synthesis. The normal range of magnesium in plasma is 1.8 to 2.4 mg/dl (1.5 to 2.0 mEq/L). One third of plasma magnesium is bound to protein. The body contains a total of about 25 g of magnesium, of which 50% is present in the skeleton and almost all the rest is present in the intracellular fluid. The usual daily intake of magnesium ranges from 300 to 500 mg. On average, 40% of this ingested magnesium is absorbed. In a steady state, the same amount, 120 to 200 mg, is excreted in the urine.

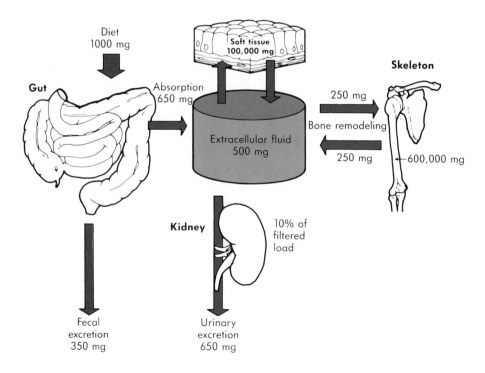

■ **Fig. 48-2**   Average daily phosphate turnover in humans. Note both the external balance between intake and excretion and the internal balance between entry into and exit from bone.

Serious magnesium depletion results from intestinal malabsorption, alcoholism, or diuretic overuse. Neuromuscular irritability, as described for calcium depletion, may result. In rare cases, dangerous ventricular arrhythmias may occur.

■ *Bone Dynamics*

A detailed account of the development of the skeleton, its structural properties, and its mechanical function is beyond the scope of endocrine physiology. However, a brief review of the organization of bone in relation to its function as a mineral reservoir is essential to an understanding of hormonal regulation of calcium and phosphate metabolism.

About 80% of the bone mass consists of **cortical bone.** The dense, concentric outer layers of the appendicular skeleton (long bones) and the thinner outer layer of the flat bones are the major components of cortical bone. About 20% of the bone mass consists of **trabecular bone:** bridges of bone spicules that make up the larger inner parts of the axial skeleton (skull, ribs, vertebrae, and pelvis) and the smaller interior of the shafts of long bones (Fig. 48-3). *Although of lesser mass, trabecular bone has five times as much total surface area as cortical bone. Because of its greater accessibility, trabecular bone is more important than cortical bone in calcium turnover.*

Throughout life, the bone mass is continuously being renewed by the well-regulated coupling of the processes of bone formation and resorption. This coupling occurs within individual microscopic units, called **osteons** or **bone modeling units,** that are present in all types of bone. The exact chemical and/or mechanical signals that coordinate local rates of formation and resorption are incompletely understood. During the growth years, formation exceeds resorption, and skeletal mass increases. Linear growth occurs at the ends of long bones by replacement of cartilage in specialized areas known as **epiphyseal plates.** These growth plates close off at the end of puberty when adult height is reached. Increase in bone width occurs by addition to the *periosteum,* or the outer surfaces of cortical bone located under the connective tissue covering. Once adult bone mass is achieved, equal rates of formation and resorption maintain the peak bone mass until age 30 to 40 years. At this time, resorption begins to exceed formation, and the total mass slowly decreases.

The process of bone turnover in the adult is known as *remodeling,* which is also one of the major mechanisms for maintaining calcium homeostasis. About 10% of the total adult bone mass normally turns over each year in the remodeling process. Endocrine diseases that disrupt the coupling of formation and resorption have severe consequences on bone. The dysfunction is more pronounced if these diseases occur during the early phase of growth and the late phase of senescence, when a natural disequilibrium already exists between bone formation and resorption. *Women also more often experience severe consequences of such diseases than do men, because women have a 25% smaller peak bone mass and an accelerated rate of loss during the first 5 years after the menopause.*

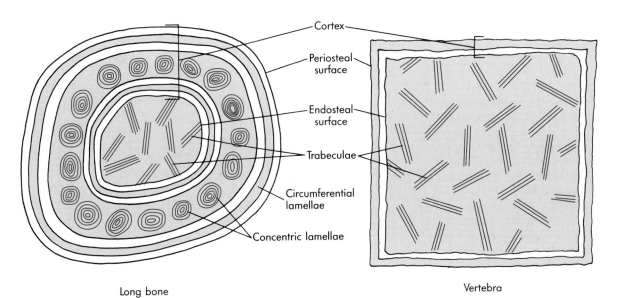

Long bone   Vertebra

■ **Fig. 48-3**   Schematic cross-sectional representations of a long bone, primarily cortical, and a vertebra, primarily trabecular. The long bone is distinguished by a thick outer cortex containing circumferential rings (lamellae) within which concentric lamellae known as haversian canals are present. These contain nutrient vessels. The inner portions of long bones and vertebrae consist of bridging spicules of bone or trabeculae in organized lamellar arrays. Between the trabeculae are bone marrow elements and connective tissue cells.

Three major cell types are recognized in histologic sections of bone: **osteoblasts, osteocytes,** and **osteoclasts** (Fig. 48-4). The first two bone cell types arise from primitive cells, called *osteoprogenitor cells,* within the connective tissue of the mesenchyme. A variety of local bone proteins, which act as skeletal growth factors, attract osteoprogenitor cells. Along with several hormones, these skeletal growth factors direct the differentiation of precursors into osteoblasts and stimulate their growth. The osteoclasts, which are much fewer in number, originate from the same precursors as circulating monocytes and tissue macrophages (i.e., promonocytes or monoblasts).

■ Bone Formation

Bone formation is carried out by active osteoblasts, which synthesize and extrude collagen into the adjacent extracellular space. The collagen fibrils line up in regular arrays and produce an organic matrix known as **osteoid,** within which calcium is then deposited as amorphous masses of calcium phosphate. About 10 days elapse between osteoid formation and mineralization. Once mineralization is initiated, however, most of the calcium phosphate is deposited within 6 to 12 hours. Thereafter, hydroxide and bicarbonate ions are gradually added to the mineral mixture, and mature **hydroxyapatite** crystals are slowly formed. These crystals have a calcium/phosphate ratio of 2.2 by weight and 1.7 by moles. As this completely mineralized bone accumulates and surrounds the osteoblast, this cell decreases its synthetic activity and it becomes an interior osteocyte (Fig. 48-4). Osteoblastic activity, therefore, is usually observed only along the surfaces of bone—the concentric **lamellae** of cortical bone or the linear lamellae of the interior bridging trabeculae (Fig. 48-3). Resting osteocytes or osteoblasts are arranged along these surfaces, and these cells may initiate the cycle of remodeling in each osteon.

The mineralization process requires adequate plasma concentrations of calcium and phosphate and is dependent on vitamin D. The enzyme **alkaline phosphatase** and possibly other macromolecules from the osteoblast also participate in this process. Of note are **osteonectin,** a protein of 32,000 molecular weight, and **osteocalcin,** a protein of 6000 molecular weight. These two proteins form 1% to 2% of all bone protein. Osteonectin binds to collagen, and the resultant complex in turn binds hydroxyapatite crystals. Osteocalcin is distinguished by the presence of γ-carboxyglutamate residues, which have an affinity for calcium and a strong avidity for uncrystallized hydroxyapatite. Alkaline phosphatase and osteocalcin also play roles in bone formation, and their plasma levels are standard markers of osteoblastic activity.

Specific peptide derivatives of procollagen that are excreted in the urine also serve as indices of bone formation.

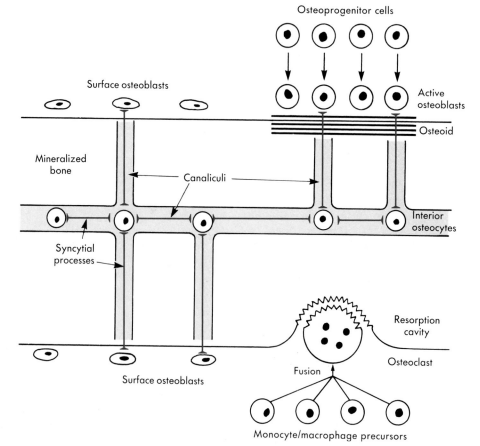

■ **Fig. 48-4** The relationships between bone cells and bone surfaces. The canaliculi provide a huge interface between the interior surfaces of mineralized bone and intercellular fluid. This permits efficient osteolysis with transfer of calcium and phosphate to the exterior via syncytial processes connecting interior and surface osteocytes. (Redrawn from Avioli LV et al: *Bone metabolism and disease.* In Bondy PK, Rosenberg LE, editors: *Metabolic control and disease,* Philadelphia, 1980, WB Saunders.)

Within each bone unit, minute fluid-containing channels, called **canaliculi,** traverse the mineralized bone. Through these channels, the interior osteocytes remain connected with surface cells via syncytial cell processes (Fig. 48-4). This arrangement permits transfer of calcium from the enormous surface area of the interior to the exterior of the bone units and thence into the extracellular fluid. This transfer process, which is carried out by the osteocytes, is known as **osteocytic osteolysis.** It probably does not actually decrease bone mass but simply removes calcium from the most recently formed crystals.

■ *Bone Resorption*

In contrast to osteocytic osteolysis, the process of resorption of bone does not merely extract calcium; it also destroys the entire matrix of bone and thereby diminishes the bone mass. The cell responsible for bone resorption is the osteoclast. This giant (up to 100 microns) multinucleated (10 to 20 nuclei) cell is formed by fusion of several precursor cells (Fig. 48-4). The osteoclast contains large numbers of mitochondria and lysosomes. It attaches to the endosteal and periosteal surfaces of bone modeling units, a process mediated by **integrins.** At the point of attachment, a ruffled border is created by infolding of the plasma membrane. Within this zone, the process of bone dissolution is carried out by type 4 collagenase, phosphatase, lysosomal enzymes, and creation of a local acidic environment. Thus, the osteoclast literally tunnels its way into the mineralized bone. Calcium, phosphate, the amino acids **hydroxyproline** and **hydroxylysine** that are unique to collagen, and fluorescent products of collagen cross-linkages, known as **pyridinolines,** are all released into the extracellular fluid during resorption. Urinary excretion rates of the organic products provide quantitative indices of bone resorption.

■ *Coordination of Resorption and Formation*

As noted previously, resorption and formation are closely coordinated within each bone modeling unit. The remodeling process begins with a chemical signal from resting osteoblasts (Fig. 48-5). This paracrine signal stimulates recruitment and differentiation of osteoclast precursors and activation of the mature osteoclasts. These osteoclasts then resorb a segment of bone as described, after which macrophages "clean up" the residue of the resorption process. Osteoblasts are then recruited to the same site and fill in the newly created resorption cavity. Thus, the first phase of the remodeling cycle is actually resorption, which lasts about 10 days. The second phase, formation, takes about 3 months to complete.

All aspects of the remodeling cycle are influenced by a large array of hormones and growth factors, as well as by cytokines from immune cells (Table 48-1). These molecules can affect one or more of the various steps either positively or negatively, or even both, depending on the concentration of each regulatory factor and the duration of exposure. The process of bone modeling is one example of coordinated function of the endocrine and immune systems.

Bone remodeling is ordinarily regulated to compensate for change. For example, if the primary effect of a hormone is to stimulate formation, this effect will be at least partially balanced by a secondary increase in resorption. This compensation occurs by the mechanism of coupling.

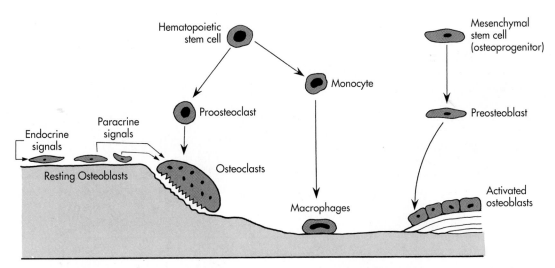

■ **Fig. 48-5**   Process of bone remodeling. Endocrine signals to resting osteoblasts generate local paracrine signals to nearby osteoclasts and osteoclast precursors. The osteoclasts resorb an area of mineralized bone, and local macrophages complete the clean-up of dissolved elements. The process then reverses to formation as osteoblast precursors are recruited to the site and differentiate into active osteoblasts. These lay down new organic matrix and mineralize it. Thus, new bone replaces the previously resorbed mature bone. (Modified from Raisz LG: *N Engl J Med* 318:820, 1988.)

Therefore, the net effect of any endocrine abnormality depends on the degree to which the total bone mass is defended by the compensatory process of coupling.

The total bone mass of humans peaks at 25 to 35 years of age. At this time, men have a larger bone mass than women. A gradual decline occurs in both genders with aging, but women undergo an accelerated phase of bone loss, caused by increased resorption in the perimenopausal period. Although the rate of bone remodeling actually increases with age, the osteoblasts do not refill cavities with normal speed; that is, bone resorption exceeds formation. The reduced bone density (Fig. 48-6) and mass, **osteoporosis,** creates a susceptibility to wrist and vertebral fractures, particularly in women in the sixth and seventh decades of life.

By the eighth and ninth decades, hip fractures become prevalent in both genders. A generous calcium intake, habitual exercise, and avoidance of smoking and excessive alcohol intake throughout life reduce the risk of osteoporosis.

■ **Table 48-1**   Major effects of various hormones on bone

Bone formation	Bone resorption
Stimulated by	**Stimulated by**
Growth hormone (constant)	Parathyroid hormone (constant)
Insulin-like growth factors	Vitamin D
Insulin	Cortisol
Estrogen	Thyroid hormone
Androgen	Prostaglandins
Vitamin D (mineralization)	Interleukin-1
Transforming growth factor-β	Interleukin-6
Skeletal growth factor	Tumor necrosis factor α
Bone-derived growth factor	Tumor necrosis factor β
Platelet-derived growth factor	
Calcitonin	
Parathyroid hormone (intermittent)	
Inhibited by	**Inhibited by**
Cortisol	Estrogen
	Androgen
	Calcitonin
	Transforming growth factor-β
	γ-Interferon
	Nitric oxide

■ *Vitamin D*

Vitamin D, after its activation to the hormone 1,25-$(OH)_2$-D, is one of the two major regulators of calcium metabolism. 1,25-$(OH)_2$-D *increases calcium absorption from the intestine and the calcium resorption from bone. Both actions raise or sustain the plasma calcium concentration.* Vitamin 1,25-$(OH)_2$-D has similar effects on phosphate.

■ *Vitamin D Production*

Humans acquire vitamin D from two sources. Vitamin D is produced in the skin by ultraviolet irradiation (D_3) and is ingested in the diet (D_3 and D_2). In this sense, vitamin D itself is not a "classic hormone" because it is not produced by an endocrine gland. However, vitamin D under-

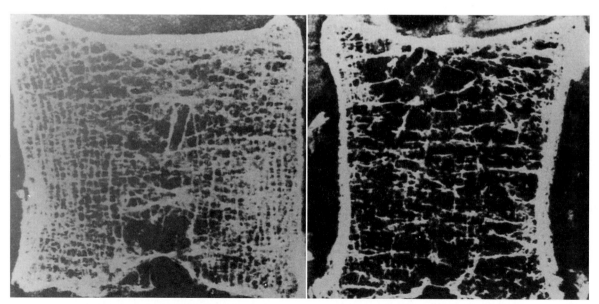

■ **Fig. 48-6**   **A,** Radiograph of a normal vertebra from a 40-year-old woman. **B,** Radiograph of a vertebra from a 92-year-old woman. Note the marked loss of trabeculae with relative preservation of cortex. (From Atkinson P: *Calcif Tissue Res* 1:24, 1967.)

goes molecular modification to yield a metabolite that then acts on distant target cells, and its mechanism of action is similar to that of thyroid and steroid hormones. These actions justify its classification as a hormone.

The structures of vitamin D_3, its precursors, and its metabolites are shown in Fig. 48-7. Vitamin D_2, which differs from vitamin D_3 only in an additional double bond at the 21 to 22 position, is derived from the plant sterol ergosterol by ultraviolet radiation. Vitamin D_2 is a major dietary source in many countries. Because vitamin D_2 has biological actions identical to those of vitamin D_3, the term *vitamin D* is used to indicate both forms.

Vitamin D_3 synthesis occurs primarily in specialized skin cells, **keratinocytes,** which are located in the epidermis. Under the influence of summer sunlight (ultraviolet [UV] radiation at 290 to 315 nm), **7-dehydrocholesterol** is photoconverted to **previtamin D_3** (Fig. 48-7). A minimum of 20 mJ radiation energy per square centimeter of skin is required. The amount of previtamin D_3 formed is related in exponential fashion to the UV input. Previtamin D_3 is then spontaneously converted over 3 days to vitamin D_3 in a reaction driven by thermal energy from sunshine. Continuous exposure to sunlight also causes photodegradation of previtamin D_3 to inactive products in reactions catalyzed by UV radiation at 315 to 330 nm. *Thus, although sunlight stimulates vitamin D_3 production, it also restrains overproduction,* so that excessive exposure to sunlight does not cause systemic vitamin D toxicity. Synthesis of vitamin D_3 is inhibited by 1,25-$(OH)_2$-D and stimulated by PTH.

In winter or in sunlight-poor climates, dietary vitamin D may be essential for health. The most important sources are fish, liver, and irradiated milk. The minimal daily dietary requirement of vitamin D is approximately 2.5 μg, and the recommended daily intake is 10 μg (400 Units). Because of its fat solubility, absorption of vitamin D from the intestine is mediated by bile salts and occurs via the lymphatic glands. Excesses are efficiently stored in adipose tissue and liver and can take several months to be dissipated.

Vitamin D has very little, if any, intrinsic biological activity. It must undergo successive hydroxylations in order to act as a hormone (Fig. 48-7). In the liver, it is hydroxylated by a microsomal and mitochondrial enzyme to 25-OH-D. This reaction requires NADPH and O_2. From the liver, 25-OH-D is transported to the kidney (and possibly to other sites), where it undergoes further alteration (Fig. 48-7). Although 25-OH-D can be shown to have intrinsic activity in vitro, it is essentially inactive in the absence of the kidneys. Its physiological function in calcium regulation appears to be that of a precursor to much more highly active metabolites.

The alteration that 25-(OH)-D undergoes in the kidneys yields two metabolites. Hydroxylation of 25-(OH)-D in the 1 position to 1,25-$(OH)_2$-D occurs in the mitochondria of the proximal convoluted and straight tubules of the kidneys. The 1-α-hydroxylase enzyme is a mixed

function P-450 steroid hydroxylase that requires NADPH, O_2, and a flavoprotein known as **renoredoxin** or **ferredoxin.** Vitamin 1,25-$(OH)_2$-D is the most potent vitamin D metabolite in vivo, and it expresses all the currently well-defined activities of vitamin D. Alternatively, 25-OH-D may be hydroxylated in the 24 position to 24,25-$(OH)_2$-D in a mitochondrial reaction that again requires NADPH and O_2. Whether 24,25-$(OH)_2$-D has significant biological activity remains controversial. However, it is far less potent than 1,25-$(OH)_2$-D in most assay systems, and it probably represents only a means of inactivating excess vitamin D. Recent evidence nevertheless suggests that 24,25-$(OH)_2$-D could play a separate role in expressing particular vitamin D actions.

Regulation of 1,25-$(OH)_2$-D production largely occurs in the kidney. (The rate of 25-OH-D synthesis in the liver is decreased by 1,25-$(OH)_2$-D via product inhibition.) Regulation primarily occurs at the alternative 1- or 24-hydroxylase step (Fig. 48-8). Vitamin 25-OH-D is preferentially directed toward the active metabolite 1,25-$(OH)_2$-D when vitamin D, calcium, or phosphate is lacking. In vitamin D–deficient states, it is partly the lack of 1,25-$(OH)_2$-D itself that enhances 1-hydroxylation, because 1,25-$(OH)_2$-D suppresses 1-hydroxylase synthesis and activity.

Even when the amount of vitamin D is sufficient, the 1-hydroxylase enzyme is still subject to regulation by calcium and phosphate levels. Calcium deprivation leads to hypocalcemia, which in turn stimulates PTH hypersecretion. The decreased plasma calcium concentration and the increased PTH concentration both independently stimulate 1-hydroxylase synthesis and activity. Phosphate deprivation leads to hypophosphatemia and a lowered renal cortical phosphate content, which also directly increases 1-hydroxylase activity. *Thus, the supply of active 1,25-$(OH)_2$-D is augmented whenever the mobilization of calcium or phosphate from intestine and bone into the extracellular fluid is needed.* Conversely, the supply of inactive 24,25-$(OH)_2$-D is augmented when 1,25-$(OH)_2$-D and phosphate are plentiful and bone formation can be sustained.

Vitamin D, 25-OH-D, 1,25-$(OH)_2$-D, and 24,25-$(OH)_2$-D all circulate bound to an α-globulin. The concentrations, approximate half-lives, and estimated daily production rates for these three key metabolites in humans are shown in Table 48-2. Vitamin 1,25-$(OH)_2$-D has the shortest half-life of the three and by far the lowest concentration, which befits its potency.

Certain relationships among the plasma concentrations of the three metabolites are also physiologically significant. Vitamin 1,25-$(OH)_2$-D concentration is ordinarily independent of 25-OH-D concentration. Except in severe vitamin D deficiency or toxicity states, the regulatory factors previously described are able to maintain the appropriate concentration of active metabolite, irrespective of the supply of precursor. In contrast, 24,25-$(OH)_2$-D concentration is ordinarily directly proportional to 25-

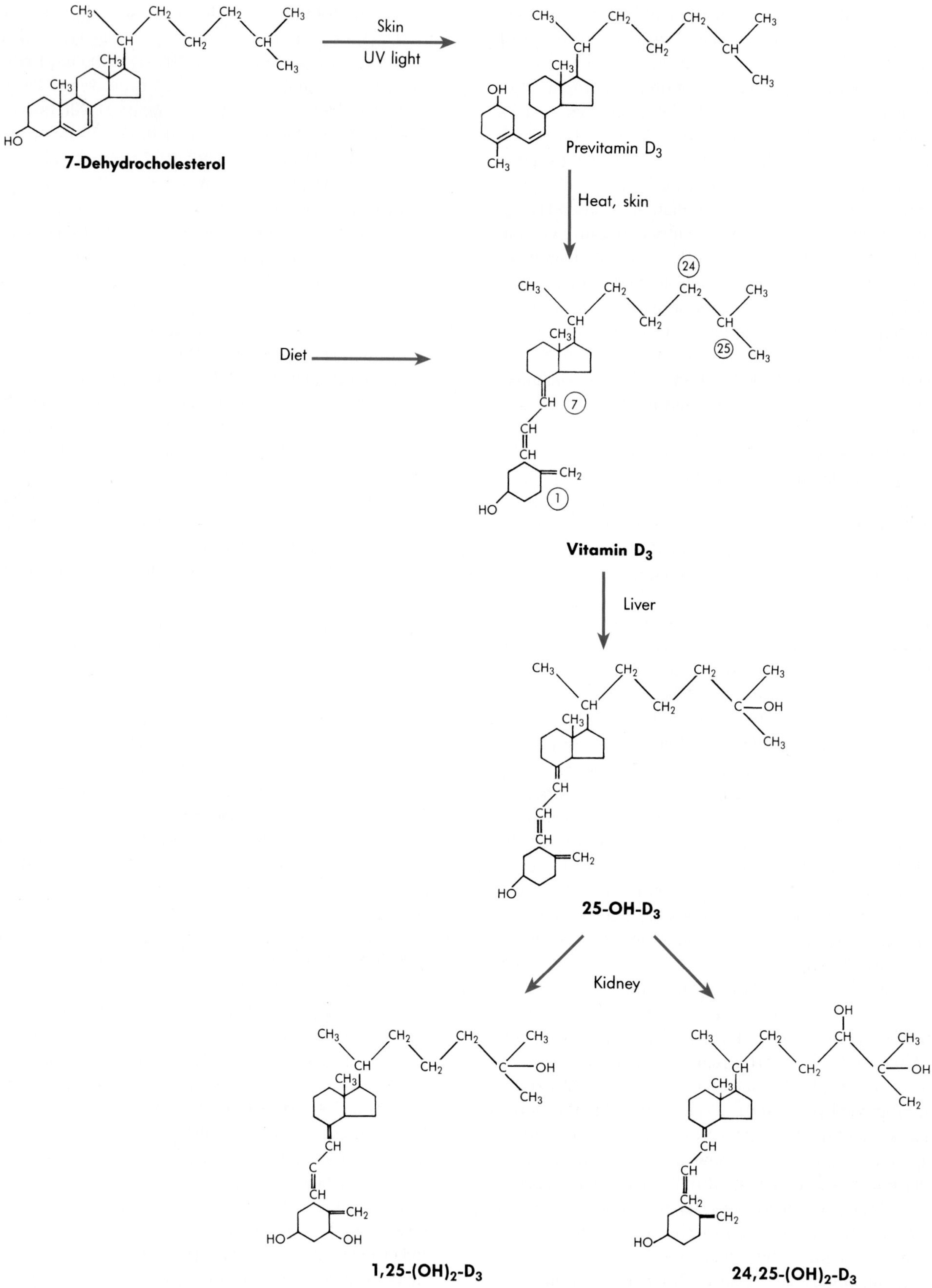

■ **Fig. 48-7**   Structures of vitamin D_3, its precursor, and its metabolites.

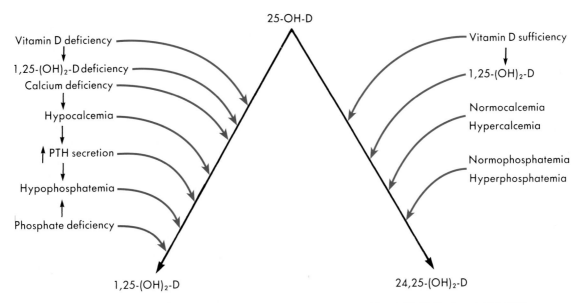

■ **Fig. 48-8** Factors that regulate conversion of 25-OH-D₃ to either 1,25-(OH)₂-D or 24,25-(OH)₂-D. The former is increased by either calcium or phosphate lack.

■ **Table 48-2** Vitamin D metabolism in humans

	Plasma concentration (µg/L)	Plasma half-life (days)	Estimated production rate (µg/day)
1,25-(OH)₂-D₃	0.03	0.25	1
24,25-(OH)₂-D₃	2	15 to 40	1
25-OH-D₃	30	15	10

OH-D concentration. This proportional relationship reflects the role of 24-hydroxylation as a key sluicing mechanism for disposing of excess precursor. Vitamin 1,25-(OH)₂-D can be further hydroxylated to 1,24,25-(OH)₃-D, a compound that has little activity. Thus, if an excess of 1,25-(OH)₂-D should develop, it can still be inactivated by 24-hydroxylation. Many other hydroxylated vitamin D₃ metabolites without apparent function have been described. Both active and inactive vitamin D metabolites undergo biliary excretion and enterohepatic recycling.

Vitamin D deficiency results from inadequate access to sunlight and/or inadequate dietary sources. Preterm black infants who live in air-polluted cities (inadequate UV radiation) and who are breast fed (inadequate ingestion of the vitamin) are at increased risk for **rickets**, a disease characterized by bone deformation (e.g., bowlegs). Intestinal diseases that cause malabsorption of fats and decreased enterohepatic recycling of vitamin D and its critical metabolites also lead to deficiency states. Vitamin D is the replacement therapy used for all of these vitamin D–deficient states. Hepatic disease, kidney failure, and defective genes that encode the 25-hydroxylase or 1-hydroxylase enzyme prevent normal conversion to 1,25-(OH)₂-D and can be treated with the specific deficient metabolite.

■ *Vitamin D Actions*

Vitamin 1,25-(OH)₂-D acts through the general nuclear mechanism outlined for steroid hormones (see Fig. 45-13). The vitamin D receptor is found in both the cytoplasm and nucleus. Binding of 1,25-(OH)₂-D induces receptor phosphorylation, and the resultant complex attaches to 1,25-(OH)₂-D regulatory elements in target DNA molecules. An accessory protein is required to facilitate this attachment. Heterodimers between the vitamin D receptor and retinoid receptors also play a role in induction or suppression of target gene transcription.

Table 48-3 lists some of the important genes involved in vitamin D actions. The vitamin D receptor is up-regulated by 1,25-(OH)₂-D. It is also up-regulated by PTH, insulin-like growth factors, estrogen, and cortisol.

One major product of 1,25-(OH)₂-D action is a series of calcium binding proteins of various molecular weights, called **calbindins.** These proteins bind calcium ions in various stoichiometric proportions and exhibit significant homology with calmodulin and myosin light chain. In contrast to the slowly developing nuclear effects via its receptor (and not through a transcriptional mechanism), 1,25-(OH)₂-D also has rapid membrane effects that involve an increase in cGMP and intracellular calcium levels.

■ **Table 48-3**   Target genes of vitamin D

Gene	Transcription
Vitamin D receptor	Increased
Calcium-binding proteins	Increased
(calbindins)	Increased
Calcium pump	Increased
Osteocalcin	Increased
Alkaline phosphatase	Increased
24-Hydroxylase	Increased
Parathyroid hormone	Decreased
1-Hydroxylase	Decreased
Collagen	Decreased
Interleukin-2	Decreased
γ-Interferon	Decreased

The major action of 1,25-(OH)$_2$-D is to stimulate absorption of calcium from the intestinal lumen against a concentration gradient. A rapid phase of action is evident within minutes to 6 hours; a slower phase takes 24 to 96 hours. Vitamin 1,25-(OH)$_2$-D localizes to the nuclei of intestinal villus and crypt cells, but not to goblet or submucosa cells. There, it acts on the brush border and increases the number of calcium pump molecules in the basolateral membrane. Hours after calcium entry from the intestinal lumen to the capillaries has been rapidly stimulated, the calbindin concentration rises. These molecules may act to ferry calcium across the intestinal cell or to buffer the high calcium concentrations that result from initial entry of the ion. The rate of calcium absorption across the duodenum is proportional to the cell content of calbindin. Vitamin 1,25-(OH)$_2$-D is responsible for the adaptation, described previously, whereby intestinal calcium absorption can be adjusted to alterations in the amount of dietary calcium. In addition to calcium absorption, 1,25-(OH)$_2$-D stimulates the active absorption of phosphate and magnesium across the intestinal cell membrane. The mechanisms for the absorption of phosphate and magnesium are independent of and less well defined than those in the absorption of calcium.

Another major target organ of 1,25-(OH)$_2$-D is bone, where it causes complex effects. Osteoblasts, but not osteoclasts, have 1,25-(OH)$_2$-D receptors. Nonetheless 1,25-(OH)$_2$-D stimulates bone resorption, probably by stimulating a paracrine signal that originates in the osteoblast. In this way, 1,25-(OH)$_2$-D increases the recruitment, differentiation, and fusion of precursors into active osteoclasts, which carry out their resorptive missions. Vitamin 1,25-(OH)$_2$-D also increases osteocytic osteolysis.

Vitamin D also plays a role in bone formation. The normal mineralization of newly formed osteoid along a calcification front is critically dependent on vitamin D. In its absence, excess osteoid accumulates from lack of 1,25-(OH)$_2$-D repression of osteoblastic collagen synthesis (Table 48-3). The bone formed in the absence of 1,25-(OH)$_2$-D is weak. It is still unclear whether this action of vitamin D is entirely accounted for by augmentation of the supply of calcium and phosphate in the fluid bathing the osteoblast, or whether 1,25-(OH)$_2$-D also acts in a direct manner on the bone matrix or cells to hasten mineralization. A direct effect on bone formation is supported by the fact that 1,25-(OH)$_2$-D induces the synthesis of osteocalcin and fibronectin. In any case, the first observable effect of vitamin D replacement on the bone in vitamin D–deficient animals and humans is the reappearance of a normal mineralized calcification front. Vitamin D (possibly through its 24,25-(OH)$_2$-D metabolite) may also stimulate cartilage development at some stage.

Vitamin D–related abnormalities may play a role in the senescent bone loss described above. Aging is associated with decreases in exposure to sunlight, synthesis of vitamin D from 7-dehydrocholesterol (Fig. 48-7), dietary intake of vitamin D, synthesis of 1,25-(OH)$_2$-D, D receptors in the intestine, and calcium absorption. Lack of calcium impairs bone formation.

An important feedback action of 1,25-(OH)$_2$-D is to directly repress the gene responsible for the synthesis of PTH. This action is facilitated by 1,25-(OH)$_2$-D induction of its own receptor, as well as by a calbindin in parathyroid cells.

Vitamin 1,25-(OH)$_2$-D weakly stimulates renal calcium reabsorption by increasing the number of calcium pumps. It also stimulates calcium transport into skeletal and cardiac muscle; muscle weakness and cardiac dysfunction can result from vitamin D deficiency.

The same skin cells (keratinocytes) that synthesize vitamin D, as well as other epidermal cells, also produce 1,25-(OH)$_2$-D from 25-OH-D. In a paracrine and autocrine manner, 1,25-(OH)$_2$-D stimulates differentiation and inhibits proliferation of these cells. Thus, formation of the outer cornified layer of the epidermis, with its appropriate content of enzymes and structural proteins, is regulated by vitamin D.

A new role for vitamin D in immunomodulation has also emerged. Macrophages, monocytes, and transformed lymphocytes can synthesize 1,25-(OH)$_2$-D from 25-OH-D. Promyelocytes, monocytes, and activated T lymphocytes also express the 1,25-(OH)$_2$-D receptor, and binding of vitamin D can decrease their production of interleukin-2, γ-interferon, and other cytokines. The proliferation of T and B lymphocytes as well as immunoglobulin synthesis by β-lymphocytes are decreased by 1,25-(OH)$_2$-D. Thus, vitamin D participates in autocrine and paracrine actions important in the regulation of immune responses, which are diminished in vitamin D–deficient states.

Macrophages and osteoclasts also have common ancestors. Therefore, 1,25-(OH)$_2$-D probably mediates an integrated endocrine, paracrine, and autocrine system whereby osteoclasts and tissue macrophages are recruited sequentially when they are needed for bone resorption and for clean-up of the resultant waste products.

In diseases characterized by formation of granulomas that contain mononuclear inflammatory cells (e.g., **sarcoidosis** and **tuberculosis),** these cells can synthesize excess 1,25-(OH)$_2$-D. Symptomatic hypercalcemia may result.

Finally, vitamin D receptors are also found in the pancreatic islets, anterior pituitary, hypothalamus, placenta, ovary, aortic endothelium, and skin fibroblasts. The presence of these receptors accounts for a variety of other vitamin D actions that involve calcium, such as enhancement of insulin (see Chapter 47) and prolactin (see Chapter 49) secretion.

Vitamin D actions can be lost as a result of mutant receptors (e.g., in vitamin D–resistant **rickets),** hormone antagonists, and hormone deficiency. In children, the epiphyseal growth centers are affected by defective mineralization of bone, and this defect leads to the typical manifestations of rickets (Fig. 48-9), which include bowing of the extremities and collapse of the chest wall. In adults, pain, vertebral collapse, and fractures along stress lines characterize the condition known as **osteomalacia.** In children and adults, excess osteoid accumulates in the bone. Plasma calcium and phosphate levels are decreased, whereas alkaline phosphatase and PTH levels are increased. Therapy requires the appropriate form of vitamin D in amounts that range from physiological to pharmacological.

Excessive vitamin D action causes overabsorption of calcium from the diet and increased bone resorption. Hypercalcemia, hypercalciuria, and kidney stones often result. Hyperphosphatemia is also present because of increased phosphate influx and suppression of PTH secretion (see below). The duration of toxicity is greatest in vitamin D excess, because of its large storage capacity, and is least in 1,25-(OH)$_2$-D excess, because of rapid removal of the active hormone. Treatment consists of blocking the effects of the vitamin D excess with calcitonin or with cortisol analogues.

■ *Parathyroid Hormone*

The parathyroid glands secrete **parathyroid hormone (PTH),** the other major regulator of calcium and phosphorus metabolism. *The paramount effect of PTH is to increase plasma calcium levels by stimulation of bone resorption, renal tubular calcium reabsorption, and 1,25-(OH)$_2$-D synthesis. At the same time, PTH decreases plasma phosphate concentration by inhibition of renal tubular phosphate reabsorption.*

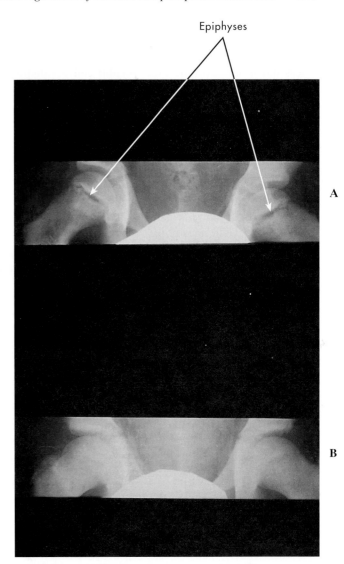

Epiphyses

A

B

■ **Fig. 48-9** **A,** Radiograph of the hips of a child with deficient 1,25-(OH)$_2$-D action because of renal failure and reduced production from 25-(OH)-D. Note the widened irregular epiphyseal growth areas. **B,** The same hips after treatment with vitamin D has mineralized the epiphyses.

Four parathyroid glands develop at 5 to 14 weeks of gestation from the third and fourth branchial pouches. Normally, they descend to lie posterior to the thyroid gland, but ectopic locations in the neck and mediastinum can also occur. The total weight of adult parathyroid tissue is about 130 mg, and that of any one gland is 30 to 50 mg. The blood supply of the parathyroid glands is from the thyroid arteries and is easily interrupted during thyroid surgery. Samples drawn from the left and right thyroid veins can localize the site of unilateral parathyroid gland hyperfunction, when necessary.

The histologic appearance of the parathyroid glands changes with age. The predominant cell, known as the **chief cell,** is present throughout life and is the normal source of PTH. Resting chief cells have abundant glycogen, an involuted Golgi apparatus, and a few clusters of secretory granules. Activated cells have little glycogen, a large convoluted Golgi apparatus with vacuoles and vesicles, and a granular endoplasmic reticulum. A second, less numerous cell type—the **oxyphil cell**—is distinguished by an eosinophilic cytoplasm and first appears at puberty. Either of these cells may hypersecrete PTH pathologically.

■ *Synthesis and Release of PTH*

PTH is a single-chain protein of 9000 molecular weight. It contains 84 amino acids (Fig. 48-8). The biological activity of PTH resides in the N-terminal portion of the molecule within amino acids 1 to 27. The larger C-terminus portion may carry out other functions that are unrelated to calcium metabolism.

PTH is synthesized from a precursor molecule called *prepro-PTH* (Fig. 48-10), which contains 115 amino acids. As the peptide chain of prepro-PTH grows to its complete length on the ribosomes, the N-terminal signal sequence is enzymatically removed in two steps, leaving pro-PTH. The prohormone is transported to the Golgi apparatus, within which the processing of pro-PTH to PTH is completed very efficiently. Consequently, the parathyroid glands normally contain much less pro-PTH than PTH. Some PTH is packaged for storage in mature secretory granules and is later released by exocytosis. In addition, some newly synthesized PTH may be trans-ported, still in Golgi vesicles, directly through the cell for immediate release. Cleavage of PTH between amino acids 33 and 40 (Fig. 48-10) also occurs within the gland and prevents release of the intact hormone into the circulation.

The dominant regulator of parathyroid gland activity is the plasma calcium level. PTH and calcium form a negative feedback pair. Secretion of PTH is inversely related to the plasma calcium concentration in a sigmoidal fashion (Fig. 48-11). Maximal secretory rates of PTH are achieved below a total calcium concentration of 7 mg/dl (ionized calcium, 3.5 mg/dl). As total calcium concentration increases to 11 mg/dl (ionized calcium, 5.5 mg/dl), PTH secretion is progressively diminished to a persistent low basal rate that is not suppressible by further elevation of plasma calcium. It is actually the ionized fraction of plasma calcium that regulates PTH secretion. PTH secretion responds to small alterations in the concentration of ionized plasma calcium within seconds even if total calcium concentration is kept constant. The dose-response curve is steep, with a set point for half-maximal secretion at an ionized calcium level of about 4.5 mg/dl (Fig. 48-11). The greater the *rate of fall* in the concentration of ionized calcium, the larger is the PTH secretion response. This relationship suggests that the parathyroid cells possess an "anticipatory" capability.

Suppression of PTH secretion by an increased concentration of ionized calcium represents a notable exception to the usual rule that calcium influx into the cytoplasm of

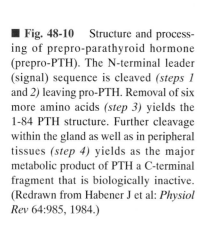
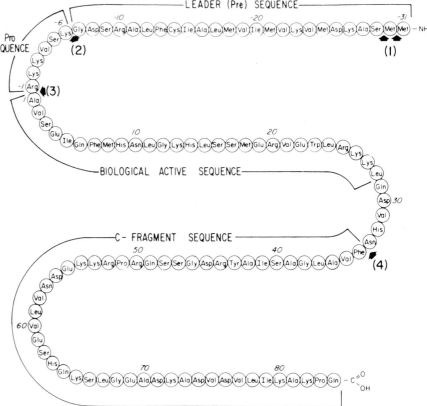

■ **Fig. 48-10**   Structure and processing of prepro-parathyroid hormone (prepro-PTH). The N-terminal leader (signal) sequence is cleaved (*steps 1* and *2*) leaving pro-PTH. Removal of six more amino acids (*step 3*) yields the 1-84 PTH structure. Further cleavage within the gland as well as in peripheral tissues (*step 4*) yields as the major metabolic product of PTH a C-terminal fragment that is biologically inactive. (Redrawn from Habener J et al: *Physiol Rev* 64:985, 1984.)

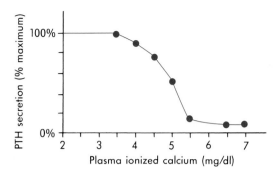

■ **Fig. 48-11** The inverse relationship between PTH and plasma ionized calcium concentration in humans. (Redrawn from Brent GA et al: *J Clin Endocrinol Metab* 67:944, 1988. From The Endocrine Society.)

endocrine cells stimulates protein hormone secretion by exocytosis (see Fig. 45-3). However, *a unique calcium receptor within the parathyroid cell plasma membrane senses changes in the extracellular fluid concentration of ionized calcium* (Fig. 48-12). This typical G protein–linked receptor (see Figs. 45-8 to 45-10) possesses a hydrophilic extracellular domain of 141 amino acids, a seven-span transmembrane portion of 250 amino acids, and an intracellular tail of 222 amino acids. *An increase in binding of Ca⁺⁺ to the extracellular component of the receptor activates phospholipase C and inhibits adenylyl cyclase. The resultant rise (via generation of inositol trisphosphate) in intracellular calcium levels and fall in cAMP levels stops exocytosis of the PTH-containing secretory granules* (Fig. 48-12).

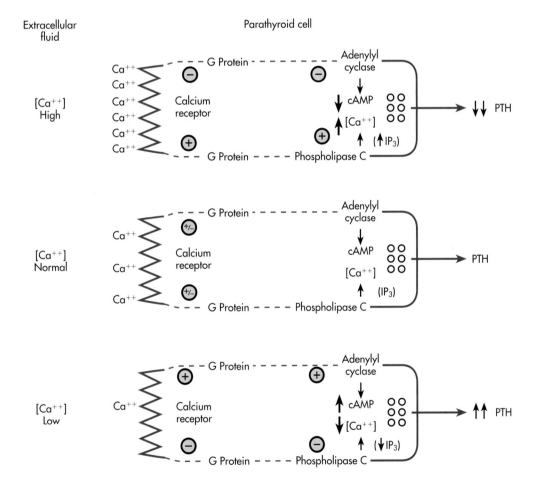

■ **Fig. 48-12** Mechanism of regulation of PTH secretion by changes in extracellular fluid ionized calcium [Ca⁺⁺] concentration. An increase in [Ca⁺⁺] is sensed by a plasma membrane [Ca⁺⁺] receptor in the parathyroid cell *(top tier)*. The activated receptor is linked to an inhibitory G protein, which inhibits adenylyl cyclase. As a result, intracellular cAMP levels fall. The activated receptor is also linked to a stimulatory G protein that stimulates phospholipase C. As a result, inositol trisphosphate (IP₃) levels increase and transduce a rise in intracellular [Ca⁺⁺]. Exocytosis of PTH secretory granules and PTH release are *decreased*. The opposite sequence occurs when there is a decrease in extracellular fluid [Ca⁺⁺]; in that case, exocytosis of PTH secretory granules and PTH release are increased. *IP₃,* Inositol trisphosphate; ⊕, disinhibited or stimulated; ⊖, inhibited or unstimulated; ⊘, balanced between inhibited and stimulated.

When the binding of Ca^{++} to the receptor decreases, the suppression of granule exocytosis is lifted and PTH secretion increases (Fig. 48-12).

Activation of the calcium receptor by hypocalcemia also leads to an increase in PTH synthesis and a decrease in PTH degradation within the parathyroid cells. Exposure to a high calcium concentration for hours to days represses PTH gene transcription but does not affect processing of prepro-PTH to PTH. Chronic exposure to a high calcium concentration eventually also decreases proliferation of parathyroid cells. *Thus, hypercalcemia decreases PTH synthesis, stores, and release, as well as (ultimately) parathyroid cell mass. Conversely, hypocalcemia increases PTH synthesis, stores, and secretory rates and ultimately stimulates growth of the glands.*

The divalent cation Mg^{++} acutely modulates PTH secretion in a manner analogous to that of Ca^{++}, that is, a decrease in magnesium levels stimulates PTH secretion. Because Mg^{++} is less effective on a molar basis, it is much less important than calcium in its normal physiological range (1.5 to 2.5 mEq/L). In contrast, *chronic hypomagnesemia strongly inhibits PTH synthesis,* and in severely magnesium-depleted individuals, the rate of PTH release is reduced. In addition, hypomagnesemia impairs the response of target tissues to PTH. Both of these effects lead to concurrent hypocalcemia.

Despite the close physiological relation of phosphate to calcium, no direct effects of phosphate on the parathyroid glands have been demonstrated. However, a rise in plasma phosphate concentration causes an immediate fall in ionized calcium concentration, which in turn stimulates PTH secretion.

Vitamin 1,25-(OH)$_2$-D inhibits transcription of the PTH gene and decreases PTH secretion. It also inhibits proliferation of parathyroid cells. These actions, coupled with the stimulatory effect of PTH on 1,25-(OH$_2$)-D synthesis, constitute yet another negative feedback loop that regulates calcium metabolism.

PTH secretion is also pulsatile. In addition, PTH secretion increases at night and with aging, and bone resorption is especially active under both conditions. The nocturnal peak is independent of plasma calcium concentration.

Phosphodiesterase inhibitors (by increasing cAMP), epinephrine (via its β-adrenergic receptor), dopamine, and histamine (via H$_2$ receptors) all stimulate PTH secretion. α-Adrenergic agonists and prostaglandins inhibit PTH secretion by decreasing cAMP levels. Cosecreted chromogranin and related products feed back negatively on PTH secretion; this relationship may constitute an autocrine regulatory mechanism.

An excess of aluminum, commonly present in antacids, inhibits PTH secretion. Lithium, often used to treat **manic-depressive disorders,** and thiazide diuretic drugs all stimulate PTH modestly and can cause mild hypercalcemia.

Under normal circumstances, neither prepro-PTH nor pro-PTH is secreted from the parathyroid glands. One or more products of the intraglandular degradation of PTH, however, are released. In addition, PTH undergoes rapid metabolism in the peripheral tissues. The hormone is predominantly split in the liver. The major product is a circulating 6000 molecular weight carboxy-terminal fragment that is further acted upon in the kidney. Amino terminal fragments generated during cleavage of PTH also circulate but are not biologically active. The plasma concentration of intact PTH is about 30 pg/ml (approximately 3×10^{-12} M), and its plasma half-life is 20 to 30 minutes. The carboxy-terminal fragment has a much longer plasma half-life of 6 to 12 hours. This fragment is a valid index of chronic hypersecretion, so long as renal function is normal.

■ *PTH Actions*

PTH is activated by its binding to a typical glycoprotein plasma cell membrane receptor composed of multiple subunits. The 14 to 34 region of PTH contains the receptor-binding sequence. In all target cells, hormone binding to a cell membrane receptor leads to G protein–mediated activation of adenylyl cyclase (see Fig. 45-9). The subsequent intracellular events mediated by the increased cAMP levels are not known in detail. Presumably, increased levels of cAMP trigger a protein kinase cascade that leads to phosphorylation of proteins necessary for enhanced transport of calcium and other ions. Phosphatidylinositol products may have subsidiary second messenger roles by increasing protein kinase C activity.

Independent of cAMP, PTH also stimulates the uptake of calcium into the cytosol of bone cells from the fluid that bathes them. Whether this calcium itself acts as another intracellular second messenger or whether it acts only to modulate the adenylyl cyclase response by counterregulatory inhibition remains unclear. The initial uptake of calcium by bone cells is reflected by a slight transient hypocalcemia that follows PTH administration and precedes the classic hypercalcemic response. The presence of 1,25-(OH)$_2$-D is required for the exhibition of the full spectrum of PTH actions. A sufficient intracellular concentration of magnesium is also necessary for maximal PTH responsiveness.

The overall effect of PTH is to increase the plasma calcium concentration and decrease the plasma phosphate concentration by acting on three major target organs: directly on bone and kidney, and indirectly on the gastrointestinal tract. All three actions ultimately increase calcium influx into the plasma and raise the plasma calcium concentration. In contrast, the actions of PTH on bone and intestine, which increase phosphate influx, are overwhelmed by the action on the kidney, which increases phosphate efflux, so that plasma phosphate concentration falls (Fig. 48-13).

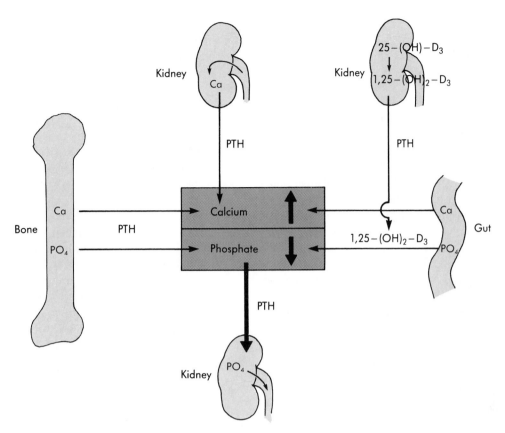

■ **Fig. 48-13**   The sites of PTH actions that lead to a net increase in serum calcium level and a net decrease in serum phosphate level. PTH stimulates calcium and phosphate resorption from bone. In contrast, PTH stimulates calcium reabsorption but inhibits phosphate reabsorption in the kidney. PTH stimulates renal formation of 1,25-(OH)$_2$-D, and the latter in turn increases absorption of both minerals from the intestine.

Bone. PTH receptors are present in both osteoblasts and osteoclasts. PTH accelerates removal of calcium from bone by two processes. Its initial effect is to stimulate osteolysis. This process causes calcium to be transferred from the bone canalicular fluid into the osteocyte, and thence out the opposite side of the cell into the extracellular fluid. The canalicular fluid is probably replenished with calcium from the surface of partially mineralized bone. Phosphate does not appear to be mobilized with calcium in this process.

A second, more slowly developing effect of PTH is to stimulate the osteoclasts to resorb completely mineralized bone. In this process, both calcium and phosphate are released for transfer into the extracellular fluid, and the organic bone matrix is hydrolyzed by increased activity of collagenase and lysosomal enzymes. PTH initially increases the ruffled border of the osteoclast and the clear resorptive zone that develops between it and the mineralized bone. Increases in osteoclast size, RNA synthesis, and the number of osteoclast nuclei then follow. In a later phase of PTH action, differentiation of precursor cells to osteoclasts and their proliferation is stimulated. The giant osteoclasts create large resorption cavities in both cortical and trabecular bone. PTH also induces increases in acid phosphatase and carbonic anhydrase and accumulation of lactic acid and citric acid. The resultant increase in protons lowers the ambient pH and contributes to the resorptive process. As a consequence, various products of bone destruction are released into the plasma and then excreted in the urine.

Although PTH receptors are present on osteoclasts, the resorptive effects of PTH cannot be demonstrated in vitro unless osteoblasts are also present as intermediary cells. Osteoblasts, and particularly a larger variety termed **proosteoblasts,** respond to the hormone in a number of ways. One response is an early alteration in osteoblast shape and cytoskeletal arrangement, probably by cAMP-induced phosphorylation of myosin light chains. PTH also inhibits the synthesis of collagen by osteoblasts, probably at the level of transcription. The proosteoblast has long syncytial processes that extend through the bone matrix and intertwine with other cells and vascular structures. Thus, they may mediate the resorptive effects of PTH by stimulating secretion of osteoblast products, such as interleukin-6 or macrophage colony-stimulating factor, which have paracrine effects on neighboring osteoclasts and their precursors. The resorptive effects of PTH on bone are achieved by the elevated concentrations of hormone that result from chronic stimulation of the parathyroid glands by hypocalcemia; thus the resorption of bone completes a negative feedback loop that restores the plasma calcium level to normal. Bone resorptive effects seen on histologic examination reflect continuous exposure to PTH.

However, PTH also has anabolic actions on bone. In culture, PTH causes an increase in the number of osteoblasts and in collagen synthesis. *When given in lower doses and intermittently, PTH stimulates bone formation in humans.* The plasma level of alkaline phosphatase, an osteoblastic enzyme whose activity parallels bone formation, is often increased by PTH. These anabolic actions are mediated by increases in local insulin-like growth factors and transforming growth factors, the synthesis of which PTH stimulates. The net effect of sustained increases in PTH may be either a decrease or an increase in total skeletal mass. Trabecular bone may be preserved by PTH at the expense of cortical bone. Whether total skeletal mass increases or decreases probably depends on concomitant factors that affect bone remodeling; these factors include mechanical stress, the level of exercise, and the availability of calcium, phosphate, vitamin D, and many other hormones with endocrine or paracrine actions (Table 48-1).

Primary hyperparathyroidism usually results from a benign parathyroid neoplasm (adenoma). Hypercalcemia, hypophosphatemia, hypercalcinuria, and renal calculi (stones) are typical manifestations. This condition seldom causes clinically evident bone disturbances, because the hallmark hypercalcemia is usually discovered early by health screening tests. However, long-term secondary massive overproduction of PTH, typical of slowly developing renal failure, causes major bone effects. Areas of osteoclastic hyperactivity and rampant bone resorption are present next to areas of excessive and disorganized trabecular bone formation. Pain, fractures, and deformity result. Plasma alkaline phosphatase and osteocalcin levels are elevated. In **hypoparathyroidism,** bone mass is generally increased.

Kidney. PTH increases the reabsorption of calcium from the ascending loop of Henle and the distal tubule of the kidney (see also Chapter 43). By this action, the PTH secreted in response to hypocalcemia immediately helps raise the decreased plasma calcium concentration. Reabsorption of calcium is mediated by PTH stimulation of cAMP production at the capillary surface of the renal tubular cell. The cAMP is transported to the luminal surface of the cell, where it activates protein kinases that are located in the brush border and are involved in calcium reabsorption. (The previously described calcium-sensing receptor is also present in and modulates calcium reabsorption by these cells). The relationship between urinary calcium excretion and plasma calcium concentration is

shifted to the right by PTH (Fig. 48-14). *Therefore, acute stimulation of PTH secretion by calcium deficiency helps prevent hypocalcemia by causing the kidney to reabsorb a greater fraction of the filtered calcium.*

In **hyperparathyroidism,** the plasma calcium level can become high enough from the direct actions of PTH on bone and the indirect actions on intestine for the hormone's primary renal calcium-conserving action to be overwhelmed by the increased filtered load of calcium. The result is **hypercalcinuria** and an increased frequency of renal calcium stone formation.

An interesting cause of familial hypercalcemia is a mutant calcium receptor. In individuals with this receptor, the plasma PTH concentration is inappropriately normal or even slightly elevated because the mutant parathyroid gland calcium receptor is relatively insensitive to calcium. The same insensitivity in the renal tubular cell calcium receptor (in the capillary side plasma membrane) causes inappropriate reabsorption of calcium in the presence of hypercalcemia. Thus, these patients have **hypocalcinuria** with hypercalcemia.

The most dramatic effect of PTH on the kidney is to inhibit the reabsorption of phosphate in the proximal tubule and thereby increase urinary phosphate excretion (see also Chapter 43). *cAMP excretion into the urine also increases, as expected, just before that of phosphate. The*

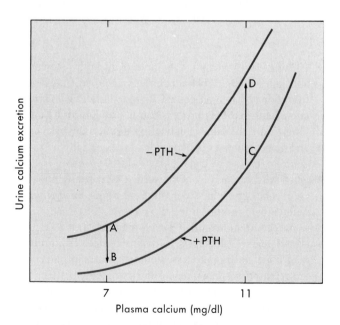

■ **Fig. 48-14**   Effect of PTH on the relationship between urine calcium excretion and plasma calcium level. At a low plasma calcium level, PTH secretion is stimulated, and the hormone shifts urine calcium excretion from point *A* to point *B,* thus conserving calcium. At a high plasma calcium level, PTH secretion is suppressed, and urine calcium excretion is shifted from point *C* to point *D,* thus disposing of excess calcium. (Redrawn from Nordin BEC et al: *Lancet* 2:1280, 1969.)

important phosphaturic effect of PTH allows disposition of the extra phosphate released by PTH-stimulated bone resorption. Without this effect, simultaneous plasma elevation of calcium and phosphate concentration could occur, with the potential danger of precipitating calcium-phosphate complexes in critical tissues. In contrast, under circumstances of primary phosphate deprivation, the plasma calcium concentration tends to rise and thus suppress PTH secretion. A lower level of PTH in turn allows more tubular phosphate reabsorption and conserves this essential mineral.

PTH also inhibits the reabsorption of sodium and bicarbonate in the proximal tubule in a manner parallel to that of phosphate reabsorption inhibition (see also Chapter 44). This action may prevent the occurrence of metabolic alkalosis, which could result from the release of bicarbonate during the dissolution of hydroxyapatite crystals in bone. In addition, PTH stimulates reabsorption of magnesium by the renal tubules, which helps to conserve this important cation.

A most important action of PTH in the kidney is to stimulate the synthesis of vitamin $1,25\text{-}(OH)_2\text{-}D$. This activity occurs via increased levels of cAMP; protein kinase A phosphorylates and activates a protein phosphatase, which then dephosphorylates the ferroprotein renoredoxin. In its dephosphorylated active form, renoredoxin is essential to the activity of the renal 1-hydroxylase enzyme. In addition, the decrease in plasma and renal cortical phosphate caused by PTH enhances 1-hydroxylation of $25\text{-}OH\text{-}D_3$. *Thus, PTH increases the level of available $1,25\text{-}(OH)_2\text{-}D$, and in this indirect but critical way increases calcium absorption from the intestine.*

All the above additional renal effects help to explain hyperparathyroidism is often accompanied by **hypophosphatemia,** a mild **hyperchloremic metabolic acidosis,** and elevated plasma $1,25\text{-}(OH)_2\text{-}D$ levels. The reverse findings are seen in hypoparathyroidism.

Overall action of PTH. The outcome of all the major biochemical effects of PTH is illustrated in Fig. 48-15, which demonstrates the results of administering the hormone to a hypoparathyroid patient. As shown, there is a prompt increase in plasma calcium concentration and a decrease in plasma phosphate concentration. The renal tubular reabsorption of phosphate falls. Urinary excretion of calcium initially declines as its tubular reabsorption increases. However, as the plasma calcium concentration continues to increase, the filtered load increases and urinary calcium excretion then rises. Urinary excretion of hydroxyproline increases as a result of PTH-stimulated bone resorption.

Hypoparathyroidism is usually caused by inadvertent surgical removal of the glands; less often, the cause is autoimmune destruction. Both conditions are marked by hypocalcemia, hyperphosphatemia, and low plasma PTH concentrations. Rarely, patients have mutant G proteins that cannot effectively transduce the PTH-receptor signal. Although plasma calcium concentration is low in this form of hypoparathyroidism, fractional urine calcium excretion is increased and plasma PTH concentration is high (because of negative feedback). The clinical consequences of hypocalcemia were described above. Because PTH therapy is still not available, oral calcium and $1,25\text{-}(OH)_2\text{-}D$ must be used to treat all forms of hypoparathyroidism and return plasma calcium concentration to normal. The result (ironically) can be hypercalcinuria with the threat of kidney stones.

■ *PTH-Related Protein*

PTH-related peptide or protein (PTH_{rp}) was originally discovered as a product of human cancers that were of squamous cell origin and that were associated with hypercalcemia. It is now known that normal tissues also express this molecule. These tissues include skin keratinocytes, lactating mammary epithelium, placenta, and fetal parathyroid glands.

The gene for PTH_{rp} and the gene for PTH are on paired chromosomes and evolved from a common ancestor. Three products of amino acid length 139 to 173 are expressed by alternate splicing of the PTH_{rp} gene primary transcript. As a result of the striking homology between the N-terminal amino acids of PTH_{rp} and of PTH, PTH_{rp} exhibits most of the actions of PTH on bone and kidney. PTH_{rp} exerts these actions by binding to the PTH receptor, although interestingly the amino acids in the receptor binding sequences of the two hormone molecules are not homologous. One action of PTH, stimulation of renal 1-hydroxylase, is not shared by PTH_{rp}. Hence, patients with hypercalcemia caused by PTH_{rp} do not have elevated plasma $1,25\text{-}(OH)_2\text{-}D$ levels.

There is likely a normal physiological role for PTH_{rp} during intrauterine life and early infancy. This role is probably carried out by paracrine actions. PTH_{rp} in the placenta and the fetus is thought to function in maintaining the 30% to 40% increased ionized calcium concentration gradient that exists between fetal and maternal plasma. PTH_{rp} present in mammary tissue may regulate calcium concentration in breast milk. It may also function in the gastrointestinal tract of the infant, or it may escape degradation and play a systemic role in calcium homeostasis early in neonatal life. PTH_{rp} in skin contributes to regular cellular differentiation. The recent discovery of a mutant gene for the PTH_{rp}/PTH receptor that is constitutively overactive and causes severe abnormalities in the growth plate structure of affected individuals also suggests a role for PTH_{rp} in regulation of the transformation of cartilage to bone (see p 851).

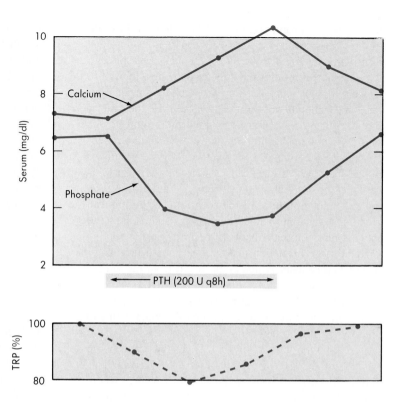

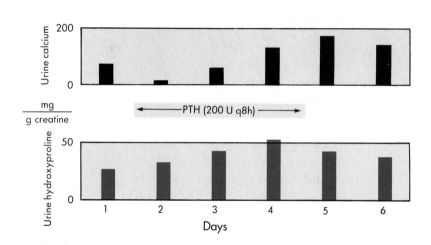

■ **Fig. 48-15** Effect of PTH administration to a PTH-deficient human who begins with a low plasma calcium and a high plasma phosphate level. The plasma calcium level increases and plasma phosphate level decreases. Urine calcium initially declines because of PTH action on the renal tubule; urine calcium excretion subsequently increases as the plasma calcium level rises and the filtered load of calcium rises in parallel. Urine hydroxyproline increases because of enhanced bone resorption. The initially very high tubular resorption of phosphate *(TRP)* falls so that urine phosphate *(not shown)* excretion increases.

■ *Calcitonin*

■ *Synthesis and Release of Calcitonin*

The parafollicular, or C, cells of the thyroid gland secrete another protein hormone, **calcitonin,** which influences calcium metabolism. *Whereas PTH acts to increase the plasma calcium concentration, calcitonin acts to lower it.* The parafollicular cells are of neural crest origin. In humans, they are concentrated in the lateral lobes of the thyroid gland, where they constitute 0.1% of the epithelial cells. They are distinguished from ordinary thyroid hormone–producing cells (see Chapter 50) by their large size, pale cytoplasm, and small secretory granules.

Calcitonin is a straight-chain peptide composed of 32 amino acids. The hormone contains a seven-membered disulfide ring at the N terminus and prolineamide at the

C terminus. Both fish and animal calcitonins are active in humans. The biologically active core of the molecule probably resides in its central region.

Calcitonin synthesis proceeds from a large preprohormone. The hormone is packaged in granules along with N-terminal and C-terminal copeptides. The gene for calcitonin illustrates the significant relationship that exists between the endocrine and nervous systems. In some cells, the primary RNA transcript encodes preprocalcitonin and directs synthesis of calcitonin. However, in other cells (in both thyroid and nervous tissue), the same primary RNA transcript encodes the precursor for and directs the synthesis of an entirely different peptide. This molecule, known as **calcitonin gene-related peptide (CGRP),** circulates in human plasma and probably arises from perivascular nerves. CGRP is a potent vasodilator and cardiac inotropic agent. The evolutionary path by which a hormone and a neuropeptide arose from *alternate* expression of the same gene and the functional significance of this relationship remain to be determined.

The major stimulus of calcitonin secretion is a rise in the plasma calcium concentration. However, the degree of response seen in various species is related to their need to prevent hypercalcemia. Vertebrates that originated in fresh water (of low calcium concentration) but migrated into the sea (with a calcium concentration of 40 mg/dl) were the first to require and develop a calcium-lowering hormone. When vertebrates moved to land, the emphasis in calcium economy shifted away from defense against hypercalcemia toward defense against hypocalcemia. PTH was developed, and the importance of calcitonin in regulatory plasma calcium concentration probably declined.

Calcitonin circulates in humans at concentrations of 10 to 20 pg/ml (5×10^{-12}) and increases twofold to tenfold after an acute increase in the plasma calcium concentration of as little as 1 mg/dl. Much larger responses of the hormone to calcium infusion are elicited in patients with calcitonin-secreting tumors. Conversely, in such patients, a sharp reduction in the ionized calcium concentration lowers the plasma calcitonin concentration. The calcium-stimulating effect on calcitonin secretion is mediated by the calcium-sensing receptor found in parathyroid and renal cells and involves an increase in intracellular cAMP levels. Ingestion of food stimulates calcitonin secretion without elevating the plasma calcium concentration. Food-stimulated calcitonin secretion is mediated by several gastrointestinal hormones, of which gastrin is the most potent. Excessive responses to gastrin provide a useful diagnostic test for states of calcitonin hypersecretion. Circulating calcitonin is heterogeneous, and it is largely degraded and cleared by the kidney.

■ *Calcitonin Actions*

The target cell of calcitonin is the osteoclast. Binding of calcitonin to its plasma membrane receptor is followed by an elevation of the intracellular concentration of cAMP, the second messenger for calcitonin in all target cells. The affected osteoclasts lose their ruffled borders, undergo cytoskeletal rearrangement, exhibit reduced motility, detach from bone surfaces, and are thus deactivated.

The major effect of calcitonin administration is a rapid fall in the plasma calcium concentration caused by inhibition of bone resorption. The magnitude of this decrease is proportional to the baseline rate of bone turnover. In normal adults, the effect is minimal. However, in individuals with diseases that cause high rates of bone resorption, significant hypocalcemia can result. These individuals also display an escape from the calcitonin effect, possibly caused by down-regulation of calcitonin receptors. Nevertheless, continued provision of calcitonin eventually decreases the number of osteoclasts as well as their activity. More dense bone with fewer resorption cavities eventually results.

Calcitonin is clearly a physiological antagonist to PTH with respect to calcium. However, with respect to phosphate, it has the same net effect as PTH; that is, it decreases the plasma phosphate level. This decrease is caused by inhibition of bone resorption, promotion of phosphate entry into bone, and a small increase in urinary phosphate excretion. This hypophosphatemic effect is independent of the hypocalcemic effect.

The importance of calcitonin to normal human calcium economy is still unclear. Ordinarily, the absorption of dietary calcium loads produces little, if any, elevation of the plasma calcium concentration. Whether the calcitonin increase provoked by eating helps prevent the development of postprandial hypercalcemia is not clear. Calcitonin deficiency that results from complete removal of the thyroid gland does not lead to significant hypercalcemia. A chronic excess of calcitonin generated either by tumor of the thyroid gland or by exogenous administration does not produce hypocalcemia. At present, it may be most reasonable to conclude that any effects of calcitonin deficiency or excess are easily offset by appropriate adjustment of PTH and vitamin D concentration.

On the other hand, the possibility that calcitonin significantly regulates bone remodeling cannot be easily excluded. It could participate in fetal skeletal development. The fact that plasma calcitonin is lower in women than in men and also declines with aging may suggest a functional role for the hormone in the development of accelerated bone loss after the menopause.

Calcitonin is used in the acute treatment of hypercalcemia and in certain bone diseases in which a sustained reduction in osteoclastic resorption is therapeutically beneficial. Finally, the discovery of calcitonin in a number of locations throughout the body—in the pituitary gland and hypothalamus and within cells of neural crest origin—has raised the possibility that calcitonin may also have paracrine and neurotransmitter functions. In this regard, calcitonin does exhibit analgesic properties independent of the opioid system.

■ *Integrated Hormonal Regulation of Calcium and Phosphate*

From the previous discussion, it should be clear that a complex interplay of several hormones that act on a number of tissues is responsible for maintenance of normal concentrations of calcium and phosphate in body fluids. This integrated system is best visualized by tracing the compensatory responses to deprivation of calcium and of phosphate (Figs. 48-16 and 48-17).

Calcium deprivation causes hypocalcemia, which acts as a signal for the stimulation of PTH secretion (Fig. 48-

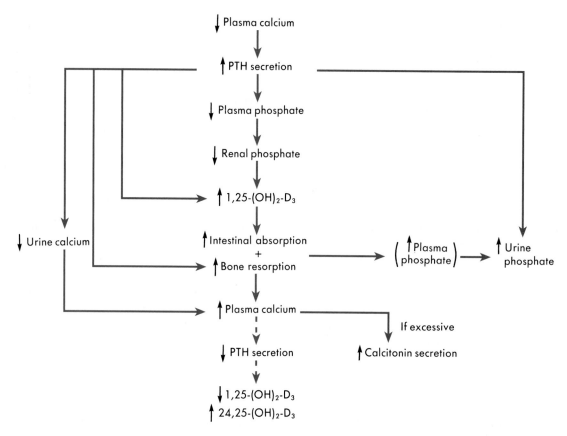

■ **Fig. 48-16** The compensatory response to calcium deprivation. See text for explication.

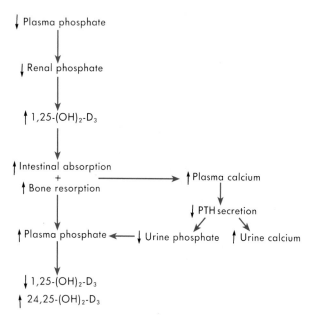

■ **Fig. 48-17** The compensatory response to phosphate deprivation. See text for explication.

16). PTH increases bone resorption and renal tubular calcium reabsorption, and thereby raises plasma calcium concentration. PTH also increases urinary phosphate excretion, and thereby decreases the plasma phosphate concentration and renal cortical phosphate content. All three factors—hypocalcemia, excess PTH, and hypophosphatemia—act to stimulate the production of 1,25-(OH)$_2$-D. The latter steroid hormone raises the plasma calcium concentration toward normal by increasing absorption of calcium from the gastrointestinal tract and, in concert with PTH, by increasing osteocytic and osteoclastic bone resorption. Thus, this beautifully integrated response to calcium deprivation increases the flux of calcium into the extracellular fluid. Simultaneously, the extra phosphate that enters with the calcium from the bone and intestine is eliminated by excretion in the urine. The recovery of plasma calcium concentration to normal shuts off PTH hypersecretion by negative feedback, augmented by a suppressive effect of 1,25-(OH)$_2$-D on PTH synthesis. 1,25-(OH)$_2$-D synthesis will then decline and 24,25-(OH)$_2$-D synthesis will increase; thus, the whole sequence will diminish. As a further safety valve, should the compensatory rise in plasma calcium greatly exceed the normal concentration, stimulation of calcitonin secretion would moderate it as well.

In a contrasting sequence, phosphate deprivation via hypophosphatemia directly stimulates 1,25-(OH)$_2$-D production (Fig. 48-16). Vitamin 1,25-(OH)$_2$-D increases the flux of phosphate into the extracellular fluid by stimulating its absorption from the intestine and by stimulating bone resorption. The extra calcium that simultaneously enters with phosphate raises the plasma calcium concentration, and this increase suppresses PTH secretion. The absence of PTH causes the kidney tubules to increase reabsorption of phosphate. Urinary phosphate is conserved, and thus aids in the restoration of plasma phosphate concentration to normal. At the same time, the lack of PTH permits easier disposal of the extra mobilized calcium. This process diminishes the renal tubular reabsorption of calcium and increases its excretion in the urine. As plasma phosphate returns to normal, 24,25-(OH)$_2$-D production is favored, 1,25-(OH)$_2$-D concentrations decline, and the whole process is reversed.

The combined arrangement of dual hormone regulation and dual hormone action permits selective defense of either the plasma calcium or plasma phosphate concentration, without creating a circulatory excess of the other. The same principles apply in reverse to imposition of excess calcium or excess phosphate loads of either endogenous or exogenous sources.

Certain characteristics of these homeostatic systems for adjustment of body calcium and phosphate stores deserve emphasis. The renal responses of PTH provide the most rapid (within minutes) defense against perturbations in both calcium and phosphate stores. As PTH secretion ranges from very high to very low concentrations, the rate of urinary calcium excretion can rise 25-fold from approximately 0.05 to 1.2 mg/min, and that of phosphate can fall from 2 to 0 mg/min. A sudden 2 to 3 mg/dl increase in either calcium or phosphate concentration in the extracellular fluid can be corrected within 24 hours by the kidney, acting under the appropriate alteration in PTH concentration. In response to complete phosphate and calcium deprivation, renal conservation of phosphate is complete, whereas that of calcium is not.

The gastrointestinal component of this homeostatic system is both slower and narrower in range than the renal component. As a result of variations in 1,25-(OH)$_2$-D, the absorption of dietary calcium increases from 20% to 70% as calcium intake decreases from 2000 to 200 mg/day. Thus, absorbed calcium can effectively range from 140 to 400 mg/day. Hormonal effects on phosphate absorption are even less striking, because the latter is virtually a linear function of dietary intake.

Bone responses to regulatory fluctuations in both PTH and 1,25-(OH)$_2$-D are rapid when produced by osteocytic osteolysis and relatively slow when caused by osteoclastic resorption. However, the capacity for compensatory calcium and phosphate uptake and release is enormous. In humans, tenfold variations in calcium turnover have been observed.

Finally, an important difference between renal and gastrointestinal mechanisms on the one hand and bone mechanisms on the other hand must be considered. The compensatory responses of the kidney and the intestine are able to defend total body *and bone* stores of calcium and phosphate against erosion or inundation. In contrast, the skeletal mechanisms of defense against perturbations in plasma calcium and phosphate concentrations eventually sacrifice the chemical and structural integrity of the bone mass if they are employed for long periods.

■ *Summary*

1. Calcium participates critically in a myriad of biological functions, including neurotransmission, hormone secretion and action, enzyme activities, muscle contraction, and blood clotting. Calcium is also the chief mineral that contributes to the structural integrity of the skeleton and teeth.

2. Extracellular Ca^{++} concentration (approximately 10^{-3} M) is closely controlled in order to regulate the wide, transient swings in the much lower intracellular Ca^{++} concentration (approximately 10^{-7} M).

3. Phosphate is critical to all major enzymatic pathways involved in energy generation, substrate disposition, and synthesis of protein and other macromolecules. Phosphate is also the anion partner of calcium in bone structure.

4. Calcium balance and plasma calcium homeostasis depend on dietary intake, fractional gastrointestinal absorption, regulation of renal excretion, and internal movement of calcium into and out of skeletal reservoirs.

5. Phosphate balance and plasma phosphate homeostasis reflect dietary intake, renal excretion, and internal shifts among extracellular fluid, large soft tissue contents, and the skeletal reservoir.

6. Bone is a complex organ with cells specifically devoted to a continuous process of remodeling. In this process, mineralized bone is reabsorbed by osteoclasts (releasing calcium and phosphate) and is then re-formed by osteoblasts (assimilating calcium and phosphate). This process is augmented during growth periods. With aging, resorption exceeds formation and bone mass declines.

7. Vitamin D is a steroid molecule either synthesized from cholesterol in the skin by ultraviolet light or absorbed from the diet. The basic structure is modified successively in the liver and kidney to 1,25-(OH)$_2$-D, the active metabolite.

8. Vitamin 1,25-(OH)$_2$-D acts via its osteoblast nuclear receptor to increase calcium (and phosphate) absorption from the gastrointestinal tract. The hormone is therefore critical to maintaining the supply of calcium for bone formation and growth, as well as other calcium-dependent processes. It also enhances bone resorption. Overall, 1,25-(OH)$_2$-D increases plasma calcium and plasma phosphate concentrations.

9. Parathyroid hormone (PTH) is a straight-chain peptide synthesized from a prohormone in the four parathyroid glands. PTH is released by exocytosis in response to a decrease in plasma calcium concentration that is sensed by a calcium receptor in the plasma membrane of the parathyroid cell. PTH synthesis and secretion are suppressed by calcium and 1,25-(OH)$_2$-D.

10. PTH acts via a plasma membrane receptor and cAMP (1) to increase osteoclastic bone resorption, (2) to increase renal tubular reabsorption of calcium, (3) to increase 1,25-$(OH)_2$-D synthesis in the kidney, and (4) to decrease renal tubular reabsorption and increase urinary excretion of phosphate. Overall, PTH increases plasma calcium and decreases plasma phosphate concentrations.

11. Calcium deficiency evokes a synergistic sequence that increases PTH and 1,25-$(OH)_2$-D secretion. The combined actions of these two hormones increase the inflow of calcium and restore plasma concentrations to normal, and they simultaneously dispose of the inflow of extra phosphate by enhancing its renal excretion.

12. In contrast, phosphate deprivation evokes a synergistic sequence that increases 1,25-$(OH)_2$-D secretion but suppresses PTH secretion. The result is to restore the plasma phosphate concentration toward normal while disposing of the inflow of extra calcium by increasing its renal excretion.

13. Calcitonin is a peptide hormone synthesized in C cells within the thyroid gland. It is a PTH antagonist in bone and is secreted in response to hypercalcemia. Thus, it acts to lower the plasma concentration of calcium.

■ *Self-Study Problems*

1. A victim of accidental trauma requires emergency surgery, goes into shock in the operating room, and receives 10 pints of whole blood rapidly. The citrate in the blood binds calcium and decreases the plasma ionized calcium level. Describe the endocrine responses and the mechanism of their actions in restoring the ionized calcium level to normal.

2. How are the mechanisms of bone formation and resorption linked? Does this linkage contribute to calcium homeostasis?

■ *Bibliography*

Journal articles

Bell NH: Vitamin D metabolism, aging, and bone loss (editorial), *J Clin Endocrinol Metab* 80:1051, 1995.

Bikle DD, Pillai S: Vitamin D, calcium, and epidermal differentiation, *Endocr Rev* 14:3, 1993.

Bouillon R, Okamura WH, Norman AW: Structure-function relationships in the vitamin D endocrine system, *Endocr Rev* 16:200, 1995.

Brown EM: Extracellular Ca^{2+} sensing, regulation of parathyroid cell function, and role of Ca^{2+} and other ions as extracellular (first) messengers, *Physiol Rev* 71:371, 1991.

Brown EM et al: Cloning and characterization of an extracellular Ca^{2+}-sensing receptor from bovine parathyroid, *Nature* 366:575, 1993.

Chattopadhyay N, Mithal A, Brown EM: The calcium-sensing receptor: a window into the physiology and pathophysiology of mineral ion metabolism, *Endocr Rev* 17:289, 1996.

Dempster DW et al: Anabolic actions of parathyroid hormone on bone, *Endocr Rev* 14:690, 1993.

Epstein S: Serum and urinary markers of bone remodeling: assessment of bone turnover, *Endocr Rev* 9:437, 1988.

Fitzpatrick LA: Differences in the actions of calcium versus lanthanum to influence parathyroid hormone release, *Endocrinology* 127:711, 1990.

Gambacciani M et al: The relative contributions of menopause and aging to postmenopausal vertebral osteopenia, *J Clin Endocrinol Metab* 77:1148, 1993.

Gross M, Kumar R: Physiology and biochemistry of vitamin D–dependent calcium binding proteins, *Am J Physiol* 259:195, 1990.

Holick MF: Skin: site of the synthesis of vitamin D and a target tissue for the active form, 1,25-dihydroxyvitamin D_3, *Ann NY Acad Sci* 548:14, 1988.

Ishimi Y et al: Regulation by calcium and 1,25-$(OH)_2$-D_3 of cell proliferation and function of bovine parathyroid cells in culture, *J Bone Miner Res* 5:755, 1990.

Mahonen A et al: Effect of 1,25-$(OH)_2$-D_3 on its receptor mRNA concentration and osteocalcin synthesis in human osteosarcoma cells, *Biochem Biophys Acta* 30:1048, 1990.

Mallette LE: The parathyroid polyhormones: new concepts in the spectrum of peptide hormone action, *Endocr Rev* 12:110, 1991.

Munson PL, Hirsch PF: Importance of calcitonin in physiology, clinical pharmacology, and medicine, *Bone Miner* 16:162, 1992.

Nemeth EF, Scarpa A: Are changes in intracellular free calcium necessary for regulating secretion in parathyroid cells? *Ann NY Acad Sci* 493:542, 1987.

Nissenson RA et al: Synthetic peptides comprising the amino-terminal sequence of a parathyroid hormone–like protein from human malignancies: binding to parathyroid hormone receptors and activation of adenylate cyclase in bone cells and kidney, *J Biol Chem* 263:12866, 1988.

Orloff JJ et al: Parathyroid hormone–like proteins: biochemical responses and receptor interactions, *Endocr Rev* 10:476, 1989.

Raisz LG: Local and systemic factors in the pathogenesis of osteoporosis, *N Engl J Med* 318:818, 1988.

Reichel H et al: The role of the vitamin D endocrine system in health and disease, *N Engl J Med* 320:980, 1989.

Roodman GD: Advances in bone biology: the osteoclast, *Endocr Rev* 17:308, 1996.

Ross TK, Darwish HM, and Deluca HF: Molecular biology of vitamin D action, *Vitam Horm* 49:281, 1994.

Rouleau MF et al: Characterization of the major parathyroid hormone target cell in the endosteal metaphysis of rat long bones, *J Bone Miner Res* 10:1043, 1990.

Schipani E et al: Constitutively activated receptors for parathyroid hormone and parathyroid hormone–related peptide in Jansen's metaphyseal chondrodysplasia, *N Engl J Med* 335:708, 1996.

Schmid C: IGFs: function and clinical importance to the regulation of osteoblast function by hormones and cytokines with special reference to insulin-like growth factors and their binding proteins, *J Intern Med* 234:535, 1993.

Shigeno C et al: Parathyroid hormone receptors are plasma membrane glycoproteins with asparagine-linked oligosaccharides, *J Biol Chem* 263:3872, 1988.

Stern PH: Vitamin D and bone, *Kidney Int* 29:S17, 1990.

Walters MR: Newly identified actions of the vitamin D endocrine system, *Endocr Rev* 13:719, 1992.

Webb AR et al: Sunlight regulates the cutaneous production of vitamin D_3 by causing its photodegradation, *J Clin Endocrinol Metab* 68:882, 1989.

Yamamoto M et al: Hypocalcemia increases and hypercalcemia decreases the steady-state level of parathyroid hormone messenger RNA in the rat, *J Clin Invest* 83:1053, 1989.

Books and monographs

Bringhurst FR: *Calcium and phosphate distribution, turnover, and metabolic actions.* In DeGroot LJ, editor: *Endocrinology,* ed 3, Philadelphia, 1995, WB Saunders.

Coleman DT, Fitzpatrick LA, Bilezikian J: *Biochemical mechanisms of parathyroid hormone action.* In Bilezikian J, editor: *The parathyroids: basic and clinical concepts,* New York, 1994, Raven Press.

Kronenberg HM, Bringhurst FR, Segre GV, Potts JT Jr: *Parathyroid hormone biosynthesis and metabolism.* In Bilezikian J, editor: *The parathyroids: basic and clinical concepts,* New York, 1994, Raven Press.

Martin TJ, Moseley JM: *Parathyroid hormone–related protein.* In DeGroot LJ, editor: *Endocrinology,* ed 3, Philadelphia, 1995, WB Saunders.

MacIntyre I: *Calcitonin: physiology, biosynthesis, secretion, metabolism, and mode of action.* In DeGroot LJ, editor: *Endocrinology,* ed 3, Philadelphia, 1995, WB Saunders.

Potts JT Jr et al: *Parathyroid hormone: physiology, chemistry, biosynthesis, secretion, metabolism, and mode of action.* In DeGroot LJ, editor: *Endocrinology,* ed 3, Philadelphia, 1995, WB Saunders.

The Hypothalamus and Pituitary Gland

The hypothalamus-pituitary unit forms the most complex and, in some respects, the most dominant component of the entire endocrine system. Its internal anatomic and functional relationships are elaborate and subtle. *The output of the hypothalamus-pituitary unit regulates the function of the thyroid, adrenal, and reproductive glands and is directly responsible for somatic growth and lactation and milk secretion. It also helps maintain body fluid homeostasis.*

Numerous hormones are synthesized, stored, and released by the hypothalamus-pituitary unit. Two hormones, **antidiuretic hormone (ADH) (arginine vasopressin)** and **oxytocin,** are synthesized by neurons in the hypothalamus but are stored and secreted by the posterior pituitary gland, or **neurohypophysis.** A group of tropic hormones—**adrenocorticotropic hormone (ACTH), thyroid-stimulating hormone (TSH), luteinizing hormone (LH), follicle-stimulating hormone (FSH), growth hormone (GH),** and **prolactin**—are synthesized, stored, and secreted by mostly hormone-specific endocrine cell types in the anterior pituitary gland, or **adenohypophysis.** A set of **releasing** and **inhibiting hormones** that are produced in the hypothalamus and travel to the adenohypophysis regulates the synthesis and secretion of these adenohypophyseal tropic hormones. All of these hormones emanate from a mass of only 500 mg of pituitary tissue in association with 10 g of adjacent hypothalamus.

■ *Anatomy*

A knowledge of the embryologic development of the pituitary gland is crucial to an understanding of its anatomy and function. *The fully developed gland is actually an amalgam of hormone-producing glandular cells (the adenohypophysis, or anterior pituitary) and neural cells with secretory function (the neurohypophysis, or posterior pituitary).* The anterior endocrine portion of the pituitary develops from an upward outpouching of ectodermal cells from the roof of the oral cavity (Rathke's pouch). This pouch eventually pinches off and becomes separated from the oral cavity by the sphenoid bone of the skull. The lumen of the pouch is reduced to a small cleft. The posterior neural portion of the pituitary develops from a downward outpouching of ectoderm from the brain in the floor of the third ventricle. The lumen of this pouch is obliterated inferiorly as the sides fuse into the infundibular process. Superiorly, the lumen remains contiguous with, and forms a recess in, the adult third ventricle. The upper portion of this neural stalk expands to invest the lowest portion of the hypothalamus and is called the **median eminence.** The cleftlike remnant of Rathke's pouch demarcates the interwoven anterior and posterior portions of the pituitary. In some animals, but not in humans, cells in the area of Rathke's pouch and adjacent to the neurohypophysis form a distinct intermediate lobe.

The entire pituitary gland sits in a socket of sphenoid bone called the **sella turcica.** A reflection of the dura mater, called the *diaphragm,* extends across the top of the sella turcica and separates the bulk of the pituitary gland from the brain. However, the neural stalk penetrates the diaphragm, maintaining its continuity with the hypothalamus. These anatomic relationships are shown in Fig. 49-1, *B.* The human pituitary gland can be visualized by computed tomography (CT) and nuclear magnetic resonance imaging (MRI) (Fig. 49-1, *A*). The volume of the pituitary decreases with aging and increases during pregnancy.

The blood supply to this amalgam of neural and endocrine tissue is complex. In the posterior pituitary, the neural tissue of the infundibular process is supplied with blood mostly from the **inferior hypophyseal artery.** The capillary plexus of this artery drains into the dural sinus. The neural tissue of the upper stalk and of the median eminence is supplied largely by the **superior hypophyseal artery.** After investing the axons in these areas, the capillary plexus that emanates from this artery forms a

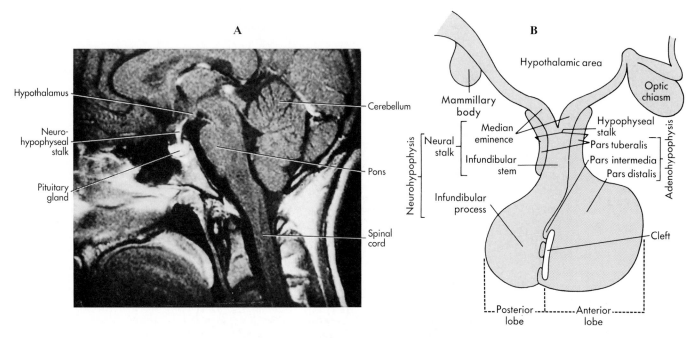

■ **Fig. 49-1**   **A,** Magnetic resonance image of the head shows the proximity of the hypothalamus and pituitary gland and their connection by a neurohypophyseal stalk. (Courtesy of Steven Wiener, MD.) **B,** Diagram of the pituitary gland shows its division into the adenohypophysis and neurohypophysis. (Adapted from an original painting by Frank H. Netter, MD, from The CIBA Collection of Medical Illustrations, Division of CIBA-Geigy Corporation.)

set of long portal veins that carry the blood downward into the anterior pituitary. There, these **portal veins** give rise to a second capillary plexus that supplies the anterior pituitary endocrine cells with most of their blood supply, which is then drained off into the dural sinus. The anterior pituitary also receives blood via a set of short portal veins that originate in the capillary plexus of the inferior hypophyseal artery within the neural stalk. Thus, very little or no direct arterial blood supply reaches the adenohypophyseal cells. Furthermore, it should be noted that the anterior pituitary gland lies outside the blood-brain barrier.

The implications of the anatomic arrangement of the hypothalamus-pituitary complex and its blood supply become apparent when the functional relationships are examined in Fig. 49-2. The neurohypophysis represents a collection of axons whose cell bodies lie in the hypothalamus. Peptide hormones synthesized in the cell bodies of these hypothalamic neurons travel down their axons in neurosecretory granules to be stored in the nerve terminals lying in the posterior pituitary gland. These terminals consist of neurosecretory vesicles invested with modified astroglial cells known as *pituicytes.* Upon stimulation of the cell bodies, the granules are released from the axonal terminals by exocytosis; the peptide hormones then enter the peripheral circulation via the capillary plexuses of the inferior hypophyseal artery. Thus, a single neural cell performs the entire process of hormone synthesis, storage, and release in the classic example of neurocrine function.

In contrast, the adenohypophysis is a collection of endocrine cells regulated by blood-borne stimuli that originate in neural tissue. Cell bodies of particular hypothalamic neurons synthesize releasing hormones and inhibiting hormones, which travel in packets down their axons only as far as the median eminence. Here, they are stored within neurosecretory granules in the nerve terminals. After these hypothalamic neurons are stimulated by nerve impulses, the releasing or inhibiting hormones are discharged into the median eminence and enter the capillary plexus of the superior hypophyseal artery. From here, they are transported down the long portal veins and exit from the secondary capillary plexus to reach their specific endocrine target cells in the adenohypophysis. The endocrine cells respond to the releasing or inhibiting hormones by increasing or decreasing their output of tropic hormones that are stored in secretory granules. These hormones enter the same second capillary plexus through which they ultimately reach the peripheral circulation. Thus, two cells—one neural and one endocrine—participate in the processes that lead to synthesis and release (by exocytosis) of the anterior pituitary tropic hormones, a combination of neurocrine and endocrine function. Key evidence in support of this functional arrangement includes the following observations:

1. Neural tracts that contain hypothalamic peptides can be traced by immunohistochemical techniques down to the median eminence, where they end in proximity to capillaries (Fig. 49-3).

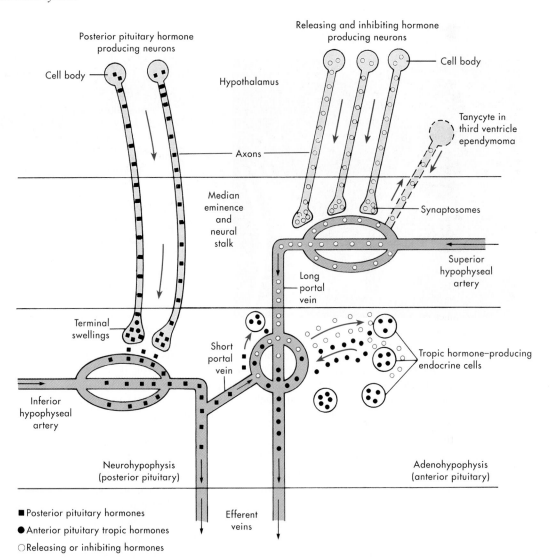

Posterior pituitary hormone
producing neurons

Releasing and inhibiting hormone
producing neurons

Cell body

Hypothalamus

Cell body

Tanycyte in
third ventricle
ependymoma

Axons

Synaptosomes

Median
eminence
and
neural
stalk

Superior
hypophyseal
artery

Long
portal
vein

Terminal
swellings

Short
portal
vein

Tropic hormone–producing
endocrine cells

Inferior
hypophyseal
artery

Neurohypophysis
(posterior pituitary)

Adenohypophysis
(anterior pituitary)

Efferent
veins

■ Posterior pituitary hormones
● Anterior pituitary tropic hormones
○ Releasing or inhibiting hormones

■ **Fig. 49-2** Anatomic and functional relationships between the hypothalamus, the pituitary gland, and their blood supply. Note that the adenohypophysis has no direct arterial supply but receives blood from the median eminence, which contains hypothalamic releasing and inhibiting hormones. Arrows indicate direction of movement of hormone molecules. Posterior pituitary hormones reach their storage and release area by axonal transport from the neuron cell bodies where they are synthesized. Anterior pituitary hormones are synthesized and stored in situ. They are secreted in response to hypothalamic peptides that reach the anterior pituitary by axonal transport followed by blood transport via portal veins.

2. Direct measurement of hypothalamic peptides reveals that the concentrations of these peptides are tenfold to twentyfold higher in pituitary portal venous blood than in peripheral blood.
3. Exposure of anterior pituitary tissue in perfusion systems or in tissue culture to individual hypothalamic peptides causes specific patterns of stimulation or inhibition of the release of corresponding tropic hormones.

The above description implies an entirely unidirectional arrangement. However, not all the venous drainage from the anterior pituitary necessarily empties directly into the systemic circulation. The short portal veins may act as conduits for a reverse flow of blood from the anterior pituitary cells through the neurohypophyseal capillary plexus back up to the axons or cell bodies in the median eminence or the hypothalamus. This direction of flow would permit high concentrations of anterior pituitary tropic hormones to bathe these neurons without impedance from the blood-brain barrier, and thus allows short-loop feedback from endocrine to neural cells.

It is also possible that two-way traffic between the cerebrospinal fluid and both the neurohypophysis and adenohypophysis may exist. Specialized ependymal cells in the interior recess of the third ventricle send down long processes that interdigitate with blood vessels in the

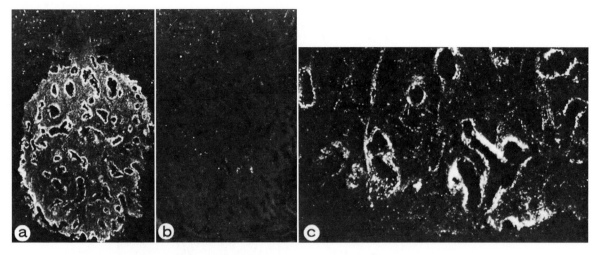

■ **Fig. 49-3** Immunohistochemical localization of growth hormone–releasing hormone (GHRH) in the median eminence of the squirrel monkey. **A,** Section stained with fluorescent-labeled antibody to GHRH shows localization of GHRH around capillaries of the median eminence. **B,** Section stained with fluorescent-labeled control serum shows little reaction, demonstrating specificity of the antibody to GHRH. **C,** Higher power of **A** showing GHRH in axonal tracts ending in the vicinity of the capillaries. (From Bloch B et al: *Nature* 301:607, 1983. From Macmillan Journals.)

median eminence and infundibular stalk (Fig. 49-2). These cells, known as **pituitary tanycytes,** could facilitate transfer of regulatory substances from the cerebrospinal fluid to the pituitary. They could also allow posterior pituitary peptide hormones, hypothalamic releasing or inhibiting hormones, or even anterior pituitary tropic hormones to have access to the brain via the cerebrospinal fluid.

■ *Hypothalamic Function*

The hypothalamus clearly plays a key role in regulating pituitary function. It can be considered a central relay station for collecting and integrating signals from diverse sources and funneling them to the pituitary (Fig. 49-4). The hypothalamus receives afferent nerve tracts from the thalamus, the reticular activating substance, the limbic system (amygdala, olfactory bulb, hippocampus, and habenula), and the eyes and remotely from the neocortex. Some of the connections to the hypothalamus are multisynaptic. Through this input, pituitary function can be influenced by pain, sleep or wakefulness, emotion, fright, rage, olfactory sensations, light, and possibly even thought. It can be coordinated with patterned behavior and mating responses of neural origin. The proximity of other hypothalamic nuclei that govern thirst, appetite, energy stores, temperature regulation, and autonomic nervous system function also allows coordination between the output of pituitary hormones and a wide variety of basic functions.

The proximity of these various areas of the hypothalamus to each other has functional logic. For example, hormones of the thyroid gland increase energy expenditure,

metabolic rate, and thermogenesis. The neurons that ultimately control thyroid gland output are anatomically close to neurons that regulate energy intake via appetite control and also temperature. As the hypothalamus-pituitary unit is systematically studied, other similar examples are becoming apparent.

Hypothalamohypothalamic tracts can integrate multiple simultaneous pituitary responses with each other and regulate pituitary function in accordance with change in temperature, energy needs, or fluid balance. The neurotransmitters involved in afferent impulses to the hypothalamus are largely norepinephrine, acetylcholine, and serotonin. Dopamine, acetylcholine, γ-aminobutyric acid (GABA), and the opioid peptide β-endorphin act as neurotransmitters for efferent impulses to the median eminence. These impulses regulate the discharge of releasing hormones or inhibiting hormones into the adjacent capillaries (Fig. 49-2). In addition, neurotransmitters such as dopamine from the hypothalamus may reach the portal vein blood and, via receptors in the endocrine cells, directly influence the output of anterior pituitary tropic hormones. Dopamine and β-endorphin also modulate efferent hypothalamic outflow by transmitting signals between different areas of the hypothalamus.

The hypothalamus-pituitary axis is also under the influence of blood-borne substances from the periphery. Virtually all the tropic hormones from the adenohypophysis cause changes in the concentrations either of peripheral target gland hormones (thyroid, adrenal, gonadal) or of substrates, such as glucose or free fatty acids. Conditions exist for at least three levels of humoral feedback, as illustrated in Fig. 49-5. Peripheral gland hormones or substrates that arise from tissue metabolism can exert feedback control on both the hypothalamus and the

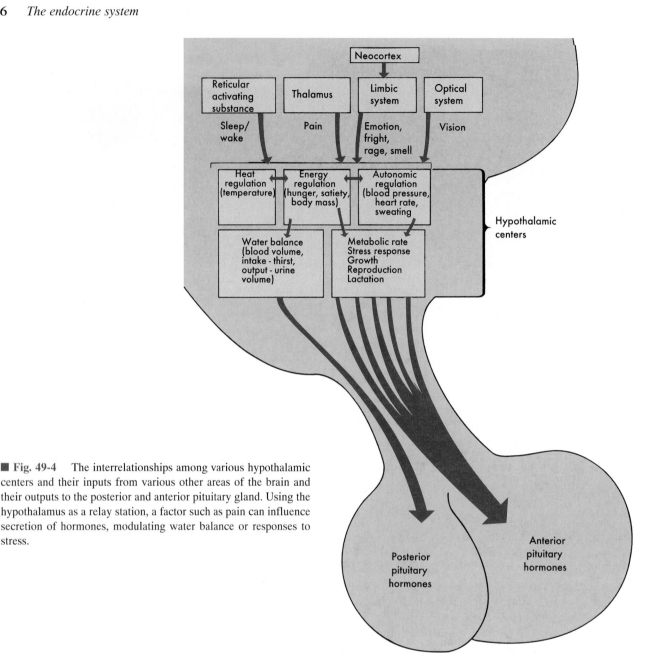

■ **Fig. 49-4**   The interrelationships among various hypothalamic centers and their inputs from various other areas of the brain and their outputs to the posterior and anterior pituitary gland. Using the hypothalamus as a relay station, a factor such as pain can influence secretion of hormones, modulating water balance or responses to stress.

anterior pituitary gland. This mechanism is known as **long-loop feedback** and is usually negative, although it can occasionally be positive. Negative feedback can also be exerted by the tropic hormones themselves through effects on the synthesis or discharge of the related hypothalamic releasing or inhibiting hormones. This mechanism is known as **short-loop feedback.** Because tropic hormones do not ordinarily cross the blood-brain barrier, short-loop feedback may occur either by specialized transport across fenestrated endothelial cells of the capillaries that bathe hypothalamic neurons, or by reverse flow through the short portal veins, as previously described. Finally, hypothalamic releasing hormones may even inhibit their own synthesis by stimulating the discharge of a paired hypothalamic inhibiting hormone. This mechanism, called **ultra-short-loop feedback,**

could occur in two ways: by neurotransmission between two hypothalamic cells, or by transport of the releasing hormone via the pituitary tanycytes to the cerebrospinal fluid and then back to the hypothalamus.

The anterior pituitary gland is the central point of the hypothalamic pituitary-peripheral gland axis. At this level, *hypothalamic releasing hormones and peripheral target gland hormones are usually antagonists: one accelerates while the other brakes anterior pituitary hormone secretion.* The short- and ultra-short-loop feedback mechanisms help maintain the balance finally achieved.

Table 49-1 lists the currently known or suspected hypothalamic releasing or inhibiting hormones.

The hypothalamus can be subdivided somewhat imprecisely into endocrinologically distinct functional areas. In general, the lateral hypothalamus receives affer-

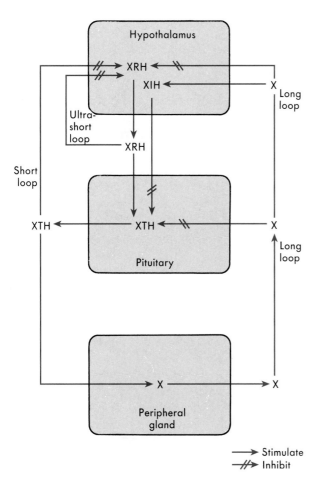

■ Fig. 49-5   Negative feedback loops regulating hormone secretion in a typical hypothalamus-pituitary-peripheral gland axis. *X*, Peripheral gland hormone; *XTH*, pituitary tropic hormone; *XRH*, hypothalamic releasing hormone; *XIH*, hypothalamic inhibiting hormone.

ent impulses and relays them to the neurosecretory nuclei of the anterior and medial basal portions of the hypothalamus. The anterior segment of the hypothalamus contains two well-defined collections of large (magnocellular) neurons, the supraoptic and paraventricular nuclei. These nuclei are responsible for the synthesis of the two posterior pituitary peptide hormones (oxytocin and ADH). Their axons project primarily to the posterior pituitary, although some fibers also project to the median eminence and to other neurons in the floor of the third ventricle and the brainstem. Clustered immediately beneath the third ventricle, in the arcuate nucleus and the periventricular nucleus of the medial basal hypothalamus, are small (parvicellular) neurons responsible for synthesis of the various hypothalamic releasing and inhibiting hormones. Some of these neurons are also located in the paraventricular nucleus. The axons of these small neurons project to the median eminence. However, cells that also contain hypothalamic releasing hormones are scattered in numerous other areas of the hypothalamus. In these neurons, the hypothalamic peptide hormones may have particular neurotransmitter roles related

to or distinct from their known endocrine functions. Immunohistochemical mapping has shown a sufficient anatomic separation between dense collections of hypothalamic peptides to indicate that, in general, only one cell type produces each neurohormone. However, in at least one instance, two peptide hormones (corticotropin-releasing hormone [CRH] and ADH) are co-localized within certain hypothalamic neurons.

The names of all the hypothalamic peptides are based on the anterior pituitary hormone whose secretion they were originally discovered to influence. It was initially presumed that each tropic hormone was controlled by a unique hypothalamic releasing or inhibiting hormone and that each hypothalamic hormone had only one target anterior pituitary cell. However, the actual physiology is more complex. **Thyrotropin-releasing hormone (TRH)** can also stimulate secretion of prolactin. **Somatostatin,** discovered as a GH-inhibiting factor, can also inhibit the secretion of TSH.

Pathologically functioning adenohypophyseal cells in pituitary tumors may have receptors for hypothalamic regulatory peptides that the normal adenohypophyseal cells do not. For example, **anterior pituitary adenomas** that secrete GH may have TRH receptors. These tumor cells respond to this hypothalamic peptide with secretion of GH, and this aberrant response is a useful diagnostic test for the presence of these adenomas. Tumor cells from types other than the GH-secreting line may have receptors for the peptide somatostatin, which inhibits GH. The presence of somatostatin receptors on the tumor cells makes possible the use of analogs of this peptide to treat such adenomas by reducing the size of these tumors and stopping hypersecretion of their hormone product.

Hypothalamic peptide hormones have also been found outside the hypothalamus, in such diverse areas as the cerebral cortex, limbic area, spinal cord, autonomic ganglia, sensory neurons, and pancreatic islets and throughout the gastrointestinal tract. In these areas, these peptides serve neuromodulatory roles related to or independent of their endocrine function.

The hypothalamic peptides are synthesized via preprohormones, as described in Chapter 45. Many common features characterize their functional behavior (Box 49-1).

The secretion of hypothalamic releasing and inhibiting hormones into the pituitary portal veins is pulsatile. This pulsatile pattern apparently depends on intrinsic neural oscillators within the cells that release these hormones. Pulsatile secretion of these hormones is critical for maintenance of the appropriate pattern and level of secretion of their target anterior pituitary hormones. Pulsatility may also determine whether the receptors for hypothalamic peptides are up- or down-regulated.

To exert their effects, releasing and inhibiting hormones first bind to plasma membrane receptors in the

■ **Table 49-1**   Hypothalamic hormones and factors

Hormone	Predominant hypothalamic localization	Structure	Target pituitary hormones
Thyrotropin-releasing hormone (TRH)	Paraventricular	pGLU-HIS-PRO-NH$_2$	Thyrotropin Prolactin Growth hormone (pathological)
Gonadotropin-releasing hormone (GnRH)	Arcuate	pGLU-HIS-TRP-SER-TYR-GLY-LEU-ARG-PRO-GLY-NH$_2$	Luteinizing hormone Follicle-stimulating hormone Growth hormone (pathological)
Corticotropin-releasing hormone (CRH)	Paraventricular	SER-GLN-GLU-PRO-PRO-ILE-SER-LEU-ASP-LEU-THR-PHE-HIS-LEU-LEUARG-GLU-VAL-LEU-GLU-MET-THR-LYS-ALA-ASP-GLN-LEU-ALA-GLN-GLN-ALA-HIS-SER-ASN-ARG-LYS-LEU-LEU-ASP-ILE-ALA-NH$_2$	Adrenocorticotropin β- and γ-Lipotropin β-Endorphins
Growth hormone–releasing hormone (GHRH)	Arcuate	TYR-ALA-ASP-ALA-ILE-PHE-THR-ASN-SER-TYR-ARG-LYS-VAL-LEU-GLY-GLN-LEU-SER-ALA-ARG-LYS-LEU-LEU-GLN-ASP-ILE-MET-SER-ARG-GLN-GLN-GLY-GLU-SER-ASN-GLN-GLU-ARG-GLY-ALA-ARG-ALA-ARG-GLY-ALA-ARG-ALA-ARG-LEU-NH$_2$	Growth hormone
Growth hormone–inhibiting hormone (somatostatin)	Anterior periventricular	ALA-GLY-CYS-LYS-ASN-PHE-PHE-TRP-LYS-THR-PHE-THR-SER-CYS	Growth hormone Prolactin Thyrotropin, adrenocorticotropin Adrenocorticotropin (pathological)
Prolactin-inhibiting factor (PIF)	Arcuate	Dopamine	Prolactin, thyrotropin Growth hormone (pathological)
Prolactin-releasing factor (PRF)	Not known	Not established	Prolactin

---

Box 49-1   *Characteristics of hypothalamic releasing hormones*

1. Secretion in pulses.
2. Action on specific plasma membrane receptors.
3. Transduction of signals through calcium, membrane phospholipid products, and cyclic AMP (cAMP) as second messengers.
4. Stimulation of release of stored target anterior pituitary hormones via exocytosis.
5. Stimulation of synthesis of target anterior pituitary hormones at the transcriptional level.
6. Modification of the biological activity of target anterior pituitary hormones by post-translational effects such as glycosylation.
7. Stimulation of hyperplasia and hypertrophy of target cells.
8. Modulation of effects by up- or down-regulation of their own receptors.

---

anterior pituitary cells. The cytosolic calcium concentration, and then the cAMP concentration, increases. In addition, diacylglycerols, inositol phosphates, and arachidonic acid from membrane phospholipids help mediate the intracellular effects that follow. Specific proteins are presumably phosphorylated by activated protein kinase A or C. Granule exocytosis is rapidly stimulated with release of stored tropic hormones. In addition, tropic hormone synthesis is stimulated or inhibited by increasing or decreasing transcription of their genes. In some instances, the biological activity of the target pituitary hormones may also be increased after translation by

■ **Table 49-2** Anterior pituitary cells and hormones

Cell	Pituitary population (%)	Products/molecular weight	Targets
Corticotroph	15-20	Adrenocorticotropin (ACTH), 4500 β-Lipotropin, 11,000	Adrenal gland Adipose tissue Melanocytes
Thyrotroph	3-5	Thyrotropin (TSH), 28,000	Thyroid gland
Gonadotroph	10-15	Luteinizing hormone (LH), 28,000 Follicle-stimulating hormone (FSH), 33,000	Gonads
Somatotroph	40-50	Somatotropin, growth hormone (GH), 22,000	All tissues
Mammotroph	10-25	Prolactin, 23,000	Breasts Gonads

modifying their content of sugars or sialic acid or by phosphorylation.

The anterior pituitary contains at least five endocrine cell types (Table 49-2) that arise from a common precursor in the following order: corticotrophs, thyrotrophs, gonadotrophs, somatotrophs, and mammotrophs. A specific protein transcription factor, called **Pit-1,** is involved in specifying the differentiation and proliferation of somatotrophs, mammotrophs, and possibly thyrotrophs. The synthesis of Pit-1 in the precursor cells is induced by cAMP, the level of which is raised or lowered by the appropriate hypothalamic peptides.

A nonsense mutation in the Pit-1 gene results in **hypoplasia** of the anterior pituitary gland and deficient secretion of GH, prolactin, and thyrotropin (Table 49-2).

Anterior pituitary cells cannot be completely distinguished from each other by conventional histologic staining and are not localized to exclusive areas. However, immunohistochemical techniques that employ hormone-specific antisera have permitted each type to be specifically identified. In addition, "null cells," which contain no known hormones, are present in the anterior pituitary. The distribution of cell types within the gland is not random. Certain cell types tend to associate with each other, intertwine, or even form junctional complexes. Growth factors and even hypothalamic peptides are also localized within certain anterior pituitary cells. Thus, paracrine interactions and even autocrine effects are likely characteristics of anterior pituitary function.

Mathematical modeling of the plasma profiles of human anterior pituitary hormones suggests that tonic secretion of these hormones is negligible. Rather, secretion is episodic, prompted by pulses of hypothalamic releasing hormones. Secretion bursts probably last only a few minutes. The longer duration of the resultant plasma peaks (90 to 140 minutes) reflects the relatively slow metabolic clearance rates of the anterior pituitary hormones.

■ *Anterior Pituitary Hormones*

■ *Thyrotropic Hormone (Thyroid-Stimulating Hormone [TSH])*

TSH is a glycoprotein hormone whose function is to regulate the growth and metabolism of the thyroid gland and the secretion of its hormones, **thyroxine (T_4)** *and* **triiodothyronine (T_3).** The TSH-producing cells normally form 3% to 5% of the adult human anterior pituitary population, and they are found predominantly in the anteromedial area of the gland. These cells develop at about 13 weeks of gestation, at the same time that the fetal thyroid gland begins to secrete thyroid hormone.

TSH has a molecular weight of 28,000 and contains carbohydrate units bound covalently to the peptide chains. The hormone consists of two subunits tightly associated by noncovalent forces. The α subunit consists of 96 amino acids. This subunit is nonspecific, as it is also a component of two other anterior pituitary hormones (FSH and LH), as well as of a placental hormone (human chorionic gonadotropin [HCG]). The β subunit of 110 amino acids confers the specific biological activity on the TSH molecule. Nevertheless, both α and β subunits are required for receptor binding and subsequent hormone action.

TSH synthesis. Separate genes, located on different chromosomes, code for the individual α and β subunits. A signal N-terminal peptide is eliminated from each primary translation product (termed a **prehormone**). Subsequently, the N-glycoside–linked sugar moieties that are rich in mannose and protect the nascent molecule from premature proteolysis are added. During transport from the rough endoplasmic reticulum and packaging in the Golgi apparatus, the carbohydrate units are further modified, sialic acid and sulfate are added, and intramolecular disulfide bonds are formed. These changes ensure the proper conformation that permits the two individual subunits to combine in the mature TSH molecule, which is stored in secretory granules. Expression of the α and β subunit genes is separately regulated, but in coordination with each other. Ordinarily, an excess of the nonspecific α subunit is produced, but selective addition of an extra O-linked oligosaccharide renders the excess α subunits incapable of combining with β subunits. Transcription of both TSH subunit genes is stimulated by the hypothalamic TRH and is suppressed by thyroid hormone. In addition, TRH and thyroid hormone modulate the glycosylation process to increase or decrease biological activity, respectively. Transcription of the α-subunit gene is also regulated by cAMP.

TSH secretion. The secretion of TSH is reciprocally regulated by two major factors. TRH increases the rate of secretion, whereas thyroid hormone decreases the rate of secretion by negative feedback (Fig. 49-6). As a result of this balance, TSH is secreted in a relatively steady, but somewhat pulsatile, fashion. This pattern is congruent with that of its target gland, whose own output is steady and whose hormones' actions slowly wax and wane.

TRH is a tripeptide, pyroglutamine-histidine-proline-amide. Its synthesis in the hypothalamus is directed by a gene that codes for a large precursor molecule that contains the small sequence of glutamine-histidine-proline-glycine. After translation, glutamine undergoes cyclization, and the terminal glycine is replaced with an amino group. TRH is stored in the median eminence and reaches its target cells via the pituitary portal vein. There, TRH interacts with specific plasma membrane receptors on thyrotroph cells. This interaction triggers an influx of calcium and increases in phosphatidylinositol products, which act as second messengers. TSH is then released by exocytosis. TRH eventually down-regulates its own receptors, and the releasing hormone loses effectiveness.

After intravenous administration of TRH, plasma TSH levels rise as much as tenfold and return toward baseline levels by 60 minutes (Fig. 49-7). With repeated TRH injections, the TSH response diminishes over time, mainly because the secondarily stimulated thyroid gland increases its output of T_4 and T_3 (Fig. 49-7). This clinical experiment demonstrates vividly the negative feedback regulation of TSH secretion depicted in Fig. 49-6. Small increases in thyroid hormone concentration suppress TSH secretion by blocking the stimulatory action of TRH; conversely, small decreases of thyroid hormone augment TSH responsivity to TRH. Significant modulation of TSH secretion is associated with variations in plasma thyroid hormone concentrations of only 10% to 30% above or below the individual's baseline level. The thyrotroph's response to continuous TRH stimulation is also limited by down-regulation of the TRH receptor.

The intracellular mediator of thyroid hormone's effect on TSH is probably T_3. Furthermore, T_3 generated within the pituitary cell from T_4 is more effective and important in this regard than is T_3 that enters from the circulation. The suppressive effect of thyroid hormone on TSH release has a half-life of days and may be mediated by the induction of a protein with TSH-suppressing properties. In addition, T_3 decreases the number of TRH receptors. A minor hypothalamic effect of T_3 also reduces the synthesis or release of TRH.

Because of negative feedback, in individuals who have thyroid diseases that result in deficiency of thyroid hormone (**hypothyroidism**), TRH actions are relatively unrestrained. As a result, these individuals have very high plasma TSH levels and hyperplasia of the thyrotrophs. Return of plasma TSH to normal is the most useful indicator that the dose of thyroid hormone replacement therapy is correct.

Physiological modulation of TSH secretion (and consequently of thyroid hormone output) occurs in at least two circumstances: fasting and exposure to cold. TSH responsiveness to TRH (and possibly TRH release itself) are diminished during fasting. This downward regulation coincides with a decrease in metabolic rate that helps the fasting individual adapt to the absence of energy intake. In animals, TSH secretion is augmented by exposure to cold, but this effect is difficult to demonstrate conclusively in adult humans. Because TSH increases thermogenesis via stimulation of the thyroid gland, this response to cold is logical.

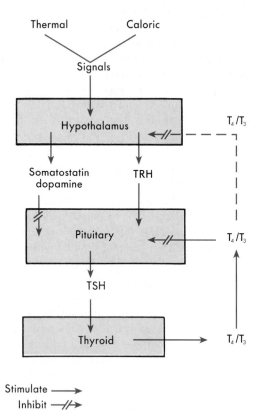

Fig. 49-6 Regulation of thyroid-stimulating hormone (TSH) secretion. Thyroxine (T_4) and triiodothyronine (T_3) from the thyroid gland exert negative feedback on the pituitary by blocking the action of thyroid-releasing hormone (TRH). Negative feedback of T_4 and T_3 at the level of the hypothalamus is less well established. Somatostatin and dopamine each inhibit TSH secretion tonically.

Other hormonal and neural influences have been noted. TSH secretion exhibits a slight diurnal variation, with the highest levels occurring at night. A tonic inhibitory effect on TSH secretion is exerted by the hypothalamic peptide somatostatin and the neurotransmitter dopamine. **Cortisol** (a hormone from the adrenal cortex) decreases both TRH and TSH secretion; GH also reduces TSH secretion.

TSH normally circulates in plasma at a concentration of 0.3 to 5 μU/ml, which approximates a concentration of 10^{-11} M. Daily TSH production (about 165,000 μU) is approximately equivalent to the entire content of one normal pituitary gland. The metabolic clearance rate of TSH is 50 L/day and is inversely related to the degree of glycosylation of the molecule. In normal individuals, the α subunit is also secreted and circulates at low levels.

When TSH secretion is chronically hyperstimulated in response to deficient function of the thyroid gland, both β and α subunits circulate in elevated amounts. Plasma levels of α units are also elevated in patients who appear to have nonfunctioning pituitary tumors. These tumors probably arise from less differentiated precursor cells or from dedifferentiated cells in the thyrotroph or gonadotroph lines.

TSH actions. TSH binds to a plasma membrane receptor, and cAMP is the second messenger for many of the hormone's effects. The only important TSH actions are those exerted on the thyroid gland, where it promotes growth and differentiation of the gland and stimulates all steps in thyroid hormone secretion. These steps include glandular uptake of iodide, its organification, the completion of thyroid hormone synthesis, and the subsequent release of thyroid gland products (Fig. 49-5). These effects are described in detail in Chapter 50.

■ *Adrenocorticotropic Hormone (ACTH)*

ACTH is an anterior pituitary polypeptide hormone whose function is to regulate the growth and secretion of the adrenal cortex. Its most important target gland hormone is cortisol. The corticotrophs form 20% of the anterior pituitary population. Although these cells are primarily found in the pars distalis of the anterior lobe (Fig. 49-1, *B*), ACTH-producing cells may also exist in a vestigial human intermediate lobe in pathological situations. In the human fetus, ACTH synthesis and secretion begin at 10 to 12 weeks of gestation, just before the development of the adrenal cortex.

ACTH is a straight-chain peptide with 39 amino acids and a molecular weight of 4500. The N-terminal 1 to 24 sequence contains full biological activity, and sequence 5 to 10 is critical for stimulating the adrenal cortex. The remaining C-terminal portion probably only prolongs the hormone's action by protecting it from enzymatic degradation.

Synthesis of ACTH. The synthesis of ACTH illustrates the principle that the primary gene product in peptide hormone synthesis may yield several biologically active molecules. As shown in Fig. 49-8, the mature messenger RNA

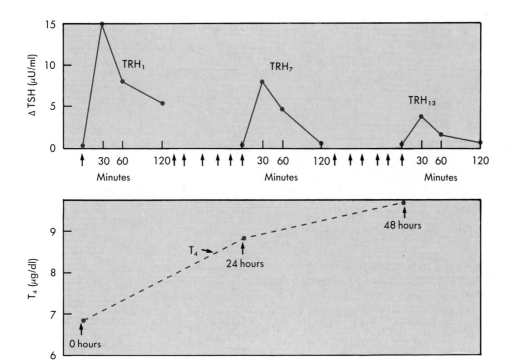

■ **Fig. 49-7** Pituitary and thyroid gland responses to repetitive injections of TRH every 4 hours for 48 hours in humans. Note that as plasma thyroxine (T$_4$) increases as a result of stimulation of the thyroid gland by TSH, the pituitary TSH responses to TRH are progressively blunted. *TRH$_1$*, First injection; *TRH$_7$*, seventh injection; *TRH$_{13}$*, thirteenth injection. (Redrawn from Snyder PJ: *J Clin Invest* 52:2305, 1973. From The American Society for Clinical Investigation.)

transcript of the gene directs the synthesis of a 31,000-molecular-weight protein known as **preproopiomelanocortin.** Sequential processing of this primary gene product in humans gives rise to ACTH, along with several other products that are cosecreted into the plasma. These include β-lipotropin, γ-lipotropin, β-endorphin, and the N-terminal peptide. Some ACTH molecules may undergo post-translational phosphorylation or glycosylation.

Melanocyte-stimulating hormone (MSH) activity resides within several of these peptides: α-MSH within ACTH; β-MSH within γ-lipoprotein; and γ-MSH within the N-terminal peptide. In extrapituitary sites (brain, hypothalamus, gastrointestinal tract, pancreatic islets, and adrenal medulla), the various MSH molecules, their parent molecules, and ACTH are also produced from proopiomelanocortin and may subserve different signaling functions.

Finally, the N-terminal pentapeptide of β-endorphin is identical to metenkephalin, with which it shares analgesic and mood-modifying effects of opioids. The brain enkephalins, however, do not arise by cleavage of β-endorphin but are synthesized from an entirely different precursor directed by a separate gene.

Secretion of ACTH. *The regulation of ACTH secretion is among the most complex of all the pituitary hormone regulatory patterns* (Fig. 49-9). *ACTH exhibits circadian rhythms, cyclic bursts, and feedback control and it responds to a wide variety of stimuli* (Table 49-3). Hypothalamic CRH is the important final mediator of the regulatory inputs. CRH is a peptide with 41 amino acids that originates in small cells of the paraventricular nucleus (Table 49-1). It stimulates the synthesis and release by exocytosis of ACTH and its proopiomelanocortin coproducts via calcium and cAMP as second messengers. ADH also exhibits corticotropin-releasing activity, and under particular physiological circumstances, such as stress, it augments the effect of CRH. The gene that directs the synthesis of prepro-CRH has considerable homology with the genes for prepro-ADH; this homology suggests a common evolutionary starting point for these molecules.

CRH receptors are also found throughout the brain and spinal cord, and the peptide is synthesized in many peripheral cells, including immune cells. The widespread distribution of CRH receptors indicates that CRH has other important central nervous system functions related to or independent of stimulating ACTH release. CRH causes central arousal, increased sympathetic nervous system activity, and increased blood pressure. In contrast, CRH decreases reproductive function by decreasing the synthesis of gonadotropin-releasing hormone (GnRH) and gonadotropins and by inhibiting sexual behavior. CRH also decreases feeding activity and growth. CRH may also regulate β-endorphin and its analgesic action. Finally, in immune cells, CRH stimulates release of cytokines and also augments their activity on target cells. CRH circulates at very low plasma levels bound to a specific protein.

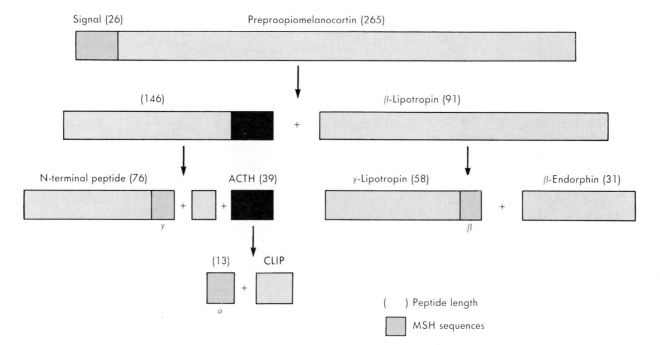

■ **Fig. 49-8**   The processing of preproopiomelanocortin. In the anterior lobe of the human pituitary, adrenocorticotropic hormone (ACTH), β-lipotropin, γ-lipotropin, β-endorphin, and a 76-amino acid N-terminal fragment are end products that are released. In other species, ACTH is further cleaved to α-melanocyte-stimulating hormone (α-MSH) and corticotropin-like intermediate peptide *(CLIP)* in the neural intermediate lobe. In humans, MSH activity is provided by MSH sequences within larger molecules such as ACTH.

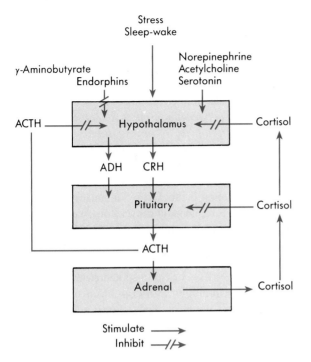

■ Fig. 49-9 Regulation of ACTH secretion. Corticotropin-releasing hormone (CRH) and antidiuretic hormone (ADH) stimulate ACTH secretion. Cortisol from the adrenal glands exerts negative feedback (1) at the pituitary level by blocking CRH action and (2) at the hypothalamus level by inhibiting CRH release. Norepinephrine, acetylcholine, and serotonin are positive modulators, whereas endorphins, ACTH itself, and γ-aminobutyric acid are negative modulators of CRH release.

ACTH secretion has a markedly diurnal pattern. As shown in Fig. 49-10, a large peak occurs 2 to 4 hours before awakening. Thereafter, the average level decreases to virtually zero, just before or after the subject falls asleep. A rise and fall in the major adrenocortical hor-

■ Table 49-3 Regulation of ACTH secretion

Stimulation	Inhibition
Corticotropin-releasing hormone	Cortisol increase
Cortisol decrease	Enkephalins
Adrenalectomy	Opioids
Metyrapone	ACTH
Sleep-wake transition	Somatostatin
Stress	γ-Aminobutyric acid (GABA)
Hypoglycemia	
Anesthesia	
Surgery	
Trauma	
Infection	
Pyrogens	
Psychiatric disturbance	
Anxiety	
Depression	
Antidiuretic hormone	
α-Adrenergic agonists	
β-Adrenergic antagonists	
Serotonin	
Acetylcholine	
Interleukins	
Gastrointestinal peptides	

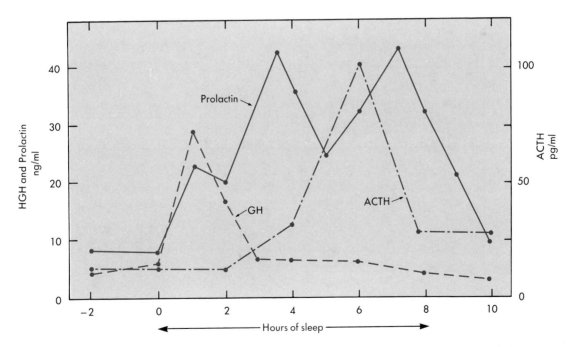

■ Fig. 49-10 Nocturnal release of ACTH, growth hormone (GH), and prolactin. Note the distinctive pattern for each hormone. (Redrawn from Takahashi Y et al: *J Clin Invest* 47:2079, 1968; Berson SA et al: *J Clin Invest* 47:2725, 1968, from The American Society for Clinical Investigation; and Sassin JF et al: *Science* 177:1205, 1972, from The American Association for the Advancement of Science.)

mone, cortisol, is entrained in this ACTH pattern. The timing of the diurnal pattern can be shifted by systematically altering the sleep-wake cycle for a number of days; however, the ACTH peak is not entrained with a specific stage of sleep. Quite the opposite, in fact, is true: slow-wave sleep decreases the ACTH and cortisol response to CRH irrespective of the time of day. The circadian rhythm is diminished or abolished by loss of consciousness, blindness, or constant exposure to either dark or light.

The nocturnal ACTH surge is primarily generated in the suprachiasmatic nucleus of the hypothalamus by CRH release. Although this peak is not directly caused by negative feedback from its target adrenal gland hormone, cortisol, the nocturnal peak is augmented by previous cortisol deficiency. Conversely, this peak can be completely suppressed by excess cortisol, which decreases expression of the CRH gene. The diurnal pattern is composed of pulses of ACTH release with little or no tonic or constitutive secretion. Up to three pulses occur per hour, with each pulse lasting about 20 minutes. Major ACTH peaks appear to be caused by increased amplitude rather than increased frequency of secretory bursts. As would be expected, pulses of cosecreted β-endorphin occur simultaneously with those of ACTH, whereas cortisol pulses follow 10 minutes later. Men exhibit both a greater frequency and a greater amplitude of ACTH pulses than do women. Age has little effect on ACTH secretion.

Negative feedback inhibition of ACTH secretion is produced by cortisol, or by any synthetic analog with a potency proportional to its other cortisol-like activity (Fig. 49-9). The suppressive action of cortisol may outlive the duration of cortisol exposure. Conversely, when (1) cortisol action is blocked by an antagonist, (2) cortisol secretion is reduced by disease, or (3) cortisol release is pharmacologically inhibited (Fig. 49-11), ACTH secretion is stimulated. Cortisol suppresses ACTH secretion at the pituitary level by blocking the stimulatory action of CRH (Fig. 49-12). Cortisol also decreases the synthesis of ACTH by inhibiting transcription of preproopiomelanocortin and blocking hypothalamic release of CRH. The negative feedback effects of cortisol on diurnal and stress-induced ACTH release are also indirectly mediated

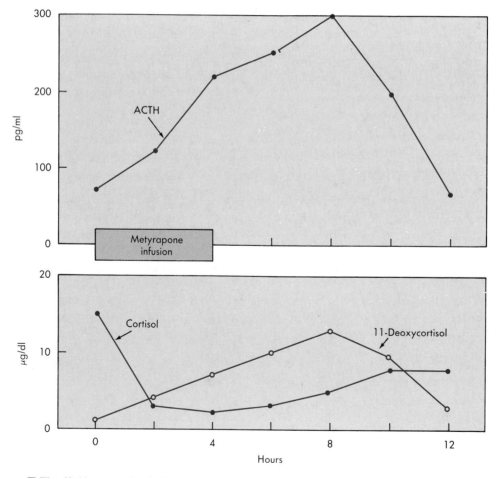

■ **Fig. 49-11** Negative feedback stimulation of ACTH release by metyrapone, a drug that blocks the conversion of 11-deoxycortisol to cortisol in the adrenal gland. Note that plasma ACTH increases as plasma cortisol decreases. The biologically inactive precursor-11-deoxycortisol increases as a result of ACTH action on the adrenal gland. (Redrawn from Jubiz W et al: *Arch Intern Med* 125:468, 1970. From The American Medical Association.)

by neural input from the hippocampus to the CRH neurons of the hypothalamus. Two distinct cortisol receptors in the hippocampus provide a range of affinities to accommodate the usual range of plasma cortisol levels.

> Overactivity of the hypothalamic-pituitary-adrenal axis is characteristic of some types of depressive illness. The pituitary corticotrophs are superresponsive to stimulation by CRH and underresponsive to suppression by cortisol. Hence, cortisol is secreted in mild excess. These features suggest a primary overdrive of the system by CRH neurons in the hypothalamus.

ACTH may also inhibit its own secretion by decreasing CRH release, an example of short-loop feedback. Chronic deficiency of cortisol leads to persistent elevation of the plasma ACTH concentration, but the diurnal and pulsatile patterns are preserved, indicating their basic nonfeedback origin.

> Chronic autonomous hypersecretion of cortisol or long-term therapeutic administration of cortisol analogs for various diseases leads to functional atrophy of the CRH-ACTH-adrenal axis. Complete recovery of this axis after the suppressive influence has been removed may take up to 1 year. During that time, the individual often requires exogenous cortisol if a stressful medical or surgical situation arises, because a normal adrenal gland response to the stress cannot be assured.

ACTH secretion responds most strikingly to stressful stimuli, a response that is critical to survival. Numerous factors that elicit the stress reaction in humans are noted in Table 49-3. The response to insulin-induced hypoglycemia is illustrated in Fig. 49-13. In some circumstances, such as major abdominal surgery or severe psychiatric disturbance, the stress-induced hypersecretion of ACTH completely overrides negative feedback. The hypersecretion cannot be suppressed even if the adrenal cortex secretes cortisol at its maximal level. Stress also often obliterates the diurnal variation of ACTH levels, although pulsatility persists. The pathways vary by which each particular stress signals, senses, and then stimulates CRH (and ADH) secretion. For example, hypothalamic sensitivity to glucose levels per se, which is augmented by both norepinephrine (via α-adrenergic receptors) and serotonin input, induces the ACTH response to hypoglycemia.

However, in its most general sense, stress is a life-threatening situation that usually evokes both CRH secretion and activation of the sympathetic nervous system (see Fig. 51-27). As detailed in Chapter 51, CRH secretion and sympathetic nerve activation have mutually reinforcing actions.

ACTH circulates unbound in plasma with a half-life of 15 minutes. Basal concentrations at 6 AM range from 20 to 100 pg/ml (average 50 pg/ml or 10^{-11} M). Daily production is less than one third of average adult human pituitary content. Because the bulk of the ACTH is

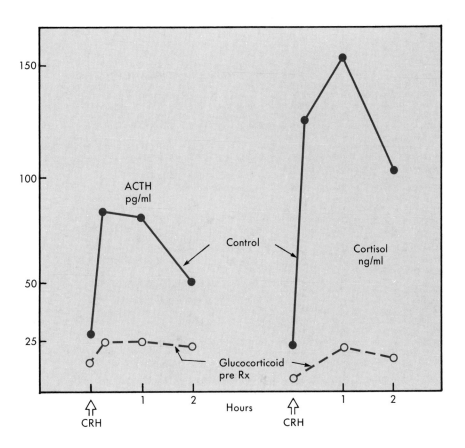

■ **Fig. 49-12** Plasma ACTH and cortisol responses to administration of CRH. Pretreatment with a synthetic glucocorticoid (an analog of cortisol) suppresses the action of CRH on the pituitary. The diminished ACTH response leads secondarily to a diminished secretion of cortisol by the adrenal glands. (Redrawn from Copinschi G et al: *J Clin Endocrinol Metab* 57:1287, 1983.)

secreted during a limited period in each day, there is sufficient time for ACTH stores to be replenished.

Action of ACTH. ACTH combines with its adrenal cell plasma membrane receptor to evoke an increase in cAMP as its principal second messenger (see Fig. 51-7). *ACTH stimulates the growth of specific zones of the adrenal cortex, and the synthesis and secretion of cortisol and other steroid hormones.* ACTH increases the size rather than the number of adrenal cells; in the absence of ACTH, profound atrophy of the relevant adrenal zones occurs. All steps in the synthesis of adrenal steroids are stimulated by ACTH, which are detailed in Chapter 51. Adrenal responsiveness to ACTH is attenuated and delayed by previous chronic underexposure to the tropic hormone; conversely, responsiveness is accentuated by previous chronic overexposure.

ACTH synthesis and receptors for ACTH are located in the brain and gastrointestinal tract, where the peptide may have neuromodulatory or paracrine functions. A relationship also exists between ACTH and the immune system. ACTH receptors and ACTH secretion occur in lymphocytes, and cytokines released by lymphocytes stimulate ACTH release by corticotrophs.

Because of its MSH sequences, ACTH increases skin pigmentation. MSH acts on melanocytes and causes the dispersal of melanin pigment granules within these cells and their dendrites. MSH also stimulates the key enzyme in melanin synthesis (tyrosinase) and the transfer of melanin from the melanocytes to epidermal cells (keratinocytes). These actions, which are mediated by specific plasma membrane MSH receptors and cAMP, cause the skin to darken. Skin keratinocytes express the proopiomelanocortin gene and its various translation products (see above). Therefore, these MSH actions may occur in paracrine rather than endocrine fashion under normal circumstances.

Hyperpigmentation of the skin characterizes diseases in which very large increases in ACTH secretion chronically occur. ACTH excess and MSH effects result from negative feedback when the adrenal cortex is destroyed (**Addison's disease,** or primary adrenocortical insufficiency) or from ectopic production of ACTH by malignant neural crest cells.

Secretion and actions of other proopiomelanocortin peptides. The remaining peptides in proopiomelanocortin are under the same transcriptional and translational control as ACTH. The functional significance of this fact is still not well understood, although it

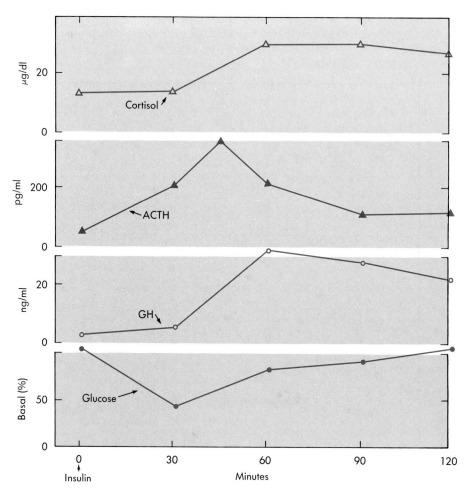

■ **Fig. 49-13** Stimulation of ACTH, cortisol, and GH secretion by insulin-induced hypoglycemia in humans. (Redrawn from Ichikawa Y et al: *J Clin Endocrinol Metab* 34:895, 1972.)

could reflect a coordinated physiological response. The plasma level of each peptide rises and falls in parallel with the ACTH level in feedback and stress situations. The molar ratios of these levels differ from 1.0 because of differences in metabolic clearance rates.

The proopiomelanocortin products were named **lipotropins** because of their lipolytic activity, but their role in mobilizing fatty acids from human adipose tissue is unknown. Similarly, the low plasma levels—or even all of the sources—of circulating β-endorphin are of uncertain endocrine significance. When administered to humans, β-endorphins (like opioids) inhibit ACTH secretion, as well as gonadotropin secretion. These observations point to neurocrine actions of β-endorphin generated in the hypothalamus.

■ Gonadotropic Hormones (Luteinizing Hormone [LH] and Follicle-Stimulating Hormone [FSH])

LH and FSH are glycoproteins whose function is to regulate the development, growth, pubertal maturation, reproductive processes, and sex steroid hormone secretion of the gonads of either sex. Both hormones are usually secreted by a single cell type, the gonadotroph. Gonadotrophs make up about 10% to 15% of the anterior pituitary cell population and are scattered throughout the gland. Small subclasses of gonadotrophs secrete only LH or only FSH. Gonadotrophs also appear to go through cycles in which differential expression of the two gonadotropins occurs at different times. Both hormones are present by 10 to 12 weeks of fetal life; however, neither is absolutely required for initial intrauterine development of the gonads or for the initial steps in sexual differentiation.

LH, with a molecular weight of 28,000, and FSH, with a molecular weight of 33,000, have similar structures. Each is composed of the common pituitary hormone α subunit (molecular weight, 14,000; 92 amino acids) and a unique β subunit. The unique β subunit differentiates the two hormones from each other, as well as from TSH and HCG (Fig. 49-14). The α and β subunits are held together by noncovalent forces, and disulfide bridges create tertiary structures. The carbohydrate moieties (15% to 25% by weight) contain oligosaccharides composed of mannose, galactose, fucose, galactosamine, acetylglucosamine, and sialic acid. The carbohydrate groups function in receptor binding and responses, whereas the sialic acid residues decrease the rate of hormone degradation. The α subunit is required for binding of gonadotropins to their receptors; neither the β subunit of LH nor that of FSH is biologically active by itself.

The details of LH and FSH biosynthesis are similar to those already described for TSH. Individual genes code for the α and two β subunits; transcription of the β-subunit genes is rate limiting for gonadotropin synthesis. The addition and later modification of the carbohydrate moieties allows considerable variation of the bioactivity of secreted LH and FSH molecules in different physiological circumstances, such as throughout the menstrual cycle. In women, the pituitary stores of both LH and FSH also fluctuate, and are highest just before ovulation. The patterns of release also suggest more than one intracellular pool of LH.

Secretion of LH and FSH. *The regulation of LH and FSH secretion is even more complex than that of ACTH. Regulation embodies pulsatile, periodic, diurnal, cyclic, and stage-of-life elements.* Regulation is also different in women and men. The main factors that control secretion of the gonadotropins are discussed in this chapter; their reproductive function is reviewed and discussed in detail in Chapter 52. Both the secretion of LH and that of FSH are stimulated mainly by a single hypothalamic hormone, known either as **gonadotropin-releasing hormone (GnRH)** or **luteinizing hormone–releasing hormone (LHRH).** As the latter alternate name implies, this hormone causes a much greater increase in LH than in FSH secretion. Whether a separate hypothalamic releasing hormone exists with a greater specificity for FSH remains uncertain. GnRH is a decapeptide (Table 49-1) that is synthesized from a large prohormone that also gives rise to other products. The cells of origin of GnRH are predominantly in the arcuate nucleus and the preoptic area of the hypothalamus. After transport to the median eminence, GnRH is stored in small granules.

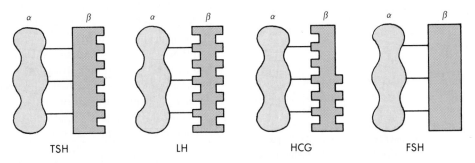

■ **Fig. 49-14** Structural similarities among TSH, luteinizing hormone (LH), human chorionic gonadotropin (HCG), and follicle-stimulating hormone (FSH) are depicted schematically. Note that all share the same α subunit.

A variety of influences regulate the release of GnRH. GnRH neurons are under dopaminergic, serotonergic, noradrenergic, and endorphinergic influence (Fig. 49-15). In particular, GnRH neurons are closely associated with dopamine neurons within the arcuate nucleus of the hypothalamus. Dopamine inhibits LH secretion by decreasing GnRH release and also by acting directly on the gonadotrophs. Endorphins also inhibit GnRH release and LH secretion. Neural input from the retina to the hypothalamus accounts for the influence of light-dark cycles on GnRH release. In some species, **melatonin** from the pineal gland mediates the seasonal variations in gonadotropin secretion and reproductive activity that are related to daylight length. The production of melatonin, which inhibits gonadotropin release, is itself suppressed by light and stimulated by darkness. Although melatonin levels and gonadotropin secretion are inversely related in humans, the role of melatonin in the *regulation* of human reproduction has not yet been conclusively established. Stress is also a well-noted influence on reproductive functions. Menstrual function in women and sperm production in men are commonly lost during prolonged physical or psychic stress. These effects may be mediated by CRH, which inhibits GnRH release.

Another influence of interest are **pheromones,** which are airborne or waterborne chemical exciters or inhibitors. After perception of these chemical signals by the sense of smell, connections from the olfactory bulb to the hypothalamus probably transfer reproductive signals from the environment and from other individuals.

GnRH-triggered release of LH and FSH begins with the binding of GnRH to a gonadotroph 7 span plasma membrane receptor. After this binding, calcium-calmodulin and phosphatidylinositol products are generated as principal second messengers. The exocytosis of gonadotropin secretory granules is rapidly stimulated. Intracellular signaling molecules are generated by protein kinase C activation, and they feed back on GnRH signal transduction to regulate the length and amplitude of the response. GnRH both down-regulates and up-regulates its receptor. GnRH stimulates transcription of the LH and FSH β-subunit genes. The bioactivity of LH and FSH is also increased by modification of their carbohydrate composition.

Intravenous infusion of GnRH causes a biphasic response in plasma LH. An initial peak of LH is reached at 30 minutes, followed by a secondary rise that begins at 90 minutes and continues for hours thereafter (Fig. 49-16). In contrast, GnRH causes only a uniphasic progressive rise in FSH (Fig. 49-16). In women, LH is secreted in pulses characterized by a 15-minute upsurge and a downslope with a half-life of 60 minutes. These peaks of plasma LH have a periodicity varying from 1 to 7 hours, depending on the phase of the menstrual cycle. The amplitude of the pulses can be equivalent to 100% changes in the plasma LH level, except at the time of ovulation, when it is much greater. Men also exhibit eight to ten secretory bursts of LH per day (Fig. 49-17).

Pulsatile secretion of LH, which is due mainly to pulsatile secretion of GnRH (Fig. 49-18), does not depend on the presence of sex steroid hormones from target glands; agonadal individuals and postmenopausal women exhibit even sharper spikes of the plasma LH level. Pulsatile secretion of LH is dampened in young children, but the pulse amplitude increases sharply as puberty approaches. At first, these higher amplitude pulses increase only at night, coincident with a modest reduction in melatonin levels from childhood to puberty. Thus, during the initial stages of puberty, LH peaks sharply at night. Although this diurnal pattern lasts only 1 or 2 years and disappears as puberty is completed, the heightened amplitude of LH pulses becomes fixed. The most striking feature of LH secretion in women, as opposed to men, is its monthly cyclicity. The menstrual cycle results from a complex interaction between the GnRH neuron-gonadotroph unit and sequential changes in ovarian steroid secretion, which is detailed in Chapter 52.

Some women are infertile because disordered hypothalamic regulation fails to produce proper pituitary gonadotroph function and ovulation. Normal men-

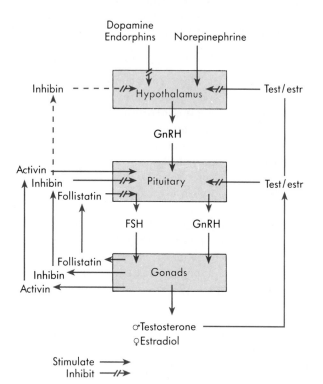

■ **Fig. 49-15** Regulation of gonadotropin secretion. Gonadotropin-releasing hormone (GnRH) stimulates LH and FSH release. The gonadal steroids, estradiol in women and testosterone in men, exert negative feedback (1) at the pituitary level by blocking GnRH action and (2) at the hypothalamic level by inhibiting GnRH release. Negative modulation by endorphins and dopamine may mediate some of the steroid hormone feedback. Separate gonadal protein products selectively suppress (inhibin and follistatin) or stimulate (activin) FSH release.

strual cycles and ovulation can be restored only if exogenous GnRH is administered to these women in pulses that mimic the timing, amplitude, and frequency of the normal hypothalamic generator. The same is true for spermatogenesis in infertile men. In contrast, continuous administration of GnRH to either gender down-regulates the GnRH receptor and produces gonadotropin deficiency, with consequent loss of gonadal function. This technique is employed therapeutically to suppress painful menses in women with endometriosis or to inhibit growth of prostate cancer in men.

FSH secretion also exhibits a pulsatile pattern that is usually synchronized with the pattern of LH secretion, but is of lesser magnitude (Fig. 49-17). Because the ratio of FSH to LH levels in plasma can fluctuate considerably, it has been suggested that a separate hypothalamic releasing hormone exists for FSH. However, the frequency of GnRH pulses may be a factor in these fluctuations,

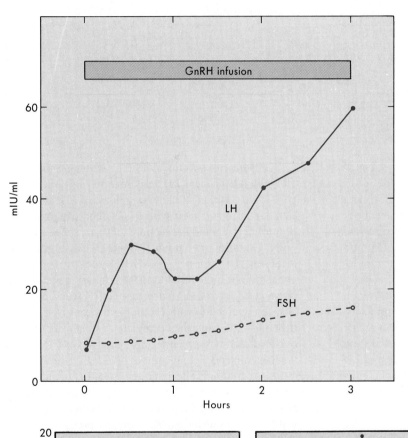

■ **Fig. 49-16** Stimulation of gonadotropin release by GnRH. Note the biphasic response of LH and uniphasic response of FSH. The initial LH response represents immediate release from a subset of secretory granules. The later response is from other secretory granules and augmented synthesis of LH. *LHRH,* Luteinizing hormone–releasing hormone. (Redrawn from Wang CF et al: *J Clin Endocrinol Metab* 42:718, 1976.)

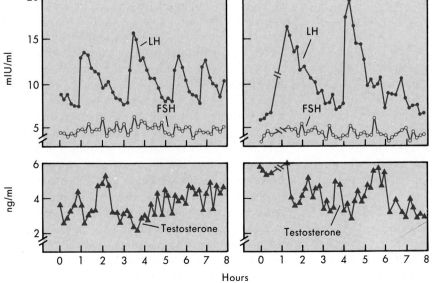

■ **Fig. 49-17** Pulsatile fluctuations in plasma LH levels are reflected in pulsatile fluctuations in its target hormone, testosterone, in men. (Redrawn from Naftolin F et al: *J Clin Endocrinol Metab* 36:285, 1973.)

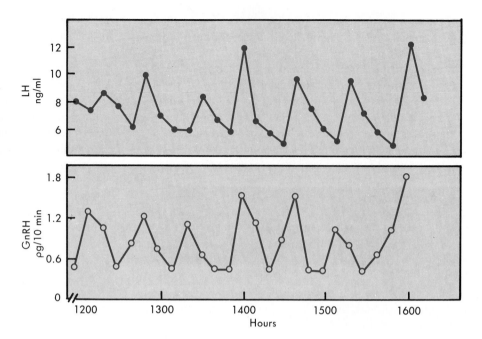

because a decreased LH pulse frequency is associated with an increased FSH:LH ratio. In addition, the sensitivity of the individual FSH- and LH-secreting gonadotrophs may be differentially affected by feedback from gonadal sex steroid and protein hormones. Furthermore, fluctuations in the plasma FSH to LH ratio could also result from differential changes in the metabolic clearance rates of the two hormones.

Feedback regulation of gonadotropins. The secretion of both LH and FSH is regulated by gonadal products. However, the patterns and mechanisms are more complex than those that have been described thus far for TSH and ACTH. In general, the basic regulatory mechanism of LH and FSH secretion is classic negative feedback. Thus when the gonads are functionally inactive or surgically removed, the plasma levels of FSH and LH become elevated. FSH, however, usually increases proportionally more than does LH. A number of gonadal products from at least two gonadal cell types normally act to restrain the secretion of each gonadotropin by negative feedback. The basic schema is depicted in Fig. 49-15.

The gonadal steroid hormones, **testosterone** in men and **estradiol** in women, are the most important of these negative feedback signals. The major androgen, testosterone, from the Leydig cells of the testis and the interstitial cells of the ovary, inhibits the release of LH. The major estrogen, estradiol, which arises from the granulosa cells of the ovary and the Leydig and Sertoli cells of the testis (as well as by conversion from testosterone in peripheral tissues and in the hypothalamus), also inhibits the release of LH. Both the amplitude and the frequency of the LH pulses are affected; such changes indicate pituitary and hypothalamic sites of feedback.

Both estradiol and testosterone administration blunt the response of the gonadotroph to a single pulse of GnRH.

Conversely, in estradiol-deficient women and testosterone-deficient men, LH responses to GnRH are exaggerated. In addition to inhibiting release of LH (and FSH), estradiol decreases their synthesis by repressing transcription of their common α subunit and their specific β subunits. Estradiol may produce some of these effects by altering the number of GnRH receptors on the gonadotroph. In addition to these pituitary effects, estradiol and testosterone also decrease GnRH secretion, probably via interaction with endorphin neurons in the hypothalamus. The latter then complete this pathway of negative feedback by suppressing discharge of GnRH from the median eminence into the portal blood (Fig. 49-2).

FSH secretion is also inhibited by estradiol and testosterone, which block the pituitary response to GnRH. However, feedback inhibition of FSH secretion is specifically carried out by another gonadal product, a glycoprotein called **inhibin** (Chapter 52). Secreted by ovarian granulosa cells and testicular Sertoli cells, inhibin suppresses FSH β-subunit synthesis, GnRH-stimulated FSH release, and possibly GnRH secretion. In contrast to its effects on FSH secretion, inhibin has much less effect on LH secretion.

In addition to exerting negative feedback on LH and FSH secretion, estradiol also exerts positive feedback effects. Regulation of LH and FSH secretion is complex. When estradiol is administered to women in an appropriate dose range and for a sufficient number of days, LH response to GnRH is *augmented* rather than reduced. Furthermore, if GnRH is administered repetitively to properly estradiol-primed women, the cumulative increments in plasma LH are amplified. This response signifies that both the sensitivity of the gonadotroph (perhaps by an increase in the number of its GnRH receptors) and its LH stores have been enhanced by estradiol treatment.

Moreover in women so treated, a rapid further increase in estradiol itself causes a significant rise in plasma levels of LH.

Some aspects of this positive and negative feedback can be observed simultaneously. For example, when estradiol-deficient, agonadal women are given initial estradiol replacement therapy, the originally elevated basal levels of LH (and FSH) decline (negative feedback) after 7 days of treatment. However, the capacity to respond to subsequent repetitive doses of GnRH actually increases (positive feedback).

Progesterone, another major steroid product of the ovary, also modulates LH release. Administered acutely, progesterone can increase plasma LH levels 24 to 48 hours later. Progesterone can also either enhance or blunt the positive feedback effects of estradiol on GnRH responsiveness. The effect on feedback depends on the timing of administration of the two hormones. However, continuous administration of progesterone (or analogs) inhibits gonadotropin secretion.

Oral contraceptives utilize the negative feedback effects of estradiol (or its analogs) plus progesterone (or its analogs) to interfere with the normal timing and quantities of LH and FSH secretion. As a result, the delicately balanced stimulation of the ovaries by the two gonadotropins is lost, and ovulation is prevented.

Other protein products of the gonads influence FSH secretion. **Activin,** related structurally to inhibin, stimulates FSH synthesis and release. Activin is also synthesized within pituitary cells and may have autocrine and paracrine actions as well. **Follistatin** inhibits FSH secretion, probably by binding activin. **Prolactin,** a mammotropic hormone from the anterior pituitary, also inhibits GnRH release and lowers basal secretion of LH and FSH. Finally, LH can inhibit secretion of its own releasing hormone via short-loop negative feedback.

LH and FSH both circulate unbound to plasma proteins. The average concentrations of both hormones are in the range of 4 to 20 mIU/ml in men and in reproductive-age women. In the latter, the levels of both hormones are higher in the first half of the menstrual cycle than in the second half; in addition, both hormones show sharp, single-day peaks at the time of ovulation. Basal plasma concentrations of each hormone are of the order of 10^{-11} M. The metabolic clearance rates of LH and FSH, respectively, are 36 and 20 L/day, and their half-lives in plasma are approximately 1 and 3 hours. The slower rate of degradation of FSH reflects its high sialic acid content. In contrast to the trivial excretion of other peptide hormones, 10% of the daily production of LH and FSH appears in the urine. This relatively large amount permits employment of urinary gonadotropin measurements as a reflection of integrated plasma concentrations. Such measurements are particularly useful when plasma levels of the hormones are low, as in children.

Home measurements of urinary LH by women can help them anticipate ovulation and assist in conception. Measurement of HCG, the pregnancy gonadotropin, can detect early pregnancy.

The common α subunit is secreted to a small extent by normal gonadotrophs. In contrast, the individual β subunits of LH and FSH are secreted only by hyperstimulated or neoplastic gonadotrophs.

Actions of gonadotropins. LH and FSH bind to specific plasma membrane receptors; in each case, cAMP is generated as the primary second messenger. FSH stimulates ovarian granulosa cells and testicular Sertoli cells to synthesize and secrete estradiol and a variety of protein products essential to oogenesis and spermatogenesis, respectively. LH stimulates ovarian interstitial (thecal) cells and testicular Leydig cells to secrete testosterone and other products that play roles in reproduction. The actions of gonadotropins are discussed in detail in Chapter 52.

■ *Growth Hormone (Somatotropin, GH)*

GH stimulates postnatal somatic growth and development and helps to maintain normal lean body mass and bone mass in adults. In addition, it has numerous actions on protein, carbohydrate, and fat metabolism. The hormone originates in anterior pituitary somatotrophs that make up 40% to 50% of the adult gland. It is stored in large, dense granules. In humans, somatotrophs can form tumors that secrete excess GH and produce a highly distinctive disease called **acromegaly.**

GH is a single-chain polypeptide with a usual molecular weight of 22,000. It contains 191 amino acids and two disulfide bridges (Fig. 49-19). GH is a member of a large family of "helix bundle proteins." In the GH molecule, the amino acids form four helixes that are connected by thin loops. This structure is important for binding with its receptor.

Synthesis of GH. The normal pituitary GH gene is one of a five-gene cluster from a gene family that also directs the synthesis of the structurally related hormones prolactin, human placental lactogen, and a GH variant produced exclusively in the placenta. A tissue-specific constitutive protein transcription factor (Pit-1) that binds to the promotor region of the GH gene is essential to that gene's selective expression in the pituitary gland. Four additional genes capable of directing synthesis of slightly larger GH molecules are present, but these genes are not normally expressed. The GH gene transcribes a messenger RNA that directs synthesis of a prehormone. Subsequently, a signal peptide is removed and the hormone in final form is stored in granules. The synthesis of GH is increased by its specific hypothalamic **growth hormone–releasing hormone (GHRH)** and is decreased by **somatostatin,** its hypothalamic inhibitor (Table 49-1).

Thyroid hormone and cortisol synergistically induce GH synthesis by transcriptional mechanisms.

Secretion of GH. GH release is stimulated by GHRH to its plasma membrane receptor. cAMP and Ca^{++} are primary mediators of GH release, and phosphatidylinositol products are secondary mediators of GHRH action. Prostaglandins are also potent stimulators of GH release in vitro.

The hypothalamic peptide somatostatin (Table 49-1) is a powerful inhibitor of GH release. Somatostatin blocks GHRH stimulation in a noncompetitive manner. It acts through its own plasma membrane receptor, in part by decreasing intracellular cAMP and calcium levels. GH is secreted in pulses, which are caused by pulsatile release of GHRH into the portal blood. Somatostatin diminishes the degree to which the somatotroph is able to respond to the GHRH pulses and also reduces the frequency of those pulses.

As seen in Table 49-4, GH secretion is under many different influences. An acute fall in plasma levels of either of the major energy-yielding substrates, glucose or free fatty acids (FFAs), produces an increase in GH. For example, when insulin is administered intravenously, the plasma level of GH increases up to tenfold 30 to 60 minutes after the plasma glucose level has fallen to below 50 mg/dl (Fig. 49-13). Conversely, a carbohydrate-rich meal or a pure glucose load causes a prompt decrease in the plasma GH level of at least 50%. Responses to similar alterations in FFA levels are slower and smaller. Both glucose and FFAs mainly suppress GH release by increasing somatostatin.

A high-protein meal or the infusion of a mixture of amino acids raises the plasma GH level; arginine is the most consistent amino acid stimulator. However, prolonged protein calorie deprivation or total fasting also stimulates GH secretion, by decreasing negative feedback from a peripheral product of GH action. Exercise and various stresses, including blood drawing, anesthesia, fever, trauma, and major surgery, are rapid stimulators of GH secretion. In addition to GH spikes produced by these factors, GH is secreted episodically at 2-hour intervals. A regular nocturnal GH peak occurs 1 hour after the onset of deep stage 3 or 4 sleep (Fig. 49-10). Although this GH peak is preceded by a nocturnal plasma GHRH peak, somatotroph responsiveness to GHRH is also increased by sleep.

The neurotransmitters dopamine, norepinephrine, acetylcholine, and serotonin all increase GH secretion by stimulating release of GHRH. The GH responses to

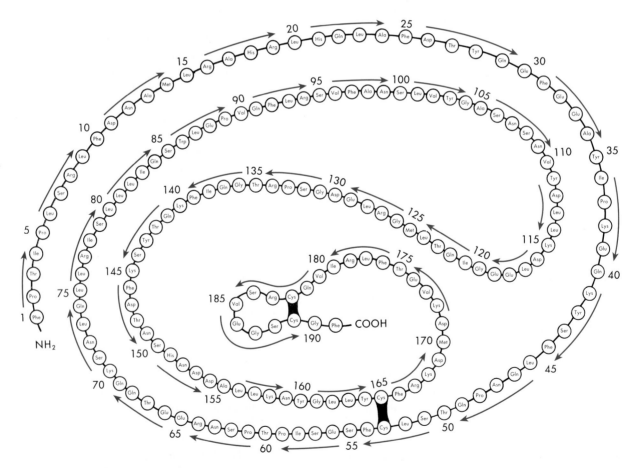

■ **Fig. 49-19**   Structure of HGH. Although consisting of nearly 200 amino acids and containing two disulfide bridges, growth hormone (GH) is a single polypeptide chain. It does form a helical tertiary structure. (From Li C et al: *Proc Natl Acad Sci* 74:1016, 1977.)

exercise, stress, hypoglycemia, and arginine administration are augmented by α-adrenergic stimulation and are reduced by β-adrenergic stimulation of receptors in GHRH and somatostatin releasing neurons. The sleep-induced rise in GH and the response to hypoglycemia are enhanced by serotonergic pathways from the brainstem. Cholinergic pathways augment GH response to GHRH and to all other stimuli by inhibiting somatostatin release.

GH secretion is greater in women than in men and is greatest just before ovulation. The gender difference is explained by the stimulating effect of estradiol on GH secretion. However, testosterone also increases GH secretion. Daily GH production is slightly increased in children, rises further during the period of puberty, and then declines to adult levels (Fig. 49-20) after puberty is completed. A further late reduction in GH secretion in response to GHRH and other stimuli occurs with aging. This decline is GH secretion may be partly responsible for the decline in lean body mass, protein synthesis, and

metabolic rate, as well as the increase in adipose mass that characterizes elderly humans.

During puberty, the increase in GH pulses and daily secretion correlates with the rate of increase in height. Furthermore, especially tall adults demonstrate greater responses to GHRH than do adults of average height. Thus, the final height of humans may be partly determined by their inherent GH secretory capacity. In some otherwise normal children of short stature, a subtle deficiency in integrated 24-hour GH secretion has been observed. It is not known whether treatment with exogenous GH increases the final achieved height or only accelerates the growth process.

Like the regulation of other anterior pituitary hormones, feedback regulation of GH is also complex (Fig. 49-21). For example, GH inhibits its own secretion. Administration of exogenous GH dampens subsequent endogenous GH responsiveness to a number of stimuli, including hypoglycemia and stage four sleep. The mechanisms for this self-regulation may involve short-loop feedback, because GH stimulates the synthesis and release of its inhibitor, somatostatin (Fig. 49-21). However, somatostatin synthesis and release are also increased by **somatomedins,** which are circulating **insulin-like-growth factor** peptides (IGF-1 and IGF-2) that are generated outside the pituitary and mediate many actions of GH. Somatomedins also act at the pituitary level to decrease responsiveness to GHRH (Fig. 49-21). Finally, GHRH itself, in doses too small to stimulate the somatotrophs but administered in a manner that allows access to the hypothalamus, may decrease rather than increase GH secretion. This ultra-short-loop paradoxical effect probably results from a stimulation of somatostatin release and may reflect the existence of axonal connections between GHRH neurons and somatostatin neurons.

Other negative regulatory influences have also been noted. Although basal cortisol levels stimulate GH gene expression, an excess of this steroid decreases GH

■ **Table 49-4**   Regulation of growth hormone secretion

Stimulation	*Inhibition*
Growth hormone–releasing hormone	Somatostatin
Glucose decrease	Glucose increase
Free fatty acid decrease	Free fatty acid
Amino acid increase (arginine)	increase
Fasting	Somatomedins
Prolonged caloric deprivation	Growth hormone
Stage IV sleep	β-Adrenergic
Exercise	agonists
Stress (Table 49-3)	Cortisol
Puberty	Senescence
Estrogens	Obesity
Androgens	Pregnancy
Dopamine	
Acetylcholine	
Serotonin	
α-Adrenergic agonists	
γ-Aminobutyric acid	
Enkephalins	

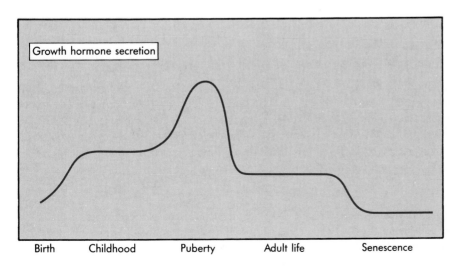

Growth hormone secretion

Birth   Childhood   Puberty   Adult life   Senescence

■ **Fig. 49-20**   Lifetime pattern of GH secretion. GH levels are higher in children than in adults, with a peak period during puberty. GH secretion declines with aging.

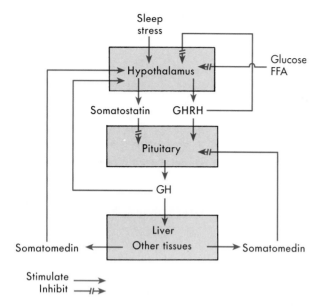

■ **Fig. 49-21** Regulation of GH secretion. The hypothalamic peptide *(GHRH)* stimulates growth hormone release, whereas the hypothalamic peptide somatostatin inhibits it. Negative feedback is by the peripheral mediators of GH action: somatomedins, also known as insulin-like growth factors. Negative feedback occurs both via somatomedin inhibition of GHRH action and by somatomedin stimulation of somatostatin release. GH inhibits its own secretion by short-loop feedback. In addition, GHRH inhibits its own release via ultra-short-loop feedback. In both these cases, the negative feedback is probably effected by increasing the release of inhibitory somatostatin. Likewise, glucose and free fatty acids (FFA) inhibit GH secretion at the hypothalamic level.

responses to GHRH. Insulin also represses GH gene expression. A decline in pituitary GH secretion occurs during the latter part of pregnancy, perhaps in response to production of placental GH and placental lactogen. Obese individuals exhibit dampened GH responses to all stimuli, including GHRH itself. These responses are restored to normal by weight reduction.

The normal basal plasma GH concentration is 1 to 5 ng/ml (about 10^{-10} M). This concentration may increase up to fiftyfold in response to various stimuli. Circulating GH is bound to a plasma protein whose structure is virtually identical to the extracellular portion of the hepatic plasma membrane GH receptor. One molecule of GH binds two of the circulating binding protein molecules. The plasma half-life of GH is 20 minutes and the metabolic clearance rate is 350 L/day. Daily secretion in normal adults is 300 to 500 μg, which is only 5% of the large pituitary store. Although only 0.002% of secreted GH is excreted unchanged by the kidney, daily urinary GH excretion correlates well with the integrated 24-hour plasma GH profile.

Actions of GH. *GH is a hormone with profound anabolic action. In its absence, growth is stunted in humans. When the hormone is administered to unequivocally GH-deficient individuals, it causes prompt nitrogen retention and hypoaminoacidemia. Decreased urea production also results because the amino acids are diverted from oxidation to protein synthesis as growth ensues.* Many GH actions are carried out by the peripherally generated mediators, somatomedins (IGF-1 and IGF-2).

The various major GH targets and effects are indicated in Fig. 49-22. The most striking and specific effect of GH is the stimulation of linear growth that results from GH action on the epiphyseal cartilage or growth plates of long bones. All aspects of the metabolism of the cartilage-forming cells, the chondrocytes, are stimulated. These metabolic effects include the incorporation of the amino acid proline into collagen and its conversion to hydroxyproline, and the incorporation of sulfate into the proteoglycan chondroitin. Together, chondroitin and collagen form the resilient extracellular matrix of cartilage. GH also stimulates the proliferation of chondrocytes, as well as their synthesis of DNA, RNA, and proteins. GH also supports protein synthesis by stimulating cellular uptake of amino acids.

Other tissues participate in the anabolic response to GH. GH increases the activity and probably the number of bone modeling units. After GH administration, urinary hydroxyproline and calcium excretions initially increase, indicating activation of osteoclastic bone resorption (see Chapter 48). However, plasma osteocalcin levels subsequently rise, indicating osteoblastic responses that reflect bone formation (see Chapter 48). Ultimately, total bone mass and mineral content are increased by GH.

Visceral organs (liver, kidney, pancreas, intestines), endocrine glands (adrenals, parathyroids, pancreatic islets), skeletal muscle, heart, skin, and connective tissue all undergo hypertrophy and hyperplasia in response to GH. In most instances, the functional capacity of the enlarged organ is enhanced. For example, GH increases renal plasma flow, glomerular filtration, cardiac output, and hepatic clearance of test substances. GH also increases cardiac muscle size and contractility (see also Chapter 23), and it induces muscle enzymes involved in contraction. The net result is an increase in cardiac output. In addition to stimulating height increase during puberty, GH sensitizes the gonads to LH and FSH and thereby promotes pubertal sexual maturation.

GH exerts several actions on carbohydrate and lipid metabolism. Normal levels of GH are required to sustain normal pancreatic islet function; in the absence of GH, insulin secretion declines. However, an excess of GH causes decreased glucose uptake by insulin-sensitive tissues, such as muscle, and increased hepatic glucose output. Insulin secretion then rises to compensate for the GH-induced insulin resistance. GH is also lipolytic; this characteristic leads to increases in plasma FFAs and ketoacids, especially when insulin secretion cannot compensate adequately. The increased FFA levels may themselves contribute to GH-induced insulin resistance. Increased oxidation of fat and decreased oxidation of glu-

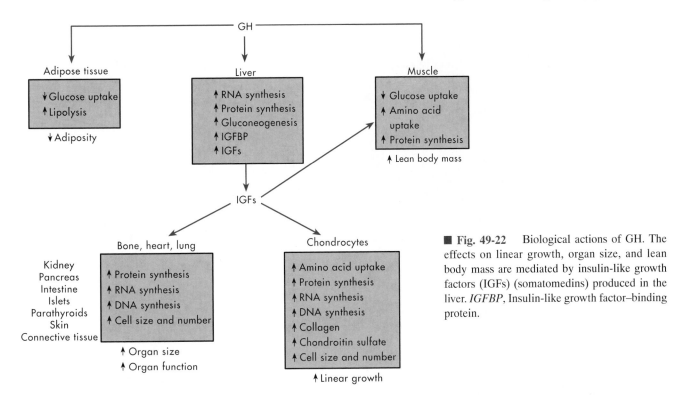

■ **Fig. 49-22** Biological actions of GH. The effects on linear growth, organ size, and lean body mass are mediated by insulin-like growth factors (IGFs) (somatomedins) produced in the liver. *IGFBP*, Insulin-like growth factor–binding protein.

cose are reflected in a decreased respiratory quotient; total metabolic rate is also usually increased. *On balance, GH is a diabetogenic hormone.*

GH increases the volume of extracellular fluid by stimulating the renin-angiotensin-aldosterone axis (see Chapter 51), by suppressing atrial natriuretic peptide (ANP), and by the action of its mediator somatomedin on renal tubules. Proximal tubular phosphate reabsorption, and thus the plasma phosphate concentration, are increased by GH. Calcium absorption from the intestine is enhanced, probably by GH stimulation of $1,25\text{-}(OH)_2$-vitamin D_3 production.

Deficiency of GH in children can result from hypothalamic dysfunction, pituitary destruction, a biologically incompetent GH or GH receptor molecule, failure to generate somatomedins normally, or GH receptor deficiency. Short stature and correspondingly delayed bone and sexual maturation are the consequences of GH deficiency. Mild obesity is common and puberty is usually delayed. In adults, decreased muscle and total lean body mass, decreased muscle strength and exercise performance, and decreased bone density occur. The diagnosis of GH deficiency is established by demonstrating low plasma GH levels, which fail to rise during the night or after a variety of stimuli, and low levels of somatomedins. Replacement treatment with GH causes nitrogen retention, increased lean body mass, increased muscle performance, decreased adipose mass, and a greater sense of well-being. In children, growth velocity increases, pubescence occurs, and fertility is established.

Sustained hypersecretion of GH results from pituitary tumors and produces a unique syndrome called **acromegaly.** If hypersecretion of GH begins before puberty is completed, the individual grows very tall and has long arms and legs. If hypersecretion occurs after puberty, only periosteal bone growth can be increased by GH. This bone growth causes widened fingers, toes, hands, and feet; prominent bony ridges above the eyes; and a prominent lower jaw (Fig. 49-23). Facial features are coarsened by accumulation of excess soft tissue and a bulbous nose (Fig. 49-23). The tongue is enlarged and the skin is thick, whereas subcutaneous fat is sparse. Virtually all organ sizes are increased. Enlargement of the heart, hypertension, and accelerated atherosclerosis often lead to a shortened lifespan. The insulin antagonistic effect of GH produces an abnormal tolerance to carbohydrate or even frank diabetes mellitus that requires treatment with insulin. The diagnosis is confirmed by demonstrating elevated plasma GH levels, which are not suppressed when glucose is administered. Plasma levels of somatomedins are also high. Definitive treatment requires surgical removal of the tumor. Somatostatin analogs that diminish GH hypersecretion are also useful.

Mechanisms of GH action. Plasma membrane GH receptors of varying sizes are present in target cells found in many tissues, including the liver and adipose tissue. GH receptors belong to a family of receptors composed of glycoprotein disulfide–linked subunits that span the plasma membrane. The length of the intracellular cyto-

A   B   C

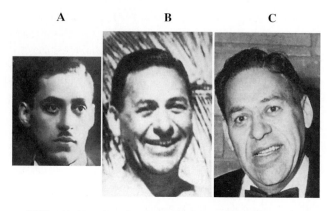

■ **Fig. 49-23** **A** to **C,** A patient with acromegaly, a GH excess syndrome. Note the gradual coarsening of the face over many years before diagnosis.

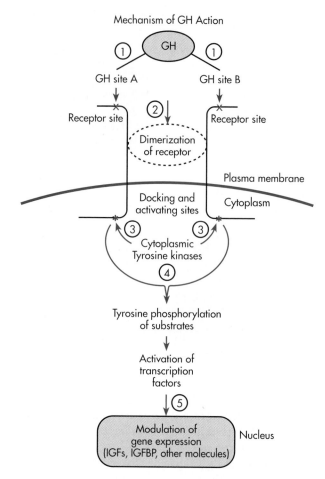

■ **Fig. 49-24** Transduction of GH signals. *1,* One GH molecule binds two plasma membrane GH receptor molecules to different sites on the hormone. *2,* This causes dimerization of the two receptor molecules, which activates them. *3,* The intracytoplasmic portions of the receptors attract, dock, and activate tyrosine kinases. *4,* These phosphorylate transcription factors that *(5),* induce or repress expression of GH target genes such as IGFs.

plasmic receptor tail varies from tissue to tissue and among the hormone ligands. The latter include prolactin, erythropoietin, interleukins, and granulocyte-macrophage colony-stimulating factors. As shown in Fig. 49-24, one GH molecule binds two GH receptor molecules; the receptor dimer then initiates GH actions by attracting a set of intracytoplasmic tyrosine kinases, docking them, and activating them. The substrates and products remain to be identified. Two different amino acid sequences in GH bind the identical amino acid sequence in each of the two receptor molecules. For this reason, an excess of GH may inhibit the hormone's actions, because two receptor monomers may each bind a GH molecule at the same GH site. This binding prevents formation of the active receptor dimer, and nullifies hormone action. Synthesis of GH receptors requires the presence of GH itself, but an excess of GH down-regulates synthesis of its receptors. The GH receptor is also induced by insulin and estrogens and is repressed by fasting.

Many hours must elapse after administration of GH before its anabolic, growth-promoting effects become evident. It is now apparent that most, if not all, of these effects require the generation of a family of peptide hormone intermediaries, the somatomedins or IGFs.

These compounds have a molecular weight of about 7000 and are structurally related to proinsulin. IGF-1 is a 70-amino acid straight-chain peptide with 50% homology to the A-chain and B-chain domains of proinsulin (see Fig. 46-3). IGF-2 has 70% homology with IGF-1 in these same domains. Both somatomedins, however, have distinctive C-chain domains. Circulating somatomedins originate primarily as a result of GH-stimulated production in the liver. In contrast to the sharp and rapid fluctuations of plasma GH, IGF-1 and IGF-2 concentrations are relatively stable. For example, they do not increase after hypoglycemia as GH does. In general, the plasma concentration of IGF-2 is threefold to fourfold higher than that of IGF-1.

The plasma half-life of the IGF molecules is much longer than that of GH, because they circulate bound to at least six carrier proteins. Circulating **insulin growth factor binding proteins (IGFBP$_{1-6}$)** are synthesized in the liver, but local synthesis in other tissues also occurs. IGFBP$_1$ is increased by fasting but decreased by insulin. IGFBP$_1$ may serve to transfer IGF molecules out of the plasma so that they can act on certain target cells. IGFBP$_3$ (the most prevalent IGFBP) forms a large ternary complex with IGF-1 or IGF-2 and an acid-labile protein. This complex serves as a large reservoir that keeps IGF molecules from leaving plasma and protects them from degradation. The hepatic synthesis of IGFBP$_3$ is increased by GH. The presence of the binding proteins in many tissues suggests that they also have important modulating effects on the actions of locally produced IGF molecules.

The growth-promoting effects of GH can be largely accounted for by the IGFs. These factors have been shown to stimulate typical GH responses in cartilage, muscle, adipose tissue, fibroblasts, and tumor cells in vitro. IGF molecules also stimulate nitrogen retention and enhance renal function in vivo. IGF molecules that are generated locally within clones of GH target cells (e.g., osteoblasts) and that act in an autocrine or paracrine fashion may be even more important than IGF molecules that are derived from the plasma.

Somatomedins bind to specific plasma membrane receptors. The receptor for IGF-1 is a dimer, structurally similar to the insulin receptor (see Figs. 45-12 and 47-10), and has intrinsic tyrosine kinase activity. IGF-1 also binds both insulin and IGF-2 receptors, although with lower affinities. The receptor for IGF-2 is a monomer that does not resemble those of IGF-1 and insulin. It binds IGF-1 with lower affinity, but it does not bind insulin at all. The IGF receptor tyrosine kinases phosphorylate cytoplasmic protein substrates. These in turn set up mitogenic signals probably in the same manner as that described for insulin in Chapter 47.

These cross-reactivities may assume biological importance when very high concentrations of either somatomedins or insulin exist. For example, some patients with tumors that secrete IGF-2 develop spontaneous hypoglycemia because the IGF-2 activates the insulin receptor in the liver and elsewhere. In other patients who have insulin receptor deficiency and who have (in compensation) extremely high plasma insulin levels, the soft tissues grow excessively because of activation of the IGF receptors and their downstream mitogenic pathways by insulin.

Plasma somatomedins are increased by administration of GH, with a time lag of 12 to 18 hours, and they are absent in GH-deficient individuals. IGF-1 synthesis is GH dependent, and its plasma levels are very sensitive to changes in GH availability. In contrast, IGF-2 levels do not reflect GH status nearly as well. During adolescence, the augmented secretion of GHRH and of GH increases the plasma levels of IGF-1. The levels of IGF-1 correlate well with the progression of pubertal growth.

Although GH itself is not absolutely necessary for fetal growth, one or more of the somatomedins produced in the embryo or placenta may be. IGF-2 and its receptor are expressed very early in fetal development (at the two-cell stage in mice). IGF-2 stimulates placental growth and is found in trophoblast cells (see Chapter 52). IGF-2 also stimulates growth of both the preimplantation and postimplantation embryo. In contrast, IGF-1 and its receptor are expressed later in life. Both IGF-1 and IGF-2 stimulate progression through the G_1 phase of the cell cycle that leads up to the phase of DNA synthesis. In newborns, plasma IGF-2 levels decline while those of IGF-1 increase. IGF-1 stimulates neuronal development during early postnatal life.

GH and IGF-1 are also important for normal development and function of the immune system. Both molecules are produced by monocytes-macrophages. In addition, IGF-1 stimulates functioning of neutrophils.

Somatomedin production is reduced by factors that can override GH. Fasting, low energy or low protein intake, and insulin deficiency all lead to diminished liver production of IGFs and to a decrease in their plasma levels, despite increases in GH secretion. In fact, in these pathophysiological states, the lack of somatomedin is the likely cause of the elevated GH levels through negative feedback. Estrogens and cortisol also decrease somatomedin production, which may account for their antagonism to GH action, despite their stimulation of GH secretion.

Overall role of GH in substrate flow. It is useful to review the interactions between GH and insulin in common physiological circumstances, as presented in Fig. 49-25. When protein and energy intake are both ample, the absorbed amino acids are used for protein synthesis and to stimulate growth. Hence, both GH and insulin secretion are stimulated by amino acids, and together they augment the production of somatomedins. The latter in turn stimulate accretion of lean body mass. (These actions are probably directly enhanced by insulin also.) The insulin antagonistic effect of the GH molecule itself on carbohydrate metabolism is also useful at this time; it helps to prevent hypoglycemia, which might result from insulin stimulation in the absence of carbohydrate.

On the other hand, when a carbohydrate load is ingested and insulin secretion is correspondingly increased, GH secretion is decreased (and $IGFBP_1$). In this circumstance, accelerated generation or actions of somatomedins are not needed, because protein anabolism is not advantageous in the absence of amino acid inflow. Neither is insulin antagonism necessary. On the contrary, unrestrained expression of insulin action permits efficient storage of the excess carbohydrate calories.

Finally, when an individual is fasting, insulin secretion falls, partly because of a fall in plasma glucose levels. Although this decline in insulin increases GH secretion (and $IGFBP_3$), the calorie deficit and significant deficiency of insulin lead to a decrease in somatomedin production. Again, these effects are appropriate in a situation in which an increase in protein anabolism is disadvantageous and protein catabolism is essential. However, the increase in GH may still be beneficial during fasting, because it enhances lipolysis, decreases peripheral glucose use, and increases glucose production.

■ *Prolactin*

In humans, prolactin is a protein hormone principally concerned with stimulating breast development and milk production. In addition, it exerts an influence on reproductive function and immune responses. Prolactin originates in specific anterior pituitary cells that make up 10% to 25% of the pituitary population. They increase in number during pregnancy and lactation, and with estrogen treatment.

Prolactin is a single-chain protein of molecular weight 23,000. The molecule contains 198 amino acids and three disulfide bridges. Its gene and structure are homologous to those of GH (Fig. 49-19), but the molecule has a major midportion loop. Synthesis of prolactin proceeds from a prehormone. The N-terminal signal peptide is cleaved, and transient N-glycosylation takes place before the compound arrives in the Golgi apparatus. There, the hormone molecules subsequently destined to be stored in granules and released by acute stimuli (or secreted during pregnancy) are deglycosylated. However, some of the N-glycosylated molecules escape complete processing and are secreted constitutively. These molecules form a major part of circulating prolactin in nonpregnant women, and they have lower biological activity. Transcription of the prolactin gene is regulated by factors that also regulate secretion of the hormone. Thus, TRH increases prolactin messenger RNA, whereas dopamine decreases it.

Secretion of prolactin. Table 49-5 lists the most important influences on prolactin secretion. Consistent with its essential role in lactation, prolactin secretion increases steadily during pregnancy. This increase is probably mediated by the large increase in estrogen, which stimulates hyperplasia of prolactin-producing cells and synthesis of the hormone by inducing transcription of the gene. In addition, although estrogen does not itself stimulate the release of prolactin, it enhances responsiveness to other stimuli. If a new mother does not nurse her child, the plasma level of prolactin declines 3 to 6 weeks after delivery to the normal (nonpregnant) range. However, suckling (or any other form of nipple stimulation) maintains elevated levels of prolactin secretion, especially for the first 8 to 12 weeks after birth (Fig. 49-26).

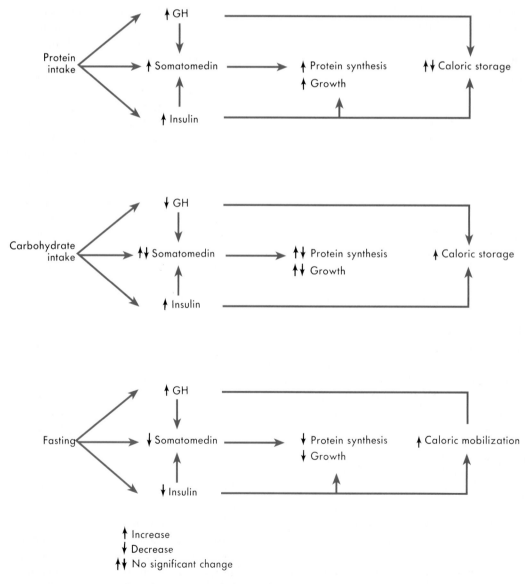

↑ Increase
↓ Decrease
↑↓ No significant change

■ **Fig. 49-25** Complementary regulation of GH and insulin secretion coordinate nutrient availability with anabolism and either caloric storage or mobilization. Note that both hormones are increased by protein, and both stimulate protein synthesis.

Prolactin secretion from mammotrophs is also stimulated in paracrine fashion by the presence of neighboring gonadotrophs, which are themselves responding to GnRH. These gonadotrophs, which release **angiotensin II,** increase prolactin release by nearby mammotrophs.

Like other tropic hormones, prolactin secretion rises at night (Fig. 49-10). The first peak appears 60 to 90 minutes after the onset of slow-wave sleep, and subsequent peaks occur later, after cycles of REM (rapid eye movement) sleep. Stresses, including anesthesia, surgery, insulin-induced hypoglycemia, fear, and mental tension, all cause prolactin release. The function of sleep- or stress-induced prolactin release is unknown.

The details of the pathways for regulating prolactin release in each physiological circumstance remain incompletely known. *However, uniquely among the pituitary hormones, prolactin secretion is tonically inhibited by the hypothalamus* (Fig. 49-27). Disruption of the hypothalamic-pituitary connection induces prompt and enduring increases in plasma prolactin levels. **Dopamine** has many characteristics that qualify it for the role of primary **prolactin-inhibiting factor (PIF),** although it is not a hypothalamic peptide. This catecholamine strongly inhibits prolactin release, either when generated within the brain in vivo or when applied to pituitary tissue in vitro. After binding to dopamine receptors on the mammotrophs, its inhibiting action is mediated by lowering the levels of calcium and cAMP.

A dopaminergic tract runs from the hypothalamus to the median eminence, and dopamine concentrations in the pituitary portal veins are elevated to levels capable of inhibiting prolactin release in vitro. In addition, dopamine from the posterior pituitary (arriving via short portal veins) and dopamine generated or concentrated in adjacent anterior pituitary cells (by paracrine or autocrine action) contribute to chronic inhibition. Somatostatin and a peptide that results from the processing of the gene transcript of GnRH are other hypothalamic inhibitors of prolactin secretion.

The inhibitory effect of dopamine on prolactin secretion is useful therapeutically. Pathological prolactin hypersecretion, for example, from tumors, is readily suppressed by dopamine agonists. They may even

■ **Table 49-5** Regulation of prolactin secretion

Stimulation	Inhibition
Pregnancy	Dopamine
Estrogen	Dopaminergic agonists
Nursing—breast manipulation	Somatostatin
Sleep	GnRH-associated peptide
Stress (Table 49-3)	Prolactin
TRH	γ-Aminobutyric acid
Dopaminergic antagonists	(GABA)
Opioids	
Serotonin	
Histamine antagonists (H$_2$)	
Adrenergic antagonists	
Candidate prolactin-releasing factors	
Vasoactive intestinal peptide	
Peptide histidine-isoleucine	
Oxytocin	
Angiotensin II	
Neurotensin	
Galanin	
Neurophysin II	
Intermediate lobe product	

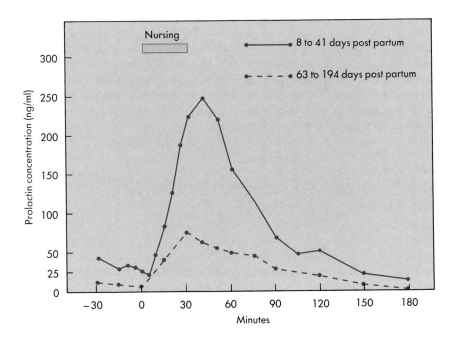

■ **Fig. 49-26** Stimulation of prolactin secretion by nursing. Note the decreased responses with an increasing interval of time from delivery. (Redrawn from Noel GL et al: *J Clin Endocrinol Metab* 38:413, 1974.)

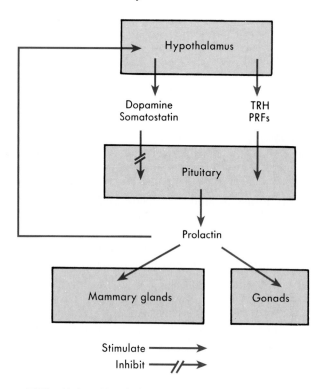

■ **Fig. 49-27**   Regulation of prolactin secretion. The predominant mode of hypothalamic regulation is tonic inhibition by dopamine with a contribution from somatostatin. TRH and a number of prolactin-releasing factor *(PRF)* candidates stimulate prolactin release, but their relative roles are uncertain. Prolactin itself exerts negative feedback by stimulating secretion of its inhibitor dopamine.

shrink such tumors. In contrast, numerous dopaminergic analogs used to treat psychiatric disorders cause elevated prolactin levels and biological effects of the hormone.

Prolactin inhibits its own secretion via a short-loop feedback. It does so by directly increasing the synthesis and release of dopamine, its hypothalamic inhibitor. The hypothalamus has positive as well as negative effects on prolactin secretion. A number of candidates exist for the role of prolactin-releasing hormone (PRH) (Table 49-5). TRH, for example, stimulates prolactin synthesis and release; it acts through specific membrane receptors in the mammotroph, and phosphatidylinositol products are generated as second messengers. When TSH secretion is chronically increased as a result of negative feedback from the thyroid gland, prolactin also tends to increase modestly, probably because of increased endogenous TRH. However, TRH is probably not the sole or the most important stimulator of prolactin release. Suckling, for example, does not produce a simultaneous, acute rise in plasma levels of TSH, as would be expected if TRH mediated the plasma prolactin increase. Some evidence links oxytocin to this particular prolactin-stimulating function. A number of other peptides that are found in the

hypothalamus or median eminence and that have receptors in the anterior pituitary have prolactin-releasing activity (Table 49-5), but their functional roles are unclear.

Normal basal plasma concentrations of prolactin are about 10 ng/ml (5×10^{-10}) and are similar in women and men. The half-life of the hormone is 20 minutes, and the daily production is around 350 μg. The kidney is a likely organ of prolactin degradation, because patients with renal failure often have high plasma prolactin levels. Prolactin is also present in amniotic fluid; its source is pregnancy-modified cells of the uterus stimulated by a placental prolactin-releasing factor.

Biological effects of prolactin. *Prolactin participates in stimulating the original development of breast tissue and its further hyperplasia during pregnancy. It is the principal hormone responsible for lactogenesis.* Before and after puberty, prolactin, together with estrogens, progesterone, cortisol, and GH, stimulates the proliferation and branching of ducts in the female breast. During pregnancy, prolactin, along with estrogen and progesterone, causes the development of lobules of alveoli within which milk is produced. Finally, after parturition, prolactin, together with insulin and cortisol, stimulates milk synthesis and secretion.

To exert these effects, prolactin binds to plasma membrane receptors homologous to those of GH in their extracellular binding domains (Fig. 49-28). The intracytoplasmic tails of prolactin receptors are different from and shorter than those of GH receptors. Signal transduction is effected via activation of cytoplasmic tyrosine kinases, as described for GH. As a result of binding to its receptor, prolactin induces transcription of genes for the milk proteins casein, lactalbumin, and β-lactoglobulin, and also stabilizes their messenger RNAs. Galactosyl transferase and *N*-acetyllactosamine synthetase are also induced. These enzymes are necessary for synthesis of lactose, the major sugar in milk. The synthesis of fatty acids and phospholipids is also stimulated by prolactin, specifically in breast tissue. Prolactin up-regulates the number of its own receptors. Estrogen also increases the number of prolactin receptors. However, estrogen and progesterone directly antagonize the stimulatory effect of prolactin on milk synthesis.

Prolactin has both stimulating and inhibiting effects on reproduction, depending in part on the phase of the reproductive process during which it acts. Excess prolactin blocks the synthesis and release of GnRH; this action causes the loss of normal GnRH pulses and prevents ovulation in females and normal sperm production in males. Prolactin can both induce and repress gene transcription for certain enzymes essential to gonadal steroid hormone production. Whether induction or repression occurs depends on which cell type is affected and, in females, on the stage of the menstrual cycle. In addition, certain reproductive behavioral effects of prolactin have been described, such as inhibition of libido in humans and

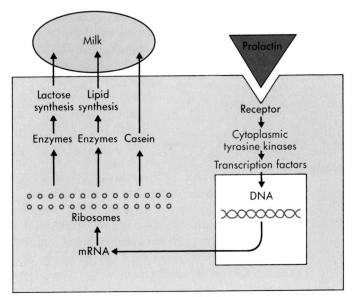

Mammary gland

■ **Fig. 49-28**   Mechanism of prolactin action. After binding to a plasma membrane receptor, cytoplasmic tyrosine kinase second messengers phosphorylate transcription factors that stimulate expression of genes. These genes direct synthesis of the milk protein casein and of enzymes essential for production of milk components: lactose, casein, and lipids.

stimulation of parental protective behavior toward the newborn in animals.

Interest is increasing in certain effects of prolactin on cell growth and proliferation. Although the effects resemble GH effects, they are expressed through prolactin receptors. In addition, prolactin, like GH, may induce an intermediary growth molecule, **synlactin,** synthesized and released by the liver, in analogy to the somatomedins. Prolactin, like GH, is synthesized by immune cells and also by maternal uterine cells during pregnancy. These observations suggest a role for the hormone in the immunologic balance required for acceptance of fetal tissues by the mother and protection of maternal tissues from fetal invasion. During pregnancy, locally produced prolactin may also participate in the osmoregulatory function of amniotic fluid.

In women, prolactin deficiency, caused by destruction of the anterior pituitary, results in inability to lactate. Prolactin excess results from hypothalamic dysfunction or from pituitary tumors. In women, prolactin hypersecretion causes infertility and even complete loss of menses. Less often, lactation unassociated with pregnancy (**galactorrhea**) occurs. In men, decreased testosterone secretion and sperm production result from prolactin excess. Stimulation of breast development is uncommon and lactation is rare. In both sexes, libido is decreased. The diagnosis of excess prolactin is established by demonstrating a high plasma prolactin level. If surgical removal of a mammotrophic tumor is not required, dopaminergic drugs reduce prolactin secretion to normal levels and restore fertility.

■ *Posterior Pituitary Hormones*

Two nonapeptides of homologous structure (Fig. 49-29), **antidiuretic hormone (ADH),** also known as **arginine vasopressin (AVP),** and **oxytocin (OCT),** are secreted from the posterior pituitary gland. *The primary role of ADH is to conserve body water and regulate the tonicity of body fluids. The primary role of oxytocin is to eject milk from the lactating mammary gland.* Although their primary human functions are different, the synthesis, storage, and mode of secretion of the two hormones are similar and are discussed together.

Both hormones are synthesized in the cell bodies of hypothalamic neurons. ADH originates largely in the supraoptic nucleus, and oxytocin largely in the paraventricular nucleus of the hypothalamus. However, each hormone is also synthesized in the alternate site. The genes that direct synthesis of the respective preprohormones are remarkably similar and are close together on the same chromosome (Fig. 49-30). The hormone sequences are contained within exon-1.

In addition to ADH or oxytocin, the products from these genes include distinctive proteins, known as **neurophysins,** of molecular weight 10,000. Neurophysin I for oxytocin and neurophysin II for ADH are virtually identical in their large central cores (corresponding to exon-2 in each gene). The two neurophysins differ in their N-terminal portions, which are coded for by exon-1 (Fig. 49-30) and in their C-terminal portions, which are coded for by exon-3. In the case of ADH, an additional glycopeptide is coded for by exon-3. After processing of the preprohormones, ADH and oxytocin are packaged together with their respective neurophysins in neurosecretory granules. The neurophysins may serve as carrier proteins in the process of transport of the neurohormones down the axons. The latter end in the posterior pituitary as terminal swellings, known as **Herring bodies.**

ADH and oxytocin are released when a nerve impulse is transmitted from the cell body in the hypothalamus

Antidiuretic hormone (ADH)

cys-tyr-phe-gln-asn-cys-pro-arg-gly-NH₂

Oxytocin

cys-tyr-ile-gln-asn-cys-pro-leu-gly-NH₂

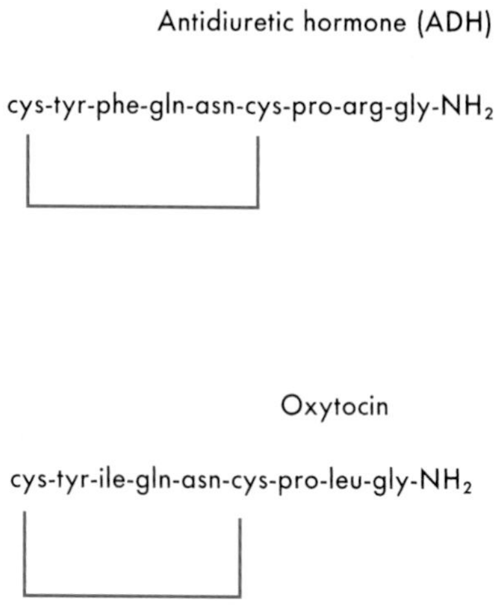

■ **Fig. 49-29**   Structures of posterior pituitary peptides. The alternative term for ADH is arginine vasopressin (AVP).

down the axon, where it depolarizes the neurosecretory vesicles within the terminal Herring body (Fig. 49-2). An influx of calcium into the neurosecretory vesicle then results in hormone secretion by exocytosis. During this process, the hormone dissociates from its neurophysin, and each separately enters the closely adjacent capillary. Subsequent passage of the hormone into the bloodstream is accomplished by endocytosis into the endothelial cell and then by diffusion through pores in the fenestrated capillary endothelium.

Mechanical disruption of the neurohypophyseal tract by trauma, tumor, or surgery temporarily causes ADH deficiency, which can disappear with regeneration of the axons. However, if disruption occurs at a high enough level, the cell bodies in the hypothalamus die and ADH deficiency is permanent.

■ *Secretion of ADH*

Consistent with its role in water metabolism, *secretion of ADH is primarily regulated by osmotic and volume stimuli* (Table 49-6). Water deprivation increases the osmo

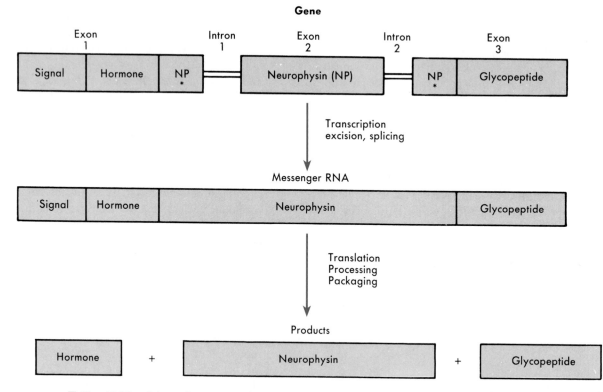

■ **Fig. 49-30**   Schematic representation of the synthesis of the two posterior pituitary peptides, ADH and oxytocin. The two gene structures are similar. In each case, exon 1 codes for the signal peptide, the hormone, and a variable portion of its corresponding neurophysin. Exon 2 is virtually identical in the two genes and codes for the homologous large central core of each neurophysin. In the case of ADH only, exon 3 contains a base sequence extension that codes for a C-terminal glycopeptide, which is coreleased with ADH. (Redrawn from Richter D, Ivell R: *Gene organization, biosynthesis, and chemistry of neurohypophyseal hormones.* In Imura H: *The pituitary gland,* New York, 1985, Raven Press.)

lality of plasma and hence of the fluids bathing the brain. This hyperosmolality induces a loss of intracellular water from osmoreceptor neurons in the hypothalamus. Although these neurons could be identical with the magnocellular neurons that secrete ADH, evidence favors the existence of a distinct population of osmoreceptor neurons with connections to the ADH neurons. In either case, the shrinkage of neuronal cell volume or increase in intracellular osmolality causes ADH to be released. Conversely, water ingestion suppresses osmoreceptor firing and consequently shuts off ADH release. ADH is initially suppressed by reflex neural stimulation shortly after water is swallowed; the plasma ADH level then declines further after the water is absorbed from the intestine and plasma osmolality falls.

If plasma osmolality is directly increased by administration of solutes, only those solutes that do not freely or rapidly penetrate cell membranes, such as sodium, cause ADH release. Substances that enter cells rapidly, such as urea, do not stimulate ADH secretion because they do not produce osmotic disequilibrium between extracellular and neuronal intracellular fluids. A selective increase in sodium concentration of the cerebrospinal fluid also increases ADH secretion. The hypothalamic osmoreceptors are extraordinarily sensitive and respond to changes in osmolality of only 1% to 2% (Fig. 49-31). An increase in plasma osmolality of 1 mOsm/kg increases the ADH level by 0.2 to 0.3 pg/ml. If water deprivation is prolonged, ADH synthesis is also increased.

In response to plasma hyperosmolality, osmoreceptor neurons also stimulate thirst. In humans, the threshold for this action is close to or somewhat higher than the threshold for ADH release of around 280 mOsm/kg (Fig. 49-31). Therefore, ADH secretion is at least as important as thirst in maintaining normal body water content.

■ **Table 49-6**   Regulation of ADH secretion

Stimulation	Inhibition
Extracellular fluid osmolality increase	Extracellular fluid osmolality decrease
Volume decrease	Volume increase
Pressure decrease	Temperature decrease
Cerebrospinal fluid sodium increase	α-Adrenergic agonists
Angiotensin II	γ-Aminobutyric acid (GABA)
Pain	Ethanol
Nausea and vomiting	Cortisol
Stress (Table 49-3)	Thyroid hormone
Hypoglycemia	Atrial natriuretic peptide
Cytokines	
Temperature increase	
Senescence	
Drugs	
Nicotine	
Opiates	
Barbiturates	
Sulfonylureas	
Antineoplastic agents	

ADH release is also stimulated by a decrease of 5% to 10% in total circulating blood volume, central blood volume, cardiac output, or blood pressure (Fig. 49-32). Hemorrhage is a potent stimulus of ADH release (see also Chapter 31). Quiet standing, tilting, or positive-pressure breathing also reduce central blood volume; therefore, they increase ADH secretion, particularly if blood pressure falls. Conversely, administration of blood or isotonic saline solution, which increases total circulating blood volume, or immersion up to the neck in water, which increases central blood volume, suppresses ADH release.

Hypovolemia is perceived by a number of pressure sensors in the body (see Chapters 24 and 28). These sensors include carotid and aortic baroreceptors, stretch receptors in the walls of the left atrium and pulmonary veins, and possibly the juxtaglomerular apparatus of the kidney. The afferent impulses of this neurohumoral arc are carried by the ninth and tenth cranial nerves to their respective nuclei in the medulla. From the medulla, the impulses are carried by way of the midbrain via adrenergic neurotransmitters to the supraoptic nuclei of the

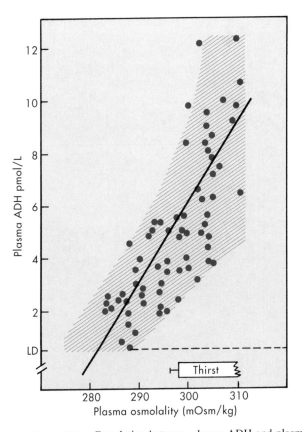

■ **Fig. 49-31**   Correlation between plasma ADH and plasma osmolality in humans. As plasma osmolality is increased by infusing hypertonic sodium chloride, ADH secretion is stimulated, and plasma ADH rises over a linear concentration range. This response to hyperosmolality just precedes the response of thirst. Both ADH release and thirst lead to increases in body water that limit further increments in the osmolality of body fluids. (From Baylis P: *Clin Endocrinol Metab* 12:747, 1983.)

hypothalamus. Normally, the pressure receptors *tonically inhibit* ADH release by modulating an inhibitory flow of adrenergic impulses from the medulla to the hypothalamus. A decrease in pressure increases ADH secretion by reducing the flow of neural impulses from the baroreceptors to the brainstem. The reduced neural input to the baroreceptors relieves the source of tonic inhibition on the hypothalamic cells that secrete ADH.

Hypovolemia also stimulates the generation of renin and angiotensin directly within the brain. This local angiotensin II enhances the release of ADH, in addition to stimulating thirst. Furthermore, volume regulation of ADH is partly mediated or reinforced by **atrial natriuretic peptide (ANP).** When circulating volume is increased, ANP is released by cardiac myocytes; this ANP, along with ANP generated locally in supraoptic hypothalamic neurons (brain ANP), acts to inhibit ADH release (see also Chapter 42). Plasma ADH rises to much higher levels in response to hypotension than in response to hyperosmolarity (compare Fig. 49-32 with Fig. 49-31). This exaggerated response reflects the fact that the vascular system is less sensitive to ADH than is the kidney.

The two major stimuli of ADH secretion interact. Increases or decreases in circulating volume reinforce the osmolar responses by raising or lowering, respectively, the threshold for osmotic release of ADH. Thus, hypovolemia sensitizes the ADH response to hyperosmolarity. However, if hypovolemia is severe, baroregulation overrides osmotic regulation, and ADH secretion is stimulated, even though plasma osmolality may be below 270 mOsm/kg (see also Chapter 31).

Secretion of ADH is also influenced by a number of other conditions (Table 49-6). Pain, emotional stress, heat, and a variety of drugs are stimulators; nausea and vomiting are especially potent. Inflammatory cytokines, such as interleukin-6, also stimulate ADH release. Elderly individuals secrete more ADH then younger individuals, probably in compensation for a lesser ability of their kidneys to concentrate urine. Ethanol is a commonly encountered inhibitor of ADH secretion. As little as 30 to 90 ml of whiskey is sufficient to suppress ADH secretion. Cortisol and thyroid hormones restrain ADH release; in their absence, ADH may be secreted even though plasma osmolality is low.

ADH circulates at an average basal concentration of 1 pg/ml (10^{-12} M). The plasma half-life is 8 minutes, although the half-life of biological action may be up to 20 minutes. Metabolic clearance of ADH increases with its plasma level and averages 600 ml/min at plasma concentrations of 10 pg/ml. Urinary clearance of ADH consistently averages 5% of total metabolic clearance and 50% of the glomerular filtration rate. Therefore, urinary excretion rates are a valid index of ADH secretion. The latter is normally about 1 mg/day.

During water deprivation, secretion of ADH increases threefold to fivefold. Transient fiftyfold increases can occur with hemorrhage (see Chapter 31), severe pain, or nausea. Neurophysin II also circulates in plasma, and its levels rise and fall parallel with ADH. The C-terminal glycopeptide of prepro-ADH origin is also present in plasma. No functional role for these peptides in peripheral tissues has yet been identified.

■ Actions of ADH

The major action of ADH is on renal cells that are responsible for reabsorbing free (i.e., osmotically unencumbered) water from the glomerular filtrate (Chapter 42). These ADH-responsive cells line the distal convoluted tubules and collecting ducts of the renal medulla. *ADH increases the permeability of these cells to water.* ADH binds to a specific plasma membrane receptor (known as the V_2 receptor) on the capillary (basal) side of the cell, where it activates adenylyl cyclase. The increase in intracellular cAMP activates a protein kinase on the opposite luminal (apical) side of the cell. The activated protein kinase phosphorylates membrane and other proteins. As a result, microtubular and microfilamentous elements of the cell cytoskeleton transport vesicles that contain water channels to the luminal membrane. The vesicles fuse with the plasma membrane and create channels through which water rapidly moves from the tubular lumen into the collecting duct cell. Through a separate mechanism, urea is likewise reabsorbed.

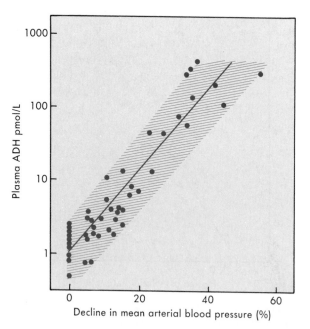

■ **Fig. 49-32** Correlation between plasma ADH and declining blood pressure in humans. As blood pressure is decreased by infusing an agent that blocks sympathetic ganglion function, ADH secretion is stimulated. In this response, plasma ADH rises over an exponential concentration range (compare Fig. 49-31). (From Baylis P: *Clin Endocrinol Metab* 12:747, 1983.)

The increase in membrane permeability to water permits back diffusion of water along an osmotic gradient, from the hypotonic tubular urine that emerges from the loop of Henle to the hypertonic interstitial fluid of the renal medulla. The mechanisms for establishing this gradient are discussed in Chapter 42. ADH also acts on the ascending limb of the loop of Henle to enhance sodium transport into the medullary interstitium. The resultant increase in the osmolality of the interstitium helps create the osmotic gradient for water reabsorption. The net result of ADH action is to increase the osmolality of urine to a maximum that is fourfold greater than that of the glomerular filtrate or plasma (Fig. 49-33). In other words, ADH significantly reduces free-water clearance by the kidney.

Water deprivation stimulates ADH secretion and thereby decreases free-water clearance and enhances water conservation. A water load decreases ADH secretion and thus results in increased free-water clearance and more efficient excretion of the load. Thus, ADH and water form a negative feedback loop. The sigmoidal dose-response relationship between plasma levels of ADH and urine osmolality is shown in Fig. 49-33. Most of the renal effect occurs at plasma ADH levels between 2 and 5 pg/ml. In this range, urine osmolality correlates directly with plasma ADH concentrations. An increase in plasma ADH concentration of only 0.3 pg/ml increases urine osmolality from 60 to 300 mOsm/kg in water-loaded humans. At 5 pg/ml, a maximal ADH effect of 900 mOsm/kg is achieved.

ADH deficiency is caused by destruction or dysfunction of the supraoptic and paraventricular nuclei of the hypothalamus. The inability to produce concentrated urine is the hallmark of ADH deficiency, a condition called **diabetes insipidus.** In normal individuals, water deprivation can be compensated for by an increase in urine osmolality to 1000 to 1400 mOsm/kg. Individuals who lack ADH cannot achieve osmolalities higher than that of plasma (290 mOsm/kg) and in severe cases not higher than 50 mOsm/kg. Because a typical diet generates up to 900 mOsm of solute per day that must be excreted by the kidney, urine volumes may be as high as 12 L/day in patients with diabetes insipidus, in contrast to the usual 1 to 3 L. Patients therefore urinate frequently both day and night, and they must also drink excess fluids to replace the loss of water. Despite this water intake, chronic elevation of serum osmolality (>290 mOsm/kg) and of serum sodium (>145 mEq/L) can occur. Replacement with ADH or long-acting analogs relieves the frequent urination and thirst and prevents disastrous dehydration.

A number of factors blunt the action of ADH on the tubular cell: solute diuresis, chronic water loading (which reduces medullary hyperosmolarity), prostaglandin E (which interferes with ADH activation of adenylyl cyclase), ANP, cortisol, potassium deficiency, calcium excess, and lithium (which is used in the treatment of psychiatric disorders). Certain sulfonylureas, used in the treatment of diabetes mellitus, and a tetracycline antibiotic enhance ADH action.

ADH subserves other functions in addition to its primary role in water metabolism. In response to hemorrhage, ADH contributes to increasing vascular tone by binding to arteriolar smooth muscles via the V_{1a} receptor and causing them to constrict. This action is mediated by Ca^{++} and phospholipase C–generated second messengers. In contrast, a V_2 receptor–mediated vasodilator effect of ADH may prevent blood pressure from changing too much when ADH secretion is in the physiological range. However, when ADH is administered systemically in large doses, it elevates the blood pressure and constricts the coronary and splanchnic beds. The latter effect has been exploited therapeutically in controlling serious gastrointestinal bleeding.

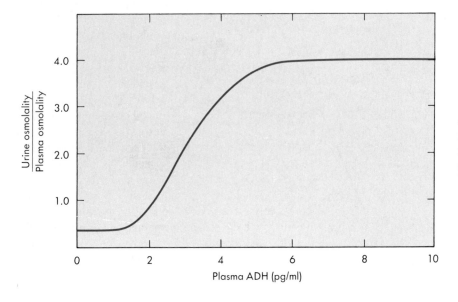

■ **Fig. 49-33**   Dose-response curve for the effect of ADH in increasing renal tubular reabsorption of free water, expressed as the ratio of urine to plasma osmolality. A maximal ratio of 4.0 is reached. (Data from Moore WW: *Fed Proc* 30:1387, 1971.)

ADH excess, inappropriate to either the osmolarity or volume of the body fluids, can result from (1) increased secretion caused by central nervous system disease, trauma, or psychosis; (2) increased secretion in response to cytokines released during infections or other medical or surgical stress; (3) ectopic production of the hormone by tumors; or (4) potentiation of hormone secretion or action by drugs. The reduction in free-water clearance caused by ADH, combined with voluntary or involuntary water intake, leads to water retention. Plasma sodium concentration and osmolality are significantly lowered, whereas urine osmolality is increased. Characteristically, sodium excretion in the urine is also increased, despite the hyponatremia, as a result of a compensatory increase in ANP secretion. Both intracellular and extracellular fluid volumes are expanded. The swelling of brain cells and hypoosmolality can cause headache, nausea, lethargy, somnolence, convulsions, and coma when plasma osmolality declines to below 250 mOsm/kg and plasma sodium to below 125 mEq/L. Water restriction is a logical and effective acute treatment. Occasionally, this treatment must be supplemented with drugs that induce a hypotonic diuresis or with hypertonic sodium chloride solutions to raise osmolality more rapidly.

ADH also functions as a corticotropin-releasing factor via axons that transmit the peptide to the median eminence (see section on ACTH, p 881). From there, it travels via the portal veins to the anterior pituitary, where it interacts with a V_{1b} receptor. In addition, ADH may serve as a neurotransmitter in the brain to facilitate memory. Finally, ADH, present locally in high concentrations and acting via a V_1 receptor in a paracrine manner, stimulates smooth muscle contraction in the human spermatic cord. This effect may facilitate ejaculation of sperm.

■ Oxytocin Secretion

Oxytocin (OCT) is known as the milk letdown factor. *Suckling is an immediate and the major stimulus for OCT release.* Afferent neural impulses are carried from sensory receptors in the nipple to the spinal cord, where they ascend in the spinothalamic tract. From relays in the brainstem and midbrain, they reach the paraventricular nuclei of the hypothalamus. From there, via a cholinergic synapse, they trigger OCT release from the neurosecretory vesicles in the posterior pituitary. As suckling is continued, OCT synthesis and transfer down the hypothalamic axon are also stimulated. As shown in Fig. 49-34, the stimulus of suckling is specific for OCT, because little release of ADH is noted. Likewise, the various stimuli for ADH secretion stimulate little or no OCT release in humans. Opioid (endorphinergic) input to the hypothalamus inhibits OCT responses to stimuli. OCT circulates unbound and exhibits a plasma half-life of 3 to 5 minutes. It is degraded by the kidneys and liver.

■ Oxytocin Actions

OCT binds to plasma membrane receptors distinct from those of ADH. Increases in calcium levels and in phosphatidylinositol products mediate OCT actions. *The unique effect of OCT is to cause contraction of the myoepithelial cells of the alveoli of the mammary glands.*

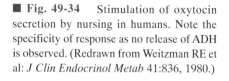

■ **Fig. 49-34** Stimulation of oxytocin secretion by nursing in humans. Note the specificity of response as no release of ADH is observed. (Redrawn from Weitzman RE et al: *J Clin Endocrinol Metab* 41:836, 1980.)

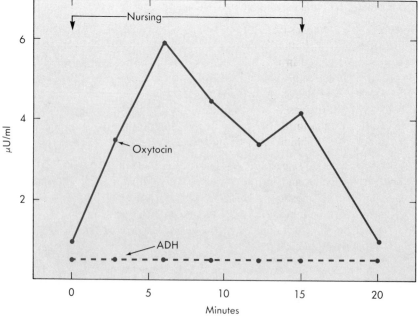

As a result, milk is forced from the alveoli into the ducts, from where it is evacuated by the infant. Estrogens augment and catecholamines block the action of OCT. Men have about the same basal plasma OCT levels as do women. Although the levels rise acutely during orgasm, the function of OCT in men is not clear.

OCT also has a powerful action on smooth muscle in the uterus. Rhythmic contractions of the myometrium are stimulated by very small doses, which act by lowering slightly the threshold for membrane depolarization. Large doses lower the threshold still further, prevent repolarization and spiking discharges, and induce a sustained tetanic contraction. Neither maternal plasma OCT levels nor fetal OCT availability bears a consistent relationship to the progress of labor during childbirth. Therefore, despite the ability to stimulate rhythmic uterine contractions, secreted OCT seems to be more a contributing factor than an essential hormone of human parturition (see Chapter 52). However, after delivery, it may play an important role in the sustained contractions that help to maintain hemostasis after evacuation of the placenta. OCT is used to induce labor in women who are physiologically ready, and it is also used therapeutically to decrease immediate postpartum bleeding. OCT and its receptor are also present in the ovary, where OCT may have a paracrine role in terminating the corpus luteum at the end of the menstrual cycle (see Chapter 52).

■ *Summary*

1. The hypothalamic-pituitary unit regulates growth; lactation; fluid homeostasis; and the functions of the thyroid gland, adrenal glands, and gonads. This unit receives input from the thalamus, reticular activating substance, the limbic system, and from olfactory and visual stimuli. These signals are then relayed to various parts of the endocrine system.

2. Peptide hormones that are synthesized in the cell bodies of certain hypothalamic neurons pass down their axons to be stored in and released into the circulation from the posterior pituitary gland. Other hypothalamic peptides travel down axons to the median eminence, from which they are released into a portal venous circulation that carries them to the anterior pituitary gland. There, they stimulate or inhibit release of target hormones.

3. Hypothalamic releasing and inhibiting peptides are secreted in pulses and induce effects via cAMP, Ca++, and phosphatidylinositol products as second messengers. They stimulate or inhibit transcription, modulate translation, and stimulate or inhibit secretion of the target anterior pituitary hormones.

4. The anterior pituitary gland contains five functional cell types that are in close proximity and thus capable of paracrine interactions. These cell types are thyrotrophs, adrenocorticotrophs, gonadotrophs, somatotrophs, and mammotrophs. Each secretes a hormone or hormones in response to hypothalamic stimulation. Peripheral target gland hormones or other peripheral products of hormonal action feed back negatively to inhibit their respective anterior pituitary hormones.

5. Thyrotropin (TSH) is a glycoprotein that contains α and β subunits. TSH stimulates secretion and growth of the thyroid gland. It is released in response to thyrotropin-releasing hormone (TRH) and to thyroid hormone deficiency.

6. Adrenocorticotrophin (ACTH) is a peptide that stimulates the secretion and growth of the adrenal cortex. It is synthesized from a multifunctional precursor and is secreted in bursts in response to corticotropin-releasing hormone, to cortisol deficiency, and to various stresses, such as trauma and hypoglycemia.

7. Both follicle-stimulating hormone (FSH) and luteinizing hormone (LH) are made primarily by a single gonadotrophic cell type. These glycoprotein hormones share common α subunits with each other and with TSH, but have distinctive β subunits.

8. In women, FSH stimulates the development of ovarian follicles and estradiol secretion, and in men spermatogenesis. LH stimulates steroid hormone secretion in both genders, primarily estradiol and its precursors in women, and testosterone in men. LH also stimulates ovulation. Estradiol and testosterone, as well as secreted gonadal protein hormones, feed back on FSH and LH secretion in complex ways.

9. Growth hormone (GH) is a large protein that stimulates cartilage development and growth, bone growth, and accretion of lean body mass. It acts primarily via peptide mediators (insulin-like growth factors, or somatomedins) produced in the liver and in many GH target cells. GH also acts to antagonize insulin, stimulate lipolysis, and increase the metabolic rate. GH is secreted in response to growth hormone–releasing hormone (GHRH), hypoglycemia, amino acids, and stress. Its secretion is inhibited by somatostatin from the hypothalamus, somatomedin, and glucose.

10. Prolactin is structurally similar to GH, but it specifically stimulates growth of the mammary glands and production of milk. Prolactin is normally tonically inhibited by dopamine from the hypothalamus. Its synthesis is markedly increased during pregnancy and is augmented by estrogens. Its release is stimulated by suckling.

11. Antidiuretic hormone (ADH) is a small peptide that acts on the renal tubules via cAMP as messenger. ADH increases the reabsorption of free water and the final urine osmolality. ADH also acts as a vasoconstrictor via a separate plasma membrane receptor. ADH is secreted from the posterior pituitary in response to an increase in plasma osmolality or to a decrease in plasma volume or blood pressure.

12. Oxytocin (OCT) is structurally very similar to ADH, but it acts specifically on the mammary gland to release milk. It is secreted in response to suckling. OCT also causes contraction of the uterus and plays a role in the overall process of parturition.

■ *Self-Study Problems*

1. What is the functional significance of the blood supply of the pituitary gland and its anatomic relationship to the hypothalamus?

2. How is ACTH secretion mainly controlled?

3. Describe the sequence in major growth hormone actions.

4. A patient undergoes major abdominal surgery, during which there were several decreases in blood pressure that required extra administration of fluid intravenously. He is found to have a serum sodium level of 122 mEq/L and a serum osmolality of 250 mOsm/kg 24 hours later. He shows no evidence of dehydration. Describe the sequence that led to this abnormality and its possible consequences.

■ *Bibliography*

Journal articles

Amato G et al: Body composition, bone metabolism, and heart structure and function in growth hormone (GH)–deficient adults before and after GH replacement therapy at low doses, *J Clin Endocrinol Metab* 77:1671, 1993.

Argetsinger LS, et al: Identification of JAK2 as a growth hormone receptor-associated tyrosine kinase, *Cell* 74:237, 1993.

Bjerknes R, Aarskog D: Priming of human polymorphonuclear neutrophilic leukocytes by insulin-like growth factor I: increased phagocytic capacity, complement receptor expression, degranulation, and oxidative burst, *J Clin Endocrinol Metab* 80:1948, 1995.

Brixen K et al: A short course of recombinant human growth hormone treatment stimulates osteoblasts and activates bone remodeling in normal human volunteers, *J Bone Miner Res* 5:609, 1990.

Chin WW: Hormonal regulation of thyrotropin and gonadotropin gene expression, *Clin Res* 36:484, 1988.

Chou JL et al: In vitro and in vivo growth and casein gene expression of mouse mammary tumor epithelial cells in response to hormones, *Exp Cell Res* 186:250, 1990.

Conn PM, Crowley WF Jr: Gonadotropin-releasing hormone and its analogues, *N Engl J Med* 324:93, 1991.

Cooke NE, Liebhaber SA: Molecular biology of the growth hormone–prolactin gene system, *Vitam Horm* 50:385, 1995.

Corpas E, Harman SM, Blackman MR: Human growth hormone and human aging, *Endocr Rev* 14:20, 1993.

Daughaday WH, Rotwein P: Insulin-like growth factors I and II: peptide, messenger, ribonucleic acid and gene structures, serum, and tissue concentrations, *Endocr Rev* 10:68, 1989.

deBoer H, Blok G-J, Van der Veen EA: Clinical aspects of growth hormone deficiency in adults, *Endocr Rev* 16:63, 1995.

English DE et al: Evidence for a role of the liver in the mammotrophic action of prolactin, *Endocrinology* 126:2252, 1990.

Gharib SD et al: Molecular biology of the pituitary gonadotropins, *Endocr Rev* 11:177, 1990.

Giraldi A et al: Oxytocin and the initiation of parturition, a review, *Dan Med Bull* 37:377, 1990.

Gitay-Goren H et al: Effects of prolactin on steroidogenesis and cAMP accumulation in rat luteal cell cultures, *Mol Cell Endocrinol* 65:195, 1989.

Giudice LC et al: Insulin-like growth factors and their binding proteins in the term and preterm human fetus and neonate with normal and extremes of intrauterine growth, *J Clin Endocrinol Metab* 80:1548, 1995.

Hirsch AT et al: Vasopressin-mediated forearm vasodilation in normal humans; evidence for a vascular vasopressin V_2 receptor, *J Clin Invest* 84:418, 1989.

Holl RW et al: Thirty-second sampling of plasma growth hormone in man: correlation with sleep stages, *J Clin Endocrinol Metab* 72:854, 1991.

Horseman ND, and Yu-Lee L-Y: Transcriptional regulation by the helix bundle peptide hormones: growth hormone, prolactin, and hematopoietic cytokines, *Endocr Rev* 15:627, 1994.

Hunt G: Melanocyte-stimulating hormone: a regulator of human melanocyte physiology, *Pathobiology* 63:12, 1995.

Iannotti JP: Growth plate physiology and pathology, *Orthop Clin North Am* 21:1, 1990.

Iranmanesh A et al: Intensive venous sampling paradigms disclose high frequency adrenocorticotropin release episodes in normal men, *J Clin Endocrinol Metab* 71:1276, 1990.

Jacobson L, Sapolsky R: The role of the hippocampus in feedback regulation of the hypothalamic-pituitary-adrenocortical axis, *Endocr Rev* 12:118, 1991.

Jones MT, Gillham B: Factors involved in the regulation of adrenocorticotropic hormone/beta lipotropic hormone, *Physiol Rev* 68:743, 1988.

Kelly PA et al: The prolactin/growth hormone receptor family, *Endocr Rev* 12:235, 1991.

Kerrigan JR, Rogol AD: The impact of gonadal steroid hormone action on growth hormone secretion during childhood and adolescence, *Endocr Rev* 13:281, 1992.

LaBarbera AR, Rebar RW: Reproductive peptide hormones, generation, degradation, reception, and action, *Clin Obstet Gynecol* 33:576, 1990.

Lamberts SW, Macleod RM: Regulation of prolactin secretion at the level of the lactotroph, *Physiol Rev* 70:279, 1990.

Magner JA: Thyroid stimulating hormone: biosynthesis, cell biology and bioactivity, *Endocr Rev* 11:354, 1990.

Miller N et al: Short-term effects of growth hormone on fuel oxidation and regional substrate metabolism in normal man, *J Clin Endocrinol Metab* 70:1179, 1990.

Moller J et al: Expansion of extracellular volume and suppression of atrial natriuretic peptide after growth hormone administration in normal man, *J Clin Endocrinol Metab* 72:768, 1991.

Norsk P, Epstein M: Effects of water immersion on arginine vasopressin release in humans, *J Appl Physiol* 64:1, 1988.

Pelletier G et al: Identification of human anterior pituitary cells by immunoelectron microscopy, *J Clin Endocrinol Metab* 46:534, 1978.

Salomon F et al: The effects of treatment with recombinant human growth hormone on body composition and metabolism in adults with growth hormone deficiency, *N Engl J Med* 321:1797, 1989.

Samuels MH et al: Pathophysiology of pulsatile and copulsatile release of thyroid-stimulating hormone, luteinizing hormone, follicle-stimulating hormone, and alpha-subunit, *J Clin Endocrinol Metab* 71:425, 1990.

Seeman TE, Robbins RJ: Aging and hypothalamic-pituitary-adrenal response to challenge in humans, *Endocr Rev* 15:233, 1994.

Southworth MB et al: The importance of signal pattern in the transmission of endocrine information: pituitary gonadotropin responses to continuous and pulsatile gonadotropin-releasing hormone, *J Clin Endocrinol Metab* 72:1286, 1991.

Spencer SA et al: Growth hormone receptor and binding protein, *Recent Prog Horm Res* 46:165, 1990.

Theill LE, Karin M: Transcriptional control of growth hormone expression and anterior pituitary development, *Endocr Rev* 14:670, 1993.

Thissen JP, Ketelslegers JM, Underwood LE: Nutritional regulation of the insulin-like growth factors, *Endocr Rev* 15:80, 1994.

Thompson CJ et al: Reproducibility of osmotic and nonosmotic tests of vasopressin secretion in men, *Am J Physiol* 260:R533, 1991.

Veldhuis J et al: Twenty-four-hour rhythms in plasma concentrations of adenohypophyseal hormones are generated by distinct amplitude and/or frequency modulation of underlying pituitary secretory bursts, *J Clin Endocrinol Metab* 71:1616, 1990.

Wells JA et al: The molecular basis for growth hormone-receptor interactions, *Recent Prog Horm Res* 48:253, 1993.

Wennink JM et al: Growth hormone secretion patterns in relation to LH and testosterone secretion throughout normal male puberty, *Acta Endocrinol (Copenh)* 123:263, 1990.

Werner H, Adamo M, Roberts CT Jr, LeRoith D: Molecular and cellular aspects of insulin-like growth factor action, *Vitam Horm* 48:1, 1994.

Winer LM et al: Basal plasma growth hormone levels in man: new evidence for rhythmicity of growth hormone secretion, *J Clin Endocrinol Metab* 70:1678, 1990.

Books and monographs

Baylis PH: *Vasopressin and its neurophysin.* In DeGroot LJ, editor: *Endocrinology,* ed 3, Philadelphia, 1995, WB Saunders.

Cooke NE: *Prolactin: basic physiology.* In DeGroot LJ, editor: *Endocrinology,* ed 3, Philadelphia, 1995, WB Saunders.

Kato Y et al: *Regulation of prolactin secretion.* In Imura H, editor: *The pituitary gland,* New York, 1985, Raven Press.

Keith LD, Kendall JW: *Regulation of ACTH secretion.* In Imura H, editor: *The pituitary gland,* New York, 1985, Raven Press.

Müller EE: *Role of neurotransmitters and neuromodulators in the control of anterior pituitary hormone secretion.* In DeGroot LJ, editor, *Endocrinology,* ed 3, Philadelphia, 1995, WB Saunders.

Pfaff DW, Lauber AH: *Hypothalamus and hormone-regulated behaviors.* In DeGroot LJ, editor: *Endocrinology,* ed 3, Philadelphia, 1995, WB Saunders.

Pickering BT: *Oxytocin.* In DeGroot LJ, editor: *Endocrinology,* ed 3, Philadelphia, 1995, WB Saunders.

Reeves WB, Anderoli TE: *The posterior pituitary and water metabolism.* In Foster D, Wilson J, editors: *Williams textbook of endocrinology,* ed 8, Philadelphia, 1992, WB Saunders.

Reichlin S: *Neuroendocrinology.* In Foster D, Wilson J, editors: *Williams textbook of endocrinology,* ed 8, Philadelphia, 1992, WB Saunders.

Riskind PN, Martin JB: *Functional anatomy of the hypothalamic-anterior pituitary complex.* In DeGroot LJ, editor: *Endocrinology,* Philadelphia, 1989, WB Saunders.

Thorner MO et al: *The anterior pituitary.* In Foster DF, Wilson JD, editors: *Williams textbook of endocrinology,* ed 8, Philadelphia, 1992, WB Saunders.

The Thyroid Gland

The thyroid gland was the first endocrine gland to be recognized as such on the basis of the symptoms associated with excess or deficient function. Physicians had previously speculated that deficiency of an internal secretion caused the clinical state associated with atrophy of the gland. This speculation was borne out when crude thyroid extracts successfully reversed the symptoms associated with thyroid atrophy; these extracts were the first example of successful hormonal therapy. Soon thereafter, *the most important mission of the thyroid gland was discovered to be regulation of the overall rate of body metabolism, including its most fundamental component—oxygen utilization. In addition, the gland was found to be critical for normal growth and development.*

The thyroid gland develops from endoderm associated with the pharyngeal gut. The gland descends to the anterior part of the neck, where it divides into two halves that lie on either side of the trachea (Fig. 50-1, *A*). Abnormal descent may locate the thyroid anywhere from the base of the tongue to the anterior mediastinum. By 11 to 12 weeks of gestational age, the gland is capable of synthesizing and secreting thyroid hormones under the stimulus of fetal thyroid-stimulating hormone (TSH). Both fetal TSH and thyroid hormone are required for subsequent normal intrauterine development of the central nervous system and skeleton (although not for body growth) because only small amounts of this needed thyroid hormone reach the fetus from the maternal circulation.

Together, the two lobes of the adult thyroid gland weigh approximately 20 g. They receive a rich blood supply from the thyrocervical arteries and innervation from the autonomic nervous system. The basic histologic structure of the thyroid gland is shown in Fig. 50-1, *B*. A single layer of hormone-producing, cuboidal epithelial cells forms a circular follicle 200 to 300 μm in diameter. Within the lumen of the follicle, newly synthesized hormone is stored in the form of a **colloid** material. The base of each epithelial cell is covered by a basement membrane, and tight junctions connect adjacent cells at both their basal and apical (luminal) portions. When the gland is intensely stimulated, the endocrine cells enlarge and assume a more columnar shape, and their nuclei move toward the base of the cell (Fig. 50-1, *C*). The lumens of the follicles then appear scalloped because of endocytic resorption of the hormone-containing colloid (Fig. 50-1, *C*). Evidence suggests that the epithelial cells are polyclonal and that their capacity to perform various steps in hormone synthesis in response to stimulation differs from cell to cell.

The thyroid gland contains another type of cell in addition to epithelial cells. Scattered within the gland, in close association with the epithelial cells, are parafollicular cells, called **C cells.** These cells are the source of the polypeptide hormone **calcitonin,** which is discussed in Chapter 48.

■ *Synthesis and Release of Thyroid Hormones*

The secretory products of the thyroid gland are **iodothyronines** (Fig. 50-2), a series of compounds resulting from the coupling of two iodinated tyrosine molecules. Approximately 90% of the thyroid output is **3,5,3′,5′-tetraiodothyronine (thyroxine, or T$_4$);** 10% is **3,5,3′-triiodothyronine (T$_3$);** and less than 1% is **3,3′,5′-triiodothyronine (reverse T$_3$, or rT$_3$).** Normally, these three compounds are secreted in the same proportions as they are stored in the gland. *However, T$_3$ is the molecule responsible for most of the tissue actions of thyroid hormone.*

Because of the unique role of iodide in thyroid physiology, a description of thyroid hormone synthesis properly begins with a consideration of iodide turnover (Fig. 50-3). An average of 400 μg of iodide per person is ingested daily in the United States. In a steady state, virtually the same amount is excreted in the urine. Iodide is actively concentrated in the thyroid gland, salivary glands, and gastric glands. About 70 to 80 μg of iodide is taken up daily by the thyroid gland from a circulating pool that contains approximately 250 to 750 μg of iodide. If this extrathyroidal iodide pool is labeled with a small dose of radioactive iodine (^{123}I or ^{131}I), the percentage of thyroid uptake of this tracer in 24 hours (8%

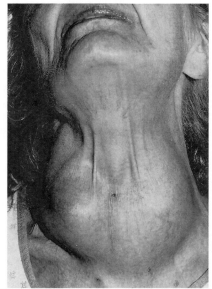

A

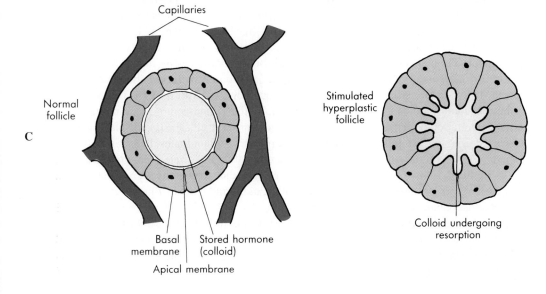

■ **Fig. 50-1**   **A,** The thyroid gland is located in the anterior neck, where it is easily visualized and palpated when it is enlarged (goiter). **B,** Photomicrograph of a thyroid gland follicle. **C,** Schematic drawing of a normal thyroid gland follicle and a follicle stimulated by thyrotropin (TSH). Note the change in cellular shapes from cuboidal to columnar, the relocation of the nuclei to the base of the cells, and the scalloped appearance of the follicle lumen.

B

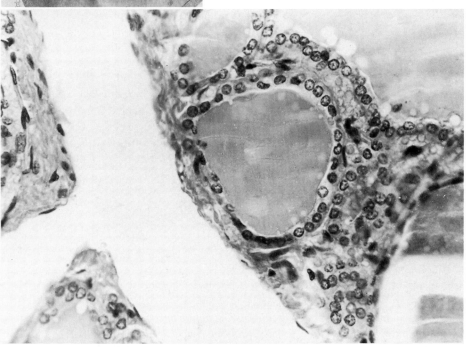

C

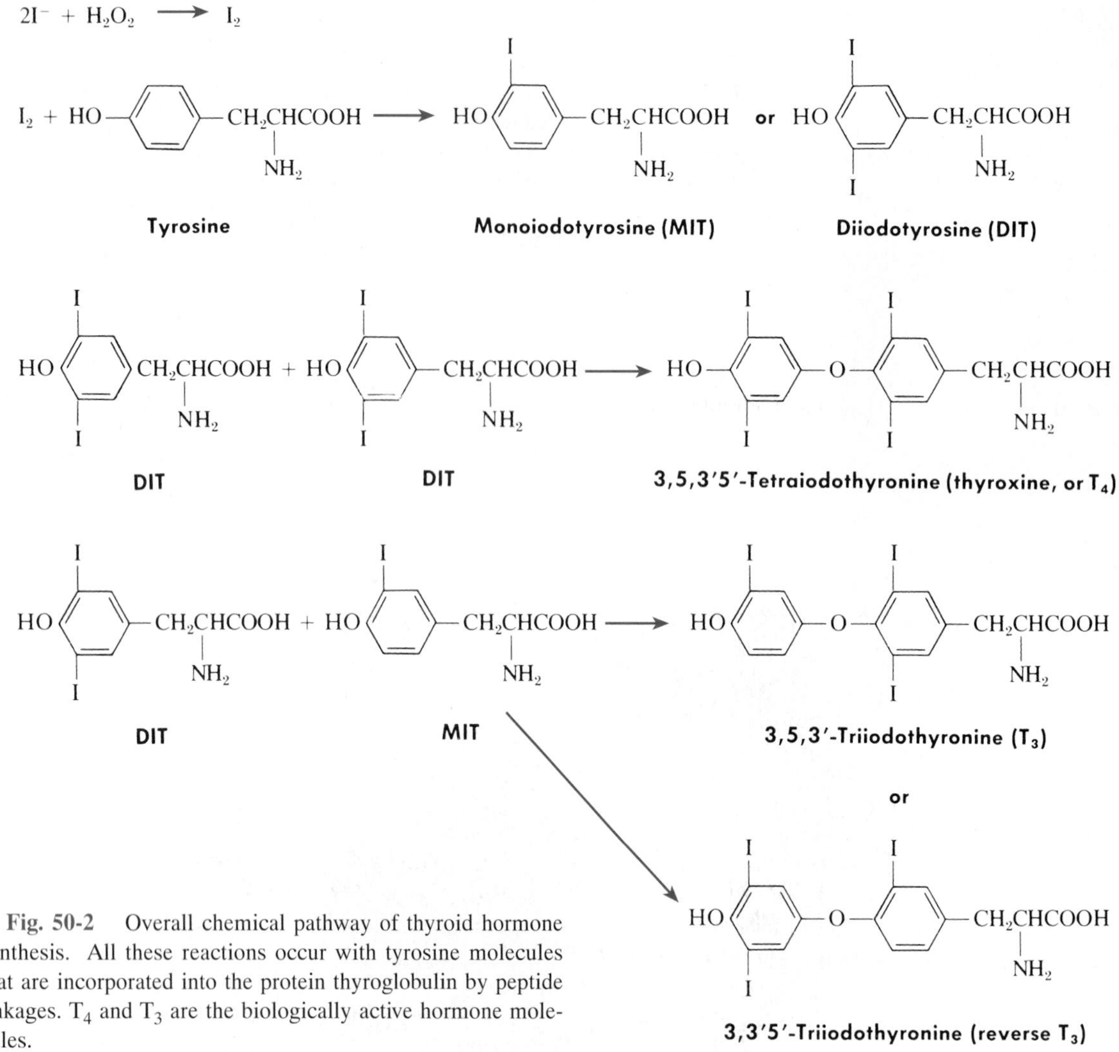

$$2I^- + H_2O_2 \longrightarrow I_2$$

$$I_2 + HO-\text{⟨⟩}-CH_2CHCOOH \longrightarrow HO-\text{⟨⟩}-CH_2CHCOOH \quad \text{or} \quad HO-\text{⟨⟩}-CH_2CHCOOH$$

Tyrosine   **Monoiodotyrosine (MIT)**   **Diiodotyrosine (DIT)**

DIT   DIT   3,5,3'5'-Tetraiodothyronine (thyroxine, or T₄)

DIT   MIT   3,5,3'-Triiodothyronine (T₃)

or

3,3'5'-Triiodothyronine (reverse T₃)

■ **Fig. 50-2** Overall chemical pathway of thyroid hormone synthesis. All these reactions occur with tyrosine molecules that are incorporated into the protein thyroglobulin by peptide linkages. T₄ and T₃ are the biologically active hormone molecules.

to 35%) gives a dynamic index of thyroid gland activity. The total iodide content of the thyroid gland averages 7500 μg, virtually all of which is in the form of iodothyronines. In a steady-state condition, 70 to 80 μg of iodide, or about 1% of the total, is released from the gland daily. Of this amount, 75% is secreted as thyroid hormone and the remainder is free iodide. The large ratio (100:1) of iodide stored in the form of hormone to the amount turned over daily protects the individual from the effects of iodide deficiency for about 2 months. Iodide is further conserved by a marked reduction in iodide renal excretion as the circulating concentration and filtered load fall.

A deficiency of iodide is a major cause of **hypothyroidism** in such varied areas of the world as China and the Peruvian Andes. This tragic form of endemic **cretinism** (see below) can be easily prevented by public health programs that provide yearly injections of a slowly absorbed iodide preparation.

Iodide is actively transported into the gland against chemical and electrical gradients by a Na⁺-I⁻ cotransport (symport) system located in the basal membrane of the thyroid epithelial cells (see Chapter 1). Normally, a thyroid/plasma-free iodide ratio of 30 is maintained. This so-called **iodide trap** requires energy generation by oxidative phosphorylation and is linked to a Na⁺, K⁺-ATPase. The iodide trap is markedly stimulated by TSH, mediated through cyclic AMP (cAMP). This stimulation may also require the synthesis of a specific protein, possibly the iodide carrier itself. The trap displays saturation kinetics. A primary reduction in dietary iodide intake depletes the circulating iodide pool and greatly enhances the activity of the iodide trap. Under these circumstances, the percentage of thyroid uptake of iodide can reach 80% to 90%.

A number of anions, such as thiocyanate (CNS_4^-), perchlorate ($HClO_4^-$), and pertechnetate (TcO_4^-) act as competitive inhibitors of active iodide transport. If iodide cannot be rapidly incorporated into tyrosine after its

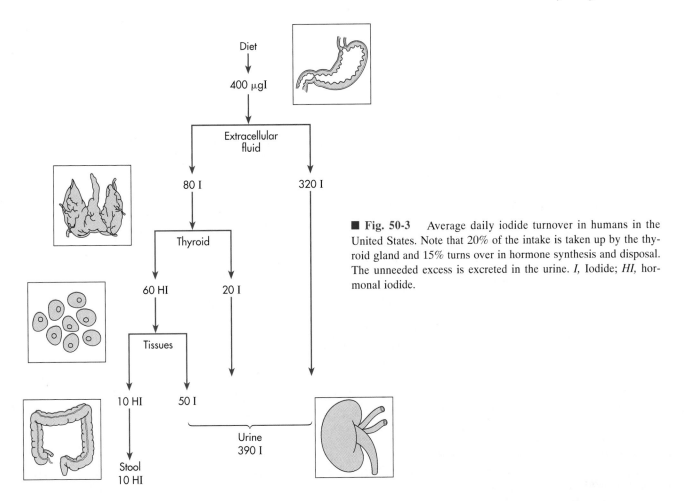

■ **Fig. 50-3** Average daily iodide turnover in humans in the United States. Note that 20% of the intake is taken up by the thyroid gland and 15% turns over in hormone synthesis and disposal. The unneeded excess is excreted in the urine. *I*, Iodide; *HI*, hormonal iodide.

uptake by the cell, administration of one of these competitive anions will, by blocking further uptake, cause a rapid discharge of the iodide from the gland. This discharge occurs as a result of the high thyroid/plasma concentration gradient.

Rapid iodide discharge can be demonstrated by monitoring the thyroid gland in vivo after the iodide pool is labeled with radioactive iodine. This procedure assists in the diagnosis of biosynthetic defects in hormone synthesis. In its radioactive form as $^{99m}TcO_4$, pertechnetate is a useful substitute for radioactive iodide in the measurement of the trapping function and in the visualization of thyroid gland anatomy by external isotope scanning with a photon detector.

The steps in thyroid hormone synthesis subsequent to entry of iodide into the gland are shown in Fig. 50-2 and depicted in Fig. 50-4. Once within the gland, iodide rapidly moves to the apical surface of the epithelial cells and into the lumen of the follicles. Iodide (I^-) is immediately oxidized to iodine (I^0) and incorporated into tyrosine molecules (Fig. 50-2). The latter are not free in solution but are incorporated by peptide linkages within **thyroglobulin.** Thyroglobulin is a large glycoprotein that also contains covalently bound phosphate and sulfate residues. Thyroglobulin is synthesized on the rough endoplasmic reticulum of thyroid epithelial cells as peptide units of molecular weight 330,000 (the primary translation product of its messenger RNA). These units combine, after which carbohydrate moieties are added as the molecule moves to the Golgi apparatus. The completed protein is contained in small vesicles, which move to the apical plasma membrane and into the adjacent lumen of the follicle (Fig. 50-4).

Immediately within the follicle at the apical membrane-colloid interface, thyroglobulin is iodinated to form both **monoiodotyrosine (MIT)** and **diiodotyrosine (DIT)** (Fig. 50-2). After iodination, two DIT molecules are coupled to form T_4, or one MIT and one DIT molecule are coupled to form T_3. Very little rT_3 is synthesized. This entire sequence of reactions is catalyzed by **thyroid peroxidase,** an enzyme complex largely localized to the apical membrane. The immediate oxidant (electron acceptor) for the reaction iodide $\rightarrow$ iodine is hydrogen peroxide. The mechanism whereby hydrogen peroxide is itself generated in the thyroid gland likely involves reduction of oxygen by NADPH via NADPH oxidase.

A closer look at the formation of MIT and DIT reveals that a single tyrosine, located at the fifth position from the N terminus of both MIT and DIT (site A), is a preferential but not an exclusive site of synthesis of T_4 or T_3.

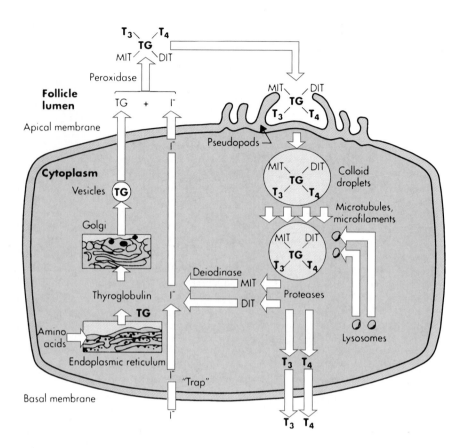

■ **Fig. 50-4** Overall schema of thyroid hormone synthesis and release. T_4 and T_3 synthesis occurs within the protein molecule thyroglobulin *(TG)* at the border of the cytoplasm and the follicle lumen. Retrieval of stored hormone requires endocytosis of the colloid followed by intracytoplasmic proteolysis by lysosomes. Iodide in the precursor molecules monoiodotyrosine *(MIT)* and diiodotyrosine *(DIT)* is recovered by the action of the enzyme deiodinase.

About 10% of all tyrosines in thyroglobulin are iodinated. Both iodide and tyrosines are complexed to sites on the peroxidase enzyme; they undergo oxidation by H_2O_2 and are then combined to form MIT or DIT. The next step, coupling, may be facilitated by the three-dimensional structure of thyroglobulin, which brings an MIT or DIT molecule at site A next to a second MIT or DIT molecule that is buried deeper within thyroglobulin. The second MIT or DIT donates its iodinated phenolic ring to the first MIT or DIT at site A. Depending on the pairing, this process produces T_4 or T_3 at site A and leaves dehydroalanine in peptide linkage within the deeper portion of thyroglobulin.

Thyroglobulin iodination occurs rapidly; labeled iodide appears in hormone molecules 1 minute after in vivo administration. After 1 hour, 90% to 95% of iodide is organically bound. The usual distribution of iodoaminoacids, as residues per molecule of thyroglobulin, is MIT, 7; DIT, 6; T_4, 2; and T_3, 0.2. Approximately one third of the iodine in thyroglobulin is in the form of calorigenic hormone (T_4 and T_3). Certain factors regulate the ratio of T_3 synthesis to T_4 synthesis. When iodide availability is restricted, the formation of T_3 is favored. Because T_3 is three times as potent as T_4, this response provides more active hormone per molecule of organified iodide. The proportion of T_3 is also increased when the gland is hyperstimulated by TSH or other activators.

Once thyroglobulin has been iodinated, it is stored in the lumen of the follicle as colloid (Fig. 50-4). Release of the peptide-linked T_4 and T_3 into the bloodstream

requires proteolysis of the thyroglobulin. Histochemical and radiographic studies have demonstrated that the colloid is retrieved from the lumen of the follicle by the epithelial cell through endocytosis. A thyroglobulin receptor in the apical membrane may facilitate this process. Endocytosis starts when the plasma cell membrane forms pseudopods that engulf a pocket of colloid. After this portion of the luminal content has been pinched off by the plasma cell membrane, it appears as a colloid droplet within the cytoplasm (Fig. 50-5). The droplet moves through the cytoplasm toward the basal membrane, probably as a result of microtubule and microfilament function. At the same time, lysosomes move from the base toward the apex of the cell and fuse with the colloid droplets. The action of the lysosomal proteases then releases free T_4 and T_3, which leave the cell through the plasma membrane at the basal end and enter the bloodstream via the adjacent rich capillary plexus.

The MIT and DIT molecules, which also are released during proteolysis of thyroglobulin, are rapidly deiodinated within the follicular cell by the enzyme **deiodinase** (Fig. 50-4.) Because MIT and DIT are metabolically useless and would be lost in the urine if secreted, their deiodination retrieves the iodide for recycling into T_4 and T_3 synthesis. Only minor amounts of intact thyroglobulin leave the follicular cell under normal circumstances.

In acute and subacute inflammations of the thyroid gland, disruption of thyroid follicles leads to leakage

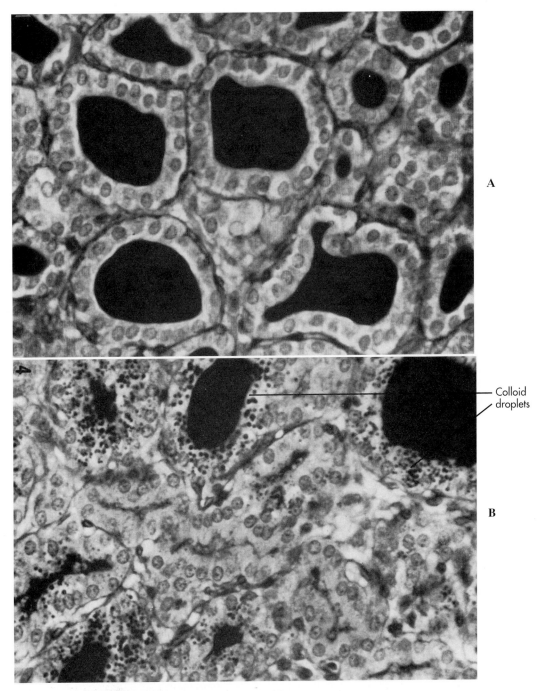

Colloid droplets

■ **Fig. 50-5**   Histologic demonstration of the process of resorption of colloid. **A,** Unstimulated follicles. **B,** Within minutes of TSH administration, colloid droplets are seen inside the follicular cells. (From Wollman SH et al: *J Cell Biol* 21:191, 1964. From The Rockefeller University Press.)

of thyroglobulin into the circulation. The elevated plasma levels of thyroglobulin can be diagnostic of such diseases. In cases of thyroid cancer, total surgical removal of the gland and subsequent ablation of any gland remnants by radioactive iodine are usually performed. After such treatment, the presence of significant levels of thyroglobulin in the plasma indicates the existence of persistent or recurrent cancer cells somewhere in the body.

■ *Regulation of Thyroid Gland Activity*

The most important regulator of thyroid gland function and growth is the hypothalamic-pituitary TRH-TSH axis (see Chapter 49 and Fig. 49-6). Because the diurnal (within a day) variation of TSH secretion is small, thyroid hormone secretion and plasma concentrations are also relatively constant. Only small nocturnal increases in secretion of TSH and release of T_4 occur. *TSH stimulates the synthesis of thyroglobulin, the process of iodide trapping, and each of the subsequent steps in T_4 and T_3 synthesis. It also stimulates endocytosis of colloid, the proteolysis of thyroglobulin, and the release of T_4 and T_3 from the gland.* Sustained TSH stimulation leads to hypertrophy and hyperplasia of the follicular cells. The enlarged cells show an increased volume of endoplasmic reticulum, increased numbers of ribosomes, a larger and more complex Golgi apparatus, and an increase in DNA synthesis. Proliferation of capillaries is also observed, and thyroid blood flow increases. In the absence of TSH, marked atrophy of the gland occurs. However, in humans, a low basal level of thyroid hormone production and release can continue seemingly independent of TSH.

The regulatory effects of TSH are exerted through multiple actions (Fig. 50-6). The initial step is binding of TSH to a plasma transmembrane receptor of 764 amino acids. The extracellular α subunit of the receptor binds the α and β subunits of TSH. The β subunit of the receptor probably winds through the plasma membrane seven times and is functionally linked to adenylyl cyclase by a G protein. The β subunit ends in a short intracellular tail of about 80 amino acids. Although the β subunit of TSH confers its specificity for the TSH receptor, it is the α subunit of TSH (common to LH and FSH) that initiates the messenger cascade. This subunit of the TSH molecule binds to the N terminus of the extracellular domain of the receptor. The binding triggers a conformational change in the receptor and causes the C terminus of its extracellular domain to contact the transmembrane sites in the receptor. The latter then interact with neighboring G proteins that activate adenylyl cyclase. The resultant increases in cAMP levels mediate TSH stimulation of iodide uptake by the cell, as well as many of its other actions on T_4 and T_3 synthesis. The phosphatidylinositol second messenger system helps to mediate some TSH effects.

Within minutes of thyroid cell exposure to TSH, thyroglobulin, which is stored within the follicular lumen, undergoes endocytosis, and colloid droplets appear in the cytoplasm (Fig. 50-5). Shortly thereafter, iodide uptake and peroxidase activity increase. Currently, TSH also stimulates glucose oxidation, especially via the hexose monophosphate shunt. This reaction may be the means for generating the NADPH needed for the peroxidase reaction.

Further effects of TSH on the thyroid gland occur after a delay of hours to days. TSH stimulates transcription of the thyroglobulin and peroxidase genes, an action medi-

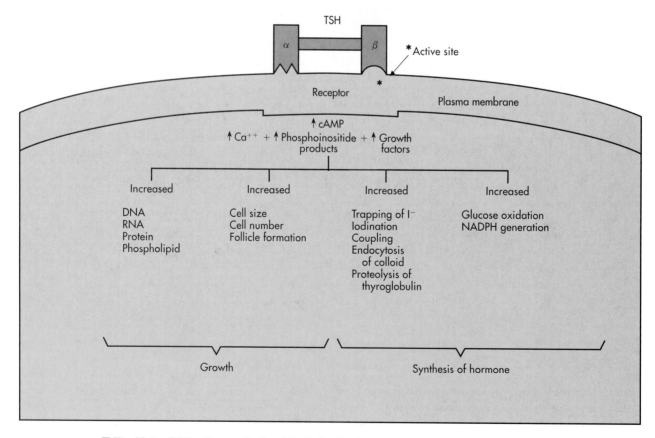

■ **Fig. 50-6**   TSH actions on the thyroid cell. Cyclic adenosine monophosphate (cAMP) along with calcium ions (Ca++) and phosphoinositol products act as second messengers generated by TSH binding to its receptor. All steps in thyroid hormone production, as well as many aspects of thyroid cell metabolism and growth, are stimulated by TSH. Growth factors are important intermediaries in cell proliferation and in synthesis of some proteins such as thyroglobulin.

ated by a specific protein transcription factor. Both insulin and insulin-like growth factors (IGFs) are also required for thyroglobulin synthesis to proceed. Nucleic acid and protein synthesis are also generally increased, via effects on both transcription and translation. These actions, which underlie the growth-promoting effects of TSH on the gland, are supported by local production of IGFs and epidermal growth factor in response to TSH.

The regulation of thyroid hormone secretion by TSH is under exquisite feedback control (see Fig. 49-6). Circulating T_4 and T_3 each produce feedback to the pituitary to decrease TSH secretion; if the levels of T_4 and T_3 fall, TSH secretion increases. It is free T_4 and T_3, not the protein-bound portions, that regulate pituitary TSH output. The pituitary gland is capable of deiodinating T_4 to T_3, and the latter acts as the final effector molecule in turning off TSH.

Mutant TSH receptors that are constitutively activated without hormone binding are one cause of thyroid adenomas and **hyperthyroidism.** These adenomas secrete T_4 and T_3 autonomously, that is, independent of TSH. The excessive production of T_4 and T_3 suppresses TSH secretion by negative feedback. The lack of TSH then leaves the remaining normal thyroid tissue atrophied and functionless. In another form of hyperthyroidism, **Graves' disease,** autoantibodies to the TSH receptor are produced. These immunoglobulins react with the TSH receptor and activate adenylyl cyclase, just as TSH does. The results are again a stimulated, TSH-independent gland and very low plasma TSH levels. Only rarely is hyperthyroidism caused by excess TSH from an adenoma of the pituitary thyrotrophs.

Another important regulator of thyroid gland function is iodide itself, which has a biphasic action. At relatively low levels of iodide intake, the rate of thyroid hormone synthesis is directly related to iodide availability. However, if the intake of iodide exceeds 2 mg/day, the intraglandular concentration of iodide (or some organic iodine product) reaches a level that inhibits the iodide trap and the mechanism of hormone biosynthesis. Thus, hormone production declines to normal. This autoregulatory phenomenon is known as the **Wolff-Chaikoff effect.** In unusual instances, the inhibition of hormone synthesis by iodide can be great enough to induce thyroid hormone deficiency.

Other modes of autoregulation may help prevent excessive responses to TSH stimulation. Thyroglobulin inhibits binding of TSH to its receptors, as well as the response of adenylyl cyclase to the tropic hormone. In addition, T_4 and T_3 also directly inhibit the thyroid gland in vitro. The thyroid also receives adrenergic, VIPergic, and cholinergic innervation. Epinephrine and vasoactive intestinal polypeptide (VIP) stimulate T_4 release via increased cAMP, and acetylcholine inhibits it via

increased cGMP. Prostaglandins also mimic some of the effects of TSH. The physiological roles of the above influences are not clear.

Thyroid hormones increase oxygen utilization, energy expenditure, and heat production. Therefore, it is logical to expect that the availability of active thyroid hormone correlates with changes in the body's caloric and thermal status. In fact, ingestion of excess calories, particularly in the form of carbohydrate, increases the production and plasma concentration of T_3 as well as the individual's metabolic rate, whereas prolonged fasting leads to corresponding decreases. However, similar fluctuations in T_4 do not occur. Therefore, because most T_3 arises from circulating T_4 (Table 50-1), peripheral mechanisms are more important in mediating these changes than are alterations in thyroid gland secretion.

In animals, exposure to cold increases thyroid gland activity. Humans living in cold polar zones also increase T_3 production and modestly increase TSH responsiveness to TRH. In the neonatal period, when the infant suddenly becomes responsible for maintenance of its own body temperature, an acute rise in TSH secretion is followed by a rise in plasma T_4 to levels well above those of adults. Over the ensuing weeks or months, plasma T_4 then subsides to a range that remains stable in adult life until a small decline occurs with senescence.

Pharmacologic inhibition of thyroid gland activity is of major therapeutic importance. A class of drugs known as **thiouracils** suppresses the synthesis of T_4 and T_3 by inhibiting peroxidase activity. Because organification is blocked, iodide taken up by activity of the iodide trap is rapidly discharged again, as can be shown by studies with radioactive iodine (see above). After administration of thiouracils has continued for weeks, the stores of thyroid hormone (and of iodide) become depleted. These drugs are effective in the treatment of **hyperthyroidism.**

Lithium, frequently used to treat manic-depressive illness, inhibits the release of thyroid hormones and, secondarily, their synthesis, probably by blocking adenylyl cyclase and cAMP accumulation. Thus,

■ Table 50-1   Average thyroid hormone turnover

	T_4	T_3	rT_3
Daily production (μg)	90	35	35
From thyroid (%)	100	25	5
From T_4 (%)	—	75	95
Extracellular pool (μg)	850	40	40
Plasma concentration			
Total (μg/dl)	8.0	0.12	0.04
Free (ng/dl)	2.0	0.28	0.20
Half-life (days)	7	1	0.8
Metabolic clearance (L/day)	1	26	77
Fractional turnover per day (%)	10	75	90

lithium can cause **hypothyroidism.** Finally, a large excess of iodide, in addition to the effects previously noted, can also promptly inhibit thyroid hormone release. Although this action is transient, the administration of iodide for several weeks may benefit individuals with severe hyperthyroidism.

■ *Metabolism of Thyroid Hormones*

Table 50-1 shows the average daily production rates, pool sizes, plasma concentrations, half-lives, metabolic clearances, and fractional turnovers of T_4, T_3, and rT_3. *T_4 is clearly the dominant secreted and circulating form of thyroid hormone.* In contrast, the major portion of T_3 and virtually all of rT_3 are derived secondarily from circulating T_4, rather than primarily from thyroid gland secretion. *Thus, T_4 serves primarily as a prohormone for T_3, in addition to probably providing some intracellular action of its own.* This "storage" function of plasma T_4 is also reflected in its much lower metabolic clearance and fractional turnover rates, compared with those of T_3 or rT_3. The small amount of intact thyroglobulin that is secreted circulates at an average plasma concentration of 5 ng/ml.

Most conversion of T_4 to T_3 occurs in tissues with high blood flows and rapid exchanges with plasma, such as the liver and possibly the kidneys. This process supplies circulating T_3 for uptake by other tissues in which local T_3 generation is too restricted to provide sufficient thyroid hormone action. Aging is associated with a decrease in TSH secretion, which in turn leads to a decrease in T_4 production. Because this decrease in the T_4 level is balanced by a reduction in T_4 degradation, plasma T_4 levels are essentially unchanged. However, plasma T_3 levels decline slightly.

Secreted T_4 and T_3 circulate in the bloodstream almost entirely bound to proteins. Normally, only about 0.03% of total plasma T_4 and 0.3% of total plasma T_3 exist in the free state (Table 50-1). However, free T_4 and T_3 are the critical fractions that are *biologically active*, not only in exerting thyroid hormone effects on peripheral tissues but in pituitary feedback as well. The major binding protein is **thyroxine-binding globulin (TBG).** TBG is a glycoprotein α globulin that is synthesized in the liver. Each TBG molecule binds one molecule of T_4; at the normal TBG concentration of 1.5 ng/dl, 20 μg of T_4 can be bound per deciliter.

About 70% of circulating T_4 and T_3 is bound to TBG; 10% to 15% is bound to another specific thyroid-binding protein called **transthyretin (TTR).** Albumin binds 15% to 20%, and 3% is bound to lipoproteins. Compared with TBG, TTR and albumin have much lower affinities but much higher capacities for binding T_4 and T_3. Ordinarily, however, only alterations in TBG concentration significantly affect total plasma T_4 and T_3 levels.

Two biological functions have been ascribed to TBG. First, it maintains a large circulating reservoir of T_4,

which buffers any acute changes in thyroid gland function. Even the instant addition to the plasma of the amount of calorigenic hormone needed for an entire day would cause a barely perceptible increase in the total T_4 concentration (Fig. 50-7). Conversely, after removal of the thyroid gland, it would take 1 week for the plasma T_4 concentration to fall as much as 50%. Second, the binding of plasma T_4 and T_3 to large proteins prevents the loss of these relatively small hormone molecules into the urine, and thereby helps conserve iodide. The roles of TTR and perhaps also of albumin are to deliver T_4 and T_3 to cells; TTR, in particular, may provide thyroid hormones to the central nervous system.

The reservoir function of TBG is best understood by examining the chemical equilibrium between T_4 and TBG. This equilibrium governs the distribution of the hormone between the free (T_4) and bound ($T_4 \cdot$ TBG) forms.

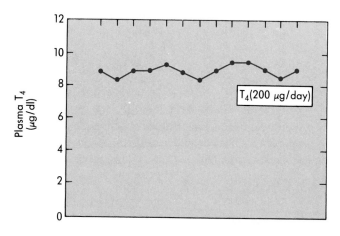

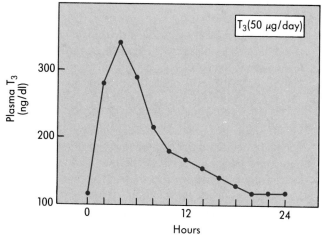

■ **Fig. 50-7** Effect of administering a single day's supply of thyroid hormone by mouth to hypothyroid individuals. Note that 50 μg of T_3 elevates plasma T_3 levels for many hours, whereas 200 μg of T_4 causes no significant change in plasma T_4 (or T_3). This occurs because of the much larger pool size and tighter protein binding of T_4 than of T_3. (Redrawn from Saberi M et al: Serum thyroid hormone and thyrotropin concentrations during thyroxine and triiodothyronine therapy, *J Clin Endocrinol Metab* 39:923, 1974.)

$$T_4 + TBG \rightleftharpoons T_4 \cdot TBG \qquad (50\text{-}1)$$

$$Keq = \frac{[T_4 \cdot TBG]}{[T_4]\,[TBG]} \qquad (50\text{-}2)$$

$$\frac{[T_4]}{[T_4 \cdot TBG]} = \frac{Free\ T_4}{Bound\ T_4} = \frac{1}{Keq\,[TBG]} \qquad (50\text{-}3)$$

$$[T_4] = [T_4 \cdot TBG] \times \frac{1}{Keq\,[TBG]} \qquad (50\text{-}4)$$

A temporary decrease in free T_4, caused by a decrease in thyroid gland output or accelerated uptake by target cells, can be rapidly compensated for by dissociation of bound T_4 ($T_4 \cdot TBG$), until the new ratio of $T_4/(T_4 \cdot TBG)$ returns to that required by Keq (equation 50-3). A temporary increase in free T_4, caused by endogenous secretion or exogenous administration, can be rapidly compensated for by association of the excess T_4 with TBG, because normally only 30% of the available T_4-binding sites on TBG are occupied. Of course, *sustained decreases or increases in T_4 supply that are caused by thyroid disease, eventually lead to sustained decreases or increases in free T_4*, because the latter is directly proportional to $T_4 \cdot TBG$ (equation 50-4).

Note also that a primary change in TBG concentration will also disturb the ratio of free to bound T_4 (equation 50-3). In this situation, the normal thyroid gland must increase or decrease its rate of hormone secretion appropriately, until the new equilibrium state restores the free T_4 level to normal.

TBG concentration can decrease because of reduced hepatic synthesis (liver disease) or excessive loss in the urine (kidney disease). The free T_4 concentration will then increase temporarily. In compensation, pituitary TSH secretion will be suppressed by negative feedback. T_4 output by the thyroid gland will then decrease until the new, lower steady-state level of bound $T_4 \cdot TBG$ yields a normal level of free T_4 (equation 50-4). TBG levels can also increase, most commonly because of estrogen administration or pregnancy. In this situation, free T_4 will decrease temporarily; this decrease will stimulate pituitary secretion of TSH. Consequently, T_4 output by the thyroid gland will increase. T_4 output will continue until the elevated level of bound $T_4 \cdot TBG$ is sufficient to restore the free T_4 level to normal in a new steady-state condition.

Although major alterations in TBG are not usually caused by thyroid gland disease, TBG levels must be considered when plasma total thyroid hormone concentrations are measured for diagnostic purposes.

Identical considerations govern the circulating levels of free and bound T_3. However, the buffering action of TBG is less effective for T_3 (Fig. 50-7), because the Keq for T_3 is an order of magnitude lower than that for T_4 (2×10^9 versus 2×10^{10}, respectively) and because the total extrathyroidal pool of T_3 is much smaller than that of T_4 (Table 50-1). Thus, rapid addition of T_3, in an

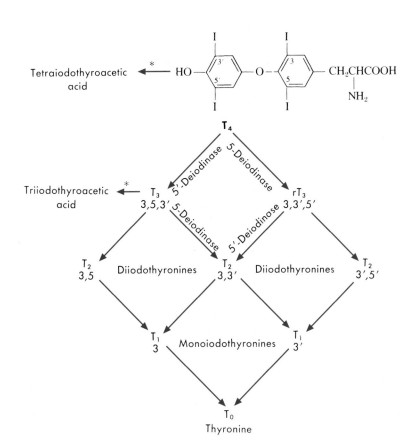

■ **Fig. 50-8**   Peripheral metabolism of thyroxine *(T₄)* is largely by successive deiodinations. A key regulatory step is the proportion of T_4 undergoing the initial deiodination to metabolically active T_3 versus metabolically inactive rT_3. Asterisks signify oxidative deamination and decarboxylation. T_4 and T_3 sulfates and glucuronides are also formed in small amounts.

amount equivalent to the calorigenic hormone needed for an entire day, produces greater swings in the concentrations of total and free T_3 (Fig. 50-7).

The major pathways of peripheral metabolism of circulating thyroid hormones are outlined in Fig. 50-8. Most of the T_4 that is released by the gland daily undergoes deiodination. However, approximately 15% is irreversibly excreted in the bile as the various iodothyronines in glucuronide or sulfate conjugates. Tetraiodoacetic acid and triiodoacetic acid are less important metabolites. The liver, kidney, and skeletal muscle are the major sites of T_4 degradation. The overall rate of disposal of T_4 is directly related to the free T_4 concentration in the plasma. Thus, T_4 increases its own degradative metabolism. The entire cascade of products—T_3, T_2, and T_1—of the sequential deiodination steps is regularly increased in the plasma in hyperthyroidism (T_4 excess) and is usually decreased in hypothyroidism (T_4 deficiency).

Relationship between Hormone Metabolism and Hormone Action

The initial step in T_4 metabolism—the intracellular conversion of T_4 to either T_3 or rT_3—is of critical importance to thyroid hormone action. T_3 is the hormone of greatest biological activity, whereas rT_3 has no significant calorigenic action. Therefore, factors that regulate the relative rates of outer ring versus inner ring monodeiodination (Fig. 50-8) also determine the quantitative biological effect of secreted T_4. The T_3 generating activity, **5′- monodeiodination,** is supplied by several tissue-specific types of the enzyme 5′ monodeiodinase. In the pituitary gland and certain areas of the brain, the affinity of the isoenzyme for T_4 is high, a characteristic that strongly favors local T_3 generation. The liver and kidney have a different isoenzyme with a lower affinity but a higher capacity for T_4; this same isoenzyme also has a high affinity and capacity for rT_3. In these organs, regulation of the circulating T_3 supply, as well as disposition of unneeded excess T_4, is favored. This deiodinase isoenzyme is distinguished by the presence of the rare amino acid selenocysteine in its composition. The essential trace element, selenium, therefore plays a role in thyroid physiology.

In humans, the normal distribution of T_4 products is approximately 45% T_3 and 55% rT_3. An increase in T_4 concentration leads to a decrease in its conversion to T_3. Thus, the biological effects of T_4 excess or deficiency are automatically slightly mitigated by accelerated or retarded metabolic inactivation, respectively.

Certain clinical states and factors are associated with reduced conversion of T_4 to T_3 and often with a reciprocally enhanced conversion of T_4 to rT_3. These conditions include the gestational period, fasting, major medical and surgical stress, catabolic diseases, hepatic disease, renal failure, thiouracil drugs, and β-adrenergic blockade. In many cases, inhibition of the hepatic 5′-monodeiodinase isoenzyme appears to explain this switch. As seen in Fig. 50-8, inhibition of 5′ monodeiodinase decreases production of T_3 from T_4 (reducing plasma T_3) and simultaneously decreases degradation of rT_3 to $3,3'T_2$ (increasing plasma rT_3). The reduction of 5′ monodeiodinase activity may also result from decreased glucose metabolism, increased free fatty acid (FFA) metabolism, and excess secretion of the stress hormone cortisol. When 5′ monodeiodinase activity is reduced, sulfation of T_4 and T_3 increases and sulfation greatly diminishes the biological activity of whatever T_3 is produced.

The biological effects of T_4 are largely a result of its intracellular conversion to T_3. T_3 has 10 times the affinity for the thyroid receptor for (TR) as T_4 (and 100 times the affinity as rT_3). When administered exogenously, T_3 is three to four times more potent than T_4 in humans. However, evidence continues to favor some intrinsic biological activity of T_4 itself. For example, in hypothyroid individuals, a low plasma T_4 level (and high TSH level) can be accompanied by a state of biological thyroid deficiency, despite a normal plasma T_3. Conversely, a clinically normal state can exist with a normal plasma T_4 concentration despite a low plasma T_3. In the absence of endogenous thyroid gland function, the maintenance of a euthyroid (normal) state requires exogenous doses of T_3 that sustain supranormal plasma T_3 levels, whereas only doses of T_4 that sustain normal plasma T_4 levels are required. A possible explanation for this phenomenon is that the T_3 that has been generated from T_4 *intracellularly* might be more efficient than the T_3 that reaches its intracellular sites of action from the circulation.

Intracellular Actions of Thyroid Hormone

Free T_4 and T_3 enter cells by a carrier-mediated, energy-dependent process. Within the cell, most, if not all, of the T_4 is converted to T_3 (or rT_3). T_3 and T_4 bind to a nuclear receptor protein of the steroid hormone–vitamin D family (Fig. 50-9) (see also Chapter 45 and Fig. 45-13). This thyroid receptor (TR) is associated with chromatin, usually template inactive. At least three forms of TR exist, and these forms are expressed in a tissue-specific manner by separate genes. One form, the *unliganded* TR, is usually found bound to thyroid regulatory elements (TREs) in target genes. *TR constitutively represses most gene expression, although certain genes may be constitutively activated.* Binding of T_3 (or possibly T_4, see below) to TR relieves the repression exerted through the TRE, and thus gene expression is induced.

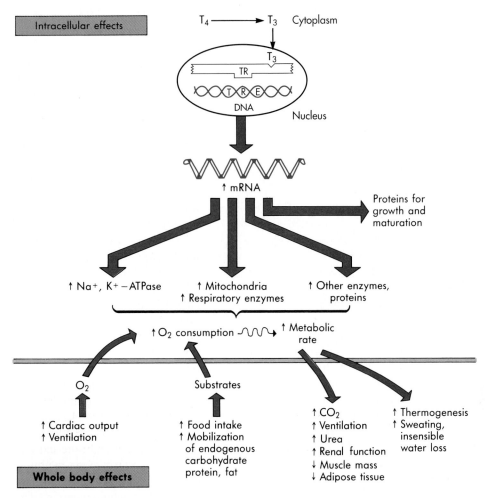

Fig. 50-9 Overall schema of thyroid hormone effects. The upper portion represents intracellular actions resulting from T_3 binding to its nuclear receptor *(TR)*, which is linked to thyroid regulatory elements (TREs) in target DNA molecules. The lower portion catalogs all the various whole body effects of thyroid hormone that sustain increased oxygen consumption and permit disposal of the excess CO_2, heat, and metabolic products.

TREs have two half-sites with the nucleotide base sequence AGGTCA. Two TRs can form a homodimer that binds to both TRE half-sites, but more often one TR molecule and one retinoid receptor molecule form a heterodimer that, when bound to T_3, activates the target gene. The two TRE half-sites can function as direct repeats of each other, palindromes, reverse palindromes, or even as single sites themselves. One endogenous molecule analogous to the T_3 receptor also exists that does not bind T_3 but can bind to the TRE and block T_3 action. A host of T_3 target genes exist, including those for growth hormone, osteocalcin, myosin chains, malic enzyme, TSH, and the T_3 receptor itself. An additional cell-specific, constitutive basal factor is necessary to permit T_3-receptor complex action on certain genes in some cells and at some stages of development. Subsequent to T_3-TR-TRE interactions, a large number of messenger RNA levels are increased or decreased, and the synthesis of the related proteins is altered accordingly.

In addition to nuclear receptors, thyroid hormone–binding sites have been identified by some investigators in ribosomes, mitochondria, and the plasma membrane. Binding of thyroid hormone to these sites may mediate post-transcriptional and pretranslational events, such as association of messenger RNA with ribosomes, or post-translational processes, such as membrane transport. These mechanisms may explain some thyroid hormone actions that are not presently accounted for by modulation of gene expression.

The responsiveness of tissues to T_3 correlates with their nuclear receptor number and with the degree of receptor saturation, although not always in a linear manner. In humans, ordinarily about half the available T_3 receptor sites are occupied. In some tissues, T_3 may down-regulate its own receptor by inhibiting its synthesis; this action provides still another means for receptor modulation of T_3 action. Because thyroid hormone appears to act largely through influencing transcription, many of its effects can be blocked by inhibitors of protein synthesis. Usually, there is a 12- to 48-hour delay before most of the hormone's effects become evident in vivo. Indeed, several weeks of T_4 replacement are required before all the consequences of the hypothyroid state in humans are eliminated.

The multitude of thyroid hormone actions is still difficult to explain exactly on an intracellular basis. A large catalog of changes in enzymes, structural and functional proteins, and substrates—all induced by thyroid hormone—can be listed (Table 50-2). However, a single final common pathway that serves as a unifying mechanism of the hormone's actions, particularly on oxygen utilization, has not yet been incontrovertibly established. The hormone acts at multiple loci, which vary in different tissues. General effects in the nucleus include stimulation of RNA polymerase and phosphoprotein kinases and the synthesis of other nuclear proteins. These nuclear effects are followed or paralleled by an increase in the biogenesis of mitochondria and their rate of respiration. The number and size of the inner membrane components and the areas of mitochondria, as well as protein synthesis and RNA synthesis of these organelles, are all increased by thyroid hormone. These effects could also involve, at least secondarily, mitochondrial DNA. Key respiratory enzyme activities, such as NADPH cytochrome C reductase and cytochrome oxidase, are increased by thyroid hormone. α-Glycerophosphate dehydrogenase and pyridine nucleotide transhydrogenases, which are important in regulating the levels of pyridine nucleotide cofactors, are likewise increased. Clearly, these actions of thyroid hormone are relevant to increases in oxygen uptake and CO_2 production.

■ **Table 50-2** Selected molecules whose concentration, activity, and/or gene expression is modulated by thyroid hormone

Increased	Decreased
Na+, K+-ATPase (in some tissues)	TSH (thyrotropin)
Cytochrome oxidase	Thyroid hormone
α-Glycerophosphate	receptor
dehydrogenase	Myosin heavy chain-β
Pyridine nucleotide	Creatine kinase
transhydrogenases	Inhibitory G protein
Urea	Total and LDL
Malic enzyme	cholesterol
Ca-ATPase	
Myosin heavy chain-α	
Glucose transporters	
β-Adrenergic receptor	
Stimulatory G protein	
cAMP	
Erythropoietin	
Tyrosine	
Osteocalcin	
Alkaline phosphatase	
Hydroxyproline	
Growth hormone	
Antidiuretic hormone	
Sex steroid–binding globulin	
Metabolites of cortisol	

The level of malic enzyme involved in providing NADPH for fatty acid synthesis is greatly augmented by T_3. In this interesting example, T_3 acts synergistically with large amounts of ingested carbohydrate to multiply an original carbohydrate-generated signal and to provide an enzyme important in converting an excess of glucose to triglycerides. Because this process requires energy, more oxygen is used. Induction of another thyroid-specific protein (labeled S_{14}) in the liver precedes an increase in fatty acid synthase activity, which is another essential enzyme in this whole process.

The clinical observation that thyroid hormone increases the rate of oxygen use without necessarily increasing useful work output suggested that the hormone causes a decrease in the efficiency with which high-energy phosphate bonds are formed during aerobic respiration. Early studies with supraphysiological doses of thyroid hormone supported such a theory. However, this hypothesis has not been borne out. The normal P/O ratios of approximately 3 (fixation of phosphate/O_2 uptake) observed in muscle from hyperthyroid humans and animals have weakened support for this theory.

Another explanation for thyroid hormone's ability to increase oxygen consumption arose from the observation that the hormone increases the activity and amount of plasma membrane Na+, K+-ATPase, an enzyme essential for membrane cation transport (see also Chapter 1). Ouabain, an inhibitor of this enzyme, also blocks the action of thyroid hormone on respiration. Because the sodium pump is responsible for up to 80% of energy turnover in some tissues, large amounts of ADP would be generated by augmenting its activity. The extra ADP that results from the increased Na+, K+-ATPase activity would then stimulate oxygen utilization in the mitochondria.

In keeping with this mechanism is a report that T_3 binds to the inner mitochondrial membrane enzyme adenine nucleotide translocase, which is responsible for transporting adenosine diphosphate (ADP) into and adenosine triphosphate (ATP) out of the mitochondria. However, in some thyroid-sensitive tissues, Na+, K+-ATPase accounts for only 15% of total oxygen utilization. Hence, this unified mechanism of thyroid hormone action is dubious. Another suggestion is that thyroid hormone simultaneously stimulates fatty acid synthesis and fatty acid oxidation and thereby operates a futile thermogenic energy cycle in order to produce heat for temperature regulation.

In tissues such as brain, in which oxygen consumption is not stimulated at all, thyroid hormones still increase the synthesis of specific structural or functional proteins. In brain and other tissues, thyroid hormones also stimulate the transport of amino acids across the cell membrane and thereby facilitate protein synthesis. On the other hand, proteolytic and lysosomal enzyme activities in muscle are also increased by thyroid hormone.

■ Whole Body Actions of Thyroid Hormone on Metabolism

■ General Effects

The most obvious in vivo effect of thyroid hormone is to increase the basal rate of oxygen consumption and heat production (Fig. 50-9). This action is demonstrated in all tissues except the brain, gonads, and spleen. Resting oxygen use in humans ranges from about 150 ml/min in the hypothyroid state to about 400 ml/min in the hyperthyroid state (normal, 225-250 ml/min). When standardized to body surface area, the basal metabolic rate ranges from −40% to +80% of normal at the clinical extremes of thyroid function. The respiratory quotient (RQ), which reflects the fuel mix being oxidized (see Chapter 46), is not affected. Glucose and fatty acid oxidation are both increased, as are lactate-glucose recycling and fatty acid–triglyceride recycling. Thyroid hormone does not specifically augment diet-induced oxygen utilization, and it may not change the efficiency of energy use with exercise.

Thermogenesis must also increase concomitantly with oxygen use. Thus, changes in body temperature parallel fluctuations in thyroid hormone availability. The potential increase in body temperature, however, is moderated by a compensatory increase in heat loss through appropriate thyroid hormone–mediated increases in blood flow, sweating, and ventilation.

■ Respiratory Effects

Thyroid hormone could not stimulate oxygen utilization for long without also enhancing oxygen supply. Thus, T_4 and T_3 increase resting respiratory rate, minute ventilation, and ventilatory responses to hypercapnia and hypoxia (see Chapters 33 and 37). These actions maintain a normal arterial PO_2 when O_2 utilization is increased and a normal PCO_2 when CO_2 production is increased. Additionally, the red blood cell mass increases slightly and thereby enhances the oxygen-carrying capacity. This increase in red blood cell mass results from stimulation of erythropoietin production, which arises directly by alteration of its gene expression and indirectly by way of the renal tissue hypoxia that results from increased O_2 use.

■ Cardiac Effects

Most important, thyroid hormone increases cardiac output, ensuring sufficient oxygen delivery to the tissues (Fig. 50-10). The resting heart rate and the stroke volume are both increased. The speed and force of myocardial contractions are enhanced. Systolic blood pressure is modestly augmented and diastolic blood pressure is decreased. The resultant widened pulse pressure reflects the combined effects of the increased stroke volume and the reduction in total peripheral vascular resistance that result from blood vessel dilation in skin, muscle, and heart. These effects in turn are secondary to the increase in tissue production of heat and CO_2 that thyroid hormone induces (see Chapters 26 and 29).

The cardiac inotropic effects are partly indirect, via adrenergic stimulation, and partly direct (Fig. 50-10). Myocardial calcium uptake and adenylyl cyclase activity are increased and enhance contractile force. Thyroid hormone induces the myosin heavy-chain alpha gene and represses the beta gene, thereby increasing the velocity of myocardial contraction. The calcium-ATPase of the sarcolemmal reticulum is increased, which facilitates sequestration of calcium during diastole and shortens the relaxation time.

> The cardiac effects of thyroid hormone are particularly important when aging individuals develop hyperthyroidism. The only clinical manifestation may be the development of rapid **atrial arrhythmias,** such as **flutter** or **fibrillation.** Alternatively, otherwise unexplained heart failure may occur or symptoms of coronary insufficiency may develop or worsen if the aging heart cannot meet the increased tissue oxygen demands.

Normal function of skeletal muscles also requires normal amounts of thyroid hormone. This requirement may well be related to the regulation of energy production and storage in this tissue. Concentrations of creatine phos-

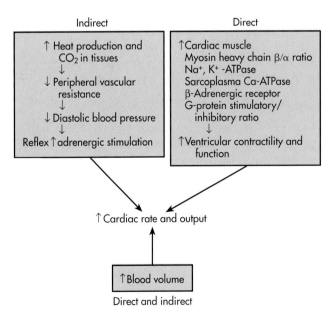

■ **Fig. 50-10** Mechanisms by which thyroid hormone increases cardiac output. The indirect mechanisms are probably quantitatively more important.

phate are reduced by an excess of T_4 and T_3; the inability of muscle to take up and phosphorylate creatine leads to its increased urinary excretion.

■ *Metabolic Effects*

Increased oxygen use ultimately depends on an increased supply of necessary substrates for oxidation. Thyroid hormone stimulates provision of these substrates. T_4 and T_3 augment glucose absorption from the gastrointestinal tract. They increase glucose turnover (glucose uptake, oxidation, and synthesis), lipid turnover (FFA release from adipose tissue and oxidation), plasma triglycerides and FFA, and protein turnover (release of muscle amino acids, protein degradation, and, to a lesser extent, protein synthesis and urea formation). Multiple enzymes in these pathways are also increased by thyroid hormone. T_4 and T_3 potentiate the respective stimulatory effects of epinephrine, norepinephrine, glucagon, cortisol, and growth hormone on gluconeogenesis, lipolysis, ketogenesis, and proteolysis of the labile protein pool. *The overall metabolic effect of thyroid hormone has therefore been aptly described as accelerating the response to starvation.* In addition, thyroid hormone stimulates the synthesis of cholesterol, but more so its oxidation and biliary secretion. The net effect is a decrease in the body pool and plasma levels of total and low-density lipoprotein cholesterol. The synthesis of bile acids is decreased.

The metabolic disposal of adrenal and gonadal steroid hormones, some B vitamins, and some administered drugs is increased by thyroid hormone. Therefore, the endogenous secretion rates of hormones such as cortisol, the dietary requirements of vitamins such as riboflavin, and the doses of drugs such as digoxin that are necessary to maintain normal or effective plasma levels of these substances are all increased by thyroid hormone.

■ *Thyroid Hormone and the Sympathetic Nervous System*

One of the prominent but incompletely understood features of thyroid hormone is its interaction with the sympathetic nervous system. Certain effects of thyroid hormone, such as the increases in metabolic rate, heat production, heart rate, motor activity, and central nervous system excitation, are also produced by the adrenergic catecholamines epinephrine and norepinephrine. An indisputable explanation for this striking similarity remains to be found. Thyroid hormone does not increase the levels of catecholamine hormones or their metabolites in blood, urine, or tissues. Indeed, norepinephrine levels—a marker of sympathetic nervous system activity—are reduced by thyroid hormone. However, increased levels of cAMP, a β-adrenergic second mes-

senger, are found in plasma, urine, and muscle. Furthermore, the cAMP response to epinephrine in cultured myocardial cells is augmented by T_3. At least one mechanism for this important effect is that T_3 induces the increase in the number of β-adrenergic receptors in heart muscle. Synergism between catecholamines and thyroid hormones is also required for maximal thermogenesis, lipolysis, glycogenolysis, and gluconeogenesis to occur. For example, in brown adipose tissue, T_3 amplifies the induction of **thermogenin,** the uncoupling protein, by norepinephrine (see Chapter 46). Catecholamines in turn increase the 5′-monodeiodinase activity of this tissue and thereby increase the local production of the active T_3 molecule.

Hyperthyroidism has a number of causes. Most commonly, the entire gland undergoes hyperplasia as a result of autoimmune stimulation (**Graves' disease**). In this condition, antibodies formed against the TSH receptor bind to it and mimic TSH actions on thyroid growth and hormone synthesis. The next most common cause of hyperthyroidism is the formation of benign neoplasms in one or more areas of the thyroid. These neoplasms have escaped from normal hypothalamic-pituitary regulation and secrete thyroid hormone autonomously. Least common causes are inflammation of the thyroid, excessive pituitary secretion of TSH, or ingestion of exogenous T_4 or T_3.

The patient with an excess of thyroid hormone presents one of the most striking pictures in clinical medicine. *The large increase in metabolic rate causes the highly characteristic combination of weight loss despite an increased intake of food.* The increased heat production causes discomfort in warm environments, excessive sweating, and a greater intake of water. The increase in adrenergic activity is manifested by a rapid heart rate, hyperkinesis, tremor, nervousness, and a wide-eyed stare. Weakness is caused by a loss of muscle mass as well as impairment of muscle function. Other symptoms include a labile emotional state, breathlessness during exercise, and difficulty swallowing or breathing due to compression of the esophagus or trachea by the enlarged thyroid gland (**goiter**).

The diagnosis of hyperthyroidism is established by demonstrating an elevated serum T_4 or T_3 level (appropriately corrected for any abnormalities in TBG concentrations). In most cases, the thyroid uptake of iodine (labeled with ^{131}I or ^{123}I) is excessive. Serum TSH levels are low, because the pituitary is inhibited by the high levels of T_4 and T_3. In rare cases an adenoma of the pituitary thyrotrophs causes hyperthyroids, and TSH levels are high. The most definitive treatment of hyperthyroidism is ablation of thyroid tissue, either by radiation effects of ^{131}I or by surgery. Alternatively, thiouracil drugs are administered.

■ *Effects on Growth and Tissue Development*

Another major effect of thyroid hormone is on growth and maturation. The most spectacular example is the process of metamorphosis in nonhuman vertebrates. Endogenous thyroid hormone levels are very low in amphibians until just before the major stage of metamorphosis. At this point, the hormone levels increase sharply and parallel the rapid change from the larval to the adult form, after which the levels again decline. Thyroid hormone accelerates all aspects of tadpole metamorphosis, including limb growth, tail resorption, shortening of the gastrointestinal tract, and induction of hepatic ureagenesis. These effects are accomplished by thyroid hormone–induced increases in protein and nucleic acid synthesis in the limb buds, proteolytic and hydrolytic enzyme activities in the tail, and the hepatic content of carbamyl phosphate synthase, the rate-limiting enzyme in the urea cycle.

In humans, thyroid hormone stimulates endochondral ossification, linear growth of bone, and maturation of the epiphyseal bone centers (see Chapter 48). T_3 enhances the maturation and activity of chondrocytes in the cartilage growth plate, in part by increasing local somatomedin production and action (see Chapter 49). Although thyroid hormone is not required for linear growth until after birth, it is already essential for normal maturation of growth centers in the bones of the developing fetus. T_3 also stimulates adult bone remodeling, and T_3 receptors are present in osteoblasts. Increased osteoid and bone formation are manifested by increases in plasma levels of alkaline phosphatase and osteocalcin; increased resorption is apparent from increases in urinary excretion of hydroxyproline and pyridinium cross-link compounds (see Chapter 48).

A reduction in bone mass (**osteoporosis**) is recognized as one of the potential consequences of long-term exposure to excess thyroid hormones. Therefore, to prevent this initially silent complication, thyroid hormone replacement therapy for hypothyroid individuals must be carefully titrated.

The regular progression of tooth development and eruption depends on thyroid hormone, as does the normal cycle of growth and maturation of the epidermis, its hair follicles, and nails. The normal degradative processes in these structural and integumentary tissues are also stimulated by thyroid hormone. Thus, either too much or too little thyroid hormone can lead to hair loss and abnormal nail formation.

Thyroid hormone alters the characteristics of subcutaneous tissue by inhibiting the synthesis and increasing the degradation of mucopolysaccharides (glycosoaminoglycans) in the intercellular ground substance as well as that of **fibronectin**, a fibroblast product that causes adherence.

■ *Effects on the Nervous System*

Thyroid hormone performs a critical set of actions on the timing and pace of development of the central nervous system. *If thyroid hormone is deficient in utero and early infancy, growth of the cerebral and cerebellar cortex, proliferation of axons, and branching of dendrites, synaptogenesis, myelinization, and cell migration are all decreased. Irreversible brain damage can result when the deficiency of thyroid hormone is not recognized and treated promptly after birth.* The above structural defects are paralleled by biochemical abnormalities. In various areas of the brain of hypothyroid embryos, the cell size, RNA and protein content, the amount of tubulin- and microtubule-associated protein, the protein and lipid content of myelin, the local production of critical growth factors, and the rates of protein synthesis are found. Enzymes such as succinic dehydrogenase, which is essential for energy generation, and galactosyl sialyl transferase, which is essential for myelin formation, as well as biosynthetic enzymes and receptors for neurotransmitters, are also diminished.

The crucial role of thyroid hormone in central nervous system development is underscored by a number of adaptive phenomena that occur specifically in the neonatal brain and increase the biological effectiveness of thyroid hormone at this critical time. In the cortex and other areas of the brain, brain-specific T_3 receptor is increased. *The activity of a specific brain 5′-monodeiodinase is augmented,* and it enhances the local conversion of T_4 to T_3. Conversely, *the activity of brain 5′-monodeiodinase is diminished,* and it reduces the local degradation of T_3 to $3,3′$ T_2 (see Fig. 50-7). These latter two factors are very important because only T_4—and not T_3—is effectively taken up by immature brain tissue.

Thyroid hormone also enhances wakefulness, alertness, responsiveness to various stimuli, auditory sense, awareness of hunger, memory, and learning capacity. Normal emotional tone also depends on proper thyroid hormone availability. Furthermore, the speed and amplitude of peripheral nerve reflexes are increased by thyroid hormone, as is the motility of the gastrointestinal tract.

In both women and men, thyroid hormone plays an important permissive role in the regulation of reproductive function. The normal ovarian cycle of follicular development, maturation, and ovulation; the homologous testicular process of spermatogenesis; and the maintenance of the healthy pregnant state are all disrupted by significant deviations of thyroid hormone from the normal range. In part, these deleterious effects may be caused by alterations in the metabolism or availability of steroid hormones; for example, thyroid hormone stimu-

A　　　　　　　　　　B　　　　　　　　　　C

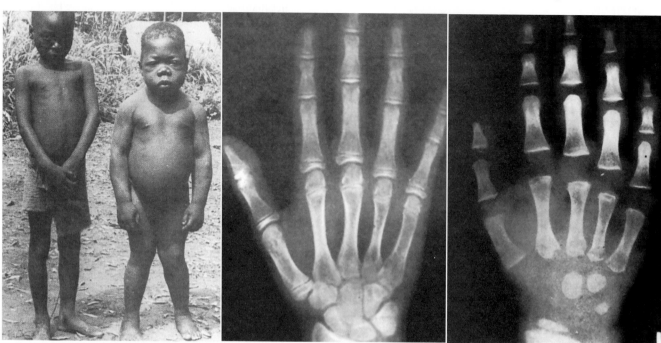

■ **Fig. 50-11** **A,** A normal 6-year-old child *(left)* and a congenitally hypothyroid 17-year-old child *(right)* from the same village in an area of endemic cretinism. Note especially the short stature, obesity, malformed legs, and dull expression of the mentally retarded hypothyroid child. Other features are a prominent abdomen, a flat broad nose, a hypoplastic mandible, dry scaly skin, delayed puberty, and muscle weakness. (From Delange FM: *Endemic cretinism.* In Braverman LE, Utiger RD, editors: *Werner and Ingbar's the thyroid,* ed 7, Philadelphia, 1996, Lippincott-Raven.) Hand x-ray films of a 13-year-old normal child **(B)** and a 13-year-old hypothyroid child **(C)**. Note that the hypothyroid child has a marked delay in development of the small bones of the hands, in growth centers at either end of the fingers, and in the growth center of the distal end of the radius. **(B** from Tanner JM et al: *Assessment of skeletal maturity and prediction of adult height (TW2 method),* New York, 1975, Academic Press. **C** from Andersen HJ: *Nongoitrous hypothyroidism.* In Gardner LI, editor: *Endocrine and genetic diseases of childhood and adolescence,* Philadelphia, 1975, WB Saunders.)

lates hepatic synthesis and release of sex steroid–binding globulin. T_3 also promotes differentiation of prepubertal testicular *Sertoli cells* (see Chapters 49 and 52).

Thyroid hormone also has significant effects on other parts of the endocrine system. Pituitary production of growth hormone is increased by thyroid hormone, while that of prolactin is decreased. Adrenocortical secretion of cortisol, as well as metabolic clearance of this hormone, is stimulated, but plasma free cortisol levels remain normal. The ratio of estrogens to androgens (see Chapter 52) is increased in men (in whom breast enlargement may occur with hyperthyroidism). Decreases in both parathyroid hormone and 1,25-$(OH)_2$-vitamin D production are compensatory consequences of the effects of thyroid hormone on bone, as described above.

Kidney size, renal tubular epithelium, renal plasma flow, glomerular filtration rate, and tubular transport maximums for a number of substances are also increased by thyroid hormone.

Hypothyroidism in adults most often results from idiopathic atrophy of the gland, which is thought to be preceded by a chronic autoimmune inflammatory reaction. In this form of **lymphocytic thyroiditis,** the antibodies that are produced may block hormone synthesis and/or thyroid gland growth or may have cytotoxic properties. Other causes of hypothyroidism include radiation damage, surgical removal, nodular goiters, and hypothalamic or pituitary destruction. In children, iodide deficiency, biosynthetic defects, and resistance to the action of thyroid hormones caused by mutant thyroid receptors can also cause hypothyroidism.

The clinical picture of hypothyroidism is in many respects the exact opposite of that seen in hyperthyroidism. *The lower-than-normal metabolic rate leads to weight gain without an appreciable increase in caloric intake.* The decreased thermogenesis lowers body temperature and causes intolerance to cold,

■ **Table 50-3** Some congenital defects in thyroid hormone synthesis

Defect	Diagnostic pattern
Iodide trap	Decreased uptake of radioactive iodine; decreased salivary/blood ratio of radioactive iodine
Peroxidase	Increased early uptake of radioactive iodine*; rapid discharge by perchlorate
Deiodinase	Increased uptake of radioactive iodine*; increased MIT and DIT in urine
Coupling	Increased uptake of radioactive iodine*; increased MIT and DIT and decreased T_4 and T_3 in thyroid tissue

*Radioactive iodine uptake is increased because of increased TSH secretion, which stimulates the iodine trap.

decreased sweating, and dry skin. Adrenergic activity is decreased and therefore bradycardia may occur. Movement, speech, and thought are all slowed, and lethargy, sleepiness, and a lowering of the upper eyelids (ptosis) occur. An accumulation of mucopolysaccharides—ground substance—in the tissues causes an accumulation of fluid also. This **myxedema** produces puffy features; an enlarged tongue; hoarseness; joint stiffness; effusions in the pleural, pericardial, and peritoneal spaces; and entrapment of pressure on peripheral and cranial nerves, with consequent dysfunction. Constipation, loss of hair, menstrual dysfunction, and anemia are other signs.

Notably, hypothyroidism in infancy or childhood causes marked retardation of growth (Fig. 50-11, *A*) and even greater slowing in the maturation of the epiphyseal growth centers of the bone (Fig. 50-11, *B* and *C*). If hypothyroidism is present at birth and remains untreated for even 2 to 4 weeks, the central nervous system will not normally mature in the first year of life. Developmental milestones, such as sitting, standing, and walking, will be late, and severe irreversible mental retardation can result. Such individuals are known as **cretins** (Fig. 50-11, *A*).

Hypothyroidism is diagnosed by finding a low serum T_4 level. (The exception would be in cases caused by thyroid hormone receptor abnormalities.) Serum TSH is elevated because of negative feedback, unless the hypothyroidism is caused by hypothalamic or pituitary disease. If the pituitary is at fault, TSH levels will be low and will not respond to administration of TRH. Replacement therapy with T_4 is curative. T_3 is not needed, because it will be generated intracellularly from the administered T_4. Furthermore, giving T_3 raises plasma T_3 to unphysiological levels (Fig. 50-7).

The stepwise nature of thyroid hormone synthesis offers multiple possible causes of congenital hypothyroidism that result from specific enzyme deficiencies. These syndromes are characterized by the symptoms of hypothyroidism noted previously, plus thyroid gland enlargement (congenital goiter) (Fig. 50-1) that results from persistent hypersecretion of TSH. Table 50-3 lists the best understood of these rare syndromes, with the biochemical findings that point to the lesion. Replacement therapy with T_4 corrects the hormone deficiency in each instance and reduces the size of the goiter. Large amounts of iodine alone can be used successfully if the iodide trap is defective.

■ *Summary*

1. The thyroid gland is the source of tetraiodothyronine (thyroxine, T_4) and triiodothyronine (T_3). The basic endocrine unit in the gland is a follicle that consists of a single circular layer of epithelial cells surrounding a central lumen that contains colloid or stored hormone.

2. T_4 and T_3 are synthesized from tyrosine and iodide by the enzyme complex peroxidase. Tyrosine is incorporated in peptide linkages within the protein thyroglobulin. After iodination, two iodotyrosine molecules are coupled to yield the iodothyronines.

3. Secretion of stored T_4 and T_3 requires retrieval of thyroglobulin from the follicle lumen by endocytosis. To support hormone synthesis, iodide is both actively concentrated by the gland and conserved within it by recycling the iodotyrosine molecules that escape coupling within thyroglobulin.

4. Thyrotropin (TSH) acts on the thyroid gland via its plasma membrane receptor and cAMP to stimulate all steps in the production of T_4 and T_3. These steps include iodide uptake, iodination and coupling, and retrieval from thyroglobulin. TSH also stimulates glucose oxidation, protein synthesis, and growth of the epithelial cells. This last effect is partly mediated by insulin growth factors.

5. More than 99.5% of the T_4 and T_3 circulates bound to the proteins thyroid-binding globulin (TBG), transthyretin, and albumin. Only the free fractions of T_4 and T_3 are biologically active. Changes in TBG levels require corresponding changes in thyroid hormone secretion to maintain normal concentrations of free T_4 and T_3.

6. T_4 functions largely as a prohormone. Monodeiodination of the outer ring yields 75% of the daily production of T_3, which is the principal active hormone. Alternatively, monodeiodination of the inner ring yields reverse T_3, which is biologically inactive. Proportioning of T_4 between T_3 and reverse T_3 regulates the availability of active thyroid hormone.

7. T_3 and, to a much lesser extent, T_4 bind to a thyroid hormone receptor (TR) that itself exists linked to thyroid regulatory elements (TREs) in target DNA molecules.

As a result, induction or repression of gene expression increases or decreases a large number of enzymes, as well as structural and functional proteins.

8. Thyroid hormone increases and is a major regulator of the basal metabolic rate. Oxygen utilization and CO_2 production are stimulated by mechanisms that include increases in the size and number of mitochondria, Na^+, K^+-ATPase activity, and the rates of glucose and fatty acid oxidation and synthesis.

9. Additional important actions of thyroid hormone are to increase heart rate, cardiac output, and ventilation and to decrease peripheral resistance. These actions subserve the increased tissue oxygen demand. The corresponding increase in heat production leads to increased sweating. Substrate mobilization and disposal of metabolic products are enhanced.

10. Other thyroid hormone effects on the central nervous system and skeleton are crucial to normal growth and development. In the absence of the hormone, brain development is retarded and cretinism results. The stature shortens and the bones fail to mature. In adults, thyroid hormone increases the rates of bone resorption and of degradation of skin and hair.

11. Hyperthyroidism and hypothyroidism are usually diagnosed easily. Both are very amenable to therapy, which is usually medical.

■ *Self-Study Problems*

1. A 45-year-old woman has the left lobe of her thyroid gland removed for a thyroid neoplasm that proves to be benign. Describe the subsequent responses that will return her serum T_4 level to normal after the initial decrease.

2. A high school wrestler has grown out of his weight class and is no longer confident of competing successfully. He surreptitiously ingests a daily excess of T_4 in order to lose 10 pounds of weight. However, he notes a decline in strength and stamina, and during exercise conditioning he notes breathlessness and a racing heart. His academic performance declines. His physician notes hyperkinesis and a very forceful heartbeat. Describe the reasons for these consequences.

■ *Bibliography*

Journal articles

Acheson K et al: Thyroid hormones and thermogenesis: the metabolic cost of food and exercise, *Metabolism* 33:262, 1984.

Brent GA: Mechanisms of disease: the molecular basis of thyroid hormone action, *N Engl J Med* 331:847, 1994.

Brown D et al: Amphibian metamorphosis: a complex program of gene expression changes controlled by the thyroid hormone, *Recent Prog Horm Res* 50:309, 1995.

Contempre B et al: Detection of thyroid hormones in human embryonic cavities during the first trimester of pregnancy, *J Clin Endocrin Metab* 77:1719, 1993.

Dillmann WH: Biochemical basis of thyroid hormone action in the heart, *Am J Med* 88:626, 1990.

Izumo S et al: All members of the MHC multigene family respond to thyroid hormone in a highly tissue-specific manner, *Science* 231:597, 1986.

Klein I: Thyroid hormone and the cardiovascular system, *Am J Med* 88:631, 1988.

Kohn LD et al: The thyrotropin receptor, *Vitam Horm* 50:287, 1995.

Larsen PR et al: Relationships between circulating and intracellular thyroid hormones, physiological and clinical implications, *Endocr Rev* 2:87, 1981.

Lazar MA: Thyroid hormone receptors: multiple forms, multiple possibilities, *Endocr Rev* 14:184, 1993.

Lazar MA et al: Nuclear thyroid hormone receptors, *J Clin Invest* 86:1777, 1990.

Mariotti S, Franceschi C, Cossarizza A, Pinchera A: The aging thyroid, *Endocr Rev* 16:686, 1995.

Misrahi M et al: Cloning, sequencing and expression of human TSH receptor, *Biochem Biophys Res Commun* 166:394, 1990.

Murata Y et al: Thyroid hormone inhibits fibronectin synthesis by cultured human skin fibroblasts, *J Clin Endocrinol Metab* 64:334, 1987.

Mutvei A et al: Thyroid hormone and not growth hormone is the principal regulator of mammalian mitochondrial biogenesis, *Acta Endocrinol (Copenh)* 121:223, 1989.

Nelson BD: Thyroid hormone regulation of mitochondrial function. Comments on the mechanism of signal transduction, *Biochem Biophys Acta* 1018:275, 1990.

Oppenheimer JH et al: Advances in our understanding of thyroid hormone action at the cellular level, *Endocr Rev* 8:288, 1987.

Piolino V et al: Thermogenic effect of thyroid hormones: interactions with epinephrine and insulin, *Am J Physiol* 259:E305, 1990.

Porterfield SP, Hendrich CE: The role of thyroid hormones in prenatal and neonatal neurological development—current perspectives, *Endocr Rev* 14:94, 1993.

Reed HL et al: Changes in serum triiodothyronine (T_3) kinetics after prolonged Antarctic residence: the polar T_3 syndrome, *J Clin Endocrinol Metab* 70:965, 1990.

Roger PO et al: Thyrotropin is a potent growth factor for normal human thyroid cells in primary culture, *Biochem Biophys Res Commun* 149:707, 1987.

Samuels HH et al: Regulation of gene expression by thyroid hormone, *Annu Rev Physiol* 51:623, 1989.

Sterling K: Direct thyroid hormone activation of mitochondria: identification of adenine nucleotide translocase (AdNT) as the hormone receptor, *Trans Assoc Am Physicians* 100:284, 1987.

Taylor T, Weintraub B: Thyrotropin (TSH)-releasing hormone regulation of TSH subunit biosynthesis and glycosylation in normal and hypothyroid rat pituitaries, *Endocrinology* 116:1968, 1985.

Vulsma T et al: Maternal-fetal transfer of thyroxine in congenital hypothyroidism due to a total organification defect or thyroid agenesis, *N Engl J Med* 321:13, 1989.

Books and monographs

Delange FM: *Endemic cretinism.* In Braverman LE, Utiger RD, editors, *Werner and Ingbar's the thyroid,* ed 7, Philadelphia, 1996, Lippincott-Raven.

Dunn AD: *Release and secretion of thyroid hormone.* In Braverman LE, Utiger RD, editors: *Werner and Ingbar's the thyroid,* ed 7, Philadelphia, 1996, Lippincott- Raven.

Klein I, Levey GS: *The cardiovascular system in thyrotoxicosis.* In Braverman LE, Utiger RD, editors, *Werner and Ingbar's the thyroid,* ed 7, Philadelphia, 1996, Lippincott-Raven.

Oppenheimer JH, Schwartz HL, Strait KA: *The molecular basis of thyroid hormone actions.* In Braverman LE, Utiger RD, editors: *Werner and Ingbar's the thyroid,* ed 7, Philadelphia, 1996, Lippincott-Raven.

Scanlon MF, Toft AD: *Regulation of thyrotropin secretion.* In Braverman LE, Utiger RD, editors: *Werner and Ingbar's the thyroid,* ed 7, Philadelphia, 1996, Lippincott-Raven.

Schwartz HL: *Effect of thyroid hormone on growth and development.* In Oppenheimer JH, Samuels HH: *Molecular basis of thyroid hormone action,* New York, 1983, Academic Press.

Smallridge RD: *Metabolic, physiologic and clinical indexes of thyroid function.* In Braverman LE, Utiger RD, editors: *Werner and Ingbar's the thyroid,* ed 7, Philadelphia, 1996, Lippincott-Raven.

Taurog A: *Hormone synthesis: thyroid iodine metabolism.* In Braverman LE, Utiger RD, editors: *Werner and Ingbar's the thyroid,* ed 7, Philadelphia, 1996, Lippincott-Raven.

The Adrenal Glands

The adrenal glands are complex, multifunctional endocrine organs that are essential for life. Severe illness results from their atrophy, and death follows their complete removal.

Each adrenal gland consists of two distinct functional parts (Fig. 51-1). The outer zone, or **cortex,** makes up 80% to 90% of the gland and is derived from mesodermal tissue. The cortex is the source of corticosteroid hormones. The inner zone, or **medulla,** makes up the other 10% to 20% of the adrenal gland and is derived from neuroectodermal cells of the sympathetic ganglia. The medulla is the source of catecholamine hormones.

The adrenal glands are located in the retroperitoneum, just above each kidney. Their total weight is 6 to 10 g. The adrenal glands have one of the body's highest rates of blood flow per gram of tissue. They receive arterial blood from branches of the aorta, the renal arteries, and the phrenic arteries. Arterial blood enters sinusoidal capillaries in the cortex and then drains into medullary venules. This arrangement exposes the medulla to relatively high concentrations of corticosteroids from the cortex. The right adrenal vein drains directly into the inferior vena cava, whereas the left adrenal vein drains into the renal vein on that side. The human adrenals can be visualized radiographically by computed tomography (CT) or magnetic resonance imaging (MRI), and each adrenal vein can be catheterized for blood sampling.

■ *The Adrenal Cortex*

The major hormones secreted by the adrenal cortex are (1) the **glucocorticoids, cortisol** and **corticosterone,** *which are critical to life because of their effects on carbohydrate and protein metabolism;* (2) a **mineralocorticoid, aldosterone,** *which is vital to maintaining sodium and potassium balance and extracellular fluid volume;* and (3) precursors to the **sex steroids, androgens** and **estrogens,** *which contribute to establishing and maintaining secondary sexual characteristics.* The discovery of the potent anti-inflammatory effects of glucocorticoids generated intense medical interest in cortisol and its glucocorticoid analogs, which have wide therapeutic usefulness.

The cortical portion of the adrenal gland differentiates by 8 weeks of gestation and is initially much larger than the adjacent kidney. At this time, the cortex contains two zones. The **peripheral neocortex,** making up 15% of the cortex, is undifferentiated and relatively inactive. The inner 85%, known as the **fetal cortex,** is highly active and produces fetal adrenal steroids throughout almost all intrauterine life. Shortly after birth, the fetal cortex begins to involute, and it disappears completely in 3 to 12 months. At the same time, the thin outer zone of the fetal cortex enlarges and differentiates into the permanent three-layered adrenal cortex of the mature human. Each layer or zone mainly secretes one of the three types of corticosteroids (Fig. 51-1).

The three mature cortical zones differ in their histologic appearances. The outermost **zona glomerulosa** is very thin and consists of small cells that have numerous elongated mitochondria with lamellar cristae. The middle **zona fasciculata** is the widest zone and consists of columnar cells that form long cords. The cytoplasm is highly vacuolated and contains lipid droplets. The mitochondria of the zona fasciculata cells are distinguished by their large size and numerous vesicular cristae within their membranes. The innermost **zona reticularis** contains networks of interconnecting cells. These cells contain fewer lipid droplets than fasciculata cells but have similar mitochondria. When stimulated by **adrenocorticotropic hormone (ACTH),** the size and number of cells in the fasciculata and reticularis increase. In addition, their mitochondria become larger and more numerous, and they develop central ribosomes and vesicular cristae. The mitochondria also develop polylamellar membranes that extend to nearby cholesterol-containing vacuoles. The endoplasmic reticulum also increases. These changes relate to ACTH effects on steroid hormone synthesis, as detailed later.

■ *Synthesis of Adrenocortical Hormones*

All hormones of the adrenal cortex represent chemical modifications of the steroid nucleus shown in Fig. 51-2. Potent glucocorticoids require the presence of a ketone at

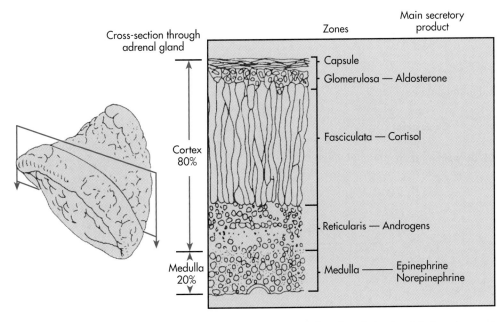

■ **Fig. 51-1**   Schematic representation of the zones of the adrenal gland and their main secretory products.

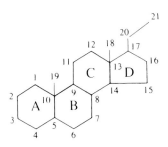

■ **Fig. 51-2**   The adrenocorticosteroid nucleus.

the 3 position and hydroxyl groups at the 11 and 21 positions. Potent mineralocorticoids require an oxygenated carbon at the 18 position. Potent androgens are characterized by the elimination of the C_{20-21} side chain and the presence of an oxygenated carbon at the 17 position. Estrogens are characterized by aromatization of the A ring. In the course of adrenal development, adrenocortical cells migrate inward from the outermost layer; during this migration, they gain 17-hydroxylating activity and lose 18-hydroxylating activity. Those that migrate farthest inward also lose 11-hydroxylating activity.

The precursor for all adrenocortical hormones is cholesterol, which is actively taken up from the plasma by adrenal cells. Specific adrenal plasma membrane receptors bind both circulating low-density (LDL) and high-density (HDL) lipoproteins, which are rich in cholesterol. After transfer into the cell by endocytosis, microtubules move the cholesterol to cytoplasmic vacuoles, within which most of the cholesterol is esterified and then stored. A small amount of cholesterol is also synthesized in adrenal cells from acetyl coenzyme A (acetyl CoA) by the usual biochemical pathway. Under basal conditions, free cholesterol from plasma is the major source used for

adrenocortical hormone synthesis. When production of corticosteroids is stimulated by ACTH, however, the stored esterified cholesterol becomes the most important precursor.

Most of the synthetic reactions from cholesterol to active hormones involve **cytochrome P-450 enzymes,** which are **mixed oxygenases** that catalyze steroid hydroxylations. These hydrophobic hemoproteins are located in the lipophilic membranes of the endoplasmic reticulum and mitochondrial cristae. Molecular oxygen is split so that one of its oxygen atoms is inserted between the carbon and hydrogen of the steroid site, while the other oxygen atom is reduced by hydrogen to H_2O. NADPH and, to some extent, NADH, which are generated by oxidation of a variety of substrates, are the ultimate donors of the hydrogen. A flavoprotein enzyme, **adrenoxin reductase,** and an iron-containing protein, **adrenoxin,** are intermediates in the transfer of hydrogen from NADPH to the P-450 enzymes.

Glucocorticoids. The synthesis of glucocorticoids occurs largely in the zona fasciculata, with a smaller contribution from adjoining cells in the zona reticularis. **Cortisol** is the dominant glucocorticoid in humans. However, if cortisol synthesis is blocked but the pathway to **corticosterone** is open, increased synthesis of corticosterone can provide the glucocorticoid activity necessary for maintaining health.

The sequence of reactions in glucocorticoid synthesis is shown in Fig. 51-3. The intracellular localization and mediating activators of the various reactions are illustrated in Fig. 51-4. Cortisol synthesis can be described in five steps. First, esterified cholesterol is hydrolyzed, and free cholesterol is actively transported from the storage vacuoles to the mitochondria (Fig. 51-5). Second, the

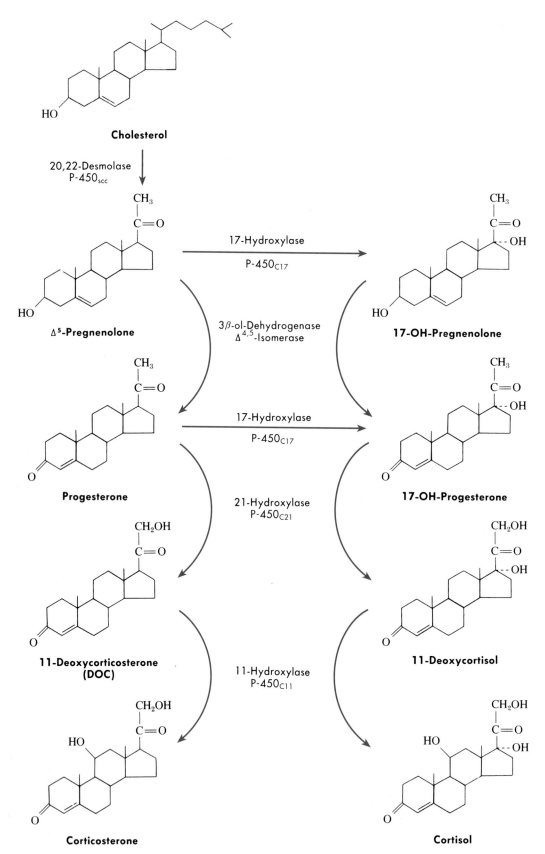

Cholesterol

20,22-Desmolase
P-450$_{scc}$

CH$_3$
C=O

HO

Δ^5-Pregnenolone

17-Hydroxylase
P-450$_{C17}$

CH$_3$
C=O
--OH

HO

17-OH-Pregnenolone

3β-ol-Dehydrogenase
Δ^{4,5}-Isomerase

CH$_3$
C=O

O

Progesterone

17-Hydroxylase
P-450$_{C17}$

CH$_3$
C=O
--OH

O

17-OH-Progesterone

21-Hydroxylase
P-450$_{C21}$

CH$_2$OH
C=O

O

**11-Deoxycorticosterone
(DOC)**

CH$_2$OH
C=O
--OH

O

11-Deoxycortisol

11-Hydroxylase
P-450$_{C11}$

CH$_2$OH
C=O

HO

O

Corticosterone

CH$_2$OH
C=O
HO   --OH

O

Cortisol

■ **Fig. 51-3**   Synthesis of glucocorticoids in the zona fasciculata. Cortisol is the major glucocorticoid in humans. When cortisol cannot be synthesized, corticosterone is an adequate endogenous alternative.

cholesterol is then transported across the outer mitochondrial membrane to the inner mitochondrial membrane, where the first enzyme, as well as adrenoxin reductase and adrenoxin, is localized. Third, the initial reaction that converts cholesterol to Δ^5-pregnenolone is catalyzed by a side chain cleavage enzyme P-450$_{scc}$, also known as 20,22-desmolase. This intramitochondrial complex carries out successive hydroxylations, followed by cleavage of the cholesterol side chain. Fourth, the Δ^5-product, pregnenolone, is then converted to 11-deoxycortisol by

successive steps within the endoplasmic reticulum (Figs. 51-3 and 51-4). Fifth, 11-deoxycortisol is transferred back to the mitochondria and hydroxylated in the 11 position. The end product, cortisol, rapidly diffuses out of the cell. The last and most critical step in glucocorticoid synthesis, 11-hydroxylation, is efficient in humans; 95% of the 11-deoxycortisol formed is converted to cortisol.

The order of hydroxylations from Δ^5-pregnenolone to 11-deoxycortisol can vary. Even the 3β-ol-dehydrogenase and $\Delta^{4,5}$-isomerase reactions can occur after all the

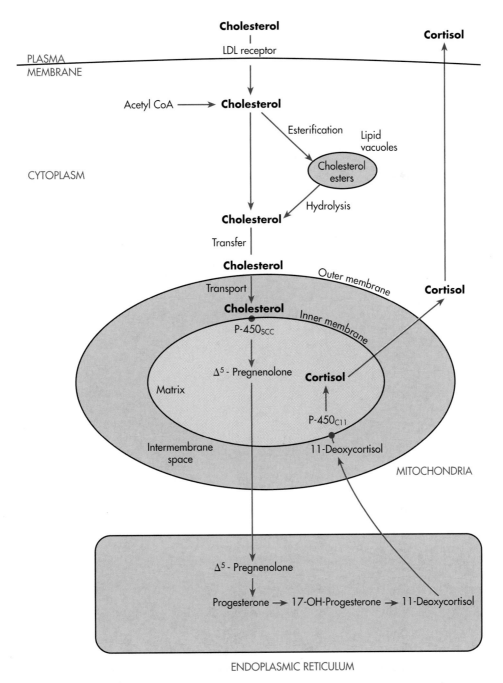

■ **Fig. 51-4** Intracellular localization of the steps involved in cortisol biosynthesis. Note the importance of making cholesterol available to the mitochondria.

hydroxylations, rather than before. However, the sequences presented in Fig. 51-3 (17-21-11) show the usual pattern of precursor accumulation that occurs when the various hydroxylases are either chemically blocked or congenitally deficient. A limited degree of 18-hydroxylation in the zona fasciculata also produces small amounts of 18-OH-cortisol, 18-OH-deoxycorticosterone (18-OH-DOC), and 18-OH-corticosterone.

Cortisol is not stored appreciably in the adrenocortical cell. Hence, an acute need for increased amounts of circulating cortisol requires rapid activation of the entire synthetic sequence from cholesterol.

Androgens and estrogens. The synthesis of sex steroid precursors occurs largely in the zona reticularis.

The 17-hydroxylated derivatives of Δ^5-pregnenolone and progesterone are the starting points for androgen and estrogen synthesis. Removal of the C_{20-21} side chain by a microsomal desmolase-like reaction is the key step, yielding dehydroepiandrosterone (DHEA) and androstenedione, respectively, as shown in Fig. 51-5. This reaction is catalyzed by the same enzyme, P-450$_{c17}$, that catalyzes the previous 17-hydroxylation step. DHEA is sulfated by a specific enzyme; the sulfate donor is 3'-phosphoadenosine 5'-phosphosulfate. Dehydroepiandrosterone sulfate (DHEA-S), DHEA, and androstenedione are the major androgen precursor products of the adrenal glands. Although they are weak androgens themselves, they are converted to the more potent androgen

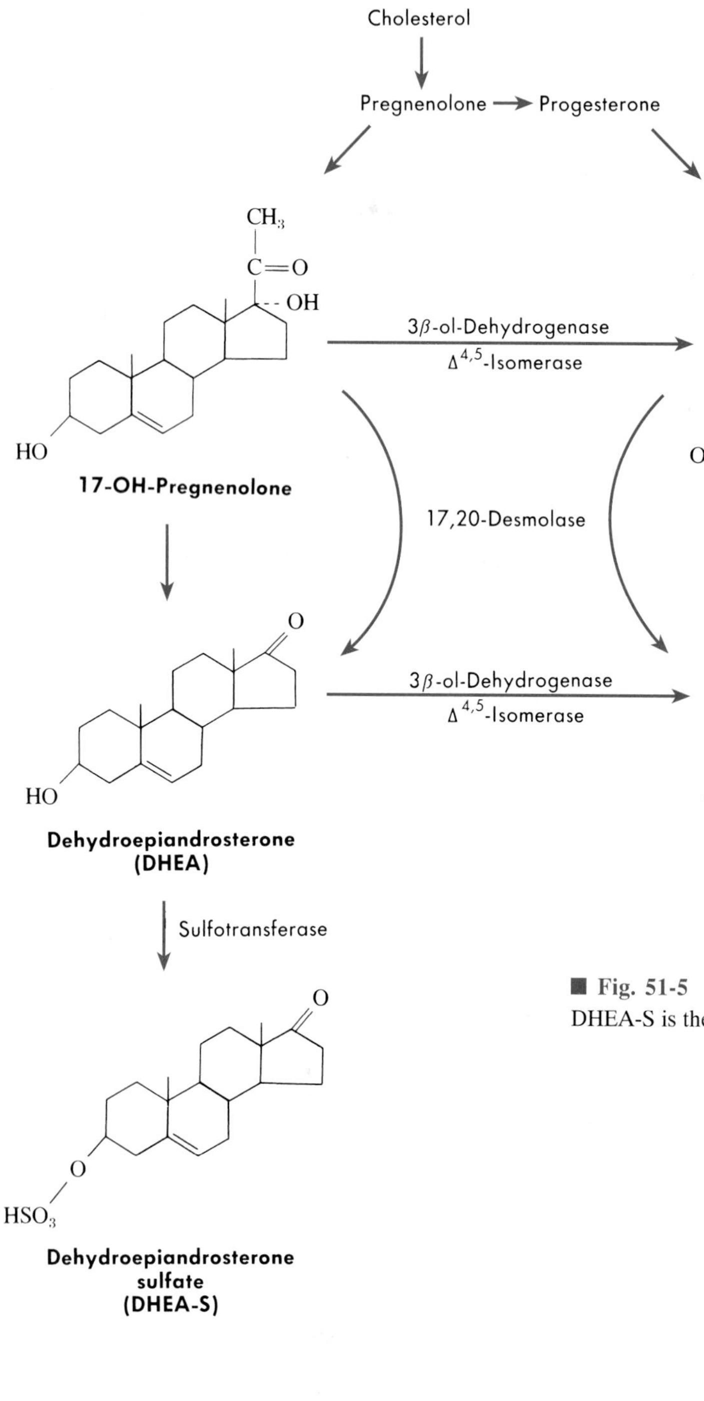

■ **Fig. 51-5**   Synthesis of androgen precursors in the zona reticularis. DHEA-S is the major product.

testosterone (see Chapter 52) in peripheral tissues. Only tiny amounts of testosterone itself are secreted by the zona reticularis. The same is true for the potent estrogen **estradiol** (see Chapter 52).

In women, the adrenal glands ultimately supply 50% to 60% of the androgenic hormone requirements. In contrast, adrenal androgen precursors are of little biological importance to men, because the testes produce a large quantity of testosterone. The further conversion of androgen precursors to estrogens within the adrenal cortex is not significant in women until the ovaries cease to function. After the menopause, estrogens secreted directly by the adrenal glands or arising in peripheral tissues from adrenal androgen precursors become important sources of estrogenic activity. Note that 17-hydroxylation is the last reaction common to the synthesis of cortisol and the adrenal androgens (compare Fig. 51-3 with Fig. 51-5). When cortisol synthesis is impaired at any point beyond this step, the accumulation of 17-hydroxypregnenolone and 17-hydroxyprogesterone leads to greatly increased androgen synthesis.

Mineralocorticoids. The synthesis of **aldosterone,** the major mineralocorticoid, is carried out exclusively by the zona glomerulosa (Fig. 51-6). The sequence of synthesis—from cholesterol to corticosterone—is identical to that in the zona fasciculata. The C18 methyl group of corticosterone is then hydroxylated and converted to an aldehyde by a mitochondrial P-450 mixed oxygenase to yield aldosterone, which is rapidly released. 18-OH corticosterone is not a direct intermediate but a byproduct of the enzymatic reaction. The 11-hydroxylase and 18-methylcorticosteroid oxidase enzymes are 95% homologous in their amino acid sequences. They are coded for by separate genes; one is expressed in both the zonae fasciculata and glomerulosa, the other exclusively in the glomerulosa. The two genes are also regulated independently (see below). DOC and 18-OH DOC have some mineralocorticoid activity. However, only rarely are they secreted in physiologically significant amounts by the zona fasciculata under ACTH stimulation.

Genetic defects in cortisol biosynthesis have important and varied consequences. A defect in either the 21- or 11-hydroxylase enzyme gene leads to overproduction of androgenic steroids from the accumulated precursors, 17-OH progesterone and 17-OH pregnenolone (Fig. 51-3). Excess androgens cause masculinization of female fetuses in utero and early sec-

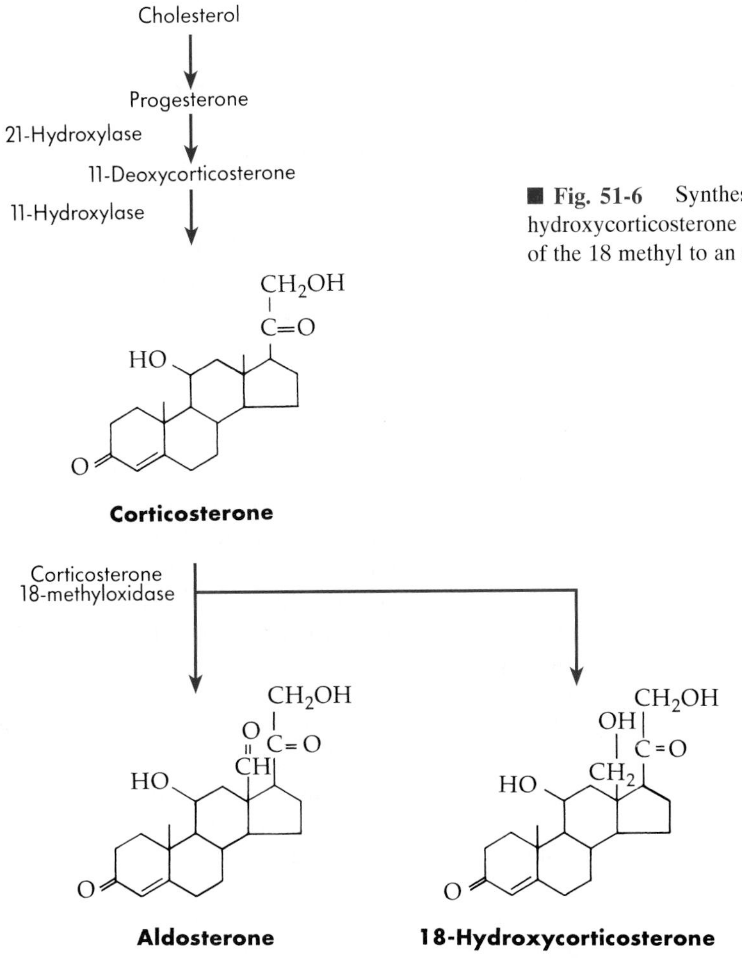

■ **Fig. 51-6** Synthesis of aldosterone in the zona glomerulosa. Note that 18-hydroxycorticosterone is a byproduct rather than an intermediate of the oxidation of the 18 methyl to an aldehyde.

ondary sexual changes in male infants and young boys. Severe deficiency of 21-hydroxylase activity may also cause manifestations of cortisol (glucocorticoid) and aldosterone (mineralocorticoid) deficiency. Deficiency of 11-hydroxylase leads to overproduction of 11-deoxycorticosterone (Fig. 51-3), large amounts of which cause excess mineralocorticoid activity. Deficiency of 17-hydroxylase/17,20-desmolase activity leads to absent androgens and estrogens. Men and women who lack androgens and estrogens have absent secondary sexual characteristics, and women are without menses. Corticosterone provides normal glucocorticoid activity, but overproduction of 11-deoxycorticosterone causes excess mineralocorticoid activity. The diagnosis of each specific enzyme defect is made by demonstrating low plasma levels of the missing hormone product and elevated levels of the hormone precursors. Plasma ACTH levels are also elevated by negative feedback (see Fig. 49-9 and below).

Inhibitors of adrenocortical hormone synthesis. A number of drugs that block steroid synthesis at various steps have diagnostic and therapeutic usefulness. **Metyrapone** inhibits 11-hydroxylation, the last and critical step in cortisol synthesis. Administration of this drug creates acute cortisol deficiency and thereby stimulates ACTH secretion via negative feedback. As a result of the increase in ACTH, adrenal production of the immediate precursor to cortisol, 11-deoxycortisol (Fig. 51-3), markedly increases. This adrenal response demonstrates the reserve capacity of the normal hypothalamic-pituitary ACTH axis (see Fig. 49-11). Failure to respond to this drug indicates a hypothalamic-pituitary disease that has abolished this function.

Aminoglutethimide is a potent inhibitor of the desmolase reaction, and it thereby decreases all adrenal steroid synthesis. This drug has been used to treat women with breast cancer to diminish estrogen production. **Ketoconazole,** an antifungal agent, also inhibits several steps in adrenocorticosteroid synthesis, and thus it is effective in treating states of cortisol excess.

■ *Regulation of Zona Fasciculata and Zona Reticularis Functions*

The secretion of cortisol by the zona fasciculata is exclusively controlled by the hypothalamic-pituitary corticotropin-releasing hormone (CRH)-ACTH axis (see Chapter 49 and Figs. 49-9 to 49-13). The secretion of adrenal androgens is likewise regulated by ACTH, but some evidence suggests that a separate pituitary tropic hormone may act specifically on the zona reticularis. In the absence of ACTH, adrenocortical secretion virtually ceases.

ACTH initiates its regulatory action by binding to its plasma transmembrane receptor, a step that requires calcium (Fig. 51-7). This binding is followed by G-protein activation of adenylyl cyclase and a rise in cAMP levels as the principal second messenger. Phosphatidylinositol products play adjunctive second messenger roles. Protein kinases A and C then probably phosphorylate various protein mediators of ACTH action. A **steroidogenesis activator protein** mediates immediate hydrolysis of stored cholesterol esters. A **sterol transfer protein** transports the released cholesterol to the outer mitochondrial membrane (Fig. 51-5). A **steroidogenic acute regulatory protein** chaperones the cholesterol to the inner mitochondrial membrane, where it can react with the P-450_{scc}, adrenoxin reductase–adrenoxin complex. Later, a **steroid hormone–inducing protein** increases transcription of the genes for P-450_{scc}, P-450_{c17}, P-450_{c11}, adrenoxin, and the LDL receptor. *Thus, all steps in corticosteroid hormone synthesis, from cholesterol entry to the generation of final products, are activated by ACTH.* In addition, ACTH acts on the cytoskeleton to bring cholesterol-containing vacuoles into intimate association with the mitochondria. The rate-limiting step in the entire sequence is the transfer of cholesterol to the first mitochondrial enzyme. Perhaps by stimulating local insulin-like growth factor (IGF) generation, ACTH administered chronically increases the size and number of adrenal cells and their mitochondria. This trophic effect is enhanced because ACTH up-regulates its own receptor, and both ACTH and IGF up-regulate each other's receptors.

As seen in Fig. 51-8, plasma levels of cortisol, adrenal androgens, and their precursors rise within minutes of intravenous ACTH administration to humans. ACTH induces a sustained, twofold to fivefold increase in cortisol secretion. Plasma ACTH concentrations of about 300 pg/ml, or six times the basal level, are maximally effective in stimulating cortisol secretion in the short term. However, when the adrenal gland is chronically hyperstimulated by ACTH, the gland undergoes hyperplasia, and its capacity for cortisol secretion rises up to twentyfold.

All the factors that influence ACTH secretion, as detailed in Chapter 49, likewise affect cortisol secretion; plasma levels of the latter generally follow those of the former by 15 to 30 minutes. Thus, cortisol secretion, like that of ACTH, exhibits distinct diurnal variation, with a peak just before the subject awakens in the morning. The lowest levels of cortisol secretion (near zero) occur just after the subject falls into slow-wave sleep (Fig. 51-9), which independently blunts the response of corticotrophs to CRH. The diurnal curve of total and free plasma cortisol includes 7 to 13 pulses or episodes of cortisol secretion per day. Half of the total daily cortisol is secreted within the major predawn burst.

The plasma peaks of cortisol are determined by the frequency and duration of secretory bursts rather than by gradual changes within a range of cortisol secretion rates.

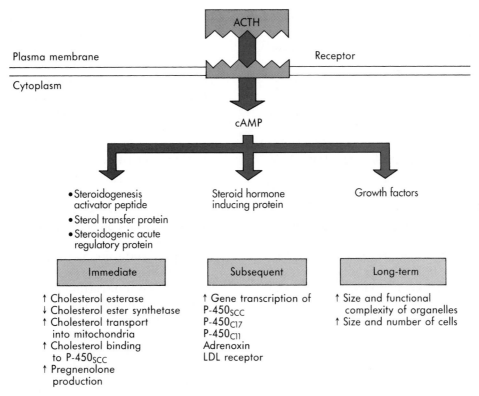

■ **Fig. 51-7**   Overview of adrenocorticotropic hormone *(ACTH)* actions on target adrenocortical cells. Note that the major second messenger, cyclic adenosine monophosphate *(cAMP),* activates immediate protein mediators and also induces production of later protein mediators. *LDL,* Low-density lipoprotein.

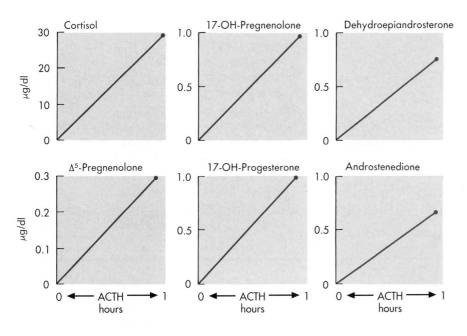

■ **Fig. 51-8**   Increments in plasma adrenocortical hormones in response to a 1-hour infusion of ACTH in humans. Note the increase of both precursors and hormonally active products. These changes indicate that ACTH activates the entire biosynthetic sequence. (Redrawn from Lachelin GCL et al: *J Clin Endocrinol Metab* 49:892, 1979.)

Thus, the basal unstimulated rate of secretion is actually near zero, and acute ACTH pulses produce essentially all-or-none adrenal responses. The reason for each of the daytime bursts of cortisol is unknown. A consistent burst after lunch suggests that cortisol secretion may be entrained with feeding patterns, although not necessarily in response to plasma substrate fluctuations. The plasma profiles of other adrenal steroids, such as DHEA, parallel that of cortisol; any disparities reflect differences in their metabolic clearance rates.

Plasma cortisol levels are increased by the stress of surgery, burns, infection, fever, psychosis, electroconvul-

sive therapy, acute anxiety, prolonged and strenuous exercise, and hypoglycemia. If attendant pain is prevented by disruption of the sensory input to the hypothalamus or by opioid analgesia, the cortisol response is blocked because CRH and ACTH do not increase. Plasma cortisol levels are decreased promptly by the administration of synthetic glucocorticoids, such as dexamethasone (Table 51-1), which suppresses ACTH secretion by negative feedback (see Fig. 49-12). A single dose of dexamethasone that is biologically equivalent to twice the daily secretion rate of cortisol is sufficient to completely eliminate the nocturnal ACTH peak and the subsequent morning rise in plasma cortisol level. However, major stress may override feedback suppression, and eliminate the diurnal pattern of cortisol secretion.

The average normal 8 AM plasma levels of cortisol and other adrenal steroids in humans, as well as their estimated secretion rates, are given in Table 51-2. The dominance of cortisol over corticosterone as a glucocorticoid is evident. Under severe stress, the maximal rate of cortisol secretion is 300 to 400 mg/day. Therefore, this amount is usually provided to patients who lack adrenal function and are either acutely ill or must undergo surgery; without the steroid, they may not survive. Plasma cortisol concentration varies little from childhood

to senescence, but secretion rates are correlated with lean body mass. In contrast, DHEA and DHEA-S increase to adult levels during late childhood and puberty. These adrenal steroids then decline significantly as an individual ages. Because ACTH secretion does not vary throughout life, the selective change in DHEA vs. cortisol with age suggests that intra-adrenal factors may be responsible for these differences. Epidemiologic evidence suggests that low plasma levels of DHEA are correlated with a tendency to weight gain and an increased risk of cardiovascular disease later in life.

■ *Metabolism of Adrenocorticosteroids*

Most of the cortisol (75% to 80%) that circulates in plasma is bound to a specific corticosteroid-binding α2-globulin called **transcortin.** Each molecule of this glycoprotein binds a single molecule of cortisol. The normal plasma concentration of transcortin is 3 mg/dl, and its binding capacity is 20 μg cortisol/dl. An additional 15% of plasma cortisol is bound to albumin, and only 5% to 10% is free. The concentration of transcortin, and therefore of total cortisol, is increased during pregnancy and by estrogen administration. The physiological effects of increased cortisol binding are determined by principles similar to those that characterize thyroxine binding (see Chapter 50).

Transcortin may have functions of its own when bound to cortisol, because cellular receptors for the transcortin-cortisol complex have been found that activate adenylyl cyclase. Transcortin is also cleaved by a leukocyte enzyme, a process that could increase free cortisol concentration at sites of inflammation. The plasma half-life of cortisol is about 70 minutes, and the metabolic clearance rate averages 200 L/day. The cortisol circulating free in plasma is filtered by the kidney, but only about 0.3% of the total daily secretion, or approximately 50 μg, is excreted in the urine.

Cortisol is in equilibrium with its biologically inactive 11-keto analog, **cortisone,** via the enzyme 11β-OH dehy-

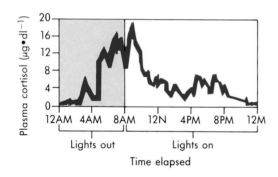

■ **Fig. 51-9** Pulsatile and diurnal nature of cortisol secretion. (Redrawn from Weitzman ED et al: *J Clin Endocrinol Metab* 33:14, 1971. The Endocrine Society.)

■ **Table 51-1**   Relative glucocorticoid and mineralocorticoid potency of natural corticosteroids and some synthetic analogs in clinical use*

	Glucocorticoid	*Mineralocorticoid*
Cortisol	1.0	1.0
Cortisone (11-keto)	0.8	0.8
Corticosterone	0.5	1.5
Prednisone (1.2 double bond)	4	<0.1
6α-Methylprednisone (Medrol)	5	<0.1
9α-Fluoro-16α-hydroxyprednisolone (triamcinolone)	5	<0.1
9α-Fluoro-16α-methylprednisolone (dexamethasone)	30	<0.1
Aldosterone	0.25	500
Deoxycorticosterone	0.01	30
9α-Fluorocortisol	10	500

*All values are relative to the glucocorticoid and mineralocorticoid potencies of cortisol, which have each been set at 1.0 arbitrarily. Cortisol actually has only 1/500 the potency of the natural mineralocorticoid aldosterone.

drogenase (Fig. 51-10). This enzyme, which is present in many tissues, renders exogenous cortisone an effective source of cortisol activity (Table 51-1).

Most cortisol and cortisone is metabolized in the liver; the reduced metabolites are conjugated and excreted in the urine as glucuronides. About half of these excretory products are normally derived from cortisol and half from cortisone (Fig. 51-10).

The measurement of urinary metabolites of cortisol provides a reliable index of cortisol secretion as long as hepatic and renal functions are normal. Particularly useful is the 17,21-dihydroxy-20-ketone configuration of tetrahydrocortisol and tetrahydrocortisone (Fig. 51-10). The excretion of these so-called **17-hydroxycorticoids** represents up to 50% of total daily cortisol secretion. Normal excretion rates of 17-hydroxycorticoids range from 2 to 12 mg/day, and they are slightly higher in men than in women, as are cortisol secretion rates. Adrenocortical responsiveness to ACTH (or metyrapone) or suppressibility by exogenous synthetic glucocorticoids can be assessed by daily measurements of urinary 17-hydroxycorticoids.

The cortisol precursors progesterone and 17-hydroxyprogesterone are metabolized to the cortols known as *pregnanediol* and *pregnanetriol,* respectively. In adult females, these urinary metabolites reflect both adrenal and ovarian secretion. In prepubertal children, however, elevation of urinary pregnanetriol specifically indicates increased secretion of adrenal 17-hydroxyprogesterone, and it is therefore a valuable marker for particular congenital defects in cortisol secretion.

The metabolism of androgens, in general, involves reduction of the 3-ketone group and the A ring in the liver. The two isomers formed, androsterone and etiocholanolone, are then excreted in the urine. However, these metabolites are not specific for the adrenal gland, because they arise from gonadal androgens also. DHEA-S is entirely excreted directly in the urine and is virtually adrenal specific.

Androsterone, etiocholanolone, and DHEA-S together constitute the major part of a urinary fraction called **17-ketosteroids.** Normal 17-ketosteroid values range from 5 to 14 mg/day in women and 8 to 20 mg/day in men. Two thirds of this fraction is normally derived from adrenal and one third from gonadal androgen secretions. In virilized children or adult women, a large increase in urinary 17-ketosteroid excretion almost always indicates an adrenal abnormality. Similar information can be more readily obtained by measurement of plasma or urinary DHEA-S.

■ *General Actions of Glucocorticoids*

Cortisol is essential for life. Although provision of carbohydrate and of a pure mineralocorticoid or sodium chloride can postpone death, human beings cannot survive removal of both adrenal glands for long without glucocorticoid replacement. Cortisol maintains glucose production from protein, facilitates fat metabolism, supports responsiveness of the vascular tree, modulates central nervous system function, and profoundly affects the immune system. In addition, cortisol affects skeletal turnover, muscle function, and renal function. The net effect of its metabolic actions is catabolic or antianabolic. The term *permissive* has been used to describe many of cortisol's actions, implying that the hormone may not directly *initiate* so much as *allow* certain processes to occur. Several examples may serve to better define this permissive role:

1. Cortisol may amplify the effect of another hormone on a process that it does not affect directly. For example, cortisol does not itself stimulate glycogenolysis, but it augments the stimulation of glycogenolysis by glucagon.
2. Cortisol and glucagon individually increase the activity of the enzyme phosphoenolpyruvate carboxykinase (see Fig. 47-13). However, their combined effect on this important regulatory step of gluconeogenesis is synergistic rather than additive.
3. The enzyme tyrosine transaminase is inducible by cortisol. It is not normally inducible by its substrate, tyrosine. However, in the presence of small doses of cortisol, tyrosine administration will now induce the enzyme.

Intracellular actions of glucocorticoids. In vitro and in vivo, the effects of cortisol may be evident within 30 minutes (inhibition of ACTH release). However, cortisol effects more usually require hours (increase in plasma glucose) or days (induction of glucose-6-phosphatase) to be expressed. Cortisol enters target cells freely and is then bound to a glucocorticoid receptor (GR), also known as the type II GR. Without its ligand, this receptor may shuttle back and forth between the cytoplasm and the nucleus. GR consists of four identical subunits. It belongs to the superfamily of steroid, thyroid, vitamin D, and retinoid receptors (see Chapter 45). GR is found in many tissues, including numerous areas of the brain. Although GR appears to be the same molecule in all cells, its concentration varies with cell type, degree of

■ Table 51-2   Average 8 AM plasma concentration and secretion rates of adrenocortical steroids in adult humans

	Plasma concentration (μg/dl)	*Secretion rate (mg/dl)*
Cortisol	13	15
Corticosterone	1	3
11-Deoxycortisol	0.16	0.40
Deoxycorticosterone	0.07	0.20
Aldosterone	0.009	0.15
18-OH Corticosterone	0.009	0.10
Dehydroepiandrosterone sulfate	115	15

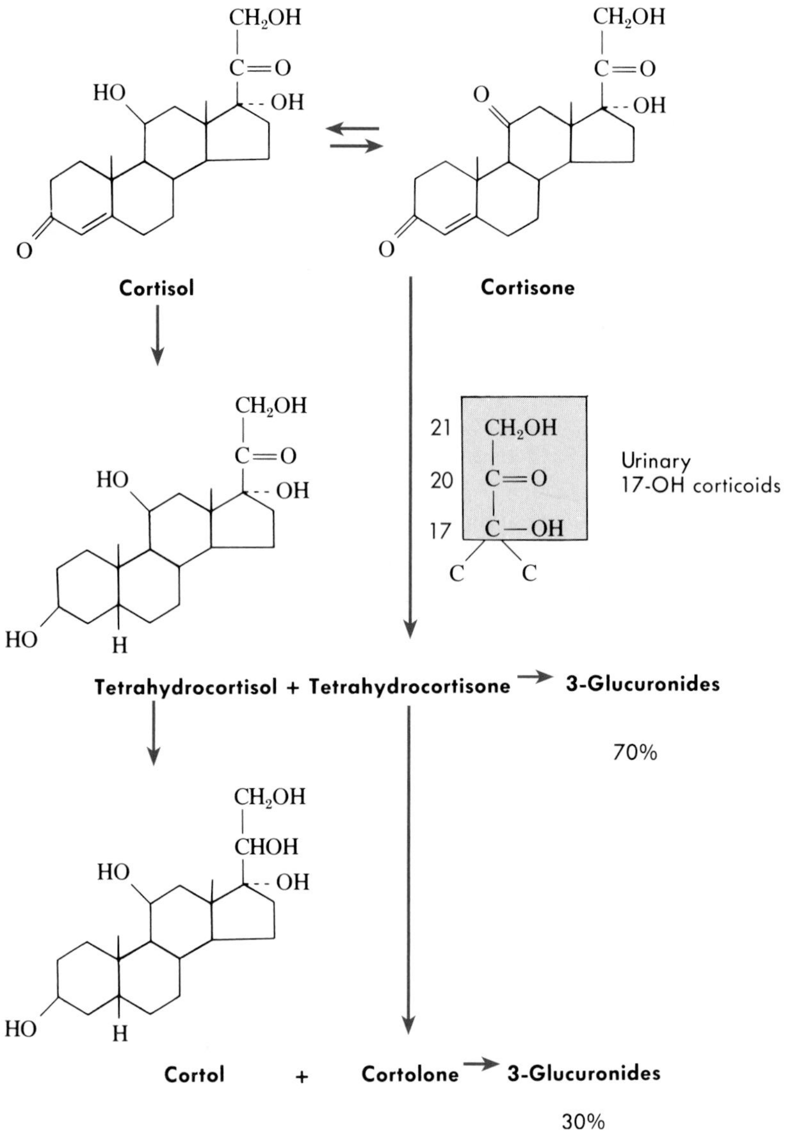

■ **Fig. 51-10** Major pathways of cortisol metabolism. The analogous compounds are formed from cortisone. The ratio of cortisol to cortisone metabolites is normally about 1:1.

cellular differentiation, and phase of the cell cycle (lowest in G-I and M, highest in S and G-II). The GR concentration is also down-regulated by glucocorticoids.

In the cytoplasm, cortisol combines noncovalently but strongly with its receptor. Binding of cortisol transforms the receptor into a molecule that is capable of moving into the nucleus and binding to specific glucocorticoid regulatory elements (GREs) on target DNA molecules (Fig. 51-11). Binding of cortisol to the C-terminal portion of GR displaces an inhibitory heat shock protein complex from a nearby site on the receptor. This displacement changes the receptor conformation; hyperphosphorylation of the receptor ensues, and C-terminus sites are exposed that facilitate translocation of the hormone-receptor complex into the nucleus. There, two liganded GRs combine to form a *homodimer* unit, which latches on with zinc fingers to 2 GRE half-sites (AGAACA are the bases).

The GRE sequences are palindromes separated by three nucleotides. GREs are usually located upstream from the gene promotor, but they may be downstream or may even exist within the gene. A single gene may have more than one type of paired GRE half-sites. Constitutive protein transcription factors may also be required to facilitate binding of a cortisol-GR complex to a GRE. Other transcription factors (even induced by other hormones) may block the interaction of the GR with the GRE.

Once the cortisol-GR complex has bound to a GRE, initiation or repression of gene transcription takes place. Repression may sometimes occur by displacement of activating factors from the DNA molecule, as is the case when cortisol inhibits certain inflammation-related genes that lack GREs. In other instances, a negative GRE exists within the gene, as is the case when cortisol suppresses transcription of the proopiomelanocortin gene (see Chapter 49).

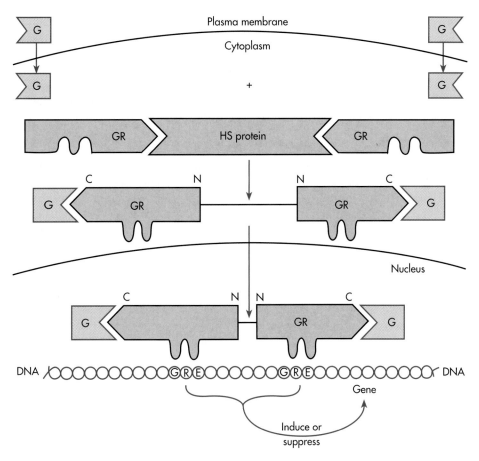

■ **Fig. 51-11** Mechanism of glucocorticoid (cortisol) action. The hormone *(G)* enters the cytoplasm and displaces a heat shock *(HS)* protein from the ligand-binding portion of the glucocorticoid receptor *(GR)*. This changes the GR's conformation so that it can readily enter the nucleus. There, complexed to G in the form of homodimers, GR then interacts with glucocorticoid regulatory elements *(GRE)* in target DNA molecules. Of note, not all GREs on DNA molecules share exactly the same consensus sequence of base pairs. *G,* Glucocorticoid; *GR,* glucocorticoid receptor; *GRE,* glucocorticoid regulating element; *HS,* heat shock.

In any one target cell type, only certain genes are affected. For example, in the anterior pituitary gland, the growth hormone gene is induced by cortisol, but the gene for the enzyme tyrosine aminotransferase is not. The opposite is true in the liver. GR can also bind other steroids. For example, progesterone and GREs can bind other steroid receptors, such as the progesterone receptor. However, only the simultaneous combination of glucocorticoid plus GR plus GRE produces the conformation necessary to induce the unique glucocorticoid effect on the expression of a gene.

Mutant GRs with deficient activity have been found in families who are resistant to cortisol action. Such individuals have compensatory increases in plasma cortisol levels because of inadequate negative feedback on CRH and ACTH secretion. Some AIDS patients appear to have acquired altered GRs with a markedly reduced affinity for cortisol. As a result, the number of GRs per cell is increased owing to the inadequate repression of the GR gene itself by cortisol. When the GR is severely defective, cortisol action may be so impaired that the patient is clinically cortisol deficient (see below).

The mineralocorticoid receptor (MR) shows strong homology to GR in its C-terminus and midmolecule domains; therefore, it is also known as the type I GR. Although this receptor exerts its physiological function mainly by binding mineralocorticoids, it actually binds cortisol ten times more strongly than does GR or type II GR. Thus, MR may mediate some cortisol actions when the basal concentrations of cortisol are low, whereas GR may mediate actions when stimulated cortisol concentrations are high. The selective central nervous system distribution of MR also suggests that it specifically mediates certain actions of cortisol in the brain.

Other intracellular mechanisms of cortisol action also probably exist. Cortisol does not generally alter intracellular cAMP levels. It does, however, synergize with the nucleotide in many situations, and cAMP can mimic some actions of cortisol. Cortisol may also act by altering cGMP levels and the phospholipid component of various intracellular membranes. Even within a single cell type, various enzyme changes produced by cortisol are not necessarily simultaneous or proportional in magnitude. This observation suggests multiple mechanisms of action.

Effects on metabolism. *Cortisol acts permissively to facilitate the mobilization of fuels. The nocturnal surge in cortisol supports the enhancement of gluconeogenesis, lipolysis, and ketogenesis necessary for overnight metabolic stability. The most important overall action of cortisol is to facilitate the conversion of protein to glycogen* (Fig. 51-12). Cortisol enhances the mobilization of muscle protein for gluconeogenesis by accelerating protein degradation and inhibiting protein synthesis. In fasted humans, the rates of entry of essential and nonessential amino acids into the blood are increased by cortisol. This change indicates that proteins are being broken down

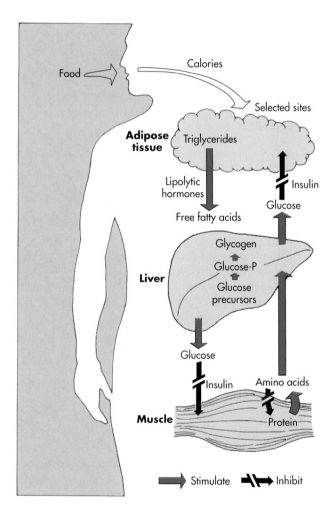

■ **Fig. 51-12** Effect of cortisol on the overall flow of fuels facilitates release of amino acids from muscle, their use for gluconeogenesis, storage and release of glucose, and release of free fatty acids from adipose tissue.

(Fig. 51-13). The plasma concentrations of the branched-chain amino acids increase; however, alanine levels do not rise, because the conversion of alanine to glucose is also markedly increased by cortisol (Fig. 51-13).

Although the combined catabolic and antianabolic action of cortisol in normal amounts is physiologically beneficial, a continuous excess of glucocorticoid action can drain the body's protein stores, most notably in muscle, bone, connective tissue, and skin. Dietary protein cannot make up for this drain, because protein synthesis is inhibited. Cortisol further stimulates the transformation of the proteolytically derived amino acids into glucose precursors, and thence into glucose (Fig. 51-12). Table 51-3 lists enzymes that are induced by cortisol and that are important to glucose production and to the disposition of ammonia released from gluconeogenic amino acids.

Glucocorticoids are critical for the survival of a fasting animal or human. Without glucocorticoids, proteolysis does not increase much, as evidenced by lack of increase in urinary nitrogen excretion (see Chapter 46). Therefore, when liver glycogen stores are depleted, deficient gluconeogenesis from protein may lead to death from hypoglycemia. The secretion of cortisol is modestly increased by fasting, but it is the *previous* exposure to normal levels of cortisol that permits initial augmentation of amino acid mobilization.

Cortisol plays a similar role in the defense against hypoglycemia that is evoked by insulin. Although the rapid release of the glycogenolytic hormones glucagon and epinephrine is mainly responsible for the rapid recovery of plasma glucose levels, the *previous* action of cortisol leads to the build-up of sufficient glycogen stores on which the other hormones can act. The critical enzyme that catalyzes glucose release from the liver, glucose-6-phosphatase, is also cortisol dependent. During the late phase of recovery from hypoglycemia, cortisol also decreases peripheral glucose utilization.

Although the major impact of cortisol is on liver glycogen, an excess of the hormone eventually increases plasma glucose levels. *This increase occurs because cortisol powerfully antagonizes the actions of insulin on glucose metabolism, and thereby inhibits insulin-stimulated glucose uptake in muscle and adipose tissue and reverses insulin suppression of hepatic glucose production.* As shown in Fig. 51-14, cortisol decreases tissue sensitivity, but not maximal responsiveness, to insulin. This antagonism takes place largely at postreceptor steps; for example, insulin represses, whereas cortisol induces, transcription of the gene for phosphoenolpyruvate carboxykinase. Cortisol also demobilizes glucose transporters from the plasma membrane to intracellular sites, thus directly reducing glucose uptake. As is the case with another insulin antagonist, growth hormone (see Chapter 49), cortisol eventually potentiates the increased insulin secretion that compensates for the insulin resistance produced by cortisol.

Cortisol also plays a somewhat analogous and permissive role in fat metabolism (Fig. 51-12). Although cortisol itself has some lipolytic activity, its presence is necessary for epinephrine, growth hormone, and other lipolytic substances to stimulate hydrolysis of stored triglycerides at maximal rates. Thus, during fasting, cortisol permits accelerated release of stored energy in the form of fatty acids and of glycerol for gluconeogenesis.

Cortisols actions on body fat are complex. The hormone increases appetite and caloric intake, probably by

■ **Table 51-3** Enzymes whose activities are increased by cortisol

Provide carbon precursors	*Convert pyruvate to glycogen*	*Release glucose*	*Dispose of ammonia liberated from amino acids in urea cycle*
Alanine transaminase	Pyruvate carboxylase	Glucose-6-phosphatase	Arginine synthetase
Tyrosine transaminase	Phosphoenolpyruvate carboxykinase		Argininosuccinase
Tryptophan pyrrolase	Phosphoglyceraldehyde dehydrogenase		Arginasenase
Threonine dehydrase	Aldolase		
Serine dehydrase	Fructose 1,6-biphosphatase		
	6-Phosphofructo-2-kinase/ fructose 2,6-biphosphatase		
	Phosphohexoisomerase		
	Glycogen synthase		

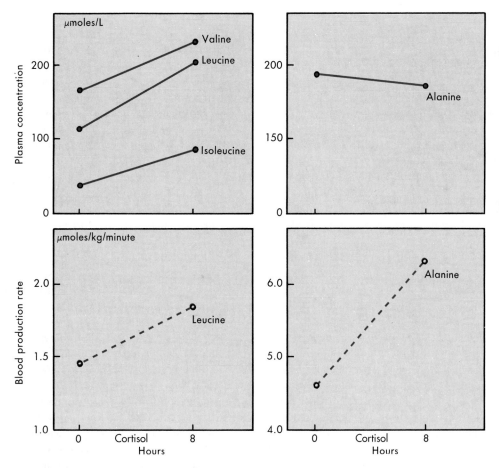

■ **Fig. 51-13**   Effect of cortisol infusion for 8 hours in normal humans on the plasma concentrations and blood production rates of several amino acids. The plasma concentrations of leucine and two other essential branched-chain amino acids increase. The increase of leucine is accomplished by an increase in its production rate and therefore indicates that cortisol stimulates proteolysis. Although the blood production rate of alanine also increases, its plasma concentration does not, because (in contrast to the nongluconeogenic leucine) cortisol simultaneously stimulates alanine use by augmenting its conversion to glucose. (Redrawn from Simmons PS et al: *J Clin Invest* 73:412, 1984.)

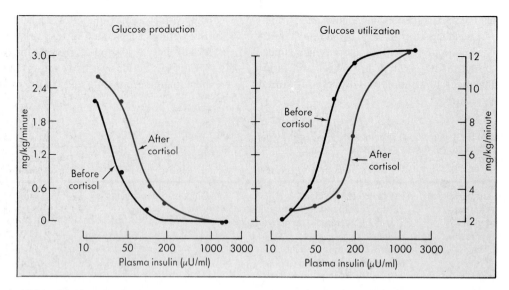

■ **Fig. 51-14**   Effect of cortisol on glucose turnover in response to increasing levels of insulin in a human. Cortisol decreases the sensitivity to insulin (the dose-response curve is shifted to the right) with regard to both insulin inhibition of glucose production and insulin stimulation of glucose use. (Redrawn from Rizza RA et al: *Am J Med* 70:169, 1981.)

inducing neuropeptide Y synthesis in the hypothalamus and by suppressing CRH release (see Chapter 46). It also increases differentiation of adipose tissue cells from preadipocytes to adipocytes, and stimulates lipogenesis by increasing adipocyte lipoprotein lipase and glucose-6-phosphate dehydrogenase activity. These actions vary in different regions of the body. *Therefore, an excess of cortisol finally results in obesity, with a peculiar distribution of fat that favors the abdomen, trunk, and face but spares the extremities* (Fig. 51-15). Because cortisol also induces **leptin** synthesis in adipocytes, the gain in fat mass is eventually limited by the negative feedback action that leptin exerts on the appetite center in the hypothalamus (see Chapter 46).

In short, cortisol is an important diabetogenic, anti-insulin hormone. Its primary hyperglycemic and lipolytic and secondary ketogenic actions are usually exhibited only when its secretion is greatly stimulated by stress. Cortisol then potentiates and extends the duration of the hyperglycemia evoked by glucagon, epinephrine, and growth hormone and accentuates loss of body protein. These diabetogenic and catabolic actions are markedly amplified when insulin secretion is deficient.

Cortisol also affects numerous organs and systems throughout the body, as depicted in Fig. 51-16.

Effects on muscle. Cortisol maintains the contractility and work performance of skeletal and cardiac muscle. This inotropic action of cortisol on skeletal muscle may be exerted at the myoneural junction via an increase in acetylcholine synthesis. In addition, cortisol increases myocardial Na^+, K^+-ATPase and β-adrenergic receptors. However, an excess of cortisol decreases muscle protein synthesis, increases muscle catabolism, and consequently reduces muscle mass and muscle strength. The ratio of

the insulin-sensitive, slow oxidative type I muscle fibers to the fast glycolytic type II-B muscle fibers is decreased by cortisol. This effect adds to the insulin resistance.

Effects on bone. *Cortisol inhibits bone formation by several mechanisms.* First, cortisol reduces the synthesis of type I collagen, the fundamental component of bone matrix. Second, cortisol decreases the rate of differentiation of osteoprogenitor cells to active osteoblasts (see Chapter 48). Third, cortisol decreases the absorption of calcium from the intestinal tract by antagonizing the action of 1,25-$(OH)_2$-vitamin D_3; it may also diminish the synthesis of this active vitamin D metabolite. The result of these actions is a reduction in the availability of calcium for bone mineralization. Cortisol additionally increases the rate of bone resorption. Thus, one major consequence of cortisol excess is an overall reduction in bone mass **(osteoporosis).**

Effects on connective tissue. Inhibition of collagen synthesis by cortisol produces thinning of the skin and the walls of capillaries. The resultant fragility of the capillaries leads to their easy rupture and to intracutaneous hemorrhage.

Effects on the vascular system. *Cortisol is required for the maintenance of normal blood pressure.* In addition to sustaining myocardial performance, the hormone permits normal responsiveness of arterioles to the constrictive action of catecholamines and angiotensin II. The mechanism for this effect may be inhibition of the membrane sodium–calcium exchanger, which would prolong the transient calcium increases produced by the vasoconstrictors. Cortisol decreases production of vasodilator prostaglandins and helps to maintain blood volume by decreasing the permeability of the vascular endothelium.

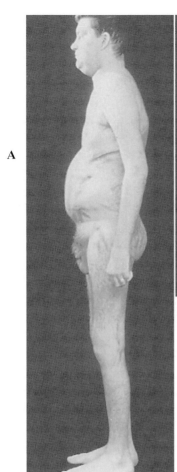

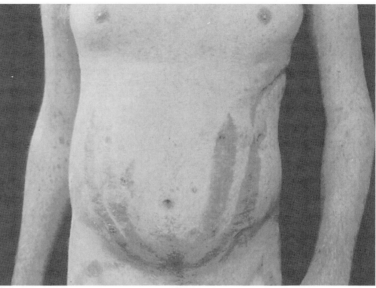

■ **Fig. 51-15** An individual suffering from cortisol excess (Cushing's syndrome). **A,** Note the loss of muscle mass in extremities and selective accumulation of fat in the abdomen and above the clavicles. **B,** The extremely thin skin reveals blood flowing through vessels just below.

Effects on the kidney. *Cortisol increases the rate of glomerular filtration* by decreasing preglomerular resistance and increasing glomerular plasma flow. *The hormone is also essential for rapid excretion of a water load.* In the absence of cortisol, the synthesis and secretion of antidiuretic hormone (ADH) are increased (by negative feedback on hypothalamic neurons), and its action on renal tubules is enhanced. Therefore, free-water clearance is diminished and dilution of the urine is limited (Fig. 51-17). Cortisol is also required for generation of ammonium ion from glutamate in response to acid loads. The hormone also increases phosphate excretion by decreasing its reabsorption in the proximal tubules.

Effects on the central nervous system. Cortisol modulates excitability, behavior, and mood of individuals; the electrical activity of neurons is influenced. Both type I and type II GRs are present in various areas of the brain, particularly in the limbic system and the hippocampus. Cortisol decreases rapid eye movement (REM) sleep but increases both slow-wave sleep and time spent awake. The nocturnal rise in ACTH and cortisol generally precedes S_1, or light, sleep. In excess, cortisol can cause insomnia, strikingly elevate or depress moods, decrease memory and hippocampal volume and memory function, and lower the threshold for seizure activity. Cortisol also specifically decreases the ability to detect a salty taste

and dampens acuity to gustatory, olfactory, auditory, and visual stimuli. On the other hand, cortisol improves the ability to integrate those sensations that are perceived and to organize appropriate responses.

Effects on the fetus. *Cortisol facilitates in utero maturation of the central nervous system, retina, skin, gastrointestinal tract, and lungs.* The latter two effects have been best studied. The digestive enzyme capacity of the intestinal mucosa changes from a fetal pattern to a mature adult pattern under the influence of cortisol. This maturation process permits the newborn to use disaccharides present in milk. Timely preparation of the fetal lung to permit satisfactory breathing immediately after birth is facilitated by cortisol, which increases the rate of development of the alveoli, flattening of the lining cells, and thinning of the lung septa. Most important, during the last weeks of gestation, the synthesis of surfactant, a phospholipid vital for maintaining alveolar surface tension, is increased (see Chapter 33). This last effect is mediated by increasing the activity of key enzymes, such as phosphatidyl acid phosphatase and choline phosphotransferase, which are involved in the surfactant biosynthetic pathway.

Effects on inflammatory and immune responses. *Cortisol has a profound influence on the complex set of reactions evoked by tissue trauma, chemical irritants, infection, or foreign proteins* (Fig. 51-18). The immedi-

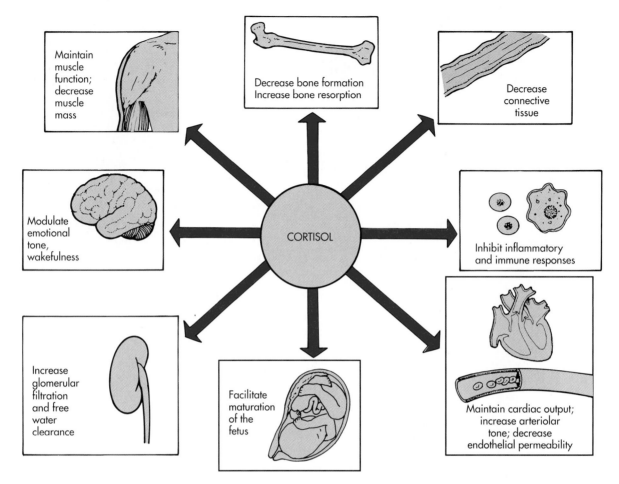

■ Fig. 51-16   Overview of cortisol effects on various tissues, organs, and systems other than its effects on general metabolism as noted in Fig. 51-12.

ate local reaction to injury consists of dilation of capillaries and changes in the endothelial cell membranes that increase microvascular permeability and enhance the trapping of circulating leukocytes at the site of injury. These reactions, mediated by **prostaglandins, thromboxanes, leukotrienes, nitric oxide,** and **platelet-activating factor,** are profoundly inhibited by cortisol and all currently available synthetic glucocorticoids that are used therapeutically. The inhibition of these reactions by cortisol stems mainly from the hormone's suppression of the synthesis and release of **arachidonic acid,** which is a precursor of many of the immune mediators. Cortisol decreases the availability of arachidonic acid by inducing **lipocortin,** a phosphoprotein that inhibits the activity of the enzyme phospholipase A_2. This phospholipase releases arachidonic acid from its linkage to phosphatidyl choline. Arachidonic acid is the immediate precursor to the proinflammatory prostaglandins, thromboxanes, and leukotrienes, and its production is the rate-limiting step in their synthesis. In addition, cortisol decreases the expression of the gene that codes for cyclooxygenase 2, an enzyme that directs prostaglandin synthesis toward inflammatory products. Cortisol also decreases the expression of the gene that encodes nitric oxide synthase. In addition, glucocorticoids stabilize lysosomes and

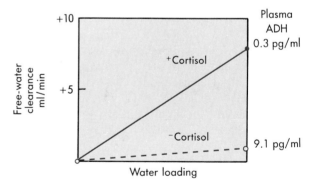

■ Fig. 51-17   Effect of cortisol on the response of adrenalectomized dogs to water loading. In the absence of the hormone, there is little increase in free-water clearance, and antidiuretic hormone *(ADH)* levels remain high (because of negative feedback on ADH neurons). Cortisol replacement allows a normal suppression of ADH levels and a sharp increase in free-water clearance. (Modified from Boykin J et al: *J Clin Invest* 62:738, 1978. From the American Society for Clinical Investigation.)

thereby reduce the local release of proteolytic enzymes and hyaluronidase, other substances that contribute to tissue swelling. The differentiation and proliferation of local inflammatory mast cells (but not their release of histamine) are also inhibited by cortisol.

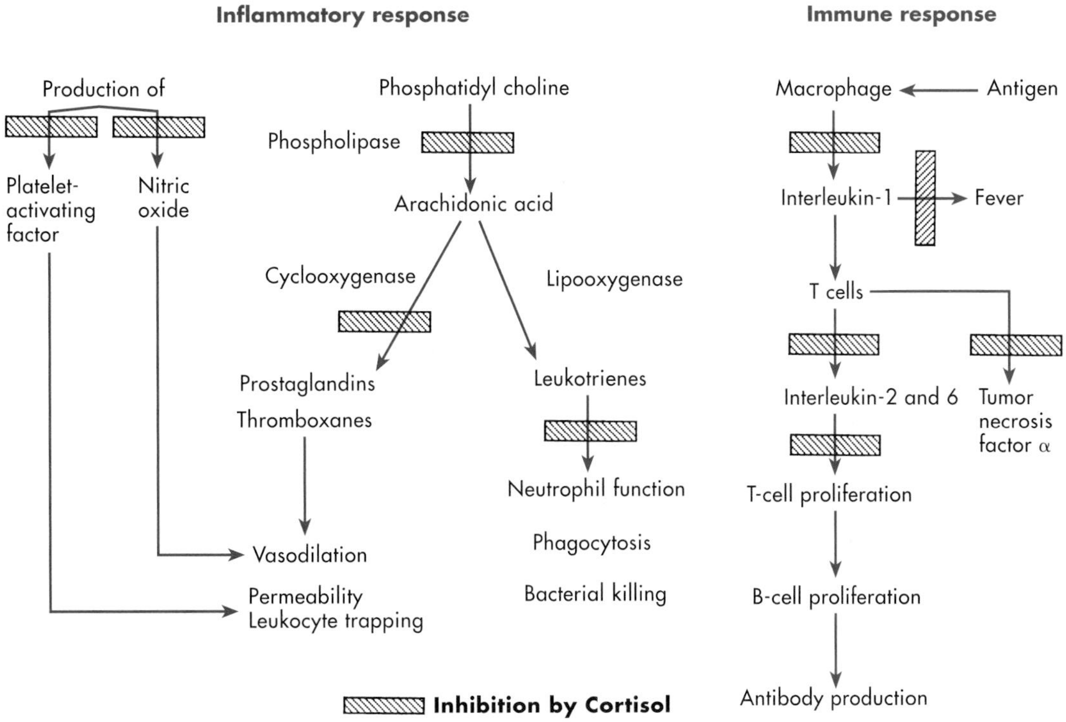

Inflammatory response   **Immune response**

■ **Fig. 51-18**   Mechanisms whereby cortisol inhibits many steps in the processes involved in inflammation and immune system responses. Inhibition of the enzymes phospholipase and cyclooxygenase and the synthesis of nitric oxide and platelet-activating factor impairs the vascular component of inflammation. Inhibition of leukotriene actions impairs neutrophil phagocytosis and bactericidal abilities. Inhibition of antigen presentation and macrophage cytokine release impairs proliferation and cytokine release of T cells. Ultimately, B-cell function is reduced so that both cellular and humeral immunity are decreased.

Cortisol inhibits the recruitment of circulating leukocytes to the site of trauma or infection. The hormone also decreases margination of leukocytes from blood vessels and their adherence to capillary endothelium. This process requires interaction between **chemotactic peptides** that attract the leukocytes and specific endothelial cell surface receptors. Cortisol inhibits the production and binding of these peptides to their receptors. Cortisol also decreases the phagocytic and bactericidal activity of neutrophils and the leukotriene-stimulated respiratory burst that accompanies these activities. *Because cortisol increases the release of neutrophils from bone marrow, the circulating number of these cells actually increases (Fig. 51-19), although their effectiveness decreases.* In contrast, *cortisol decreases the number of circulating eosinophils by stimulating their programmed death, called* **apoptosis.**

Cortisol also decreases the proliferation of fibroblasts and their synthesis and deposition of fibrils. This process forms the basis for the chronic inflammatory response to injury. *The net result of inhibiting fibroblast function is to impede the local responses to irritants or invading microorganisms and thus to prevent the walling off of an infection.*

Cortisol also profoundly suppresses the immune system responses to foreign substances. The hormone decreases the number of circulating thymus-derived lymphocytes (T cells), especially the proportion of type 1 helper T_4 lymphocytes, by stimulating apoptosis (Fig. 51-19). In addition, their transport to the site of antigenic stimulation, and their functions, are decreased. *Thus, cell-mediated immunity, as typified by the rejection of transplanted tissue of nonself origin, is markedly inhibited by the hormone.*

The mechanism of this inhibition by cortisol is multifactorial (Fig. 51-18). When a foreign protein, or **antigen,** enters the body, it is engulfed by a monocyte/macrophage. This cell "presents" the antigen to T cells and simultaneously elaborates **interleukin-1 (IL-1),** a peptide lymphokine that activates a subset of T cells with helper or inducer function. In turn, the helper T cells secrete a variety of interleukins that produce a cascade of still more T cells and cytokines of various functions. Cortisol inhibits the initial presentation of antigen and the production of IL-1, IL-2, IL 6, gamma interferon, and other macrophage and lymphocyte products. Cortisol affects resting immune cells more than those that are already activated by antigens, and lymphocyte proliferation is arrested in cell stages G_0 and G_1. Even the differentiation of monocytes to macrophages is inhibited by cortisol.

One of the results of T-cell activation is the recruitment and activation of B lymphocytes, which produce neutral-

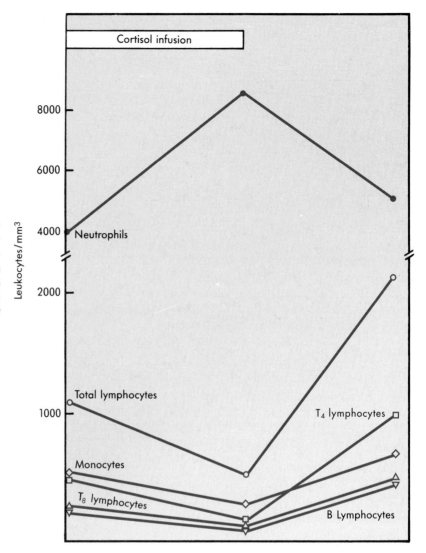

■ Fig. 51-19 Effects of cortisol on circulating leukocytes. Note the increase in neutrophils and decrease in monocytes and lymphocytes of all types. T_4 helper lymphocytes were disproportionately reduced. Eosinophils *(not shown)* also decrease. (Data from Calvano SE et al: *Surg Gynecol Obstet* 164:509, 1987.)

izing **antibodies** directed against specific antigens. Thus, the proliferation and differentiation of B lymphocytes and their production of antibodies are influenced at least indirectly by cortisol. However, the specific reaction of antibodies with antigen molecules is not affected by glucocorticoids, nor is the degradation of the antibodies.

The anti-inflammatory action of glucocorticoids also includes the suppression of the febrile response to infections or tissue injury. This action probably occurs from decreased production of IL-1, which acts as an endogenous pyrogen.

A negative feedback relationship between the hypothalamic-pituitary-adrenal axis and the immune system also exists. Immune reactivity varies in a diurnal pattern that is opposite to that of cortisol secretion. *Whereas cortisol inhibits immune responses as described above, inflammatory cytokines stimulate cortisol release.* IL-1, IL-6, and tumor necrosis factor$_\alpha$ (TNF$_\alpha$) all stimulate CRH and thence ACTH secretion; this in turn stimulates the adrenal zona fasciculata to synthesize and secrete cortisol. In addition, CRH and ACTH genes are expressed by

some immune cells, and therefore these two peptides may also exert autocrine or paracrine effects on the immune response.

It has been repeatedly stressed that cortisol is essential to the survival of the severely stressed, traumatized, or infected individual. However, many of the defense mechanisms incorporated in the response to injury are inhibited by elevated levels of glucocorticoids. To explain this paradox, it has been suggested that permissive basal or modestly elevated levels of cortisol are required for the initial metabolic (and possibly some of the immunologic) beneficial responses to stress. However, if a local inflammatory reaction becomes too intense or spreads to adjacent uninjured tissue, the reaction may create local pressure or ischemia. Furthermore, if the initially selective immune system reaction broadens to include responses to nonspecific antigens or even self-antigens, these defensive processes could become more damaging than the original injury. Thus, the later and more greatly elevated cortisol levels produced by cytokine feedback on the hypothalamus-pituitary-adrenal axis serve to limit cellular and tissue responses so that they do not destroy normal structure and function, for example, by autoimmune reactions.

The anti-inflammatory and immunosuppressive actions of glucocorticoids are used in treating nonendocrine diseases. Administered in high doses, they represent a double-edged sword. When the symptoms of tissue injury that result from disease are functionally disabling or life threatening or when the rejection of transplanted vital organs (kidney, heart, liver) must be prevented, glucocorticoids are dramatically beneficial. However, if glucocorticoids are administered therapeutically for very long, they may increase the susceptibility to bacterial, fungal, and viral infections or allow their dissemination. They may also prevent or delay normal wound healing after injury or surgery. These serious adverse effects, along with diabetes, osteoporosis, and psychiatric disorders, enjoin physicians to prescribe glucocorticoids only when no safer form of treatment can succeed. This injunction obviously does not apply to the use of cortisol as replacement therapy in individuals who have lost adrenocortical function.

■ *Action of Adrenal Androgens*

The adrenal steroids DHEA-S, DHEA, and androstenedione are relatively weak androgens. Their physiological function is largely expressed by their peripheral conversion to the potent androgen testosterone (see Chapter 52). In females, testosterone derived from adrenal androgen precursors sustains normal pubic and axillary hair. It may also possibly contribute to the maintenance of red blood cell production. In males, the amount of testosterone produced in the testicle far exceeds that produced in the adrenal glands, and thus the latter is unimportant physiologically. Estradiol of direct or indirect adrenal origin is an important source of estrogen activity after the menopause.

The most common cause of endogenous cortisol excess is bilateral hyperplasia of the adrenal cortex that results from hypersecretion of ACTH. Tumors that autonomously secrete cortisol also occur. The major manifestations of endogenous hypercortisolism include (1) obesity, with a peculiar distribution of fat in the cheeks, the supraclavicular areas, the posterior cervicothoracic junction, the trunk, and the abdomen (the extremities are spared) (Fig. 51-15); (2) loss of bone mass (osteoporosis), vertebral fractures, and necrosis of the hips; (3) loss of connective tissue integrity, associated with fragile capillaries, easy bruisability, and thin skin through which the underlying blood vessels may be seen (purple **striae**) (Fig. 51-

15); (4) increased protein catabolism, which results in atrophy and weakness of the muscles of the trunk and extremities, poor wound healing, and stunted growth in children; (5) abnormal carbohydrate metabolism, or even overt diabetes; (6) impaired wound healing and response to infections; and (7) insomnia, euphoria, or depression. All these pathological consequences can also be produced by large therapeutic doses of synthetic glucocorticoids.

Endogenous glucocorticoid excess is diagnosed by demonstrating elevated plasma cortisol or urinary free cortisol levels, loss of normal cortisol diurnal variation, and loss of normal suppressibility of cortisol secretion by potent exogenous glucocorticoids, such as **dexamethasone** (Table 51-1). If the pituitary gland causes cortisol hypersecretion, plasma ACTH is elevated. If autonomous adrenal tissue has developed, negative feedback decreases the levels of plasma ACTH and inhibits the normal rise in plasma ACTH produced by CRH administration (see Fig. 49-12).

Adrenal androgen hypersecretion is clinically silent in adult males but is detectable in females by their signs of masculinization. This includes loss of regular menses, regression of breast tissue, increased body hair, acne, deepening of the voice, enlargement of the clitoris, increased muscularity, and heightened libido. Plasma and urinary DHEA-S and, in women, testosterone levels are elevated.

■ *Aldosterone Regulation of Zona Glomerulosa Function*

The principal function of aldosterone, the major mineralocorticoid, is to sustain extracellular fluid volume by conserving body sodium. Hence, aldosterone is largely secreted in response to signals that arise from the kidney when a reduction in circulating fluid volume is sensed. As shown in Fig. 51-20, when body sodium is depleted (e.g., by dietary restriction), the fall in extracellular fluid and plasma volume decreases renal arterial blood flow and pressure. The juxtaglomerular cells of the kidney respond to this change by secreting the enzyme **renin** into the peripheral circulation. As detailed in Chapter 42, renin acts on its substrate, **angiotensinogen** (an α_2-globulin of hepatic origin), to form the decapeptide **angiotensin I**. This decapeptide is then further cleaved by an angiotensin converting enzyme to the octapeptide **angiotensin II**. This potent vasoconstrictor binds to specific adrenal zona glomerulosa cell plasma membrane receptors; through G-protein linkages, calcium and phosphatidylinositol products are generated as second messengers. Protein kinase C is translocated to the plasma membrane and is activated. Subsequently, the transfer of cholesterol to the mitochondria and the desmolase and 18-methylcorticosteroid oxidase steps in the synthesis of

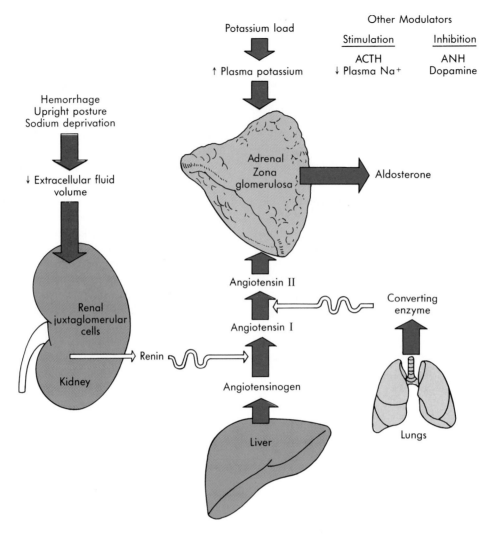

■ Fig. 51-20   Regulation of aldosterone secretion. Activation of the renin-angiotensin system in response to hypovolemia is the predominant stimulus to aldosterone production. Elevation of plasma potassium is the other major stimulus. ACTH has a minor tonic role. *ANH,* Atrial natriuretic hormone.

aldosterone are stimulated (Fig. 51-6). Minute increases in plasma angiotensin II are sufficient to stimulate maximal aldosterone release.

During several days of only a 10 mEq sodium intake, aldosterone secretion rates increase fourfold to eightfold. The renin and aldosterone responses to hypovolemia are also rapidly evoked by hemorrhage, assuming an upright posture for several hours, or an acute diuresis (see also Chapters 31 and 42). Such maneuvers increase plasma aldosterone twofold to fourfold. Conversely, when excess sodium is ingested and extracellular fluid volume expands, renin release, angiotensin II generation, and aldosterone secretion all are suppressed. *Thus, the juxtaglomerular cells and the zona glomerulosa form a negative feedback system. Sodium deprivation induces aldosterone hypersecretion via renin and angiotensin. When the additional aldosterone has caused sufficient sodium retention and the extracellular fluid and plasma volume are restored to normal, the extra renin release is shut off*

and aldosterone hypersecretion ceases. In this manner, daily aldosterone secretion ranges from 50 μg (with a dietary sodium intake of 150 mEq) to 250 μg (with a dietary sodium intake of 10 mEq).

The release of renin is enhanced by increased sympathetic neural activity, which is induced by hypovolemia, via norepinephrine and β-adrenergic receptors in the kidney. The release of renin is also stimulated by certain local prostaglandins; therefore, prostaglandin synthesis inhibitors (e.g., nonsteroidal anti-inflammatory agents) can reduce aldosterone responses. Short-loop feedback inhibition of renin release is exerted by angiotensin II, but there is no direct feedback on the juxtaglomerular cells by aldosterone.

The actions described above form part of the physiological basis for the therapy of **hypertension**. β-adrenergic antagonists lower blood pressure in part by reducing the sodium retention caused by renin-aldosterone activity. In a similar way, inhibitors of **angiotensin converting enzyme** or angiotensin II receptor blockers also lower blood pressure. Antagonists of aldosterone at the renal tubule cell level directly prevent sodium reabsorption and reduce hypertension.

Atrial natriuretic peptide (ANP) reinforces the effects of the renin-angiotensin system on aldosterone secretion. In response to volume expansion, atrial myocytes release ANP, which binds to specific receptors in the zona glomerulosa and inhibits the synthesis and release of aldosterone. This direct inhibitory effect is mediated by decreased cAMP and increased cGMP levels. ANP also reduces aldosterone secretion indirectly by decreasing renin release.

Aldosterone also participates in a vital negative feedback relationship with potassium (Fig. 51-20). *The hormone facilitates the clearance of potassium from the extracellular fluid, and in physiological concordance, potassium acts to stimulate aldosterone secretion.* In humans, an increase of plasma potassium of only 0.5 mEq/L immediately raises plasma aldosterone threefold, and an increase in dietary potassium from 40 to 200 mEq/day increases plasma aldosterone sixfold. Conversely, potassium depletion lowers aldosterone secretion. Potassium stimulates aldosterone release by depolarizing the adrenal cell membrane. As a result, voltage-dependent calcium channels open and the intracellular calcium concentration increases. Accordingly, calcium channel blockers may inhibit aldosterone release.

ACTH, in doses and in a manner similar to those that increase cortisol secretion, also stimulates aldosterone secretion (Fig. 51-7). However, this stimulatory effect of ACTH in vivo wanes after several days. Because of the increased action of aldosterone, sodium is retained and extracellular fluid volume rises above normal; therefore, the release of renin and angiotensin is suppressed and ANP release is stimulated. Together, these compensatory responses to overhydration return aldosterone levels to baseline and prevent further fluid retention.

The physiological role of ACTH in maintaining aldosterone output is a tonic one; that is, when ACTH is deficient, the zona glomerulosa is less able to respond to its primary stimulus of sodium depletion. This debility is seldom critical in patients with **hypopituitarism.** ACTH also stimulates the secretion of deoxycorticosterone (DOC) and 18-OH-DOC from the zona fasciculata. Under rare circumstances, these steroids can generate clinical syndromes of mineralocorticoid excess.

The major factors that stimulate aldosterone secretion act in an interrelated way. A low sodium intake or a low plasma sodium level potentiates aldosterone responsiveness to angiotensin, potassium, and ACTH. The increased sensitivity to angiotensin is explained by increased binding of angiotensin II to its receptors and by enhanced activity of the biosynthetic pathway. Conversely, if the potassium content of the adrenal cell is depleted, the responses to angiotensin and ACTH are diminished. The neural transmitters acetylcholine and serotonin also stimulate aldosterone secretion, whereas dopamine decreases it via an inhibitory G protein and lowered levels of cAMP.

In humans, the plasma aldosterone level fluctuates diurnally; the highest concentration occurs at 8 AM and the lowest at 11 PM. Although this profile correlates with similar directional changes in plasma renin and plasma cortisol levels, the diurnal pattern of aldosterone seems to arise independently of these levels. It is not affected by variation in sodium intake, posture, ACTH suppression by exogenous glucocorticoids, or plasma potassium levels.

Aldosterone circulates in plasma bound to a specific aldosterone-binding globulin, to transcortin, and to albumin. Overall binding to these proteins is weaker than for cortisol. Hence, the plasma half-life is only 20 minutes and the metabolic clearance rate is 1600 L/day. Ninety percent of aldosterone is cleared by the liver in a single passage. There, aldosterone is reduced to tetrahydroaldosterone, the major metabolite that is excreted in the urine as its 3-glucuronide conjugate. A smaller portion of aldosterone is excreted simply as its own 18-glucuronide conjugate. The latter metabolite, however, is most commonly measured in the urine for diagnostic purposes. The values of aldosterone 18-glucuronide in subjects with a normal sodium diet range from 5 to 20 μg/day.

■ *Actions of Aldosterone and Other Mineralocorticoids*

Aldosterone binds to the mineralocorticoid receptor in target cells, and the complex affects gene transcriptional changes in a manner similar to that described for cortisol. Various proteins that mediate the hormone's effects are induced or suppressed, but their exact identity remains to be established. A lag of 1 to 2 hours is required between exposure to aldosterone and its onset of action.

The kidney is the major site of mineralocorticoid activity (Fig. 51-21). Aldosterone stimulates the active reabsorption of sodium from the tubular urine back into the nearby capillaries by collecting duct and late distal convoluted tubule cells (see also Chapter 42). Thus, net urinary sodium excretion is diminished and this vital extracellular cation is conserved. Because water is passively reabsorbed with the sodium, there is little increase in plasma sodium concentration. Hence, extracellular fluid volume expands in a virtually isotonic fashion. Although only 3% of total sodium reabsorption is regulated by aldosterone, its deficiency produces a significant negative sodium balance.

Aldosterone acts at the following locations: (1) at the apical (luminal) surface of renal tubular cells to increase the number of membrane channels through which sodium enters the cell along an electrochemical gradient;

(2) at the basal (capillary) surface of the cell to increase Na⁺,K⁺-ATPase, which pumps the sodium out; (3) in the mitochondria, stimulating Krebs cycle reactions, such as citrate synthase, that help generate the needed energy for extrusion of sodium into the interstitial fluid and capillary blood; and (4) in the cytosol to increase phospholipase activity and synthesis of fatty acids, possibly for membrane generation.

Aldosterone stimulates the active secretion of potassium out of the tubular cell and into the urine (Fig. 51-21) *concurrently with sodium reabsorption.* However, this coincidence of effects does not constitute a direct and stoichiometric exchange of potassium for sodium. Nonetheless, the active reabsorption of sodium makes the tubular lumen electronegative, which may facilitate the transfer of potassium into the tubular urine. The ability of the tubules to excrete a potassium load depends on distal nephron flow and sodium delivery. Aldosterone allows a small secretion of potassium, even when sodium intake is restricted. However, the extent of kaliuresis increases in parallel with the rate of delivery of sodium to the distal tubule. Thus, a high sodium intake will greatly exacerbate urinary potassium losses caused by aldosterone.

Most of the potassium that is excreted daily results from distal tubular secretion. *Hence, aldosterone is criti-cal for disposal of the daily dietary potassium load at a normal plasma potassium concentration.* However, unlike what occurs with sodium flux, potassium flux does not cause an osmotically balancing movement of water. Therefore, in the absence of aldosterone, potassium retention can cause a dangerous rise in the plasma potassium concentration. An excess of the hormone decreases the plasma potassium level.

Continued administration of aldosterone when sodium intake is normal (ad libitum) produces sodium retention, weight gain (Fig. 51-22), and an increase in blood pressure as a result of the expanded extracellular fluid volume. However, after several days and an accumulation of 200 to 300 mEq of sodium, retention ceases, balance is achieved, and body weight stabilizes. This eventual escape from sodium retention is probably caused by a decrease in proximal tubule sodium reabsorption, which in turn results from expansion of the extracellular fluid and subsequent release of ANP. Nonetheless, aldosterone-induced potassium loss continues because a high rate of sodium delivery to the distal tubule is maintained.

In addition to its effects on potassium secretion, aldosterone enhances tubular secretion of hydrogen ions as sodium is reabsorbed. Therefore, aldosterone excess leads to the development of mild systemic metabolic alkalosis, which can be further aggravated by the depletion of potassium (see Chapters 43 and 44). Ammonium excretion is also increased. The final urine pH is usually alkaline, however, because the expansion of extracellular fluid volume inhibits bicarbonate reabsorption. In contrast, a deficiency of aldosterone produces a hyperchloremic non–anion gap metabolic acidosis. Finally, aldosterone also stimulates the excretion of magnesium.

Aldosterone also affects mineral transport in other organs. The hormone stimulates sodium reabsorption from the colon while enhancing potassium excretion in the feces. Similarly, the hormone decreases the ratio of sodium to potassium in perspiration and saliva. These actions, however, have little importance in overall cation balance. Aldosterone significantly affects sodium and potassium exchange between the extracellular fluid and intracellular fluid. The net result is to increase the potassium content of the intracellular space.

A clinically important effect is the increased blood pressure that results from an excess of aldosterone. In part, hypertension is an indirect consequence of the retention of sodium, expansion of the extracellular fluid volume, and a slight increase in cardiac output. In addition, the sodium and water content of the arteriolar cells may increase; the resultant swelling narrows the arteriolar lumen and increases peripheral resistance. Finally, arterial smooth muscles possess mineralocorticoid receptors (including a novel one that resides in the plasma membrane and triggers an increase in cytoplasmic inositol trisphosphate). Aldosterone antagonists lower peripheral resistance; thus, aldosterone probably has a direct vasoconstrictor action.

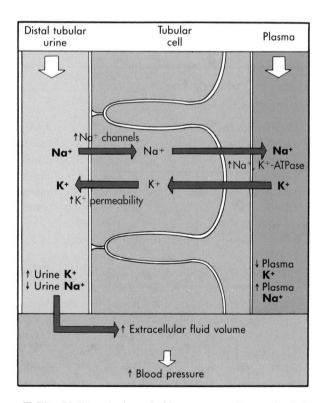

■ **Fig. 51-21** Action of aldosterone on the renal tubule. Sodium reabsorption from tubular urine into the tubular cell is stimulated. Simultaneously, potassium secretion from the tubular cell into the tubular urine is increased. At the capillary surface, Na⁺, K⁺-ATPase activity is increased so that sodium exits the cell into the capillary and potassium enters the cell from the capillary.

An excess of aldosterone (**hyperaldosteronism**) or any other mineralocorticoid produces a clinical syndrome characterized by hypertension, a slightly expanded extracellular fluid volume, hypokalemia with metabolic alkalosis, and slight hypernatremia. The diagnosis is established by demonstrating that plasma and urinary aldosterone (or rarely, DOC or 18-OH-DOC) are elevated even when the patient has a high sodium intake. If the secretion of aldosterone is autonomous, plasma renin levels are low, because of the expanded extracellular volume. Obstructive lesions of the renal arteries, which reduce perfusion pressure, stimulate excess renin secretion and, secondarily, hypersecretion of aldosterone. Treatment of hyperaldosteronism caused by zona glomerulosa tumors is accomplished by removal of the neoplasm and/or by treatment with drugs that antagonize aldosterone action (see below).

Although cortisol binds well to the mineralocorticoid receptor, it is normally prevented from contributing significantly to renal mineralocorticoid action because the kidney has very high levels of **11-β-hydroxysteroid dehydrogenase.** This enzyme inactivates cortisol locally by converting it to cortisone (Fig. 51-10). Aldosterone actions in the kidney are blocked by high concentrations of progesterone and 17-hydroxyprogesterone. An important inhibitor, which is used clinically as a diuretic and antihypertensive agent, is **spironolactone.** This drug is a competitive antagonist that binds to the mineralocorticoid receptor.

Complete destruction of the adrenal cortex, or **Addison's disease,** results from autoimmune, infectious, and malignant processes. Addison's disease usually progresses slowly as cortisol, aldosterone, and adrenal androgen deficiencies develop. A lack of cortisol leads to anorexia, weight loss, malaise, lethargy, fatigue, muscle weakness, nausea and vomiting, abdominal pain, fever, poor tolerance of minor medical or surgical stress, fasting hypoglycemia, an increase in circulating lymphocytes and eosinophils, and a reduction in neutrophils. A loss of adrenal androgens may contribute to anemia and, in females, a loss of pubic and axillary hair. Because of negative feedback, the secretion of ACTH and all proopiomelanocortin products increases as cortisol levels decline; the melanocyte-stimulating activity of ACTH and its coproducts produces striking hyperpigmentation of the skin. The diagnosis of Addison's disease is confirmed by demonstrating low plasma cortisol levels and decreased urinary excretion of 17-hydroxycorticoids and elevated plasma ACTH. If exogenous ACTH is administered, the levels of cortisol and its urinary metabolites fail to increase normally.

Deficiency of aldosterone is marked by polyuria, which is caused by natriuresis. Dehydration, hypotension, hyperkalemia, hyponatremia, and metabolic acidosis are characteristic. Plasma and urinary aldosterone levels are low, whereas plasma renin and angiotensin levels are elevated consequent to the stimulus of sodium depletion.

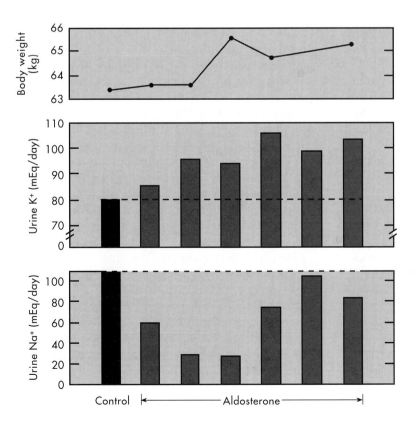

■ **Fig. 51-22**   Effects of aldosterone administration in a normal human. Note the eventual escape from sodium retention with stabilization of body weight after a small gain. However, potassium continues to be lost in the urine. Dashed lines represent levels of sodium and potassium intake. (Redrawn from August JT et al: *J Clin Invest* 37:1549, 1958. From The American Society for Clinical Investigation.)

When adrenal insufficiency is caused by ACTH deficiency (resulting from disease of the hypothalamus or pituitary), the clinical picture is the same as that described for loss of cortisol and adrenal androgen. However, plasma aldosterone and plasma potassium remain normal, because renin-angiotensin II stimulation is intact. Hyperpigmentation does not occur, because ACTH and copeptides are not present in excess.

Treatment of acute adrenal insufficiency (adrenal crisis) requires doses of intravenous cortisol that produce plasma cortisol levels typical of stress, and by sufficient isotonic sodium chloride infusion to restore normal extracellular fluid volume and lower plasma potassium levels. For maintenance, patients require oral cortisol or cortisone and a synthetic mineralocorticoid, such as **9α-fluorocortisol** (Table 51-1).

■ *The Adrenal Medulla*

The adrenal medulla is the source of the circulating catecholamine hormone **epinephrine.** It also secretes small amounts of **norepinephrine**, nominally a neurotransmitter, which in select circumstances may also function as a hormone. These compounds have diverse effects on metabolism as well as on virtually all organ systems in the body. *The adrenal medulla essentially represents an enlarged and specialized sympathetic ganglion. However, the neuronal cell bodies of the medulla do not have axons; instead, they discharge their catecholamine hormones directly into the bloodstream, and thus function as endocrine rather than nerve cells.* The adrenal medulla is formed in parallel with the peripheral sympathetic nervous system. At about 7 weeks of gestation, neuroectodermal cells from the neural crest invade the anlage of the primitive adrenal cortex. There, these cells develop into the medulla, which begins to secrete catecholamines during gestation and by birth is completely functional. The development of sympathetic nervous tissue and induction of neural hormone synthesis are stimulated by **nerve growth factor.**

Adrenomedullary tissue in the adult weighs about 1 g and consists of **chromaffin cells** (so named for their affinity for chromium stains). These cells are organized in cords and clumps in intimate relationship with venules that drain the adrenal cortex and with nerve endings from *cholinergic preganglionic fibers* of the sympathetic nervous system. Within the chromaffin cells are numerous granules 100 to 300 nm in diameter, similar to those found in postganglionic sympathetic nerve terminals. These granules contain the catecholamine hormones, epinephrine and norepinephrine (20% by weight), adenosine triphosphate and other nucleotides (15%), protein (35%),

and lipid (20%). They also contain enkephalins, β-endorphin, other proopiomelanocortin peptides, neuropeptide Y, and chromogranin.

The adrenal medulla is often activated in association with the rest of the sympathetic nervous system and acts in concert with it. Some actions of the neurotransmitter norepinephrine (which is released locally at the effector site of the postganglionic sympathetic nerve endings) are duplicated and amplified by the hormone epinephrine, which reaches similar sites via the circulation. However, epinephrine has unique effects of its own, some of which modulate those of norepinephrine. Furthermore, under certain circumstances (e.g., during hypoglycemia), the adrenal medulla is probably activated selectively, without the sympathetic nervous system.

■ *Synthesis and Storage of Catecholamine Hormones*

The catecholamine hormones are synthesized within the chromaffin cell by the series of reactions shown in Fig. 51-23. The first reaction, catalyzed by the enzyme **tyrosine hydroxylase,** is the rate-limiting step in the sequence and occurs in the chromaffin cell cytoplasm. The conversion of tyrosine to dihydroxyphenylalanine (dopa) requires molecular oxygen, the cofactor tetrahydrobiopterin, and NADPH. The subsequent catecholamine products through norepinephrine all inhibit this initial reaction. The conversion of dopa to dopamine is catalyzed by a nonspecific aromatic L-amino acid decarboxylase that uses pyridoxal phosphate as a cofactor. The dopamine thus formed in the cytoplasm must be taken up by the chromaffin granules before it can be acted on further.

The next enzyme in the sequence, **dopamine β-hydroxylase,** is found only in the granules. In the presence of molecular oxygen and a hydrogen donor, it catalyzes the formation of norepinephrine from dopamine. In approximately 15% of the granules, the sequence ends here and the norepinephrine is stored. In the rest of the granules, norepinephrine diffuses back into the cytoplasm. There, it is *N*-methylated by **phenylethanolamine *N*-methyltransferase,** which uses *S*-adenosylmethionine as the methyl donor. The resultant epinephrine is then taken back up by the chromaffin granules, in which it is stored as the predominant adrenomedullary hormone. The uptake of dopamine, norepinephrine, and epinephrine by the secretory granules is an active process that requires adenosine triphosphate (ATP) and magnesium. The storage of the catecholamine hormones at such high intragranular concentrations also requires energy in the form of ATP. In the granules, ATP is stored in a complex consisting of 1 mole of ATP with 4 moles of catecholamine and chromogranin.

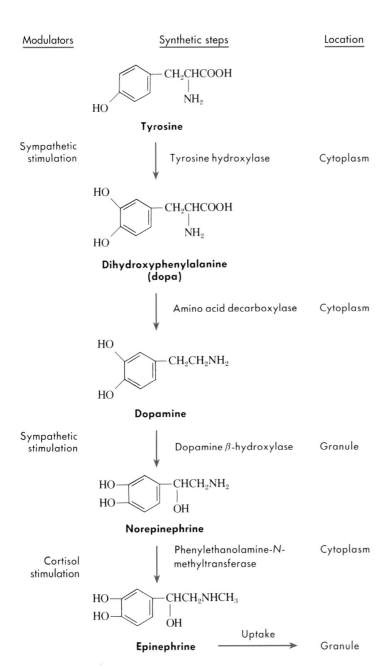

Modulators   Synthetic steps   Location

Tyrosine

Sympathetic stimulation   Tyrosine hydroxylase   Cytoplasm

Dihydroxyphenylalanine (dopa)

Amino acid decarboxylase   Cytoplasm

Dopamine

Sympathetic stimulation   Dopamine β-hydroxylase   Granule

Norepinephrine

Phenylethanolamine-N-methyltransferase   Cytoplasm

Cortisol stimulation

Epinephrine —— Uptake ——▶   Granule

■ **Fig. 51-23**   Pathway of catecholamine hormone synthesis in the adrenal medulla. Note that the dopamine β-hydroxylase reaction occurs within the secretory granule in which norepinephrine and epinephrine finally reside. Note also the stimulatory effects of sympathetic nerve impulses and of cortisol to which the adrenal medulla has preferred vascular access (see text).

Several factors regulate the synthesis of epinephrine and norepinephrine. Acute sympathetic stimulation activates tyrosine hydroxylase, possibly by decreasing cytoplasmic catecholamine levels and relieving product inhibition. Chronic stimulation of the preganglionic fibers induces increased concentrations of both tyrosine hydroxylase and dopamine β-hydroxylase and thus helps to ensure maintenance of the output of both catecholamines when the demand is continuous. The mechanism of induction may involve a cAMP-dependent protein kinase. ACTH acts directly and helps to sustain the levels of the same two enzymes under stressful conditions. By contrast, cortisol specifically induces the *N*-methyltransferase and therefore selectively stimulates

epinephrine synthesis. The anatomic relationship between the medulla and the cortex subserves this action, because blood from the cortex with a high concentration of cortisol directly perfuses the chromaffin cells.

■ *Regulation of Adrenomedullary Secretion*

Secretion from the adrenal medulla is an integral part of the "fight-or-flight" reaction evoked by stimulation of the sympathetic nervous system (Fig. 51-24). Thus, perception or even anticipation of danger or harm (anxiety), trauma, pain, hypovolemia from hemorrhage or fluid loss, hypotension, anoxia, extremes of temperature, hypoglycemia, and

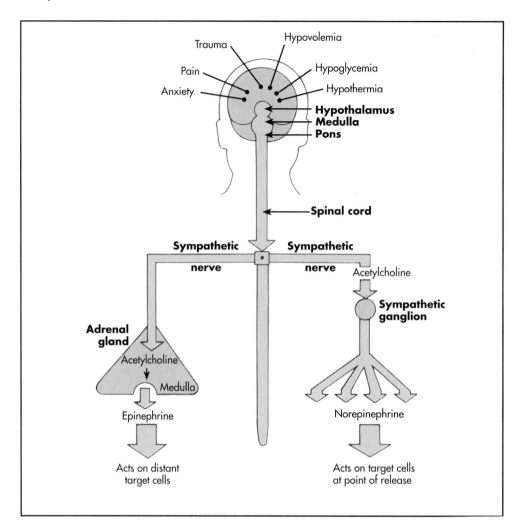

■ **Fig. 51-24**   Stimuli to activation of catecholamine effects and their pathways. The adrenal medulla is homologous to a sympathetic ganglion. The latter releases norepinephrine into synaptic clefts. The adrenal medulla releases primarily epinephrine into the bloodstream, where it acts on distant targets.

severe exercise cause rapid secretion of epinephrine (and probably norepinephrine) from the adrenal medulla. These stimuli are sensed at various higher levels in the sympathetic nervous system, and responses are initiated in the hypothalamus and brainstem (see Chapter 15). Usually, activation of the adrenal medulla follows activation of the sympathetic nervous system, and the adrenomedullary responses are activated by more intense stimuli.

The final common effector pathway that activates the adrenal medulla consists of cholinergic preganglionic fibers in the greater splanchnic nerve. When these fibers are stimulated, acetylcholine is released from the nerve terminals. This neurotransmitter depolarizes the chromaffin cell membrane by increasing its permeability to sodium. Depolarization in turn induces an influx of calcium ions, which stimulate exocytosis of the secretory granules. Epinephrine, norepinephrine, ATP, the enzyme dopamine β-hydroxylase, and other constituents (see above) are released into the circulation. The membranous

material of the granule is retained in the chromaffin cell and probably recycled.

Basal plasma epinephrine levels are 25 to 50 pg/ml (6×10^{-10} M). The estimated daily basal delivery rate of epinephrine is 150 μg. The rate of epinephrine release can increase greatly with physiological stimuli (Table 51-4). For example, with a modest fall in plasma glucose concentration to 55 to 60 mg/dl, epinephrine concentrations rise to approximately 250 pg/ml. If epinephrine is infused exogenously at a rate sufficient to achieve this epinephrine concentration, the plasma glucose level rises. Hence, the adrenal medulla secretes enough epinephrine to contribute to glucose homeostasis.

The same relationship between epinephrine secretion and its effects characterizes the cardiovascular responses. An increase in heart rate and systolic blood pressure can be produced by the concentrations of epinephrine that are generated endogenously when an individual assumes an upright position (Table 51-4). In addition, the high con-

■ **Table 51-4** Comparison of circulating concentrations of catecholamine hormones with biologically effective concentrations

Physiological state	Relevant biological action	Plasma epinephrine (pg/ml)		Plasma norepinephrine (pg/ml)	
		Observed	*Effective range for relevant biological action*	*Observed*	*Effective range for relevant biological action*
Basal	—	34	—	228	—
Upright position	↑ Heart rate and blood pressure	73	50-125	526	1800
↓ Plasma glucose	↑ Plasma glucose	230	150-200	262	1800
Severe hypoglycemia	—	1500	—	770	—
Diabetic ketoacidosis	↑ Lipolysis and ketosis ↓ Insulin	510	100-400	1270	1800

Based on data from Clutter WE et al: *J Clin Invest* 66:94, 1980; Silverberg AB et al: *Am J Physiol* 234:E252, 1978; and Christensen NJ: *Diabetes* 23:1, 1974.

centrations of epinephrine that occur in illnesses such as diabetic ketoacidosis (see Chapter 47) can contribute to the pathological state by stimulating glycogenolysis, lipolysis, and ketosis. Thus, epinephrine functions as a true hormone in all these situations.

In contrast, circulating norepinephrine levels do not generally increase to levels sufficient to produce relevant biological actions (Table 51-4). Therefore, norepinephrine does not usually function in an endocrine fashion, although it may do so in severe, stressful illnesses such as myocardial infarction. Instead, the effects of norepinephrine on metabolic processes, such as glucose production or lipolysis, result from its role as a neurotransmitter. The necessary high concentrations of norepinephrine are thus generated locally at the effector site.

■ *Metabolism of Catecholamines*

Essentially all the epinephrine that circulates in the body is derived from the adrenal medulla. In contrast, most of the circulating norepinephrine is derived from sympathetic nerve terminals and from the brain, having escaped immediate local reuptake from synaptic clefts. However, the metabolic fate of epinephrine and norepinephrine merges into one or two major excretory products (Fig. 51-25).

Epinephrine and norepinephrine have extremely short lifespans in the circulation; this feature allows rapid turnoff of their dramatic effects. Half-lives are in the range of 1 to 3 minutes, and their metabolic clearance rates range from 2.0 to 6.0 L/min. The clearance rates of both hormones can be further increased by the hormones themselves by activation of β-adrenergic receptors, another mechanism that helps to limit the actions of these hormones. Only 2% to 3% of catecholamines is excreted unchanged in the urine. The normal total daily excretion is about 50 μg, of which 20% is epinephrine and 80% is norepinephrine. Another 100 μg is excreted as sulfate or glucuronide conjugates. Most epinephrine is metabolized within the adrenomedullary chromaffin cell when synthesis exceeds the capacity for storage. Circulating epinephrine and norepinephrine are metabolized predominantly in the liver and kidney.

The catecholamine hormones are metabolized by the reaction sequences shown in Fig. 51-25. The key enzymes are **catecholamine O-methyltransferase** and the combination of **monoamine oxidase** and **aldehyde oxidase.** O-Methylation and oxidative deamination can be carried out in either order; these reactions give rise to several products that are then excreted in the urine. O-Methylation alone yields an average daily excretion of metanephrine (from epinephrine) plus normetanephrine (from norepinephrine) of 300 μg. In contrast, the excretion of the common deaminated products, vanillylmandelic acid (VMA) and methoxyhydroxyphenylglycol (MOPG), averages 4.0 mg and 2.0 mg, respectively. Normally, epinephrine accounts for only a minor fraction of urinary VMA and MOPG; the majority is derived from norepinephrine and largely reflects activity of the sympathetic nervous system. *Activity of the adrenal medulla can be assessed specifically only by measurement of urinary free epinephrine or plasma epinephrine levels.*

■ *Actions of Catecholamines*

Intracellular actions. Epinephrine and norepinephrine exert their effects on a group of plasma membrane receptors designated β_1, β_2, β_3, α_1, and α_2. The relative potency of the two catecholamines varies with each receptor type. Epinephrine tends to react more strongly with β receptors, and norepinephrine with α receptors, but overlap is considerable. Specific agonists and antagonists have been developed for each receptor type.

The β_1, β_2, and α_2 receptors are structurally similar. All three of these receptors are single-unit transmembrane glycoproteins (see Fig. 5-5). α_1 receptors differ from these receptors and have higher molecular weights. β_1, β_2, and β_3 receptors are coupled to and stimulate adenylyl cyclase; thus, cAMP is the second messenger for these biological effects. Protein kinase A is then activated, and a cascade of changes in enzyme activities follows. The α_2 receptor, in contrast, is coupled to an inhibitory G protein; thus, hormone binding decreases cAMP levels and protein kinase A activity. The α_1 receptor is coupled to the phosphatidylinositol membrane system; calcium, along with protein kinase C, mediates the hormone effects.

Continuous stimulation of catecholamine release or exposure to catecholamine agonists down-regulates the number of adrenergic receptors and induces partial refractoriness to hormone action. Conversely, sympathectomy increases the number of receptors and enhances sensitivity to catecholamines. Acute exposure to catecholamine hormones produces rapid desensitization to subsequent doses. This effect is caused by phosphorylation of the various receptors by the hormone-activated protein kinase A or C. Phosphorylation renders the receptors inaccessible to further hormone binding. Receptor desensitization is a form of rapid intracellular negative feedback, which limits hormone actions.

β Agonists are used clinically to relieve bronchial constriction in patients with asthma. However, overuse leads to a state of refractoriness to such therapy by the mechanisms detailed above.

Effects on metabolism. A list of epinephrine and norepinephrine actions is presented in Table 51-5. The overall effects on metabolism are depicted in Fig. 51-26. Both catecholamine hormones increase glucose production. They stimulate glycogenolysis in the liver by binding to β-receptors and activating phosphorylase through the same cAMP-initiated cascade produced by glucagon. Glycogen synthase activity is concurrently restrained. The adrenomedullary epinephrine response to hypoglycemia is not needed as long as glucagon secretion is intact. However, in the absence of glucagon, epinephrine becomes essential for recovery from hypoglycemia.

Epinephrine and norepinephrine also stimulate gluconeogenesis by activation of α and β receptors on the liver cells. In addition, they stimulate muscle glycogenolysis, which increases plasma lactate levels and provides additional gluconeogenetic substrate to the liver. Simultaneously, epinephrine inhibits insulin-mediated glucose uptake by muscle and adipose tissue. By activating α receptors, the catecholamines also stimulate glucagon secretion and inhibit insulin secretion. *All these*

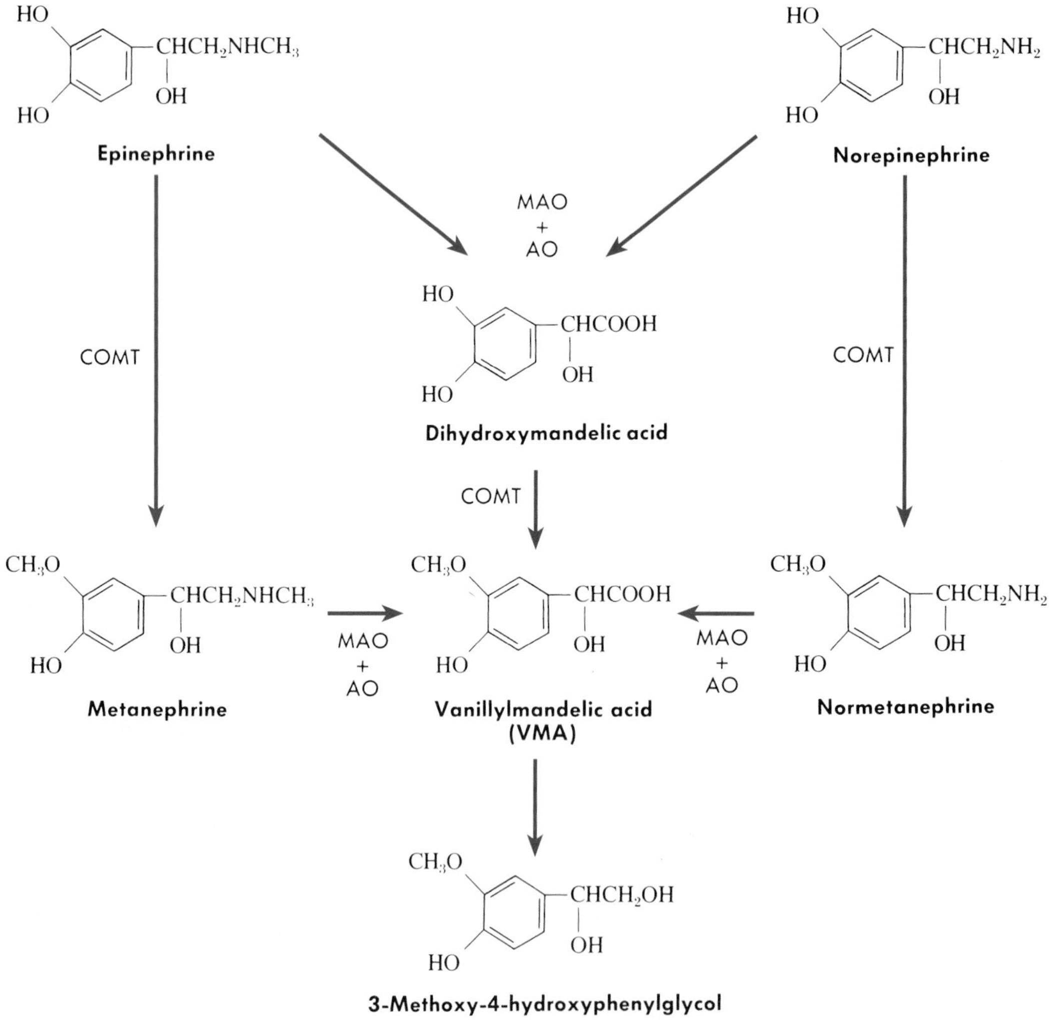

■ **Fig. 51-25**   Metabolism of catecholamine hormones. VMA is quantitatively the main product. *MAO,* Monoamine oxidase; *AO,* aldehyde oxidase; *COMT,* catecholamine-*O*-methyltransferase.

catecholamine actions help prevent hypoglycemia or restore plasma glucose and glucose delivery to the central nervous system. At the same time, epinephrine activates adipose tissue lipase and thereby increases plasma free fatty acid levels, their β oxidation in muscle and liver, and ketogenesis.

When the catecholamine hormones are secreted during exercise, they promote (1) use of muscle glycogen stores by stimulating phosphorylase, (2) efficient hepatic reutilization for gluconeogenesis of lactate released by the exercising muscle, and (3) provision of free fatty acids as alternative fuels. When epinephrine secretion is stimulated by "stress," such as during illness or surgery, its actions on fuel turnover contribute significantly to induction of hyperglycemia and ketosis; that is, it is a diabetogenic hormone.

Epinephrine also increases the basal metabolic rate by 7% to 15%, as well as increasing nonshivering thermogenesis and diet-induced thermogenesis. Therefore, epinephrine is an important part of the response to cold exposure and helps to regulate overall energy balance and stores. In neonates of many species, brown adipose tissue* is an important site where catecholamines increase heat production (see Chapter 46). Here, they stimulate proton conductance into the mitochondria and thereby uncouple ATP synthesis from oxygen utilization.

In most metabolic effects, epinephrine is more potent than norepinephrine. The latter nonetheless contributes to the regulation of metabolism via the activity of the sympathetic nervous system. For example, sympathetic nervous system activity, with norepinephrine as the mediator, decreases with fasting and increases after feeding. By modulating thermogenesis, norepinephrine thus helps to adapt total energy utilization to energy availability. In contrast, epinephrine secretion increases modestly during prolonged fasting and also 4 to 5 hours after a meal, in both cases in response to a declining plasma glucose level. This increase in epinephrine levels helps to sustain glucose production for use by the central nervous system.

Effects on the cardiovascular system. The cardiovascular effects of epinephrine reinforce its metabolic actions. Heart rate, contractile force, and cardiac output increase; on the other hand, arteriolar constriction is selectively produced in the renal, splanchnic, and cutaneous beds. Systolic blood pressure increases, whereas diastolic blood pressure remains unchanged or decreases

■ **Table 51-5** Some actions of catecholamine hormones

β *Epinephrine > norepinephrine*	α *Norepinephrine > epinephrine*
↑ Glycogenolysis	↑ Gluconeogenesis (α_1)
↑ Gluconeogenesis (β_2)	↑ Glycogenolysis (α_1)
↑ Lipolysis (β_3) (β_2)	
↑ Calorigenesis (β_1)	
↓ Glucose utilization	
↑ Insulin secretion (β_2)	↓ Insulin secretion (α_2)
↑ Glucagon secretion (β_2)	
↑ Muscle K$^+$ uptake (β_2)	↑ Cardiac contractility (α_1)
↑ Cardiac contractility (β_1)	
↑ Heart rate (β_1)	
↑ Conduction velocity (β_1)	
↑ Arteriolar dilation: ↓ BP (β_2) (muscle)	↑ Arteriolar vasoconstriction; ↑ BP (α_1) (splanchnic, renal, cutaneous, genital)
↑ Muscle relaxation (β_2)	↑ Sphincter contraction (α_1)
Gastrointestinal	Gastrointestinal
Urinary	Urinary
Bronchial	Platelet aggregation (α_2)
	Sweating ("adrenergic")
	Dilation of pupils (α_1)

BP, Blood pressure.

*The role of this specialized adipose tissue in human physiology is controversial.

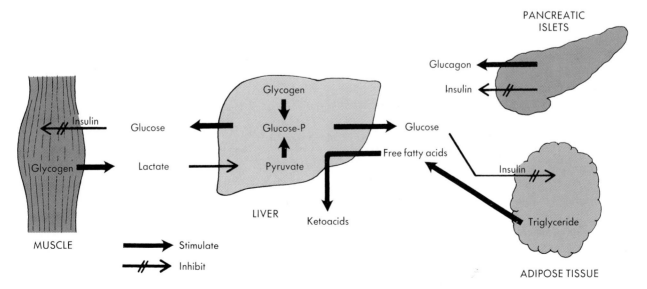

■ **Fig. 51-26** Metabolic actions of epinephrine. The hormone stimulates glucose production and inhibits glucose use. It also stimulates lipolysis and ketogenesis. Insulin secretion is inhibited. The net effect is a rise in plasma glucose, free fatty acids, and ketoacids.

slightly. During exercise, the net effect of these changes is to shunt blood toward the active muscles while maintaining coronary and cerebral blood flow (see Chapters 30 and 31). These changes guarantee delivery of substrate for energy production to the critical organs in the fight-or-flight situation. During exposure to cold, constriction of cutaneous vessels helps to conserve heat and thereby reinforces the thermogenic action of epinephrine.

The cardiovascular responses to catecholamines also initially benefit an individual who has suffered major trauma, circulatory failure, or hypoxia. Without them, death might rapidly ensue. However, prolonged secretion of catecholamines eventually becomes deleterious. Reduced blood flow to the kidneys leads to renal failure; reduced blood flow to the splanchnic bed leads to hepatic failure, as well as intestinal paralysis and necrosis; and reduced blood flow to many tissues leads to decreased oxygenation with increased lactate production. In the face of decreased lactate utilization in the liver, increased lactate production produces metabolic (lactate) acidosis (see Chapter 44).

Effects on other systems. Catecholamines exert other diverse effects. Inhibition of gastrointestinal and genitourinary motor activity, relaxation of bronchioles to prevent expiratory airway obstruction and improve gas exchange, and dilation of pupils to permit better distant vision are of benefit to the endangered individual. Catecholamines modulate ADH release (β receptors stimulate and α receptors inhibit). They increase renin release by stimulation of β receptors in the kidney. The increase in renin increases aldosterone secretion, which in turn enhances sodium retention. This action is augmented by local catecholamine effects in the kidney on the distribution of blood flow and on tubular function. Epinephrine stimulates influx of potassium into muscle cells via β_2 receptors. The movement of potassium into the intracellular space helps to prevent hyperkalemia. The important interaction between catecholamine and thyroid hormone function is reviewed in Chapter 50. Thyroid hormone secretion is enhanced by catecholamines under some circumstances, and the peripheral conversion of T_4 to T_3 is stimulated via β_2 receptors.

Catecholamine agonists and antagonists are used widely in medicine. A group of agonists called **amphetamines** are used as nasal decongestants, appetite suppressants, and general stimulants. Amphetamines may be prescribed or sold over the counter, but their illicit availability has also become a public health problem. They may cause hypertension; exacerbate tachycardia, palpitations, and nervousness in hyperthyroid patients; or increase plasma glucose in diabetic patients. In large doses, they can produce life-threatening "highs." Certain β agonists are used to quiet premature uterine contractions in pregnancy.

β-Adrenergic antagonists, α_1 antagonists, and α_2 agonists are used to treat hypertension. β Antagonists relieve symptoms and extend life in coronary artery disease. They also counteract the hyperactive adrenergic state in hyperthyroid patients.

■ *Pathological Secretion of Catecholamines*

Spontaneous deficiency of epinephrine is unknown as an adult disease, and adrenalectomized patients do not require epinephrine replacement. Hypersecretion of epinephrine and norepinephrine from tumors of the chromaffin cells (**pheochromocytoma**) results in a well-defined syndrome. Dramatic clinical episodes are caused by spurts of catecholamine release. These bursts can result from stress or from a rapid change in posture. Sudden severe headache, palpitations, chest pain, extreme anxiety with a sense of impending death, and cold perspiration may occur. Blood pressure may rise to extremely high levels, for example, to 250/150. If epinephrine is mainly being secreted, the heart rate will be increased; if norepinephrine is the predominant hormone, the heart rate will decrease in a reflex response to the marked hypertension. In addition to these episodes, chronic catecholamine excess may produce weight loss, as a result of an increased metabolic rate and decreased appetite. Hyperglycemia can result from inhibition of insulin secretion.

The diagnosis is established by detecting high plasma levels of epinephrine or norepinephrine when the patient is recumbent and at rest. In addition, urinary excretion of free catecholamines, metanephrines, and VMA is usually increased.

Definitive treatment requires removal of the adrenomedullary tumor. Symptomatic treatment is provided by α-adrenergic antagonists, which lower the elevated blood pressure, and β-adrenergic antagonists, which reduce dangerous tachycardia.

■ *Integration of the Response to Stress*

The intimate anatomic relationship between the adrenal medulla and the adrenal cortex mirrors a fundamental functional relationship between the adrenergic nervous system and the CRH-ACTH-cortisol axis. Both the adrenal cortex and the adrenal medulla are major participants in adaptation to stress. In addition, interactions between these two physiological entities and the immune system add further complexity to this adaptative response, particularly when stress is produced by foreign substances or invading organisms. Thus, it is useful to present an integrated overview of the adaptation to stress (Fig. 51-27).

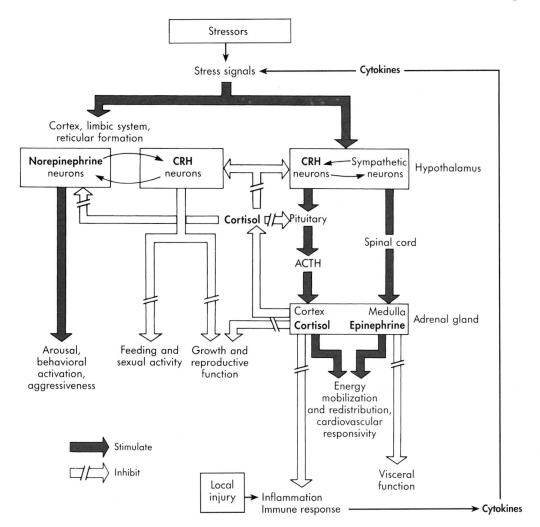

■ **Fig. 51-27** Integrated responses to stress. Responses mediated by the sympathetic nervous system (SNS) and the hypothalamic-pituitary-adrenocortical axis (HPA) are mutually reinforcing, at both the central and peripheral levels. Negative feedback by cortisol can also limit an overresponse that might be harmful to the individual. A feedback relationship between local immune responses to injury and the HPA-SNS consortium also exists. Cytokines stimulate the central responses, and cortisol inhibits excessive cytokine production. *Colored arrows,* Stimulation; *open arrows,* inhibition; *CRH,* corticotropin-releasing hormone; *ACTH,* adrenocorticotropic hormone.

Stress is perceived by many areas of the brain, from the cortex down to the brainstem. Major stresses activate CRH and ADH neurons in the paraventricular nucleus and adrenergic neurons elsewhere in the hypothalamus. The activation is mutually reinforcing, because norepinephrine increases CRH release and CRH increases adrenergic discharge (Fig. 51-27). CRH and ADH release stimulates ACTH release and ultimately elevates plasma cortisol levels; adrenergic stimulation elevates plasma epinephrine and norepinephrine levels. Together, these hormones increase glucose production. Catecholamines do so rapidly by activating glycogenolysis, and cortisol acts more slowly by providing amino acid substrate for gluconeogenesis. Together, they shift glucose utilization toward the central nervous system and away from peripheral tissues. Epinephrine also rapidly augments free fatty acid supply to the heart and to muscles, and cortisol facil-itates this lipolytic response. Both hormones raise blood pressure and cardiac output and improve delivery of substrates to tissues that are critical to the immediate defense of the organism.

The neurotransmitter norepinephrine and the neuropeptide CRH can produce other adaptive responses to stress. A general state of arousal and vigilance, an activation of defensively useful behavior, and appropriate aggressiveness result from adrenergic stimuli to the pertinent brain centers. At the same time, CRH input to other hypothalamic neurons inhibits growth hormone and gonadotropin release, as well as sexual activity, presumably because growth and reproduction are not useful functions during stress. These actions are reinforced by the excess of cortisol, which also suppresses growth and ovulation. In addition, CRH inhibits appetite and feeding behavior, which again are inappropriate when the organism perceives itself to be in immediate serious danger. CRH input into the arcuate nucleus of the hypothalamus, hindbrain, and spinal cord increases awareness of pain; in contrast, proopiomelanocortin peptide products related to ACTH (see Chapter 49) produce analgesia and feedback to dampen excessive CRH and norepinephrine release caused by stress.

At the same time, a variety of cytokines are released at local sites of injury. These immune system "hormones" stimulate cellular and humoral defenses that repel, neutralize, or eliminate harmful organisms or foreign molecules. However, a balance is needed between these useful local responses and their possibly counterproductive systemic spread. If plasma cytokine concentrations (such as IL-1, IL-6, and TNF_α) become greatly elevated, they stimulate CRH release, which ultimately raises plasma cortisol (Fig. 51-27). As the level of plasma cortisol becomes progressively elevated, the production of these same cytokines is inhibited.

Individuals who respond strongly to stress with CRH, and therefore with cortisol, have less chance of activating any underlying autoimmune disease process but may increase their risk of disseminating an infection. The reverse is true in individuals who are unable to mount even a "normal" stress response.

In short, the hypothalamic CRF-pituitary ACTH-adrenal cortisol axis and the sympathetic nervous system operate jointly in adaptation to stress. They reinforce each other's actions to promote life-saving behavior and inhibit activities that divert individuals and their resources from defensive responses to danger. They also interact with the immune system to produce a balance between useful local cytokine production and potentially dangerous systemic effects of these immune products.

■ *Summary*

1. The two adrenal glands consist of an outer three-layered cortex and an inner medulla. The cortex secretes three types of steroid hormones: cortisol, a glucocorticoid; aldosterone, a mineralocorticoid; and androgen precursors. The medulla secretes the catecholamine hormones epinephrine and norepinephrine. The adrenal glands are richly vascularized and essential to survival because of the cortisol they produce.

2. All adrenocorticosteroids are synthesized from cholesterol by sequential enzymatic steps, which consist of side-chain cleavage and hydroxylation of key sites in the steroid nucleus. Cortisol specifically requires an 11-hydroxyl group; aldosterone, an 18-hydroxyl group; and androgens, a 17-hydroxyl group for respective activities. The mitochondrial and microsomal enzymes involved are P-450 mixed oxygenases. Steroid hormones are not stored directly. Rather, increased secretory demands require rapid synthesis from stored cholesterol.

3. Cortisol and androgen secretion are regulated by adrenocorticotropic hormone (ACTH). The pituitary hormone acts through a plasma membrane receptor with cAMP as the main second messenger. ACTH stimulates cellular uptake of cholesterol, its movement from storage vacuoles into mitochondria, and all subsequent biosynthetic steps.

4. Cortisol has major effects on protein, glucose, and fat metabolism. The hormone binds to its receptor, and the complex links to a glucocorticoid regulatory element on target DNA molecules. Modulation of gene expression of numerous enzymes and proteins follows. Cortisol increases muscle proteolysis and stimulates hepatic conversion of the liberated amino acids into glucose, which is then released into the circulation or stored in the liver as glycogen. Cortisol also inhibits insulin-stimulated glucose uptake by muscle. Cortisol stimulates caloric intake and favors deposition of fat in selected sites. By inhibiting collagen synthesis, cortisol reduces bone formation and impairs the integrity of capillaries and skin.

5. Cortisol strongly inhibits the entire process of inflammation, including the recruitment of neutrophils and the release of numerous inflammatory mediators. It also inhibits the immune system and prevents proliferation of thymus-derived lymphocytes and production of lymphokines. These actions underlie the broad therapeutic use of synthetic analogs of cortisol as anti-inflammatory and immune suppressant agents.

6. Aldosterone is a major regulator of sodium, potassium, and fluid balance. Aldosterone secretion is regulated mainly by the renin-angiotensin system. In response to sodium deprivation, production of angiotensin II is increased. This hormone stimulates aldosterone secretion via Ca^{++} and phosphatidylinositol second messengers. Aldosterone secretion is also directly stimulated by potassium.

7. Aldosterone acts on the renal tubule via a specific nuclear receptor and gene expression. Sodium reabsorption is increased with concomitant expansion of extracellular fluid. Potassium excretion is simultaneously increased and plasma potassium concentration is lowered.

8. The adrenal medulla is an enlarged, specialized sympathetic ganglion. It synthesizes epinephrine and norepinephrine from tyrosine and stores these catecholamine hormones in granules. They are released in response to stimulation of preganglionic cholinergic sympathetic nervous system fibers. Hypoglycemia, hypovolemia, hypotension, stress, and pain are major stimuli.

9. Epinephrine (and to a lesser extent norepinephrine) act as true hormones to increase glycogenolysis in liver

and muscle and lipolysis in adipose tissue. Epinephrine also decreases insulin-stimulated glucose uptake and increases the metabolic rate. cAMP and Ca^{++} are second messengers. Epinephrine increases plasma glucose, free fatty acids, and ketoacids. Numerous vascular and visceral actions of the sympathetic nervous system are also reinforced by circulating epinephrine.

■ *Self-Study Problems*

1. A patient who receives a glucocorticoid to prevent rejection of a renal transplant suffers staphylococcal contamination of an accidental penetrating wound of the abdomen. How will the glucocorticoid influence his defensive response to the infection?

2. How does aldosterone help mediate the process of acclimatization that occurs when a Scandinavian soldier is abruptly sent by the United Nations to a trouble spot in the Sahara desert?

3. A tourist from Kenya hiking in Yellowstone Park suddenly encounters an adult bear who advances toward her. Describe the useful catecholamine responses that could facilitate her avoidance of the danger.

■ *Bibliography*

Journal articles

Allison AC, Lee SW: The mode of action of anti-rheumatic drugs. I. Anti-inflammatory and immunosuppressive effects of glucocorticoids, *Prog Drug Res* 33:63, 1989.

Bamberger CM, Schulte HM, Chrousos GP: Molecular determinants of glucocorticoid receptor function and tissue sensitivity to glucocorticoids, *Endocr Rev* 17:245, 1996.

Barbarino A et al: Corticotropin-releasing hormone inhibition of gonadotropin release and the effect of opioid blockade, *J Clin Endocrinol Metab* 68:523, 1989.

Barrett PQ et al: Role of calcium in angiotensin II-mediated aldosterone secretion, *Endocr Rev* 10:496, 1989.

Bergendahl M et al: Fasting as a metabolic stress paradigm selectively amplifies cortisol secretory burst mass and delays the time of maximal nyctohemeral cortisol concentrations in healthy men, *J Clin Endocrinol Metab* 81:692, 1996.

Born J et al: Influences of cortisol on auditory evoked potentials (AEPs) and mood in humans, *Neuropsychobiology* 20:145, 1989.

Burnstein KC, Cidlowski JA: Regulation of gene expression by glucocorticoids, *Annu Rev Physiol* 51:603, 1989.

Cato ACB, Wade E: Molecular mechanisms of anti-inflammatory action of glucocorticoids, *BioEssays* 18:371, 1996.

Chrousos GP: The hypothalamic-pituitary-adrenal axis and immune-mediated inflammation, *Semin Med Beth Israel Hosp Boston* 332:1351, 1995.

Chrousos GP, Gold PW: The concepts of stress and stress system disorders, *JAMA* 267:1244, 1992.

Cidlowski JA et al: The biochemistry and molecular biology of glucocorticoid-induced apoptosis in the immune system, *Recent Prog Horm Res* 51:457, 1996.

Darmaun D et al: Physiological hypercortisolemia increases proteolysis, glutamine, and alanine production, *Am J Physiol* 255:E366, 1988.

DeFeo P et al: Contribution of cortisol to glucose counterregulation in humans, *Am J Physiol* 257:E35, 1989.

Estaban NV et al: Daily cortisol production rate in man determined by stable isotope dilution/mass spectrometry, *J Clin Endocrinol Metab* 72:39, 1991.

Goodfriend TL, Elliott ME, Catt KJ: Angiotensin receptors and their antagonists, *N Engl J Med* 334:1649, 1996.

Gustafsson J et al: Biochemistry, molecular biology and physiology of the glucocorticoid receptor, *Endocr Rev* 8:185, 1987.

Hauner H et al: Glucocorticoids and insulin promote the differentiation of human adipocyte precursor cells into fat cells, *J Clin Endocrinol Metab* 64:832, 1987.

Horber FF et al: Differential effects of prednisone and growth hormone on fuel metabolism and insulin antagonism in humans, *Diabetes* 40:141, 1991.

Horrocks PM et al: Patterns of ACTH and cortisol pulsatility over twenty-four hours in normal males and females, *Clin Endocrinol (Oxf)* 32:127, 1990.

Kirkham BW, Panayi GS: Diurnal periodicity of cortisol secretion, immune reactivity and disease activity in rheumatoid arthritis: implications for steroid treatment, *Br J Rheumatol* 28:154, 1989.

Lundgren JD et al: Mechanisms by which glucocorticosteroids inhibit secretion of mucus in asthmatic airways, *Am Rev Respir Dis* 141:S52, 1990.

Mastorakos G, Chrousos GP, Weber JS: Recombinant interleukin-6 activates the hypothalamic-pituitary-adrenal axis in humans, *J Clin Endocrinol Metab* 77:1690, 1993.

Matthews DE et al: Effect of epinephrine on amino acid and energy metabolism in humans, *Am J Physiol* 258:E948, 1990.

Miller WL: Molecular biology of steroid hormone synthesis, *Endocr Rev* 9:295, 1988.

Norbiato G et al: Cortisol resistance in acquired immunodeficiency syndrome, *J Clin Endocrinol Metab* 74:608, 1992.

Peers SH, Flower RJ: The role of lipocortin in corticosteroid actions, *Am Rev Respir Dis* 141:S18, 1990.

Penhoat A et al: Synergistic effects of corticotropin and insulin-like growth factor I on corticotropin receptors and corticotropin responsiveness in cultured bovine adrenocortical cells, *Biochem Biophys Res Commun* 165:355, 1989.

Prummel MF et al: The course of biochemical parameters of bone turnover during treatment with corticosteroids, *J Clin Endocrinol Metab* 72:382, 1991.

Rebuffe-Scrive M et al: Muscle and adipose tissue morphology and metabolism in Cushing's syndrome, *J Clin Endocrinol Metab* 67:1122, 1988.

Rosner W: The functions of corticosteroid-binding globulin and sex hormone-binding globulin: recent advances, *Endocr Rev* 11:80, 1990.

Schenker Y: Atrial natriuretic hormone and aldosterone regulation in salt-depleted state, *Am J Physiol* 257:E583, 1989.

Schleimer RP: Effects of glucocorticosteroids on inflammatory cells relevant to their therapeutic applications in asthma, *Am Rev Respir Dis* 141:S59, 1990.

Simpson ER, Waterman MR: Regulation of the synthesis of steroidogenic enzymes in adrenal cortical cells by ACTH, *Annu Rev Physiol* 50:427, 1988.

Smith JB, Lee H-W, Smith L: Regulation of expression of sodium-calcium exchanger and plasma membrane calcium ATPase by protein kinases, glucocorticoids, and growth factors, *Ann NY Acad Sci* 779:258, 1996.

Stocco DM, Clark BJ: Regulation of the acute production of steroids in steroidogenic cells, *Endocr Rev* 17:221, 1996.

Taylor AL, Fishman LM: Corticotropin-releasing hormone, *N Engl J Med* 319:213, 1988.

Umeki S, Soejima R: Hydrocortisone inhibits the respiratory burst oxidase from human neutrophils in whole-cell and cell-free systems, *Biochem Biophys Acta* 1052:211, 1990.

Vamvakopoulos NC, Chrousos GP: Hormonal regulation of human corticotropin-releasing hormone gene expression: implications for the stress response and immune/inflammatory reaction, *Endocr Rev* 15:409, 1994.

Veldhuis JD et al: Amplitude modulation of a burstlike mode of cortisol secretion subserves the circadian glucocorticoid rhythm, *Am J Physiol* 257:E6, 1989.

Wick G, Hu Y, Schwarz S, Kroemer G: Immunoendocrine communication via the hypothalamo-pituitary-adrenal axis in auto-immune diseases, *Endocr Rev* 14:539, 1993.

Wong MM et al: Long-term effects of physiologic concentrations of dexamethasone on human bone-derived cells, *J Bone Miner Res* 5:803, 1990.

Young DB: Quantitative analysis of aldosterone's role in potassium regulation, *Am J Physiol* 255:F811, 1988.

Books and monographs

Keiser HR: *Pheochromocytoma and related tumors.* In DeGroot LJ, editor: *Endocrinology,* ed 3, Philadelphia, 1995, WB Saunders.

Lansberg L, Young JB: *Catecholamines and the adrenal medulla.* In Wilson JD, Foster DW, editors: *Williams textbook of endocrinology,* Philadelphia, 1992, WB Saunders.

Meikle AW: *Secretion and metabolism of the corticosteroids and adrenal function and testing.* In DeGroot LJ, editor: *Endocrinology,* Philadelphia, 1989, WB Saunders.

Mortensen RM, Williams GH: *Aldosterone action. Physiology.* In DeGroot LJ, editor: *Endocrinology,* ed 3, Philadelphia, 1995, WB Saunders.

Munck A, Náray-Fejes-Tóth A: *Glucocorticoid action. Physiology.* In DeGroot LJ, editor: *Endocrinology,* ed 3, Philadelphia, 1995, WB Saunders.

Orth DN, Kovacs WJ, Debold CR: *The adrenal cortex.* In Wilson JD, Foster DW, editors: *Williams textbook of endocrinology,* Philadelphia, 1992, WB Saunders.

The Reproductive Glands

The endocrine glands that have been discussed in previous chapters are essential to the maintenance of the life and the well-being of the individual. *The endocrine function of the reproductive glands, or gonads, is primarily concerned with the preservation and the well-being of the species.* The evolution of sexual reproduction has required the development of highly complex patterns of gonadal function. The gonads govern the development, maturation, and nutritional support of the individual male and female germ cells and their successful union in reproduction. They also assist in the early growth and development of the offspring within the body of the mother. Although many obvious differences exist between the functioning of the testes and the ovaries, there are also important basic conceptual similarities and operational homologies. Therefore, this chapter presents human gonadal endocrinology as a single unit in the following sequence: (1) sexual differentiation, (2) homologous aspects of gonadal structure and function, (3) testicular function, (4) ovarian function, and (5) endocrine aspects of pregnancy.

■ Sexual Differentiation

The process of sexual differentiation (i.e., the pattern of development of the gonads, genital ducts, and external genitalia) produces the most fundamental and obvious differences between the genders. However, during the first 5 weeks of gestation, the gonads of males and females are indistinguishable and their genital tracts are unformed. Between this stage of the "indifferent gonad" and that of the mature individual of either gender, the process of sexual differentiation (Figs. 52-1 to 52-3) takes place. Before this process is described, it is useful to consider the gonadal cell lines and functions that are common to both genders (Fig. 52-1).

Primordial germ cells generate the **oogonia** and **spermatogonia,** which undergo eventual reductional division and maturation into large numbers of ova and sperm, respectively. Only a few of each eventually unite with each other to reproduce the species, in a manner that guarantees an almost infinite variety of individual characteristics.

One cell line of the indifferent gonad becomes the **granulosa cells** of the **ovarian follicle** and the **Sertoli cells** of the **testicular seminiferous tubules.** The function of these cells is homologous: to sustain or "nurse" the germ cells, foster their maturation, and guide their movement into the genital duct system. This cell line is also the main source of estrogenic hormones in females. Another cell line of the indifferent gonad, the **interstitial cells,** gives rise to **theca cells** in the ovary and **Leydig cells** in the testis. The primary function of this cell line is to secrete androgenic hormones. These hormones are essential to the development of masculine sex characteristics and sperm production and, in females, as precursors for estrogen synthesis.

The final maleness or femaleness of individuals is best characterized in terms of differences in genetic sex (genotype), gonadal sex, and genital sex (phenotype).

■ Genetic Sex

The normal male chromosome complement is 44 autosomes and two sex chromosomes, X and Y. *The presence of the Y chromosome is a positive and the single most constant determinant of maleness.* Without a Y chromosome (or critical material translocated from a Y to an X chromosome), neither testes nor a masculine genital pattern can develop.

The Y chromosome contains the 14-kilobase segment known as the SRY gene (sex determining region of the Y). This gene, located on the distal part of the short arm of the human Y chromosome (Y_p), encodes the **testis-determining factor (TDF),** a transcription factor protein with a "zinc finger" configuration that binds to DNA molecules. A gene identical to the SRY gene, or that is close by and linked to it, encodes a histocompatibility antigen known as H-Y. This glycoprotein antigen is one of two present on the surface of all male cells (except diploid germ cells). Both antigens are involved in rejection of male tissue by female recipients. A receptor for this protein has been found in gonadal tissue. When H-Y antigen is added to a culture of indifferent gonads from normal female embryos, the gonads undergo masculinization, and dissociated ovarian cells reaggregate in a testicular pattern. At least one other antigen encoded by DNA located on the long arm of the Y chromosome (Y_q) is involved in the development of normal spermatogenesis.

Although the SRY gene is essential for masculinization, it is not sufficient for complete maleness. Autosomal and X-chromosomal genes also play roles. Virilization of the genital ducts and external genitalia requires the presence of an androgen hormone receptor, which is encoded by genes on the X chromosome. In addition, a TDF allele may be present on the X chromosome. Hence, a dose effect of TDF (X and Y alleles), rather than a qualitative effect, may determine maleness.

The normal female chromosome complement is 44 autosomes and two sex chromosomes, XX. *Both of the X chromosomes are active in germ cells. The genesis of a normal ovary is dependent on the presence of two X chromosomes and the absence of a Y chromosome* (Fig. 52-1). In addition, autosomes participate in ovarian development, because individuals with a normal complement of XX sex chromosomes can still inherit defective gonads as an autosomal recessive trait. The second X chromosome of an XX female is normally inactivated early in all extragonadal tissues. However, differentiation of feminine genital ducts and external genitalia requires that only the remaining single X chromosome be active in directing transcription within the cell. *Therefore, if an abnormality of meiosis or mitosis produces an individual with only a single X chromosome and no Y chromosome (XO karotype), the phenotype will still be female although the gonads will be defective* (Fig. 52-1).

■ *Gonadal Sex*

Before any gonad appears, primordial germ cells differentiate in the 5-day-old blastocyst. At 22 to 24 days of gestation, the germ cells are present within the yolk sac endoderm. They then migrate to the genital ridge, where they associate with mesonephric tissue to form an indifferent gonad that is present for only 7 to 10 days. The primitive gonad consists of coelomic epithelium, the precursors of granulosa (female) and Sertoli (male) cells; mesenchymal stromal cells, the precursors of theca (female) and Leydig (male) cells; and the germ cells (Fig. 52-1). The entire assembly of the primitive gonad is organized as an outer **cortex** and inner **medulla.**

In a normal genetic male at 6 to 7 weeks' gestational age, the **seminiferous tubules** begin to form as the Sertoli cells enclose the germ cells. The Leydig cells appear at 8 to 9 weeks. At that point, there is a recognizable testis that initiates secretion of **testosterone,** the hormone critical for further male development. The synthesis of estrogen may be prevented by another SRY gene product that inhibits expression of the crucial enzyme, **aromatase** (see later). The medulla of the testis dominates anatomically, whereas the cortex regresses.

In the normal genetic female, differentiation of the indifferent gonad into an ovary does not start until 9 weeks of age. At this time, *both X chromosomes* within the germ cells become activated (Fig. 52-1). Activation of

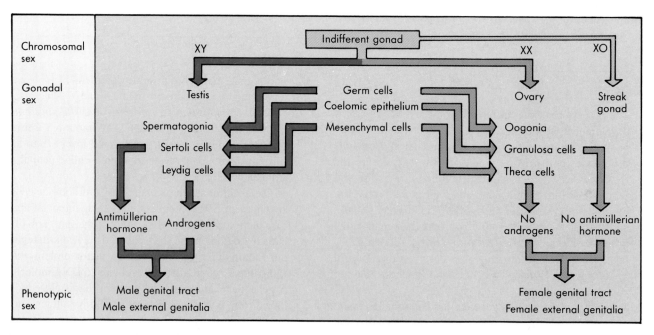

■ **Fig. 52-1**   Overview of the development of the cells of the ovary and testis from the primitive indifferent gonad. The hormonal products from the testis and the absence of these products from the ovary determine the gender differences in the internal genital tracts and the external genitalia.

both X chromosomes is an absolute requirement for the further development and survival of the germ cells. These germ cells begin to undergo mitosis, giving rise to oogonia, which continue to proliferate. Shortly thereafter, meiosis is initiated in some of the oogonia, and they become surrounded by granulosa cells and stroma; interstitial cells subsequently appear from the stroma. The germ cells, now known as **primary oocytes,** remain in the diplotene or late prophase stage of meiosis until possible ovulation many years later. In contrast to the male gonad, the cortex predominates in the developed ovary, while the medulla regresses. The ability of the primitive ovary to synthesize estrogenic hormones develops at about the same time that testosterone synthesis begins in the testis. The estrogens may contribute to further female development by blocking the masculinizing actions of any available androgens (see below).

■ *Genital (Phenotypic) Sex*

Up to this point in fetal development, sexual differentiation does not require any known hormonal products. However, differentiation of the genital ducts and of the external genitalia does require hormones. *The guiding principle is that positive hormonal influences, normally arising from the gonad, are required to produce male genitals. In the absence of any gonadal hormonal input, female genitals will develop.*

During the sexually indifferent stage, from 3 to 7 weeks' gestational age, two genital ducts develop on each side of the embryo. In the male at about 9 to 10 weeks, the **wolffian,** or **mesonephric, ducts** begin to grow and eventually give rise to the epididymis, the vas deferens, the seminal vesicles, and the ejaculatory duct (Fig. 52-2). This system is responsible for delivering sperm from the testis to the penis and thence into the vagina for reproduction. The differentiation of the wolffian ducts is preceded by the appearance of the testosterone-secreting Leydig cells in the testis. Testosterone stimulates the growth and differentiation of the wolffian ducts in the male. Furthermore, *the testosterone produced by each testis acts unilaterally on its own wolffian duct* (Fig. 52-2), as shown by gonadal transplantation experiments or testosterone implantations. Testosterone does *not* have to be converted to its hormonally active product, **dihydrotestosterone,** to act within the wolffian duct cells, as it does in some other tissues (described later). Indeed, these cells do not develop the 5α-reductase activity necessary for this conversion until after they have fully differentiated. In the female, the wolffian ducts begin to regress at 10 to 11 weeks because the ovary does not secrete testosterone.

The müllerian ducts arise parallel to and in part from the wolffian ducts on each side. In the male, these ducts begin to regress at 7 to 8 weeks' gestational age, about the same time that the Sertoli cells of the testis appear. These cells produce a glycoprotein hormone called **müllerian-inhibiting factor (MIF),** or **antimüllerian hormone (AMH),** which causes the **müllerian ducts** to atrophy. AMH is a glycoprotein composed of two identical subunits. It is encoded by a gene from a superfamily of

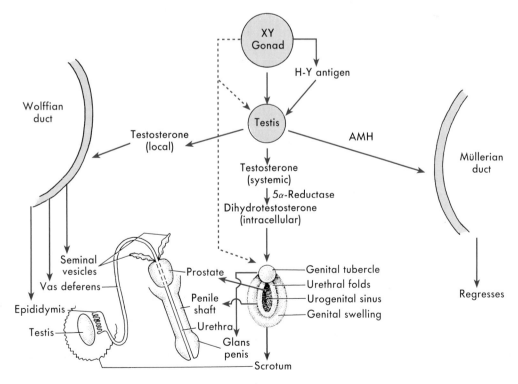

■ **Fig. 52-2**   Development of the human male reproductive organs and tract. Note the *dependence* on hormone products of the gonad (testosterone, dihydrotestosterone, and antimüllerian hormone [AMH]).

growth-regulating factors, including **transforming growth factors α and β, epidermal growth factor, inhibin,** and **activin.** A product of the SRY gene may greatly boost early AMH production in males. AMH probably acts by blocking the stimulatory effect of epidermal growth factor on the müllerian system. In addition, AMH may participate in organizing the testis into seminiferous tubules, stimulating development of Leydig cells, and initiating descent of the testis into the inguinal area. Although AMH is found in the postnatal testis and in plasma of male infants and children, its function after birth remains unclear.

AMH is not produced constitutively by granulosa cells until late in gestation or after birth, and it is present at much lower levels in female than in male infants and children. Therefore, in females, who lack early substantial amounts of AMH, the müllerian ducts continue to grow. They differentiate into fallopian tubes at the upper ends, whereas at the lower ends they join to form the uterus, cervix, and upper vagina (Fig. 52-3). This *differentiation* is completed at 18 to 20 weeks of gestational age and does not require any known ovarian hormone or even the presence of ovaries. However, if estradiol is lacking, *hypoplasia* (e.g., of the uterus) can result.

The external genitalia of both sexes begin to differentiate at 9 to 10 weeks of gestation. They are derived from the same anlage: the genital tubercle; the genital swelling; the urethral, or genital, folds; and the urogenital sinus. In males, testosterone must be secreted into fetal circulation and then be converted to dihydrotestosterone within the cells of the anlage tissues for the external genitalia to differentiate normally. As a result of dihy-

drotestosterone stimulation, the genital tubercle grows into the glans penis, the genital swellings fold and fuse into the scrotum, the urethral folds enlarge and enclose the penile urethra and corpora spongiosa, and the urogenital sinus gives rise to the prostate gland (Fig. 52-2). In addition to androgen hormone activity, the presence of the androgen receptor is required in these target tissues.

In normal females or in the absence of any gonads, the anlage tissues develop into the clitoris, labia majora, labia minora, and lower vagina, respectively (Fig. 52-3). Hormones are not essential for this development to occur. Growth to normal size (e.g., of the labia) requires estrogen. *However, if the normal female fetus is exposed to an excess of testosterone or other androgens (e.g., from the adrenal glands) during the period of differentiation of the external genitalia, a male pattern can result.* Once the female pattern of differentiation has been achieved, androgen exposure cannot change it to the male pattern, although it can cause enlargement of the clitoris.

The androgen production necessary for early sexual differentiation does not depend on fetal pituitary gonadotropins (see Chapter 49). A luteinizing hormone (LH)–like hormone from the placenta, called **chorionic gonadotropin,** stimulates testosterone production by the fetal Leydig cells. However, placental steroid hormone precursors, such as pregnenolone, might serve as a source of fetal androgens. Such placental precursors might obviate the necessity for gonadotropin stimulation of the reactions from cholesterol to pregnenolone (see later discussion). The *growth* of the male external genitalia in the last 6 months of gestation does require fetal pituitary LH to stimulate the necessary quantity of androgen.

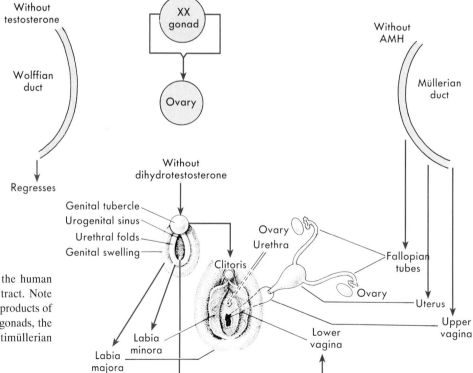

■ **Fig. 52-3**   Development of the human female reproductive organs and tract. Note the *independence* from hormonal products of the gonad. In the absence of any gonads, the female format results. *AMH,* Antimüllerian hormone.

Similarly, the final molding and size of the female external genitalia in utero may be affected by estrogens whose secretion depends on pituitary LH stimulation of the ovaries.

Other aspects of phenotypic sexual differentiation are not evident until well after birth, such as differences between the relatively constant pattern of gonadotropin secretion in the male versus the monthly cyclic pattern in the female, the different degree of breast development, and the psychological identification with a unique gender. The factors that imprint or regulate these traits in humans have not been conclusively established. In rodents, circulating androgens induce the fetal hypothalamus to set a constant pattern of gonadotropin secretion in the postpubertal male. To do so, androgens (paradoxically) require metabolism to estrogens within the target neurons. In the absence of androgens, the cyclic pattern of the female rodent ultimately results. Here is yet another instance in which the female pattern is the "neutral pattern," whereas the male pattern requires an action ultimately derived from the Y chromosome. Whether the same mechanism operates in humans is not certain.

Mammary gland development in the rodent embryo also is clearly regulated by hormones. In the absence of testosterone, a normal female breast develops; in its presence, the breast ductal system is suppressed. However, in humans, male or female differences in breast development are not apparent before puberty. At that time, the estrogenic milieu in the female induces growth and differentiation of breast tissue, whereas the androgenic milieu in the male suppresses it.

Some clinical evidence supports the interpretation that psychological gender identification is largely independent of hormonal regulation or even the phenotype of the genitalia. Instead, it appears to depend more on rearing cues and other factors. However, exceptions have been noted. In certain cases of genetic male pseudohermaphrodites who are raised as girls, pubertal testosterone stimulation may cause significant growth of the penis and may reverse the psychosocial gender from female to male. This reversal could partly result from a change in the way the individual is viewed by family and social associates.

■ Abnormalities of Sexual Differentiation

Anatomic aberrations that result from certain genetic errors are listed in Table 52-1. Sexual differentiation can be distorted by abnormalities in either sex chromosomes or autosomes.

Individuals with the XO chromosomal karyotype have a vestigial gonadal streak, because they lack the ovarian organizational input of two active X chromosomes or the testicular organizational input of the Y chromosome. The absence of AMH and testosterone secretion in turn leads to müllerian duct development, female external genitalia, and wolffian duct regression.

XY individuals who cannot respond to androgenic hormones because of receptor deficiency (the X-linked **testicular feminization syndrome**) still develop testes because of the presence of the Y chromosome. They demonstrate müllerian duct regression, caused by the presence of AMH. However, they show no growth or development of the wolffian ducts nor masculinization of the external genitalia because the lack of androgen receptors prevents effective testosterone or dihydrotestosterone action. The external genitalia are feminine.

XY individuals who have genetic defects in testosterone biosynthesis develop testes because of the presence of the Y chromosome, and the müllerian ducts regress because of the presence of AMH. However, depending on the degree of testosterone deficiency, the wolffian duct structures are variably underdeveloped, and the external genitalia may show effects ranging from a failure of complete fusion of the urethral folds to an entirely female pattern.

XY individuals who cannot adequately convert testosterone to dihydrotestosterone have a normal testis because of the presence of the Y chromosome. Their müllerian ducts regress because of the presence of AMH. The development of the epididymis, vas deferens, and seminal vesicles is normal because of the presence of testosterone. However, the external genitalia vary from a partial to a complete female pattern, depending on the degree of deficiency of dihydrotestosterone.

■ **Table 52-1**   Examples of abnormal development of the reproductive system

Genetic state	Gonad	Müllerian duct	Wolffian duct	External genitalia
XY, normal ♂	Testis	Regressed	Developed	♂
XX, normal ♀	Ovary	Developed	Regressed	♀
XO, Turner's syndrome	Streak*	Developed	Regressed	♀
XY, loss of X-linked gene for androgen receptor	Testis	Regressed	Regressed	♀
XY, deficient testosterone synthesis	Testis	Regressed	Regressed to variably developed	♀/♂
XY, deficient 5α-reductase	Testis	Regressed	Developed	♀/♂
XXY, Klinefelter's syndrome	Dysgenetic testis	Regressed	Developed	♂
XX, adrenal 21- or 11-hydroxylase deficiency	Ovary	Developed	Regressed	♀/♂

*A fibrous streak essentially devoid of germ cells.

XX individuals who overproduce adrenal androgens in utero (see Chapter 51) have ovaries because of the presence of two X chromosomes, and the müllerian ducts develop normally because of the absence of AMH. The wolffian structures regress because of the absence of local gonadal testosterone and the relatively late exposure to adrenal androgen excess. However, depending on the severity of androgen hypersecretion, the external genitalia show variable degrees of the male pattern, ranging from mild enlargement of the clitoris to complete scrotal fusion of the labia and a persistent urogenital sinus.

Individuals with more than two X chromosomes develop testes if a Y chromosome is also present, and they develop ovaries if a Y chromosome is not present. Their genital ducts and external genitalia develop normally. However, spermatogenesis and seminiferous tubule development are markedly deficient in XXY males (**Klinefelter's syndrome**). XXX females may have shortened reproductive lives. The mechanisms by which extra X chromosomes damage germ cell function are unknown.

■ *Common Aspects of Gonadal Function*

■ *Pathway of Gonadal Steroid Synthesis*

Both genders use the same pathway of steroid hormone biosynthesis in gonadal tissue (Fig. 52-4). The steroid hormone biosynthetic pathway in the gonads starts with cholesterol and is essentially identical to that of the adrenal cortex. The enzyme genes and characteristics, cofactor requirements, and localizations are also the same as those described in Chapter 51 for the adrenal glands. In the gonads, more in situ cholesterol from acetyl CoA may be synthesized than in the adrenal glands.

Although two parallel synthetic pathways lead to testosterone, the Δ_5 pathway from pregnenolone is favored (Fig. 52-4). Oxidation of the A ring by the 3-β-ol-dehydrogenase–isomerase complex can take place at any point from pregnenolone to androstenediol. Only a small quantity of testosterone undergoes 5α-reduction to dihydrotestosterone. A further α-reduction of the 3-ketone position to 5α-androstanediol also takes place within the testis (Fig. 52-4).

Androgens are the obligate precursors of estrogens. The key step in conversion to estrogen is aromatization of the A ring, a reaction heavily favored in the ovary and placenta. The aromatase enzyme complex is a cytochrome P-450 localized in the endoplasmic reticulum. It sequentially hydroxylates the 19-methyl group, oxidizes it to the aldehyde, hydroxylates the 2 position, and then creates a 1-2 double bond by reduction. Following these steps, the 19-carbon is removed by decarboxylation, and the characteristic benzene ring is formed. Estradiol and estrone are formed from testosterone and androstenedione, respectively. The two estrogens may also be interconverted by 17-hydroxysteroid dehydrogenase.

■ *Other Gonadal Products*

Testicular Sertoli and Leydig cells and ovarian granulosa cells synthesize and secrete numerous peptide and protein products that act in endocrine, paracrine, and even autocrine fashion to modulate the process of gametogenesis. Inhibins and activins are members of the same superfamily of growth regulating factors as AMH. They are constructed by combining three basic subunits in various combinations, as shown in Fig. 52-5. **Inhibin** is a glycoprotein that circulates in plasma and inhibits gonadotropin-releasing hormone (GnRH)–stimulated follicle-stimulating hormone (FSH) secretion by the pituitary gland. **Activin** has the opposite action and stimulates FSH secretion. Each also has intragonadal actions (described later). Activin also stimulates development of some embryonic tissues. **Follistatin** is another FSH-suppressing protein, but its structure is entirely unrelated to that of inhibin. It acts by binding and neutralizing activin. Insulin-like growth factor-1 (IGF-1 or somatomedin C) and transforming growth factors α and β are also synthesized by these cell lines, and they modulate cell growth and hormonal responses by paracrine effects within the gonads.

Leydig cells synthesize and secrete proopiomelanocortin products (see Chapter 49) and oxytocin. A peptide that functionally resembles GnRH but is structurally dissimilar to it is also present in the gonads. A variety of trace metal–binding proteins, steroid-binding proteins, IGF-binding proteins (see Chapter 49), proteases, prostaglandins, immune cytokines, and extracellular matrix molecules, such as laminin, integrins, collagen types I and IV, and proteoglycans, are also produced by gonads. These substances have local functions in the nurture and development of the germ cells and in the later exodus of ova and sperm from the gonads.

■ *Gonadotropin Actions in the Gonads*

The general framework for the hypothalamic-pituitary-gonadal axis is presented in Chapter 49 (see Fig. 49-15). *Luteinizing hormone (LH) and follicle-stimulating hormone (FSH) are the coordinate pituitary regulators of gonadal function. Through negative feedback, their synthesis and secretion are increased by decreases in gonadal steroids.* LH stimulates the interstitial cell line of male and female gonads (Leydig and thecal cells) mainly to secrete androgens. LH also acts on female granulosa cells.

LH binds to a plasma membrane receptor, a single polypeptide that associates in oligomers. The receptor has a large extracellular portion, spans the plasma mem-

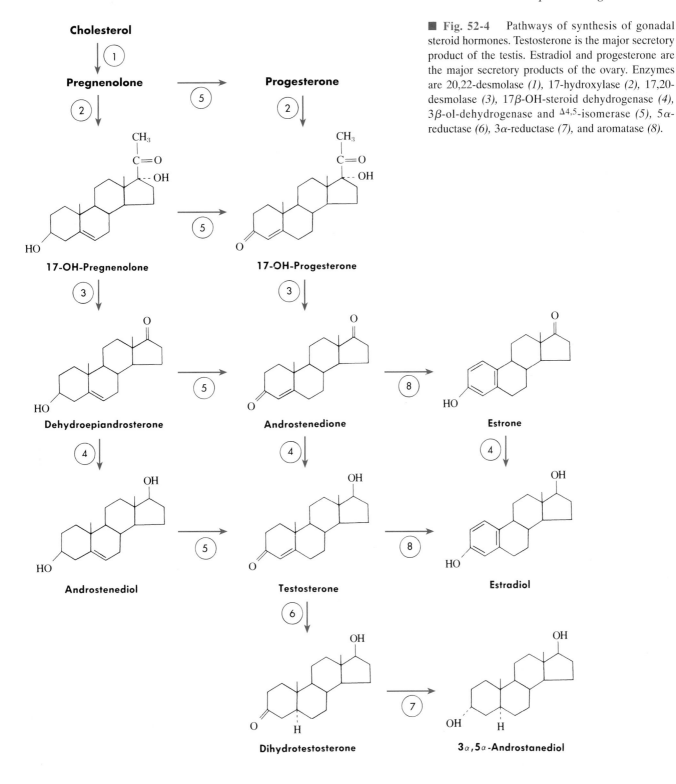

■ **Fig. 52-4** Pathways of synthesis of gonadal steroid hormones. Testosterone is the major secretory product of the testis. Estradiol and progesterone are the major secretory products of the ovary. Enzymes are 20,22-desmolase *(1)*, 17-hydroxylase *(2)*, 17,20-desmolase *(3)*, 17β-OH-steroid dehydrogenase *(4)*, 3β-ol-dehydrogenase and $^{\Delta 4,5}$-isomerase *(5)*, 5α-reductase *(6)*, 3α-reductase *(7)*, and aromatase *(8)*.

brane seven times, and terminates in an intracellular carboxy tail. It acts by means of a G protein, adenylyl cyclase, and cAMP as a second messenger.

The interaction of LH with its receptor is exquisitely sensitive. As little as 1% receptor occupancy by LH molecules can be sufficient for stimulation of some responses, and 5% to 10% occupancy can produce maximal cellular responses. Continued stimulation of gonadal cells by LH leads to down-regulation of its receptors and reduced

responsivity to the hormone. Prostaglandins are additional intermediaries in LH action, and they may potentiate the cAMP effects. LH increases the uptake and mobilization of cholesterol and its conversion to pregnenolone by stimulating the P-450 reaction. It also stimulates transcription of the gene for the enzyme 17-hydroxylase-17,20-desmolase (Fig. 52-4) and the cofactor adrenoxin.

FSH acts on ovarian granulosa cells and testicular Sertoli cells by binding to a plasma membrane receptor.

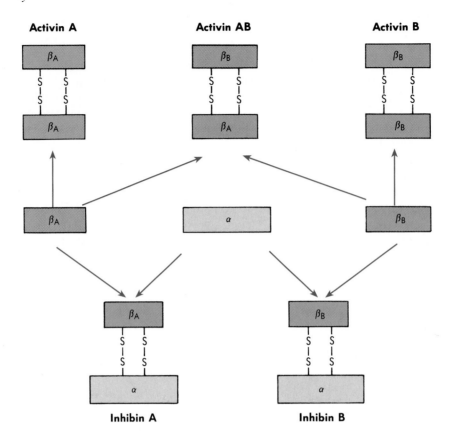

Fig. 52-5   Synthesis of inhibin A and B from a common α subunit and two distinct β subunits. Activins are synthesized by combining the β subunits into 2 homodimers (A-A and B-B) and 1 heterodimer (A-B).

The FSH receptor shares partial homology with the LH receptor. The increase in cAMP concentration that follows FSH-receptor binding results in an increase in transcription of the aromatase gene and a marked stimulation of estrogen synthesis. FSH also stimulates synthesis of inhibin and numerous other protein products of Sertoli and granulosa cells. Another important effect of FSH is to increase the number of LH receptors in granulosa cells, thereby amplifying their sensitivity to LH.

In addition to their actions on steroidogenesis, LH and FSH produce diverse metabolic effects in their target gonadal cells. Glucose oxidation and lactic acid production are increased, effects that may lead to local vasodilation. The long-term tropic effects of the two hormones depend on stimulation of amino acid transport, RNA synthesis, and general protein synthesis.

■ *Age-Related Changes in Gonadotropin Secretion*

The hypothalamic-pituitary-gonadal axis is unique in that it changes throughout the human lifespan. Although the patterns of change in females and males differ, there are certain common aspects.

■ *Intrauterine and Childhood Patterns*

In humans, GnRH is present in the hypothalamus by 4 weeks of gestation, and FSH and LH are present in the pituitary gland by 10 to 12 weeks. A broad peak of gonadotropin concentrations occurs in fetal plasma at midgestation (Fig. 52-6). After the concentrations drop to low levels before birth, they increase transiently again at about 2 months of age (this increase is more prolonged in females). For the rest of childhood, both gonadotropins are secreted at very low but detectable levels. These changes are mirrored by fluctuations of plasma testosterone in males and of plasma estradiol in females.

■ *Puberty*

The transition from a nonreproductive to a reproductive state during puberty requires maturation of the entire hypothalamic-pituitary-gonadal axis. *Before this maturation occurs, plasma LH and FSH levels are low despite low concentrations of gonadal steroids and inhibin. Therefore, either the negative feedback system is inoperative or the hypothalamus and pituitary gland are exquisitely sensitive to testosterone, estradiol, and inhibin.*

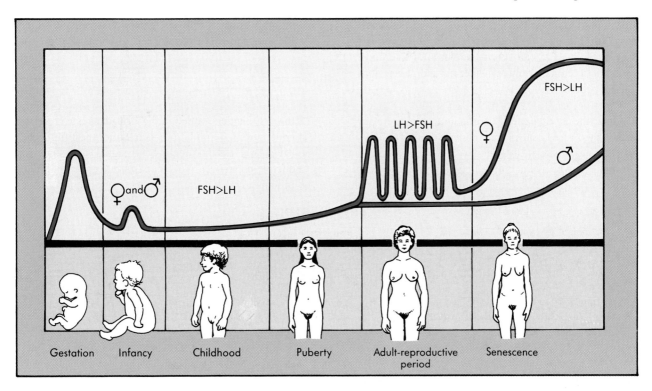

■ **Fig. 52-6** Pattern of gonadotropin secretion throughout life. Note transient peaks during gestation and early infancy and low levels thereafter in childhood. Women subsequently develop monthly cyclic bursts, with luteinizing hormone *(LH)* exceeding follicle-stimulating hormone *(FSH);* men do not. Both genders show increased gonadotropin production after age 50 years, with FSH exceeding LH.

Even removal of opioid inhibition does not increase plasma LH and FSH.

The gradual maturing of hypothalamic neurons during puberty leads to an increased synthesis and release of GnRH. The time and rate of onset of this maturational process may be genetically preprogrammed, because familial patterns are apparent. Other central nervous system components may influence this process. Nocturnal secretion of melatonin from the pineal gland declines from childhood to adult life, and destruction of the gland may cause premature puberty. Conversely, nocturnal melatonin levels are elevated in children with delayed puberty. However, it has not yet been finally established that in humans melatonin is the normal suppressor of gonadotropins during childhood or that the rate of decline of melatonin is the normal regulator of the onset of puberty. A role for adrenal dehydroepiandrosterone (DHEA) in GnRH neuron maturation is suggested by the typical rise in DHEA secretion that precedes puberty. The achievement of an adequate adipose tissue mass may be another determinant of the time of onset of reproductive function.

As puberty approaches, the low-level pulsatile pattern of LH and FSH secretion becomes more pronounced. The ratio of plasma LH to FSH rises as the pulse frequency increases. During early and middle puberty, a barely detectable childhood nocturnal peak in LH secretion is greatly amplified. The nocturnal LH peak then dis-

appears when adult status is reached (Fig. 52-7). *The gonad itself is not necessary for these changes in GnRH and gonadotropins to occur.*

During early puberty, LH exceeds FSH output. More LH is synthesized and stored in the pituitary in response to amplified pulsatile GnRH secretion, perhaps because the pulsatility allows better maintenance of GnRH receptors. Although the gonadal target cells respond to LH in childhood, their responsiveness is augmented by puberty. Therefore, testosterone levels in males and estradiol levels in females increase sharply. In addition, FSH stimulates a pubertal rise of inhibin levels in both genders. Thus, early puberty can be viewed as a cascade of increasing maturation from the hypothalamic to the pituitary to the gonadal level. The increasing levels of the appropriate sex steroid in each gender potentiate growth hormone secretion, an effect that contributes to the acceleration of linear growth and secondarily to maturation of the reproductive organs and processes.

In both genders, it is often difficult to distinguish between a late onset of what will eventually be normal puberty and a disease of the hypothalamus or pituitary gland that prevents the expected increase in gonadotropins. Because failure to show physical signs of puberty by age 13 or 14 (see below) is psychologically distressing, treatment with sufficient testosterone or estradiol to induce such changes and a growth spurt may be warranted. Such hormonal support does not cause fertility and can be withdrawn after an appropriate period to determine whether normal puberty has finally begun.

Once the adult pattern of gonadotropin secretion is established, the basal plasma concentrations of LH and FSH (approximately 10^{-11} molar) are similar in men and women. However, an important distinguishing feature between the genders is the establishment of a dramatic monthly gonadotropin cycle in females only, in which the LH bursts greatly exceed the FSH bursts (Fig. 52-6).

■ *Climacteric*

In both genders, a decline in gonadal responsiveness to gonadotropin stimulation occurs after the fifth decade of life. In males, this decline is gradual, and some reproductive capacity usually persists into the eighth decade. In females, normal full reproductive capacity is lost com-

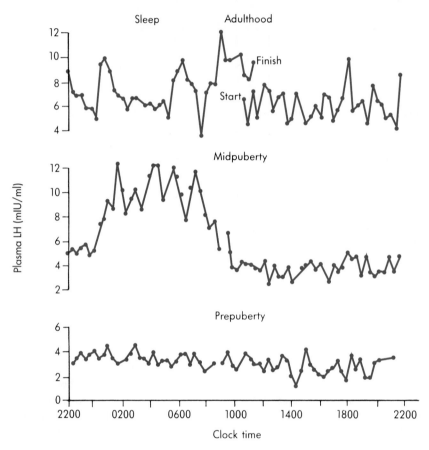

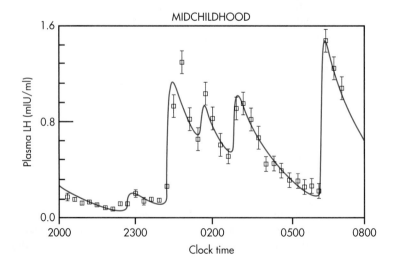

■ **Fig. 52-7**   LH secretion in childhood, puberty, and adult life. During puberty, the pattern of LH secretion becomes much more pulsatile. In addition, a nocturnal peak in LH is greatly amplified in early and middle puberty. This peak disappears when puberty is completed. Males and females both show these changes. As seen in the inset, nocturnal peaking is demonstrable even in childhood when a very sensitive LH assay is used. (Redrawn from Boyar RM et al: *N Engl J Med* 287:582, 1972. Inset redrawn from Wu FC et al: *J Clin Endocrinol Metab* 81:1798, 1996.)

pletely over a period of several years, and menopause occurs. In both genders, however, continued negative feedback leads to elevated plasma gonadotropin levels. The FSH level rises more than the LH level, and the increase is more distinct in females (Fig. 52-6).

■ *The Testes*

■ *Anatomy*

The human testes are normally situated in the scrotum, where they are maintained at a temperature 1° to 2° C below that of the body core temperature. *This lower temperature is essential for normal sperm production.* A lower temperature is partly maintained by the intertwined coiling of arteries and veins to facilitate heat exchange between them. Each testis weighs about 40 g and has a long diameter of 4.5 cm in adults. The testes receive blood from the spermatic arteries, which arise directly from the aorta.

Eighty percent of the adult testis is made up of the **seminiferous tubules;** the remaining 20% is composed of supportive connective tissue, throughout which Leydig cells are scattered (Fig. 52-8). The seminiferous tubules are a coiled mass of loops; each loop begins and ends in a single duct, the tubulus rectus. The tubuli recti in turn anastomose in the rete testis and eventually drain via the ductuli efferentes into the **epididymis.** The epididymis serves as a storage and maturation depot for spermatozoa. From the epididymis the spermatozoa are carried via the vas deferens and ejaculatory duct into the penis, to be emitted during copulation.

The structure of the adult seminiferous tubule is complex (Fig. 52-8). Each tubule is bounded by a basement membrane that separates it from the Leydig cells, the peritubular (myoid) cells, and the surrounding connective tissue. Gap junctions connect adjacent Leydig cells. Located immediately beneath the basement membrane are **spermatogonia** and Sertoli cells. As the spermatogonia divide and develop successively into **spermatocytes** and **spermatids,** a column of germ cells is formed that reaches from the basement membrane to the lumen of the tubule, culminating in the spermatozoa.

In contrast, the cytoplasm of each Sertoli cell extends all the way from the basement membrane to the lumen of the tubule. This cytoplasm invests the spermatogonia and its germ cell line successors (Fig. 52-8). *Special processes of the Sertoli cell cytoplasm fuse into tight junctions, which create two compartments of intercellular space between the basement membrane and the lumen of the tubule.* The spermatogonia and early primary spermatocytes lie within the proximal **basal compartment,** whereas the later spermatocytes and their gradually maturing descendents that lead to spermatozoa lie in the distal **adluminal compartment.** This separation maintains a barrier between the blood and these compartments that is begun by the basement membrane and overlapping peritubular cells (Fig. 52-8). In even more discriminating fashion, the cytoplasm of the adjacent Sertoli cells excludes a variety of circulating substances from the intercellular fluid that bathes the maturing germ cells and from the seminiferous tubular fluid that bathes the spermatozoa. This barrier also prevents late spermatogenic products from reaching the bloodstream, where, if recog-

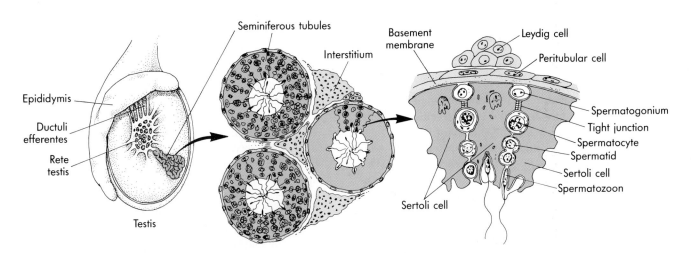

■ **Fig. 52-8**   Schematic representation of the architecture of the testis. Note that the Leydig cells and peritubular cells are separated from the spermatogenic tubules by a basement membrane. Within the tubules, the germ cell line is completely invested by cytoplasm of the surrounding Sertoli cells. Tight junctions between adjacent Sertoli cells separate the ancestral spermatogonia from their descendent spermatocytes, spermatids, and spermatozoa. Thus, a blood testis barrier effectively filters plasma, permitting only selected substances to reach the developing germ cells from Sertoli cell cytoplasm. (Redrawn from Skinner MK: Cell-cell interactions in the testis, *Endocr Rev* 12:45-77, 1991. From The Endocrine Society.)

nized as foreign substances, they could evoke immune rejection mechanisms.

In short, the testis consists of separate but interacting functional elements (Figs. 52-8 and 52-9). The Leydig cells (the first element) are pure steroid-secreting cells. Their major product, testosterone, has both important local effects on germ cell replication as well as on distant target cells. Peritubular myoid cells (the second element) (Fig. 52-8) secrete paracrine regulatory products and may produce contractile effects on the tubules and the vasculature. The seminiferous tubules (the third element) are the site where spermatogenesis take place. These tubules are bathed in Sertoli cell products and are exposed to locally generated testosterone.

■ *The Biology of Spermatogenesis*

The production of sperm takes place continuously throughout the reproductive life of the male. Approximately 100 to 200 million sperm are produced daily. Generating this large number of sperm requires the spermatogonia to renew themselves by cell division. This situation differs fundamentally from that in the female, who at birth has a fixed number of oocytes that decreases throughout her life.

Each spermatogonium can give rise to 64 spermatozoa. The extraordinary metamorphosis from human spermatogonium to spermatozoon is depicted in Fig. 52-10. The first two mitotic divisions of a spermatogonium give rise to four cells: a single resting cell *(Ad)* that will eventually serve as the ancestor of a later generation of sperm and three active cells *(Ap)*. The Ap cells divide by further mitoses to yield type B spermatogonia, which then give rise to a number of primary spermatocytes. These cells enter the prophase of meiosis, the first reduction division, in which they remain for about 20 days. This process occurs within the basal compartment of the seminiferous tubule.

Meiosis is a complex process of chromosomal reduplication, synapsis, cross-over, division, and cell separation. This process is reflected histologically in the changing appearance of the **primary spermatocytes** up through the pachytene stage (Fig. 52-10). Their daughter cells, the **secondary spermatocytes,** immediately divide again by mitosis in the adluminal compartment. These daughter cells, now called *spermatids,* each contain 22 autosomes and either an X or a Y sex chromosome. The spermatids lie near the lumen of the seminiferous tubule. *They are attached to the abutting Sertoli cells by specialized junctions. The spermatocytes and spermatids of each generation are connected with each other through intercellular bridges.*

The next process in spermatogenesis is called **spermiogenesis.** In this process, spermatids undergo nuclear condensation, shrinkage of cytoplasm, formation of an **acrosome,** and development of a tail to emerge as flagellated spermatozoa (Figs. 52-10 and 52-11). The spermatozoa are then extruded into the lumen of the tubule by a process called **spermiation,** during which most of the cytoplasm of the spermatozoa is ejected as the **residual body** and remains embedded in the cytoplasm of a Sertoli cell.

Once in the seminiferous tubules, the spermatozoa appear as linear structures with several components (Fig. 52-11). The **head** contains the nucleus and an acrosomal cap in which hydrolytic and proteolytic enzymes are concentrated. These enzymes facilitate penetration of the ovum and possibly also the mucous plug of the female cervix. The **middle piece,** or body, contains mitochondria, which generate the motile energy of the spermatozoon. The **chief piece** of the tail contains stored adenosine triphosphate (ATP) and pairs of contractile microtubules down its entire length; one pair lies in the center, and nine pairs are located around the circumference. Cross-bridging arms contain **dynein,** a magnesium-dependent ATPase, which catalyzes the conversion of ATP energy into a sliding movement between the microtubules. *This sliding movement imparts flagellar motion to the spermatozoa.* Both cAMP and Ca^{++} regulate sperm motility.

In a human, the entire sequence of development from spermatogonia to spermatozoa takes 60-70 days. *However, individual resting spermatogonia do not enter the process of spermatogenesis randomly. Cycles of spermatogenesis exist with distinct cycle times.* Groups of adjacent resting spermatogonia initiate a new cycle about every 16 days, thus constituting one "generation." At about the same time that the primary spermatocytes of one cycle enter prophase, a second cycle of spermatogonia is activated. A third cycle begins at approximately the same time that spermatids appear from the first cycle. By the time these spermatids are completely transformed into spermatozoa, a fourth cycle of spermatogonia development has been started.

Several spermatogenic cycles are often in process simultaneously, around the circumference of any individual seminiferous tubule. Within each cycle, specific stages of cellular development can be identified histologically. Thus, several cellular constellations can exist side by side. In some mammals, but possibly not in humans, spermatogenic cycles are repeated in a defined topographic relationship to each other along the length of each seminiferous tubule. This phenomenon has been termed the **wave of spermatogenesis.**

The individual germ cells that make up the successive descendants of type B spermatogonia lying within the adluminal compartment of the tubule are not totally separated. Continuity of cytoplasm and cell-to-cell intercommunication may exist. Because of these possibilities and because of the regular topographic association of particular stages of spermatogenesis in neighboring cycles, products of germ cells in one stage of spermatogenesis might initiate or regulate events in other stages.

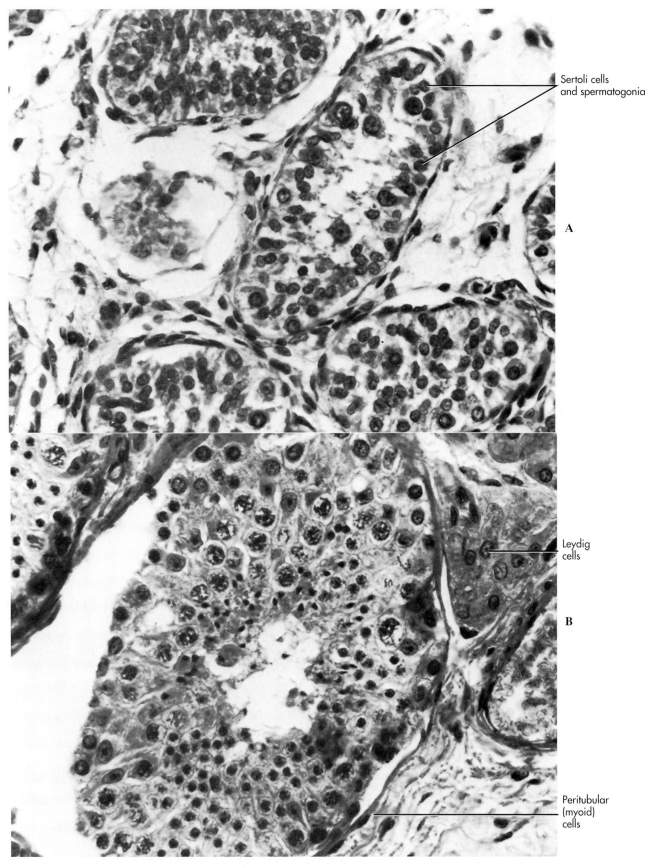

Sertoli cells
and spermatogonia

A

Leydig
cells

B

Peritubular
(myoid)
cells

■ **Fig. 52-9**   Histologic sections of the testis from prepubertal **(A)** and postpubertal **(B)** males. Note the absence of Leydig cells and active spermatogenesis before puberty. (Courtesy of Dr. Howard Levin.)

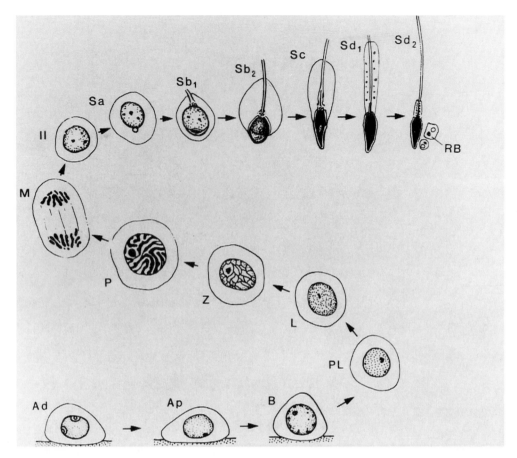

■ **Fig. 52-10** Development of spermatozoa from spermatogonia in the human. *Ad,* Dark spermatogonium; *Ap,* pale spermatogonium; *B,* type B spermatogonium; *PL,* preleptotene primary spermatocyte; *L,* leptotene spermatocyte; *Z,* zygotene spermatocyte; *P,* pachytene spermatocyte; *M,* meiotic division; *II,* secondary spermatocyte; *Sa, Sb, Sc, Sd,* spermatids; *RB,* residual body. (Redrawn from DeKretser DM et al. In DeGroot LJ, editor: *Endocrinology,* ed 3, vol 3, Philadelphia, 1995, WB Saunders, p 2309.)

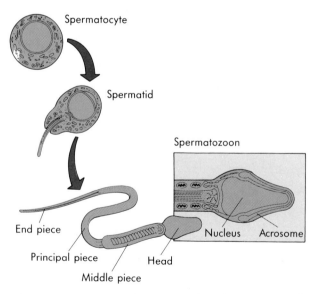

■ **Fig. 52-11** Schematic representation of the morphologic alterations in the development of the spermatozoon from the spermatocyte.

After spermiation, the spermatozoa reach the epididymis, which they traverse in a period of 2 to 4 weeks. During this time, the spermatozoa undergo further maturation, gaining motility and losing all their cytoplasm.

Spermatozoa are initially transported into the epididymis by seminiferous tubular fluid currents generated by the peritubular myoid cells or by contraction of the testicular capsule. The epididymis is lined by specialized epithelial cells and is surrounded by contractile muscle cells. The growth and differentiation of the epididymis, as well as the motility and fertility of the sperm that migrate through it, depend on androgens. Marked changes in fluid osmolality, electrolytes, and the concentrations of many small molecules occur progressively within the length of the epididymis. These changes suggest homologies with the function of the renal tubules.

Proteins provided by epididymal and seminiferous tubular fluid bind to the membranes of sperm and enhance their motility and fertilizing ability. These proteins include a forward-mobility protein, an acrosomal stabilizing or inhibiting factor, and a protein that binds to the outer membrane of the ovum. The amount of sperm contained in the epididymis is about the equivalent of a single ejaculate or a single day's production. After reaching the vas deferens, sperm may be stored viably for several months between ejaculations.

■ *Sexual Functioning*

Delivery of spermatozoa into the female genital tract for reproductive purposes occurs by ejaculation from the vas deferens. To this initial ejaculate, successive fluids are added by various structures. The first secretions are added from the prostate gland and contain citrate, calcium, zinc, and acid phosphatase. The alkalinity of prostatic fluid helps neutralize the acid pH of the semen and the vaginal and cervical secretions. The later secretions are from the seminal vesicles. These secretions contain fructose, an important oxidative substrate for the spermatozoa, and prostaglandins, which may stimulate contractions of the uterus and fallopian tubes and thereby help propel the spermatozoa toward the ovum.

Seminal fluid also contains LH, FSH, prolactin, testosterone, estradiol, inhibins, endorphins, oxytocin, kallikreins, relaxin (see later discussion), proteases, plasminogen activator, and sperm-coating proteins. Because the concentrations of these substances are usually higher than those in plasma, they have probably entered from cells of the genital tract (e.g., epididymal cells).

Ejaculation requires preceding penile erection, which is caused by blood filling the venous sinuses of the corpora cavernosa and spongiosa. An eightfold increase in blood content converts the flaccid penis into a firm organ for penetration. This process may be initiated in the brain or may begin with afferent sensory impulses from the penis carried by the **pudendal nerve.** The process is further mediated by impulses in the pelvic nerves, which contain both parasympathetic and sympathetic fibers. During the **flaccid phase,** sympathetic neural tone dominates and the cavernosa are kept empty by constriction of smooth muscle and of the supplying arterioles. During the initial **filling phase,** parasympathetic stimuli dominate, anteriolar constriction diminishes, and the penis elongates without a change in cavernosa pressure. During the next **tumescence phase,** release of nitric oxide and prostaglandin E_1 causes relaxation of the cavernosa smooth muscle and an increase in its compliance, which allows easy entry of blood and engorgement. In the **full erection phase,** output of blood from the penis is markedly decreased by pressure on the veins from the engorged cavernosa. In this phase, the pressure of the engorged cavernosa rises to just below that of the systolic blood pressure. In the final **rigid phase,** cavernosa pressure exceeds systolic blood pressure. Ejaculation, which occurs during this phase, results from sympathetic stimuli that cause contraction of the ischiocavernosa and bulbocavernosa muscles.

Inability to ejaculate, or impotence, is a common problem. It may be caused by structural and functional disorders, including neuropathies and spinal cord lesions, or by psychogenic complications. New detailed knowledge about the physiology of erection has led to improved pharmacologic therapy. Direct self-injection of α-adrenergic antagonists or appropriate prostaglandins into the cavernosa at the base of the penis generates erections that last 1 to 3 hours, permiting satisfactory intercourse. In other instances, a simple mechanical pump creates a vacuum in an airbag placed around the penis; transmission of the negative pressure to the cavernosa results in their engorgement and in adequate erection.

A typical ejaculate contains 200 to 400 million spermatozoa in a volume of 2 to 4 ml. The first 1 ml has the highest concentration of sperm. Once within the vagina, the spermatozoa's rate of flagellated movement is up to 44 mm/min. However, to reach the ovum, sperm require assistance by smooth muscle contractions in the female genital tract. The lifespan of the spermatozoa within the female genital tract is approximately 2 days.

Ejaculated sperm cannot immediately fertilize an ovum. In vivo fertilization can take place only after the sperm have been acted upon by the milieu of the female reproductive tract for 4 to 6 hours. This process is termed **capacitation.** In vitro human fertilization can take place after the spermatozoa have been washed free of seminal fluid. This suggests that seminal fluid contains substances that coat the sperm surface and that prevent union of a sperm with an ovum. Materials in the female genital tract may either remove or neutralize these substances. In the course of capacitation, cholesterol is withdrawn from the sperm membrane, and the surface proteins of the membrane redistribute. In addition, calcium influx occurs and sperm motility becomes more whiplike.

Although the process of capacitation is incompletely understood, it results in unique patterns of sperm motility that may enhance the penetration of the ovum. Most importantly, capacitation permits the **acrosomal reaction.** In this reaction, the acrosomal membrane fuses with that of the outer sperm membrane (Fig. 52-11). Pores are created through which the acrosomal hydrolytic and proteolytic enzymes can escape. These enzymes then create a path through the protective membranes of the ovum for penetration of the sperm.

■ *Hormonal Regulation of Spermatogenesis*

The endocrine mechanisms that govern human spermatogenesis are not completely understood. Clearly, adult functioning of the GnRH–LH/FSH–testicular axis, as illustrated in Fig. 49-15, is essential for spermatogenesis to occur at all. *Of critical importance is the pulsatile release of GnRH and resultant arrival of LH and FSH at their target cells.* Men with congenital GnRH deficiency can be made fertile only if exogenous GnRH is given in appropriately sized pulses and timed intervals, not if it is given continuously.

The prepubertal testis contains only resting spermatogonia and quiescent Sertoli cells. These cells do not exhibit cyclic alterations in structure or biochemical functioning. Neither Leydig cells nor peritubular cells of the adult myoid character are present (Fig. 52-9). Pubertal activation of gonadotropin secretion leads to dramatic and complex changes. The proximity of several stimulated endocrine cell types (with multiple secretory products) to each other and to the germinal cell line creates many potential and observed paracrine effects, and possibly also autocrine effects. These effects are in addition to central feedback actions. The specific or critical nature of each effect and the point in spermatogenesis at which it operates are still difficult to determine.

During fetal life, the transient midgestation surge of pituitary FSH, LH, and testosterone release may stimulate the transformation of the primordial germ cells into resting spermatogonia. Withdrawal of fetal gonadotropins then leaves the spermatogonia in suspended development throughout childhood, possibly through operation of a local meiosis inhibitor. Both AMH and inhibin have been proposed for this role. Shortly after FSH secretion begins to rise at the onset of puberty, the spermatogonia are activated.

The most immature germ cells have FSH receptors. FSH also certainly stimulates the Sertoli cells, whose functions are in turn required for initial germ cell mitotic and early meiotic activity. These cells are described in detail

later. LH stimulates the Leydig cells to secrete testosterone, which presumably diffuses across the basement membrane and can enter the Sertoli cells, which contain androgen receptors. The high local concentration of testosterone (50- to 100-fold greater than in plasma) is essential for completion of the later stages of spermatogenesis. In men who lack LH, for example, testosterone administration to attain normal systemic plasma levels, even if given with FSH, cannot sustain spermatogenesis. It is possible that testosterone or its active metabolite, dihydrotestosterone, may also enter and act within the germ cells; rodent germ cells contain both dihydrotestosterone and the 5α-reductase enzyme necessary for its production from testosterone (Fig. 52-4). Conversion of small amounts of testosterone to estradiol within the Leydig and Sertoli cells makes this estrogen available as another possible local spermatogenesis modulator that is ultimately derived from LH action. *The trophic effect of LH on Leydig cells is absolutely essential to spermatogenesis,* and FSH may also contribute to a full Leydig cell response.

Once regular spermatogenesis has been established during puberty, it can continue to a small extent in adults who have very low levels of FSH and LH (Fig. 52-12), provided that testosterone is present in high amounts. Under these circumstances, the number of sperm is markedly reduced, but the sperm are normal in appearance. Selective restoration of either FSH alone or LH alone can increase sperm numbers (Fig. 52-12), but both are required for normal levels to be reached. In some men, after a suitable period of exposure to FSH, LH alone can sustain sufficient sperm production (15 to 60 million per ejaculate) to permit fertility. FSH and LH appear to maintain all but a critical first step in sper-

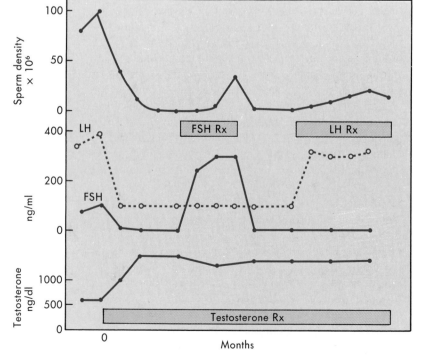

■ **Fig. 52-12**   Individual effects of FSH and LH on human sperm production. Normal men were given sufficient testosterone to suppress endogenous FSH and LH secretion by negative feedback. As a result, sperm density declined to very low but detectable levels. Selective restoration of either FSH or LH individually raised sperm levels. However, neither gonadotropin alone could return sperm production to normal. (Redrawn from Matsumoto AM et al: *J Clin Invest* 72:1005, 1983; and Matsumoto AM et al: *J Clin Endocrinol Metab* 59:882, 1984.)

matogenesis by acting on the intervening Sertoli and Leydig cells, respectively.

Other pituitary hormones are also involved in spermatogenesis. Prolactin receptors are present on Leydig cells; prolactin increases the number of LH receptors and synergizes with LH to stimulate androgen production. Growth hormone is essential for the normally timed onset of reproductive function. The role of growth hormone may be to stimulate local production of insulin-like growth factors by Sertoli cells.

Despite the cycles of spermatogenesis within each seminiferous tubule, the testis as a whole is continuously releasing spermatozoa. Furthermore, although gonadotropin release is pulsatile, the daily *mean* plasma levels of FSH and LH vary little in adult men. However, temporal or topographic differences may exist in the density of gonadotropin receptors or in the peritubular myoid cell control of capillary blood flow. Such variations could modulate gonadotropin availability and thereby be responsible for the cyclic and topographic nature of the spermatogenic process. In general, spermatogenesis is obviously different from that of oogenesis, in which a clear phasic pattern of gonadotropin secretion, highlighted by a single distinct burst, produces the monthly release of a single ovum.

The Sertoli cells and their responses to FSH and testosterone are crucial to spermatogenesis. Between fetal life and puberty, Sertoli cell function is unknown; after puberty, the Sertoli cells do not undergo any further cell divisions. Each remains in contact with up to five other Sertoli cells and with an estimated 47 germ cells in different stages of development. Ectoplasmic processes from Sertoli and germ cells invaginate into each other's plasma membranes. In close association with the cycle of spermatogenesis, Sertoli cells undergo regular changes in the activity and shape of the nucleus; the size, shape, and branching of the cytoplasmic processes; the concentrations of lipid and glycogen; mitochondrial function; and enzyme content. These changes relate to the processing of the germ cells in an intimate and regular manner, which suggests that the Sertoli cells may be responding in part to signals from the germ cells. One candidate signal is the cytokine, tumor necrosis factor-α (TNF-α), which is secreted by spermatids. Sertoli and Leydig cells have TNF-α receptors, and Sertoli cells secrete inhibin in response to TNF-α.

The cytoplasmic processes of the Sertoli cells extend from the basement membrane to the lumen of the seminiferous tubule. These processes act as conduits, between which the various stages of germ cells move in their passage to the lumen (Fig. 52-8). As spermatocytes mature, new tight junctions between the investing Sertoli cells develop behind them while the old tight junctions ahead of them "unzip." In this way, spermatocytes pass from the basal to the adluminal compartment without breaking the integrity of the blood-testis barrier formed by Sertoli cell cytoplasm. The Sertoli cell cyto-

plasm acts as a filter, permitting only certain substances to reach the spermatocytes.

Many products are synthesized and secreted by the Sertoli cells in response to FSH. Some of these secretions are directed into the lumen of the seminiferous tubule (Fig. 52-8). FSH induces the enzyme aromatase and stimulates estradiol production by Sertoli cells from androgen precursors of Leydig cell origin. In response to FSH and testosterone acting synergistically, an **androgen-binding glycoprotein (ABP)** with an amino acid sequence identical to that of the circulating sex steroid–binding globulin (SSBG) (see below) is synthesized. ABP binds testosterone, dihydrotestosterone, and estradiol with high affinity. In this way, ABP regulates the availability of these hormones to germ cells in the seminiferous tubular fluid (Figs. 52-8 and 52-13). ABP is also secreted into epididymal fluid, where it prevents reabsorption of sex steroids and ensures their continued presence for sperm needs. ABP may also regulate the inhibitory effect of estradiol on Leydig cell testosterone synthesis (Fig. 52-13).

Inhibin B, activin, and various growth factors are also synthesized under the influence of FSH and testosterone. Destruction or spontaneous loss of the spermatogenic cells suppresses inhibin secretion, which suggests that a signal from spermatogenic cells stimulates synthesis of inhibin by the Sertoli cells (Fig. 52-13). In addition to their central feedback roles of inhibiting and stimulating FSH secretion, respectively, inhibin and activin may also have reciprocal local actions on the neighboring cells (Fig. 52-13). For example, inhibin increases, whereas activin decreases, testosterone secretion by the Leydig cells. Thus, FSH can also influence Leydig cell function indirectly by modulating production of inhibin and activin. FSH promotes the availability of iron, copper, vitamin A, and crucial sphingolipids to the germ cells by stimulating synthesis of their binding proteins. Binding proteins then extract their respective ligands from plasma and transfer them to the germ cells. FSH also increases the glucose metabolism of Sertoli cells, and the resultant pyruvate and lactate are available energy substrates for the spermatogenic cells.

FSH-stimulated proteases and plasminogen activator are probably involved in the process of spermiation. Either by mechanical or chemical means, the Sertoli cell facilitates the spermatozoa into the tubular lumen. In this process, the nucleus of the spermatozoon is oriented toward the base of the tubule. The bulk of the cytoplasm is then squeezed out past the nucleus and shed as the residual body (Fig. 52-10), while the spermatozoon is cast free. The residual body and other fragments are then phagocytosed by the Sertoli cells and subsequently degraded.

Other paracrine interactions may be important in maintaining the proper testicular environment to support spermatogenesis (Fig. 52-13). Thus, testosterone from the Leydig cells stimulates differentiation and proliferation of the peritubular myoid cells. The peritubular myoid cells secrete a protein that stimulates some functions of Sertoli cells. A positive feedback loop exists between Leydig and Sertoli cells in that testosterone stimulates inhibin secretion and inhibin stimulates testosterone secretion. However, activin and estradiol from Sertoli cells reduce testosterone synthesis by Leydig cells. Each of these interactions may vary in functional significance at different points in the cycle of spermatogenesis.

■ *Secretion and Metabolism of Androgens*

Testosterone, the major androgenic hormone, is synthesized as described previously (Fig. 52-4). Its synthesis and release by the Leydig cells are regulated by LH; therefore, plasma testosterone levels undergo small coordinate pulses throughout the day (see Fig. 49-17). In addition, the plasma testosterone level follows a superimposed diurnal trend: plasma testosterone is about 25% lower at 8:00 PM than at 8:00 AM. When exogenous LH is supplied for a prolonged period, the plasma testosterone level initially rises, then briefly declines, and then rises again. The temporary decrease may be caused by downregulation of LH receptors by the peak concentrations of

gonadotropin; the later upswing may reflect stimulation of the expression of enzyme genes involved in testosterone synthesis and of Leydig cell growth.

Testosterone gives rise to two other potent androgens: **dihydrotestosterone (DHT)** and **5α-androstanediol** (Fig. 52-4). The major portion of each of these two androgens is formed from the reduction of testosterone in peripheral tissues. The plasma levels, blood production rates, and metabolic clearances of these androgens are shown in Table 52-2. The testosterone precursor, androstenedione, is also secreted in major amounts by the Leydig cells (Fig. 52-4), but it contributes little per se to androgen action.

The two estrogens—estradiol and estrone—are produced in significant amounts in men. However, only a trivial fraction of the daily production is provided directly by testicular secretion. Most is derived from circulating testosterone and androstenedione by aromatization, which takes place largely in the adipose tissue and liver.

Leydig cell function varies distinctively during the lifespan of males. As shown in Fig. 52-14, plasma testosterone rises to levels of 400 ng/dl in the fetus when the external genitalia are undergoing differentiation to the masculine pattern. By birth, however, these

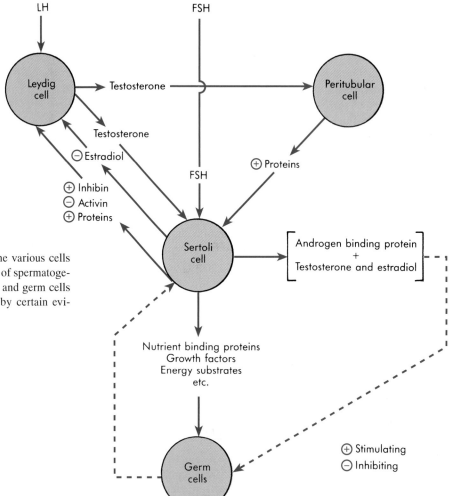

■ **Fig. 52-13** Interactions among the various cells of the testis in the hormonal regulation of spermatogenesis. Dotted lines to and from Sertoli and germ cells represent plausible effects suggested by certain evidence.

levels have declined to less than 50 ng/dl. Soon thereafter, plasma testosterone again begins to rise, reaching a peak of 150 to 200 ng/dl at 4 to 8 weeks of age. The physiological significance of this elevation in testosterone concentration is not known. Plasma testosterone again falls to low levels and remains so throughout childhood; these low plasma levels correspond to the absence of Leydig cells (Fig. 52-9).

At about age 11 years, the plasma testosterone level begins to rise steeply, reaching the adult plateau of about 600 ng/dl at about age 17 (Fig. 52-14). This level is sustained for about 50 years. During the seventh and eighth decades of life, the plasma testosterone level gradually declines owing to the loss of Leydig cell responsiveness to stimulation. Although decreasing testosterone levels may be associated with a decline in libido and a decrease in bone and muscle mass, spermatogenesis itself is remarkably well preserved in most octogenarians.

Only 1% to 2% of circulating testosterone is in the free form; 65% of testosterone is bound to a liver-derived glycoprotein called **sex steroid–binding globulin (SSBG),** also known as testosterone-estradiol–binding globulin. SSBG differs from ABP only in its carbohydrate content.

Most of the remaining testosterone is bound to albumin and other proteins. SSBG also binds dihydrotestosterone and 5α-androstanediol. The SSBG-bound fractions serve as circulating reservoirs of androgens, similar to those of thyroid hormone and cortisol. In general, only the free and the loosely bound albumin fractions of testosterone and the other androgens reach cells and are biologically active. However, receptors exist for SSBG itself in target tissues; therefore, SSBG may have actions of its own or it may serve as a delivery molecule for androgens in certain cases.

The concentration of SSBG is increased by thyroid hormone and estrogens and is decreased by androgens. Reciprocally, then, estrogen reduces the percentage of free testosterone, whereas androgen increases it. About 1% of the daily production of testosterone (70 μg) is excreted daily in the urine as a glucuronide. Most of the remainder is metabolized to two 17-ketosteroid products that are excreted in the urine (Fig. 52-15). Because most of the 17 ketosteroids arise from adrenal androgen precursors, measurement of plasma total and free testosterone (and occasionally urine testosterone) is the mainstay for assessing Leydig cell function.

■ Table 52-2　Turnover of gonadal steroids in adult men

Steroid	Plasma concentration (ng/dl)	Blood production rate (μg/day)	Metabolic clearance rate (L/day)
Testosterone	650	7000	1100
Dihydrotestosterone	45	300*	600
5α-Androstanediol	12	200*	1800
Androstenedione	120	2400	2000
Estradiol	3.0	50†	1700
Estrone	2.5	60†	2500

*About 60% to 80% produced peripherally from testosterone.

†About 80% to 90% produced peripherally from testosterone and androstenedione, respectively.

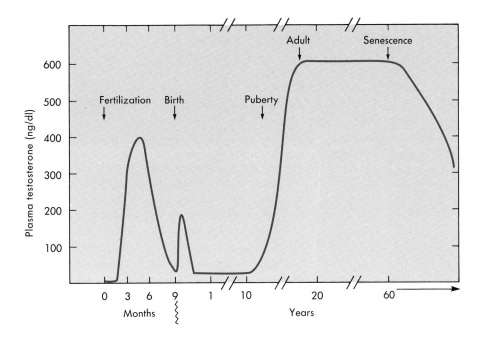

■ **Fig. 52-14** Plasma testosterone profile during the lifespan of a normal male. (Based on data from Griffin JE et al: *The testis.* In Bondy PK, Rosenberg LE, editors: *Metabolic control and disease,* Philadelphia, 1980, WB Saunders; and Winter JSD et al: Pituitary-gonadal relations in infancy, *J Clin Endocrinol Metab* 42:679, 1976.)

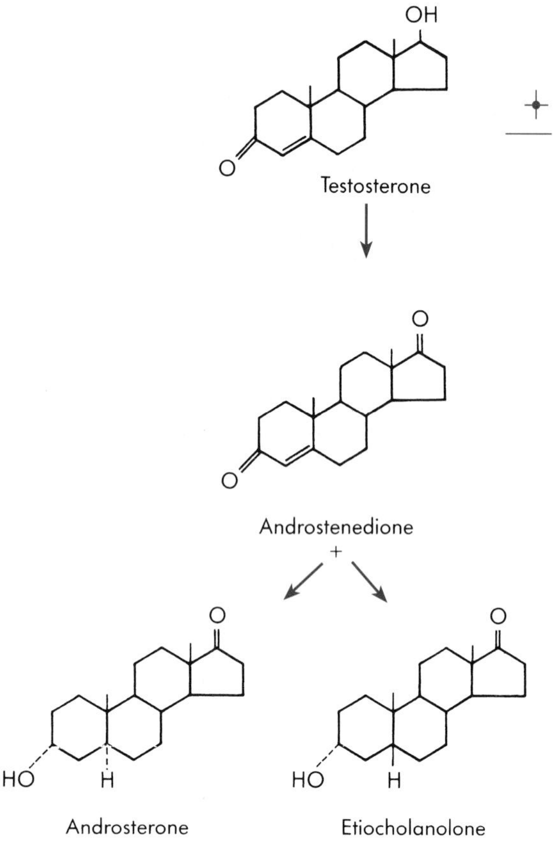

■ **Fig. 52-15**   Metabolism of testosterone to very weak androgens excreted in the urine as 17-ketosteroids.

Inhibin B (Fig. 52-5) circulates in the plasma of males and its level correlates inversely with FSH levels. This inverse relationship supports the idea that inhibin B functions to suppress FSH secretion. Inhibin A (Fig. 52-5) is not detectable in males.

■ *Androgen Actions*

The extratesticular effects of testosterone and related androgens can be divided into two major categories: (1) effects that pertain specifically to reproductive function and secondary sexual characteristics and (2) effects that pertain more generally to stimulation of nonreproductive tissue growth and maturation. Similar intracellular mechanisms are involved in both categories of effects. In general, the model for steroid hormone effects is applicable (see Fig. 45-13).

Testosterone diffuses freely into cells. In many, but not all, target cells, it rapidly undergoes reduction to DHT and, in some cells, to 5α-androstanediol (Fig. 52-4). The relevant hydroxysteroid dehydrogenases are located in microsomes and use NADPH as the reductant. DHT is much more potent than testosterone in some biological actions. However, all three steroids bind to a single cytoplasmic receptor of the steroid receptor superfamily (see Fig. 45-13).

The androgen hormone–receptor complex formed in the cytoplasm then dimerizes and moves into the nucleus, where it interacts with target DNA molecules and nuclear transcription factors. As a result of this interaction, RNA polymerase, various messenger RNAs, and the synthesis of proteins are stimulated. In addition, the activities of enzymes that play roles in DNA synthesis, such as thymidine kinase and DNA polymerase, are increased. Virtually all androgen actions can be blocked by inhibitors of RNA or protein synthesis. Therefore, these actions require the induction of new enzyme molecules, as opposed to allosteric or covalent activation of existing enzyme molecules.

In androgen target tissues, such as the prostate gland and seminal vesicles, polyamine (e.g., spermine and putrescine) synthesis is stimulated by testosterone, and these compounds in turn increase RNA synthesis. Androgens also stimulate the remarkable growth of these accessory organs of reproduction. This growth is characterized by hypertrophy and hyperplasia of the epithelial cells, stromal components, and blood vessels. In the prostate gland, a steroid-binding protein and a **prostate-specific antigen (PSA)** are induced.

The major circulating androgen by far is testosterone (Table 52-2). This hormone can be considered in part a prohormone for DHT and 5α-androstanediol, much as thyroxine is a prohormone for triiodothyronine. However, testosterone also has a definite intrinsic hormonal activity of its own in fetal and adult tissues that lack the enzyme 5α-reductase. For example, males who have congenital 5α-reductase deficiency cannot produce DHT. Although these individuals have feminized external genitalia at birth, during puberty they undergo selective masculinization in response to the rising testosterone secretion, and they produce sperm.

The effects of androgens according to the probable actual effector molecule are classified in Fig. 52-16. DHT is specifically required in the fetus for differentiation of the genital tubercle, genital swellings, genital folds, and urogenital sinus into the penis, scrotum, penile urethra, and prostate, respectively. DHT is required again during puberty for growth of the scrotum and prostate and for stimulation of prostatic secretions.

The mitogenic effects of androgens (and specifically of DHT) on the prostate gland are of great clinical importance. The conditions known as **benign prostatic hypertrophy (BPH)** and **prostate cancer** are common after age 50. BPH interferes with bladder function and can even cause renal failure by obstruction. Treatment with an inhibitor (**finasteride**) of the enzyme 5α-reductase reduces DHT concentrations in the prostate, causing the gland to shrink. Prostate cancer can be detected early by screening; its presence is

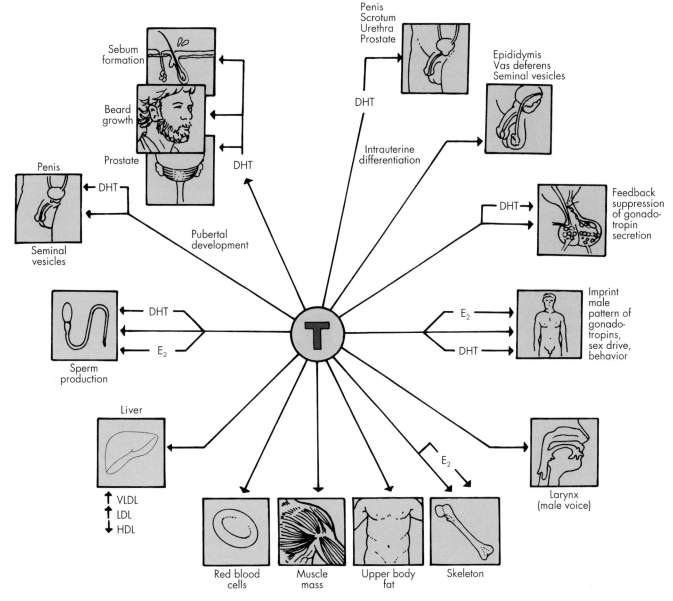

■ **Fig. 52-16**　The spectrum of testosterone *(T)* effects. Note that some effects result from the action of T itself, whereas others are mediated by dihydrotestosterone *(DHT)* and possibly estradiol *(E₂)* after they are produced from testosterone. *VLDL, LDL, HDL:* Very-low-density, low-density, and high-density lipoproteins, respectively.

suggested by an elevated serum level of PSA (see above). Growth of prostate cancer is at least partly androgen dependent, and therefore complete removal of androgen action is a mainstay of treatment. Methods include excision of the testes; markedly reducing LH and hence testosterone secretion with long-acting continuous GnRH agonists; and inhibiting testosterone and DHT actions with a receptor blocker (**flutamide**) or estrogens.

DHT or 5α-androstanediol stimulates the hair follicles and produces the typical male pattern of hair growth characterized by beard growth, a diamond-shaped pubic escutcheon, relatively large amounts of body hair, and

the recession of the temporal hairline, which in some men culminates in baldness. DHT or 5α-androstanediol is also responsible for increased production of sebum by the sebaceous glands, and the consequent development of acne, especially during puberty.

Testosterone, on the other hand, specifically stimulates the differentiation of the wolffian ducts into the epididymis, vas deferens, and seminal vesicles. During puberty, testosterone, with or without DHT, causes enlargement of the penis and the seminal vesicles. It also causes enlargement of the larynx and thickening of the vocal cords, which results in a deeper voice. Also, as noted, testosterone is the major local hormone required for initiation and maintenance of spermatogenesis.

Testosterone itself also first stimulates the pubertal growth spurt. It then terminates linear growth by closing the epiphyseal growth centers. Androgen receptors in osteoblasts transduce testosterone-stimulated increases in levels of transforming growth factors. Also, estradiol is an essential partner of testosterone or a mediator of testosterone's action on bone maturation in males.

Recently, XY males have been discovered who either lack estrogen receptors or have mutant genes for the enzyme aromatose and are therefore estradiol deficient. In both instances, the adult individuals are tall and their epiphyses are unfused. Plasma LH levels are elevated despite normal or increased testosterone levels. These findings suggest a normal role for estradiol in epiphyseal function in males and in gonadal feedback on the male hypothalamus.

Testosterone causes enlargement of the muscle mass in boys during puberty. In subsequent adult life, administration of testosterone in either sex causes nitrogen retention, which reflects protein anabolism. It is noteworthy that the hypothalamus lacks significant 5α-reductase activity. Thus, androgen suppression of gonadotropin secretion by negative feedback is largely a direct function of testosterone, with a possible small additional effect from circulating DHT. Estradiol produced from testosterone in the hypothalamus also contributes.

Testosterone has important actions on lipid metabolism. It increases levels of circulating low-density lipoprotein (LDL) cholesterol and decreases levels of circulating high-density lipoprotein (HDL) cholesterol (see Chapter 46). It also favors accumulation of upper body, abdominal, and visceral fat. These lipid effects are associated with a greater risk of cardiovascular disease in men than in premenopausal women.

Certain other diverse androgenic actions can be ascribed to testosterone. These include (1) stimulation of erythropoietin synthesis and maturation of erythroid precursors, which help maintain a normal red blood cell mass; (2) stimulation of renal sodium reabsorption; (3) suppression of hepatic synthesis of SSBG, cortisol-binding globulin, and thyroxine-binding globulin; (4) suppression of mammary gland growth; (5) initiation of sexual drive (libido) and the ability to achieve a physiologically complete erection (potency); and (6) stimulation of aggressive behavior. The latter two effects are controversial, as many other factors may outweigh the contribution of testosterone.

■ *Male Puberty*

Beginning at an average age of 10 to 11 years, and ending at an average age of 15 to 17 years, males develop full reproductive function, Leydig cell proliferation, and adult levels of androgenic hormones (Figs. 52-9 and 52-14). They achieve adult size and function of the accessory organs of reproduction, complete secondary sexual characteristics, and adult musculature. They undergo a linear growth spurt, and the epiphyses close when they attain adult height. A composite picture of the measurable and visible portions of this sequence is shown in Fig.

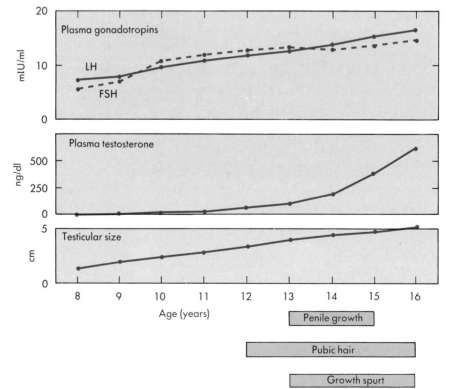

■ **Fig. 52-17** Average chronological sequence of hormonal and biological events in normal male puberty. (Based on data from Marshall WA, Tanner JM: *Arch Dis Child* 45:13, 1970; and Winter JSD et al: *Pediatr Res* 6:126, 1972.)

52-17. It must be stressed that this process can start as early as age 8 and as late as age 20, without any evidence of disease. The mechanisms of pubertal onset were described previously (Fig. 52-7).

Enlargement of the testis is the first and most important clinical sign of puberty. This enlargement signals an increase in the volume of the seminiferous tubules, and it is preceded by small increases in plasma FSH levels. As plasma LH levels increase, Leydig cells appear, and testosterone secretion is stimulated. The plasma testosterone level then climbs rapidly over a 2-year period, during which time pubic hair appears, the penis enlarges, and linear growth achieves peak velocity (Fig. 52-17). Sometime during this interval, at a median age of 13 years, sperm production begins. In about one third of boys, breast growth and tenderness appear transiently. These signs probably reflect increased production of estradiol secondary to LH stimulation. As testosterone levels continue to climb, the breast tissue regresses. One to 2 years after adult testosterone levels are reached, closure of the epiphyseal growth centers ends puberty. The plasma AMH level decreases from childhood levels, in response to an inhibiting effect of pubertal testosterone on this Sertoli cell product. Testosterone, via conversion to estradiol as an intermediate active molecule, also recruits increases in growth hormone secretion during puberty.

■ *The Ovaries*

The ovaries, fallopian tubes, and uterus make up the internal reproductive organs of the female and are situated in the pelvis. Each adult ovary weighs approximately 15 g, and is attached to the lateral pelvic wall and to the uterus by ligaments, through which run the ipsilateral ovarian artery, vein, lymphatic vessels, and nerve supply.

The ovary consists of three zones (Fig. 52-18). The dominant zone is the **cortex,** which is lined by germinal epithelium and contains the **oocytes.** Each oocyte is enclosed within a *follicle.* Follicles in various stages of development and regression are present throughout the cortex during the reproductive years (Fig. 52-18).

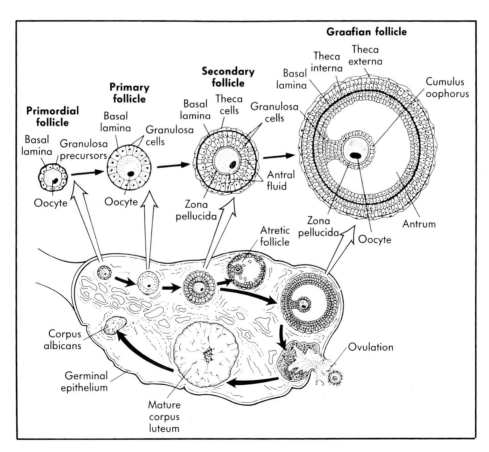

■ **Fig. 52-18**   Schematic representation (not to scale) of the structure of the ovary, showing the various stages in the development of the follicle and its successor structure, the corpus luteum. The follicle grows from a primordial size of 25 μm to an ovulatory size of 10 to 20 mm. The oocyte is shielded from indiscriminate exposure to interstitial fluid contents by the basal lamina and the cytoplasm of the surrounding granulosa cells. The hormones and other constituents of the antral fluid are critical regulators of follicular development. (Redrawn from Ham AW, Leeson TS: *Histology,* ed 4, Philadelphia, 1968, JB Lippincott.)

Interposed between the follicles is the stroma, which is composed of supporting connective tissue elements and interstitial cells. The other two zones of the ovary are the **medulla,** which consists of a heterogeneous group of cells, and the **hilum,** at which the blood vessels enter. These zones contain scattered steroid-producing cells, whose normal function is unknown. During physical examination, the ovaries can be felt through the abdominal wall and can also be well visualized by ultrasonography and computed tomography (CT).

As a hormone-secreting organ, the ovary functions in two ways. First, the ovarian sex steroids and protein hormones function locally to modulate the complex events in the development and extrusion of the ova (a process called *ovulation*). Second, ovarian hormones are secreted into the circulation and act on diverse target organs, including the uterus, fallopian tubes, vagina, breasts, hypothalamus, pituitary gland, adipose tissue, bones, kidney, liver, and vascular system. Many, but not all, of these distant effects are closely related to the reproductive sequence.

The fundamental reproductive unit in the female is the single ovarian follicle, which is composed of one germ cell completely surrounded by a cluster of endocrine cells. When fully developed and functional, the follicle (1) maintains and nurtures the resident oocyte, (2) matures the oocyte and releases it at the right time, (3) prepares the vagina and fallopian tubes to assist in fertilization, (4) prepares the lining of the uterus to accept and implant a zygote, and (5) maintains hormonal support for the fetus until the placenta can take over this function.

■ *The Biology of Oogenesis*

The primordial germ cells migrate from the yolk sac of the embryo to the genital ridge at 5 to 6 weeks of gestation. There, in the developing ovary, they produce oogonia by mitotic division until 20 to 24 weeks of gestation, when the total number of oogonia has reached a maximum of 7 million. Beginning at 8 to 9 weeks of gestation, some oogonia start into the prophase of meiosis and become primary oocytes. This process continues until 6 months after birth, when all oogonia have been converted to oocytes. At this time, oocytes are 10 to 25 μm in diameter. They grow to 50 to 120 μm at maturity, the size of the nucleus and cytoplasm having increased proportionately. The first meiotic division is not completed until the time of ovulation; thus, primary oocytes have lifespans of up to 50 years. The lengthy suspension of the oocyte in prophase apparently depends on the hormonal milieu provided by its surrounding sustaining cells. Both X chromosomes are required in the ovary for oocyte meiosis and survival.

From the start of oogenesis, however, a process of oocyte attrition also occurs. By birth, only 1 to 2 million primary oocytes remain, and by the onset of puberty the number falls to 400,000. Thus, in contrast to the male, who continuously produces spermatogonia and primary spermatocytes, the female cannot manufacture new oogonia and must function with a continuously declining number of primary oocytes from which ova can mature. At or soon after menopause, few, if any, oocytes are left, and reproductive capacity ends. The development of ovarian follicles from their primordial state to the point at which an ovum is launched can be divided into three stages.

Stage 1. Follicles begin to form in the fetal ovary at 12 to 16 weeks of gestation. The first stage of development of the ovarian follicle parallels the prophase of the oocyte. This stage progresses slowly, over a period that is usually not less than 13 years but may be as long as 50 years. As an oocyte enters meiosis, it induces a single layer of spindle cells from the stroma to surround it completely. These cells are the precursors of the **granulosa cells.** Cytoplasmic processes from these cells attach to the plasma membrane of the oocyte. In addition, a membrane called the **basal lamina** forms outside the spindle cells, delimiting the complex from the surrounding stroma. The resultant structure constitutes the **primordial follicle,** which is about 25 μm in diameter (Fig. 52-18).

Beginning at 21 to 31 weeks of gestation, some of these follicles enter the next phase of development. The spindle-shaped cells change to a cuboidal shape and become granulosa cells and thus a **primary follicle** is formed. As the granulosa cells divide and form several layers around the oocyte, a **secondary follicle** is created. The granulosa cells secrete mucopolysaccharides, which form a protective halo, the **zona pellucida,** around the oocyte (Fig. 52-18). The cytoplasmic processes of the granulosa cells, however, continue to penetrate the zona pellucida, creating conduits through which these cells can selectively provide nutrients and chemical signals to the maturing primary oocyte within. Thus, the cytoplasm of the granulosa cells, like that of the male Sertoli cells, forms a filter through which plasma substances must pass before reaching the germ cell.

The secondary follicle continues to grow and reaches a diameter of 150 μm. At this point, the oocyte has reached its maximal size, on average 80 μm in diameter. Two other developments take place concurrently: (1) another layer of spindle interstitial cells is recruited outside the basal lamina and forms the **theca interna** and (2) the granulosa cells begin to extrude small amounts of fluid that form collections between them. The first stage of follicular development is now complete. With rare exceptions, this first stage is the maximal degree of development found in the prepubertal ovary.

Stage 2. In contrast to the first stage, the second stage of follicular development is much more rapid, requiring only 70 to 85 days. This stage takes place mainly after **menarche** (i.e., after the onset of menses). Past the midpoint of each menstrual cycle, a small cohort of secondary follicles is recruited to enter the next sequence. The small collections of follicular fluid coalesce into a single central area called the **antrum** (Fig. 52-18). The fluid in the antrum contains mucopolysaccharides, plasma proteins, electrolytes, glycosoaminoglycans, proteoglycans, gonadal steroid hormones, FSH, LH, inhibin, activin, several growth factors, oxytocin, arginine vasopressin, and proopiomelanocortin products. The steroid hormones reach the antrum by direct secretion from granulosa cells and by diffusion from the theca cells outside the basal lamina. A nonsteroidal substance made by granulosa cells that can inhibit oocyte meiosis is also secreted into the antral fluid. AMH or inhibin may be this factor.

The granulosa cells continue to proliferate, and gap junctions develop between them. These gap junctions form a syncytium of electrical and chemical communication. They displace the oocyte into an eccentric position on a stalk, where it is surrounded by a distinctive granulosa cell layer, called the **cumulus oophorus,** which is two to three cells thick. The theca cells also proliferate, and those nearest the basal lamina are transformed into cuboidal, steroid-secreting cells of the theca interna. Additional peripheral layers of spindle cells from the stroma form around the theca interna and, together with an ingrowth of blood vessels, make up the **theca externa.** The new vessels give the follicle direct access to blood-borne molecules such as gonadotropins. By the end of this second stage, the entire complex, called a **graafian follicle** or **antral follicle** (Fig. 57-18), has reached an average diameter of 2 to 5 mm. Although graafian follicles may occasionally be found in prepubertal ovaries, they are relatively small and in an early phase of development.

Stage 3. The third and final stage of follicular development is the most rapid and occurs only in the postpubertal reproductive ovary. *Five to 7 days after the onset of menses, a single graafian follicle is selected from its cohort and becomes the **dominant follicle** of that cycle.* With rare exceptions, this process occurs in only a single ovary each month. In addition to further cellular growth, the production of antral fluid is significantly increased. The colloid osmotic pressure of the fluid also increases because of depolymerization of the mucopolysaccharides, but the total intrafollicular pressure remains at 16 to 20 mm Hg. The granulosa cells spread apart and the cumulus oophorus loosens. At the same time, the vascularity of the theca increases greatly. With exponential growth, the total size of this follicle reaches 20 mm in the final 48 hours before ovulation, which takes place at the midpoint of the menstrual cycle. The portion of the basal lamina adjacent to the surface of the ovary then undergoes proteolysis. The follicle gently ruptures and releases the oocyte with its adherent cumulus oophorus into the peritoneal cavity. At this time, the initial meiotic division is completed. The resultant secondary oocyte is drawn into the closely approximated fallopian tube. The other daughter cell, called the **first polar body,** is discarded. In the fallopian tube, penetration by a sperm stimulates the completion of the second meiotic division and yields the haploid (23 chromosome) ovum and the **second polar body.**

Corpus luteum formation. After ovulation, the remaining elements of the ruptured follicle next form a new endocrine structure, the **corpus luteum** (Fig. 52-18). *This new endocrine unit provides the necessary balance of gonadal steroids that optimizes conditions for implantation of a fertilized ovum, and for subsequent maintenance of the zygote until the placenta can assume this function.* The corpus luteum is made up of granulosa cells, theca cells, thecal capillaries, and fibroblasts. The granulosa cells comprise 80% of the corpus luteum. They undergo hypertrophy to a diameter of 30 μm and become arranged in rows. The mitochondria develop dense matrices with tubular cristae, numerous lipid droplets form within the cytoplasm, and the smooth endoplasmic reticulum proliferates. These changes reflect the marked increase in the capacity of the cells to produce steroid hormones, as described in Chapter 51. This process, called **luteinization,** is precipitated by the exit of the oocyte from the follicle.

The remaining 20% of the corpus luteum consists of theca cells arranged in folds along its outer surface. The theca cells exhibit similar, although less dramatic, luteinization changes. The basal lamina between the theca and granulosa cells disappears, which allows direct vascularization of the granulosa cells.

The antrum may become engorged temporarily with blood from hemorrhaging thecal vessels, but a clot quickly forms and is subsequently lysed. If fertilization and pregnancy do not ensue, the corpus luteum begins to regress after a 14-day lifespan. In this process, known as **luteolysis,** the endocrine cells undergo necrosis and the structure is invaded by leukocytes, macrophages, and fibroblasts. Gradually, the former corpus luteum is replaced by an avascular scar, known as the **corpus albicans** (Fig. 52-18).

Atresia of follicles. During the reproductive lifespan of the average woman, only 400 to 500 oocytes (one per month) undergo the complete sequence of events that culminate in ovulation. The remaining millions of oocytes disappear. Some are lost each month because they enter into a growth phase with other follicles, but they do not become dominant follicles. Most, however, undergo the process called **atresia,** which begins almost as soon as the first primordial follicles appear in the fetal ovary.

Atresia is caused by **apoptosis,** or programmed cell death. Apoptosis is characterized by increased free radical formation and DNA cleavage by the enzyme endonuclease. In first-stage follicles, atresia appears to be a relatively simple process precipitated by oocyte degeneration. The oocyte becomes necrotic, its nucleus becomes pyknotic, and the granulosa cells also degenerate. This simple type of atresia accounts for the disappearance of most follicles. In more advanced follicles, atresia is more complex. In some of these follicles, the granulosa cells furthest from the oocyte first undergo necrotic changes. Loss of their function may actually cause the oocyte to resume meiosis to the point of extrusion of the first polar body. Eventually, however, the granulosa cells in the cumulus oophorus also die, the protective zona pellucida disappears, and the oocyte degenerates. Fibroblasts then invade the follicle, and everything inside the basal lamina collapses into an avascular scar. Outside the basal lamina, the theca cells dedifferentiate and return to the pool of interstitial cells from which they came.

■ *Hormonal Patterns during the Menstrual Cycle*

The menstrual cycle is divided physiologically into three sequential phases. The **follicular phase** begins with the onset of menstrual bleeding and averages 15 days (range, 9 to 23 days). The **ovulatory phase** lasts 1 to 3 days and culminates in ovulation. The **luteal phase** has a more constant length of about 13 days and ends with the onset of menstrual bleeding. The overall duration of a normal menstrual cycle averages 28 days, but it can vary from 21 to 35 days, depending mostly on the length of the follicular phase.

A series of cyclic changes in gonadal steroid and protein hormone production characterize adult ovarian function (Fig. 52-19, Table 52-3). This monthly hormone profile results from cyclic changes in pituitary gonadotropins (Fig. 52-19) coupled with paracrine and autocrine effects on the follicle. Critical changes in FSH and LH secretion reflect changes in pituitary sensitivity to GnRH (Fig. 52-20, *A*) and changes in the pulsatility of the hypothalamic GnRH generator. However, the pattern of gonadotropin secretion is also critically regulated by both negative and positive feedback from gonadal steroids and is influenced by inhibin and activin. These interactions are described in detail in Chapter 49 and presented in Fig. 49-15.

Toward the end of the luteal phase (a few days before the onset of menstrual bleeding), plasma FSH and LH are at their lowest levels (Fig. 52-19). The LH/FSH ratio is slightly greater than 1. One or 2 days before the onset of menses, FSH levels begin to rise, followed somewhat later by a rise in LH levels. *The estrogen (estradiol and estrone) levels increase gradually, stimulated by the rise in the FSH level in this first half of the follicular phase.* Progesterone, 17-hydroxyprogesterone, and the androgens androstenedione and testosterone remain at relatively low, constant levels.

During the second half of the follicular phase, FSH levels fall modestly, whereas LH levels continue to rise very slowly. The LH/FSH ratio therefore increases to about 2. *Concurrently, estradiol and estrone production and plasma levels rise sharply, and just before the ovulatory phase, they reach peaks that are fivefold to ninefold*

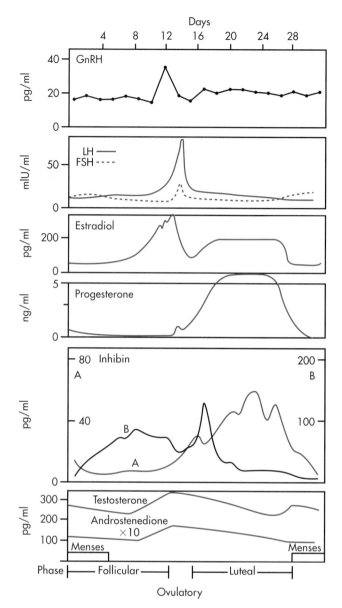

■ **Fig. 52-19**   Plasma hormone levels throughout the menstrual cycle. Note the increases of estradiol and gonadotropin-releasing hormone *(GnRH)* preceding ovulatory surges of LH and FSH. The later broad peaks of progesterone and estradiol are produced by corpus luteum secretion. The earlier inhibin B peak results from follicle production; the later inhibin A peak results from corpus luteal production.

higher. The estradiol is secreted directly by the dominant follicle, In contrast, estrone is produced largely by peripheral conversion from estradiol and androstenedione. Progesterone, largely secreted by the adrenal cortex, and 17-hydroxyprogesterone remain at low levels until just before the ovulatory phase, when the progesterone level begins to increase as a consequence of ovarian secretion. Androstenedione and testosterone also rise modestly in parallel with 17-hydroxyprogesterone. About half the androgenic steroids are derived from ovarian secretion and half are derived from adrenal secretion.

■ **Table 52-3** Turnover of gonadal steroids in adult women

Steroids	Plasma concentration (ng/dl)	Production rate (µg/day)	Metabolic clearance rate (L/day)
Estradiol			
Early follicular	6	80	1400
Late follicular	50	700	
Middle luteal	20	300	
Estrone			
Eary follicular	5	100	2200
Late follicular	20	500	
Middle luteal	10	250	
17-Hydroxyprogesterone			
Early follicular	30	600	2000
Late follicular	200	4000	
Middle luteal	200	4000	
Progesterone			
Follicular	100	2000	2200
Luteal	1000	25,000	
Testosterone	40	250	700
Dihydrotestosterone	20	50	400
Androstenedione	150	3000	2000
DHEA	500	8000	1600

Modified from Lipsett MB: In Yen SSC, Jaffe RB, editors: *Reproductive endocrinology,* Philadelphia, 1978, WB Saunders. *DHEA,* Dehydroepiandrosterone.

The ovarian contribution results from LH stimulation of the theca cells in the dominant follicle.

The succeeding ovulatory phase is characterized by a very sharp spike in plasma gonadotropin levels. The LH level increases much more than the FSH level (Fig. 52-19), and hence the LH/FSH ratio rises to about 5. It takes an average of 14 hours for this surge to be achieved, and the doubling time is 5 hours. The plateau lasts 14 hours, and LH and FSH levels then decline over 20 hours. Plasma estradiol levels plummet from their peak at the same time that LH and FSH are on their ovulatory upswing. Estrone, 17-hydroxyprogesterone, androstenedione, and testosterone also now decrease, but much more gradually than estradiol. In contrast, a small but significant rise in progesterone begins during the ovulatory phase.

After ovulation, LH and FSH both continue to decline during the luteal phase, and they reach their lowest points toward the end of the cycle, before the onset of menses. *The most distinctive and important feature of the luteal phase is a tenfold increase in the progesterone level, which emanates from the corpus luteum.* Levels of estradiol, estrone, and 17-hydroxyprogesterone also increase, and broad second peaks of each occur through the middle of the luteal phase. Levels of androstenedione and testosterone, however, continue to decline during the luteal phase.

Inhibin levels also fluctuate systematically throughout the cycle (Fig. 52-19). Inhibin B (Fig. 52-5) levels rise during the follicular phase in parallel with FSH, and they display a periovulatory phase peak. The levels become very low during the luteal phase. In contrast, inhibin A (Fig. 52-5) levels are low during the follicular phase, but they increase markedly in parallel with the progesterone level during the luteal phase. Thus, inhibin B comes from the dominant follicle, whereas inhibin A comes predominantly from the corpus luteum. Inhibin B plus estradiol feed back on the pituitary to reduce FSH secretion during the latter part of the follicular phase. Inhibin A plus estradiol and progesterone feed back on the pituitary to suppress FSH and LH secretion throughout the luteal phase. If pregnancy does not occur, the menstrual cycle ends as estrogen and progesterone levels decrease dramatically to their lowest values. FSH levels again begin to rise, and bleeding signals the start of a new cycle.

■ *Hormonal Regulation of Oogenesis and the Stages of Follicular Development*

Stage 1. The initial growth of the primordial follicle appears to be a local phenomenon. It is independent of gonadotropins, but factors from the oocyte stimulate early granulosa cell development. In turn, granulosa cell products initiate formation of the theca and then stop maturation of the oocyte once it reaches 80 µm in diameter. The transient surge of FSH and LH release that occurs midway through gestation and even the normally low levels of gonadotropins secreted during childhood are necessary for an adequate rate of follicular growth throughout the rest of life. Without any gonadotropin stimulation, follicular growth is greatly impaired. Nonetheless, the first stage, from primordial to primary follicle, continues until menopause; its occurrence does not appear to depend on the presence or the state of reproductive cycling.

Thus, the exact mechanism by which a particular group of resting primordial follicles is recruited to descend from the cortex into the interstitium toward the medulla and to initiate development into primary follicles is unknown. However, the most "selectable" follicles are those whose theca interna begins to develop during the periovulatory phase of that cycle when the surge of gonadotropin release increases the vascularity of the follicles and helps protect them from atresia.

Stage 2. After the menarche, recruitment of a cohort of primary follicles for second-stage development occurs in the early luteal phase of the menstrual cycle. Each cohort gradually develops further over a period of 60 to 70 days, until the late luteal phase two cycles later. At this point, a total of about 20 follicles in both ovaries have reached the size of 2 to 4 mm and are capable of responding further to the FSH increase in the follicular phase of the next cycle.

Before their selection, primary follicles show evidence of only the faint presence of steroid hormone–producing enzymes. *The initial action of FSH on primary follicles is to stimulate growth of the granulosa cells* (Fig. 52-21). *However, aromatase activity is progressively increased*

■ **Fig. 52-20** **A,** Increased responsiveness of pituitary gonadotrophs to GnRH in the late follicular phase of the menstrual cycle when endogenous estradiol levels are increased. **B,** Plasma LH and FSH after exogenous estradiol administration. After the initial decrease caused by negative feedback, plasma LH rebounds well above the baseline when estradiol is discontinued. This positive effect of estradiol is also accentuated as the follicular phase of the menstrual cycle progresses. (**A** redrawn from Wang CF et al: The functional changes of the pituitary gonadotrophs during the menstrual cycle, *J Clin Endocrinol Metab* 42:718, 1976. **B** redrawn from Yen SSC et al: *Causal relationship between the hormonal variables.* In Ferin M et al, editors: *Biorhythms and human reproduction,* New York, 1974, John Wiley.)

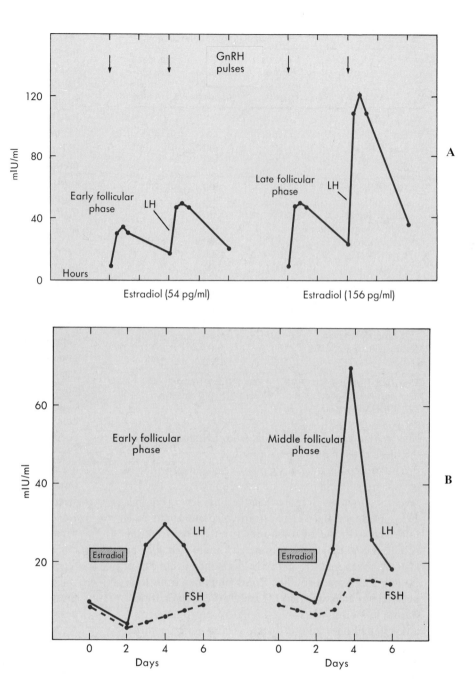

by FSH, and hence estrogen synthesis from androgen precursors is enhanced. The increasing local estradiol concentration causes proliferation of its own receptors and those of growth factors. It also reinforces FSH actions by increasing FSH receptors and by synergizing with the gonadotropin to stimulate further granulosa cell hyperplasia and hypertrophy (Fig. 52-21). These effects in turn further boost estradiol production. Local synthesis of IGF-1 and IGF-2, in response to FSH, further amplifies the primary FSH signals for proliferation and steroidogenesis. In contrast, epidermal growth factor and transforming growth factor-α decrease FSH-induced estradiol synthesis but reinforce granulosa cell proliferation. Thus, the initiation of second-stage follicular development may be viewed as a self-propelling mechanism that involves

fine coordination between the pituitary gland and ovary and that yields successively increasing rates of follicular growth and estradiol production.

Three other important actions, which develop somewhat later in the second stage, contribute to this autocatalytic process. First, FSH, along with estradiol, induces LH receptors on the granulosa cells. Second, the slowly rising plasma estradiol levels condition the hypothalamic gonadotropin axis, which maintains or slightly increases plasma LH while plasma FSH is decreasing. Furthermore, pituitary LH stores are enhanced by estradiol. This enhancement is reflected by the fact that administration of exogenous pulses of GnRH produces greater LH responses in the second half of the follicular phase than in the first half (Fig. 52-20, *A*). Thus, pituitary

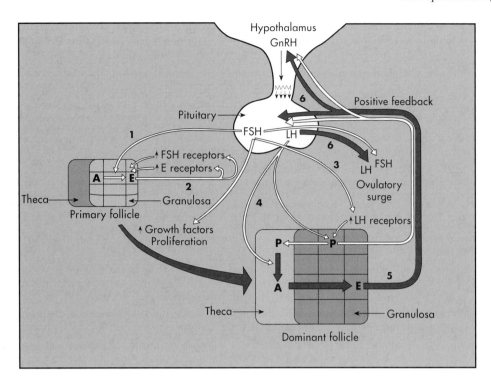

■ **Fig. 52-21**   Hormonal regulation of follicular development. *1,* FSH stimulates granulosa cell growth and estradiol *(E)* synthesis in certain primary follicles. *2,* The local estradiol increases its own receptors and FSH receptors, amplifying both hormones' effects. Thus, a self-propelling mechanism is set into motion. *3,* FSH also stimulates growth factor production and granulosa cell proliferation. FSH later increases LH receptors, augmenting granulosa and theca cell responsiveness to LH. *4,* LH stimulates theca cell growth and androgen *(A)* production. Androgen is then converted to estradiol in the granulosa cells. LH also stimulates progesterone *(P)* production in the granulosa cells. *5,* As a result of two-way steroid traffic, the dominant follicle emerges as a very efficient secretor of estradiol. *6,* Rising estradiol, with late potentiation by progesterone, feeds back positively on the pituitary gland and hypothalamus to evoke the preovulatory surge of LH and FSH.

stores of LH are built up for the coming essential ovulatory surge. Third, estradiol increases the number of LH receptors in theca cells.

The rising LH level stimulates the theca cells to produce increasing amounts of androgens, with androstenedione production predominating over testosterone production. These steroids diffuse across the basal lamina, where they serve as substrates for granulosa cell aromatase and sustain the augmented estradiol production (Figs. 52-4 and 52-21). In addition, LH stimulates the granulosa cells to produce progesterone, some of which diffuses back into the theca cells to serve as a substrate for androgen synthesis (Fig. 52-21). Thus, although granulosa cells and theca cells can individually synthesize both androgens and estrogens to some extent, their proximity and the two-way traffic of steroids between them greatly increase the overall efficiency of the follicle.

The gonadal protein hormones also contribute paracrine effects to this process. Inhibin B from granulosa cells, together with IGF-1 stimulated by growth hormone action, augments androgen production by theca cells. Although activin inhibits this production, this inhibition may be offset by activin enhancement of FSH and

LH receptors. Follistatin also inhibits activin actions and directly stimulates progesterone synthesis.

FSH also stimulates production of a variety of other molecules by the granulosa cells, which probably have paracrine effects. The situation is analogous to that of the Sertoli cell and spermatogenesis. Thus, transferrin and ceruloplasmin pick up iron and copper, respectively, from their plasma-binding analogs and transfer these vital elements to the oocyte. FSH also stimulates granulosa cell metabolism and provides lactic acid and 2-ketoisocaproic acid as energy sources for the oocyte. IGFs and transforming growth factors may modulate oocyte development. Locally produced plasminogen activator and cytokines are involved in ovulation. Concentrations of renin and angiotensin, oxytocin, and GnRH-like peptides are all elevated in the follicular fluid, but their functions are obscure.

Stage 3. By days 5 to 7 of the follicular phase, only one follicle has reached a size greater than 11 mm. This **dominant follicle** selects itself by outstripping the others. Its key characteristic is increased aromatase activity and therefore more efficient synthesis of estradiol. The increased aromatase activity may result from greater vascularity, and therefore from greater accessibility to

FSH. Because FSH is more available to this follicle and it has an increased number of FSH receptors, the dominant follicle is not as dependent on the waning FSH supply in the middle to late follicular phase. A greater production of inhibin, a lesser production of activin, and a more favorable array of growth factors at this crucial time may increase cAMP and/or LH receptors and thereby increase the supply of precursor androgens from the theca cells. *Whatever the mechanism, its greater production of estradiol permits the dominant follicle to inhibit further substantive growth of its sister follicles, to prime the GnRH-gonadotropin axis for generating the ovulatory LH surge, and to alter the tissues of the genital tract to favor conception* (Fig. 52-22).

The remaining follicles undergo atresia, the largest of them in the midluteal phase when the FSH level is low. These follicles have a decreased number of FSH receptors as well as a low FSH concentration, and a high androgen/estrogen ratio in the follicular fluid. Also, the fact that cohort follicles are stunted more severely in the ovary that contains the dominant follicle than in the contralateral ovary suggests greater secretion of a specific paracrine inhibitor, such as activin, by the dominant follicle.

The sharply increasing estradiol release from the dominant follicle triggers the ovulatory surge of gonadotropins (Figs. 52-20, *B*, and 52-23). A critical plasma estradiol level of at least 200 pg/ml, sustained for at least 2 days, is required to elicit this positive feedback effect on LH, an effect that is more pronounced later than earlier in the follicular phase (Fig. 52-2, *B*). Although the much smaller periovulatory increase in progesterone is not absolutely required for ovulation, it does synergize with estradiol by amplifying and prolonging the gonadotropin surge. The loci of this positive feedback on gonadotropin secretion are both the pituitary and the hypothalamus. The mechanism involves decreasing the inhibitory activity of dopaminergic and endorphinergic neurons on GnRH neurons (Fig. 49-15). The pituitary gonadotrophs, appropriately primed by the preceding

pattern of gonadal steroid exposure, respond to GnRH with heightened sensitivity at this time (Fig. 52-20, *A*). The LH molecules released are more bioactive, probably because of posttranslational modulation of their sialic acid content by estradiol. In addition, a peak of peripheral plasma GnRH levels probably precedes the LH/FSH peak (Fig. 52-19). This peak likely indicates an augmented flow of GnRH from the hypothalamus to the pituitary, an effect that is also attributable to gonadal estrogens (Fig. 52-23).

The surge of LH with FSH then triggers ovulation by a multicomponent mechanism. LH stimulation of the granulosa cell neutralizes the action of an oocyte maturation inhibitor. Release from inhibition allows meiosis to be completed. Stimulation of progesterone levels enhances proteolytic enzyme activity and increases the distensibility of the follicle. As a result, follicular fluid volume rapidly increases. The LH surge also induces the enzyme **prostaglandin endoperoxidase synthase** in granulosa cells. This enzyme increases the synthesis of prostaglandins, thromboxanes, and leukotrienes and thereby causes a pseudoinflammatory response that leads to follicular rupture. Mucification of the cumulus oophorus, and possibly contraction of the follicular wall stimulated by oxytocin, contribute to extrusion of the oocyte. Plasminogen activator, stimulated by FSH, generates the proteolytic enzyme plasmin, which catalyzes breakdown of the follicular wall. Increases in the concentrations of histamine, bradykinins, platelet-activating factor, and blood flow then follow. FSH also stimulates the process whereby the oocyte-cumulus complex becomes detached and free-floating just before extrusion. Finally, immediately after the LH surge, the numbers of LH receptors are temporarily reduced by down-regulation. This reduction in LH receptors desensitizes the granulosa and thecal cells to LH. The resultant rapid fall in androgen and estradiol production contributes to loss of integrity of the follicle. The LH surge also neutralizes the activity of the luteinization-inhibiting factor found in preovulatory fluid, and thereby stimulates luteinization of the granulosa cells.

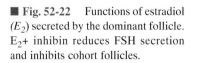

■ **Fig. 52-22** Functions of estradiol (*E₂*) secreted by the dominant follicle. E₂+ inhibin reduces FSH secretion and inhibits cohort follicles.

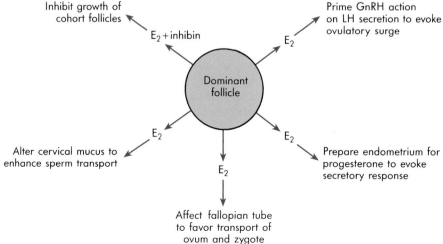

Corpus luteum function. Once the oocyte leaves the ovary, it is not under any other immediate hormonal influence. However, the organization and growth of the corpus luteum and its secretory pattern are under hormonal control. In humans, LH is essential for luteinization of the granulosa cells. Their subsequent high rate of progesterone production is facilitated by increased activity of the enzymes 3β-hydrogenase and $^{\Delta 4,5}$ isomerase (Fig. 52-4). Luteinization requires restoration and maintenance of LH receptors, which in turn depends on proper exposure to FSH and LH pulses in the preceding follicular phase. Prolactin may help sustain progesterone output by increasing the LH receptors. However, plasma prolactin levels vary only slightly throughout the menstrual cycle, and corpus luteum function has been observed in prolactin-deficient women. Estradiol also may play an autocrine role in maintaining the corpus luteum, possibly by facilitating vascular ingrowth.

During the luteal phase, low-frequency/high-amplitude LH pulses replace the high-frequency/low-amplitude pulses of the follicular phase. This change in pulse characteristics may result from conditioning of the GnRH generator by the high progesterone concentrations. In addition, the steadily increasing progesterone, estradiol, and inhibin A output of the corpus luteum exerts negative feedback on the pituitary gland. As a result, the levels of LH and FSH (Fig. 52-19) gradually decline. If the declining LH levels of the late luteal phase are not replaced by the equivalent placental hormone, **human chorionic gonadotropin (HCG),** the corpus luteum regresses, and its secretion of progesterone and estradiol ceases completely in 14 days.

In the nonpregnant female who lacks HCG, the corpus luteum begins to regress by the eighth day after ovulation. The breakdown of the corpus luteum (luteolysis) is associated with decreasing LH receptors, steroidogenic enzymes, and vascularity. This process is also marked by increasing concentrations of cholesterol in the corpus luteum as progesterone synthesis declines. Luteolysis is probably mediated by prostaglandins made within the corpus luteum. By the twelfth postovulatory day, progesterone, estradiol, and inhibin A levels have fallen to levels low enough to release the pituitary gland from negative feedback inhibition. FSH then begins to rise in the next cycle.

Extraordinary coordination between the various elements of the female hypothalamic-pituitary-ovarian axis is required for ovulation and conception. This creates numerous possibilities for failure, and infertility often arises from dysfunction of this system. Disease or conditions that disrupt GnRH release or impair the gonadotroph responsiveness prevent the necessary initial FSH pattern from recruiting a dominant follicle, and complete loss of menses (**amenorrhea**) may result. A dominant follicle may produce enough estrogen for uterine bleeding to occur (see below) but not enough to induce a midcycle peak of the LH level. **Anovulatory cycles** result. An elevated ratio of LH to FSH levels in the follicular phase is associated with excessive theca cell production of androgens, which results in the formation of numerous atretic and cystic follicles. This condition is known as the **polycystic ovary syndrome.** Even if ovulation occurs, inadequate progesterone production

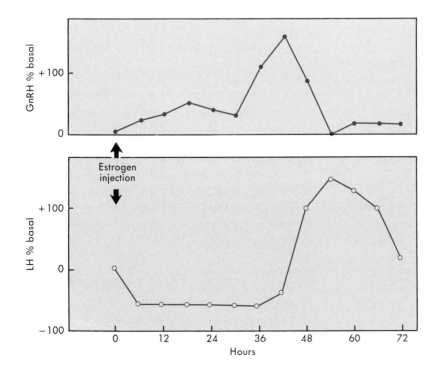

■ **Fig. 52-23** Effect of exogenous administration of estrogen on plasma GnRH and LH levels. After an initial phase of suppression, the positive feedback action of estrogen on LH secretion is seen at 48 hours. This delayed rise in LH levels is preceded by an increase in GnRH levels, suggesting a hypothalamic locus of estrogen action. (Redrawn from Miyake A et al: *J Clin Endocrinol Metab* 56:1100, 1983.)

by the corpus luteum may lead to poor preparation of the reproductive tract for either fertilization or implantation.

Various medical therapies are available for female infertility. For example, the drug **clomiphene** is an estrogen receptor antagonist that acts in the hypothalamus. By simulating estrogen deficiency and producing negative feedback, clomiphene increases GnRH and gonadotropin secretion in women who have a hypothalamic origin of infertility. Alternatively, endogenous pituitary function can be suppressed with a long-acting GnRH superagonist, and ovulation can then be induced by carefully timed doses of exogenous FSH and LH. LH is provided in the form of HCG.

The hormonal regulation of the female reproductive cycle, as just described, has left open an important question: *what ultimately determines the monthly cyclicity of the LH/FSH surge and the resultant ovulation?* Although the concept of a primary central nervous system clock is inherently attractive, considerable evidence suggests that in humans it is the ovary that principally determines the basic rhythm. Five observations support this point:

1. Cyclic release of gonadotropins is not observed in women whose ovaries never functioned or whose ovaries were removed during the reproductive years, or in postmenopausal women after follicular development has ceased.
2. During the reproductive years, the ovulatory gonadotropin surge does not occur until the dominant follicle has reached the appropriate stage of development, however long that may take.
3. When the antiestrogen, hypothalamic stimulator clomiphene is given for 5 to 7 days to treat infertility, a *spontaneous* LH/FSH surge and ovulation can occur several days after the drug is stopped, provided that a dominant follicle has emerged and grown.
4. Administration of estrogen with or without progesterone in a format that resembles the normal preovulatory estradiol rise can induce an LH surge (Fig. 52-23), even in postmenopausal women.
5. In monkeys whose pituitary glands have been completely severed from the hypothalamus, central nervous system regulation of gonadotropin secretion is disrupted. However, if GnRH is replaced intravenously in a physiological pulsatile pattern to reinstitute and sustain basal FSH and LH secretion, subsequent cyclic ovarian function occurs with an LH/FSH surge that does not require any change in the rate or pattern of the GnRH infusion.

Such observations suggest that a GnRH pulse generator in the central nervous system is required to initiate and sustain follicular development. However, it is the developing pattern of ovarian events and secretions, most critically in the dominant follicle, that conditions this pulse generator and the pituitary gonadotrophs to respond at a later time with an ovulatory LH/FSH surge. Perhaps no other phenomenon so clearly illustrates the intricate nature of the interactions among endocrine, paracrine, autocrine, and neural mechanisms of regulation.

The close coordination between the emergence of a single dominant follicle and the ovulatory signal it recruits makes multiple pregnancies unlikely in humans. For example, the natural rate of occurrence of **dizygotic twins** is less than 1% of live births. By contrast, a much higher rate (15%) results from the multiple ova produced by cycles in which follicular development and ovulation are stimulated artificially "from above" by administration of exogenous FSH and LH in superimposed profiles.

Ovarian signals can be either overridden or reinforced by other influences on and from the hypothalamus. Loss of cyclic gonadotropin secretion can occur in situations that suggest that the hypothalamus is responding to a caloric or adipose mass, thermal, photic, olfactory, emotional, or inflammatory signal. Cyclic gonadotropin secretion can cease in women who are calorically deprived and who therefore lose considerable amounts of adipose tissue and lean body mass, and also in women who exercise excessively. This also occurs in women who undergo physical translocation, climatic change, or emotional deprivation or who suffer from chronic inflammatory diseases. Such inhibitory influences may be mediated by hypothalamic endorphins, corticotropin-releasing hormone (CRH), or even leptin.

Well-known examples of anovulation or even complete amenorrhea occur in women with **anorexia nervosa,** in ballet dancers, or in marathon runners. The ovarian dysfunction can be so serious that it causes profound estrogen deficiency with consequent **osteoporosis.**

Alterations in the levels of adrenal androgen, cortisol, or thyroid hormone can also inhibit ovulation. Seasonal variation in reproductive activity suggests modulation by melatonin, because human conception rates are lowest in the winter months (when darkness is most prevalent and the secretion of inhibitory melatonin is highest). It has also been observed that women who live close to one another can adopt a common timing of their menstrual cycles, possibly because of chemical signals **(pheromones)** emitted by one individual that affect a nearby individual. In humans, no evidence exists that ovulation is stimulated by sexual behavior. However, female-initiated sexual activity is reportedly increased around the time of ovulation; this increase in libido is possibly caused by increased androgen levels at that time (Fig. 52-19).

■ Gonadal Steroid Effects

Intracellular actions. Estradiol, estrone, other estrogens, and progesterone all enter cells freely and bind to cytoplasmic receptors of the steroid-thyroid superfamily (see Fig. 45-13). The **estrogen receptor (ER)** contains 595 amino acids and is variably phosphorylated. After the hormone binds to the receptor, the resultant cytoplasmic complex is transformed into an active state and translocated into the nucleus. After dimerization, the complex binds more efficiently to estrogen regulatory elements (EREs) on target genes. The structure of the ERE resembles that of the thyroid regulatory element. As a result of the estrogen-ER complex binding to the ERE, gene expression is enhanced or suppressed, and various proteins are increased or decreased in genital and other tissue. The relatively early and rapid target cell responses to estrogen are likely due to protooncogenes, such as c-jun and c-fos, which are activated. These transcription factors may then facilitate later actions of ER via its EREs within more specific target DNA molecules, such as those that regulate synthesis of ovalbumin, ovomucoid, and growth factors. In addition, estradiol can stabilize mRNA levels of certain gene products, such as vitellogenin.

The **progesterone receptor (PR)** contains 934 amino acids. Its interaction with progesterone and progesterone regulatory elements (PREs) on DNA molecules resembles the cortisol format (see Fig. 55-11). Indeed, these interactions overlap in such a manner that a progesterone inhibitor that binds to PR (mifepristone, an abortifacient drug) also inhibits the binding of cortisol to its receptor. Not surprisingly, mifepristone is used to treat endogenous hypercortisolism.

One of estradiol's important actions is to increase the synthesis of ER and PR. In this way, estradiol amplifies its own effects on growth of the follicle and on proliferation of the endometrium. This action also prepares target tissues for subsequent efficient progesterone action. Conversely, progesterone decreases the synthesis of ER. This action accounts for the inhibition by progesterone of further endometrial proliferation during the luteal phase.

Several synthetic compounds have important pharmacologic actions by virtue of their ability, as antagonists or as partial agonists, to bind to ER and PR. **Tamoxifen** binds to ER and suppresses the growth of estrogen-responsive breast cancer tumors. **Clomiphene** binds especially well to hypothalamic ERs, and as already noted it can induce ovulation by negative feedback. **Mifepristone** binds to the PR and blocks its actions. This effect induces early abortion by removing the progesterone support for the conceptus.

The cyclic changes in estradiol and progesterone secretion produce effects on the uterus, fallopian tubes, vagina, and breasts (Fig. 52-24). These effects coordinate precisely with the expectation of conception and the institution of a pregnancy.

Uterus. The function of the uterus is to house and nurture the developing fetus until birth. The uterus is a muscular organ that encloses a cavity lined with stromal cells and a special mucous membrane called the **endometrium.** At the beginning of the follicular phase of each menstrual cycle, the uterus is shedding its lining (menstruation) and is therefore incapable of receiving a conceptus. The endometrium is only 1 to 2 mm thick and its glands are sparse and straight. The lumen of the glands is narrow and the glands themselves exhibit few mitoses (Fig. 52-24). After the menstrual endometrial slough ceases, the increase in estradiol secretion during the follicular phase causes a threefold to fivefold increase in endometrial thickness to a maximum of 8 to 10 mm just before ovulation. Mitoses appear in the glands and stroma, the glands become tortuous, and the spiral arteries that supply the endometrium elongate. This stage is termed the **proliferative phase** of the endometrium. The mucus elaborated by the cervix also changes dramatically during this phase from a scant, thick, viscous material to a copious, more watery, but more elastic substance that can be stretched into a long, fine thread. The mucus also produces a characteristic fernlike pattern when dried on a glass slide. In this estrogen-stimulated condition, the cervical mucus creates a myriad of channels in the opening of the cervix that facilitate the entrance of the sperm and direct their motion forward into the uterine cavity.

Shortly after ovulation, the rise in the plasma progesterone level produces marked alterations (Fig. 52-24) in the endometrium. Its rapid proliferation slows, mitotic activity is reduced, and the endometrial thickness decreases to 5 to 6 mm. The uterine glands become much more tortuous and begin to accumulate glycogen in large vacuoles at the base of each cell. As the luteal phase of the cycle progresses, these vacuoles move toward the lumen of the glands, and the mucus secretion of these glands greatly increases. These secretions contain glycogen, glycoproteins, and glycolipids that sustain and facilitate attachment of a conceptus. The stroma of the endometrium becomes edematous, and the originally straight spiral arteries elongate further and become coiled. These changes constitute the **secretory phase** of the endometrium. During this phase, progesterone decreases the quantity of the cervical mucus and causes it to return to its original thick, nonelastic state; the ferning pattern is not seen.

If pregnancy does not occur and the corpus luteum regresses, lymphocytes and neutrophils appear. The abrupt loss of estradiol and progesterone causes spasmodic contractions of the spiral arteries and uterine muscles. These effects are probably mediated by local production of leukotrienes and prostaglandins. The resultant ischemia produces necrosis, the stroma condenses and degenerates, and the superficial endometrial cells are sloughed along with sludged blood. These changes constitute the **menstrual period.**

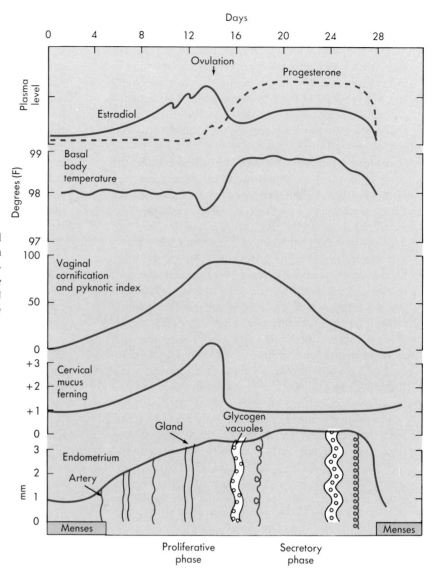

■ **Fig. 52-24** Correlation of biological changes throughout the menstrual cycle with the profiles of plasma estradiol and progesterone levels. (Redrawn from Odell WD: *The reproductive system in women.* In DeGroot LJ et al, editors: *Endocrinology,* vol 3, New York, 1979, Grune & Stratton.)

Fallopian tubes. The fallopian tubes are the normal site of fertilization. These bilateral structures, 10 cm long, emerge from the uterus. Each tube ends in finger-like projections called **fimbriae,** which lie close to the ipsilateral ovary. The fallopian tube consists of a muscular layer surrounding a mucosa lined by an epithelium that contains both ciliated and secretory cells. The cilia beat toward the uterus. During the follicular phase, estradiol increases the number of cilia and their rate of beating, as well as the number of actively secreting epithelial cells. Estradiol also stimulates tubal secretions that provide a mucoid medium in which the sperm may move efficiently upstream against the ciliary beat. In addition, the fimbria become more vascularized.

As ovulation approaches, tubal contractions increase, and the fimbria undulate so as to draw the shed ovum into the tube. During the luteal phase, progesterone probably maximizes the ciliary beat and enhances the movement of any fertilized ovum toward the uterus. Progesterone also increases the secretion of materials nutritious to the

ovum, to any incoming sperm, and to the zygote, should fertilization occur.

Vagina. The vaginal canal is lined with a stratified squamous epithelium that is highly sensitive to estradiol. In the absence of estradiol, only a thin layer of basal and parabasal cells is present. For the first few days of the follicular phase of the menstrual cycle, the vaginal epithelium is thin. Smears taken from the surface show cells, identified by their vesicular nuclei, that arise from the layer beneath the epithelium.

As the cycle progresses to the ovulatory phase, more layers of epithelium are added, and the maturing cells accumulate glycogen. Vaginal smears at this time show many large, eosinophilic-staining, cornified cells with small pyknotic or absent nuclei. The percentage of these cells on a vaginal smear is a sensitive index of estrogenic activity (Fig. 52-24). Progesterone, on the other hand, reduces the percentage of cornified cells. Vaginal secretions are increased by estradiol, and they too form an important element in the events that lead to fertilization.

Breasts. The mammary glands consist of a large series of lobular ducts lined by an epithelium that is capable of secreting milk. These ducts empty into larger milk-conveying ducts that converge at the nipple. These glandular structures are embedded in supporting adipose tissue, and the breasts are separated into lobules by connective tissue.

The development of adult-sized mammary glands depends absolutely on estrogens. Before puberty, the breasts grow only in proportion to the rest of the body. After estrogen secretion increases during puberty, the growth of the lobular ducts accelerates and the area around the nipple (the areola) enlarges. These effects of estrogen on the glandular cells may be mediated by its primary action on adjacent stromal cells.

Estrogens also selectively increase the adipose tissue of the breast and give it its distinctive female shape. The lobular ducts are capable of outpouching to form numerous secretory alveoli. This process is stimulated by progesterone. In various ways, cortisol, growth hormone, prolactin, epidermal growth factor, insulin, IGF-1, and transferrin all contribute to the growth and differentiation of breast tissue. During each menstrual cycle, the lobules further proliferate, mainly in parallel with estradiol levels, but progesterone may also contribute to this process. This proliferation causes swelling of the breasts; however, by the end of the luteal phase, breast size and tenderness diminish.

Effects on other tissues. During puberty, estradiol action is to the female what testosterone action is to the male. Estradiol causes almost all the changes that result in the normal adult female phenotype. In addition to stimulating growth of the internal reproductive organs and breasts, estrogens cause pubertal enlargement of the labia majora and labia minora. Linear growth is accelerated by estradiol. However, because the epiphyseal growth centers are more sensitive to estradiol than to testosterone, they close sooner. For this reason, the average height of women is less than that of men. The hips enlarge and the pelvic inlet widens; these changes facilitate future pregnancy. The specific deposition of fat about the hips is another effect of estradiol. Because in women, estradiol predominates over testosterone, total body adipose mass is twice as large as that of men, whereas their muscle and bone mass is only two thirds that of men.

The skeleton, the kidney, the liver, and the vasculature are also target tissues of estrogens. *Estrogen inhibits bone resorption* directly by its effects on osteoclasts, and indirectly by suppressing resorptive cytokines. Bone formation may be increased by estrogens via induction of focal growth factors. Reabsorption of sodium from the renal tubules is stimulated by estradiol, which may contribute to the cyclic fluid retention noted by some women. The hepatic synthesis of a number of circulating proteins is increased by estrogens; these proteins include thyroxine-binding globulin, cortisol-binding globulin, SSBG, the renin substrate, angiotensinogen, very-low-density lipoproteins (VLDLs), and HDLs. Conversely, LDL levels are decreased by estradiol.

The effects of estrogen on the vasculature are important. In general, estradiol is vasodilatory and antivasoconstrictive. It increases the local release of vasodilators such as nitric oxide, prostaglandin E_2, and prostacyclin, and it decreases production or activity of endothelin-1, a potent local vasoconstrictor. The marked fall in estradiol secretion at the end of the luteal phase alters the endometrial balance from vasodilator to vasoconstrictor and helps initiate the ischemic necrosis of the endometrium.

Only a few systemic actions of progesterone are known. Progesterone accounts for the 0.5° C rise in body temperature that occurs shortly after ovulation (Fig. 52-24). Progesterone also acts on the central nervous system to produce an increase in appetite, a tendency to somnolence, and a heightened sensitivity of the respiratory center to stimulation by carbon dioxide. Because progesterone is an aldosterone antagonist, it can induce natriuresis (see Chapter 51). The negative feedback effect of progesterone on gonadotropin secretion requires the presence of adequate estrogen. This combination of hormonal actions is the basis for oral contraceptives used by women.

■ *Metabolism of Gonadal Steroids*

Estradiol and estrone bind to SSBG, but their affinities are much lower than that of testosterone. Therefore, the estrogens circulate bound loosely to albumin, and their metabolic clearance rates are relatively high (Table 52-3). In menstruating women, most of the circulating estradiol is derived from ovarian secretion; a minor fraction is formed from testosterone in adipose tissue, liver, and other sites. Most of the circulating estrone is derived from estradiol by peripheral 17-hydroxysteroid dehydrogenases. Estrone can also be 16-hydroxylated and then reduced to estriol (Fig. 52-25).

Sulfated and glucuronidated derivatives of all three estrogens are excreted in the urine. Values range from 20 μg during the early follicular phase to 65 μg at the preovulatory peak. An additional pathway of estrogen metabolism involves 2-hydroxylation, and it produces the so-called *catechol estrogens* (Fig. 52-25). These compounds resemble the catecholamine neurotransmitters norepinephrine and dopamine, in their hydroxylated benzene rings. Because 2-hydroxylase activity is present in the hypothalamus, the catechol estrogens generated within the brain may modulate estradiol effects on GnRH release. The catechol estrogens bind to estradiol receptors, but they do not have estradiol actions; in effect, they are natural antiestrogen agents that could increase GnRH by negative feedback.

Progesterone can bind to cortisol-binding globulin, but this binding is largely prevented by the much higher

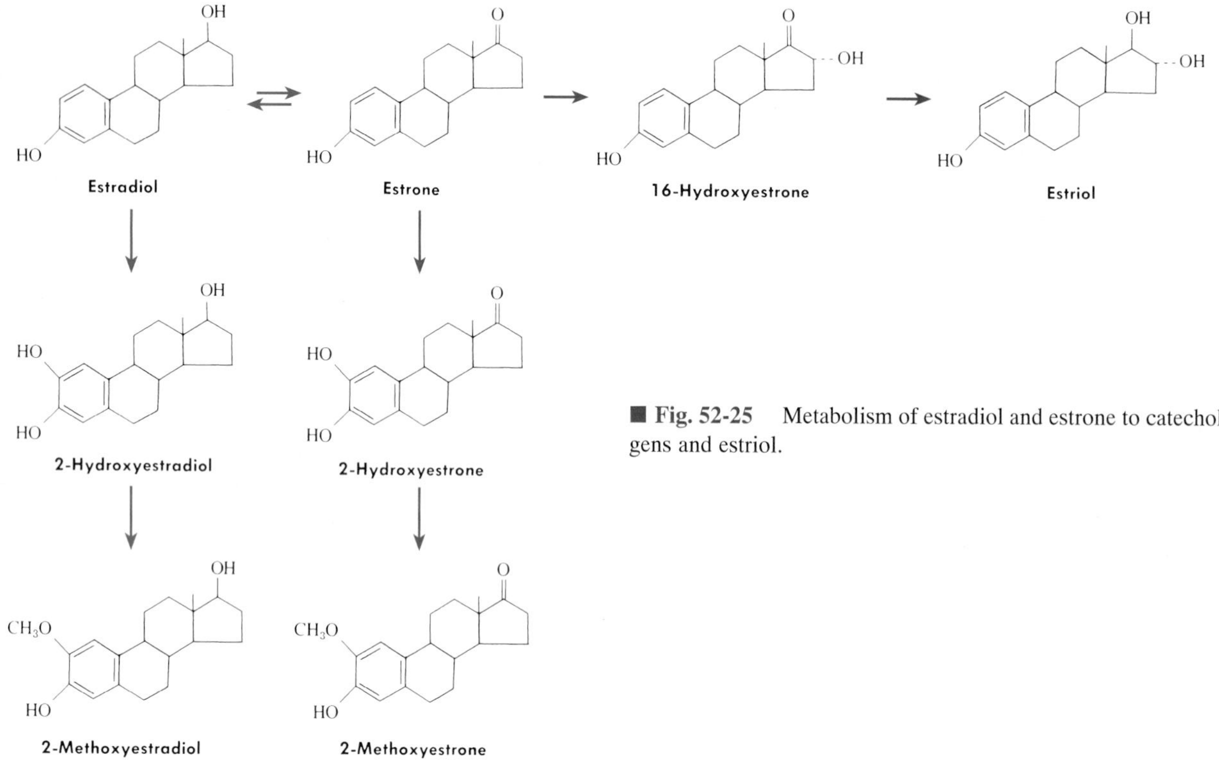

■ **Fig. 52-25** Metabolism of estradiol and estrone to catechol estrogens and estriol.

plasma cortisol concentration. Therefore, progesterone circulates loosely bound to albumin. It is reduced to the urinary metabolite pregnanediol. During the follicular phase of the cycle, about half of the circulating progesterone is secreted by the ovary and about half by the adrenal glands. During the luteal phase, however, by far most progesterone originates in the ovary.

In women, 70% to 80% of circulating testosterone is derived from peripheral conversion of DHEA and androstenedione. About half the daily production of testosterone comes from adrenal precursors and about half from ovarian precursors. In some disorders, ovarian cells can secrete sufficient testosterone to cause virilizing effects.

■ *Female Puberty*

The general process by which puberty is initiated has already been described (Fig. 52-7). Reproductive function begins after an increase in gonadotropin secretion from the low levels of childhood (Fig. 52-26). In females, however, FSH increases before LH more distinctly than in males (compare Figs. 52-17 and 52-26). Budding of the breasts is the first observable physical sign of female puberty, and it coincides with the first detectable increase in plasma estradiol, as ovarian secretion commences. The onset of menses (menarche) occurs approximately 2 years later, after LH levels have risen more sharply. Menarche correlates with both body height and bone maturation. It can be delayed by undernutrition or strenuous exercise, and it occurs later in large sibships. Menarche is accelerated by obesity and blindness.

Development of the positive feedback effect of estradiol necessary to provoke a preovulatory LH burst is the last step in the maturation of the hypothalamic pituitary ovarian unit. Therefore, ovulation usually does not occur in the first few cycles. The initial menstrual cycles are usually irregular, as the menstrual bleeding is induced by withdrawal of estrogen from graafian follicles that are undergoing atresia.

The growth spurt and the peak velocity of growth characteristically occur earlier in girls than in boys. Further increase in height usually ceases 1 to 2 years after the onset of menses. The development of pubic hair precedes menses, and it correlates most closely with rising levels of adrenal androgens, especially dehydroepiandrosterone sulfate (DHEA-S).

■ *Sexual Functioning*

The desire for sexual activity is increased by androgens. During sexual intercourse, vascular erectile tissue beneath the clitoris is activated by parasympathetic impulses. This causes the opening to the vagina to be tightened around the penis. Simultaneously, these impulses stimulate copious secretion of mucus by glands located beneath the labia minora and in the vagina. The secretions lubricate the vagina and help it produce a massaging effect on the penis. Estrogen actions maintain these glands and their secretions.

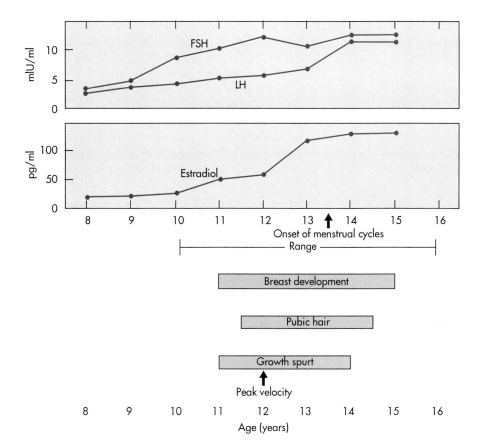

■ **Fig. 52-26** Average chronologic sequence of hormonal and biological events in normal female puberty. Note that the peak velocity of growth precedes the onset of menses, and the growth spurt ends shortly after menarche. (Redrawn from Lee PA et al: Puberty in girls, *J Clin Endocrinol Metab* 43:775, 1976; and Marshall WA, Tanner JM: *Arch Dis Child* 45:13, 1970.)

Female orgasm results from spinal cord reflexes similar to those involved in male ejaculation. Involuntary contractions of the skeletal muscle of the perineum; of the musculature of the vagina, uterus, and fallopian tubes; and of the rectal sphincter occur. The clitoris retracts against the symphysis pubis. After orgasm, the cervix remains widely patent for 20 to 30 minutes, and thereby permits sperm to enter the uterus. The first wave of sperm may reach an ovum in the fallopian tube within 10 minutes. However, these sperm, lacking capacitation, are unlikely to fertilize an ovum.

Many spermatozoa are trapped and eventually destroyed in the vagina within a few hours. The remainder reach the cervix, where they dwell in storage sites formed by the convoluted mucosa (cervical crypts) and its mucus. Here, they undergo capacitation. From this reservoir, spermatozoa migrate into the uterine cavity and fallopian tubes over 24 to 48 hours. A tremendous number of sperm are lost along the way; fewer than one in every 100,000 eventually reaches an ovum.

■ *Menopause*

The reproductive capacity of women begins to wane in the fifth decade of life, and menses completely terminate at an average age of 50. For several years before menopause, the frequency of ovulation decreases. The menses occur at variable intervals and with decreased

flow, caused by irregular peaks of estradiol secretion without adequate secretion of progesterone during the luteal phase. With the disappearance of virtually all the follicles, ovarian secretion of estrogens—and inhibins—essentially ceases. From then on, a low plasma estradiol concentration (characteristic of menopause) is maintained. Most of this estradiol comes from peripheral conversion of androgen precursors that are secreted predominantly by the adrenal glands, but some precursors come from ovarian stromal cells that remain responsive to high levels of LH. The dominant estrogen in plasma becomes estrone rather than estradiol, maintained at a 3:1 ratio.

During the last few years of reproductive life, follicular sensitivity to gonadotropin stimulation diminishes, and plasma FSH and LH levels gradually increase in compensation. Once menopause occurs, the loss of negative feedback from ovarian estradiol and inhibin causes gonadotropin levels to average four to ten times those of the normal follicular phase. The LH/FSH ratio falls to less than 1. Although the monthly cyclicity of gonadotropin secretion is lost, pulsatile secretion persists.

The programmed decline in available estrogenic biological activity causes thinning of the vaginal epithelium and loss of its secretions. Breast mass decreases also. Phenomena such as vascular flushing, which is entrained with LH pulses, and emotional lability are also related to estrogen deficiency. Because adipose tissue contains aromatase activity, this tissue is an important site of production of estrogen from adrenal and ovarian stromal androgens. Obese women may therefore have fewer symptoms of estrogen deprivation. Ovarian secretion of androgens may mildly stimulate hair growth in a male pattern.

The hormonal characteristics of the postmenopausal period are of major health importance. Loss of estrogens produces a period of increased bone resorption with accelerated bone loss for approximately 5 years **(postmenopausal osteoporosis).** Fractures of the wrist and vertebrae increase in frequency. Postmenopausal osteoporosis also sets the stage for the later but slower senescent phase of bone loss. During this phase, women are at a greater risk of hip and vertebral fractures than are men, until age 80.

The loss of estrogens after the menopause increases the risk of coronary artery disease. By age 60, death from **coronary heart disease** becomes increasingly prevalent in women. This change is partly explained by loss of the beneficial effect of estrogen on the serum lipid pattern. In addition, loss of estrogen's vasodilator effect on the endothelium of the coronary circulation may add to the increasing risk of coronary events.

For the above reasons, estrogen replacement therapy after the menopause is now frequently recommended. Estrogen replacement is especially recommended for women who have other risk factors (e.g., a sedentary life style) for osteoporosis and coronary artery disease, but who do not have a contraindication to estrogen (e.g., estrogen-sensitive breast cancer). Progesterone is usually added to protect women from estrogen-induced endometrial hyperplasia and cancer.

■ *Pregnancy*

■ *Fertilization*

After ovulation, the ovum is captured by the widened proximal portion of the fallopian tube (ampulla). Retention of the ovum within the fallopian tube is aided by adherence of the "sticky" cumulus oophorus to the cilia in the fimbria. Muscle contractions produce a to-and-fro motion, which mixes the contents of the fallopian tube and increases the chance of a random encounter between the ovum and sperm, thereby facilitating fertilization. The ovum is viable only for 12 to 24 hours. The sperm must reach the ovum within about 48 hours of ejaculation.

Once sperm are very close to the ovum, they undergo the acrosomal reaction described previously. As a result of Ca^{++} stimulation, the acrosomal cap releases a corona-dispersing enzyme, a trypsin-like enzyme (known as **acrosin**), a neuraminidase, and hyaluronidases. Together, these enzymes disperse and digest the granulosa cells of the cumulus oophorus and the corona radiata and permit attachment of sperm to the zona pellucida. Penetration of the zona is facilitated by species-specific zona receptors for sperm membrane proteins, in particular one termed

ZP_3. Many sperm bind to the zona, first reversibly and then tightly. The single successful sperm penetrates this barrier by release of the proteolytic enzyme acrosin. *Penetration of the zona pellucida by the first sperm creates a block to the entry of the other sperm.* This barrier is generated by uptake of Ca^{++} into the ovum, depolarization of its plasma membrane, and release of proteases and glycosidases that are contained in granules within the ovum. This process alters zona surface glycoproteins, such as ZP_3, so that they reject instead of attract additional sperm and prevent complete entrance of those that had partially penetrated. This important step prevents **polyploidy,** the production of an organism with more than two sets of homologous chromosomes. The polar body that results from the second reduction-division of meiosis is then released, leaving the ovum in a haploid state, that is, with 23 chromosomes. After fusion of their respective membranes, the chromatin material of the sperm head is engulfed by the ovum and forms the haploid male pronucleus. The two pronuclei generate a spindle on which the chromosomes are arranged, and a new diploid individual with 46 chromosomes is created.

The zygote, now in the blastocyst stage, traverses the fallopian tube in about 3 days. Most of this time is spent in the ampulla of the tube, where a delay at the junction with the isthmus may allow time for the endometrium to become better prepared to accept the zygote. With the early rise in luteal phase progesterone, transit time through the tube rapidly increases. *After another 2 to 3 days in the uterus, the zygote initiates implantation, which consists of three successive processes: adhesion, penetration, and invasion.* The initial requisite dissolution of the zona pellucida is brought about by alternate contraction and expansion of the blastocyst, as well as by lytic factors in the uterine secretions. These and other substances (e.g., epidermal growth factor) that facilitate implantation depend on adequate maternal progesterone levels during the luteal phase and on early paracrine signals from the zygote; such signals induce receptive endometrial responses at the site.

From the initial solid mass of blastocyst cells, a layer of trophoblasts separates. Microvilli of these cells interdigitate with those of endometrial cells, and junctional complexes form between the respective cell membranes. Endometrial molecules such as **laminin** and **fibronectin** facilitate adhesion. Once firmly attached, trophoblast cells intrude between and burrow beneath endometrial cells, lysing the intercellular matrix with a variety of enzymes. Also, the trophoblasts phagocytize and digest dead endometrial cells. Prostaglandins, probably of endometrial cell origin, and histamine may also participate in the implantation process.

Penetration by the trophoblasts is limited by concurrent changes in the stroma of the uterus. Late in the normal luteal phase, fibroblast-type stromal cells near uterine blood vessels enlarge and accumulate glycogen and lipid. These **decidual cells** disappear unless pregnancy does occurs, and the corpus luteum is maintained. If pregnancy occurs, however, continuing estrogen and especially progesterone stimulation causes widespread decidualization, which rapidly changes the entire stroma into a sheet of compact decidual cells. At the same time, the endometrial glands progressively atrophy. The decidua functions initially as a source of essential nutrients for the embryo until implantation of the embryo produces vascular connections between the mother and the embryo and a single central circulation is established. Thereafter, the decidua provides a mechanical and an immunologic barrier to further invasion of the uterine wall by the embryo. The decidua also functions as an endocrine organ; it produces prolactin, relaxin, prostaglandins, and other molecules that have paracrine actions on the muscles of the uterus and on the two fetal membranes: **chorion** and **amnion.**

Numerous locally produced factors such as IGFs, transforming growth factors, epidermal growth factor, and cytokines contribute to implantation, the growth and differentiation of trophoblast cells, the growth and development of the embryo and fetus, and the process of decidua formation. The relative importance of these factors at various times remains to be determined and integrated into a single coherent schema.

Implantation is more susceptible to mishap than is conception. Approximately 70% of all conceptions result in miscarriage. Most occur within 14 days of conception and are unrecognized by the woman, who may have only a slightly delayed menstrual period. Miscarriages later in the first trimester may still reflect suboptimal maternal-fetal attachment but are also caused by fetal anomalies

■ *Functions of the Placenta*

Pregnancy is marked by the development of a unique organ, the placenta, which has a limited lifespan. This organ has diverse functions. It serves (1) as the fetal gut in supplying nutrients, (2) as the fetal lung in exchanging oxygen and carbon dioxide, (3) as the fetal kidney in regulating fluid volumes and disposing of waste metabolites, and (4) as a versatile endocrine gland that synthesizes many steroid and protein hormones that affect both maternal and fetal metabolism. Some of these hormones can be found in maternal plasma, where they exhibit typical temporal profiles during pregnancy (Fig. 52-27), and some can also be found in fetal plasma and amniotic fluid.

Fetal trophoblasts differentiate very early into two cell types: an inner layer of **cytotrophoblasts** and, under the influence of epidermal growth factor and other stimuli, an outer layer of fused **syncytiocytotrophoblasts.** Both cell types synthesize peptide and protein hormones, many of which are identical or very similar to hypothal-

amic, pituitary, and gonadal products. The syncytiocytotrophoblasts also synthesize increasingly large amounts of steroid hormones from precursors of varied sources as pregnancy proceeds (Fig. 52-28). The adjacent arrangement of cytotrophoblast and syncytiocytotrophoblast layers forms a placental hypothalamus-pituitary–like unit. The cytotrophoblasts secrete mainly stimulatory (e.g., CRH and thyrotropin-releasing hormone [TRH]) and inhibitory hypothalamic-like peptides and gonadal growth factors, which regulate in a paracrine manner the output of pituitary-like hormones (e.g., adrenocorticotropic hormone [ACTH] and thyroid-stimulating hormone [TSH]) from the syncytiocytotrophoblast layer. However, overlap exists between the products of the two trophoblast layers.

■ *Hormones of Pregnancy*

Human chorionic gonadotropin. *Human chorionic gonadotropin (HCG) is the first key hormone of pregnancy. Secreted by the syncytiocytotrophoblast cells, it can be detected in maternal plasma and urine within 9 days of conception.* The secretion of HCG is stimulated by GnRH produced in adjacent cytotrophoblasts. HCG is a glycoprotein with a molecular weight of 39,000 and it is composed of two subunits, an α subunit and a β subunit. The α subunit is identical to that of TSH, LH, and FSH, whereas the β subunit has 80% homology with the β subunit of LH. Detection of HCG is the most commonly used and most specific test for pregnancy. The urine may be tested at home. Maternal plasma levels of HCG increase at an exponential rate, reach a peak at 9 to 12 weeks, and then decline to a stable plateau for the remainder of pregnancy (Fig. 52-27). After the fetus is delivered, HCG disappears from maternal plasma with a half-life of 12 to 24 hours.

HCG maintains the function of the corpus luteum beyond its usual lifespan of 14 days (when conception does not occur). The placental gonadotropin stimulates ovarian secretion of progesterone and estrogens by mechanisms that are essentially identical to those previously described for LH; cAMP is the second messenger. When the placenta takes over the synthesis of these steroids, thereby relieving the fetus of its dependence on the corpus luteum, HCG secretion declines. HCG that reaches the fetus stimulates essential DHEA-S production by the fetal zone of the adrenal gland and testosterone production by the Leydig cells of the testis. HCG may also stimulate the production of **relaxin** (see later discussion). In addition, HCG inhibits the maternal secretion of LH by the pituitary. Because of the structural overlap of HCG with TSH, the very high plasma concentrations of HCG that are maintained in early pregnancy can increase the maternal thyroid gland activity. In some women, this effect of HCG can even induce hyperthyroidism. HCG receptors are found in the endometrium

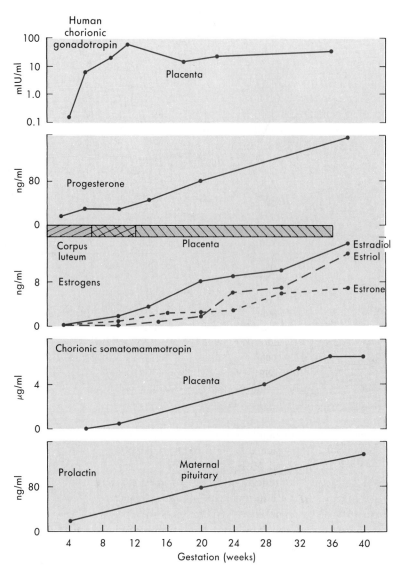

■ **Fig. 52-27** Profile of plasma hormone changes during normal human pregnancy. Note the logarithmic scale for human chorionic gonadotropin. Also note the shift from corpus luteum to placenta as the source of estrogens and progesterone between 6 and 12 weeks of gestation. (Redrawn from Goldstein DP et al: *Am J Obstet Gynecol* 102:110, 1968; Rigg LA et al: *Am J Obstet Gynecol* 129:454, 1977; Selenkow HA et al: *Measurement and pathophysiologic significance of human placental lactogen.* In Pecile A, Finzi C, editors: *The foetoplacental unit,* Amsterdam, 1969, Excerpta Medica; and Tulchinsky D et al: *Am J Obstet Gynecol* 112:1095, 1972.)

and myometrium, and the gonadotropin can inhibit the contractions produced by oxytocin. Thus, HCG may also contribute to uterine quiescence, especially in the early phase of pregnancy.

Progesterone. *Progesterone is the hormone most directly responsible for the establishment and sustenance of the fetus in the uterine cavity.* During the first 2 weeks of pregnancy, progesterone stimulates the fallopian tubal and endometrial glands to secrete the nutrients on which the zygote depends. Thereafter, it maintains the decidual lining of the uterus. Progesterone produced by the placenta is the principal substrate for synthesis of cortisol and aldosterone by the fetal adrenal gland (Fig. 52-28), which lacks the 3β-OL-dehydrogenase-$^{\Delta-4,5}$ isomerase enzyme complex necessary for progesterone synthesis. Progesterone may also modulate the secretion of HCG and human chorionic somatomammotropin (HCS) (see below).

Other actions of progesterone are important during pregnancy. *Progesterone inhibits uterine contractions, in part by inhibiting production of prostaglandins and in part by decreasing sensitivity to oxytocin.* Progesterone thus prevents premature expulsion of the fetus. It also stimulates the development of the alveolar pouches of the mammary glands and greatly increases their eventual capacity to secrete milk. Progesterone may participate in the inhibition of maternal immune responses to antigens from the fetus and thereby help prevent its rejection. Finally, progesterone stimulates the maternal respiratory center to increase ventilation, which helps to dispose of the increased carbon dioxide produced by the pregnant woman and her fetus.

The placenta begins to synthesize progesterone at about 6 weeks of gestation, and by 12 weeks it produces enough of this hormone to replace the corpus luteum for this purpose. During this transition period, the plasma progesterone level reaches a temporary plateau (Fig. 52-27). Cholesterol is extracted from maternal plasma and serves as the major precursor for placental progesterone. The synthetic pathway resembles that of the adrenal gland and the ovary. By term, progesterone production reaches a level of 250 mg/day, which is ten times greater

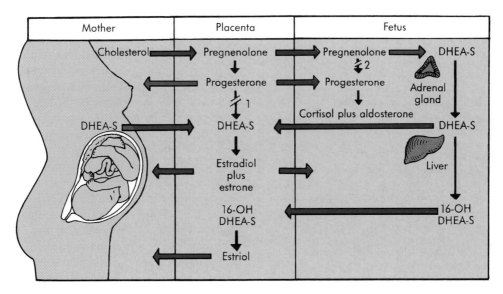

■ **Fig. 52-28**　Maternal-fetal-placental unit in steroid hormone synthesis. Progesterone is synthesized in the placenta from maternal cholesterol. In turn, this progesterone acts on the mother. Placental progesterone is transferred to the fetus, where it serves as the precursor to cortisol and aldosterone synthesis by the fetal adrenal glands. Estradiol and estrone are synthesized in the placenta from maternal and fetal dehydroepiandrosterone sulfate *(DHEA-S),* and estriol is synthesized from fetal 16α-hydroxydehydroepiandrosterone sulfate *(16-OH-DHEA-S). 1,* 17-hydroxylase/17,20-desmolase; *2,* 3β-OL-dehydrogenase-$\Delta^{4,5}$-isomerase.

than the peak rates that prevail during the luteal phase of the menstrual cycle. About 90% of the progesterone goes to the mother and 10% to the fetus. Maternal urinary pregnanediol excretion also rises markedly, reflecting the enormous increase in production of progesterone.

Estrogens. The augmented production of estrogens (estradiol, estrone, and estriol) that occurs throughout pregnancy (Fig. 52-27), results in several important actions. *Estrogens stimulate the continuous growth of the uterine myometrium, and thereby prepares it for its role in labor. Estrogens stimulate the further growth of the ductal system of the breast, from which the alveoli will develop.* In addition, estrogen, along with relaxin, causes relaxation and softening of the mother's pelvic ligaments and the symphysis pubis of her pelvic bones, allowing better accommodation of the expanding uterus.

Estrogens also play a paracrine role in placental function. They augment progesterone synthesis by increasing LDL cholesterol uptake and the activity of the P-450 enzyme. They also enhance placental conversion of cortisol to inactive cortisone (see Fig. 51-10). This inactivation may relieve inhibition of fetal pituitary corticotropin by maternal cortisol that would otherwise cross the placenta; fetal ACTH can then stimulate production of essential adrenal androgen, and later of cortisol, by the fetus.

Like progesterone, estrogens are initially produced by the corpus luteum under stimulation by HCG. The placenta then assumes this role, but it requires steroid hormone precursors from both the mother and fetus to complete the synthesis of estrogens. This unique example of coordinated maternal-placental-fetal function is depicted in Fig. 52-28. The placenta lacks significant 17-hydroxylase and 17,20-desmolase activity, and therefore it cannot generate the androgens that serve as substrates for aromatization (Fig. 52-4). Instead, the placenta extracts DHEA-S produced by the maternal and fetal adrenal glands, removes the sulfate, and synthesizes estradiol and estrone. The fetus becomes the main source of DHEA-S as pregnancy progresses. Placental synthesis of estriol, a 16-hydroxylated estrogen (Fig. 52-25), almost entirely depends on precursors from the fetus. In this process, the fetal adrenal gland synthesizes DHEA-S from placental pregnenolone, the fetal liver hydroxylates it in the 16 position, and the placenta then desulfates it and aromatizes it to estriol.

One third of the unconjugated estrogens that circulate in maternal plasma at term are accounted for by estriol. Estriol, in the form of sulfate and glucuronic acid conjugates, represents 90% of the total estrogen excreted in maternal urine. Because estriol is derived almost entirely from the fetal placental unit, maternal plasma or urine estriol levels provide one index of the well-being of the fetus.

Human chorionic somatomammotropin. Another protein hormone unique to pregnancy is **human chorionic somatomammotropin (HCS),** also called **human placental lactogen (HPL).** The synthesis of HCS by the syncytiocytotrophoblasts can be detected at about 4 weeks of gestation. The maternal plasma concentration of HCG rises steadily to a peak of 6 μg/ml at term (Fig. 52-27). The HCS production rate of 1 to 2 g/day far exceeds that of any other human protein hormone. Maternal plasma HCS levels provide another indicator of placental function. After delivery of the fetus, the hormone rapidly disappears from maternal plasma; the half-life is 20 minutes.

HCS synthesis is directed by a gene in the growth hormone family. GnRH and somatostatin produced in neighboring cytotrophoblasts probably stimulate and inhibit, respectively, HCS synthesis by syncytiocytotrophoblasts. Although HCS has 96% structural homology with growth hormone, it has only 3% of the latter's growth-promoting activity. Nonetheless, its very high plasma concentrations contribute to anabolism in the pregnant woman. HCS also has lactogenic activity, but this action may not be needed because of the high concentration of prolactin itself during pregnancy.

HCS stimulates maternal lipolysis and, like growth hormone, antagonizes insulin actions on carbohydrate metabolism. These actions tend to raise the maternal plasma glucose concentration. Maternal fasting and hypoglycemia raise plasma HCS levels. As detailed later, HCS may direct maternal metabolism to maintain a continuous flow of substrates, especially glucose, to the fetus. HCS levels in fetal plasma are far below those in maternal plasma; however, somatomedins (IGF-2), produced in the placenta as the result of HCS action, may help to stimulate fetal growth.

A **placental human growth hormone variant,** closely related to but distinct from both growth hormone and HCS, has been characterized. This variant represents the major form of growth hormone in maternal plasma, and it reaches elevated levels of 15 ng/ml by term. It is probably regulated by placental GnRH and somatostatin and, because of its high concentrations, may be as important to maternal metabolism as is HCS.

Prolactin. Another hormone secreted in excess during normal pregnancy is maternal pituitary prolactin. Plasma levels of prolactin rise linearly throughout pregnancy, and by term they reach values eight to ten times higher than those of nonpregnant women (Fig. 52-27). The prolactin synthesized during pregnancy is largely in the more bioactive nonglycosylated form (see Chapter 49). Prolactin is essential for expression of the mammotropic effects of estrogen and progesterone, and it stimulates the lactogenic apparatus (see Chapter 49, Fig. 49-28). A small amount of milk begins to be produced at about 5 months of gestation, but progressive increase in lactation is inhibited by the high levels of estrogen and progesterone.

Prolactin is also synthesized by the decidual cells of the uterus, where it helps to depress immune responses to the fetus. The decidua is the source of amniotic fluid prolactin, which may help to regulate osmolarity in fetal fluids.

Relaxin. In addition to gonadal steroids, the corpus luteum of pregnancy secretes a polypeptide hormone called **relaxin.** Its structure resembles proinsulin (see Fig. 47-3). Plasma levels of relaxin rise early in pregnancy, peak in the first trimester, and then decline somewhat. The production of relaxin by the corpus luteum is stimulated by HCG. Relaxin is also produced by decidual cells. This hormone suppresses myometrial contractions by inhibiting myosin light-chain phosphorylation. It also relaxes pelvic ligaments and increases softening, effacement, and dilation of the cervix. Thus, it may function early to ensure uterine quiescence and prevent spontaneous abortion, but later it may facilitate passage of the fetus out of the uterus.

Inhibins and related hormones. Maternal plasma inhibin levels exhibit a biphasic rise during pregnancy. Inhibin A reaches an early peak within 7 days of conception. The source of inhibin A at this point is mostly fetal trophoblasts, with some contribution from the corpus luteum in response to stimulation by HCG. A later steady rise in the inhibin A level to a peak at term represents placental production. The inhibin A level falls rapidly after delivery. In contrast, inhibin B levels remain low throughout pregnancy. One maternal role for the increased inhibin A level may be to suppress the mother's FSH secretion and unneeded ovarian follicle formation.

Both activin A and follistatin levels also increase steadily in maternal plasma. These hormones are derived from placental, decidual, and fetal membrane sources. Activin stimulates HCG and progesterone synthesis by the placenta, while follistatin interferes with this effect. The outcome of these interactions may depend on the time at which they occur and on countervailing influences from both mother and fetus.

Other maternal hormonal changes. Pregnancy induces a characteristic series of changes in a number of other endocrine functions. One of the most significant alterations occurs in pancreatic islet β-cell function. Insulin secretion, in response to glucose challenge or to meals, increases after the third month of pregnancy. This hypersecretion of insulin reaches its peak during the last trimester; the peak coincides with the peak of the plasma HCS level. Because maternal sensitivity to insulin is greatly diminished during this same period, insulin hypersecretion may be considered largely compensatory. In contrast, basal glucagon levels and responses to stimulation do not change significantly.

Aldosterone secretion increases significantly throughout pregnancy and reaches a sixfold to eightfold elevation by term. The elevation of aldosterone occurs because both the plasma renin and the renin substrate (angiotensinogen) levels are augmented by the high estrogen levels of pregnancy. Aldosterone hypersecretion may also be stimulated by a reduction in the *effective* circulating blood volume that results from the large placental blood pool. Hyperaldosteronism contributes to the positive sodium balance necessary to maintain a high total maternal plasma volume and to build the extracellular fluid of the fetus. Another mineralocorticoid, desoxycorticosterone (see Chapter 51), is also present in excess in the maternal plasma. It is synthesized in the mother's kidneys exclusively during pregnancy by 21-hydroxylation of progesterone that originates from the placenta.

The plasma total cortisol level is elevated because of the estrogen-induced increase in cortisol-binding globulin. However, plasma and urinary free cortisol also rise modestly, as do plasma levels of ACTH. The enhanced glucocorticoid activity may contribute to maternal adipose tissue gain and to mammary gland development. This enhanced activity is also probably responsible for the plethoric face, thin skin, and susceptibility to bruising of pregnant women. The ultimate cause of maternal hypercortisolism is a large increase in circulating CRH of placental origin. Although the CRH is largely protein bound and nonpulsatile, it stimulates maternal pituitary ACTH secretion and consequent cortisol secretion.

The concentration of total plasma thyroid hormones, thyroxine (T_4) and triiodothyronine (T_3), is elevated because of estrogen-induced increases in thyroid-binding globulin. Early in pregnancy, plasma free T_4 and free T_3 concentrations transiently increase above nonpregnancy levels, and they may contribute to the early phase of fetal development. The free T_4 and T_3 levels return toward baseline as pregnancy progresses. Nonetheless, the size of the maternal thyroid gland and its iodine uptake increase throughout pregnancy, as does the basal metabolic rate and resting pulse rate. These increases may all be caused by the thyrotropic activity of HCG (see above) or by secretion of a placental thyrotropin.

Maternal pituitary growth hormone secretion in response to various stimuli decreases during pregnancy, probably because its anabolic functions are carried out by HCS or by a placental growth hormone variant. Maternal LH and FSH secretion is also suppressed by the high levels of estrogen, progesterone, and inhibin from the corpus luteum initially and later from the placenta. In general, the usual circadian rhythms in maternal plasma hormone levels persist. Their transmission to the fetus may help prepare it for extrauterine life.

Calcium absorption from the diet increases during pregnancy and offsets the continuing maternal calcium drain created by the growing fetal skeleton. This increase in calcium absorption is mediated by increased maternal levels of 25-OH-vitamin D and 1,25-(OH$_2$)-vitamin D. The latter active metabolite originates in part from decidual and placental production. As a result, ionized calcium levels are maintained at normal levels, and maternal parathyroid hormone (PTH) secretion is partially suppressed, as manifested by a 50% reduction in maternal PTH levels in the plasma.

■ *Maternal-Fetal Metabolism*

During normal pregnancy, the average gain in maternal weight is 11 kg. About half of this weight gain is attributable to changes in maternal tissues, and half to the conceptus. The typical distribution of the excess weight is shown in Fig. 52-29. Approximately 250 to 300 extra kcal/day must be ingested to support this weight gain; 85% ultimately supports fetal metabolism and growth, and 15% is stored in maternal fat. An extra protein intake of 30 g/day ensures adequate supplies for maternal needs and for the accumulation of fetal protoplasm. At birth, the protein content of the fetus has reached 400 to 500 g.

From a metabolic standpoint, pregnancy can be divided into two phases. *During the first half of pregnancy, the mother herself is in an anabolic phase, and the conceptus represents an insignificant nutritional drain. During the second half of pregnancy, and especially the final third, fetal and placental weight increase at an accelerated rate. These demands cause the mother to shift into a metabolic state aptly described as "accelerated starvation."*

The initial anabolic phase is characterized by normal or even increased sensitivity to insulin. Maternal plasma levels of glucose, amino acids, free fatty acids, and glycerol are normal or slightly reduced. Carbohydrate and amino acid loads are readily assimilated. Lipogenesis is increased, and lipolysis is reduced in maternal adipose tissue. Glycogen stores are increased in the liver and

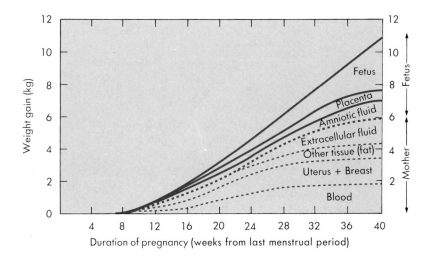

■ **Fig. 52-29** Pattern and components of maternal weight gain during normal pregnancy. (Redrawn from Pitkin RM: *Obstetrics and gynecology.* In Schneider HA, Anderson CE, Coursin DB, editors: *Nutritional support of medical practice,* New York, 1977, Harper & Row.)

muscle, and overall protein synthesis is enhanced. The net effect of these changes is to stimulate growth of the breasts, uterus, and essential musculature in the mother, while preparing her to withstand the metabolic demands of later fetal growth.

During the later catabolic phase of pregnancy, the metabolism of the mother shifts into a mode that effectively accommodates the accelerating needs of the fetus. Insulin sensitivity is replaced by maternal insulin resistance. The assimilation of dietary carbohydrate, protein, and fat by maternal tissues is slowed, resulting in elevated postprandial plasma levels of glucose and amino acids. These increases in glucose and amino acids in turn increase the rates of glucose diffusion and of facilitated amino acid transport across the placenta into the fetus. Glucose is the major fuel used by the fetus, and the amino acids are required for fetal protein synthesis. By term, the fetus, who is using glucose at a rate of 5 mg/kg/min compared with the maternal rate of 2.5 mg/kg/min, must be supplied with up to 25 g/day of glucose. During fasting intervals, maternal plasma glucose falls more rapidly than in nonpregnant women (see Fig. 46-11), as the fetus continues to siphon this vital energy substrate. Moreover, lipolysis is accelerated in the second half of pregnancy, and maternal plasma free fatty acid, glycerol, and ketoacid levels rise more rapidly than in fasting nonpregnant women (see Fig. 46-11). These changes ensure alternative oxidative fuels for the mother. In addition, ketoacids and, to a lesser extent, free fatty acids cross to the fetus, where they may be used instead of some glucose as fuel.

Placental HCS and growth hormone variant are probably the key hormones responsible for insulin resistance and for facilitating lipid mobilization during fasting in the later stage of pregnancy. The rise in the plasma free cortisol level and large increases in plasma estrogen and progesterone levels may also contribute to these actions.

Along with the other changes in maternal metabolism, plasma cholesterol and triglyceride levels rise throughout pregnancy. The cholesterol is partly used for estrogen and progesterone synthesis. The increased circulating triglycerides are largely the result of an increased hepatic synthesis of VLDL; this synthesis is stimulated by estrogens. Some of the triglycerides are stored in the breasts in preparation for milk production. The triglycerides are shifted away from less specific storage elsewhere by a marked reduction in adipose tissue lipoprotein lipase levels.

■ *Parturition*

Just as the maintenance of the pregnant state depends on a unique hormonal milieu, its termination probably also depends on specific hormonal changes. However, the exact mechanism by which parturition, or the process of giving birth, is initiated remains unclear. Cortisol, estrogen, progesterone, relaxin, oxytocin, CRH, prostaglandins, and catecholamines may all participate in the initiation and maintenance of labor and in the final uterine evacuation. Because much species variation exists, it is difficult to extrapolate directly to humans the results of studies in subhuman primates. Fig. 52-30 illustrates some current notions about the endocrine regulation of parturition.

Once the conceptus has reached a critical size, distention of the uterus itself and stretching of the muscle fibers increase their contractility. In humans, uncoordi-

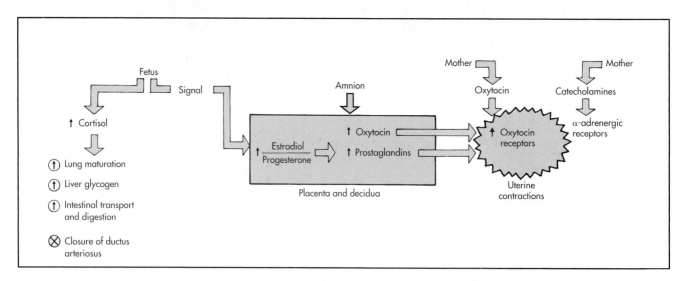

■ **Fig. 52-30** Endocrine regulation of parturition. The fetus initiates signals that decrease the ratio of effective progesterone to estrogen in the myometrium. This leads to uterine contractions, which are mainly mediated by prostaglandins. Oxytocin produced in the decidua and placenta and a small maternal contribution—combined with increased oxytocin receptors—may contribute to labor but are not essential. However, oxytocin sustains uterine contractions after expulsion of the fetus in order to minimize maternal loss of blood. Cortisol prepares the fetus to adapt to extrauterine life successfully.

nated uterine contractions, called *Braxton Hicks contractions,* begin at least 1 month before the end of gestation. Thus, the inherent contractility of the uterus in itself would probably cause eventual evacuation of the conceptus. The onset of true labor has a circadian rhythm, with a peak between 12 midnight and 5 AM. Some signal from the fetus probably initiates labor contractions. In sheep, fetal cortisol has been strongly implicated as the signal. Although gestation is prolonged in women when the fetus lacks an intact hypothalamic pituitary adrenal unit, the evidence for a *surge* of fetal cortisol secretion immediately preceding human parturition is weak at best. However, a late gestational increase in fetal cortisol secretion is important in preparing the fetus for the abrupt transition to extrauterine life (Fig. 52-30). Cortisol stimulates lung maturation, increases stores of liver glycogen, induces intestinal transport systems and digestive enzymes, and promotes closure of the ductus arteriosus.

Another recent suggestion is that the placenta acts as a clock with an alarm that is set early in gestation. The level of maternal plasma CRH, which comes from the placenta, begins to rise exponentially early in the second trimester and reaches a peak during labor. Furthermore, the high maternal levels of a CRH-binding protein fall sharply in the last month of gestation; thus, free CRH levels are very high at the end of gestation. CRH receptors are present in the uterine muscle, and CRH both potentiates the contractile response to prostaglandins and oxytocin and stimulates prostaglandin production by the decidua and amnion. In addition, an inverse correlation exists between maternal plasma CRH levels early in gestation and the absolute length of the gestational period. These observations suggest that the amount of placental CRH production early in pregnancy is at least an indicator of when parturition might begin. Conceivably, CRH may be a determinant of the time of onset of labor and may also play an active role in the process.

Even if the precise initiating signal in human parturition is unidentified, current concepts favor a multicomponent process that involves paracrine and endocrine mechanisms. *A large increase in the local concentration of prostaglandins increases myometrial cell Ca^{++} levels and triggers uterine contractions. A drop in the ratio of intrauterine progesterone to estrogen levels appears to be largely responsible for augmenting local prostaglandin levels and thereby abolishing uterine quiescence.* At term, the increased activity of the enzyme 17β,20α-hydroxysteroid dehydrogenase in the uterine tissue lowers the progesterone/estrogen ratio. This single enzyme inactivates progesterone by reducing its ketone group at position 20 of the steroid nucleus, and augments the estrogen effect by generating estradiol from estrone, by reducing the ketone at position 17. The fetal amnion and chorion may also contribute prostaglandins.

Another major stimulator of myometrial contractions is **oxytocin.** Although the concentration of oxytocin in maternal plasma does not increase consistently just before labor, the frequency of oxytocin pulses does increase. Furthermore, myometrial oxytocin receptor content rises dramatically at term, as does the local synthesis of oxytocin by the decidua and the fetal membranes. Oxytocin may therefore reinforce labor contractions, and it probably maximizes the contractions immediately after delivery, thereby minimizing maternal blood loss.

Uterine contractions may also be modulated by catecholamines; α-adrenergy is stimulatory and β-adrenergy is inhibitory. Maternal stress may release circulating catecholamines that participate in the final hormonal cascade of parturition.

In addition to uterine contractions, the rapid changes that occur in placental and cervical tissue are also important components of labor. At term, the concentration of inflammatory cytokines, such as interleukin-8, rises sharply in amniotic fluid. These cytokines are produced by maternal decidua and fetal membranes, probably under hormonal paracrine stimulation. They attract neutrophils, which then release collagenase that loosens the attachments between the maternal and fetal tissue planes and decreases the cervical resistance to pressure from the fetal head.

Once labor has begun, it proceeds in three clinically recognized stages. In the first stage, which lasts several hours, the uterine contractions, which originate at the fundus and sweep downward, force the head of the fetus against the cervix. Under this pressure, the cervix progressively widens and thins the opening to the vaginal canal. In the second stage, which lasts less than 1 hour, the fetus is forced out of the uterine cavity and through the cervix and is delivered from the vagina. In the third stage, which lasts 10 minutes or less, the placenta is separated from the decidual tissue of the uterus and forcefully evacuated. Myometrial contractions during this stage act to constrict the uterine vessels and prevent excessive bleeding. Once the placenta has been removed, all its hormonal products disappear from the maternal plasma according to their characteristic half-lives. In general, by 48 to 72 hours after birth, the steroid and protein hormone concentrations have reached nonpregnancy levels.

■ *Lactation*

Lactation is initiated after delivery by the precipitous drop in estrogen and progesterone levels. Although basal prolactin concentrations gradually decline to normal over the next 4 to 8 weeks, they are acutely elevated during each period of suckling (see Chapter 49, Fig. 49-26). This repeated transient hyperprolactinemia helps to sustain milk secretion.

Lactation, which is mediated by prolactin, also suppresses reproductive function in the nursing mother.

During the first 7 to 10 days post partum, plasma FSH and LH levels remain low. FSH then rises to above-normal follicular-phase levels, but LH remains low. The responsiveness of the ovaries to FSH is probably reduced by prolactin, and LH secretion by the pituitary is probably inhibited by prolactin.

A decrease in the circulating prolactin level, because of cessation of nursing (or by therapeutic administration of a dopaminergic agonist), plays a role in triggering LH release and in reinitiating the normal menstrual cycle.

Maternal provision of nutrients to the newborn begins within 48 hours of delivery. First, a thin fluid, known as **colostrum,** is secreted in very small quantities. This fluid contains lactose and proteins but little fat. True milk delivery follows shortly afterward. Human breast milk contains 1% protein, largely as casein, lactalbumin, and lactoglobulin. In addition, milk contains 7% lactose and 3.5% fat, which is equivalent to about 70 kcal/100 ml. By 1 week, 550 ml/day is produced; later, maximal rates of up to 2000 ml/day may be delivered. Large quantities of calcium and phosphorus are also needed by and provided to the infant in milk.

Typically, infants nurse for 6 to 12 months. The milk they receive contains a large complement of endocrine-related molecules, which includes all pituitary hormones plus their hypothalamic releasing and inhibiting hormones; insulin-like growth factors plus their binding proteins; vitamin D and thyroid and steroid hormones; PTH and PTH-related protein; and prostaglandins. The concentrations of many of these molecules are higher than those in plasma. This disparity indicates local synthesis of these substances in mammary cells or active transport into the milk. The functions of these substances may include (1) local supportive effects on breast tissues and milk secretion, (2) assistance in the development and induction of function of the immature gastrointestinal tract of the infant, (3) assistance in development of the immature infant immune system, and (4) endocrine and metabolic effects in the neonate from those substances absorbed by the immature intestinal mucosa. Milk also contains immunoglobulins, which protect the infant against infection while its own immune system matures.

Mammary cells package proteins, lactose, calcium, and phosphate in secretory vesicles and fat in droplets. Prolactin is essential to these processes (see Chapter 49). Immunoglobulins are combined with membrane receptors in vesicles when they enter the mammary cells. All of these products are then secreted into the alveoli of the breast ducts. Suckling and such anticipatory signals as the infant's cry stimulate oxytocin release via neural sensory pathways and the central **nucleus tractus solitarii.** Oxytocin causes contraction of myoepithial cells around the alveoli and smooth muscle cells in the duct walls. These contractions "let the milk down" into the areolar area, where the infant forces it out through holes in the nipple by positive pressure.

■ Endocrine State of the Fetus

Although fetal pancreatic islets are functional by 14 weeks, insulin and glucagon secretion is relatively low. Neither is critically needed for substrate metabolism, because glucose and amino acids are in plentiful supply from the mother. Fetal pancreatic β cells and α cells respond to their usual stimulators and suppressors in a blunted fashion until birth, when responsiveness rapidly increases. Fetal insulin also contributes to anabolism and to the deposition of adipose tissue.

Fetal **hyperinsulinemia** in the third trimester leads to overweight babies with increases in adipose tissue and lean body mass. This condition occurs in the 4% of pregnancies that are complicated by **gestational diabetes mellitus.** High plasma glucose levels caused by excessive maternal insulin resistance are transmitted to the fetus, where they stimulate excessive release of insulin and its anabolic actions. These babies are harder to deliver and may suffer from hypoglycemia shortly after birth.

Fetal growth hormone is not essential for linear growth; although growth hormone levels are high in plasma, growth hormone receptors are deficient in the fetus. Instead, HCS, placental growth hormone variant, and prolactin may subserve the function of growth hormone prenatally. These hormones may be responsible for the ubiquitous presence of IGF-1 and IGF-2 in fetal plasma and tissues. IGF-2 concentration is especially high, and this growth factor may mediate the most important paracrine and autocrine growth effects in fetal life, whereas IGF-1 assumes this role after birth.

Prolactin concentrations are high in fetal plasma and in amniotic fluid. Prolactin may contribute to fetal growth, osmotic regulation, and the production of cortisol and DHEA-S.

The role of fetal thyroid hormone during gestation is not completely defined. A small transfer of maternal T_4 or T_3 to the fetus may be essential for early fetal development. During the last two thirds of gestation, neither maternal nor fetal thyroid hormone may be needed for some developmental processes. At birth, the newborn's own thyroid hormone becomes critical to further central nervous system maturation and somatic growth.

Active transport of calcium across the placenta from mother to fetus is probably stimulated by PTH_{rp} from the fetal parathyroid glands and the placenta (see Chapter 48); PTH_{rp} keeps fetal plasma calcium levels high. In turn, this slight hypercalcemia inhibits fetal PTH secretion and stimulates fetal calcitonin secretion. Calcitonin, combined with 1,25-$(OH)_2$-vitamin D produced in the fetal kidney and the placenta, promotes fetal bone formation. PTH secretion increases soon after birth and assumes its regulatory role in calcium metabolism.

Fetal ACTH is probably not essential for the first 12 to 20 weeks, although later it definitely stimulates production of steroids by the fetal zone of the adrenal cortex. The newborn mounts an immediate stress response, as shown by high levels of cortisol in umbilical cord plasma. If endogenous ACTH and cortisol cannot be secreted at this time, death will ensue unless replacement therapy is provided.

■ *Summary*

1. Differences in gonadal function between the genders are derived from the process of sexual differentiation. Genetic material on the Y chromosome determines the development of a testis. Testicular antimüllerian hormone suppresses the development of female genital ducts, whereas testosterone and dihydrotestosterone induce masculinization of the genital ducts and external genitalia. Without this positive input, a female (the neutral) pattern results. Two active X chromosomes are, however, required for oogenesis.

2. Testosterone and estradiol derived from testosterone are synthesized by common pathways and enzymes in homologous cell lines in the testis and ovary. Both genders exhibit gonadotropin surges in fetal life, quiescence in childhood, activation in puberty, and increases in negative feedback late in life caused by gonadal failure. The monthly cyclic ovulatory burst of LH/FSH is unique to the female.

3. Spermatogenesis proceeds within the seminiferous tubules in a locally conditioned hormonal environment behind a blood-testis barrier. Sertoli cells, stimulated by FSH, provide growth factors, binding (carrier) proteins for testosterone and for trace metals, inhibin, and other factors to nurture and launch spermatozoa.

4. LH stimulates testosterone secretion by Leydig cells. A high local concentration of testosterone is essential to spermatogenesis. This hormone acts either indirectly, by affecting Sertoli cells, or by direct access to germ cells. Its exact mechanism of action is unknown.

5. In the ovary, oocytes stimulate formation of a follicle, which is a secluded environment analogous to the seminiferous tubules. Under the influence of FSH, a cohort of immature follicles, with their oocytes suspended in meiosis, begin to develop each month. The surrounding granulosa cells secrete estradiol, which is synthesized from androgen precursors. The precursors are provided by neighboring theca cells under LH stimulation. Other granulosa cell products, which are similar to those of the Sertoli cell, condition the oocyte.

6. A single dominant follicle emerges each month. It grows exponentially and secretes sufficient estradiol and inhibin to (1) inhibit cohort follicles, (2) prepare the uterus and fallopian tubes for fertilization, and (3) condition the GnRH-gonadotroph axis to provide an ovulatory LH/FSH surge at the appropriate time. After ovulation takes place, the endocrine cells form a corpus luteum, which secretes progesterone predominantly. The latter acts on the uterus to favor implantation of a zygote.

7. In children during puberty, testosterone in the male and estradiol in the female stimulate linear growth and skeletal maturation as well as enlargement and maturation of the accessory tissues of reproduction.

8. Male and female sexual functioning is stimulated by the autonomic nervous system. An ejaculate of 200 to 400 million sperm requires conditioning (capacitation) in the female genital tract to permit one sperm to fertilize the ovum in the fallopian tube. The zygote is subsequently maintained and protected by secretions from altered uterine cells (decidua) and from placental fetal trophoblastic cells.

9. The placenta initially produces human chorionic gonadotropin, which stimulates the corpus luteum; later, the placenta produces its own estrogen and progesterone. In addition, a variety of placental peptides and proteins are synthesized, including human chorionic somatomammotropin, insulin-like growth factors, inhibin, and molecules homologous with those secreted by the hypothalamus and pituitary gland. These hormones affect maternal and possibly fetal metabolism.

10. The mother is in an anabolic state early in pregnancy. This anabolic state facilitates growth of her energy stores and reproductive tissues. The later catabolic phase is marked by insulin resistance, and it facilitates the flow of fuels to the growing fetus.

11. The exact endocrine mechanism of human parturition is unclear, but it probably includes contributions from an increased estrogen/progesterone ratio within the uterus, from relaxin, and from oxytocin. A local increase in prostaglandins is the immediate second messenger that causes uterine contractions. A late gestational rise in the fetal cortisol level enhances extrauterine survival.

■ *Self-Study Problems*

1a. A 17-year-old girl is investigated because of short stature and somatic anomalies. She has never had a menstrual period. A chromosome analysis reveals that she has 44 normal autosomes and a single X chromosome. What sexual organs would you expect her to have and why?

1b. Would her uterus, labia, and breasts be completely normal? Why didn't she menstruate?

1c. What would her gender orientation be?

2. Which is more important to spermatogenesis, the Leydig or the Sertoli cell?

3a. A young married couple have been trying to conceive a baby for 2 years without success. The husband has a sperm count in the "fertile" range. The wife menstruates regularly. What biological and hormonal indicators could you use to determine whether the woman was ovulating?

3b. Does a normal sperm count ensure male fertility?

■ *Bibliography*

Journal articles

Adashi EY: The climacteric ovary as a functional gonadotropin-driven androgen-producing gland, *Fertil Steril* 62:20, 1994.

Andersson K-E, Wagner G: Physiology of penile erection, *Physiol Rev* 75:191, 1995.

Bryant-Greenwood GD, Schwabe C: Human relaxins: chemistry and biology, *Endoc Rev* 15:5, 1994.

Brzezinski A: Mechanisms of disease: melatonin in humans, *N Engl J Med* 336:186, 1997.

Bulun SE: Aromatase deficiency in women and men: would you have predicted the phenotypes?, *J Clin Endocrinol Metab* 81:867, 1996.

Burger HG et al: The endocrinology of the menopausal transition: a cross-sectional study of a population-based sample, *J Clin Endocrinol Metab* 80:3537, 1995.

Conn PM, Crowley WF Jr: Gonadotropin-releasing hormone and its analogues, *N Engl J Med* 324:93, 1991.

Espey LL, BenHalim IA: Characteristics and control of the normal menstrual cycle, *Obstet Gynecol Clin North Am* 17:275, 1990.

Friedman RC, Downey J: Neurobiology and sexual orientation: current relationships, *J Neuropsychiatry Clin Neurosci* 5:131, 1993.

Gharib SD et al: Molecular biology of the pituitary gonadotropins, *Endocr Rev* 11:177, 1990.

Goland RS, Jozak S, Conwell I: Placental corticotropin-releasing hormone and the hypercortisolism of pregnancy, *Am J Obstet Gynecol* 171:1287, 1994.

Gougeon A: Regulation of ovarian follicular development in primates: facts and hypotheses, *Endocr Rev* 17:121, 1996.

Groome NP et al: Measurement of dimeric inhibin B throughout the human menstrual cycle, *J Clin Endocrinol Metab* 81:1401, 1996.

Grosvenor CE, Picciano MF, Baumrucker CR: Hormones and growth factors in milk, *Endocr Rev* 14:710, 1993.

Haqq CM et al: Molecular basis of mammalian sexual determination: activation of müllerian inhibiting substance gene expression by SRY, *Science* 266:1494, 1994.

Hsueh AJW, Billig H, Tsafriri A: Ovarian follicle atresia: a hormonally controlled apoptotic process, *Endocr Rev* 15:707, 1994.

Illingworth PJ et al: Measurement of circulating inhibin forms during the establishment of pregnancy, *J Clin Endocrinol Metab* 81:1471, 1996.

Inkster S, Yue W, Brodie A: Human testicular aromatase: immunocytochemical and biochemical studies, *J Clin Endocrinol Metab* 80:1941, 1995.

Johnson MD: Genes related to spermatogenesis: molecular and clinical aspects, *Semin Reprod Endocrinol* 9:72, 1991.

Joseph DR: Structure, function, and regulation of androgen-binding protein/sex hormone-binding globulin, *Vitam Horm* 49:197, 1994.

Kalra SP: Mandatory neuropeptide-steroid signaling for the preovulatory luteinizing hormone-releasing hormone discharge, *Endocr Rev* 14:507, 1993.

Kelly RW: Pregnancy maintenance and parturition: the role of prostaglandin in manipulating the immune and inflammatory response, *Endocr Rev* 15:684, 1994.

Lee MM, Donahoe PK: Mullerian inhibiting substance: a gonadal hormone with multiple functions, *Endocr Rev* 14:152, 1993.

Liang L-F, Dean J: Oocyte development: molecular biology of the zona pellucida, *Vitam Horm* 47:115, 1993.

Lindsey J et al: Molecular mechanisms of androgen action, *Vitam Horm* 49:383, 1994.

McLean M et al: A placental clock controlling the length of human pregnancy, *Nat Med* 1:460, 1995.

Papadopoulos V: Identification and purification of a human Sertoli cell–secreted protein (HSCSP-80) stimulating Leydig cell steroid biosynthesis, *J Clin Endocrinol Metab* 72:1332, 1991.

Qu J et al: Circulating bioactive inhibin levels during human pregnancy, *J Clin Endocrinol Metab* 72:862, 1991.

Rabinovici J, Jaffe RB: Development and regulation of growth and differentiated function in human and subhuman primate fetal gonads, *Endocr Rev* 11:532, 1990.

Richards JS et al: Ovarian cell differentiation: a cascade of multiple hormones, cellular signals, and regulated genes, *Recent Prog Horm Res* 50:223, 1995.

Rossmanith WG et al: Pulsatile cosecretion of estradiol and progesterone by the midluteal phase corpus luteum: temporal link to luteinizing hormone pulses, *J Clin Endocrinol Metab* 70:990, 1990.

Saez JM: Leydig cells: endocrine, paracrine, and autocrine regulation, *Endocr Rev* 15:574, 1994.

Schwartzman RA, Cidlowski JA: Apoptosis: the biochemistry and molecular biology of programmed cell death, *Endocr Rev* 14:133, 1993.

Scott RT Jr, Hodgen GD: The ovarian follicle: life cycle of a pelvic clock, *Clin Obstet Gynecol* 33:551, 1990.

Serón-Ferré M, Ducsay CA, Valenzuela GJ: Circadian rhythms during pregnancy, *Endocr Rev* 14:594, 1993.

Skinner MK: Cell-cell interactions in the testis, *Endocr Rev* 12:45, 1991.

Sluijmer AV, Heineman MJ, DeJong FH, Evers JLH: Endocrine activity of the postmenopausal ovary: the effects of pituitary down-regulation and oophorectomy, *J Clin Endocrin Metab* 80:2163, 1995.

Southworth MB et al: The importance of signal pattern in the transmission of endocrine information: pituitary gonadotropin responses to continuous and pulsatile gonadotropin-releasing hormone, *J Clin Endocrinol Metab* 72:1286, 1991.

Steer PJ: The endocrinology of parturition in the human, *Bailliere's Clin Endocrinol Metab* 4:333, 1990.

Stojilkovic SS, Reinhart J, Catt KJ: Gonadotropin-releasing hormone receptors: structure and signal transduction pathways, *Endocr Rev* 15:462, 1994.

Tonetta SA, DiZerega GS: Intragonadal regulation of follicular maturation, *Endocr Rev* 10:205, 1989.

Turner RT, Riggs BL, and Spelsberg TC: Skeletal effects of estrogen, *Endocr Rev* 15:275, 1994.

Veldhuis JD: The hypothalamic pulse generator: the reproductive core, *Clin Obstet Gynecol* 33:538, 1990.

Wakatsuki M et al: Immunoradiometric assay for follistatin: serum immunoreactive follistatin levels in normal adults and pregnant women, *J Clin Endocrinol Metab* 81:630, 1996.

White MM et al: Estrogen, progesterone, and vascular reactivity: potential cellular mechanisms, *Endocr Rev* 16:739, 1995.

Wu FCW et al: Ontogeny of pulsatile gonadotropin releasing hormone secretion from midchildhood, through puberty, to adulthood in the human male: a study using deconvolution analysis and an ultrasensitive immunofluorometric assay, *J Clin Endocrinol Metab* 81:1798, 1996.

Zhou Z, Wong C, Sar M, Wilson EM: The androgen receptor: an overview, *Recent Prog Horm Res* 49:249, 1994.

Zirkin BR et al: Is FSH required for adult spermatogenesis? *J Androl* 15:273, 1994.

Books and monographs

Adashi EY: *The ovarian cycle.* In Yen SSC, Jaffe RB, editors: *Reproductive endocrinology,* Philadelphia, 1991, WB Saunders.

Carr BR: *The ovary.* In Carr BR, Blackwell RE, editors: *Textbook of reproductive medicine,* Norwalk, Conn, 1993, Appleton & Lange.

Carr BR: *The normal menstrual cycle: the coordinated events of the hypothalamic-pituitary-ovarian axis and the female reproductive tract.* In Carr BR, Blackwell RE, editors: *Textbook of reproductive medicine,* Norwalk, Conn, 1993, Appleton & Lange.

DeKretser DM, Risbridger GP, Kerr JB: Basic endocrinology of the testis. In DeGroot LJ, editor: *Endocrinology,* ed 3, 1995, WB Saunders.

Fisher DA: *Endocrinology of fetal development.* In Wilson JD, Foster DW, editors: *Williams textbook of endocrinology,* Philadelphia, 1992, WB Saunders.

Gooren LJG, Money J: *Normal and abnormal sexual behavior.* In DeGroot LJ, editor: *Endocrinology,* ed 3, Philadelphia, 1995, WB Saunders.

Josso N: *Anatomy and endocrinology of fetal sex differentiation.* In DeGroot LJ, editor: *Endocrinology,* ed 3, Philadelphia, 1995, WB Saunders.

Kenigsberg D, Rosenwaks Z, and Hodgen GD: *Ovarian follicular maturation, ovulation, and ovulation induction.* In DeGroot LJ, editor: *Endocrinology,* ed 3, Philadelphia, 1995, WB Saunders.

Marshall JC: *Hormonal regulation of the menstrual cycle and mechanisms of anovulation.* In DeGroot LJ, editor: *Endocrinology,* ed 3, Philadelphia, 1995, WB Saunders.

Odell WD: *Genetic basis of sexual differentiation.* In DeGroot LJ, editor: *Endocrinology,* ed 3, Philadelphia, 1995, WB Saunders.

Odell WD: *Endocrinology of sexual maturation.* In DeGroot LJ, editor: *Endocrinology,* ed 3, Philadelphia, 1995, WB Saunders.

Parker CR Jr: *The endocrinology of pregnancy.* In Carr BR, Blackwell RE, editors: *Textbook of reproductive medicine,* Norwalk, Conn, 1993, Appleton & Lange.

Reichlin S: *Neuroendocrinology.* In Foster D, Wilson J, editors: *Williams textbook of endocrinology,* ed 8, Philadelphia, 1992, WB Saunders.

Turek FW, Van Cauter E: *Rhythms in reproduction.* In Knobil E, Neil JD, editors: *The physiology of reproduction,* ed 2, New York, 1994, Raven Press.

Veldhuis JD: *The hypothalamic-pituitary-testicular axis.* In Yen SSC, Jaffe RB, editors: *Reproductive endocrinology,* Philadelphia, 1991, WB Saunders.

Word RA: *Parturition.* In Carr BR, Blackwell RE, editors: *Textbook of reproductive medicine,* Norwalk, Conn, 1993, Appleton & Lange.

Yamamoto M, Turner TT: *Epididymis, sperm maturation, and capacitation.* In Lipshultz LI, Howards SS, editors: *Infertility in the male,* St Louis, 1991, Mosby–Year Book.

Yen SSC: *The human menstrual cycle: neuroendocrine regulation.* In Yen SSC, Jaffe RB, editors: *Reproductive endocrinology,* Philadelphia, 1991, WB Saunders.

Yen SSC: *The hypothalamic control of pituitary hormone secretion regulation.* In Yen SSC, Jaffe RB, editors: *Reproductive endocrinology,* Philadelphia, 1991, WB Saunders.

APPENDIX

A

Answers to Self-Study Problems

■ *Chapter 1*

1. (a) $J = -DA\dfrac{\Delta c}{\Delta x}$

   (b) J = Net rate of diffusion in moles or grams per unit time

   D = Diffusion coefficient of the diffusing solute in the membrane

   A = Area of the membrane

   Δc = Concentration difference across the membrane

   Δx = Thickness of the membrane

   (c) The rate of diffusion of a substance across a membrane is proportional to the membrane area and to the concentration difference of the substance across the membrane and inversely proportional to the membrane thickness. The coefficient of proportionality is the diffusion coefficient.

2. (a) In general, the more lipid soluble a molecule, the more permeable are biological membranes to it. (b) For molecules of the same lipid solubility, the smaller the molecular weight, the greater is the permeability. (c) Most biological membranes are essentially impermeable to water-soluble molecules larger than about 200 molecular weight. (d) Water-soluble molecules much larger than 200 molecular weight may cross biological membranes via specific membrane transport proteins.

3. Osmosis: the flow of water across a semipermeable membrane from the side where solute is less concentrated to the side where solute is more concentrated.

   Osmotic pressure: the hydrostatic pressure that must be applied to a solution to just prevent water from entering the solution from pure water across a semipermeable membrane.

   Semipermeable membrane: a membrane permeable to water but impermeable to solutes.

4. (a) $\pi = RT\Phi ic$

   (b) $\pi = (22.4\ \text{L atm/mole}) (3) (0.01\ \text{mole/L}) = 0.672\ \text{atm}$

   (c) The more dilute the solution, the closer will Φ approach 1.0.

   (d) The osmotic coefficient (Φ) is used to correct for the nonideality of real solutions.

   (e) $\pi = RT\Phi ic = (22.4\ \text{L atm/mole}) (0.86) (3) (0.01\ \text{mole/L}) = 0.578\ \text{atm}$

5. (i) The steady-state cell volume is determined only by the concentration of impermeant solutes in the extracellular fluid.

   (ii) Permeant solutes cause only transient changes in cell volume.

   (iii) The time course of the transient is more rapid, the greater the permeability of the membrane to the permeant solute.

6. (a) Protein-mediated transport processes show saturation kinetics, chemical specificity (including stereo-specificity), competitive inhibition, and inhibition by structurally unrelated compounds (in some cases). Diffusion has none of these properties.

   (b) An active transport process can transport the transported substance from where its concentration or electrochemical potential is lower to where its concentration or electrochemical potential is higher. This requires energy. Facilitated transport systems cannot create a gradient of concentration or electrochemical potential and can only transport their particular transport substrates down their concentration or electrochemical potential gradients.

   (c) A primary active transport system depends directly on adenosine triphosphate (ATP) or some other high-energy metabolic intermediate for its energy. A secondary active transport system uses the energy in the gradient of another actively transported substance to perform active transport.

■ *Chapter 2*

1. The equation that defines the electrochemical potential difference of the ion X^+ between the two sides of a membrane, A and B, is

$$\Delta\mu(X^+) = \mu_A(X^+) - \mu_B(X^+) = RT\ln\dfrac{[X^+]_A}{[X^+]_B} + zF(E_A - E_B)$$

Concentration term: $RT\ln\dfrac{[X^+]_A}{[X^+]_B}$

Electrical term: $zF(E_A - E_B)$

2. The Nernst equation is

$$E_A - E_B = -\frac{RT}{zF}\ln\frac{[Y]_A}{[Y]_B} = \frac{RT}{zF}\ln\frac{[Y]_B}{[Y]_A}$$

where $E_A - E_B$ = electrical potential difference across membrane (side A relative to side B), R is the ideal gas constant, T is absolute temperature (°C + 273), z is the valence of the ion, F is Faraday's number, and $[Y]_A$ and $[Y]_B$ are the concentrations of the ion on sides A and B, respectively.

When an ion satisfies the Nernst equation, this means that the right hand side of the Nernst equation computed using the concentrations of the ion on the two sides of the membrane is equal to *the actual electrical potential difference that exists across the membrane*. This means that the ion is in equilibrium across the membrane. This implies that the electrochemical potential of the ion is the same on both sides of the membrane and that there is thus no net force acting on the ion.

3. The electrical potential difference, $E_A - E_B$, will be equal to -60 mV. Side A is negative with respect to side B, so side B is the electrically positive side. This is a concentration cell. Because the membrane is permeable only to K^+, the electrical potential difference across the membrane will be equal to the E_K, the equilibrium potential for K^+:

$$E_K = E_A - E_B = -\frac{RT}{zF}\ln\frac{[K^+]_A}{[K^+]_B} = -\frac{60\text{ mV}}{+1}\log\frac{1}{0.1}$$

$$= -60\text{ mV}$$

4. The Donnan relation for the ions X^+ and Y^- is $[X]_A[Y]_A = [X]_B[Y]_B$. If X^+ and Y^- are a uni-univalent ion pair that satisfy the Donnan relation on the two sides (A and B) of a membrane, then $[X]_A[Y]_A = [X]_B[Y]_B$. If the concentrations of X^+ and Y^- on the two sides of the membrane satisfy the Donnan relation, this implies that *both* ions are in electrochemical equilibrium across the membrane.

5. An electrogenic process is one that transfers net charge across a membrane. The Na^+, K^+-ATPase is an electrogenic ion pump because it transfers 3 Na^+ ions out of the cell for every 2 K^+ ions it pumps in.

6. $E_m = -81.2$ mV (inside negative). To estimate E_m, first use the Nernst equation to compute the equilibrium potentials for K^+, Na^+, and Cl^-. Then use the chord conductance equation to estimate the resting membrane potential (E_m).
   From the Nernst equation:

   $E_K = -88.6$ mV; $E_{Na} = +60$ mV; and $E_{Cl} = -88.6$ mV

   From the chord conductance equation:

   $$E_m = \frac{g_K}{\Sigma g}E_K + \frac{g_{Na}}{\Sigma g}E_{Na} + \frac{g_{Cl}}{\Sigma g}E_{Cl}$$

   $$= (0.5/1)(-88.6) + (0.05/1)(+60) + (0.45/1)(-88.6) = -81.2\text{ mV}$$

   The inside of the cell is negative with respect to the extracellular fluid.

■ *Chapter 3*

1. (a) and (b)
   (c) Resting potential = -70 mV
       Threshold = -55 mV
       Peak of overshoot = $+50$ mV
   (d) Approximate duration = 5 msec

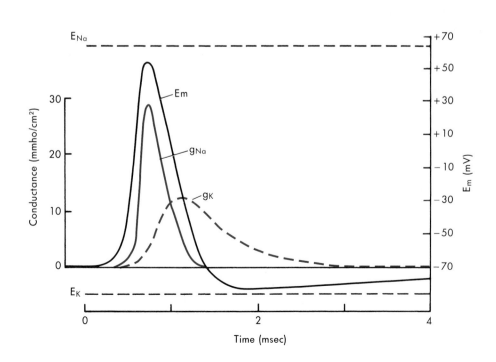

2. (a) The overshoot fails to reach E_{Na} because g_{Na} inactivates and there is a delayed rise of g_K. Both of these tend to return E_m toward the resting potential.

(b) The absolute refractory period is caused by the voltage inactivation of Na^+ channels, so that the critical number to fire another action potential cannot be recruited, no matter how strong the stimulus.

(c) Early in the relative refractory period, a larger than normal stimulus is required to trigger an action potential because some of the Na^+ channels remain voltage inactivated and the K^+ conductance is elevated. Later in the relative refractory period, during the hyperpolarizing afterpotential, refractoriness is due only to the elevated K^+ conductance.

(d) To trigger the regenerative positive feedback between depolarization and opening of Na^+ channels, it is necessary to depolarize sufficiently to bring some critical number of Na^+ channels into the open state. This critical level of depolarization required is the threshold for the action potential.

3. There is no role of the Na^+, K^+-ATPase in generating a single action potential. It does create the ion gradients that make the action potential possible, however.

4. Electrotonic conduction occurs by passive flow of electrical current between adjacent membrane areas at different electrical potentials. In this way a local depolarization is spread in both directions along the length of the cell. The length constant is the distance along the cell over which an electrotonically conducted signal decays to $1/e$ (38%) of its maximal value. The length constant depends on the ratio of the membrane resistance to the internal longitudinal resistance, and the length constant is equal to $\sqrt{r_m/r_{in}}$. For typical cells, the length constant is 1 to 2 mm.

5. In saltatory conduction, the impulse is rapidly conducted electrotonically between the nodes of Ranvier. This is because myelination greatly increases the conduction velocity in the internodal areas. The internodal plasma membrane cannot fire an action potential because the multiple layers of plasma membrane do not allow sufficient ionic currents to flow in the internodal regions. There is little decrement as an action potential is conducted through an internodal area because of the increased length constant there as the result of myelination. The action potential is conducted very rapidly, and with little decrement, between nodes and pauses to be regenerated only at the nodes; that is, it "jumps" from node to node, and for this reason is called *saltatory*.

■ *Chapter 4*

1. Action potential in motor nerve terminal $\Rightarrow$ Increase of g_{Ca} and inrush of Ca^{++} $\Rightarrow$ Release of acetyl-choline (ACh) by exocytosis $\Rightarrow$ Diffusion of ACh across junctional cleft $\Rightarrow$ Binding to ACh receptors on postjunctional membrane $\Rightarrow$ Increase in g_K and g_{Na} of postjunctional membrane $\Rightarrow$ Transient depolarization of postjunctional membrane (EPP) $\Rightarrow$ Electrotonic depolarization of adjacent areas of muscle membrane until threshold is reached $\Rightarrow$ Generation of action potential and its propagation in both directions away from neuromuscular junction.

2. The smallest amount of ACh that can be released by the presynaptic nerve terminal, the contents of a single presynaptic vesicle, is called a quantum. The size of the endplate potential varies in steps, each step corresponding to a quantum. A miniature endplate potential (MEPP) is a spontaneously occurring small depolarization of the postsynaptic membrane. MEPPs are due to the spontaneous release of individual quanta of ACh.

3. Repetitive stimulation of a motor nerve may lead to endplate potentials that increase in size with each single stimulus. This is called facilitation. When a motor nerve is tetanized (stimulated with a high-frequency volley of stimuli), the endplate potential evoked by a single stimulus may be larger after the tetanization than before. This is called post-tetanic potentiation.

4. The hydrolysis of ACh by acetylcholinesterase terminates the endplate potential. An anticholinesterase will increase both the magnitude and duration of the endplate potential.

5. We say that integration occurs at spinal motor neurons because the membrane potential of the motor neuron at any point in time is the result of the activity of its many presynaptic inputs, which may interact in a number of ways. It takes a certain number of excitatory postsynaptic potentials (EPSPs) in excess of the number of inhibitory postsynaptic potentials (IPSPs) to depolarize the cell to threshold.

■ *Chapter 5*

1. The inactive G protein is a heterotrimer of α, β, and γ subunits. It has guanosine diphosphate (GDP) in its nucleotide-binding site. When the inactive G protein interacts with a ligand-bearing receptor, the G protein undergoes a conformational change. The conformational change increases the relative affinity of the G protein for guanosine triphosphate (GTP) over GDP and diminishes the affinity of the α subunit for the $\beta\gamma$ dimer. The activated α subunit, or in some instances the $\beta\gamma$ dimer, can then interact with an enzyme or an ion channel to stimulate or inhibit its activity. The activated α subunit has GTPase activity and hydrolyzes the GTP to GDP; this causes the α subunit to revert to its inactive form, which then recombines with the $\beta\gamma$ dimer.

2. The binding of a stimulatory ligand, such as epinephrine acting through β-adrenergic receptors, results in activation of heterotrimeric G proteins with α subunits of the type called α_s (*s* for stimulatory). Activation of the G_s-type G protein by the ligand-bearing receptor causes its α_s subunit to bind GTP and then to dissociate from βγ. α_s then interacts with adenylyl cyclase to stimulate its enzymatic activity and thereby to increase the level of cyclic AMP in the cytosol.

   Substances, such as epinephrine acting at α_2 receptors and adenosine acting on α_1 receptors, inhibit adenylyl cyclase by activating G_i-type G proteins that have α subunits of a different type, called α_i (*i* for inhibitory). Binding of the inhibitory ligand to its receptor activates the G_i-type G protein and causes its α_i subunit to dissociate from the βγ dimers. The activated α_i binds to and inhibits adenylyl cyclase, thereby diminishing the concentration of cyclic AMP in the cytosol. In addition, the βγ dimers may bind to free α_s subunits and thus diminish the stimulation of adenylyl cyclase by stimulatory ligands.

3. Certain extracellular agonists bind to receptors that activate, via a G protein called G_q, the β isoform of phospholipase C. This isoform cleaves phosphatidylinositol-4,5-bisphosphate (a phospholipid present in minute quantities in the plasma membrane) into inositol-1,4,5-trisphosphate (IP_3) and diacylglycerol. IP_3 binds to specific ligand-gated Ca⁺⁺ channels in the endoplasmic reticulum and releases Ca⁺⁺ to increase its cytosolic level. When cytosolic levels of Ca⁺⁺ rise, Ca⁺⁺ binds to protein kinase C. This causes protein kinase C to bind to the inner surface of the plasma membrane, where it can be activated by the diacylglycerol that is produced by the hydrolysis of phosphatidylinositol bisphosphate. Membrane phosphatidylserine is also a potent activator of protein kinase C, once the enzyme has bound to the membrane.

4. Binding of the growth factor to its receptor results in dimerization of receptor-ligand complexes. The dimerization enhances binding affinity and activates the protein-tyrosine kinase activity of the receptor. Each monomer in a dimer phosphorylates the other monomer on multiple tyrosine residues. The activated receptor tyrosine kinase activates Ras, a monomeric GTP-binding protein. Activated Ras in turn activates a signal transduction pathway, involving the MAP kinase cascade, that ultimately turns on the transcription of certain key genes that promote cellular proliferation.

■ *Chapter 6*

1. The central nervous system is composed of the spinal cord and brain. The brain is subdivided into (1) the myelencephalon, (2) metencephalon, (3) mesen-

cephalon, (4) diencephalon, and (5) telencephalon. The corresponding adult structures are (1) medulla, (2) pons and cerebellum, (3) midbrain, (4) thalamus and hypothalamus, and (5) basal ganglia and cerebral cortex.

2. The cerebrospinal fluid (CSF) pressure would increase because CSF continues to be secreted. CSF accumulation within the closed volume of the skull would be at the expense of brain and blood volume.

3. The cells found in nervous tissue include neurons (function is neural signaling through nerve impulses and synaptic transmission), astrocytes (support, repair, and regulation of contents of extracellular space), oligodendroglia (central nervous system myelin), ependymal cells (epithelial lining of ventricles), microglia (phagocytosis), and blood vessels (exchange of nutrients and waste products).

4. Coding mechanisms include labeled lines, topographic maps, and patterns of nerve impulses.

5. Anterograde axonal transport includes both rapid and slow types. Retrograde transport is relatively fast.

■ *Chapter 7*

1. The term *receptive field* refers to the distribution of sites that, when stimulated, can alter the activity of a sensory neuron. For example, a primary afferent mechanoreceptive neuron that innervates sensory receptors in the skin can be excited by mechanical stimulation of the area of skin that contains the receptors. Mechanical spread of the stimulus may cause the receptive field to be larger than the area of the skin that actually encompasses the receptors. A central somatosensory neuron may be excited by stimulation of a region of skin, the excitatory receptive field, but also a central neuron may be inhibited by stimulation of an area of skin, the inhibitory receptive field.

2. Sensory receptors may encode the sensory modality, spatial location, threshold, intensity, frequency, and duration of a stimulus. Modality is determined by the type of receptor and its central neural connections (labeled line coding). Spatial location may depend on the location of the receptive fields of the receptors and on the relationship between the receptive fields and a spatial map of responsive neurons in the central nervous system. Threshold and intensity often depend on the thresholds of the receptors and the discharge rates evoked in the afferent nerve fibers by different intensities of stimuli. Another factor is the number of activated afferent axons. In rapidly adapting receptors, the frequency of a stimulus can be indicated by the frequency of nerve impulses generated in the afferent axons. The duration of a stimulus can be indicated by the durations of the discharge of slowly adapting

receptors or by transient discharges of rapidly adapting receptors at the beginning and end of the stimulus.

3. A motor unit consists of an α motor neuron and the skeletal muscle fibers that it innervates. When the α motor neuron discharges, all the muscle fibers of the motor unit will normally contract. The muscle fibers of a motor unit all have the same histochemical type, and the histochemical type is matched with appropriate electrophysiological properties of the α motor neuron. For example, slow-twitch muscle fibers (type S motor units with type I muscle fibers) are innervated by α motor neuron that discharge at low rates, whereas fast-twitch muscle fibers (types FF and FR, with types IIB and IIA muscle fibers) are innervated by α motor neuron that discharge at high rates.

4. The size principle is that small motor neurons are more readily activated than large motor neurons, both in reflexes and in voluntary movements. Because small motor neurons innervate slow-twitch motor units, which generate small amounts of force and which resist fatigue, the size principle ensures that the force of contraction of a muscle is appropriate for postural support and that the force increases in a suitably graded fashion as more motor units are recruited. Ordinary contractions that are used to maintain the position of a joint or to cause weak movements depend largely on the activity of small motor neurons, whereas strong movements (which are subject to fatigue) must recruit large motor neurons.

■ Chapter 8

1. The mechanoreceptors that signal flutter include Meissner's corpuscles in the glabrous skin and hair follicle afferents in the hairy skin. The receptors responsible for vibration sense are the pacinian corpuscles.

2. Cold receptors discharge in distinct bursts when the temperature of the skin is lowered by 5° to 10° C.

3. Laminae I to VI form the dorsal horn. Nociceptors end in laminae I, II (the substantia gelatinosa), and V.

4. The gate theory is based in part on the observation that tactile stimuli can reduce pain. Inhibitory interneurons of the substantia gelatinosa are proposed to gate out nociceptive signals after tactile stimuli. This theory does not take into account other inhibitory control mechanisms, such as the diffuse noxious inhibitory control system that is activated by painful stimuli.

5. Sensory maps can encode the location of stimuli on the body. Neurons are activated in a particular part of the sensory homunculus. This leads somehow to a perception of a sensation associated with the corresponding region of the body.

■ Chapter 9

1. The refractive power of the lens is variable and thereby allows the eye to focus images at various distances on the retina.

2. The iris determines the size of the pupil and thus functions like the diaphragm of a camera. When the pupil is dilated, more light can enter the eye. When the pupil is constricted, less light reaches the retina. In addition, pupillary constriction increases the depth of field, and it reduces spherical aberration by restricting the light path to the central part of the lens.

3. Glutamate acts on various glutamate receptors, including ionotropic and metabotropic receptors. When activated, the ionotropic glutamate receptors cause the opening of cation channels, and thus depolarize the neurons because of a net inward cationic current. Metabotropic receptors exert their actions through second messenger cascades. Some receptor types cause a depolarization, but others result in a hyperpolarization. In the retina, glutamate hyperpolarizes bipolar cells via its action on metabotropic receptors. Light causes hyperpolarization of photoreceptors and thereby decreases the amount of glutamate that they release. The effect on bipolar cells and eventually on retinal ganglion cells depends on changes in the amount of glutamate released by the photoreceptors.

4. A lesion of the right lingual gyrus causes a left superior homonymous quadrantanopsia (that is, blindness in the left upper part of the visual field of each eye). This occurs because the retinal ganglion cells in the lower nasal part of the left eye and in the lower temporal part of the right eye project their visual information by way of the right dorsal lateral geniculate nucleus and optic radiation to the right lingual gyrus.

5. Depending on the exact region affected, a lesion of the inferotemporal cortex could cause a loss of color vision and an inability to recognize faces. In general, form vision would be impaired.

■ Chapter 10

1. A tonotopic map is an organization of neurons in which the best frequency responses vary from low to high frequencies along a spatial gradient. For example, the hair cells and cochlear nerve fibers near the base of the cochlea have their best frequency responses at the high end of the auditory spectrum, whereas hair cells and cochlear nerve fibers near the apex respond best to low frequencies. Other structures with a tonotopic map include the cochlear nuclei, inferior colliculus, medial geniculate nucleus, and primary auditory cortex.

2. Sound waves cause an oscillation of the tympanic membrane, ossicle chain, oval window, fluid columns in the scala vestibuli, scala media and scala tympani, and secondary tympanic membrane of the round window. Movements of the scala media cause shear forces between the tectorial membrane and the stereocilia of the hair cells. Movement of the stereocilia toward the tallest of the set causes a depolarization of the hair cells, transmitter release, and activation of the relevant cochlear nerve fibers. The opposite movement results in a hyperpolarization of the hair cells and a reduction in the discharges of the cochlear nerve fibers.

3. Cochlear nerve fibers may discharge at the same frequency as the prevailing sound or at some multiple of it. Thus, the firing rate of cochlear nerve fibers can contribute to frequency encoding. However, this mechanism applies only to low-frequency sounds. The ear can discriminate much higher frequencies of sound than can be accounted for by this mechanism. Perhaps a more important factor is the location of the hair cells along the basilar membrane (place theory of hearing). Activation of hair cells near the base of the cochlea discharges the cochlear nerve fibers that represent high-frequency sound, and activation of hair cells near the apex discharges the cochlear afferents that represent low-frequency sound.

4. The superior olivary complex is involved in the spatial localization of sound. Neurons of the superior olivary complex receive excitatory or inhibitory inputs from the two ears. Sounds that originate from a particular source may reach the two ears at different times, and they may be more intense in the ear nearer the sound source and less intense in the other ear. These differences can be detected by neurons in the superior olivary complexes, and information about this discrimination is then forwarded to higher centers.

5. The firing rate of vestibular afferent fibers from the left horizontal semicircular duct decreased when the head was rotated to the right. This can be predicted by taking into account the motion of the endolymph in the horizontal ducts. A rightward rotation of the head causes a relative shift in the endolymph toward the left. This deviates the kinocilia of hair cells in the ampullary crest of the left horizontal semicircular duct away from the utricle, and hence causes a hyperpolarization and a concomitant reduction in the transmitter release and in the discharge rate of the afferent fibers that supply the hair cells.

■ *Chapter 11*

1. The cell bodies of the chemoreceptor neurons in the taste and smell pathways are located in the periphery, whereas the cell bodies of somatovisceral afferents are located in dorsal root and cranial nerve ganglia. The chemoreceptor neurons are continually replaced, along with the associated epithelial cells, because precursor neurons exist in the taste buds and olfactory epithelium of adults. On the other hand, loss of a somatovisceral sensory neuron is permanent.

2. A given chemoreceptor afferent will generally respond to several different classes of stimuli.

3. The taste pathway involves a thalamic relay in the parvocellular part of the ventral posterior medial thalamic nucleus. The olfactory bulb is a cortical structure, and its neurons project to other cortical areas. Thus, the olfactory system has a different organization from that of other sensory pathways that require a thalamic relay for information directed to the cerebral cortex. However, olfactory information is relayed by the medial dorsal nucleus of the thalamus to the prefrontal and orbitofrontal areas of cortex.

■ *Chapter 12*

1. Because the long ascending somatosensory pathways are interrupted, the individual can no longer detect touch, pressure, vibration, limb position, temperature changes, or pain in any part of the body or in the lower extremities below the level of the lesion. The lower extremities are paralyzed. After the period of spinal shock is over, the person develops hyperactive phasic stretch reflexes. These are especially evident when dynamic stimuli are applied, such as tendon taps or quick movements at joints. Clonus may be demonstrable at the ankle when the foot is briskly dorsiflexed. A Babinski sign may be elicited bilaterally. Flexor withdrawal reflexes become exaggerated, and mass reflexes may evoke bilateral flexion and evacuation of the bowel and bladder. The bladder wall becomes tonically constricted and empties reflexly. The bladder may not empty completely, and hence chronic urinary tract infections may occur.

2. The muscle spindle consists of a bundle of specialized muscle fibers known as intrafusal muscle fibers. These specialized fibers are enclosed within a connective tissue capsule, and they lie within the muscle in parallel with the regular or extrafusal muscle fibers. The intrafusal muscle fibers include the larger-diameter nuclear bag fibers and the thinner nuclear chain fibers. The nuclear bag and chain fibers are innervated at their equatorial zone by branches of a group Ia muscle spindle afferent fiber. The ending of a Ia fiber is known as a primary ending, and it involves spiral terminations about the intrafusal fibers. Nuclear chain fibers also are innervated in their juxtaequatorial

region from middle-sized myelinated group II afferent fibers. There may be one or several of these secondary endings. Stretch of the muscle spindle results in a dynamic and then a static response of the Ia fiber and a static response of the group II fiber. Dynamic responses are produced by an elastic recoil within one of the types of nuclear bag fibers. Static responses reflect the stiffness of nuclear chain fibers. Intrafusal fibers are also innervated by γ motor neurons. Dynamic γ motor neurons supply nuclear bag fibers and they function to enhance the dynamic responses of the primary endings, whereas static γ motor neurons supply nuclear chain fibers and enhance the static responses of group Ia and II fibers.

3. Muscle spindles signal the amount and rate of muscle stretch. The static response signals muscle length and the dynamic response signals the rate of muscle stretch. Golgi tendon organs signal the tension that develops in the tendon of a muscle during contraction or stretch.

4. The components of a reflex arc include an afferent limb, central connections, and an efferent limb. The afferent limb of the stretch reflex consists of groups Ia and II muscle spindle afferents. Central processing in the stretch reflex involves monosynaptic excitatory synapses of muscle spindle afferents with motor neurons that supply the same muscle that contains the muscle spindles and also that supply synergistic muscles. There is also a disynaptic pathway through group Ia inhibitory interneurons that synapse on motor neurons to antagonist muscles. Stretch reflexes that involve a given muscle result in the excitation of that muscle and in the relaxation of the antagonist muscles. Phasic stretch reflexes are produced by the dynamic responses of the primary endings of the muscle spindles, and tonic stretch reflexes are evoked by the static discharges. Phasic stretch reflexes are tested clinically by tapping the tendons of muscles with a reflex hammer to elicit a brisk reflex contraction of the muscle attached to that tendon. Tonic stretch reflexes are tested clinically by passively moving joints.

5. The afferent limb of the flexion reflex may involve low-threshold mechanoreceptors, as well as high threshold nociceptors (the flexion reflex afferents). The central mechanism consists of interneuronal pathways that cause the contraction of flexor muscles in the stimulated limb (with a concomitant relaxation of extensor muscles of the same limb) and contraction of the extensor muscles in the contralateral limb (crossed extension reflex). Sometimes, the other pair of limbs is also affected, but with the reverse pattern of contractions of flexor and extensor muscles. The flexion reflex contributes to locomotion, but it may also be part of a protective action, as in the flexor withdrawal reflex. The latter takes precedence over other reflexes.

■ *Chapter 13*

1. The lateral system controls contralateral movements, such as movements of the lower face, tongue, and distal extremities. The medial system controls bilateral movements, such as wrinkling the forehead, chewing, and moving the trunk. The lateral system includes part of the corticobulbar tract and the lateral corticospinal tract. The medial system includes the ventral corticospinal tract, the lateral and medial vestibulospinal and reticulospinal tracts, and the tectospinal tract.

2. When the corticospinal and corticobulbar tracts are interrupted at the level of the internal capsule, the contralateral upper and lower extremities and the lower face and tongue on the side opposite the lesion are paralyzed. The paralysis is of the spastic type; that is, it is characterized by hyperactive phasic stretch reflexes. Pathological reflexes, such as the sign of Babinski, may appear in the contralateral foot, and superficial reflexes, such as the abdominal and cremasteric reflexes, become weak.

3. Locomotion depends on a central pattern generator located in the spinal cord. However, this pattern generator is activated by the midbrain locomotor center and is influenced by afferent input from the periphery.

4. Cold water introduced into the left ear (with the head tilted backward so that the horizontal semicircular canal is vertical) is comparable with turning the head to the right. That is, the kinocilia in the left horizontal semicircular canal deviate away from the utricle and thereby decrease the afferent discharge from the ampullary crest of this canal. The nystagmus that develops has its fast phase to the right side. The environment appears to rotate to the left, and the subject tends to fall to the left.

5. The paralysis of gaze to the left and the right hemiplegia can be explained by a pontine lesion that destroys both the left horizontal gaze center (around the left abducens nucleus) and the left corticospinal tract.

■ *Chapter 14*

1. The primary motor cortex is the main source of motor commands for voluntary movements. The commands are executed in primates, including humans, by volleys of impulses in corticospinal and corticobulbar neurons that synapse in part directly on motor neurons and in part on interneurons in the spinal cord and brainstem. The supplementary motor cortex, which is involved in motor programming, becomes active in the planning stages and in the execution of the movement. This portion of the motor cortex may also help coordinate posture and the sequence of voluntary

movements. The premotor cortex receives sensory information from the posterior parietal cortex and so it helps transmit the somatosensory and visual sensory cues that influence the plans for movements.

2. The corticospinal neurons discharge before movements produced by the motor neurons upon which they terminate monosynaptically. This suggests that the movements result in part from the activity of the corticospinal neurons. The discharges are greatest when they occur before a movement in a preferred direction. The discharges are related to the force of contraction or to the rate of change of force of the muscle(s) activated, rather than to joint position.

3. The cerebellum regulates the rate, range, force, and direction of movements. It does this by using proprioceptive and other sensory information to compute body position, muscle length, and muscle tension. It compares the sensory information with motor commands that originate from the motor areas of the cortex, and corrects errors through its connections through the motor thalamus to the premotor and primary motor cortices. In addition to its cortical connections, the cerebellum influences cranial and spinal cord motor activity through brainstem motor relay nuclei. The cerebellum is also involved in motor learning.

4. The basal ganglia are involved in complex circuits that regulate motor activity less directly than does the cerebellum. Wide areas of the cerebral cortex connect with the basal ganglia. The basal ganglia feed information back to the supplementary motor and premotor areas through the motor thalamus. In contrast to the cerebellum, however, the basal ganglia do not receive direct input from somatosensory pathways, and they have a minimal influence on brainstem circuits. The basal ganglia also influence affective and cognitive functions.

5. (1) Some of the abnormalities that result from diseases of the cerebellum or its connections include ataxia and dysmetria, dysdiadochokinesia, decomposition of movement, intention tremor, scanning speech, and hypotonia with a pendular knee jerk. The abnormalities are expressed on the side ipsilateral to the damage.

(2) Some of the abnormalities that can result from basal ganglion disease include bradykinesia, rigidity, and pill-rolling tremor (Parkinson's disease; loss of monoaminergic neurons, especially dopaminergic neurons in the substantia nigra); chorea (as in Huntington's chorea, a genetic disorder involving the loss of cholinergic and GABAergic neurons of the striatum, as well as degeneration of the cerebral cortex); athetosis (commonly seen in cerebral palsy); ballism (due to damage to the subthalamic nucleus); and dystonia. The abnormalities are expressed on the side contralateral to the damage, because the motor dysfunction chiefly reflects changes in the output of the motor cortex.

■ *Chapter 15*

1. The functions of the sympathetic and parasympathetic nervous systems are characterized as cooperative rather than antagonistic. In some organs, the two systems exert opposite effects (e.g., pupillary dilation vs. pupillary constriction). However, the emphasis is better placed on the role of the two systems in regulating pupil size. In some organs, the two systems have comparable, although somewhat different, actions (e.g., activation of salivary glands to produce different consistencies of saliva). The body wall is supplied only by the sympathetic branch of the autonomic nervous system; the parasympathetic innervation is restricted to internal organs, which also have a sympathetic supply.

2. Visceral afferent fibers provide sensory innervation of the viscera. Some visceral afferents signal information to the central nervous system and the signal reaches consciousness, whereas others provide input that remains subconscious. Examples of visceral information that reaches consciousness include a sense of distention or flow and pain. Subconscious signals arise from baroreceptors, chemoreceptors, and other sensors, and they help in autonomic regulation of a variety of functions.

3. The afferent limb of the micturition reflex involves mechanoreceptors located in the urinary bladder wall. These receptors are sensitive to both stretch and contraction of the bladder wall musculature. These afferents activate ascending projections to the micturition center (Barrington's center) in the rostral pons, and they inhibit sympathetic preganglionic neurons that normally inhibit micturition. When sufficient activity develops in this pathway, á command is issued from the micturition center and is transmitted by reticulospinal neurons. This command further inhibits sympathetic neurons that inhibit the bladder, and it also activates parasympathetic neurons that supply the bladder and cause bladder contraction. Contraction of the bladder increases the activity in the circuit, and this activity normally results in complete emptying of the bladder.

4. The Klüver-Bucy syndrome is a behavioral disorder that results from bilateral lesions of the temporal lobes. In this syndrome, subjects are unable to use visual cues to recognize the meaning of objects, they tend to examine things by placing them in the mouth (oral tendency), they pay attention to irrelevant stimuli, they are hypersexual, their dietary habits change, and their emotionality is decreased. The visual system effects may reflect damage to visual areas of the temporal lobe. However, the changes in emotional behavior are probably caused by damage to the amygdaloid nuclei.

■ *Chapter 16*

1. The frontal lobe is involved in the planning and execution of motor behavior through actions of the primary motor, premotor, and supplementary motor areas and frontal eye fields. The motor aspects of language usage involve Broca's area, which is usually in the inferior frontal gyrus of the left frontal lobe. The prefrontal cortex is concerned with personality and emotional behavior.

   The parietal lobe processes somatosensory information in a manner that leads to the perception of touch, pressure, vibration, and position sense. It is also involved in pain and the thermal senses. The posterior parietal cortex transmits somatosensory, visual, and other sensory information to the frontal motor areas. The posterior parietal lobe in the nondominant hemisphere is involved in spatial analysis.

   The occipital lobe is largely concerned with visual processing and perception. The occipital eye field is involved in vergent eye movements, pupillary constriction, and accommodation.

   The temporal lobe functions include the processing and perception of sound and of vestibular information. There are several visual areas in this lobe. Those in the inferior temporal region are involved in color vision and in recognition of form, including that of faces. Others in the middle temporal region are involved in processing moving visual signals. Meyer's loop, a white matter structure important in visual processing, passes through the temporal lobe. Part of Wernicke's area is in the posterior part of the temporal lobe. This area is responsible for sensory processing of language. The medial temporal lobe belongs to the limbic system; part of it controls emotional behavior, and the hippocampus is involved in learning and memory.

2. The electroencephalogram (EEG) represents the summed synaptic potentials recorded extracellularly from millions of cortical neurons. It is recorded by placing one electrode against the skull and an indifferent electrode elsewhere. The EEG is strong enough to be recorded in this manner because of the orientation of many pyramidal cells perpendicular to the cortical surface. These neurons form dipoles that generate enough current to be detected at a substantial distance from their point of origin.

3. Evoked EEG potentials occur at a fixed latency after the stimulus that elicits them. The stimuli can be somatic (e.g., electrical stimulation of a peripheral nerve), visual (following a triggered flash of light), or auditory (elicited by a triggered sound). Recordings are made as with the standard EEG, although the placement of the electrode should relate to the cortical area that generates the evoked potential. The stimulus is repeated many times and the signal is stored in a device called a *signal averager*. This is a computer that stores and superimposes all of the recordings and aligns them at the time of the stimulus. The EEG is random in relation to the stimulus, and so the deflections eventually cancel out and thus yield a flat baseline. However, the evoked potential contributes a similar, if small, potential with the same waveform with each repetition of the stimulus. The summed waveforms after many recordings consist of the signal averaged evoked potential.

4. In rapid eye movement (REM) sleep, the EEG is desynchronized and resembles the EEG in the alert, awake subject. However, periodic bursts of high-voltage waves in the brain are associated with rapid eye movements (and movements of other muscles as well, as when a sleeping dog appears to be chasing rabbits). In REM sleep, muscle tone is flaccid and a number of autonomic events occur, including penile erection and transient changes in heart rate, blood pressure, and respiration. Dreams generally occur during REM sleep. In non-REM (or slow-wave sleep), the EEG is synchronized and consists of different frequency components that depend on the sleep stage. In stage 1, there are alpha and theta waves. In stage 2, slow waves are interrupted by sleep spindles and K complexes. In stages 3 and 4, there are numerous delta waves. The muscles of the body progressively relax, heart rate and blood pressure decrease, and gastrointestinal motility increases.

5. In motor aphasia, which is caused by damage to Broca's area (in the left inferior frontal gyrus), the expression of language (both spoken and written) is severely impaired. The person afflicted may only be able to utter expletives. However, comprehension is relatively intact. In sensory aphasia, which results from damage to Wernicke's area, motor expression of language is fluent. However, comprehension of written or spoken language is severely impaired, and the language expressed may include neologisms.

■ *Chapter 17*

1. Muscle 1 will develop half the force, but shorten twice as fast as muscle 2, because force is proportional to the cross-sectional area and velocity is proportional to the sum of all the sarcomeres connected in series.

2. There are important differences in the accessory, regulatory, or cytoskeletal proteins associated with thin filaments among muscle types. Presumably, this provides a role for actin isoforms. However, each actin monomer has many protein interactions (see Figs. 17-4 and 17-5, *B*). For example, in skeletal muscle, each actin monomer is associated with two adjacent actins in the same strand as well as with actins in the other strand of the polymerized actin helix, and with

tropomyosin and nebulin plus myosin during cross-bridge cycling. Any significant change in the actin conformation caused by sequence alterations will perturb one or more of these associations.

3. There must be transitions from a high actin affinity to a low affinity, and vice versa. Changes in the attached cross-bridge must alter the preferred conformation that minimizes the free energy. Structural linkages must also effectively couple the forces of individual cross-bridges and transmit them to the ends of the cells.

■ *Chapter 18*

1. (1) Neuromuscular transmission at the motor endplate causes depolarization and generation of an action potential propagated along the sarcolemma. (2) The action potential leads to a brief depolarization of the transverse tubular system. (3) Potential-dependent regulator proteins in the T-tubular membrane induce opening of closely associated Ca^{++} channels in the adjacent membrane of the sarcoplasmic reticulum. (4) Ca^{++} diffuses out of the sarcoplasmic reticulum into the myofibrils and binds to troponin, which is associated with tropomyosin in the thin filament. (5) Ca^{++} binding induces a conformational shift in the thin filament, and this shift allows cross-bridge attachment and cycling, which leads to force development or shortening. (6) The increase in the myoplasmic Ca^{++} concentration activates pumps that lower the myoplasmic Ca^{++} concentration by active transport back into the sarcoplasmic reticulum, where much of the Ca^{++} is bound to low-affinity binding sites. (7) The reduction of the myoplasmic Ca^{++} concentration allows dissociation of Ca^{++} from troponin, the thin filament returns to its "off" conformation, cross-bridge cycling ceases, and relaxation ensues.

2. The affinity of troponin for Ca^{++} is very high. Therefore, the $4Ca^{++}$-troponin complex persists during the period required for the pumps in the sarcoplasmic reticulum to reduce the myoplasmic Ca^{++} concentration to near resting levels. The result is that cross-bridges continue to cycle throughout most of the period when the free myoplasmic Ca^{++} concentration is falling.

3. They are innervated by a highly excitable (readily recruited) motor nerve with a small cell body and axon. Type I motor units contain relatively small numbers of muscle cells that have moderate cross-sectional areas and that are associated with many capillaries. Type I units have modest concentrations of glycolytic enzymes, but high mitochondrial contents that enable oxidative phosphorylation to supply ATP at a rate that matches consumption by the slow myosin isoform. The forces generated in a twitch are low, which reflects the small numbers of cells, their mod-

erate cross-sectional areas, and their slow contraction rates, causing twitch forces to be a fairly small fraction of the force in a tetanus.

4. Recruitment of more motor units and tetanization are the primary physiological factors. Changes in length are not a significant factor in most skeletal muscles, as the skeleton prevents major changes in length. In the body, contraction of antagonistic muscles in coordinated movements can modulate the expression of force by a contracting muscle.

■ *Chapter 19*

1. Imaging techniques cannot demonstrate that steady-state isometric force declines in proportion to thick and thin filament overlap at muscle lengths greater than L_o. However, the contractile system is based on isoforms of actin and myosin. Electron microscopy shows that thin filaments point away from each end of cytoskeletal structures (dense bodies), and that there is overlap between thick and thin filaments. The steady-state force-length and velocity-load relationships are qualitatively similar to those of skeletal muscle. Further, the measured single cross-bridge force and step sizes are the same as those estimated for skeletal muscle cross-bridges.

2. (1) The diverse inputs to the sarcolemma (innervation, hormones and signaling molecules generated by other cell types, and coupling between cells); (2) differences in the receptors, ion channels, and pumps in the sarcolemma that collectively allow precise regulation of the myoplasmic Ca^{++} concentration; (3) a covalent regulatory mechanism that can alter both the numbers of force-generating cross-bridges and their cycling rates; and (4) myosin heavy- and light-chain isoforms. Although myosin isoforms provide the main basis for diversity in skeletal muscle, their contributions to diversity appear to be less important than the other factors in smooth muscles.

3. (i) Four Ca^{++} ions bind to calmodulin. (ii) The $4Ca^{++}$-calmodulin complex binds and activates myosin kinase. (iii) The active $4Ca^{++}$-calmodulin-myosin kinase then phosphorylates cross-bridges at a specific site on the myosin regulatory light chain. (iv) The phosphorylated cross-bridge binds to actin and initiates a cycle.

4. Pumps and exchange mechanisms must extrude or sequester myoplasmic Ca^{++} so that its concentration in the myoplasm falls to levels at which the Ca^{++} bound to calmodulin dissociates and the myosin kinase is partially or fully inactivated. Myosin phosphatase dephosphorylates some or all of the phosphorylated cross-bridges and prevents or slows new attachments to the thin filaments, and hence force decays. Ca^{++} concentrations can fall as the result of a reduction in

excitatory signals to the sarcolemma, and/or greater inhibitory inputs that decrease membrane Ca^{++} channel permeability or stimulate Ca^{++} pumps.

5. The load is an important factor as it is in skeletal muscle. However, shortening velocities or rates of isometric force development are also proportional to crossbridge phosphorylation levels, so the level of activation is very important. Myosin isoforms appear to be less important in determining the rate of contraction in smooth muscle than in skeletal muscle.

■ *Chapter 20*

1. When small blood vessels are severed, the injury to the tissue elicits vasoconstriction of the arterioles by direct stimulation, and to some extent by stimulation of sympathetic nerve fibers in the region of the injury. Platelets adhere to the injured site of the cut vessels and release adenosine diphosphate (ADP) and thrombane A_2, which attracts more platelets, thereby "plugging up" the hole in the vessel. Finally, thromboplastin from the injured tissue initiates the cascade of clotting factors to form a clot that blocks further leakage of blood from the wound.

2. A universal donor is a person with group O blood and one whose blood can be given to any of the blood groups (O, A, B, or AB) because the blood plasma of all of these groups does not contain antibodies to group O cells. A universal recipient is a person with group AB blood and one who can receive blood from any of the blood groups because the blood plasma of people with AB blood does not have antibodies against the other blood groups. Transfusion of blood from a universal recipient to a universal donor will cause agglutination of the transfused red cells and a severe transfusion reaction that can be fatal. Other blood groups, such as Rh negative and Rh positive, must also be considered in blood transfusions.

■ *Chapter 21*

1. The arterioles have a thick, smooth muscle layer and a small internal diameter. Hence, changes in the contractile state of the vascular smooth muscle in response to alterations in sympathetic nerve activity or to the concentration of vasoactive substances can affect blood pressure when the response is widespread, and can affect the distribution of blood flow when the response is regional.

2. The venous system has a greater compliance than does the arterial system. Therefore, it takes more blood to fill the venous system than it does to fill the arterial system at any given filling pressure.

3. The velocity of the systemic circulation is greatest in the aorta and slowest in the capillaries. This is so because the total cross-sectional area of the vasculature is smallest in the aorta and largest in the capillaries, and the entire cardiac output must flow through all segments of the vascular tree per unit of time.

4. Blood is pulsatile in the arterial system because of the intermittent ejection of blood by the left ventricle. Blood flow becomes nonpulsatile (steady flow) in the capillaries because (1) the pulsations are partially damped by the elastic arteries and (2) further damping is caused by frictional resistance in the arterioles and small arteries.

■ *Chapter 22*

1. In a fast-response myocyte, the resting transmembrane potential during phase 4 remains constant (at about -90 mV). Thus, no appreciable ion flux takes place. The membrane is most permeable to K^+ during phase 4, but the ratio of extracellular to intracellular K^+ concentration is close to the equilibrium value defined by the Nernst equation for this ion. Thus, the driving force that tends to move K^+ across the cell membrane is very small. When the cell is stimulated to depolarize, the steep upstroke (phase 1) of the action potential is associated with an abrupt opening of the fast Na^+ channels. Consequently, Na^+ rushes into the cell, and the charge on the cell membrane reverses very quickly; the interior of the cell is positive to the exterior. These Na^+ channels inactivate very quickly, however, and Na^+ influx ceases. The transient outward K^+ channels are activated, and the outward flux of K^+ leads to early partial repolarization (phase 1). The Ca^{++} channels are activated during the action potential upstroke, and Ca^{++} begins to enter the cell. The influx of Ca^{++} triggers the release of Ca^{++} from the sarcoplasmic reticulum, an important step in excitation-contraction coupling of cardiac cells. For about 100 to 300 msec the influx of charge carried by Ca^{++} is counterbalanced by the efflux of charge carried by K^+. Therefore, the inside of the cell remains at a fairly constant positive potential of about $+10$ to $+20$ mV; this is the plateau (phase 2). Near the end of the plateau, the efflux of charge carried by K^+ begins to exceed the influx of charge carried by Ca^{++}, and late, full repolarization (phase 3) begins. As repolarization proceeds, K^+ conductance increases, and the rate of repolarization accelerates until the cell is fully repolarized. This constitutes phase 4 again, and the cycle is completed.

2. An atrioventricular (AV) node cell is a slow-response fiber, whereas atrial and ventricular myocytes are fast-response fibers. In a myocyte the upstroke of the action potential is much steeper and the amplitude much greater than are the respective characteristics in an AV node cell. The steep upstroke in a myocyte

reflects the rapid inrush of Na^+ through fast Na^+ channels. The rapid Na^+ flux at one point in the cell membrane of a myocyte allows a more rapid change in potential in an adjacent point in the membrane (i.e., it allows a more rapid propagation) than would prevail in the cell membrane of an AV node cell, in which the upstroke is achieved by the relatively slow influx of Ca^{++}. Furthermore, the greater amplitude of the action potential in a myocyte permits the electrotonic spread of potential to extend a greater distance down the fiber than is true for an AV node cell, which has a smaller-amplitude action potential. The greater electronic spread of excitation in the myocyte allows fibers at a greater distance from the reference point to be depolarized more expeditiously. Thus, in a cell (e.g., myocyte) whose action potential has a greater amplitude, the cardiac impulse is propagated more rapidly than in a cell (e.g., AV node fiber) whose action potential has a smaller amplitude.

3. The cardiac impulse is ordinarily generated by automatic cells in the sinoatrial (SA) node. It then passes through the perinodal tissues and radiates through the atrial tissues. When the wave front reaches the AV node, it proceeds slowly through the node and then accelerates greatly when it reaches the bundle of His, in the interventricular septum. From this bundle, it spreads rapidly through the Purkinje fiber network in the endocardial region of both ventricles, and then spreads from endocardium to epicardium via ventricular myocardial fibers.

4. The electrophysiological conditions that favor reentry are slow conduction and unidirectional block within the reentry loop. Furthermore, the refractory period of the reentered region must be less than the propagation time around the reentry loop. If conduction velocity is diminished in one region of the heart, an impulse that traverses this region will require more time to reach the more distal region. Hence, this distal region is more likely to have recovered its excitability, and therefore the tardy impulse may be able to reenter the original zone. Similarly, if one or more cardiac chambers are enlarged, the cardiac impulse has a longer path to traverse. Thus, the time required to traverse that path will be prolonged. If the path forms a loop, this longer time around the loop may allow sufficient time for the myocytes at the beginning of the loop to regain their excitability by the time the impulse completes the circuit. Reentrant rhythms do occur more commonly in enlarged ventricles or atria. Finally, unidirectional block in some region of the heart is an important factor in reentry. If two impulses traveling in opposite directions invade this region and both impulses are conducted, they would collide and extinguish each other (each would arrive at a region that was absolutely refractory as a consequence of the passage of the other impulse). However, if only one of the impulses traverses this region of unidirectional block, it might arrive at the opposite end and thus reenter that region, after the myocardial cells there had recovered their excitability.

5. First-degree AV block is characterized by an abnormally long PR interval. In second-degree AV block, not every P wave is followed by an R wave; i.e., some atrial impulses are not conducted to the ventricles. In third-degree AV block, none of the atrial impulses reach the ventricles; the P waves and R waves are independent of each other.

■ *Chapter 23*

1. Although not an anatomic syncytium, the heart behaves as if it were one; stimulation of the heart elicits an all-or-none response. Excitation spreads from cell to cell via gap junctions, and during the plateau of the action potential, some calcium enters the cells through the calcium channels and triggers the release of calcium from the sarcoplasmic reticulum. The calcium complexes with troponin C, and the Ca^{++} troponin C complex interacts with tropomyosin to unblock active sites between actin and myosin; this interaction permits enhanced cross-bridge cycling.

2. The preload is the degree of ventricular filling (distending pressure) reached by the end of diastole; the afterload is the aortic pressure during ventricular ejection. Increases in preload increase developed pressure. Increases in afterload decrease the velocity of contraction. Velocity is maximal at zero afterload.

3. Myocardial contractility can be gauged by (1) the slope of the upstroke of the ventricular pressure curve (change in pressure with time, dP/dt), (2) the initial velocity of the aortic flow curve, and (3) the ejection fraction (ratio of volume ejected per beat to the volume of blood in the ventricle at the end of diastole).

4. The pericardium restricts acute dilation of the heart but stretches with gradual enlargement of the heart or during the formation of pericardial effusion. Normally, the thin layer of fluid between the visceral and parietal layers of the pericardium serves as a lubricant for movement of the heart within the pericardial sac. In some disease states (e.g., tubercular pericarditis) the pericardium can become rigid and even calcified; such a condition can impair cardiac filling and thus reduce cardiac output.

5. In mitral stenosis the murmur is caused by the turbulence created during left ventricular filling, particularly during left atrial contraction when blood is forced through the stenotic mitral valve. Hence, the murmur just precedes the first heart sound. It is characteristically a rumbling crescendo murmur that ends with the first heart sound.

6.

$$\text{Cardiac output} = \frac{O_2 \text{ consumption/min}}{(A - V) \; O_2 \text{ difference}} = \frac{280}{0.19 - 0.12}$$

$$= 4 \text{ L/min}$$

Myocardial O_2 consumption =

$(A - V) \; O_2 \text{ difference} \times \text{coronary blood flow} = 0.14 \times 150$

$$= 21 \text{ ml/min}$$

■ *Chapter 24*

1. a. When the vagus nerves are stimulated, the heart rate diminishes promptly to a new level; it then returns very quickly to the control level when stimulation ceases. The response is so rapid because the acetylcholine (ACh)-regulated K^+ channels that help mediate the response do not require a second messenger, but these channels are activated more directly via a G protein. Also, the response decays so quickly after vagal activity ceases because acetylcholinesterase is abundant in the SA node, and it hydrolyzes the neurally released ACh very rapidly.

   b. In response to sympathetic stimulation, the heart rate rises gradually to its steady-state value, and when stimulation ceases the heart rate decays very gradually to its control level. Two factors account for the gradual rise in heart rate in response to stimulation. First, a relatively slow second messenger system (the adenylyl cyclase system) is involved in the cascade of events that lead to the change in heart rate. Second, the cardiac sympathetic nerves release norepinephrine (NE) at a relatively slow rate. The response decays gradually after cessation of stimulation because the main processes (active neuronal reuptake and diffusion into the myocardial capillaries) that remove neurally released NE from the cardiac tissues are slow.

2. When the cardiac sympathetic and vagus nerves are stimulated simultaneously, the vagal effects on heart rate usually predominate. This is because the main neurotransmitters (NE and ACh) that mediate the cardiac response are both released simultaneously, and each inhibits the neuronal release of the other. However, the neuronal action of the ACh is much more rapid than the neuronal action of the NE. Therefore, very soon after the onset of stimulation, the vagally released ACh has markedly suppressed the release of NE from the sympathetic nerves. Therefore, the response to simultaneous stimulation is often equivalent to the response to vagal stimulation alone.

3. The rise in arterial blood pressure induced by a vasoconstrictor drug stimulates the arterial baroreceptors in the carotid sinus and aortic arch. Consequently, the activity in the efferent sympathetic fibers to the heart and blood vessels diminishes, whereas the activity in the efferent vagal fibers to the heart increases.

4. Rapid intravenous infusion of blood first increases the venous return to the right ventricle. The consequent diastolic stretching of the right ventricle increases its stroke volume by the Frank-Starling mechanism. The increase in right ventricular stroke volume then increases the left ventricular end-diastolic volume, and the left ventricular stroke volume then increases. The time delay between the increments in right and left ventricular stroke volume is only the duration of two or three heartbeats.

5. Left atrial pressure usually exceeds right atrial pressure, for reasons explained in relation to Fig. 24-20. If an opening were created in the interatrial septum, the left-to-right pressure differential would cause some blood to flow from the left to the right atrium through the interatrial septal defect. Hence, right atrial pressure would tend to rise and left atrial pressure would tend to fall. Consequently, right ventricular stroke volume would increase and left ventricular stroke volume would decrease. At equilibrium, right ventricular stroke volume would exceed left ventricular stroke volume by the amount of flow shunted from the left to the right atrium with each heartbeat.

6. The stroke volume ejected by the ventricles is markedly reduced during a premature ventricular beat; sometimes the premature contraction is so feeble that the peak intraventricular pressure does not exceed the prevailing arterial pressure, and no blood is ejected by the ventricle during that contraction. Conversely, the postextrasystolic contraction is much stronger than the normal beat, and stroke volume may greatly exceed the normal stroke volume. Two major factors account for these changes in stroke volume. The first involves the Frank-Starling mechanism. With regard to the premature beat, the ventricles have insufficent time to fill adequately, and thus the subsequent contraction is weaker than normal. During the long pause between the premature and postextrasystolic beats, ventricular filling is greater than normal, and consequently the stroke volume is greater than normal. A second, less well understood mechanism also contributes to the changes in stroke volume, because substantial changes in ventricular contraction have been shown to occur in experimental isovolumic preparations, in which changes in ventricular filling are precluded (Fig. 24-23). The weak premature contraction and the strong postextrasystolic contraction are produced in part by disparities in Ca^{++} release from the sarcoplasmic reticulum; such disparities are presumed to be associated with a substantial time delay in transfer of Ca^{++} from an uptake compartment to a release compartment of the sarcoplasmic reticulum.

■ *Chapter 25*

1. The resistance to blood flow through one kidney equals the mean arterial pressure (100 mm Hg) divided by the blood flow (200 ml/min), or 0.5 mm Hg/ml/min; we shall assume that the renal venous pressure is approximately zero. The reciprocal of the resistance (R_t) to flow through both kidneys equals the sum of the reciprocals of the resistances (R_1 and R_r) of the left and right kidneys (the kidneys are aligned in parallel). That is, $1/R_t = 1/R_1 + 1/R_r$. Therefore, $R_t = 0.25$ mm Hg/ml/min. The hydraulic resistance of the two kidneys in parallel is less than the resistance of either kidney alone, because when both kidneys are being perfused, the blood can flow through twice as many parallel channels than when only one of the kidneys is being perfused.

2. A murmur in the cardiovascular system denotes that flow is turbulent in some part of the system. Reynold's number denotes some of the factors that lead to turbulence; the tendency for flow to be turbulent increases directly with the velocity of flow and inversely with the fluid viscosity. In severe anemia, the velocity of blood flow around the body is much greater than normal, and the viscosity of the blood is much less than normal.

3. The flow of blood in a blood vessel exerts a "viscous drag" on the endothelial lining of the blood vessels; it tends to pull the endothelium in the direction of the flowing blood. In a dissecting aneurysm of the aorta, a tear exists in the endothelial lining; the tear tends to be oriented at right angles to the long axis of the vessel. If a small tear exists in the endothelial lining of the aorta, the flowing blood pulls the distal lip of the tear caudally and may thereby extend the tear. This tendency will be more pronounced as the blood flow in the aorta increases. A dissecting aortic aneurysm is usually treated surgically, but before surgery the physician administers a drug (e.g., a β-adrenergic receptor antagonist) to lower the patient's arterial blood pressure and diminish the aortic flow (or cardiac output), in order to reduce the tendency to extend the tear in the aortic wall.

4. In the large arteries and veins, the suspended particles (such as red and white blood cells) are fairly evenly distributed over the cross-section of the vessel. However, in blood vessels with cross-sectional areas only a few times greater than the average diameter of the blood cells, the blood cells tend to be highly concentrated axially and the plasma is more concentrated near the vascular walls. However, the axial laminae of the bloodstream move much more rapidly than do the peripheral laminae. Because the more centrally located cells move more quickly than does the more peripherally located plasma, the ratio of cells to plasma (and therefore the hematocrit ratio) is less in the small blood vessels than in the large blood vessels.

■ *Chapter 26*

1. The arteries in patients with atherosclerosis are less compliant than in normal subjects, and hence less blood can be stored in the arteries during systole. Consequently, the heart must pump a greater flow during systole through the resistance vessels (small arteries and arterioles), and thus the heart must work harder than normal. The myocardium therefore needs a greater coronary blood flow to furnish more oxygen and nutrients than would be required in a subject with normal arteries.

2. Mean arterial pressure depends only on cardiac output and total peripheral resistance (TPR). Hence, mean arterial pressure would be the same in the two subjects. Because the cardiac outputs are the same in the two individuals, stroke volume must be much greater in the person with a heart rate of 45 beats/min than in the person with a heart rate of 75 beats/min. Therefore, the quantity of blood pumped into the aorta during the rapid ejection phase of systole would be much greater in the person with the slower heart rate. Consequently, the arterial pressure oscillation with each heartbeat about the mean arterial pressure level would be greater in the person with the greater stroke volume than in the other person; that is, the maximal arterial pressure (systolic pressure) would be greater and the minimal pressure (diastolic pressure) would be less in the former than in the latter individual.

3. Because the 20- and 70-year old subjects had the same cardiac output, heart rate, and TPR under basal conditions, their mean arterial pressures must have been the same. Because the vasoconstrictor drug elicited the same (50%) increase in TPR in the two subjects, their mean arterial pressures must have increased by 50%. A rise in arterial pressure in general tends to decrease arterial compliance, but the reduction in compliance is ordinarily much more pronounced in older than in younger subjects. After the drug had elevated the arterial pressure, therefore, a given stroke volume ejected into the less compliant aorta of the older subject would produce a greater pressure oscillation (from the diastolic to the systolic pressure level) in the older than in the younger subject. Consequently, the systolic pressure would be higher and the diastolic pressure lower in the older subject.

4. The mean arterial pressures would be identical in the normal person and in the patient with aortic valve insufficiency, because mean arterial pressure depends only on cardiac output and TPR. However, the "volume increment" (i.e., the volume of blood ejected by the left ventricle during the rapid ejection phase of systole, minus the volume of blood that leaves the arteries through the resistance vessels during this same phase of systole) would be much greater in the patient than in the normal individual. The volume

increment would be much greater in the patient because blood leaks back into the ventricle during diastole. Consequently, the greater diastolic filling leads to an augmented stroke volume (Frank-Starling mechanism). Hence, the patient's systolic pressure would be substantially greater and the diastolic pressure would be less than in the normal person.

■ *Chapter 27*

1. Capillary blood flow is influenced by mean arterial pressure, precapillary resistance, and postcapillary resistance. When the cognate arterioles dilate, as occurs with section of sympathetic nerves to the vessels, or in response to local vasodilator metabolites, greater pressure is applied to blood in the capillaries, and the velocity of flow increases; arteriolar constriction has the opposite effect. An increase in venous pressure, as may occur in heart failure, is transmitted back to the capillaries and reduces the velocity of flow. An increase in blood viscosity, as occurs in polycythemia, also slows the velocity of blood flow in the capillaries. No active changes in capillary diameter occur because capillaries cannot independently constrict or dilate.

2. The reason the capillaries in the feet do not rupture when a person stands is explained in terms of the law of Laplace: $T = Pr$, where T = wall tension, P = transmural pressure, and r = capillary radius. Although the pressure within the capillaries may reach very high levels, the small diameter of the capillaries "compensates" for the high pressure, and the increase in wall tension is very small relative to that of a large artery, like the aorta, at a similar transmural pressure.

3. The capillary will absorb fluid because the forces moving fluid from the interstitial space into the capillary lumen (plasma oncotic pressure plus tissue hydrostatic pressure) exceed the forces favoring filtration (capillary hydrostatic pressure plus tissue oncotic pressure) by 7 mm Hg.

4. Flow-limited transport means that lipid-insoluble, small solute molecules that pass through the capillary pores can move from capillary lumen to interstitial space faster than they are transported to the capillary by the flowing blood. Diffusion-limited transport means that the lipid-insoluble molecules are large enough to be partially or completely prevented from passing through the capillary pores, regardless of the rate at which they are brought to the capillaries by the flowing blood.

5. Lipid-insoluble solutes of small molecular size (e.g., NaCl, glucose) pass through capillary pores about 4 Å in diameter, whereas lipid-soluble molecules (e.g., CO_2 and O_2) pass directly through the endothelial cells as well as through the pores. Large lipid-insoluble molecules that cannot get through the capillary pores may be transported across the capillary endothelial cells by pinocytosis.

6. Albumin that has entered the interstitial space cannot be taken up directly by the capillaries because of the opposing concentration gradient and the endothelial barrier. Albumin enters the lymph capillaries, whose openings are facilitated by fine filaments that pull the lymphatic endothelial cells apart when the tissue moves, as in muscle contraction and relaxation. The albumin, along with interstitial fluid, travels through the lymphatic system. Its passage is aided by contraction of the lymphatic vessels, which have valves that prevent backflow, and by muscle contraction (squeezing of the vessels in the tissue). The lymph fluid moves through vessels of increasing size and finally enters the circulating blood at the junction of the subclavian and internal jugular veins.

■ *Chapter 28*

1. Autoregulation of blood flow describes the constancy of blood flow to an organ during alteration in perfusion pressure (blood pressure). When the metabolic activity of an organ is constant, an abrupt increase in perfusion pressure produces an immediate increase in blood flow. However, if the perfusion pressure is held at the new elevated level, blood flow gradually returns to or toward the control level within a minute. With abrupt decreases in perfusion pressure, blood flow initially decreases but then increases to or toward the control level. Studies on isolated arterioles suggest that a myogenic mechanism is responsible for autoregulation; that is, stretch of the vascular smooth muscle (increased transmural pressure) elicits contraction (increased resistance), whereas a decrease in transmural pressure elicits relaxation (decreased resistance).

2. The endothelium can synthesize vasoactive substances that act locally on the vascular smooth muscle of the resistance vessels. Known vasodilator substances that can be released by the endothelium are nitric oxide, prostacyclin, and adenosine. The endothelium is also the source of endothelin, a powerful vasoconstrictor.

3. Vascular tone refers to the partially contracted state of vascular smooth muscle in the resistance vessels. It is in part attributable to tonic activity of the sympathetic nerves that innervate the arterioles and small arteries, and also to an intrinsic factor in the vascular smooth muscle that becomes evident after interruption of the vessel innervation. The intrinsic factor causes a partial contraction that is called basal tone; its cause has not been elucidated.

4. In resting skeletal muscle, blood flow is low and largely under sympathetic neural control. The low blood flow is commensurate with the low metabolic

activity of the resting muscle. With muscle contractions, the increased metabolic activity engenders the local release of vasodilator metabolites. These metabolites dilate the resistance vessels and thereby produce an increase in blood flow in the active muscle (active hyperemia). This local mechanism can override the vasoconstriction produced by activation of the sympathetic nerves to the blood vessels.

5. When pressure within the carotid sinuses decreases, as may occur with blood loss, the number of impulses traveling up the sinus nerve and glossopharyngeal nerve to the medulla decreases. The vasomotor (vasoconstrictor) center becomes less inhibited, and the resultant increase in sympathetic activity causes arteriolar constriction and an increase in peripheral resistance. Heart rate and myocardial contractility are also increased. These factors operate to return blood pressure to the normal level. An increase in pressure in the carotid sinuses has the opposite effect.

■ *Chapter 29*

1. The answer to both questions is "Yes." Not only does preload determine cardiac performance, but also cardiac performance determines preload. The preload is the filling pressure for the ventricles, and the extent of filling is an important determinant of the mechanical performance of the ventricles. As the myocardial cells are progressively stretched, calcium sensitivity of the myofilaments is augmented, and cardiac performance is enhanced. This association (the cardiac function curve) indicates that cardiac output is directly related to the preload. It is equally true, however, that the inverse relationship also applies. As cardiac performance is enhanced, the attendant increase in cardiac output will increase the volume of blood contained in the arterial side of the vascular system. If total blood volume remains constant, any increment in arterial blood volume will induce an equivalent decrement in the venous blood volume. Hence, central venous pressure (preload) will diminish. This association (the vascular function curve) indicates that preload is inversely related to cardiac output.

2. Arterial blood pressure is not precisely equivalent to the ventricular afterload (because ventricular geometry is also a factor), but arterial blood pressure is the predominant determinant of the afterload. Arterial blood pressure is the main counterforce that opposes the ejection of blood by the contracting ventricle. This counterforce to any specific ventricular contraction has been built up as a result of the preceding ventricular contractions. Thus, the counterforce to ventricular ejection has been generated by the ventricle itself. This process is analogous to the compression of a coiled spring: as a person gradually compresses the

spring, it exerts a greater and greater counterforce to further compression.

3. Isoproterenol enhances myocardial contractility by increasing the Ca^{++} conductance of the myocyte cell membranes, and thereby augmenting the influx of Ca^{++}. Consequently, the ventricle pumps a greater cardiac output from any given filling pressure (preload). As cardiac output increases, more of the blood volume tends to be sequestered on the arterial side of the circuit, and therefore less of the blood volume is located on the venous side of the circuit. Consequently, central venous pressure diminishes, but cardiac output increases.

4. The infused blood would be distributed to the arterial and venous segments of the vascular system. The increased venous volume results in a greater ventricular filling pressure, and this increases cardiac output. The increased arterial blood volume increases afterload, but in general the inverse effect of afterload on cardiac output tends to be much less pronounced than the direct effects of preload on cardiac output. The net result of the blood transfusion is an increase in cardiac output, central venous pressure, and mean arterial pressure.

5. Cardiac output equals stroke volume (SV) times heart rate (HR). When HR is only 35 beats/min, SV usually cannot increase sufficiently (mainly because of the limitation to filling associated with the pericardium and the compliance characteristics of the ventricles). Therefore, when HR is very low, cardiac output is subnormal. A low cardiac output redistributes blood volume from the arterial to the venous segments of the vascular system, and therefore central venous pressure tends to be elevated.

6. When a person on a tilt table is rotated to the upright position, gravity increases the pressure in the vessels in the dependent regions of the body. Consequently, the pressure rises considerably in the veins of the legs and feet, and a substantial volume of blood is sequestered in the veins in this region. The hemodynamic results are similar to those that would be seen if an equivalent volume of blood were lost from the body (hemorrhage). Therefore, cardiac output, mean arterial pressure, and central venous pressure would all be diminished.

■ *Chapter 30*

1. Stimulation of the cardiac sympathetic nerves has several effects on the heart. Heart rate, contractility, and the speed of impulse conduction in the heart are all increased. The primary effect on the coronary resistance vessels is vasoconstriction. However, the increase in metabolic activity releases vasodilator substances from the myocardium. The arteriolar dila-

tion that ensues overrides the neural-mediated vasoconstriction, and the net effect is an increase in coronary blood flow. The same effects on coronary blood flow occur in the perfused fibrillating heart, in which the extravascular compression factor is eliminated.

2. Metabolic regulation of coronary blood flow means that the flow is adjusted to the metabolic (oxygen) needs of the myocardium. When the heart works harder, coronary blood flow increases even if there is no increase in coronary perfusion pressure (blood pressure). In other words, the ratio of oxygen supply to oxygen need is important in the regulation of coronary blood flow. A decrease in this ratio, caused by either a decrease in supply (e.g., hypoxemia or partial coronary occlusion) or an increase in need (e.g., exercise), elicits the release of a vasodilator substance (e.g., adenosine) that dilates the resistance vessels and tends to restore the balance between oxygen supply and demand.

3. The net effect of tachycardia on coronary blood flow is an increase in flow secondary to the enhanced metabolism of the myocardium. Opposing the "metabolic vasodilation" is the extravascular compression of the coronary vessels by the contracting cardiac muscle. In tachycardia, the heart spends more time per minute in systole (when the vessels are compressed in the left ventricular muscle) than it does at normal heart rates. However, the effect of this increase in extravascular compression (or extravascular resistance) is small relative to the effect of the metabolic vasodilation. In bradycardia, the reverse occurs. Oxygen needs are reduced, and although extravascular compression is less, the net effect is an increase in coronary resistance and a decrease in coronary blood flow.

4. If reductions in coronary blood flow are sufficiently severe and prolonged, cardiac dysfunction will be caused mainly by the necrosis (death) of myocardial cells. However, if the reduction of coronary flow is neither prolonged nor severe, the cardiac contractility may be depressed only temporarily. A relatively brief period of severe ischemia, followed by reperfusion, may be associated with a pronounced mechanical dysfunction of the heart, which eventually will fully recover. This "myocardial stunning" is produced by Ca^{++} overload of the cardiac cells during the ischemic period, combined with the generation of free radicals during the period of reperfusion. During prolonged periods of moderate ischemia, "myocardial hibernation" may prevail. The impaired mechanical function of the heart is associated with a reduction in the metabolic activity of the myocardial cells. This biochemical response tends to preserve the viability of certain cells.

5. In muscle at rest, blood flow is chiefly regulated by the sympathetic nerves to the muscle resistance vessels. In exercise, however, local (metabolic) factors supervene and blood flow increases, within limits, to meet the oxygen needs of the tissue. In skin, the major adjustments in blood flow help maintain a constant body temperature. Hence, skin blood flow (reflexly or directly) increases when there is a need to lose body heat, as in exercise or in a warm environment, and decreases when there is a need to conserve heat, as in a cold environment. Skin also serves as a blood reservoir. In hemorrhage or exhausting exercise, vasoconstriction occurs in the skin, thereby reducing the size of the total vascular bed and providing more blood to be pumped to essential organs such as the brain and heart.

6. Cerebral blood flow is remarkably constant, and because the brain is in a rigid structure, blood flow is affected by extravascular pressure, as well as by intravascular pressure. The autonomic nervous system exerts a minimal effect on cerebrovascular resistance. The primary regulatory factor is the metabolic activity of the brain tissue. An increase in brain metabolic rate (e.g., in seizures) or a decrease in oxygen supply (e.g., in hypoxia) causes an increase in cerebral blood flow by the release of a vasodilator substance (e.g., adenosine).

7. Chronic inflammation of the liver (hepatic cirrhosis) encroaches upon the blood vessels and sinusoids in the liver and elevates hepatic vascular resistance. The resultant elevation in portal venous pressure leads to esophageal varices and to extensive fluid transudation (ascites) from the splanchnic capillaries into the abdominal cavity. A portacaval shunt is often created surgically to alleviate these serious problems associated with a substantial elevation of portal venous pressure.

8. In the fetus, most of the right ventricular output passes through the ductus arteriosus and thus bypasses the lungs. When the lungs become filled with air, the resistance to blood flow through the lung vessels falls sharply. This decrease in lung vascular resistance in the newborn, in conjunction with closure of the ductus arteriosus by the higher oxygen pressure in the blood, directs right ventricular output through the pulmonary vessels.

■ *Chapter 31*

1. The primary cardiovascular change in exercise is the increase in heart rate, which facilitates the increase in cardiac output. In a sedentary person only a small increase in stroke volume occurs. In a trained individual, heart rate also increases to the same maximal level, but stroke volume is greater at rest and increases further (before heart rate reaches a maximum) during exercise. Hence, the trained athlete can achieve a greater cardiac output. Vascular resistance in the

active muscle decreases, producing a decrease in total peripheral resistance (TPR). However, despite this decrease in TPR, blood pressure increases a little because of the large increase in cardiac output. Oxygen extraction from blood perfusing the active muscles is increased, which results in an increase in the arteriovenous oxygen difference.

2. The limiting factor in the performance of whole body exercise is the pumping ability of the heart. Neither the ability of the active muscles to consume oxygen nor the oxygen-carrying capacity of the blood is limiting. Therefore, the supply of oxygen is a function of the amount of blood brought to the active muscles. Thus, with the vessels in the active muscles maximally dilated, the only way to transport more oxygen to the muscles is to increase cardiac output.

3. The arterial baroreceptor reflex is a very important mechanism for protecting the body from the effects of blood loss. When the baroreceptors signal a decline in arterial blood pressure, the reflex response is generalized arteriolar vasoconstriction, increased cardiac contractility, and increased heart rate, all of which attenuate the change in blood pressure evoked by the loss of blood. Other important mechanisms are the release of endogenous vasoconstrictors (vasopressin, angiotensin II, catecholamines), renal conservation of water and electrolytes, and the transfer of fluid from the interstitial and intracellular fluid compartments to the intravascular compartment.

4. Many factors act to aggravate the hypotension induced by blood loss. For example, the decreased arterial blood pressure tends to diminish coronary blood flow, which in turn tends to impair myocardial contractility. Diminished blood flow to the tissues generally leads to metabolic acidosis, and this in turn depresses myocardial contractility. Diminished cerebral blood flow tends to impair cerebral function, and thereby to depress the various reflex compensatory mechanisms. Aberrations of blood coagulation may lead initially to increased coagulability. The resulting disseminated intravascular clotting will then impair the circulation to the peripheral tissues. Subsequent impairment of coagulability may lead to internal hemorrhage and thereby aggravate the effects of the initiating hemorrhage. Depression of the reticuloendothelial system may allow endotoxins to invade the cardiovascular system. The subsequent induction of nitric oxide synthase in the vessels may lead to generalized vasodilation and profound hypotension.

▪ *Chapter 32*

1. The blood vessels usually accompany the airways, and each vessel is about half the diameter of the adjacent airway. The airways receive parasympathetic (cholinergic) motor innervation to their smooth muscle; the vessels receive sympathetic (adrenergic) innervation to their smooth muscle. The most important physiological difference is that ventilation is tidal (back and forth) whereas perfusion is unidirectional. Other differences are that the airways conduct a gas mixture, whereas the blood vessels conduct a non-Newtonian liquid.

2. The bronchial circulation is vital in nourishing the lung and maintaining its viability. However, a pulmonary arterial blockage is not accompanied by a venous obstruction, so blood may ebb and flow in the small pulmonary vessels with cardiac action or breathing. This movement of the blood provides some tissue nourishment. Oxygenation of lung tissue is not a problem, because the alveoli are full of gas at a high P_{O_2} of 100 mm Hg. Furthermore, the bronchial circulation provides some blood flow to the lung tissues even though pulmonary arterial vessels may be occluded.

3. This problem is crucial to an understanding of how the lung is ventilated. The entire lung moves caudally, not just that part near the diaphragm. The lower lung pulls on the upper lung as it expands. This can be seen by comparing chest x-ray films when the lungs are at functional residual capacity (FRC) and total lung capacity (TLC); the tracheal branch point (carina) moves caudally. Thus, all alveoli expand.

4. As the total barometric pressure falls, gases dissolved or chemically bound within blood or cells form bubbles and the loose interstitial connective tissue swells. In deep sea divers, this condition is called the *bends*. Because water boils at an ambient pressure of 47 mm Hg, body parts will also swell with water vapor bubbles. In some experiments conducted in the former Soviet Union on baboons, the skin ballooned up in the forearms that were exposed to explosive decompression in a special chamber. If the ambient pressure was restored quickly, the arm returned to normal size, apparently without permanent damage. Explosive decompression will almost instantly expand the gas in the lungs or intestinal tract. When an airliner decompresses, if a passenger cannot expire the pulmonary gases quickly enough, the expanding alveoli may rupture the lungs and cause a **tension pneumothorax** (the pleural space will be filled with air under pressure). The pain of gas expansion in the gut can be excruciating.

▪ *Chapter 33*

1. The problem for the skin diver is not different from the sudden decompression in a high-flying aircraft, except that in the diver the compressive pressure is 10×760 mm Hg = 7600 mm Hg. This enormous pressure will severely compress the chest and abdomen. Most of the blood volume and the abdominal contents will be

forced up into the chest, and the lung volume will be severely reduced by the high external pressure. Cardiac output will be zero, because the high external pressure will compress blood vessels throughout the body.

2. The person involved is on artificial positive end-expiratory pressure (PEEP) respiration or the airways are so narrowed that the alveolar gas cannot be expelled in the time available during expiration.

3. One need only use equation 33-10 to account for laminar and turbulent flow in an adult. Thus, P = (2.4 × 5) + (0.03 × 5²) = 12.0 + 0.75 = 12.75 cm H$_2$O. This pressure is much higher than the resting value, but it is not excessive. The turbulence factor (0.03 $\dot{V}^2$) is less than 1 cm H$_2$O.

4. The reader should use the alveolar ventilation equation and the alveolar gas equation. If one breathes very rapidly, the work of breathing is increased, and for each breath the anatomic dead space accounts for its usual fraction. With fast breathing, the tidal volume tends to decrease. Suppose the respiratory rate is 60/min. If alveolar ventilation does increase fourfold, PA$_{CO_2}$ will decrease to 10 cm H$_2$O. At the high respiratory frequency, however, alveolar ventilation will decrease substantially, because a full breath cannot be inhaled and exhaled in 1 second. Thus, much of the gas that enters the alveoli during inspiration will be dead space air.

 Breathing too slowly, of course, reduces alveolar ventilation, and PA$_{CO_2}$ will rise, unless each tidal volume increases sufficiently. However, at very slow respiratory rates, such as 1/min, each tidal volume will need to be more than 4 L to maintain normal CO$_2$ levels. The tendency will be to hypoventilate, allowing PA$_{CO_2}$ to rise and PA$_{O_2}$ to fall somewhat. One advantage of slow breathing over rapid breathing is that the anatomic dead space fraction of each breath is reduced. The deep breaths do affect alveolar surface tension also, but this is a minor factor.

Chapter 34

1. Because of partial pressure differences, the underventilated lung has a low CO$_2$ and therefore CO$_2$ diffuses into the alveoli. However, the alveolar oxygen tension is above normal and equal to the P$_{O_2}$ of arterial blood. The gradient for O$_2$ diffusion from arterial blood to alveoli is not significant.

2. If nitric oxide (NO) does not reach the involved vessels, it cannot have any effect. An obstruction of an airway would prevent the NO from reaching the pulmonary vessels to the region of the lung affected by the airway obstruction. A physical vascular obstruction, such as a pulmonary embolus, would not be affected by NO vasodilation. A fixed pulmonary

hypertension with narrowing, fibrosis, or loss of vessels is not treatable by NO.

3. The three congenital defects are (1) atrial septal defect, (2) ventricular septal defect, and (3) patent ductus arteriosus (between the aorta and pulmonary artery).

Chapter 35

1. The immediate effect of the low arterial P$_{O_2}$ is for the subject to breathe faster and deeper, which raises alveolar P$_{O_2}$ a little. The increased alveolar ventilation lowers PA$_{CO_2}$, lowers blood [H$^+$], and shifts the HbO$_2$ curve to the left, which increases the amount of oxygen that can be transported at P$_{O_2}$ = 40 mm Hg. Over time, of course, the reduced PA$_{O_2}$ increases erythropoietin secretion, stimulates red cell production, and raises hematocrit by about 10%.

2. All those cars will produce a lot of carbon monoxide and various oxides of nitrogen. To avoid pollution, methods must be devised to increase ventilation in the tunnels by using big fans and vertical ventilator shafts. If the tunnel is well ventilated, driving through it for 45 to 60 minutes will not be hazardous, especially if the drivers keep their windows shut and do not smoke. People with serious lung diseases are at risk. Maintenance workers are probably at greater risk in short, unventilated tunnels than in long, well-ventilated ones.

3. The large alveolar to arterial blood P$_{O_2}$ difference favors the $\dot{V}$/Q mechanism, because diffusion abnormalities should be corrected by high inspired oxygen. Of course, $\dot{V}$/Q maldistribution would also be corrected, except when $\dot{V}$/Q = 0, as it is in this problem (no alveolar ventilation).

4. The regulation of the number of perfused capillaries in skeletal muscle controls the mean diffusion distance to the mitochondria from the capillaries. The actual mechanisms that control the recruitment of more capillaries include the local oxygen partial pressures, local or reflex neural effects, temperature, H$^+$, accumulation of metabolites, and osmotic effects (see also Chapters 27 and 28).

5. Acetazolamide is a sulfanilamide-type chemical that can inhibit carbonic anhydrase in erythrocytes and many other cells. The respiratory consequences of complete blockade of red cell carbonic anhydrase are not serious. When the rapid hydration of CO$_2$ is prevented, the cellular and venous P$_{CO_2}$ rises because only a small quantity of the CO$_2$ that enters the capillaries will be converted to carbonic acid. Initially, as the venous blood with high P$_{CO_2}$ reaches the lungs, the alveolar P$_{CO_2}$ rises because ventilation has not yet increased. However, as the blood passes into the sys-

temic arteries and travels to the brain, the P_{CO_2} will slowly rise. Remember, the CO_2 dehydration reaction is slowed, not stopped. The rising arterial P_{CO_2} will increase the ventilation, which will increase the removal of CO_2 in the lungs. The process will eventually reach a plateau, with three net effects: venous (tissue) P_{CO_2} will increase, alveolar ventilation will rise, and arterial P_{CO_2} will increase modestly—just enough to maintain ventilation at the new level.

■ *Chapter 36*

1. Some activities involving the behavioral volitional control of breathing include talking or singing, suckling, vomiting, breathholding, coughing or sneezing, defecation or parturition, and anxiety or fear.

2. The carotid bodies in all mammals are located adjacent to the bifurcation of the common carotid arteries, which conduct blood to the brain.

3. In hemorrhage, the sympathetic nervous system increases peripheral vasoconstriction throughout the body, including the carotid bodies. The reduced blood supply to the carotid bodies activates the chemoreceptors located there. The main effect on respiration is to increase breathing frequency.

4. Because breathholding is a voluntary behavior, it will be overridden by the rising Pa_{CO_2} and to a lesser extend by the decreasing Pa_{O_2}. Even if it were possible to hold one's breath until one fainted, the loss of consciousness would immediately inhibit the breathholding, and respiration would ensue.

■ *Chapter 37*

1. Much of the motor and secretory functions of the gastrointestinal tract are directly controlled by the enteric nervous system. The enteric nervous system contains motor neurons, sensory neurons, and interneurons. Enteric sensory neurons function as the afferent arms of enteric reflex arcs by which the enteric nervous system controls motor and secretory activities of the gastrointestinal tract. The autonomic nervous system modulates the activities of the enteric nervous system. The gastrointestinal tract receives both sympathetic and parasympathetic innervation. For the most part, autonomic neurons project onto neurons of the enteric ganglia. Thus, they influence motor and secretory activities indirectly via their effects on the activities of enteric neurons. The autonomic nervous system is very important in controlling the interactions between different parts of the gastrointestinal tract. This control is apparent in such phenomena as receptive relaxation of the stomach and the gastrocolic reflex.

2. Slow waves are oscillations of the resting membrane potential of gastrointestinal smooth muscle. Their frequency varies from about 3 per minute in the stomach to 12 per minute in the duodenum. Slow waves are generated by the interstitial cells that form a thin layer located between the longitudinal and circular layers of muscularis externa. The slow waves spread, via tight junctions between cells, throughout the smooth muscle of each segment of the gastrointestinal tract.

The amplitude and, to a lesser extent, the frequency of the slow waves can be modulated by the activity of intrinsic and extrinsic nerves and by hormones and paracrine substances. If the peak of the slow wave is above threshold for the cells to fire action potentials, one or more action potentials may be triggered during the peak of the slow wave. The occurrence of action potentials enhances the contractile force. In some parts of the gastrointestinal tract, contractions may occur in response to the depolarizing phase of the slow wave even when action potentials are absent. In other parts of the gastrointestinal tract, contractions rarely occur in the absence of action potentials.

3. The regulation of gastric emptying in response to components of the contents of the duodenum is mediated by neural and hormonal mechanisms. These control mechanisms mainly slow the rate of gastric emptying, so that gastric contents are not emptied into the duodenum more rapidly than they can be dealt with in the duodenum and upper jejunum.

In response to the acid in the duodenum, the force of gastric contractions promptly decreases and duodenal motility increases. This response has neural and hormonal components. The presence of acid in the duodenum releases secretin, which diminishes the rate of gastric emptying by inhibiting antral contractions and stimulating contraction of the pyloric sphincter.

Fat-digestion products in the duodenum and jejunum decrease the rate of gastric emptying. This response results partly from the release of cholecystokinin from the duodenum and jejunum. Cholecystokinin decreases the rate of gastric emptying. Fatty acids in the duodenum and jejunum release gastric inhibitory peptide that also decreases the rate of gastric emptying.

Hyperosmotic solutions in the duodenum and jejunum slow the rate of gastric emptying. This response has both neural and hormonal components. Hypertonic solutions in the duodenum release an unidentified hormone that diminishes the rate of gastric emptying.

Peptides and amino acids release gastrin from G cells in the antrum of the stomach and the duodenum. Gastrin increases the strength of antral contractions and increases constriction of the pyloric sphincter; the net effect usually diminishes the rate of gastric emptying.

4. In a fed individual, the most frequent type of movement of the small intestine is segmentation. Segmentation is characterized by closely spaced contractions of the circular muscle layer. The maximal rate of segmentation contractions is the frequency of the slow waves. In rhythmic segmentation, the sites of the circular contractions alternate, so that a given segment of gut contracts and then relaxes. Segmental contractions may occur almost continuously, or brief intervals of relative quiescence may supervene. Peristaltic waves occur in the small intestine of a fed individual, but they usually involve only a short length of intestine.

   In a fasted individual, small intestinal motility is characterized by bursts of intense electrical and contractile activity separated by longer quiescent periods. This pattern is propagated from the stomach to the terminal ileum and is called the migrating myoelectric complex (MMC). The MMC repeats every 75 to 90 minutes. The strongest contractions of the MMC are more vigorous and more propulsive than are the contractions that occur in the fed individual.

5. Localized segmental contractions divide the colon into neighboring ovoid segments, called *haustra*. Segmentation contractions in the colon, also called *haustration*, are the most frequent contractile events. Haustral contractions are more effective in back-and-forth mixing of luminal contents than they are in propelling colonic contents.

   In the proximal colon, antipropulsive patterns commonly occur. Reverse peristalsis and segmental propulsion toward the cecum both take place. Normally the transverse and descending colon is filled with semisolid feces. Segmental haustral contractions knead the feces, and thereby facilitate absorption of the remaining salts and water. About one to three times daily, mass movements occur and sweep the feces toward the rectum. Distention of the rectum signals the urge to defecate and initiates the defecation reflex.

■ *Chapter 38*

1. According to the two-stage model of salivary secretion, the acinar cells and the cells of the striated and excretory ducts of salivary glands have different functions. The secretory endpieces (acini), perhaps with the participation of intercalated ducts, produce a primary secretion that is isotonic to plasma. The amylase concentration and the rate of fluid secretion vary with the level and type of stimulation. However, the electrolyte composition of the secretion is fairly constant, and the levels of Na^+, K^+, HCO_3^-, and Cl^- are close to plasma levels. The excretory ducts, and probably the striated ducts also, modify the primary secretion by extracting Na^+ and Cl^- from, and adding K^+ and

HCO_3^- to, the saliva. The ducts do not add to the volume of saliva. As saliva flows down the ducts, it becomes progressively more hypotonic, because the ducts remove more Na^+ and Cl^- ions from saliva than they add K^+ and HCO_3^- ions to it. The faster the flow rate of the saliva down the striated and excretory ducts, the closer to isotonicity is the saliva.

2. Parietal cells secrete HCl and intrinsic factor. Chief cells secrete pepsinogens. G cells in the antrum secrete gastrin. Surface epithelial cells secrete mucus and bicarbonate. Mucus neck cells secrete mucus. Enterochromaffin-like (ECL) cells secrete histamine. Cells near the base of gastrin glands secrete somatostatin.

3. The cephalic phase of gastric secretion is normally elicited by the sight, smell, and taste of food. Cephalic phase secretion is mediated entirely by branches of the vagus nerves. Vagal fibers stimulate enteric neurons that are predominantly cholinergic. Acetylcholine released from these neurons directly stimulates parietal cells to secrete HCl, and it also stimulates acid secretion indirectly by releasing gastrin from G cells in the antrum and duodenum and histamine from ECL cells in the gastric mucosa. Low pH in the antrum of the stomach inhibits HCl secretion by directly inhibiting parietal cells and by evoking inhibitory neural reflexes. In the absence of food in the stomach to buffer the secreted acid, the pH of the antral contents falls rapidly during the cephalic phase. Hence, the rate of HCl secretion may be considerable, but the total amount of cephalic-phase HCl secreted is low.

   The gastric phase of gastric secretion is elicited by the presence of food in the stomach. The principal stimuli are distention of the stomach and amino acids and peptides that result from the actions of pepsins. Most of the acid secreted in response to a meal is secreted during the gastric phase. When either the body or the antrum of the stomach is distended, mechanoreceptors are stimulated, which are the afferent arms of local and central reflexes. Reflexes directly stimulate parietal cells to secrete HCl and stimulate antral G cells to release gastrin. Amino acids and peptides in the antrum elicit HCl secretion by causing G cells in the antrum to release gastrin.

   During the intestinal phase, chyme in the duodenum brings about neural and endocrine responses that first stimulate and later inhibit secretion of acid by the stomach. Early in gastric emptying, when the pH of gastric chyme is greater than 3, the stimulatory influences predominate. Later, when the buffer capacity of gastric chyme is exhausted, inhibitory influences prevail. Gastric secretion is enhanced by distention of the duodenum and by protein digestion products in the duodenum. Duodenal distention brings about increased gastric acid secretion via neural reflexes that stimulate parietal cells and G cells in the gastric antrum. The duodenum and proximal jejunum contain G cells that release gastrin when stimulated by peptides and amino acids. In addition, amino acids and peptides that are absorbed in the duodenum and jejunum are carried in the blood to the gastric antrum, where they enhance gastrin release by G cells.

Several different inhibitory mechanisms are evoked by acid, fat digestion products, and hypertonicity in the duodenum and proximal part of the jejunum. Acid solutions in the duodenum inhibit acid secretion by parietal cells via enteric and vagovagal reflexes. Acid solutions in the duodenum release the hormone secretin into the bloodstream. Secretin inhibits acid secretion by inhibiting gastrin release by G cells and by decreasing the response of parietal cells to secretagogues. Acid in the duodenal bulb releases another hormone, bulbogastrone, which inhibits acid secretion by the parietal cells. Products of triglyceride digestion in the duodenum and proximal part of the jejunum release two hormones, gastric inhibitory peptide (GIP) and cholecystokinin (CCK), which inhibit acid secretion by parietal cells. Hyperosmotic solutions in the duodenum release an unidentified hormone that inhibits gastric acid secretion.

4. In the absence of stimulation by secretin, pancreatic juice consists of an enzyme component (the major stimulus for secretion of the enzyme component is CCK) and an aqueous component produced by the intralobular ducts. Secretin specifically stimulates the secretion of the extralobular ducts.

The acinar cells, and perhaps the cells of the intercalated ducts also, secrete the enzyme component of pancreatic juice. The fluid secreted by the acinar cells resembles plasma in its tonicity and in the concentrations of various electrolytes. The enzyme component contains enzymes important for the digestion of all the major classes of foodstuffs: proteases (trypsin, chymotrypsin, and carboxypeptidase), pancreatic amylase, and lipases (triacylglycerol, hydrolase, cholesterol ester hydrolase, and phospholipase A_2).

The aqueous component of pancreatic juice is elaborated by the epithelial cells that line the ducts. Pancreatic juice is isotonic to plasma. The Na^+ and K^+ concentrations of pancreatic juice are similar to those in plasma. HCO_3^- (at levels well above those in plasma) and Cl^- are the major anions. The HCO_3^- concentration increases at higher secretory rates. Under resting conditions, the aqueous component is produced primarily by the intralobular ducts. When secretion is stimulated by secretin, the additional flow comes mostly from the extralobular ducts. The secretin-stimulated secretions of the extralobular ducts have a higher bicarbonate concentration than the spontaneous secretions of the intralobular ducts.

5. Hepatocytes secrete the organic constituents of bile. Among the components of bile secreted into the bile

canaliculi by hepatocytes are bile acids, phospholipids, cholesterol, and bilirubin glucuronides. The major physiological stimuli to the hepatocytes are CCK and bile acids that return to the liver in the portal blood. Water and electrolytes are present in the bile canaliculi at about their plasma concentrations. The osmotic pressure of bile acids and other molecules secreted by the hepatocytes may cause water and electrolytes to flow into the canaliculi via the leaky tight junctions that join the hepatocytes.

The epithelial cells that line the bile ducts contribute an aqueous secretion that accounts for about 50% of the total volume of the bile. The secretion of the bile duct epithelium is isotonic and contains Na^+ and K^+ at levels similar to those of plasma, but the concentration of HCO_3^- is greater and the concentration of Cl^- is less than in plasma. The secretory activity of the bile duct epithelium is specifically stimulated by secretin.

■ *Chapter 39*

1. Glucose, galactose, and fructose are the only monosaccharides that can be absorbed. Glucose and galactose are actively taken up by the brush border epithelial cells by a transport protein known as SGLT1. SGLT1 uses the energy of the Na^+ gradient to transport glucose and galactose actively into the intestinal epithelial cells. SLGT1 transports two Na^+ ions and one glucose or galactose molecule across the brush border membrane. Fructose is not a substrate for the brush border glucose-galactose transporter. The facilitated transport of fructose across the brush border plasma membrane is mediated by GLUT5. GLUT5 is rather specific for fructose. Glucose, galactose, and fructose leave the intestinal epithelial cell at the basolateral plasma membranes via facilitated transport. The transport protein responsible for efflux of glucose, galactose, and fructose across the basolateral membrane is GLUT2.

2. Proteins and peptides are digested in the duodenum and upper small intestine by proteases secreted by the pancreas. The most important of these proteases are trypsin, chymotrypsin, carboxypeptidases A and B, and elastase. The pancreatic juice contains these enzymes in inactive, proenzyme forms. Enteropeptidase secreted by the mucosa of the duodenum and jejunum converts trypsinogen to trypsin. Trypsin acts autocatalytically to activate trypsinogen, and it also converts the other proenzymes to the active enzymes. The pancreatic proteases are present at high activities in the duodenum, and they rapidly convert dietary protein to small peptides.

The brush border of the duodenum and the small intestine contains a number of peptidases. These peptidases are integral membrane proteins whose active sites face the intestinal lumen. They reduce the peptides produced by pancreatic proteases to small peptides and amino acids.

In the epithelial cells of the small intestine, small peptides are hydrolyzed by cytosolic peptidases. Cytosolic peptidases are particularly active against dipeptides and tripeptides. Most of the small peptides that enter the intestinal epithelial cells are cleaved to single amino acids in the cell, and they are absorbed into the blood as single amino acids.

3. Mature epithelial cells near the tips of the villi are active in net absorption, whereas more immature cells in Lieberkühn's crypts function as net secretors of electrolytes and water.

Cl^- is actively taken up at the basolateral plasma membrane of crypt cells by the Na^+, K^+, $2Cl^-$ cotransporter, which uses the electrochemical potential difference of Na^+ to transport Cl^- and K^+ actively into the cell. Cl^- leaves the cell at the luminal membrane via an electrogenic Cl^- channel. Na^+ is transported into the lumen; the transport is driven by the net luminal electronegativity produced by the electrogenic Cl^- secretion into the lumen. Efflux of K^+ via K^+ channels in the basolateral membrane prevents K^+ from accumulating in the cytosol of the crypt cell. The efflux of K^+ also maintains an electrical potential difference (cytosol negative) across the luminal and basolateral membranes, and this potential difference contributes to the electrochemical driving force for the efflux of Cl^- across the luminal membrane and for the basolateral influx of Na^+ (and thus for Cl^- entry also).

4. Ca^{++} moves through Ca^{++} channels down its electrochemical potential gradient across the brush border membrane into the cytosol. An integral protein of the brush border plasma membrane called the *intestinal membrane calcium-binding protein (IMCal)* may bind Ca^{++} at the inner face of the brush border membrane.

In the cytosol of the intestinal epithelial cells, Ca^{++} is bound to calbindin. Calbindin allows large amounts of Ca^{++} to traverse the cytosol. The binding of Ca^{++} by calbindin prevents free Ca^{++} from reaching high enough concentrations to form insoluble salts with intracellular anions.

The basolateral plasma membrane contains two transport proteins capable of ejecting Ca^{++} from the cell against its electrochemical potential gradient. A Ca^{++}-ATPase in the basolateral membrane is a primary active transport protein that splits ATP and uses the energy to transport Ca^{++}. The Na^+, Ca^{++} exchanger present in the basolateral membrane uses the energy of the Na^+ gradient to extrude Ca^{++} by secondary active transport.

Ca^{++} is also transported through the cytosol of intestinal epithelial cells in membrane vesicles. Vesicular Ca^{++} is released across the basolateral membrane by exocytosis.

5. The iron-absorbing capacity of the epithelial cells is programmed when the cells are in Lieberkühn's crypts. High levels of Fe^{++} in the intestinal epithelial cells promote translation of messenger RNA for apoferritin and they diminish the stability of the message for the basolateral transferrin receptor. In an iron-replete individual, levels of apoferritin are high and the amount of transferrin receptor is low; this enhances irreversible iron storage and decreases the rate of Fe^{++} absorption. In iron deficiency, for example, after a hemorrhage, levels of apoferritin are low and the amount of transferrin receptor is high, so that less storage and more absorption of Fe^{++} occur.

6. Free fatty acids, 2-monoglycerides, cholesterol, and the other products of lipid digestion are taken up across the brush border plasma membrane so rapidly that this step does not limit the rate of their uptake. The main limitation to the rate of lipid uptake by the epithelial cells of the upper small intestine is the diffusion of the mixed micelles through an unstirred layer (200 to 500 μm thick) on the luminal surface of the brush border plasma membrane. Nutrients present in the well-mixed contents of the intestinal lumen must diffuse through the unstirred layer to reach the brush border plasma membrane.

Because of their high lipid solubility, the fatty acids, 2-monoglycerides, cholesterol, and lysolecithin can diffuse across the brush border membrane. Nevertheless, transport proteins in the brush border membrane have been shown to mediate the uptake of long-chain fatty acids and cholesterol. The brush border protein that facilitates the transport of long-chain fatty acids is known as the microvillous membrane fatty acid–binding protein. This protein uses the energy of the Na^+ gradient to power the secondary active uptake of long-chain fatty acids.

■ *Chapter 40*

1.

Before Drug	
Plasma [inulin]	1 mg/ml
Plasma [glucose]	1 mg/ml
Inulin excretion rate	100 mg/min
Glucose excretion rate	0 mg/min
Inulin clearance	100 ml/min
Glucose clearance	0 ml/min

After Drug	
Plasma [inulin]	1 mg/ml
Plasma [glucose]	1 mg/ml
Inulin excretion rate	100 mg/min
Glucose excretion rate	10 mg/min
Inulin clearance	100 ml/min
Glucose clearance	100 ml/min

Before treatment with the drug the filtered load of glucose (glomerular filtration rate [GFR] × [glucose]) is 100 mg/min (GFR calculated from inulin clearance). With this filtered load of glucose, all the glucose is reabsorbed and none is excreted. Thus, the clearance of glucose is zero. After administration of the drug, the filtered load is unchanged, but there is no glucose reabsorption. Therefore, all the glucose filtered is excreted, and the clearance of glucose equals that of inulin.

2. Structures that compose the juxtaglomerular apparatus include the macula densa of the thick ascending limb, extraglomerular mesangial cells, and renin-producing cells of the afferent and efferent arterioles. The juxtaglomerular apparatus is one component of a feedback mechanism that regulates renal blood flow and GFR. Details of this mechanism are provided in Chapter 40.

3. A spinal cord injury at the level of the twelfth thoracic vertebra will interrupt the ascending sensory fibers. Thus, there is no sensation of bladder fullness. The descending fibers that control the muscle of the external sphincter are also interrupted, as are descending fibers that modulate the micturition reflex. Voluntary control of the external sphincter is lost, resulting in the inability to control micturition (i.e., incontinence). The micturition reflex is intact, because the centers involved in this reflex arc are located in the sacral part of the spinal cord (below the injury to the spinal cord). The bladder will show spontaneous contractions as it fills (spasticity). These spontaneous contractions are normal but are usually inhibited by descending fibers from the brain. This inhibitory influence allows the bladder to fill to capacity before voiding. However, in this situation the inhibitory input is lost, and small volumes of urine are voiding frequently.

4. (A) Although red blood cells can appear in the urine as a result of damage to the glomerular filtration barrier, they may appear in the urine for other reasons. For example, they may appear in the urine as a result of bleeding in any part of the lower urinary tract. Such bleeding is seen with kidney stones, and occasionally as a result of a bacterial infection of the lower urinary tract that causes bleeding. Thus, the appearance of blood in the urine does not necessarily indicate damage to the glomerular filtration barrier.
(B) Glucose is filtered and completely reabsorbed by the proximal tubule. Thus, it is not normally found in the urine. Its presence in the urine indicates an elevated plasma glucose level such that the filtered load (GFR × [glucose]) is greater than the ability of the proximal tubule to reabsorb glucose. Because glucose is freely filtered by the normal glomerulus, damage to the ultrafiltration barrier would not increase its filtration.
(C) Na+ normally appears in the urine in healthy individuals. Like glucose, Na+ is freely filtered by the nor-

mal glomerulus. Therefore, damage to the filtration barrier does not increase the rate of Na+ excretion.
(D) This is the correct answer. Normally the urine contains essentially no protein. The glomerulus prevents the filtration of plasma proteins. However, when the glomerulus is damaged, large amounts of plasma proteins are filtered. If the amount filtered overwhelms the reabsorptive capacity of the proximal tubule, protein appears in the urine (proteinuria).

5. The equation for blood flow through an organ is Q = ΔP/R. Sympathetic agonists, angiotensin II, and prostaglandins change blood flow by altering the resistance (R). Whereas sympathetic agonists and angiotensin II increase R and thereby decrease renal blood flow (RBF), prostaglandins decrease R and thereby increase RBF.

■ *Chapter 41*

1. The glomeruli filter 25,200 mEq Na+ and 18,000 mEq Cl− each day. Over 99% is reabsorbed by the nephrons, with less than 1% appearing in the urine. Although Na+ and Cl− uptake into cells across the apical membrane and NaCl reabsorption across the paracellular pathway are passive processes (i.e., they do not require the direct input of ATP), they ultimately depend on the operation of the Na+, K+-ATPase. Accordingly, reabsorption of NaCl requires a considerable quantity of ATP. ATP synthesis by kidney cells requires large amounts of oxygen, and hence a high blood flow.

2. Passive transport always occurs down an electrochemical gradient. Diffusion of a solute (e.g., O_2) through the lipid portion of the plasma membrane occurs passively. For coupled transporters (antiport and symport), one molecule moving down its electrochemical gradient can drive its coupled molecule uphill. When this occurs, the uphill movement is termed *secondary active* transport, because the transporter is not coupled directly to the hydrolysis of ATP. Active transport occurs against an electrochemical gradient and requires the direct input of energy (i.e., ATP). Some authors refer to such transport as *primary active* transport to emphasize the direct coupling to ATP.

3. In the first phase of proximal reabsorption, Na+ enters the cell across the apical membrane by several symport and antiport mechanisms (e.g., Na+-glucose symport, Na+-amino acid symport, and Na+-H+ antiport). Na+ exits from the cell into the blood by the Na+, K+-ATPase. Therefore, Na+ is reabsorbed across the cell with glucose, amino acids, and HCO_3^-. When tubular fluid reaches the second half of the proximal tubule, the concentrations of glucose, amino acids, and HCO_3^- are greatly reduced. As a result, the tubular fluid at this point is primarily NaCl. In the second phase of proximal tubule reabsorption, NaCl uptake

across the apical membrane occurs by the parallel operation of Na+-H+ and Cl−-anion antiporters. Na+ efflux from the cell occurs via the Na+-K+-ATPase and Cl− exit occurs via KCl symport. Paracellular NaCl reabsorption also occurs. Paracellular Cl− reabsorption, in the second half on the proximal tubule, is driven by the Cl− concentration gradient across the proximal tubule. This gradient develops because relatively little Cl− is reabsorbed in the first half of the proximal tubule (i.e., Na+ is reabsorbed with other solutes). Because water reabsorption is proportionally more than Cl− reabsorption in the first half of the proximal tubule, the [Cl−] in tubular fluid increases. This increase provides the driving force for Cl− diffusion across the tight junctions. Cl− diffusion also renders the transepithelial voltage lumen positive, which in turn provides the driving force for the passive, paracellular diffusion of Na+. The transport of solutes (NaCl) across the cellular and paracellular pathways lowers the osmolality of the tubular fluid and increases the osmolality of the interstitial fluid. These changes establish a driving force for water reabsorption across the proximal tubule. Some solutes are reabsorbed with this water by the process of solvent drag. Starling forces across the wall of the peritubular capillary are important for the uptake of this interstitial fluid. These forces can regulate the rate of solute and water backflux across the tight junctions, thereby modulating net solute and water reabsorption.

4. NaCl is reabsorbed across the thick ascending limb by two mechanisms. First, transcellular transport involves Na+ and Cl− entry into the cell across the apical membrane via the 1Na+-1K+-2Cl− symporter (some Na+ is also reabsorbed by the apical membrane Na+-H+ antiporter), and exit across the basolateral membrane via the Na+, K+-ATPase (for Na+) and via a KCl symporter and Cl− channel (for Cl−: neither mechanism is shown in Fig. 41-8). Second, Na+ is also reabsorbed across the paracellular pathway because of the lumen-positive transepithelial voltage. Furosemide would have no effect on water reabsorption in the thick ascending limb because this segment of the nephron is relatively impermeable to water, and water is not reabsorbed even when NaCl reabsorptive rates are high. Furosemide increases water excretion by reducing the osmolality of the medullary interstitial fluid, which in turn reduces water reabsorption from the descending thin limb of Henle's loop.

5. Glomerulotubular balance describes the phenomenon whereby an increase in the filtered load of water and NaCl is accompanied by a parallel increase in water and NaCl reabsorption by the proximal tubule. If a constant amount of NaCl and water were reabsorbed by the proximal tubule, increases in GFR and the filtered load of NaCl and water would result in an increased delivery to more distal segments. If these

segments were not able to reabsorb the excess NaCl and water, large amounts could be lost in the urine. If such an increase in excretion were not accompanied by a corresponding rise in dietary intake, the organism would develop negative NaCl and water balance. Hence, glomerulotubular balance helps to maintain NaCl and water homeostasis despite changes in GFR and the filtered loads of water and NaCl.

■ *Chapter 42*

1. This problem illustrates the importance of effective vs. ineffective osmoles in regulating antidiuretic hormone (ADH) secretion. Although plasma osmolality is elevated, the increased osmolality is caused by urea. Because urea is an ineffective osmole with regard to ADH secretion, it is necessary to estimate the osmolality of plasma that is attributed to effective osmoles (Na+ and its anions). The effective osmolality of the plasma is estimated by doubling the plasma [Na+], which yields a value of 270 mOsm/kg H_2O. Because the effective osmolality is reduced from its normal value (280 to 290 mOsm/kg H_2O), ADH secretion is suppressed and plasma levels reduced.

2.

Nephron Site	*0-ADH*	*Max. ADH*
Proximal tubule	300	300
Beginning of thin descending limb	300	300
Beginning of thin ascending limb	1200	1200
End of thick ascending limb	≈ 100	≈ 100
End of cortical collecting duct	< 100	300
Urine	≈ 50	1200

Regardless of the presence of ADH, tubular fluid osmolality is the same in all nephron segments except the collecting duct. When ADH is present, the tubular fluid within the lumen of the collecting duct comes to osmotic equilibrium with the surrounding interstitial fluid (300 mOsm/kg H_2O in the cortex; 1200 mOsm/kg H_2O in the medulla). In the absence of ADH, solute reabsorption along the collecting duct leads to further dilution of the tubular fluid.

3. (a) *Inhibition of thick ascending limb transport:* Inhibition of thick ascending limb NaCl transport decreases the separation of solute and water that occurs at this site. Because transport by the thick ascending limb is necessary for generating the medullary interstitial osmotic gradient, the osmolality of the interstitium will fall. This impairs the reabsorption of water from the medullary collecting duct. As a result, $T^c_{H_2O}$ is reduced. The urine osmolality will approach 300 mOsm/kg H_2O, reflecting the fact that

fluid entering Henle's loop from the proximal tubule has an osmolality of this value. Thus separation of solute and water is impaired.

(b) *Nephrogenic diabetes insipidus:* In this condition, the collecting duct does not respond to ADH. As a result, it remains impermeable to water. This obviously impairs the ability of the kidneys to concentrate the urine and reabsorb solute-free water ($T^c_{H_2O}$).

4. If daily solute excretion is 800 mOsm and the individual can produce only concentrated urine that has an osmolality of 400 mOsm/kg H_2O, the minimal volume of urine required for this solute excretion is:

$$\frac{800 \text{ mOsm}}{400 \text{ mOsm/kg } H_2O} = 2 \text{ L}$$

If insensible loss is 1 L, this individual must drink at least 3 L of water (or other dilute beverage) in a 24-hour period to prevent the development of hyperosmolality. This is slightly more than the average daily intake of most individuals. For the second individual, the daily water requirement is much less, because of the ability to excrete a more concentrated urine. Minimal urine volume required in this individual would be:

$$\frac{800 \text{ mOsm}}{1200 \text{ mOsm/kg } H_2O} = 0.67 \text{ L}$$

With insensible loss of 1 L, daily water intake could be less than 2 L, and body fluid osmolality would be maintained. A corollary to these examples is that solute excretion also places constraints on the maximal volume of water that can be ingested. For example, if an individual who can dilute urine to 100 mOsm/kg H_2O excretes 800 mOsm of solute, this person could drink as much as 8 L of water without reducing body fluid osmolality. If, however, the individual excretes more solute (e.g., 1200 mOsm), 12 L of water could be ingested. Indeed, a decline in body fluid osmolality can be seen in individuals who drink large quantities of water without sufficient solute intake.

5. It is assumed that the 3-kg weight loss reflects only the loss of extracellular fluid (ECF). Because the plasma [Na$^+$] is unchanged, this represents a loss of isotonic fluid (3 L) from the ECF.
Plasma osmolality. Because the plasma [Na$^+$] is unchanged, the plasma osmolality is unchanged.
Extracellular fluid volume. The loss of fluid will decrease the ECF volume, because it is isotonic fluid loss (no change in plasma [Na$^+$]).
ADH secretion. Volume depletion will be sensed by the vascular baroreceptors, and ADH secretion will be stimulated.
Urine osmolality. The increased levels of ADH will lead to water conservation by the kidneys, and a concentrated urine will be excreted.

Sensation of thirst. Again, volume depletion will be sensed by the vascular baroreceptors and will cause an increased sensation of thirst.

6. The individual is euvolemic. To maintain Na$^+$ balance, the amount of Na$^+$ ingested in the diet must equal the amount excreted from the body. Because the kidneys are the primary route for Na$^+$ excretion, the amount of Na$^+$ excreted daily is very nearly equal to the amount ingested in the diet (small amounts of Na$^+$ are lost in perspiration and feces). Therefore, the Na$^+$ excretion rate in this individual is approximately 200 mEq/day.

7.

Regulatory factor	Volume expansion	Volume contraction
Renal sympathetic nerves	↓	↑
ANP	↑	↓
Renin-angiotensin	↓	↑
Aldosterone	↓	↑
Vasopressin	↓	↑

8. This individual has gained 4 kg. This represents the accumulation of 4 L of fluid (1 kg = 1 L) in the ECF, a portion of which will accumulate in the interstitial fluid compartment as edema. The composition of this fluid is the same as plasma and has an [Na$^+$] of 140 mEq/L. Recall that the accumulation of the fluid requires Na$^+$ retention by the kidneys. Therefore, the amount of Na$^+$ retained by the kidneys must be equal to the amount contained in 4 L of fluid having an [Na$^+$] of 140 mEq/L, or 560 mEq of Na$^+$.

■ *Chapter 43*

1. Intravenous infusion of K$^+$ into a subject with a combination of sympathetic blockade (i.e., no catecholamine release) and insulin deficiency would result in significant hyperkalemia compared with a similar infusion of K$^+$ in a normal subject. Although aldosterone secretion would be stimulated by the hyperkalemia, this hormone stimulates cell K$^+$ uptake after a 1-hour lag period. In the first hour after K$^+$ infusion, less than 50% of the infused K$^+$ is excreted by the kidneys, and because sympathetic activity and insulin release are suppressed, most of the K$^+$ remaining in the body is retained in the extracellular fluid.

2. Aldosterone deficiency would initially reduce urinary potassium excretion, and K$^+$ would be retained in the body (i.e., dietary intake would exceed excretion). This would lead to hyperkalemia, which is a potent stimulus of K$^+$ excretion. Because the individual is initially in positive K$^+$ balance, plasma K$^+$ rises until urinary K$^+$ excretion becomes equal to dietary K$^+$ intake. In the new steady state, K$^+$ intake would equal K$^+$ excretion; however, the subject has hyperkalemia. Thus, it is possible to match dietary K$^+$ intake with

excretion in the absence of aldosterone, but this occurs at an elevated plasma [K+].

3. In the first hour after a meal, the rise in plasma K+ is blunted by the rapid (minutes) uptake of K+ into skeletal muscle, liver, bone, and red blood cells. Some K+ is excreted by the kidneys, but in the first hour after the meal most K+ is sequestered in the intracellular fluid. In the ensuing hours, K+ slowly leaves the cells and is excreted by the kidneys, thus maintaining K+ balance and plasma [K+].

4. Normally, K+ excretion is determined primarily by the rate of K+ secretion by the distal tubule and collecting duct, and is largely independent of the glomerular filtration rate (GFR) and the filtered load of K+. When 50% of the nephrons are lost, the distal tubules and collecting ducts in the remaining, functioning nephrons secrete more K+ so that K+ excretion and plasma [K+] are maintained at normal levels. However, if 80% to 85% of the nephrons are lost and GFR falls to less than 15% to 20% of normal, K+ secretion by the distal tubule and collecting duct cannot increase enough to maintain urinary K+ excretion constant, and hyperkalemia ensues.

5. Approximately two thirds of Ca++ reabsorption across the proximal tubule occurs by solvent drag, a process that depends on Na+ reabsorption. Mannitol would inhibit Ca++ reabsorption by blocking solvent drag in the proximal tubule and thereby increasing urinary Ca++ excretion.

6. Furosemide would inhibit the 1Na+-1K+-2Cl− symporter and reduce the lumen-positive transepithelial voltage to 0. This in turn would inhibit passive Ca++ reabsorption via the paracellular pathway.

7. A rise in plasma [P_i] will increase the amount of P_i filtered by the glomeruli. Because normally the amount of P_i filtered is equal to the reabsorptive capacity of the kidneys, an increase in the amount of P_i filtered will increase urinary P_i excretion and reduce plasma [P_i].

■ *Chapter 44*

1. If urinary buffers were not available, the 70 mEq of acid needed to be excreted by the kidneys to maintain acid-base balance (net acid excretion = nonvolatile acid production) would have to be excreted as free H+. If the minimal urine pH = 4.0, this represents only 0.1 mEq/L of H+. Thus, to excrete 70 mEq of H+, the daily urine output would need to be:

$$\frac{70 \text{ mEq/day}}{0.1 \text{ mEq/L}} = 700 \text{ L/day}$$

This exceeds the daily glomerular filtration rate (GFR) (180 L/day). Thus, the urinary buffers are

essential for the kidney's ability to excrete sufficient quantities of H+ to maintain acid-base balance.

2.

pH	[HCO_3^-] mEq/L	Pco_2 mm Hg	Disorder
7.34	15	29	Metabolic acidosis
7.49	35	48	Metabolic alkalosis
7.47	14	20	Chronic respiratory alkalosis
7.34	31	60	Chronic respiratory acidosis
7.26	26	60	Acute respiratory acidosis
7.62	20	20	Acute respiratory alkalosis
7.09	15	50	Metabolic + respiratory acidosis
7.40	15	25	Metabolic acidosis + respiratory alkalosis

3. Carbonic anhydrase plays a critical role in the reabsorption of HCO_3^- by the cells of the proximal tubule and by intercalated cells of the collecting duct. Inhibition of this enzyme would therefore inhibit the reabsorption of HCO_3^- at these nephron sites. Because of the large fraction of the filtered load of HCO_3^- reabsorbed by the proximal tubule, the effect at this site is quantitatively more important. With decreased reabsorption, more HCO_3^- would be excreted in the urine, and urine pH would become alkaline. This loss of HCO_3^- from the body would result in the development of a metabolic acidosis.

4. The initial set of laboratory data indicates a metabolic alkalosis with appropriate respiratory compensation. Given the individual's history, the most likely cause of this simple acid-base disorder is the loss of gastric acid by vomiting. The second set of laboratory data continues to show a metabolic alkalosis with respiratory compensation. In addition, there is evidence of fluid loss (decrease in body weight by 2 kg), which indicates volume depletion. Given the worsening of this individual's metabolic alkalosis, it is somewhat surprising that the urine pH is so acidic. The appropriate renal response should be an increase in HCO_3^- excretion to correct the alkalosis. However, by decreasing the filtered load of HCO_3^- (decreased GFR) and stimulating proximal Na+ reabsorption, the volume depletion prevents the excretion of HCO_3^- (HCO_3^- reabsorption is linked to Na+). In addition, the volume depletion stimulates aldosterone secretion, which increases H+ secretion by the

intercalated cells of the collecting duct. Therefore, the urine is more acidic than expected for the degree of alkalosis. To correct this situation, euvolemia must be restored. Infusion of isotonic NaCl would accomplish this and also allow the kidneys to excrete the excess HCO_3^-, thereby restoring acid-base balance.

■ *Chapter 45*

1. Peptide hormones bind with plasma membrane receptors that either activate G proteins and effector enzymes that are membrane bound (e.g., adenylyl cyclase, phospholipase C) or that use tyrosine kinase activity within or near the intracytoplasmic tail of the receptors. Steroid and thyroid hormones bind with receptors that reside in the cytoplasm, or more often in the nucleus. Hormone binding to the receptor creates a complex that associates with a specific site on a target DNA molecule and either activates or suppresses the gene. Transcription factors may assist this process.

2. If hormone A stimulates secretion of hormone B or stimulates a rise in the concentration of a substrate such as glucose, hormone B or glucose will inhibit secretion of hormone A. If hormone B is secreted in response to a decrease in the glucose level, glucose will inhibit secretion of hormone B.

■ *Chapter 46*

1. Caloric and nutrient intake are increased by deficits in body weight and adipose mass. Appetite is increased by attractive smell and taste, sweetness of food, a decrease in plasma glucose, a reduction in serotonergic and noradrenergic tone, and an increase in the hypothalamic peptide neuropeptide Y. A decrease in fat mass decreases plasma leptin levels, leptin activity in the brain, and satiety center function. Total energy expenditure, thermogenesis, temperature, basal metabolic rate (BMR), and physical activity all then decrease. The opposite sequence occurs when energy stores become excessive as the result of a prolonged imbalance between caloric intake and expenditure.

2. (1) Free fatty acids from adipose tissue stores are mobilized and replace glucose use for all but critical functions such as a continuing activity of the citric acid (Krebs) cycle. The respiratory quotient decreases.
(2) Amino acids from muscle proteolysis and glycerol from lipolysis decrease the level of gluconeogenesis and of hepatic glucose output.
(3) Ketoacid products of fat oxidation largely replace glucose as a substrate for the brain's energy needs.
(4) Protein synthesis decreases.
(5) BMR decreases 10% to 20%.

■ *Chapter 47*

1. (1) Hepatic glycogenolysis and gluconeogenesis increase; muscle glucose uptake decreases. Plasma glucose rises.
(2) Adipose tissue lipolysis increases: adipose tissue uptake of free fatty acids (FFA) and of glucose decreases, as does triglyceride synthesis. Plasma FFAs increase.
(3) FFA delivery to liver increases. Glucagon secretion increases. Together, these increase ketogenesis. Plasma beta-hydroxybutyrate and acetoacetate increase. Metabolic acidosis ensues.
(4) Muscle proteolysis increases. The amino acids are used for gluconeogenesis instead of for protein synthesis. Urine urea and ammonia excretion increase. Negative nitrogen balance results.
(5) The catabolic state and decreased uptake of these ions cause loss of intracellular potassium, phosphate, and magnesium, which are excreted in the urine.
(6) The consequences listed in (1), (2), and (3) above are aggravated by increased secretion and actions of glucagon.

2. (1) The carbohydrate content stimulates insulin secretion and inhibits glucagon secretion. These actions favor storage of the dietary glucose intake as glycogen.
(2) The protein content stimulates insulin secretion and thus favors storage of amino acids as endogenous protein. Glucagon secretion is also stimulated, which favors conversion of some of the amino acids to glucose and prevents insulin-induced hypoglycemia.
(3) The fat content has little direct effect.
(4) The gastrointestinal hormones glucagon-like-peptide-1 (GLP-1) and gastric inhibitory peptide (GIP) are released, and they stimulate insulin secretion even before plasma glucose rises substantially. This helps to limit postprandial hyperglycemia.
(5) Somatostatin release inhibits both insulin and glucagon secretion. Because somatostatin also slows gastrointestinal motility and secretion of digestive enzymes and bile, somatostatin may act to synchronize nutrient and hormone availability and make assimilation and disposition of the nutrients optimal.

■ *Chapter 48*

1. The most immediate response is an increase in parathyroid hormone (PTH) secretion as the extracellular portion of the calcium receptor in the parathyroid gland plasma membrane senses the decrease in ionized calcium. PTH released by exocytosis acts on osteocytes to stimulate osteocytic osteolysis, with release of rapidly exchangeable calcium from bone surfaces. Osteoclastic resorption of bone is also stimulated, and this provides calcium and phosphate to the extracellular fluid. PTH also stimulates renal tubular

calcium reabsorption, which further augments circulating calcium concentration. At the same time, PTH inhibits renal tubular phosphate reabsorption. This permits the extra phosphate released from bone to be eliminated in the urine. PTH and hypocalcemia together increase production of 1,25-(OH$_2$)-vitamin D. If there is a continued need to prevent hypocalcemia after surgery, the 1,25-(OH$_2$)-D will stimulate absorption of calcium from the diet. It will also reinforce the PTH actions on bone resorption and renal tubular calcium reabsorption.

2. Bone resorption is initiated in a particular local area of bone by a paracrine signal that originates in osteoblasts and is conveyed to osteoclasts. The signal is probably a cytokine, such as interleukin-6. Osteoclasts then tunnel into trabecular or cortical bone and thereby create a "vacuum" in the bone structure. The osteoclast number is also increased in this area by recruiting and differentiating signals, such as insulin-like growth factors, that are also secreted by osteoblasts. As the area of resorbed bone grows, new osteoblasts are recruited and begin to fill in the newly created empty space. In this remodeling process, old bone is periodically replaced with new bone. Resorption releases about 500 mg of calcium a day into the extracellular fluid; the same amount is extracted from extracellular fluid by bone formation. Should the process of bone resorption be increased by an external factor (e.g., weightlessness in space), plasma calcium levels would rise, unless the coupling process ensured that bone formation also increased in tandem.

■ *Chapter 49*

1. The anterior pituitary gland receives no direct arterial blood supply. Instead, it is nourished by a set of portal veins that arise in the median eminence. The latter contains axonal terminals that store peptides transferred from hypothalamic neurons down their axons. Upon stimulation of the cell bodies, the hypothalamic peptides are released into capillaries supplied by the superior hypothalamic artery. This blood carries the peptides via the portal veins to the anterior pituitary, where they stimulate or inhibit release of anterior pituitary hormones. By contrast, the posterior pituitary gland is a direct extension of hypothalamic neurons. It receives direct arterial supply from the inferior hypophyseal artery and releases its hormones into the capillary plexus derived from the artery.

2. Corticotropin-releasing hormone (CRH) is the direct mediator that stimulates adrenocorticotropic hormone (ACTH) release. Cortisol is the adrenal cortical hormone that feeds back negatively to inhibit ACTH release. Cortisol blocks CRH action and also decreases CRH synthesis and release. In conditions of great stress (e.g., major surgery), the stimulation of CRH, augmented by antidiuretic hormone (ADH) stimulation, overcomes the inhibition by the large amounts of cortisol secreted by the adrenal cortex in response to the increased ACTH. Neural inputs to the hypothalamus also induce the CRH-mediated effects of awakening, pain, and pleasure (via endorphins) on ACTH release.

3. Growth hormone binds to its plasma membrane receptor, which transduces the hormone signal by activating cytoplasmic tyrosine kinases. Phosphorylation of transcription factors leads to induction of the synthesis of insulin-like growth factors (IFGs, somatomedins) in the liver and target cells. IGFs bind to their plasma membrane receptors, and this interaction causes autophosphorylation and induction of intrinsic tyrosine kinase activity within the receptor molecule. Phosphorylation of protein substrates in the cytoplasm activates mitogenic and metabolic pathways. In skeletal and cardiac muscle, protein synthesis is augmented, and muscle mass and contractility are increased. In cartilage and bone, osteoblastic and chondroblastic activity is induced, and bone formation exceeds bone resorption. These reactions lead to linear growth in childhood and puberty. Visceral organs, such as the kidneys, increase in size and function. In muscle, liver, and adipose tissue, insulin sensitivity is reduced by growth hormone so that a diabetogenic state can result from growth hormone excess.

4. This patient has developed a hypo-osmolar state because of excessive water retention. The major stress stimulated the release of ADH along with CRH and thereby increased ACTH and cortisol secretion. The release of ADH was also stimulated by the blood loss that decreased the arterial blood pressure. The ADH binds to its renal plasma membrane receptors, and cAMP is released as a second messenger. This stimulates sodium reabsorption by the cells of the ascending limb of the loop of Henle and reabsorption of water by the cells of the collecting ducts. The excess conservation of water dilutes the plasma constituents; hence, serum sodium concentration and osmolality decrease. This is further aggravated by increased excretion of sodium in the urine. This increased excretion is caused by two factors: (1) expansion of the plasma volume increases glomerular filtration and the filtered load of sodium; and (2) the secretion of atrial natriuretic peptide (ANP) is stimulated and sodium reabsorption is thereby inhibited. If serum osmolality falls substantially, serious overhydration of brain cells will occur as water moves down the osmotic gradient from the extracellular space to the intracellular space. Coma, convulsions, or both can result.

■ *Chapter 50*

1. Thyroid gland production of T_4 will immediately drop by about 50%. However, serum T_4 will take about 7 days to decrease 50% because of the large circulating pool of T_4 bound to thyroxine-binding globulin. As this pool nears depletion, the serum free T_4 will drop below normal. This stimulates an increase in thyroid-stimulating hormone (TSH) secretion by negative feedback, because there will be less blocking of the effect of thyrotropin-releasing hormone (TRH) on the thyrotroph cells. The higher TSH levels will stimulate iodide uptake, peroxidase activity, synthesis of thyroglobulin, and release of remaining prestored T_4. In addition, TSH will increase the size and number of the follicular cells in the remaining right lobe and will eventually restore T_4 production to normal. At this point, serum free T_4 will normalize, hypersecretion of TSH will cease, and serum TSH will return to normal.

2. The loss of weight is caused by an increase in energy expenditure ascribable to an increased basal metabolic rate and increased thermogenic "nervous" movements related to adrenergic hypersensitivity, without a sufficient compensatory increase in caloric intake. The weight loss is of both adipose tissue and muscle mass. The latter loss accounts for loss of strength. Muscle stores of creatine phosphate may also be reduced, and thus forceful contractions will be impaired. The cardiac output and rate, as well as the minute ventilation, increase to supply the extra oxygen being utilized in response to thyroxine excess. This is sensed by the patient as a racing heart (palpitations) and a feeling of shortness of breath when the normal demands of exercise are superimposed. Although cardiac contractility initially increases over the long term, cardiac output may not keep pace with demand. Therefore, lengthy exercise capacity is reduced and stamina is lost. The central nervous system effects of too much thyroxine can include insomnia and a loss of concentration and attentiveness. This can account for poor classroom performance.

■ *Chapter 51*

1. Although the circulating neutrophils may be increased, they will not be efficiently attracted to the site of bacterial invasion. The ability of those neutrophils that do reach the site to opsonize, phagocytize, and kill staphylococci will be reduced. Local vasodilation and increased capillary permeability normally caused by an invader will be inhibited. This reaction will prevent ready access of preexisting antibodies to staphylococci and their noxious products, as well as of other defense molecules and cells to the bacteria. The release of cytokines by immune cells, such as macrophages that recognize foreign antigens, will also be inhibited. Hence, proliferation of clones of lymphocytes with specific ability to target the bacteria will be reduced. Febrile response will also be diminished. As the staphylococci grow and flourish, they can disseminate to other areas of the body and cause sepsis, because the ability of fibroblasts and other connective tissue cells to enclose the bacteria with fibrous tissue is also impaired. These consequences arise from many intracellular actions of glucocorticoids. Examples include suppression of the expression of genes for the enzymes involved in prostaglandin synthesis, for interleukins-1 and -2, and for collagen.

2. Marked sweating is one of the mechanisms of disposal of extra heat that is produced by hypermetabolism in subjects who live in a greatly increased environmental temperature. The resultant loss of water (both sensible and insensible) and sodium leads to contraction of the extracellular fluid and plasma volumes. Sensors in the macula densa of the kidney stimulate increased production of renin by cells in the juxtaglomerular apparatus. This is reinforced by β-adrenergic stimuli from the sympathetic nervous system in response to stretch receptors in the vascular tree. Increased renin catalyzes release from angiotensinogen of angiotensin I, which in turn is split by angiotensin converting enzyme to angiotensin II. The latter stimulates rapid synthesis and release of aldosterone from the zona glomerulosa. Aldosterone stimulates sodium reabsorption by the distal tubules. The re-entry of sodium into the capillary blood obligates water to accompany it to maintain an iso-osmotic (isotonic) state. Thus, aldosterone preserves extracellular fluid volume and minimizes dehydration. As time passes, aldosterone also decreases sodium excretion in sweat, and eventually this limits sweat volume losses. At the same time that aldosterone stimulates sodium retention, the hormone increases renal tubular secretion of potassium into the urine and potassium uptake by peripheral cells. In this way, aldosterone decreases the risk of hyperkalemia secondary to any reduction in glomerular filtration rate that might result from dehydration.

3. Simultaneous activation of the sympathetic nervous system and the adrenal medulla greatly increases synaptic and plasma norepinephrine concentrations as well as plasma epinephrine levels. A host of β-adrenergic receptors are activated. These raise cAMP levels (and override α_2-receptor inhibitory effects on adenylyl cyclase activity). Activation of α_1-adrenergic receptors increases Ca^{++}, inositol trisphosphate, and diacylglycerol second messengers.

   The tourist's far vision is enhanced by relaxation of the ciliary muscles and by dilation of the pupils, permitting more light to enter, so she can follow and judge the bear's movements better. A sense of anxiety reinforces fear of the unknown and informs her that the situation is perilous, while enhanced alertness makes her more ready to react. Should she choose to run from this danger, she will require a burst of heavy sustained exercise. To provide energy for the initial sprint, muscle glycogenolysis is stimulated and glucose undergoes oxidation, first to lactate and then to carbon dioxide. Stimulation of liver glycogenolysis increases hepatic output of glucose and provides the exercising muscles with a sustaining plasma source of glucose. Lipolysis is also stimulated. This provides free fatty acids to the muscle as an increasingly important source of energy to the continuously active muscle. Oxidation of fatty acids in the liver produces H^+ equivalents such as NADPH and ATP, both of which are needed for reconverting lactate released by muscle and glycerol released by adipose tissue into glucose (glycogenolysis). The extra glucose also promotes the functioning of the cerebral cortex to help her think through critical decisions (e.g., whether to keep running). Bronchodilation enhances oxygen intake. Increased delivery of glucose, free fatty acids, and oxygen requires a large cardiac output and is facilitated by shunting of blood from the gut and kidneys to the muscles. Cardiac contractility and rate are increased, and the central venous pressure (cardiac preload) is augmented by an increased venous tone. Food-seeking and reproductive processes are inhibited, as usually are gastrointestinal and urinary functions. All of these would distract the escape efforts and would contribute nothing useful. The most helpful aspect of these catecholamine responses is the coordination of metabolic and cardiovascular effects that keep the energy supply from being exhausted.

■ *Chapter 52*

1. (a) Because of the absence of a Y chromosome, her gonads could not develop into testes. Lacking two active X chromosomes, her gonads could not develop into ovaries. Hence, her gonads will be only two vestigial fibrous streaks without significant endocrine function. The genital ducts could not develop into the male derivatives of the wolffian duct (epididymis, vas deferens, and seminal vesicles) because no testosterone was secreted. Instead, the female derivatives of the müllerian duct (fallopian tubes, uterus, and upper vagina) would develop because her gonads could not secrete antimüllerian hormone and suppress such development. The external genitalia would have the female pattern by default, because no testosterone or its derivative dihydrotestosterone was produced to masculinize them.

(b) Lacking any gonadal function, she would be deficient in estrogen. Therefore, those organs would be undersized and would not enlarge during puberty.

Because estrogen is lacking, the endometrium of the uterus would never build up to an amount that would cause a menstrual slough.

(c) Because of her feminine phenotype, her parents would have raised her as a girl, and these rearing cues would produce a female gender self-identification. This would be reinforced by estrogen therapy to normalize breast development, and by estrogen plus progesterone to provide menstrual cycles.

2. Both cell types are crucial for spermatogenesis. Without the function of each, spermatogenesis cannot proceed normally. The Leydig cell produces testosterone in response to stimulation by luteinizing hormone (LH). Without a very high local concentration of testosterone, the development of spermatocytes, spermatids, and spermatozoa from spermatogonia is greatly impaired. The effect of testosterone may be mediated by its actions on Sertoli cells, by conversion to estradiol within the Sertoli cell, or by eventual access of either steroid to the germ cells at various points in their descent from the base to the lumen of the tubule.

The Sertoli cell shields the male germ cell line from deleterious substances in plasma, but it permits passage of sustaining molecules. In response to follicle-stimulating hormone (FSH), the Sertoli cell produces androgen-binding protein, estradiol, and inhibin. Each of these directly or indirectly facilitates spermatogenesis by paracrine actions, or (in the case of androgen-binding protein) by also influencing the availability of testosterone and estradiol to the spermatozoa that are maturing within the epididymis. Sertoli cells also produce nutrient-binding proteins (e.g., transferrin for iron and ceruloplasm for copper) that can present essential minerals such as iron and copper to germ cells as well as substrates such as lactate for germ cell oxidation.

Products of Sertoli and Leydig cells modulate the function of their counterpart cell; for example, Sertoli cell inhibin stimulates testosterone secretion by Leydig cells. Thus, both cells and their mutual interactions are essential to creating the proper hormonal and nutrient environment for optimal sperm production.

3. (a) The most specific indicator would be daily measurement of the plasma LH level, which should increase fivefold to tenfold 12 to 24 hours before ovulation. A daily home measurement of the urinary LH level could provide similar information. Measurement of the plasma progesterone level three quarters of the way through her usual menstrual cycle would indicate whether a corpus luteum was being formed: a marked increase in the progesterone concentration to greater than 500 ng/dl would be convincing evidence that the cycles were ovulatory. Daily measurement of basal body temperature would suggest ovulation, if there were a distinct and sustained 0.5- to 10-degree rise at

some point. Likewise, examination of cervical mucus 10 to 14 days from the first day of menstrual bleeding, and again later in the cycle, would suggest ovulation if the mucus changed in character from a watery but elastic substance that dries to a fernlike pattern (estradiol dominant) to a thick, scant material that cannot fern (progesterone dominant).

(b) A normal sperm count does not ensure male fertility. Sperm need to have normal motility to reach the ovum. They need normal structure and function to penetrate the zona pellucida of the ovum; that is, they must have the ability to release enzymes from the acrosome to dispense the adherent granulosa cells and to express sperm membrane proteins that will interact with zona receptor proteins. Finally, the woman may have antibodies that are directed at sperm antigens and that prevent access of normal sperm to normal ova.

APPENDIX

B

Mini-Exam

■ Section I: Cellular Physiology

1-1. Which of the following statements about biological membranes is true?
   A. The phospholipid bilayer is quite permeable to water-soluble molecules with molecular weights between 200 and 500.
   B. Most lipid molecules are not free to move in the plane of the membrane.
   C. Flip-flop of lipid molecules from one monolayer to the other occurs infrequently.
   D. The carbohydrate chains of glycolipids and glycoproteins mostly face the cytosol.
   E. None of the above.

1-2. Which of the following statements about diffusion is true?
   A. The average time for a molecule to diffuse a particular distance is directly proportional to the first power of the distance.
   B. The rate at which substance X diffuses into a cell is proportional to the square of the area of the plasma membrane of the cell.
   C. The greater the solubility of a substance in nonpolar solvents, the smaller is its rate of permeation across biological membranes.
   D. If protein A has molecular weight 100,000 and protein B has molecular weight 200,000, the diffusion coefficient of A will be twice that of B.
   E. None of the above.

1-3. A membrane separates chambers A and B. The membrane is permeable to water but completely impermeable to NaCl. When chambers A and B are filled with water and 1 atm of hydrostatic pressure is applied to chamber A, water flows from A to B at 10 ml/min. Chamber A is then drained and refilled with a solution of NaCl with an osmotic pressure (as measured across a true semipermeable membrane) of 1 atm. Which of the following statements is true?
   A. No net water flow by osmosis will occur.
   B. A hydrostatic pressure of 1 atm applied to A would cause net water flow from A to B.

C. With no hydrostatic pressure on side A, the net osmotic flow from B to A will be 10 ml/min.
   D. If the membrane were permeable to NaCl, the osmotic water flow from B to A would be 5 ml/min.
   E. None of the above.

1-4. Which of the following statements about active transport processes is true?
   A. They always transport the transported substance against a gradient of electrochemical potential.
   B. They require a direct link to metabolic energy.
   C. The energy for secondary active transport is provided by the gradient of electrochemical potential of another solute.
   D. Only primary active transport will be inhibited by metabolic poisons.
   E. None of the above.

1-5. Which of the following statements about the Na^+, K^+-ATPase is true?
   A. It pumps 2 Na^+ out of the cell and 3 K^+ into the cell for each ATP it hydrolyzes.
   B. It is electrogenic in some but not all cells.
   C. In most cells, it pumps Na^+ and K^+ against both chemical and electrical gradients.
   D. It is driven by being phosphorylated by ATP.
   E. None of the above.

1-6. The membrane that separates chamber A from chamber B is permeable only to anions. Chamber A contains 1 M KCl, chamber B contains 0.1 M KCl. In the steady state, which of the following statements is true?
   A. The Nernst equation will apply to Cl^-, but not to K^+.
   B. The potential difference across the membrane will be 60 mV, with side A negative with respect to B.
   C. A significant amount of Cl^- (enough to diminish the concentration in A and increase it in B) will flow across the membrane to create the electrical potential difference.
   D. K^+ will flow across the membrane in proportion to the flow of Cl^-.
   E. None of the above.

1-7. The ionic distribution across the plasma membrane of a smooth muscle cell is as follows: the extracellular concentrations of K^+, Na^+, and Cl^- are 2.5, 120, and 120 mM, respectively. The cytoplasmic concentrations of K^+, Na^+, and Cl^- are 140, 10, and 12 mM, respectively. The resting membrane potential is −60 mV. Which of the following statements is true?
   A. Na^+ tends to enter the cell because of both its concentration gradient and the membrane potential.
   B. K^+ has a net tendency to enter the cell.
   C. Cl^- is not in equilibrium across the membrane.
   D. The Na^+, K^+-ATPase is not important in the steady state.
   E. None of the above.

1-8. A membrane that separates chambers A and B is permeable to K^+, Cl^-, and water but completely impermeable to X^-. Initially chamber A contains 0.1 M K^+ and 0.1 M X^- and chamber B contains 0.1 M KCl. Chamber A is pressure jacketed so that a Gibbs-Donnan equilibrium can be obtained. Which of the following statements is true?
   A. In attaining a Gibbs-Donnan equilibrium, Cl^-, but not K^+, will flow from side B to side A.
   B. The amount of K^+ that flows from B to A will be larger, by an infinitesimal amount, than the amount of Cl^- that flows.
   C. Both K^+ and Cl^- will be in equilibrium when the Gibbs-Donnan equilibrium has been attained.
   D. When the Gibbs-Donnan equilibrium has been attained, the product of the concentrations of K^+ on side A and B will equal the product of the Cl^- concentrations on side A and side B.
   E. None of the above.

1-9. Which of the following statements about resting membrane potentials is true?
   A. The electrogenicity of the Na^+, K^+-ATPase makes no contribution to the resting membrane potential of certain types of cells.
   B. The diffusion of K^+ and Na^+ down their electrochemical potential gradients contributes to the resting potential in only certain cell types.
   C. Negative fixed charge in cells does not contribute via the Gibbs-Donnan equilibrium to the resting potential of most cells.
   D. In skeletal muscle cells, the contribution of the electrogenic pump is small relative to the contribution of the ions diffusing down their electrochemical potential gradients.
   E. None of the above.

1-10. The resting conductance of the plasma membrane of a cell to K^+ is nine times that to Na^+. Cl^- is in equilibrium at the resting membrane potential. The contribution of the electrogenicity of the Na^+, K^+-ATPase is negligible. The extracellular concentrations of K^+ and Na^+ are 14 and 120 mM, respec-

tively. The cytoplasmic concentrations of K^+ and Na^+ are 140 and 12 mM, respectively. Which of the following statements is true?
   A. The resting membrane potential is about −48 mV.
   B. We cannot estimate the resting potential without knowing the relative conductance to Cl^-.
   C. Decreasing the extracellular $[K^+]$ will depolarize the cell.
   D. Increasing the K^+ conductance will depolarize the cell.
   E. None of the above.

1-11. The plasma membrane of a smooth muscle cell has a resting conductance to K^+ four times that to Na^+. The membrane Cl^- conductance is very small. The extracellular concentrations of K^+ and Na^+ are 13 and 110 mM, respectively. The cytoplasmic concentrations of K^+ and Na^+ are 130 and 11 mM, respectively. The resting membrane potential is −60 mV. Which of the following statements is true?
   A. The resting membrane potential estimated from the chord conductance equation is −48 mV.
   B. The electrogenic Na^+, K^+-ATPase might contribute the difference between the observed −60 mV and the resting potential calculated from the chord conductance equation.
   C. Inhibiting the Na^+, K^+-ATPase by treating the cell with a large dose of ouabain would have no significant effect on the resting membrane potential.
   D. If the plasma membrane were made equally conductive to Na^+ and K^+, the membrane potential would go to near −20 mV.
   E. None of the above.

1-12. For a particular cell the electrogenicity of the Na^+, K^+-ATPase makes a negligible contribution to the resting membrane potential. C^- is in equilibrium at the resting potential. The extracellular concentrations of K^+, Na^+, and Cl^- are 2.5, 120, and 120 mM, respectively. The cytoplasmic concentration of K^+ and Na^+ are 140 and 9 mM, respectively. The resting membrane potential is −60 mV. Which of the following statements is true?
   A. The intracellular $[Cl^-]$ is 3 to 4 mM.
   B. K^+ and Na^+ are in equilibrium.
   C. Increasing the conductance of the membrane to Cl^- would hyperpolarize the cell.
   D. Increasing the extracellular $[K^+]$ would depolarize the cell.
   E. None of the above.

1-13. Which of the following statements about the action potential in squid giant axons is correct?
   A. The rising phase of the action potential is due to a rapid increase in the conductance of the plasma membrane to Na^+ and K^+.
   B. The peak of the action potential reaches the equilibrium potential for Na^+.

C. The repolarizing phase of the action potential is due to a decrease in the sodium conductance and an increase in the potassium conductance.

D. The hyperpolarizing afterpotential is due to a prolonged decrease in the conductance to K^+.

E. None of the above.

1-14. Which of the following statements about the refractory periods of squid giant axons is true?

A. The absolute refractory period begins with the beginning of the action potential spike and ends when repolarization returns the cell to the resting membrane potential.

B. The relative refractory period begins near the peak of the action potential and ends when the hyperpolarizing afterpotential is over.

C. The elevated K^+ conductance is principally responsible for refractoriness during the later part of the absolute refractory period.

D. Voltage-inactivation of Na^+ channels is the major cause of the absolute refractory period.

E. None of the above.

1-15. Which of the following statements about ion channels in squid giant axons is true?

A. K^+ channels show significant voltage inactivation.

B. Na^+ channels have an activation gate and an inactivation gate.

C. The activation gate and the inactivation gate of the Na^+ channel respond with similar kinetics to a depolarization of the cell membrane.

D. The K^+ channels are blocked by tetrodotoxin.

E. None of the above.

1-16. Which of the following statements about action potentials is true?

A. Smooth muscle cells have an appreciable number of fast Na^+ channels.

B. The plateau phase of the cardiac action potential is due to opening of channels that are conductive to Ca^{++}.

C. The initial spike of cardiac ventricular action potentials is due to Na^+ channels that open and inactivate slowly.

D. The Ca^{++} that enters a smooth muscle cell during the action potential plays no important role in excitation-contraction coupling.

E. None of the above.

1-17. Which of the following statements about the conduction of a subthreshold depolarization of a nerve or muscle cell is true?

A. A subthreshold depolarization is conducted by saltatory conduction.

B. It is conducted with decrement, which means that the depolarization gets smaller as the depolarization moves along the cell.

C. The length constant is the distance over which the depolarization decreases to 50% of its maximal size.

D. The length constant is inversely related to (R_m/R_{in}) [membrane resistance/internal resistance].

E. None of the above.

1-18. Which of the following statements about conduction in a myelinated axon is true?

A. Owing to myelination, membrane resistance (R_m) is increased; this decreases the length constant.

B. Owing to myelination, membrane capacitance (C_m) is increased; this contributes to increased conduction velocity.

C. The velocity of conduction between nodes of Ranvier is very high compared with that in an unmyelinated axon.

D. The action potential is regenerated all along the axon.

E. None of the above.

1-19. Which of the following statements about neuromuscular transmission is true?

A. A miniature endplate potential occurs after an action potential in the nerve terminal.

B. Calcium influx into the nerve terminal initiates the chain of events that culminates in transmitter release.

C. The acetylcholine receptor protein is a voltage-gated ion channel that opens when it binds acetylcholine.

D. The desensitization of the acetylcholine receptor normally terminates the endplate potential.

E. None of the above.

1-20. Which of the following statements about the acetylcholine receptor protein of the neuromuscular junction is correct?

A. The acetylcholine receptor protein is a voltage-gated ion channel.

B. The acetylcholine receptor is concentrated at the neuromuscular junction.

C. The channel opened by acetylcholine is much more conductive to sodium than to potassium.

D. Depolarization of the muscle cell promotes opening of the acetylcholine receptor protein's ion channel.

E. None of the above.

1-21. Which of the following statements about synapses is true?

A. Gap junctions contain ligand-gated ion channels.

B. Synaptic delay is characteristic of chemical synapses.

C. A neurotransmitter acts to increase or decrease the conductance of the postsynaptic membrane to one or more ions.

D. Chemical synapses require influx of Na⁺ triggered by an action potential in the presynaptic nerve terminal.

E. None of the above.

1-22. Which of the following statements about synapses on cat spinal motor neurons is true?

A. An EPSP is due to opening of channels in the post-synaptic membrane that conduct primarily K⁺.

B. An IPSP is due to opening of channels in the postsynaptic membrane that conduct Cl⁻.

C. Action potentials are usually generated in dendrites.

D. Postsynaptic potentials that originate at synapses on the soma of the spinal motor neuron sum, but with significant decrement.

E. None of the above.

1-23. Which of the following statements about neurotransmitters and neuromodulators is true?

A. Acetylcholine is not a neurotransmitter in the brain.

B. α-Adrenergic synapses in the midbrain are deficient in Parkinson's disease.

C. GABA is the major inhibitory neurotransmitter in the spinal cord.

D. Glutamate is an important excitatory neurotransmitter in the brain.

E. The precursor polypeptides of neuropeptides are synthesized in nerve endings. The active neuropeptides are cleaved from the precursors by proteases.

1-24. Which of the following statements about signal transduction mechanisms is true?

A. Many signal transduction pathways involve the binding of an intracellular agonist to a membrane receptor, which directly increases the intracellular level of a second messenger.

B. Heterotrimeric GTP-binding proteins (G proteins) are inactivated by agonist-bearing membrane receptors.

C. G protein–coupled membrane receptors have seven transmembrane α-helices and make up a protein family.

D. Adenylyl cyclase is regulated positively, but not negatively, by G protein–mediated mechanisms.

E. None of the above.

1-25. Which of the following statements about heterotrimeric GTP-binding proteins is true?

A. The GDP-bound form of a G protein is the active form.

B. Low-molecular-weight GTP-binding proteins are structurally very similar to heterotrimeric G proteins.

C. In most cases the β subunit participates directly in the signal transduction cascade.

D. Hydrolysis of GTP results in inactivation of the G protein.

E. None of the above.

1-26. Which of the following statements about protein kinases is true?

A. Protein tyrosine kinases do not share significant structural homologies with serine-threonine protein kinases.

B. Protein kinase C is frequently activated by signal transduction pathways involving hydrolysis of certain membrane phospholipids.

C. All known calcium-calmodulin–dependent protein kinases have multiple substrate proteins.

D. Membrane receptors for serum growth factors are frequently serine-threonine protein kinases.

E. None of the above.

1-27. Which of the following statements is true?

A. The insulin receptor is a serine-threonine kinase.

B. Upon binding growth factor, certain growth factor receptors dimerize and dephosphorylate themselves.

C. Activated receptors for growth factors may in turn activate Ras, a heterotrimeric GTP-binding protein.

D. Activation of Ras may turn on the transcription of certain key genes that inhibit cell proliferation.

E. None of the above.

1-28. Which of the following statements is true?

A. PP-1 and PP-2 are the major classes of protein tyrosine phosphatases.

B. Serine-threonine protein phosphatases are subject to regulation via subunits that target the phosphatases to specific intracellular locations.

C. There are only three known distinct protein tyrosine kinases.

D. The receptors for atrial natriuretic peptide have adenylyl cyclase activity.

E. Nitric oxide (NO), produced by the activity of NO synthase, is an endocrine mediator

---

■ *Section II: The Nervous System*

2-1. A 67-year-old woman develops severe headaches over a period of several weeks. She has a grand mal seizure and is hospitalized. On physical examination, she is found to have papilledema. The tentative diagnosis is that she has a brain tumor. Which of the following tests would be a useful way to determine the location of the tumor?

A. Measurement of nerve conduction velocities in upper and lower extremities

B. Measurement of the intracranial pressure by inserting a transducer through a burr hole

C. Chemical analysis of cerebrospinal fluid obtained by a spinal tap

D. Imaging dye that normally does not pass through the blood brain barrier

E. Brain biopsy with the assistance of magnetic resonance imaging

2-2. A 36-year-old man has a seizure that begins with movements of his face. The movements spread to his hand and then his leg. Finally, the convulsion becomes generalized and bilateral. The sequence of the initial movements can be explained by

A. spread of seizure activity in the cerebral cortex from one somatotopic locus to another.

B. systematic changes in the pattern of seizure discharges at one cortical locus.

C. movement of seizure activity from the medulla to the cervical spinal cord and then to the lumbosacral spinal cord.

D. kindling, which is spread of seizure activity from a cortical locus to a mirror focus on the contralateral side.

E. spread of seizure activity from one thalamic nucleus to another.

2-3. Approximately how long would it take for a soluble protein molecule in the axoplasm of a lumbar motor neuron to reach the neuromuscular junction in a foot muscle by slow anterograde transport in a tall adult man?

A. Day
B. Week
C. Month
D. Year
E. Decade

2-4. Repair of myelin in multiple sclerosis, a demyelinating disease of the central nervous system, depends on the function of which cell type?

A. Astrocyte
B. Ependymal cell
C. Microglial cell
D. Oligodendrogliocyte
E. Schwann cell

2-5. Damage to a peripheral nerve is generally followed by sprouting and eventual regeneration of the interrupted axons. Upregulation of which of the following molecules helps trigger some of this regrowth?

A. Acetylcholinesterase
B. Glial fibrillary acidic protein
C. Nerve growth factor
D. Norepinephrine
E. Substance P

2-6. A hypodermic needle used to inject depot antibiotic is accidentally inserted into the sciatic nerve.

What type of nerve fibers are unlikely to be affected?

A. Autonomic preganglionic axons
B. Autonomic postganglionic axons
C. Primary afferent axons
D. Somatic motor axons from alpha motor neurons
E. Somatic motor axons from gamma motor neurons

2-7. A 56-year-old woman has severe burning pain originating from an injury of her hand. If you could record activity from nerve fibers in a peripheral nerve supplying the hand, what would you expect?

A. No nerve impulses, because pain depends on central nervous system activity

B. Very-high-frequency discharges in slowly adapting tactile afferents

C. Discharges in the axons of primary afferent C fibers

D. Nerve impulses in axons supplying thermoreceptors

E. Low-frequency activity in the axons of extensor motor neurons

2-8. A somatosensory neuron in the central nervous system is found to have a tactile inhibitory receptive field on the skin of the hand. How do you account for such an inhibitory receptive field?

A. Stimulation activates inhibitory primary afferent fibers.

B. Touching the skin reduces the activity of primary afferent fibers supplying the inhibitory field.

C. Excitation of primary afferent mechanoreceptors activates inhibitory interneurons.

D. Intense activation of the neuron by skin stimulation causes fatigue of the neuron.

E. Indentation of the skin interferes with input from the excitatory receptive field.

2-9. A 15-year-old boy injures a peripheral nerve in his arm because of a bicycle accident. He develops weakness of several muscles supplied by the nerve, and these muscles show signs of atrophy. An electromyogram taken from one of these muscles would show

A. increased numbers of motor unit potentials.
B. electrical silence.
C. only activity of slow motor units.
D. numerous fibrillation potentials.
E. motor unit potentials of intrafusal muscle fibers.

2-10. A soldier stands at attention for half an hour. What type of motor unit in the quadriceps and gastrocnemius-soleus muscles is most likely to be active?

A. FF
B. FR
C. IIA
D. IIB
E. S

2-11. A 72-year-old man develops a form (tabes dorsalis) of tertiary syphilis in which dorsal root ganglion cells are destroyed over a prolonged period of time. He has a characteristic gait in which he slaps his feet against the ground as he walks. When his eyes are closed, he tends to fall. These problems of gait and equilibrium can be attributed to the loss of what types of dorsal root ganglion cells?
A. Meissner's corpuscles
B. Muscle stretch receptors
C. Nociceptors
D. Pacininan corpuscles
E. Ruffini endings

2-12. A 25-year-old football player injures his knee when tackled on a punt return. Punctate noxious stimuli applied to the skin well away from the swollen knee hurt more than do comparable stimuli applied to the normal knee. This is a demonstration of
A. allodynia.
B. central pain.
C. nociceptive pain.
D. primary hyperalgesia.
E. secondary hyperalgesia.

2-13. An axon reflex consists of
A. a muscle contraction caused by the activity in the axon of a motor neuron.
B. antidromic invasion of a nerve impulse into another branch of a sensory axon.
C. movement of an axon caused by the activation of actin and myosin molecules in the axoplasm.
D. changes in the pattern of light reflected from an axon when the axon is activated.
E. nerve impulses originating in the terminals of sensory axons in the dorsal horn.

2-14. Stimulation of a single axon supplying a Merkel cell ending by means of a microneurography electrode in an awake human subject can elicit a sensation of
A. cold.
B. flutter.
C. pain.
D. position.
E. touch.

2-15. A patient with a peripheral nerve injury develops a pain state characterized by extreme tenderness to weak tactile stimuli. This allodynia can be accounted for by
A. excessive discharges of tactile afferent axons because of sensitization of these neurons.
B. loss of most of the tactile afferents in the injured nerve.
C. increased responses of wide-dynamic-range nociceptive neurons to tactile stimuli.

D. seizure activity in the somatotopically appropriate region of the somatosensory cortex.
E. sensitization of C nociceptors supplying the skin innervated by the injured nerve.

2-16. A boxer is repeatedly hit in the face by his opponent. Although he feels relatively little pain during the boxing match, he experiences severe pain for several days after the match. Why was his pain minimal at the time he received his injuries?
A. His trainer had given him morphine before the match.
B. The density of innervation of the skin of the face by nociceptors is low.
C. Boxers have very high pain thresholds.
D. Stress activated the endogenous analgesia systems.
E. The noxious stimuli activated the gate control mechanism.

2-17. Glaucoma can be caused by
A. hemorrhage into the vitreous humor.
B. reduced elasticity of the lens.
C. paralysis of the pupillary dilator muscle.
D. reduced drainage of aqueous humor.
E. separation of the retinal pigment cell layer.

2-18. Which of the following is a property of rods?
A. Their highest density is in the fovea.
B. They generate a "dark current."
C. They are most sensitive to red light.
D. They are depolarized by light.
E. They provide for color discrimination.

2-19. To which function is a P cell most likely to contribute?
A. Orientation to a visual target
B. Control of circadian rhythms
C. Smooth pursuit eye movements
D. Color vision
E. Movement detection

2-20. A pituitary tumor is often suspected in cases of
A. bitemporal hemianopsia.
B. central scotoma.
C. homonymous hemianopsia.
D. inferior homonymous quadrantanopsia.
E. superior homonymous quadrantanopsia.

2-21. Which of the following areas of the cerebral cortex is involved in the recognition of faces?
A. Area 7
B. Inferotemporal region
C. Middle superior temporal region
D. Middle temporal region
E. V4 region

2-22. If a Weber test reveals that sound is localized to the normal ear, the most likely cause of this condition is
A. a broken ossicular chain.
B. damage to cochlear hair cells.

C. fluid in the middle ear.
D. otosclerosis.
E. a ruptured typanic membrane.

2-23. If a Rinne test shows that bone conduction is better than air conduction in the right ear, the most likely cause of this condition is
A. a damaged right cochlear nerve.
B. a brainstem lesion that affects right cochlear nuclei.
C. otitis media on the right.
D. a stroke that involves the left primary auditory cortex.
E. a superior olivary complex lesion on the left.

2-24. A central nervous system structure that has a tonotopic organization is the
A. dorsal lateral geniculate nucleus.
B. inferior colliculus.
C. nucleus gracilis.
D. superior vestibular nucleus.
E. ventral posterior lateral nucleus.

2-25. Afferents that supply which sensory epithelium are most likely to be activated by a rapid descent in an elevator?
A. Ampullary crest of the anterior semicircular canal
B. Ampullary crest of the horizontal semicircular canal
C. Ampullary crest of the posterior semicircular canal
D. Otolithic membrane of the utricle and saccule
E. Cochlea

2-26. Neurons in which of the following structures are least likely to be affected by afferent activity that arises from the vestibular apparatus?
A. Cerebellum
B. Dorsal column nuclei
C. Oculomotor nucleus
D. Spinal cord
E. Vestibular nuclei

2-27. The taste quality detected by taste buds located on the posterior third of the tongue is
A. acid.
B. bitter.
C. salty.
D. sour.
E. sweet.

2-28. Loss of taste on the anterior two thirds of the tongue is most likely caused by a lesion that affects which cranial nerve?
A. V
B. VII
C. IX
D. X
E. XI

2-29. Which of the following odors is most likely to activate sensory nerve fibers of the trigeminal nerve?
A. Ammonia
B. Camphor
C. Eucalyptus
D. Rose
E. Rotten eggs

2-30. Which type of neuron serves as an inhibitory interneuron in the olfactory bulb?
A. Granule cell
B. Mitral cell
C. Olfactory receptor cell
D. Tufted cell
E. Uncal pyramidal cell

2-31. Neurons in which of the following central nervous system structures are least likely to process olfactory information?
A. Amygdala
B. Anterior olfactory nucleus
C. Medial dorsal thalamic nucleus
D. Nucleus of the solitary tract
E. Prepiriform cortex

2-32. Tapping the tendon of a muscle will produce a burst of nerve impulses in which type of nerve ending?
A. Golgi tendon organ
B. Group Ia muscle spindle afferent
C. Group II muscle spindle afferent
D. Muscle nociceptor
E. Merkel ending

2-33. Activation of static gamma motor neurons will have what effect?
A. Contraction of fast, fatigable muscle fibers
B. Discharge of Renshaw cells
C. Increased tonic stretch reflex
D. Initiation of flexor withdrawal reflex
E. Relaxation of nuclear chain fibers

2-34. Which reflex would explain an increased contraction of the quadriceps muscles in a soldier standing at attention long enough for tension to be reduced in the patellar tendons because of fatigue?
A. Crossed extension reflex
B. Flexion reflex
C. Inverse myotatic reflex
D. Phasic stretch reflex
E. Tonic stretch reflex

2-35. The monosynaptic reflex recorded from a ventral root after stimulation of the nerve to the medial gastrocnemius muscle is increased when the nerve to the lateral gastrocnemius muscle is also stimulated at the same time. This is an example of
A. occlusion.
B. reciprocal innervation.
C. recurrent inhibition.

D. spatial summation.

E. temporal summation.

2-36. Which one of these reflexes takes precedence over the other cited reflexes?

A. Flexion component of locomotion

B. Flexor withdrawal reflex

C. Inverse myotatic reflex

D. Phasic stretch reflex

E. Tonic stretch reflex

2-37. Which of the following muscles of the head is most likely to be paralyzed on the side opposite to a lesion of the corticobulbar tract?

A. Frontalis

B. Genioglossus

C. Masseter

D. Orbicularis oculi

E. Temporalis

2-38. Which of the following pathways that descend from the brain to the spinal cord can be considered a part of the lateral system for motor control?

A. Lateral corticospinal tract

B. Lateral vestibulospinal tract

C. Medullary reticulospinal tract

D. Tectospinal tract

E. Ventral corticospinal tract

2-39. Monoaminergic pathways that descend from the brain to the spinal cord exert a generalized form of motor control. Projections of the raphe nuclei to the spinal cord contain which monoamine?

A. Dopamine

B. Epinephrine

C. Histamine

D. Norepinephrine

E. Serotonin

2-40. If the head and body are tilted forward without bending the neck, the forelimbs will extend and the hindlimbs will flex. This is an example of which class of postural reflexes?

A. Ocular counterrolling

B. Righting reflex

C. Tonic neck reflex

D. Vestibular reflex

E. Vestibular placing reaction

2-41. The eyes of a football game spectator follow the motion of a punted football. Which class of eye movements does this illustrate?

A. Optokinetic reflex

B. Saccadic movement

C. Smooth pursuit

D. Vergence

E. Vestibulo-ocular reflex

2-42. The frontal eye fields and the superior colliculus are responsible for which type of eye movement?

A. Optokinetic

B. Saccades

C. Smooth pursuit

D. Vergence

E. Vestibulo-ocular

2-43. After a stroke, a patient believes that the left side of his body does not belong to him, but to the patient in the next bed. When asked to draw a clock-face, he places all the numbers on the right side of the drawing. The patient is likely to have a lesion of the right

A. angular gyrus.

B. inferior frontal gyrus.

C. paracentral lobule.

D. posterior parietal lobe.

E. posterior temporal gyrus.

2-44. The discharges of a corticospinal neuron

A. can be influenced by sensory input from the part of the body moved.

B. reflect joint position rather than the force of movement.

C. begin shortly after a movement occurs.

D. excite motor neurons to distal muscles strictly through disynaptic connections.

E. have no relation to the direction of movement.

2-45. Purkinje cells

A. receive inhibitory connections from climbing fibers.

B. discharge complex spikes in response to mossy fiber input.

C. excite stellate and basket cells of the molecular layer.

D. inhibit neurons in the deep cerebellar nuclei.

E. give rise to parallel fibers.

2-46. Neurons of the globus pallidus

A. are excited by neurons of the striatum.

B. excite neurons in the subthalamic nucleus.

C. are excited by neurons in the subthalamic nucleus.

D. excite neurons in the thalamus.

E. are excited by neurons in the thalamus.

2-47. Which of the following nuclei gives rise to parasympathetic preganglionic axons that travel in the glossopharyngeal nerve?

A. Dorsal motor nucleus

B. Edinger-Westphal nucleus

C. Inferior salivatory nucleus

D. Nucleus ambiguus

E. Superior salivatory nucleus

2-48. Which of the following statements about the enteric nervous system is correct?

A. The enteric nervous system is made up of only a few hundred neurons.

B. The myenteric plexus regulates fluid homeostasis.

C. There are primary afferent neurons in the myenteric plexus.

D. The submucosal plexus coordinates the contractions of the gut wall muscles.

E. Intestinal contractions cease when the gut is removed from the body.

2-49. Which receptor antagonist could be used to block fast excitatory transmission in a sympathetic ganglion?
A. Atropine
B. Bicuculline
C. Curare
D. Prazosin
E. Strychnine

2-50. Which of the following characteristics is a feature of Horner's syndrome?
A. Increased sweating on the face
B. Protrusion of the eye
C. Partial ptosis
D. Pupillary dilation
E. Vasoconstriction of facial skin

2-51. Water intake is increased by
A. hypo-osmotic extracellular fluid in the hypothalamus.
B. increased blood volume as sensed by receptors in the right atrium.
C. an action of angiotensin II on receptors in the subfornical organ.
D. inhibition of release of antidiuretic hormone.
E. activation of the area postrema.

2-52. Which cortical lobe is the most likely to be involved in a patient who has an aura of scintillations just before an epileptic seizure?
A. Frontal
B. Insular
C. Occipital
D. Parietal
E. Temporal

2-53. The oscillations in the alpha rhythm of the electroencephalogram are in which frequency range?
A. 13-30 Hz
B. 8-13 Hz
C. 4-7 Hz
D. 0.5-4 Hz
E. Less than 0.5 Hz

2-54. Which of the items below is characteristic of non-REM sleep?
A. Bursts of muscle twitches
B. Dreams
C. Profound loss of muscle tone
D. Delta waves
E. Penile erection

2-55. A boy is given a new alarm clock for Christmas. At first, the loud ticking of the clock keeps him awake at night. However, within a few days, he falls asleep soon after he gets into bed. This type of learning is called
A. classical conditioning.
B. habituation.
C. one trial.
D. operant conditioning.
E. sensitization.

2-56. Which of the following processes is least likely to be involved in the mechanism of long-term potentiation?
A. Ca^{++} efflux from the postsynaptic cell
B. Changes in neurotransmitter release
C. Activation of NMDA receptors
D. Release of retrograde messenger, such as nitric oxide
E. Activation of second messenger pathways

■ *Section III: Muscle*

3-1. Cross-bridges in smooth and skeletal muscles differ in
A. the amount of shortening that one cycle can produce.
B. the force-generating capacity.
C. the amount of ATP required by the myosin ATPase for each cross-bridge cycle.
D. the number of constituent polypeptides that make up the molecule.
E. their cycling rate for any given load.

3-2. In a relaxed skeletal muscle, the cross-bridges are
A. in a detached 45-degree conformation.
B. a complex of myosin, actin, ADP, and P_i.
C. a myosin ATP complex.
D. dissociated from the thick filaments.
E. a high-energy complex of myosin, ADP, and P_i.

3-3. When work is done on a contracting muscle by external forces,
A. it shortens.
B. it has an increased rate of ATP consumption.
C. it exhibits a reduced force-bearing capacity.
D. cross-bridge attachments to the thin filaments are formed and broken without ATP hydrolysis.
E. cross-bridges never detach from the thin filaments.

3-4. A single cross-bridge cycle can move a thin filament
A. about 10 nm (nanometers) (1 nm = 10^{-9}m).
B. about 2.5 μm (micrometers) (1 μm = 10^{-6}m).
C. to a length at which the force-generating capacity is changed by about 10%.
D. without hydrolysis of ATP.
E. by the length of an intact myosin molecule.

3-5. Troponin
   A. has one Ca^{++}-binding site.
   B. has a high affinity for myosin.
   C. binds to 6 to 7 actin monomers.
   D. is an ATPase.
   E. is present in a 1:1 molar ratio with tropomyosin.

3-6. Fine gradation of the force of contraction in a skeletal muscle is facilitated by
   A. mostly fast, glycolytic motor units.
   B. large numbers of motor units with relatively few cells.
   C. uniform excitability of motor nerves to fast and slow motor units.
   D. high ATP synthetic rates.
   E. strength training and cellular hypertrophy.

3-7. Compared with a fast motor unit, a typical slow motor unit has
   A. more cells.
   B. a higher force-generating capacity.
   C. more mitochondria.
   D. a less excitable motor nerve.
   E. a more rapid fatigue rate.

3-8. The force of contraction in a skeletal muscle is normally graded by
   A. the amount of Ca^{++} released from the sarcoplasmic reticulum by an action potential.
   B. a change in the affinity of troponin for Ca^{++}.
   C. activation of fast, glycolytic motor units instead of slow, oxidative motor units.
   D. summation of action potentials to prolong depolarization.
   E. recruitment.

3-9. Excellent performance in long distance running
   A. is accomplished by training of fast motor units.
   B. is associated with an enhanced glycolytic capacity of slow motor units.
   C. is characterized by glycogen depletion.
   D. is associated with cellular fatigue.
   E. involves contraction of mainly slow motor units.

3-10. Glycolysis is characterized by
   A. rapid rates of ATP synthesis.
   B. maximizing the amount of ATP produced per mole of glucose.
   C. the capacity to sustain prolonged, low-intensity work.
   D. creatine phosphate hydrolysis.
   E. a dependence on sustained blood supply.

3-11. The force per cross-sectional area of a smooth muscle cell is
   A. much greater than that of skeletal muscle.
   B. similar to that of skeletal muscle.
   C. low because the cells are small.
   D. attributable to phosphorylated cross-bridges.

E. independent of the myoplasmic Ca^{++} concentration.

3-12. The membrane responsible for regulating the myoplasmic Ca^{++} concentration during sustained contractions in smooth muscle is
   A. the sarcoplasmic reticulum.
   B. the caveoli.
   C. the motor end of the plate.
   D. the sarcolemma.
   E. the transverse tubules.

3-13. Sustained force maintenance (tone) in smooth muscle is characterized by
   A. a very high ratio of myosin kinase/myosin phosphatase activity.
   B. reduced ATP consumption and shortening rates.
   C. an arrested cross-bridge cycle.
   D. high myoplasmic Ca^{++} concentrations.
   E. phosphorylation of the cytoskeleton.

3-14. Increases in cell Ca^{++} concentration induce contraction in smooth muscle by
   A. binding to myosin (light-chain) kinase.
   B. producing a thin filament conformational change.
   C. formation of a complex of Ca^{++}, calmodulin, and myosin kinase.
   D. inhibiting myosin phosphatase.
   E. reducing cross-bridge phosphorylation.

3-15. The initial Ca^{++} transient induced by excitatory neurotransmitters in smooth muscle does not involve
   A. transverse tubular depolarization.
   B. activation of phospholipase C.
   C. intracellular production of inositol 1,4,5-trisphosphate.
   D. increased conductance of Ca^{++} channels in the sarcoplasmic reticulum.
   E. formation of a neurotransmitter-receptor complex in the sarcolemma.

■ Section IV: The Cardiovascular System

4-1. Which of the following is *not* essential for blood coagulation in a wound?
   A. Calcium
   B. Prothrombin
   C. Fibrinogen
   D. Platelets
   E. Thromboplastin

4-2. Intravascular clots can be dissolved by
   A. prostacyclin.
   B. plasmin.
   C. serotonin.
   D. heparin.
   E. erythropoietin.

4-3. The mean systemic arterial pressure exceeds the mean pulmonary artery pressure because
  A. the blood flow through the systemic circulation exceeds the blood flow through the pulmonary circulation.
  B. the number of systemic capillaries exceeds the number of pulmonary capillaries.
  C. the low oxygen tension in the pulmonary arterial blood causes the pulmonary resistance vessels to dilate.
  D. the compliance is greater in the systemic than in the pulmonary arteries.
  E. the resistance to blood flow is much greater in the systemic than in the pulmonary vascular bed.

4-4. An increase in left ventricular end-diastolic volume increases the stroke volume because
  A. the increased preload diminishes the ventricular compliance.
  B. the increased preload diminishes the ventricular afterload.
  C. the increased ventricular volume diminishes the stiffness of the series elastic elements.
  D. the increased myocardial fiber length enhances the responsiveness of the contractile proteins to calcium.
  E. the increased preload increases the conductance of the I_{K1} potassium channels.

4-5. In a typical capillary
  A. the pressure at the venous end exceeds that at the arterial end.
  B. the radius exceeds that of a typical arteriole.
  C. the tension in the wall increases as the hydrostatic pressure rises.
  D. the radius is more than three times as great as the radius of a red blood cell.
  E. the tension in the wall is proportional to the fourth power of the radius.

4-6. If the red blood cells in a blood vessel move at a mean velocity of 100 cm/sec and the blood flow through the vessel is 200 ml/sec, the cross-sectional area of that vessel is
  A. 2.0 cm^2.
  B. 5.0 cm^2.
  C. 20.0 cm^2.
  D. 0.20 cm^2.
  E. 0.50 cm^2.

4-7. In a normal person, most of the circulating blood is located in the
  A. systemic capillaries.
  B. systemic veins
  C. pulmonary capillaries.
  D. pulmonary veins.
  E. systemic arteries and arterioles.

4-8. The colloid osmotic pressure of the plasma is determined mainly by the plasma concentration of
  A. vitamin K.
  B. albumin.
  C. globulin.
  D. sodium.
  E. collagen.

4-9. During the resting phase of a ventricular myocardial cell, the transmembrane potential depends mostly on the conductance of the cell membrane to
  A. calcium.
  B. acetylcholine.
  C. sodium.
  D. potassium.
  E. norepinephrine.

4-10. During moderate physical exercise,
  A. stroke volume increases in proportion to the cardiac output.
  B. renal blood flow increases in proportion to the cardiac output.
  C. blood flow to the exercising muscle increases in proportion to the cardiac output.
  D. heart rate increases in proportion to the cardiac output.
  E. splanchnic blood flow increases in proportion to the cardiac output.

4-11. Arteriovenous anastomoses in the skin
  A. show basal tone and autoregulation.
  B. are responsive to metabolic activity of the skin.
  C. are insensitive to circulating epinephrine.
  D. show reactive hyperemia.
  E. close in response to sympathetic nerve activity.

4-12. If a drug is given that acts specifically to increase myocardial contractility,
  A. mean arterial pressure will decrease.
  B. arterial pulse pressure will decrease.
  C. capillary blood flow will decrease.
  D. stroke volume will decrease.
  E. central venous pressure will decrease.

4-13. Neural regulation of vascular resistance in skeletal muscle is mediated by
  A. sympathetic nerves alone.
  B. parasympathetic nerves alone.
  C. motor nerves.
  D. combined action of sympathetic and parasympathetic nerves.
  E. sympathetic cholinergic nerves.

4-14. The cardiac fibers that normally display the property of post-repolarization refractoriness are
  A. atrial myocardial fibers.
  B. ventricular myocardial fibers.
  C. atrioventricular nodal fibers.
  D. His bundle fibers.
  E. Purkinje fibers.

4-15. Velocity of shortening of myocardial fibers is greatest when
   A. preload is moderate and afterload is zero.
   B. preload is zero and afterload is moderate.
   C. preload is high and afterload is high.
   D. preload is zero and afterload is high.
   E. preload is high and afterload is moderate.

4-16. The ultrafiltration of fluid from the capillaries into the interstitial spaces increases as the
   A. tissue hydrostatic pressure decreases.
   B. oncotic pressure of the interstitial fluid decreases.
   C. hydrostatic pressure in the capillaries decreases.
   D. radius of the upstream arteriole decreases.
   E. molecular weight of the plasma proteins decreases.

4-17. The most important cause of increased blood flow through a working skeletal muscle during exercise is
   A. increased cardiac output.
   B. stimulation of sympathetic vasodilator nerves to the muscle.
   C. release of epinephrine from the adrenal medulla.
   D. vasoconstriction in the viscera.
   E. products of local metabolism.

4-18. The contribution of atrial contraction to ventricular filling is greatest
   A. when vagal activity is pronounced.
   B. at rapid heart rates.
   C. when atria and ventricles contract simultaneously.
   D. during atrial flutter.
   E. during third-degree atrioventricular block.

4-19. An increase in ventricular contractility is indicated by
   A. an increase in cardiac output accompanied by an increase in ventricular end-diastolic volume.
   B. an increase in the amplitude of the QRS complex of the electrocardiogram.
   C. an increase in cardiac output accompanied by a decrease in mean arterial pressure.
   D. a decrease in cardiac output accompanied by an increase in ventricular end-diastolic volume.
   E. an increase in cardiac output accompanied by a decrease in ventricular end-diastolic volume.

4-20. The medullary vasomotor center is stimulated most effectively by
   A. decreased arterial blood oxygen tension.
   B. decreased arterial blood hydrogen ion concentration.
   C. increased arterial blood adenosine concentration.
   D. increased arterial blood carbon dioxide tension.
   E. increased arterial blood potassium ion concentration.

4-21. In response to a substantial hemorrhage,
   A. the neural activity in the efferent vagus nerve fibers to the heart decreases.
   B. the neural activity in the carotid sinus baroreceptor nerve fibers increases.
   C. the neural activity in the efferent sympathetic nerve fibers to the heart decreases.
   D. the release of vasopressin from the posterior pituitary gland decreases.
   E. the release of renin from the kidney decreases.

4-22. During the cardiac catheterization of a person found to be normal, the blood withdrawn through the catheter had an oxygen saturation of 60%, and the recorded pressure oscillated each heartbeat between 14 and 26 mm Hg. Most likely, the catheter tip was located in the
   A. azygos vein.
   B. pulmonary artery.
   C. right atrium.
   D. foramen ovale.
   E. coronary sinus.

4-23. For a given patient, the results of laboratory and experimental studies are as follows:
   Hematocrit   55%
   Oxygen consumption   250 ml/min
   Arterial-to-mixed venous
      blood oxygen difference   25 ml/L blood
   Arterial oxygen saturation   70%
   The output of the left ventricle, L/min, is
   A. 1.25
   B. 5.0
   C. 7.5
   D. 10.0
   E. 15.0

4-24. In a physically trained person,
   A. heart rate can reach higher levels than in an untrained person.
   B. stroke volume is greater than in an untrained person.
   C. vagal tone is lower than in an untrained person.
   D. vascular resistance is higher than in an untrained person.
   E. left ventricular end-diastolic volume is less than in an untrained person.

4-25. A reduction in mean arterial pressure from 120 to 70 mm Hg causes a reflex
   A. decrease in myocardial contractility.
   B. increase in duration of the cardiac cycle.
   C. decrease in impulse conduction velocity through the atrioventricular node.
   D. increase in total peripheral vascular resistance.
   E. decrease in calcium conductance of myocytes during the action potential plateau.

4-26. If a person's resting heart rate, stroke volume, and total peripheral resistance did not change appreciably as he or she advanced from 20 to 70 years of age, but the arterial compliance did diminish substantially as the person grew older,

A. pulmonary blood flow would decrease substantially with age.

B. myocardial energy requirements would diminish with age.

C. mean arterial pressure would not change appreciably with age.

D. systemic capillary blood flow would become less pulsatile with age.

E. arterial pulse pressure would diminish with age.

4-27. In a normal resting person, the organ with the greatest oxygen consumption (per gram of tissue) and highest venous oxygen content is the

A. brain.

B. heart.

C. liver.

D. kidney.

E. skeletal muscle.

4-28. A sudden hemorrhage will cause

A. a decrease in stoke volume and a decrease in central venous pressure.

B. a decrease in arterial pressure but a rise in central venous pressure.

C. an increase in stroke volume but a decrease in central venous pressure.

D. a decrease in stroke volume but a rise in central venous pressure.

E. an increase in stroke volume and a rise in central venous pressure.

4-29. The laminar flow of a newtonian fluid through a cylindric tube varies

A. inversely with the difference in pressure at the two ends of the tube.

B. directly with the viscosity of the fluid.

C. inversely with the length of the tube.

D. inversely with the fourth power of the radius.

E. directly with the hydraulic resistance to flow.

4-30. If both the radius and the length of a cylindric tube are doubled, the resistance to the laminar flow of a newtonian fluid will

A. increase twofold.

B. remain unchanged.

C. decrease to half its previous value.

D. decrease to one fourth its previous value.

E. decrease to one eighth its previous value.

4-31. Velocity of blood flow is greatest in the

A. capillaries.

B. venules.

C. venae cavae.

D. aorta.

E. arterioles.

4-32. During the plateau of the action potential in a ventricular myocardial cell,

A. the cell is relatively refractory.

B. the efflux of calcium from the cell exceeds the influx of calcium into the cell.

C. the transmembrane potential is slightly positive.

D. the potassium conductance exceeds the potassium conductance that prevails during phase 4.

E. the influx of calcium into the sarcoplasmic reticulum exceeds the efflux of calcium from the sarcoplasmic reticulum.

4-33. Cerebral blood flow is

A. insensitive to P_{O_2}.

B. reduced by high Pa_{CO_2}.

C. characterized by autoregulation.

D. uniform throughout the brain.

E. primarily under neural control.

4-34. If a drug is given that acts specifically to constrict the arterioles in the systemic circulation,

A. cardiac output will decrease but central venous pressure will rise.

B. cardiac output and mean arterial pressure will both decrease.

C. cardiac output will increase but mean arterial pressure will not be affected.

D. cardiac output and central venous pressure will both decrease.

E. mean arterial pressure and central venous pressure will both rise.

4-35. An increase in carotid sinus pressure will

A. increase heart rate.

B. increase peripheral resistance.

C. increase capillary pressure.

D. increase myocardial contractility.

E. increase systemic blood pressure.

4-36. In a person with a prominent respiratory sinus arrhythmia,

A. efferent vagal activity decreases during inspiration.

B. efferent cardiac sympathetic activity decreases during inspiration.

C. the slope of the slow diastolic depolarization of the sinoatrial cells decreases during inspiration.

D. the arrhythmia will become more pronounced in response to hemorrhage.

E. propranolol will abolish the arrhythmia.

4-37. During isovolumic relaxation,

A. the aortic valve is closed and the mitral valve is open.

B. the aortic valve is open and the mitral valve is closed.

C. the pulmonic valve is open and the tricuspid valve is closed.

D. the pulmonic valve is closed and the tricuspid valve is open.

E. all valves are closed.

4-38. The Frank-Starling relation is essentially a restatement of
A. the force-velocity relation of cardiac muscle.
B. Poiseuille's law of the heart.
C. the length-tension diagram of cardiac muscle.
D. Laplace's law of the heart.
E. excitation-contraction coupling of cardiac muscle.

4-39. One half-hour after a brief but substantial hemorrhage,
A. the hematocrit ratio of the blood has increased.
B. the renal tubular reabsorption of sodium has decreased.
C. the secretion of epinephrine from the adrenal medulla has decreased.
D. the secretion of aldosterone from the adrenal cortex has increased.
E. the blood level of angiotensin II has decreased.

4-40. The mean pressure in the left renal artery of a normal experimental animal is 100 mm Hg but is reduced suddenly to 80 mm Hg by means of a clamp and then held at that lower level for 5 minutes. At the end of this period,
A. the blood flow to the right kidney will have increased by about 20%.
B. the oxygen consumption of the left kidney will be diminished by about 30%.
C. the blood flow to the left kidney will not be appreciably different from the control value.
D. the glomerular filtration rate of the left kidney will be decreased by about 30%.
E. the free-water clearance of the left kidney will be decreased by about 50%.

4-41. When cardiac sympathetic activity suddenly ceases, the effects of that activity subside gradually because
A. norepinephrine continues to be released from the nerve endings long after the neural activity has ceased.
B. neuropeptides coreleased with norepinephrine delay its degradation.
C. the processes that remove neurally released norepinephrine from the cardiac tissues are slow.
D. the calcium channels in the myocyte membranes are connected to the beta-adrenergic receptors by G proteins.
E. the neurally released norepinephrine alters the viscoelastic characteristic of the cardiac tissues.

4-42. When a person lying on a tilt table is shifted from a horizontal to an upright position, the cardiac output decreases because
A. arterial compliance decreases.

B. central venous pressure decreases.
C. heart rate decreases.
D. the arteriovenous shunts in the splanchnic vessels dilate.
E. sympathetic nervous activity to the heart decreases.

4-43. If the radius of a cylindric tube is tripled, the laminar flow of a newtonian fluid through the tube will
A. not be affected.
B. increase threefold.
C. increase sixfold.
D. increase ninefold.
E. increase 81-fold.

4-44. The total peripheral resistance (TPR) of a tall, stocky adult who has normal arterial blood pressure is
A. greater than the TPR of an average 10-year-old child.
B. greater than the TPR of a hypertensive adult of the same weight.
C. less during rest than during exercise.
D. less than the TPR of a normal adult of average height and build.
E. greater than the renal vascular resistance.

4-45. The pressure drop in the systemic circulation is greatest in the
A. arterioles.
B. capillaries.
C. venules.
D. aorta.
E. venae cavae.

4-46. The cardiac impulse is conducted most slowly in
A. atrial myocardial fibers.
B. atrioventricular nodal fibers.
C. His bundle fibers.
D. Purkinje fibers.
E. ventricular myocardial fibers.

4-47. In the fetus,
A. pulmonary resistance is lower than in a 1-day-old baby.
B. the left ventricle pumps more than does the right ventricle.
C. the ductus arteriosus closes in response to an increase in Pa_{CO_2}.
D. fetal hemoglobin has a greater affinity for O_2 than does adult hemoglobin.
E. the foramen ovale shunts blood from the pulmonary artery to the aorta.

4-48. If the heart rate of a resting normal person is increased from 60 to 90 beats/min by artificial atrial pacing,
A. cardiac output will increase by at least 50%.
B. stroke volume will not be affected appreciably.
C. cardiac output will not be affected appreciably.

D. arterial pulse pressure will increase.

E. central venous pressure will increase.

4-49. Hypoxia, as occurs at high altitude,

A. increases partial pressure of arterial blood CO_2 (Pa_{CO_2}).

B. decreases blood pH.

C. decreases peripheral resistance.

D. increases the respiratory rate.

E. decreases blood pressure.

4-50. When vagal activity suddenly ceases, the cardiac response to that activity disappears rapidly because the

A. cardiac cells become tachyphylactic.

B. nerve endings rapidly take up the released acetylcholine.

C. myocytes rapidly take up the released acetylcholine.

D. acetylcholine in the nerve endings is rapidly depleted.

E. abundant acetylcholinesterase rapidly degrades the released acetylcholine.

4-51. When a person is standing, the capillaries in the feet do not rupture because the

A. arterioles reflexly constrict and prevent exposure of the capillaries to high pressure.

B. tissue pressure rises and opposes an increase in capillary pressure.

C. total capillary cross-section is large enough to distribute and thereby reduce intracapillary pressure.

D. capillary diameter is so small that the wall tension is low.

E. capillaries constrict by a myogenic mechanism.

4-52. With regard to the blood supply to the normal liver,

A. more than half of the blood flow and more than half of the oxygen supply is delivered by the hepatic artery.

B. less than half of the blood flow and less than half of the oxygen supply is delivered by the hepatic artery.

C. more than half of the blood flow and more than half of the oxygen supply is delivered by the portal vein.

D. less than half of the blood flow and less than half of the oxygen supply is delivered by the portal vein.

E. less than half of the blood flow and more than half of the oxygen supply is delivered by the hepatic artery.

4-53. In a 60-year-old hypertensive person, the commonly observed increase in artrial pulse pressure is caused by

A. increased stroke volume.

B. increased myocardial contractility.

C. decreased mean circulatory pressure.

D. decreased arterial compliance.

E. increased heart rate.

4-54. The principal determinants of mean arterial pressure are

A. cardiac output and peripheral resistance.

B. arterial and venous compliance.

C. cardiac output and arterial compliance.

D. peripheral resistance and arterial compliance.

E. cardiac output and venous compliance.

4-55. The force of cardiac contraction is enhanced by

A. a reduction in preload.

B. an increase in interstitial fluid Na^+.

C. inhibition of the Na^+, K^+-ATPase.

D. phosphorylation of phospholamban.

E. administration of a beta blocker.

4-56. Cardiac Purkinje fibers

A. are located in the epicardial layers of the ventricles.

B. do not possess the property of automaticity.

C. do not display a prominent notch (phase 1) in their action potentials.

D. have a very brief plateau.

E. conduct action potentials more rapidly than do atrial or ventricular myocytes.

4-57. In severe exercise,

A. stroke volume increases proportionately more than does heart rate.

B. pulse pressure decreases.

C. capillary hydrostatic pressure decreases.

D. arterial oxygen levels fall.

E. arteriovenous oxygen difference increases.

4-58. The most important factor in the regulation of coronary blood flow is the

A. coronary perfusion pressure.

B. metabolic activity of the myocardium.

C. extravascular compression of the coronary vessels.

D. activity of the cardiac sympathetic nerves.

E. activity of the vagus nerves to the heart.

4-59. In metabolic regulation of blood flow,

A. basal vascular tone is unchanged when tissue metabolism is altered.

B. blood flow is held constant during changes in tissue metabolism.

C. blood flow and tissue metabolism are inversely related.

D. blood flow and arterial pressure are inversely related.

E. blood flow and tissue metabolism are directly related.

4-60. The less compliant arterial system in old people compared with young people

A. allows blood to flow through the capillaries at a more steady rate.

B. requires the heart to expend more energy to pump a normal cardiac output.

C. prevents the arterial systolic pressure from attaining excessively high values.

D. increases the total blood volume.

E. decreases the mean arterial blood pressure.

4-61. The ejection fraction is the

A. ratio of the blood ejected per beat by the left ventricle to the volume of blood in the left ventricle at the end of systole.

B. ratio of the blood ejected per beat by the left ventricle to the volume of blood in the left atrium in early diastole.

C. fraction of the cardiac output ejected per heartbeat.

D. stoke volume minus residual volume.

E. ratio of the blood ejected per beat by the left ventricle to the volume of blood in the left ventricle at the end of diastole.

4-62. In the coronary circulation,

A. venous oxygen content is one of the lowest in the body.

B. coronary blood flow to the left ventricle is greatest during ventricular systole.

C. autoregulation does not occur.

D. the epicardium and endocardium are equally vulnerable to reductions in coronary perfusion pressure.

E. parasympathetic effects predominate over sympathetic neural effects on the vessels.

■ *Section V: The Respiratory System*

5-1. The anatomic differences that contribute to important functional differences between the bronchi and bronchioles are that

A. bronchioles have type 1 and type 2 squamous (thin, flat, pavement) epithelial cells, whereas the bronchi have columnar epithelium with cilia.

B. the bronchiolar glands are situated directly beneath the lining epithelium (submucosa), whereas the glands of the bronchi are larger and external to the cartilage rings or plates.

C. the smooth muscle of the bronchi is arranged longitudinally (along the axis of the airway), whereas the smooth muscle of the bronchioles is arranged circularly or spirally around the lumen of the airway.

D. the bronchi are not directly attached to the connective tissue fibers of the lung tissue, whereas the bronchioles are directly embedded into the lung connective tissue structure.

E. the pulmonary arteries and veins are always adjacent to the airways leading into and out of the ventilated lungs units they subserve.

5-2. An 8-year-old normal girl (30-kg body weight) has a breathing frequency of 20/min at rest and a breath (tidal) volume of 80 ml. Her total ventilation is closest to

A. 0.25 L/min.

B. 0.6 L/min.

C. 1.6 L/min.

D. 2.4 L/min.

E. 3.2 L/min.

5-3. The principal function of the lungs is to ensure that

A. inspired air and pulmonary blood flow are distributed adequately to all lung units, so that gas exchange is accomplished with minimal energy expenditure.

B. the hemoglobin in the erythrocytes leaving each lung unit is 100% saturated with oxygen.

C. tissue cell oxygen consumption and carbon dioxide elimination are equal.

D. each lung unit is perfused in proportion to its capillary blood volume and ventilated in proportion to its gas volume.

E. diffusion into and out of blood is never rate limiting for oxygen uptake or carbon dioxide release.

5-4. Normal inspiration is limited by

A. sensory feedback to the respiratory centers in the medulla (brainstem) from mechanoreceptors in the chest wall and lung and from various chemoreceptors sensitive to oxygen and carbon dioxide.

B. the breathing frequency, about 12/min in resting adult humans, which limits each breath to 5 seconds' duration.

C. the rise of abdominal pressure as the diaphragm contracts.

D. the rise in pleural pressure as lung volume increases.

E. the mechanical limits of the chest wall.

5-5. The normal resting oxygen consumption of adult humans is determined by the

A. fact that resting cardiac output is about 5 L/min, therefore blood flow to some organs is limited.

B. ability of tissue cells to extract oxygen from the capillary blood in the time available for exchange in the capillaries.

C. ability of pulmonary capillary blood to take up oxygen from alveolar gas in the time available (less than 1 second) for exchange.

D. fact that the P_{50} of adult human blood is normally 26 to 29 mm Hg, and therefore no more than 50% of total blood oxygen concentration is available for cellular oxidative metabolism.

E. oxidative energy requirements of the body's cells.

5-6. If a patient has a lung compliance of 0.33 L/cm H_2O and chest wall compliance of 0.15 cm H_2O, the total compliance of the respiratory system is about

A. 0.05 L/cm H_2O.
B. 0.10 L/cm H_2O.
C. 0.18 L/cm H_2O.
D. 0.48 L/cm H_2O.
E. 9.70 L/cm H_2O.

5-7. A 17-year-old boy is admitted to the hospital with progressive respiratory failure caused by a viral infection in the brain. A breathing tube is inserted in his trachea. A positive pressure ventilator increases his lung volume by 0.5 L 15 times/min. At end-expiration the ventilator does not apply any pressure to the endotracheal tube. If the lung and chest wall compliances are each 0.2 L/cm H_2O over this range of lung volume change and if trans-lung pressure = 5 cm H_2O at functional reserve capacity (FRC), the

A. pleural pressure at FRC will be about +5 cm H_2O.
B. pleural pressure at end-inspiration is about −2.5 cm H_2O.
C. pleural pressure cannot be calculated without knowing the value of FRC.
D. transdiaphragm–abdominal wall pressure at end-inspiration must be about +5 cm H_2O.
E. total pressure across the lungs and chest wall at end-inspiration is about +10 cm H_2O.

5-8. In pulmonary edema caused by a toxic substance, plasma proteins enter the alveoli and inactivate the surface active material. This fixes alveolar surface tension at a constant value of 50 mN/cm. Which of the following statements regarding the pressure-volume curve of the lung best describes the new condition?

A. The deflation limb of the liquid-filled curve will be displaced to the right (greater trans-lung pressure at any given lung volume).
B. The deflation limb of the air-filled curve will be displaced to the right (greater translung pressure at any given lung volume).
C. The inflation limb of the air-filled curve will be displaced to the left (reduced translung pressure at any given lung volume).
D. The inflation limb of the air-filled curve will be normal.
E. The compliance of the respiratory system will be increased.

5-9. Given the following partial resistances of the large and small airways, R_{large} = 1.5 and R_{small} = 0.7 cm H_2O × sec/L, respectively, the total airway resistance is closest to

A. 2.2.
B. 1.6.
C. 0.8.
D. 0.5.
E. 0.4.

5-10. Given the following airway resistances of four parallel lung lobes, $Lobe_1$ = 1.8, $Lobe_2$ = 1.0, $Lobe_3$ = 0.6, $Lobe_4$ = 3.5 cm H_2O × sec/L, the total airway resistance is closest to:

A. 6.90.
B. 3.51.
C. 2.85.
D. 0.55.
E. 0.28.

5-11. Assume that the shape of the diaphragm is a portion of a sphere with a radius of curvature = 15 cm. In a supine person whose lungs are at FRC, the abdominal pressure just under the diaphragm = P_B and pleural pressure = −4 cm H_2O. The passive tension in the diaphragm (mN/cm) is about

A. 30.
B. 800.
C. 14,700.
D. 29,000.
E. 59,000.

5-12. If pulmonary arterial pressure = 40 cm H_2O, alveolar pressure = 0, left atrial pressure = 20 cm H_2O, and cardiac output = 10 L/min, which of the following estimates best the pulmonary vascular resistance and what is the overall lung perfusion zone?

A. 2.0 cm H_2O × min/L; zone 3.
B. 0.5 cm H_2O × min/L; zone 3.
C. 4.0 cm H_2O × min/L; zone 2.
D. 0.5 cm H_2O × sec/L; zone 2.
E. 2.0 cm H_2O × sec/L; zone 3.

5-13. A woman is brought to the intensive care unit at her community hospital. Chest radiographs show that her entire right lung (55% total lung mass) is consolidated (unventilated) as a result of bacterial pneumonia. Her lips, fingernail beds, and skin are blue (cyanotic). Subsequent measurements reveal arterial oxygen tension = 50 mm Hg (O_2 saturation = 85%) and mixed venous oxygen tension = 30 mm Hg (O_2 saturation = 57%), even though the patient is breathing 100% O_2. Cardiac output = 7 L/min. The patient's venous admixture is approximately (ignore any correction due to dissolved O_2 in blood)

A. 55% of cardiac output.
B. 15% of cardiac output.
C. 6.0 L/min.
D. 2.5 L/min.
E. 1.8 L/min.

5-14. The local perfusion of ventilation units is regulated mainly by

A. alveolar CO_2 tension.
B. the production and release of thromboxane.
C. alveolar O_2 tension.
D. the production and release of prostacyclin from lung endothelium.
E. the production of nitric oxide by lung endothelium.

5-15. Use Fig. 34-2, which shows idealized pressure-bloodflow curves in an adult man. Which of the following statements about curve 1 is most nearly correct? The blood flow resistance
   A. at rest is less than during exercise.
   B. at rest is greater than during exercise.
   C. during hypoxic exercise is greater than at rest at sea level.
   D. during hypoxic exercise is less than during exercise at sea level.
   E. cannot be calculated without knowing alveolar pressure.

5-16. If alveolar oxygen tension equals 100 mm Hg and if the hemoglobin-oxygen equilibrium curve is shifted 10 mm Hg to the right as a result of acidosis (increased hydrogen ion concentration in blood), which of the following is the most likely to be the systemic arterial oxygen tension? Assume that the individual is otherwise normal.
   A. 100 mm Hg.
   B. 90 mm Hg.
   C. 110 mm Hg.
   D. 99%.
   E. 95%.

5-17. The blood hemoglobin concentration is 75 g/L in a 29-year-old woman who sleeps with three children in an inadequately ventilated room heated by a small kerosene stove. Which of the following is closest to the steady state HbO_2 and $HbCO$ concentrations in her systemic arterial blood (Ca_{CO} and Ca_{O_2}), when alveolar P_{CO} and P_{O_2} are 0.4 and 100 mm Hg, respectively?
   A. Ca_{CO} = 100 ml/L; Ca_{O_2} = 0 ml/L
   B. Ca_{CO} = 0 ml/L; Ca_{O_2} = 100 ml/L
   C. Ca_{CO} = 25 ml/L; Ca_{O_2} = 75 ml/L
   D. Ca_{CO} = 50 ml/L; Ca_{O_2} = 50 ml/L
   E. Ca_{CO} = 100 ml/L; Ca_{O_2} = 100 ml/L

5-18. In the absence of carbonic anhydrase, the rate of carbonic acid (H_2CO_3) dissociation into water and CO_2 in pulmonary capillary blood is too slow to reach a steady state with respect to alveolar P_{CO_2} in the time available for blood transit (< 1 sec). Which of the following blood gas relations is most nearly correct?
   A. Arterial P_{CO_2} will fall below alveolar P_{CO_2}.
   B. Arterial P_{CO_2} will be the same as alveolar P_{CO_2}, but the blood bicarbonate concentration will be lower than the alveolar gas bicarbonate concentration.
   C. Arterial P_{CO_2} will rise above alveolar P_{CO_2}.
   D. Alveolar ventilation will remain constant.
   E. Alveolar ventilation will fall.

5-19. Normally, the venous oxygen saturation of blood leaving the myocardium in the coronary veins is about 50% (P_{O_2} = 29 mm Hg). If the systemic arterial blood P_{O_2} = 100 mm Hg and all other

blood values are normal, the mean P_{O_2} in the heart muscle capillaries is closest to
   A. 26 mm Hg.
   B. 40 mm Hg.
   C. 65 mm Hg.
   D. 75 mm Hg.
   E. 88 mm Hg.

5-20. In skeletal muscle during exercise, the number of capillaries being perfused may be three times the resting number. One major consequence of having more capillaries with blood flow is that
   A. tissue oxygen consumption is increased.
   B. tissue oxygen consumption is decreased.
   C. skeletal muscle vascular resistance is markedly decreased, which accounts for the large increase in flow.
   D. the diffusion path from blood to mitochondria is increased.
   E. the diffusing capacity of the muscle capillary network is increased at least threefold.

5-21. If the arterial blood P_{CO_2} = 80 mm Hg, $[HCO_3^-]$ = 32 mEq/L, and P_{O_2} = 100 mm Hg, it is likely that:
   A. the carotid body chemoreceptors are maximally stimulated.
   B. the carotid body chemoreceptors are not stimulated or are depressed.
   C. the medullary chemoreceptors are stimulated.
   D. the medullary chemoreceptors are not stimulated or are depressed because the bicarbonate concentration in arterial blood is high.
   E. the subject is in a coma because the reticular activating system is switched off.

5-22. A middle-aged man with chronic obstructive pulmonary disease (emphysema) has an arterial P_{CO_2} = 57 mm Hg; the predicted normal value is 40 mm Hg at an alveolar ventilation of 4.3 L/min. If we assume the patient's CO_2 production is normal (200 ml/min), alveolar ventilation is about
   A. 3.0 L/min.
   B. 8.0 L/min.
   C. 3.8 L/min.
   D. 6.1 L/min.
   E. 1.8 L/min.

5-23. Compared with the curve that depicts the normal ventilation response to CO_2 (Fig. 36-5) in an awake person, the curve for the same person when asleep can be described as
   A. having a steeper slope.
   B. being more sensitive.
   C. having a lower slope.
   D. having a lower intercept P_{CO_2}.
   E. having the same intercept P_{CO_2}.

5-24. The partial pressures of oxygen and CO_2 interact in arterial blood and brain (Fig. 36-7) in such a manner that

A. in hypoxemia, the slope of the CO_2-ventilation dose-response curve is reduced.

B. hypercapnia decreases ventilation when inspired oxygen concentration is normal.

C. in hypoxemia, the slope of the CO_2-ventilation dose-response curve is not affected.

D. hypercapnia permits ventilation to increase more when inspired oxygen is reduced than when CO_2 is absent from inspired air.

E. the threshold P_{CO_2} of the CO_2-ventilation dose-response curve is decreased when inspired oxygen concentration is increased.

5-25. If the diaphragm contracts more vigorously, it is likely that the slowly adapting lung stretch receptor activity will

A. increase inspiratory volume.

B. be greater than normal.

C. be less than normal.

D. be the same as normal.

E. cause the time for inspiration to lengthen.

■ *Section VI: The Gastrointestinal System*

6-1. In the smooth muscle of the gastrointestinal tract,

A. the electrogenic property of the Na^+, K^+-ATPase often makes a smaller contribution to the resting membrane potential than is the case in skeletal muscle.

B. cells of the circular layer have gap junctions but are not well coupled electronically.

C. resting membrane potentials are typically greater in magnitude than are those in skeletal muscle.

D. contractions are stronger when action potentials are triggered near the crests of the slow waves.

E. tone is caused by a baseline level of spontaneous action potentials.

6-2. In the enteric nervous system,

A. excitatory motor neurons from myenteric ganglia release acetylcholine, substance P, vasoactive intestinal peptide, or nitric oxide (NO) onto smooth muscle cells of the circular and longitudinal layers.

B. interneurons release substance P.

C. many stimulatory secretomotor neurons from the submucosal plexus release NO onto gland cells in the gastrointestinal tract.

D. vasodilator neurons may release norepinephrine onto mucosal blood vessels.

E. numerous sensory neurons, whose cell bodies are in the myenteric and submucosal ganglia, respond to mechanical and chemical stimuli.

6-3. In the esophagus,

A. the swallowing reflex is elicited when touch receptors on the posterior part of the hard palate are stimulated.

B. the upper esophageal sphincter opens early on in the swallowing reflex and remains open for most of the time that the esophageal peristaltic wave travels from the upper to the lower end of the esophagus.

C. if food remains in the esophagus after a swallow, a new complete swallowing reflex occurs.

D. in achalasia, the lower part of the body of the esophagus contracts spasmodically.

E. the lower esophageal sphincter remains open while the peristaltic wave traverses the length of the esophagus.

6-4. In the stomach,

A. receptive relaxation in response to gastric filling is partly mediated by the vagus nerves.

B. strong gastric contractions begin in the middle of the fundus, travel toward the antrum, and gain in strength as they travel.

C. the frequency of slow waves is about 8/min.

D. secretin and cholecystokinin (CCK) enhance the force of smooth muscle contraction.

E. contractions of the gastric smooth muscle do not occur in the absence of action potentials.

6-5. With regard to gastric emptying,

A. fats tend to be emptied during the active contractile phase of the migrating myoelectric complex (MMC).

B. acid in the duodenum elicits release of gastric inhibitory peptide, which slows the rate of gastric emptying.

C. indigestible objects tend to be emptied into the duodenum during the active contraction phase of the MMC.

D. fats and fat digestion products in the duodenum elicit the secretion of secretin, which slows the rate of gastric emptying.

E. gastrin released from duodenal G cells in response to peptides and amino acids decreases the force of gastric contractions.

6-6. In the small intestine,

A. peristalsis is the most frequent type of contractile behavior in a fed individual.

B. stimulating sympathetic nerves have very little effect on segmentation.

C. in a fasted individual, segmental contractions are more or less continuous.

D. the MMC is characterized by 75 to 90 minutes of quiescence, punctuated by 3- to 6-minute periods of intense and propulsive contractions.

E. long-range peristalsis occurs frequently.

6-7. In the colon,
  A. mass movements occur 1 to 3 times a day and they sweep the colonic contents toward the rectum.
  B. haustral contractions are controlled mainly by the parasympathetic nervous system.
  C. the gastrocolic reflex is characterized by decreased colonic motility elicited by gastric distention and other stimuli that arise in the stomach.
  D. the defecation reflex is evoked by distention of the sigmoid colon.
  E. the integrating center for the defecation reflex is in the enteric nervous system.

6-8. With regard to salivary secretion,
  A. the major control of salivary secretion is via the enteric nervous system.
  B. secretory endpieces (acini) secrete a fluid that contains salivary amylase and has HCO_3^- at levels much higher than in plasma.
  C. when salivary secretion is stimulated under physiological conditions, the concentration of bicarbonate in saliva rises.
  D. stimulation of the sympathetic nerves to salivary glands results in prolonged stimulation of salivation.
  E. agonists that elevate cyclic AMP stimulate acinar cell secretion; agonists that elevate intracellular Ca^{++} inhibit secretion of fluid and amylase.

6-9. With regard to gastric secretions,
  A. oxyntic glands that contain parietal cells are located in the body and the pylorus of the stomach.
  B. the higher the flow rate of gastric juice, the higher is its Cl^- concentration.
  C. patients with gastric ulcers secrete larger amounts of HCl than do normal individuals.
  D. glands in the pylorus contain G cells that secrete gastrin, cells that secrete mucus, and numerous chief cells and parietal cells.
  E. the rate of HCl secretion during the cephalic phase is low, but the total amount of HCl secreted may be large.

6-10. With regard to gastric acid secretion,
  A. the total amount of H^+,K^+-ATPase present in an unstimulated parietal cell is low.
  B. H^+ is secreted across the basolateral membrane of the parietal cell by the H^+,K^+-ATPase.
  C. HCO_3^- leaves the parietal cell at the basolateral membrane, and its downhill efflux powers the uphill entry of Cl^- into the parietal cell.
  D. Cl^- is secreted into the secretory canaliculus via a Cl^- active transport protein.
  E. H_2 receptor blockers inhibit HCl secretion by directly inhibiting the $H,^+K^+$-ATPase.

6-11. With regard to pancreatic secretion,
  A. the acinar cells and intralobular ducts secrete a fluid that contains the enzyme component and bicarbonate levels that are higher than in plasma.
  B. secretin stimulates the acinar cells and intralobular ducts to produce a secretion with a high bicarbonate concentration.
  C. during the gastric phase, CCK stimulates pancreatic acinar cells to secrete pancreatic enzymes.
  D. secretin does not influence the response of acinar cells to CCK.
  E. pancreatic acinar cells are stimulated to secrete by agonists that elevate intracellular cyclic AMP, but not by agonists that elevate intracellular Ca^{++}.

6-12. With regard to bile,
  A. the more phospholipid that is present in bile, the more cholesterol can be held in the bile acid-phospholipid-cholesterol mixed micelles.
  B. CCK is the most important physiological agonist of the secretions produced by epithelial cells of the bile ducts.
  C. conjugated bile acids have a higher critical micelle concentration than do unconjugated bile acids.
  D. bile acids in portal blood stimulate secretion of bile acids by hepatocytes, and they also stimulate the de novo synthesis of bile acids.
  E. the strongest physiological stimuli for emptying of the gallbladder are nerve impulses in branches of the vagus nerves that innervate the gallbladder.

6-13. With regard to the digestion and absorption of carbohydrates,
  A. the only monosaccharides absorbed to an appreciable extent are glucose and galactose.
  B. α-dextrinase (isomaltase) is the enzyme in the cytosol of jejunal epithelial cells that is responsible for cleaving the α-1,6-glycosidic linkage of branched starch molecules.
  C. certain disaccharides are taken up by intestinal epithelial cells.
  D. a small fraction of the world's adult population is lactose intolerant.
  E. sucrase and isomaltase (α-dextrinase) are synthesized as a single polypeptide chain.

6-14. With regard to the digestion and absorption of proteins,
  A. trypsinogen is activated by chymotrypsin that is secreted by the duodenal mucosa.
  B. oligopeptidases present in pancreatic juice cleave peptides to produce smaller peptides and single amino acids.
  C. neutral amino acids are transported across the brush border membrane by a single Na^+-pow-

ered secondary active transport protein with broad specificity for neutral amino acids.

    D. dipeptides and tripeptides are taken up across the brush border membrane by a single type of H+-powered secondary active transport protein.

    E. dipeptides and tripeptides are transported across the basolateral membrane and appear in portal blood.

6-15. With regard to the intestinal handling of salts and water,

    A. the enteric nervous system plays a minor role in regulation of intestinal salt and water transport.

    B. aldosterone enhances the absorption of Na+ in the colon mainly by increasing the number of Na+, K+-ATPase molecules in the basolateral membrane.

    C. cells in the crypts of Lieberkühn are stimulated to secrete Cl− into the lumen by any agonist that elevates intracellular cyclic AMP in the crypt cells.

    D. the glucose that is present in oral rehydration solution promotes the absorption of Na+, Cl−, and water by the cells in the crypts of Lieberkühn.

    E. in the jejunum and ileum, very little K+ is absorbed via the paracellular pathway.

6-16. With regard to the intestinal absorption of iron,

    A. the fraction of the ingested inorganic iron that is absorbed is larger than the fraction of the ingested heme iron that is absorbed.

    B. vitamin C inhibits iron absorption by forming a complex with ferrous (Fe++) iron.

    C. iron bound to ferritin in intestinal epithelial cells is part of the absorbable pool of iron.

    D. Fe++, but not Fe+++, is taken up across the brush border membrane by a specific transport protein.

    E. the intestinal epithelial cells of iron-deficient animals contain more apoferritin than do the intestinal epithelial cells of iron-replete individuals.

6-17. With regard to the intestinal digestion and absorption of lipids,

    A. lipid absorption may occur when bile acid–lipid mixed micelles fuse with the brush border plasma membrane.

    B. the transport of bile acid–lipid mixed micelles across the intestinal unstirred layer is the rate-limiting step in lipid absorption.

    C. triglycerides readily form mixed micelles with bile acids.

    D. resynthesis of triglycerides occurs in the lysosomes of intestinal epithelial cells.

    E. emulsification of dietary lipids by bile acids increases the rate at which brush border lipases can digest the lipids.

■ *Section VII: The Kidney*

7-1. Which of the following structures is a barrier to the filtration of proteins across the glomerulus?

    A. Capillary endothelial cells
    B. Basement membrane
    C. Lacis cells
    D. Parietal epithelial cells
    E. Mesangial cells

7-2. According to the tubuloglomerular feedback theory, an increase in the flow of tubular fluid to the macula densa will result in

    A. a decrease in the glomerular filtration rate of the same nephron.

    B. an increase in renal blood flow to the glomerulus of the same nephron.

    C. activation of the renal sympathetic nerves.

    D. an increase in proximal tubule solute and water reabsorption.

    E. an increase in renin secretion.

For questions 7-3 to 7-5 consider the following graph, which shows the relationship between plasma [PAH] and PAH secretion.

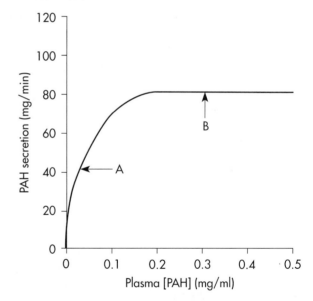

7-3. The amount of PAH filtered at the glomerulus is
    A. greater at point A than at point B.
    B. less at point A than at point B.
    C. the same at points A and B.

7-4. The amount of PAH excreted in the urine is
    A. greater at point A than at point B.
    B. less at point A than at point B.
    C. the same at points A and B.

7-5. The clearance of PAH is
    A. greater at point A than at point B.
    B. less at point A than at point B.
    C. the same at points A and B.

7-6. Some Na⁺ reabsorption in the late portion of the proximal tubule is passive through the paracellular pathway. The primary driving force for this passive reabsorption of Na⁺ is
  A. a higher luminal than peritubular hydrostatic pressure.
  B. a higher luminal than peritubular [Na⁺].
  C. a lumen-positive transepithelial voltage.
  D. a lower interstitial fluid than luminal fluid oncotic pressure.

For questions 7-7 to 7-9, the following graph shows the change in tubular fluid concentration of various substances along the length of the proximal tubule plotted as the tubular fluid to plasma concentration ratio (TF/P). Thus, the TF/P = 1 for a substance that is at the same concentration in the tubular fluid and plasma (all substances that are freely filtered have TF/P = 1 at the glomerulus).

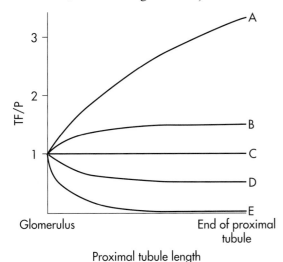

Match the following substances to the appropriate TF/P curve:

7-7. Na⁺

7-8. Inulin

7-9. Amino acids

7-10. Starling forces regulate sodium and water reabsorption by the proximal tubule. Which of the following changes in Starling forces would increase reabsorption?
  A. Increase in the capillary hydrostatic pressure
  B. Increase in capillary oncotic pressure
  C. Decrease in capillary oncotic pressure
  D. Decrease in the permeability of the peritubular capillary to sodium and water
  E. Decrease in interstitial pressure

7-11. Reabsorption of sodium and chloride in the distal tubule and collecting duct is increased by
  A. angiotensin II.
  B. peritubular Starling forces.
  C. atrial natriuretic peptide (ANP).

  D. aldosterone.
  E. urodilatin.

7-12. The daily excretion rate of total osmoles for an individual is 900 mOsm. If this individual has a urine-concentrating defect and can only produce urine having a maximal osmolality of 300 mOsm/kg H₂O, what is the minimal volume of water that must be ingested to prevent a rise in the osmolality of the body fluids? (Assume that insensible water loss is 1.5 L/day.)
  A. 1.5 L/day
  B. 3.0 L/day
  C. 4.5 L/day
  D. 6.0 L/day
  E. 7.5 L/day

7-13. Which of the following maneuvers would be expected to stimulate ADH secretion?
  A. Infusion of 1 L hypertonic NaCl
  B. Infusion of 1 L of an isoosmotic urea solution
  C. Expansion of the extracellular fluid (ECF)
  D. Infusion of 1 L of 5% dextrose in water (D5W)
  E. An acute increase in blood pressure

7-14. An individual has no urine output over a 2-day period. During this time, the body weight increases by 2 kg. The plasma [Na⁺] is unchanged. What can be concluded about the volumes and composition of the body fluids in this individual?
  A. The volume of the ICF is decreased.
  B. The volume of the ECF is increased.
  C. The total body water is normal.
  D. The plasma osmolality is decreased.
  E. The plasma volume is decreased.

7-15. A decrease in the extracellular fluid volume will
  A. increase glomerular filtration rate.
  B. increase angiotensin II levels.
  C. increase ANP levels.
  D. increase free-water clearance.
  E. increase fractional excretion of Na⁺.

7-16. A 56-year-old woman has congestive heart failure with generalized edema. Which of the following plays an important role in the formation of edema in this woman?
  A. Increased interstitial hydrostatic pressure
  B. Decreased interstitial oncotic pressure
  C. Increased plasma oncotic pressure
  D. Decreased renal excretion of Na⁺
  E. Decreased venous pressure

7-17. Vasopressin has which of the following actions?
  A. It increases water permeability of the thick ascending limb of Henle's loop.
  B. It increases urea permeability of the cortical collecting duct.
  C. It increases water permeability of the cortical collecting duct.

D. It decreases glomerular filtration rate.

E. It increases water permeability of the proximal tubule.

7-18. A reduction in dietary K^+ intake would be expected to alter K^+ transport in which segment of the nephron?

A. Proximal convoluted tubule

B. Descending limb of Henle

C. Proximal straight tubule

D. Collecting duct

E. Thick ascending limb of Henle

7-19. Urinary potassium excretion is enhanced by

A. an osmotic diuresis.

B. acute metabolic asidosis.

C. hypoaldosteronism.

D. decreased tubular flow rate.

E. a water diuresis.

7-20. Which of the following hormones plays an important role in keeping the plasma concentration of potassium within normal limits?

A. Calcitriol

B. Vasopressin

C. Parathyroid hormone

D. Insulin

E. Glucagon

7-21. A healthy individual weighing 60 kg is infused with 1 L of isotonic saline to which 20 mEq of K^+ has been added. After the infusion the plasma $[K^+]$ of this individual has increased from 3.5 to 7.8 mEq/L. What is the most likely explanation for the development of hyperkalemia in this person?

A. Shift of K^+ from the ICF into the ECF

B. Impaired renal excretion of K^+

C. Addition of 20 mEq/L of K^+ to the ECF

D. Contraction of the ECF volume

E. Development of hyperosmolality

7-22. Proximal tubule HCO_3^- reabsorption is inhibited by

A. increased P_{CO_2}.

B. volume expansion.

C. systemic acidosis.

D. decreased levels of aldosterone.

E. hypokalemia.

7-23. During a 24-hour period an individual excretes in the urine 60 mmol of NH_4^+, 40 mmol of titratable acid (TA), and 10 mmol of HCO_3^-. If this individual is in acid-base balance, how much nonvolatile acid did he or she produce from metabolism?

A. 80 mmol/day

B. 90 mmol/day

C. 100 mmol/day

D. 110 mmol/day

E. 120 mmol/day

7-24. In response to metabolic acidosis, the kidneys increase the excretion of net acid. The most important component of this compensatory response is

A. increased filtered load of HCO_3^-.

B. enhanced reabsoption of HCO_3^- by the proximal tubule.

C. increased synthesis of NH_4^+.

D. reduced H^+ secretion by the collecting duct.

E. reduced secretion of HCO_3^- by the collecting duct.

Match the acid-base disturbance with the clinical scenario and arterial blood gases described in questions 7-25 to 7-29.

A. Metabolic acidosis with respiratory compensation

B. Metabolic alkalosis with respiratory compensation

C. Respiratory acidosis with renal compensation (chronic respiratory acidosis)

D. Respiratory acidosis without renal compensation (acute respiratory acidosis)

E. Metabolic acidosis and respiratory acidosis

7-25. An individual with an asthma attack:
pH = 7.32; $[HCO_3^-]$ = 25 mEq/L; P_{CO_2} = 50 mm Hg

7-26. An individual with diabetes mellitus who forgets to take insulin:
pH = 7.29; $[HCO_3^-]$ = 12 mEq/L; P_{CO_2} = 26 mm Hg

7-27. An individual with cardiopulmonary arrest:
pH = 6.85; $[HCO_3^-]$ = 10 mEq/L; P_{CO_2} = 60 mm Hg

7-28. An individual with a gastric ulcer who ingests large quantities of antacids:
pH = 7.45; $[HCO_3^-]$ = 30 mEq/L; P_{CO_2} = 45 mm Hg

7-29. An individual with a 20-year history of smoking 3 packs/day and who has emphysema:
pH = 7.37; $[HCO_3^-]$ = 28 mEq/L; P_{CO_2} = 50 mm Hg

■ Section VIII: The Endocrine System

8-1. Each of the following hormone second messengers is generated via a G protein *except*

A. calcium.

B. cAMP.

C. inositol triphosphate.

D. tyrosine kinase.

E. diacylglycerol.

8-2. Each of the following is true about plasma membrane hormone receptors *except*

A. The intracellular C-terminus portion links to G proteins.

B. Hormone binding may result in modulation of gene transcription.

C. They may wind in and out of the plasma membrane.

D. cGMP may act as a second messenger after hormone binding.

E. cAMP may act as a second messenger after hormone binding.

8-3. Hormone secretion via exocytosis involves each of the following *except*

A. a rise in intracellular Ca++.

B. hormone storage in secretory granules.

C. cosecretion of other products of the prohormone.

D. the microtubular-microfilament system.

E. loss of nuclear membrane material.

8-4. Which of the following could decrease the *sensitivity* of a person to stimulation by a hormone?

A. A decrease in the number of target cells

B. The presence of a competitive antagonist

C. A decrease in adenylyl cyclase concentration

D. An increase in phosphodiesterase concentration

E. The presence of a noncompetitive antagonist

8-5. A single plasma level of a hormone faithfully reflects the hormone secretion rate if

A. the hormone is not excreted in the urine.

B. the hormone is secreted in a diurnal pattern.

C. the metabolic clearance rate of the hormone is normal.

D. the hormone is not metabolized by the liver.

E. the hormone is not bound to a serum protein.

8-6. Which of the following factors increases the basal metabolic rate?

A. Sleep

B. Decrease in caloric intake

C. Aging

D. Female gender

E. Gain in lean body mass

8-7. Leptin

A. is a peptide released by the hypothalamus.

B. is decreased in the plasma of obese humans.

C. is synthesized by adipose tissue cells.

D. stimulates appetite.

E. decreases energy expenditure.

8-8. High-density lipoprotein (HDL) cholesterol particles

A. are a negative risk factor for cardiovascular disease.

B. transform cholesterol esters to free cholesterol.

C. facilitate uptake of cholesterol by peripheral cells.

D. have very short half-lives (in minutes).

E. have apoproteins that inhibit the enzyme lipoprotein lipase.

8-9. Essential amino acids

A. are preferentially reabsorbed by renal tubules.

B. have carbon skeletons that cannot be synthesized by humans.

C. are required for the synthesis of particular essential proteins.

D. are those specific amino acids whose carbon skeletons are required for synthesis of glucose.

E. cannot be degraded and oxidized.

8-10. Exercise and prolonged fasting are similar in each of the following ways *except*

A. Free fatty acid mobilization is increased.

B. Glycogenolysis is increased.

C. Alanine levels in plasma fall.

D. Leucine is the principal amino acid used for gluconeogenesis.

E. Energy provided by oxidation of free fatty acids supports hepatic gluconeogenesis.

8-11. Glucagon decreases the plasma level of

A. free fatty acids.

B. amino acids.

C. beta-hydroxybutyrate.

D. acetoacetate.

E. glucose.

8-12. In the β-cell cytoplasm, insulin release is preceded by a decrease in the intracellular concentration of

A. potassium.

B. glucose-6-phosphate.

C. ATP.

D. NADPH.

E. calcium.

8-13. Which of the following is an action of insulin?

A. Inhibition of triglyceride synthesis

B. Stimulation of proteolysis

C. Stimulation of gluconeogenesis

D. Inhibition of glycolysis

E. Inhibition of ketogenesis

8-14. Which of the following effects of insulin requires the least amount of the hormone?

A. Stimulation of muscle glucose uptake

B. Stimulation of muscle glucose transport

C. Inhibition of lipolysis

D. Inhibition of hepatic glucose production

E. Stimulation of amino acid uptake

8-15. Which of the following would decrease the insulin/glucagon ratio in plasma?

A. An increase in β-adrenergic stimulation of the islets

B. Somatostatin

C. A carbohydrate meal

D. Exercise

E. A protein meal

8-16. 1,25-(OH)$_2$-vitamin D synthesis is increased by each of the following *except*

A. parathyroid hormone (PTH).

B. calcitonin.

C. calcium deficiency.

D. phosphate deficiency.

E. vitamin D deficiency.

8-17. Which of the following statements regarding trabecular bone is true?
  A. It constitutes a greater proportion of total bone mass than does cortical bone.
  B. It is mainly present in long bones.
  C. It makes up a greater proportion of total bone surface area than does cortical bone.
  D. It undergoes very little, if any, resorption in adults.
  E. It undergoes very little, if any, formation in adults.

8-18. PTH has which of the following primary actions?
  A. It increases bone resorption.
  B. It increases gastrointestinal calcium absorption.
  C. It increases 24,25-$(OH)_2$-vitamin D synthesis.
  D. It decreases urinary phosphate excretion.
  E. It decreases renal tubular calcium reabsorption.

8-19. PTH synthesis and secretion are decreased by which of the following?
  A. Increased 1,25-$(OH)_2$-vitamin D
  B. Increased cAMP
  C. Increased serum phosphate
  D. Decreased binding of calcium to its parathyroid cell plasma membrane receptor
  E. Decreased 24,25-$(OH)_2$-vitamin D

8-20. All of the following statements regarding vitamin D actions are true *except*
  A. cAMP is an intracellular second messenger.
  B. Osteoblasts have the 1,25-(OH_2)-vitamin D receptor.
  C. A calcium-binding protein is induced in target cells.
  D. Calcium transport across the intestinal brush border is increased.
  E. Bone resorption and bone formation are both facilitated.

8-21. Hypothalamic peptide hormones
  A. reach the anterior pituitary gland via the arterial blood.
  B. are synthesized within cell nuclei.
  C. reach the anterior pituitary via axonal connections to it.
  D. are secreted in pulses.
  E. cannot cross the blood-brain barrier.

8-22. ACTH secretion is inhibited by
  A. androstenedione.
  B. cortisol.
  C. ADH.
  D. norepinephrine.
  E. testosterone.

8-23. TSH, LH, and FSH are similar in that they
  A. have a common subunit in their structure.
  B. are secreted by the same anterior pituitary cell.
  C. are secreted in response to the same hypothalamic peptide–releasing hormone.
  D. are released in response to dopamine.
  E. are stored in the posterior pituitary gland.

8-24. Growth hormone actions are mediated by
  A. somatostatin.
  B. insulin.
  C. tyrosine kinases.
  D. cAMP.
  E. a nuclear receptor.

8-25. Growth hormone synthesis and release are stimulated by
  A. somatomedin.
  B. somatostatin.
  C. glucose.
  D. fatty acids.
  E. arginine.

8-26. ADH
  A. increases free-water transfer from the tubular urine to the capillary blood.
  B. decreases sodium resorption from the ascending limb of the loop of Henle.
  C. increases plasma osmolality.
  D. inhibits ACTH secretion.
  E. decreases urea reabsorption.

8-27. Prolactin secretion differs from that of other anterior pituitary hormones because
  A. it does not occur by exocytosis of secretory granules.
  B. it is stimulated by dopamine.
  C. it is stimulated by ADH.
  D. it is under tonic inhibition from the hypothalamus.
  E. it is cosecreted with growth hormone.

8-28. A 37-year-old woman presents to her physician with an enlarged thyroid gland, high levels of T_4 and T_3, and a low level of TSH in the serum. Which of the following is likely to be decreased?
  A. Heart rate
  B. Cardiac output
  C. Peripheral vascular resistance
  D. Ventilation rate
  E. Metabolic rate

8-29. By itself, a chronic increase in the concentration of thyroid-binding globulin in the serum would
  A. increase delivery of T_4 to its target cells.
  B. decrease the free T_4 level.
  C. increase T_4 conversion to T_3 in peripheral tissue.
  D. decrease TSH secretion.
  E. cause no change in the metabolic rate.

8-30. Administration of an inhibitor of thyroid peroxidase would cause an increase in the
  A. thyroid content of iodide.

B. thyroid content of monoiodotyrosine.

C. thyroglobulin content of follicular lumina.

D. serum TSH.

E. urinary excretion of diiodotyrosine.

8-31. A 40-year-old man presents with severe headaches that are found to be caused by a large pituitary mass. Serum T_4 is low. Which of the following is likely to be increased?

A. Serum TSH

B. Serum cholesterol

C. Body temperature

D. Carbon dioxide production

E. Oxygen utilization

8-32. Which of the following statements comparing T_3 with T_4 is true?

A. T_3 has a greater affinity for the thyroid receptor.

B. T_3 is secreted in greater amounts by the normal thyroid gland.

C. In equimolar amounts, T_3 administration is less likely to inhibit TSH secretion.

D. T_3 is the preferred substrate for 5'-monodeiodinase.

E. In equimolar amounts, T_3 causes a lesser increase in metabolic rate.

8-33. Aldosterone actions in the kidney lead to

A. an increase in urine sodium.

B. a decrease in plasma potassium concentration.

C. a decrease in blood pressure.

D. a decrease in atrial natriuretic hormone secretion.

E. An increase in reabsorption of free water.

8-34. Cortisol is secreted in response to each of the following *except*

A. hypoglycemia.

B. general anesthesia.

C. slow wave sleep.

D. corticotropin-releasing hormone.

E. interleukins.

8-35. A state of cortisol excess would lead to

A. increased secretion of insulin.

B. positive nitrogen balance.

C. reduction in urea synthesis.

D. decreased plasma sodium concentration.

E. increased bone formation.

8-36. The rate-limiting step in synthesis of all adrenal steroid hormones is

A. side-chain cleavage of cholesterol.

B. tyrosine uptake by secretory granules.

C. transfer of cholesterol into the mitochondria.

D. expression of the gene for 17-hydroxylase.

E. translocation of the ACTH-receptor complex into the nucleus.

8-37. Cortisol stimulates

A. secretion of cytokines by immune cells.

B. release of inflammatory prostaglandins.

C. recruitment of neutrophils to sites of bacterial invasion.

D. release of neutrophils from the bone marrow.

E. bactericidal activity of neutrophils.

8-38. Epinephrine

A. inhibits glycogenolysis in liver.

B. inhibits glycogenolysis in muscle.

C. inhibits ketogenesis.

D. stimulates lipolysis.

E. stimulates fatty acid synthesis.

8-39. The activity of the adrenal zona glomerulosa is stimulated by

A. cortisol.

B. hypernatremia.

C. atrial natriuretic peptide.

D. hypokalemia.

E. angiotensin II.

8-40. Which of the following is essential for the development of the normal female genital tract and external genitalia?

A. One X chromosome and no Y chromosome.

B. Two X chromosomes.

C. A functioning ovary.

D. Estradiol.

E. A functioning pituitary gland.

8-41. Production of sperm differs from production of ova in that the former

A. requires gonadal synthesis of androgens.

B. continues throughout the individual's lifetime.

C. occurs in an environment to which plasma constituents have free access.

D. occurs in an environment that is protected from free access of plasma constituents.

E. does not require FSH.

8-42. Testosterone has which of the following actions?

A. It increases bone resorption.

B. It increases low-density lipoprotein cholesterol levels.

C. It increases the plasma levels of sex steroid–binding globulins.

D. It decreases nitrogen balance.

E. It decreases prostate gland size and secretions.

8-43. The ovulatory surge in LH and FSH secretion is caused by a positive effect of

A. endorphins.

B. estradiol.

C. activin.

D. melatonin.

E. prolactin.

8-44. Estradiol decreases which of the following?

A. Progesterone receptors

B. The thickness of the uterine endometrium

C. The fluidity and elasticity of cervical mucus
D. FSH receptors
E. Milk secretion

8-45. Human chorionic gonadotropin
A. is produced by the corpus luteum.
B. is produced by the decidua.
C. stimulates progesterone production.
D. reaches peak levels in maternal plasma at term.
E. stimulates milk synthesis by mammary glands.

8-46. Sertoli cells and granulosa cells have which of the following in common?
A. They secrete large amounts of estradiol.
B. They secrete large amounts of testosterone.
C. They are stimulated primarily by LH.
D. They are stimulated primarily by FSH.
E. They are separated from germ cells by a basement membrane.

8-47. The metabolic milieu of the mother in the last trimester of pregnancy is characterized by
A. increased sensitivity to insulin action.
B. increased resistance to insulin action.
C. decreased lipolysis after overnight fasting.
D. decreased plasma glucose after meals.
E. increased plasma glucose after overnight fasting.

■ *Answers to Mini-Exam*
■ *Section I*

1-1. C

1-2. E

1-3. C

1-4. C

1-5. D

1-6. A

1-7. A

1-8. C

1-9. D

1-10. A

1-11. B

1-12. D

1-13. C

1-14. D

1-15. B

1-16. B

1-17. B

1-18. C

1-19. B

1-20. B

1-21. B

1-22. B

1-23. D

1-24. C

1-25. D

1-26. B

1-27. C

1-28. B

■ *Section II*

2-1. D

2-2. A

2-3. D

2-4. D

2-5. C

2-6. A

2-7. C

2-8. C

2-9. D

2-10. E

2-11. B

2-12. D

2-13. B

2-14. E

2-15. C

2-16. D

2-17. D

2-18. B

2-19. D

2-20. A

2-21. B

2-22. B

2-23. C

2-24. B

2-25. D

2-26. B

2-27. B

2-28. B

2-29. A

2-30. A

2-31. D

2-32. B

2-33. C

2-34. C

2-35. D

2-36. B

2-37. B

2-38. A

2-39. E

2-40. D

2-41. C

2-42. B

2-43. D

2-44. A

2-45. D

2-46. C

2-47. C

2-48. C

2-49. C

2-50. C

2-51. C

2-52. C

2-53. B

2-54. D

2-55. B

2-56. A

■ *Section III*

3-1. E

3-2. E

3-3. D

3-4. A

3-5. E

3-6. B

3-7. C

3-8. E

3-9. E

3-10. A

3-11. B

3-12. D

3-13. B

3-14. C

3-15. A

■ *Section IV*

4-1. D

4-2. B

4-3. E

4-4. D

4-5. C

4-6. A

4-7. B

4-8. B

4-9. D

4-10. D

4-11. E

4-12. E

4-13. A

4-14. C

4-15. A

4-16. A

4-17. E

4-18. B

4-19. E

4-20. D

4-21. A

4-22. B

4-23. D

4-24. B

4-25. D

4-26. C

4-27. D

4-28. A

4-29. C

4-30. E

4-31. D

4-32. C

4-33. C

4-34. D

4-35. C

4-36. A

4-37. E

4-38. C

4-39. D

4-40. C

4-41. C

4-42. B

4-43. E

4-44. D

4-45. A

4-46. B

4-47. D

4-48. C

4-49. D

4-50. E

4-51. D

4-52. E

4-53. D

4-54. A

4-55. C

4-56. E

4-57. E

4-58. B

4-59. E

4-60. B

4-61. E

4-62. A

■ *Section V*

5-1. D

5-2. C

5-3. A

5-4. A

5-5. E

5-6. B

5-7. B

5-8. B

5-9. A

5-10. E

5-11. D

5-12. A

5-13. D

5-14. C

5-15. D

5-16. A

5-17. D

5-18. C

5-19. B

5-20. E

5-21. C

5-22. A

5-23. C

5-24. D

5-25. B

■ *Section VI*

6-1. D

6-2. E

6-3. E

6-4. A

6-5. C

6-6. D

6-7. A

6-8. C

6-9. B

6-10. C

6-11. A

6-12. A

6-13. E

6-14. D

6-15. C

6-16. D

6-17. B

■ *Section VII*

7-1. B

7-2. A

7-3. B

7-4. B

7-5. A

7-6. C

7-7. C

7-8. A

7-9. E

7-10. B

7-11. D

7-12. C

7-13. A

7-14. B

7-15. B

7-16. D

7-17. C

7-18. D

7-19. A

7-20. D

7-21. A

7-22. B

7-23. B

7-24. C

7-25. D

7-26. A

7-27. E

7-28. B

7-29. C

■ *Section VIII*

8-1. D

8-2. A

8-3. E

8-4. B

8-5. C

8-6. E

8-7. C

8-8. A

8-9. B

8-10. D

8-11. B

8-12. A

8-13. E

8-14. C

8-15. D

8-16. B

8-17. C

8-18. A

8-19. A

8-20. A

8-21. D

8-22. B

8-23. A

8-24. C

8-25. E

8-26. A

8-27. D

8-28. C

8-29. E

8-30. D

8-31. B

8-32. A

8-33. B

8-34. C

8-35. A

8-36. C

8-37. D

8-38. D

8-39. E

8-40. A

8-41. B

8-42. B

8-43. B

8-44. E

8-45. C

8-46. D

8-47. B

Index

Page numbers in *italics* indicate illustrations. Page numbers followed by a "t" indicate tables.

WE WANT TO HEAR FROM YOU!

To help us publish the most useful materials for students, we would appreciate your comments on this book. Please take a few moments to answer the questions below, and E-mail us your comments. Thank you for your input.

Berne PHYSIOLOGY 4e
physiology.medtext@mosby.com

1. How are you using this book? Please be specific: for a first-year medical school course, as part of a clerkship rotation, to refresh the material before a Board exam, etc.

2. Was this book useful to you? Why or why not?

3. What features of textbooks are important to you?
   -color figures
   -summary tables and boxes
   -summaries
   -clinical information
   -self-assessment questions
   -price
   -what else?

4. What influenced your decision to buy this text?
   -required/recommended by instructor
   -recommendation by student
   -bookstore display
   -what else?

5. What other instructional materials did/would you find useful in this course?
   -computer-assisted instruction
   -slides
   -what else?

Are you interested in doing in-depth reviews of our textbooks?
If so, please send us your name, address and telephone number.

THANK YOU!